CONTENTS

SECTION IV
DISEASES OF NERVE AND MUSCLE

SECTION V
CHRONIC FATIGUE SYNDROME

SECTION VI
PSYCHIATRIC DISORDERS

SECTION VII
ALCOHOLISM AND DRUG DEPENDENCE

HARRISON'S
Neurology in
Clinical Medicine

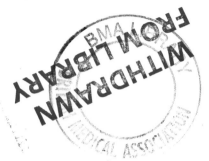

Derived from Harrison's Principles of Internal Medicine, 16th Edition

Editors

DENNIS L. KASPER, MD
William Ellery Channing Professor of Medicine,
Professor of Microbiology and Molecular Genetics,
Harvard Medical School; Director, Channing
Laboratory, Department of Medicine, Brigham and
Women's Hospital, Boston

ANTHONY S. FAUCI, MD
Chief, Laboratory of Immunoregulation; Director,
National Institute of Allergy and Infectious Diseases,
National Institutes of Health, Bethesda

DAN L. LONGO, MD
Scientific Director, National Institute on Aging,
National Institutes of Health,
Bethesda and Baltimore

EUGENE BRAUNWALD, MD
Distinguished Hersey Professor of Medicine,
Harvard Medical School; Chairman, TIMI Study Group,
Brigham and Women's Hospital, Boston

STEPHEN L. HAUSER, MD
Robert A. Fishman Distinguished Professor and Chairman,
Department of Neurology,
University of California, San Francisco, San Francisco

J. LARRY JAMESON, MD, PhD
Irving S. Cutter Professor and Chairman,
Department of Medicine,
Northwestern University Feinberg School of Medicine;
Physician-in-Chief, Northwestern
Memorial Hospital, Chicago

HARRISON'S
Neurology in Clinical Medicine

Editor

Stephen L. Hauser, MD
Robert A. Fishman Distinguished Professor and Chairman,
Department of Neurology,
University of California, San Francisco, San Francisco

Associate Editors

Scott Andrew Josephson, MD
Neurovascular and Behavioral Neurology Fellow

Joey D. English, MD, PhD
Assistant Professor

John W. Engstrom, MD
Professor and Vice-Chairman

Department of Neurology
University of California, San Francisco, California

McGraw-Hill
Medical Publishing Division

New York   Chicago   San Francisco   Lisbon   London   Madrid
Mexico City   Milan   New Delhi   Seoul   Singapore   Sydney   Toronto

Harrison's Neurology in Clinical Medicine

1234567890 DOWDOW 09876

ISBN 0-07-145745-3

This book was set in Bembo by Progressive Information Technologies. The editors were James Shanahan and Mariapaz Ramos Englis. The production supervisor was Catherine Saggese. The Index was prepared by Barbara Littlewood. Illustration manager was Charissa Baker, cover design was by Janice Bielawa, and additional text design was by Alan Barnett.

Illustration used in the Section and chapter openers was by Emantras, Inc.
Medical Illustrator: DragonFly/Media Group, Pennsylvania.

RR Donnelley was printer and binder.

Library of Congress Cataloging-in-Publication Data.

Harrison's neurology in clinical medicine / editors, Stephen L. Hauser ... [et al.].
    p. ; cm.
  Expansion of the neurology section of Harrison's principles of internal medicine.
  Includes bibliographical references and index.
  ISBN 0-07-145745-3
    1. Neurology. 2. Nervous system—Diseases. I. Title: Neurology in clinical medicine.
II. Harrison, Tinsley Randolph, 1900–. III. Hauser, Stephen L. IV. Harrison's principles
of internal medicine.
   [DNLM: 1. Nervous System Diseases. WL 140 H323 2006]
RC346.H26 2006
616.8—dc22
                                                     2005058041

CONTRIBUTORS

Numbers in brackets refer to the Sectional chapters written or co-written by the contributor.

ARTHUR K. ASBURY, MD
Van Meter Professor of Neurology Emeritus, University of Pennsylvania School of Medicine, Philadelphia [33, 35]

M. FLINT BEAL, MD
Anne Parrish Titzel Professor and Chair, Department of Neurology and Neuroscience, Weill Medical College of Cornell University; Neurologist-in-Chief, New York Presbyterian Hospital, New York [1, 23]

THOMAS D. BIRD, MD
Professor of Neurology and Medicine, University of Washington; Veterans Affairs Puget Sound Medical Center, Seattle [18, 34]

ROBERT H. BROWN, Jr., MD, DPhil
Associate Neurologist, Massachusetts General Hospital; Professor of Neurology, Harvard Medical School, Boston [21, 38]

CYNTHIA D. BROWN, MD
Department of Internal Medicine
The Johns Hopkins University School of Medicine
Baltimore (Review and Self-Assessment)

MARK D. CARLSON, MD
Professor of Medicine, Associate Vice President for Government Relations, Case Western Reserve University; Associate Dean, Case School of Medicine, Cleveland [9]

PHILIP F. CHANCE, MD
Professor of Pediatrics and Neurology, University of Washington School of Medicine; Chief, Division of Genetics and Development, Children's Hospital and Regional Medical Center, Seattle [34]

CHARLES A. CZEISLER, MD, PhD
Professor of Medicine, Harvard Medical School; Chief, Division of Sleep Medicine; Director, Sleep Disorders and Circadian Medicine, Brigham and Women's Hospital, Boston [13]

MARINOS C. DALAKAS, MD
Professor of Neurology; Chief, Neuromuscular Diseases Section, National Institute of Neurological Disorders and Stroke, National Institutes of Health, Bethesda [39]

JOSEP DALMAU, MD, PhD
Associate Professor of Neurology, Department of Neurology, University of Pennsylvania, Philadelphia [27]

ROBERT B. DAROFF, MD
Professor of Neurology and Associate Dean, Case Western Reserve University School of Medicine, Cleveland [9]

MAHLON R. DeLONG, MD
Timmie Professor of Neurology; Director of Neuroscience, Emory University School of Medicine, Atlanta [19]

WILLIAM P. DILLON, MD
Professor of Radiology, Section Chief, Neuroradiology, Vice-Chair for Research Radiology, University of California, San Francisco, San Francisco [3]

DANIEL B. DRACHMAN, MD
Professor of Neurology and Neuroscience; WW Smith Charitable Foundation Professor of Neuroimmunology; Director, Neuromuscular Unit, The Johns Hopkins University School of Medicine, Baltimore [36]

J. DONALD EASTON, MD
Professor and Chair, Department of Clinical Neurosciences, Brown Medical School and Rhode Island Hospital, Providence [17]

JOHN W. ENGSTROM, MD
Professor and Vice Chairman, Department of Neurology; Residency Program Director, University of California, San Francisco, San Francisco [6, 2]

ANTHONY S. FAUCI, MD
Chief, Laboratory of Immunoregulation; Director, National Institute of Allergy and Infectious Diseases, National Institute of Health, Bethesda [31]

HOWARD L. FIELDS, MD, PhD
Professor of Neurology and Physiology, University of California, San Francisco, San Francisco [4]

BRUCE C. GILLILAND, MD
Professor of Medicine and Laboratory Medicine, University of Washington School of Medicine, Seattle [40]

DOUGLAS S. GOODIN, MD
Professor of Neurology, University of California, San Francisco, San Francisco [28]

STEPHEN L. HAUSER, MD
Robert A. Fishman Distinguished Professor and Chairman, Department of Neurology, University of California, San Francisco, San Francisco [1,2,23,24,35]

ANNA R. HEMNES, MD
Department of Internal Medicine
The Johns Hopkins University School of Medicine
Baltimore (Review and Self-Assessment)

J. CLAUDE HEMPHILL III, MD
Assistant Professor of Neurology, University of California, San Francisco; Director, Neurovascular and Neurocritical Care Program, San Francisco General Hospital, San Francisco [15]

JONATHAN C. HORTON, MD, PhD
William F. Hoyt Professor of Neuro-Ophthalmology, Departments of Ophthalmology, Neurology, and Physiology, University of California, San Francisco, San Francisco [11]

MARK A. ISRAEL, MD
Professor of Pediatrics and Genetics, Dartmouth Medical School; Director, Norris Cotton Cancer Center, Dartmouth-Hitchcock Medical Center, Lebanon [25]

J. LARRY JAMESON, MD, PhD
Irving S. Cutter Professor and Chair, Department of Medicine, Northwestern University Feinberg School of Medicine; Physician-in-Chief, Northwestern Memorial Hospital, Chicago [26]

JAMES L. JANUZZI, JR., MD
Assistant Professor of Medicine, Harvard Medical School; Assistant Physician, Division of Cardiology and Department of Medicine, Massachusetts General Hospital, Boston [Appendix]

S. CLAIBORNE JOHNSTON, MD, PhD
Associate Professor of Neurology and Epidemiology, Director, Stroke Service, University of California, San Francisco, San Francisco [17]

JORGE L. JUNCOS, MD
Associate Professor of Neurology, Emory University School of Medicine; Director of Neurology, Wesley Woods Hospital, Atlanta [19]

WALTER J. KOROSHETZ, MD
Vice-Chair, Neurology Service, Massachusetts General Hospital, Associate Professor of Neurology, Harvard Medical School, Boston [30]

ALEXANDER KRATZ, MD, PhD, MPH
Assistant Professor of Pathology, Harvard Medical School; Director, Clinical Hematology Laboratory, Massachusetts General Hospital [Appendix]

ANIL K. LALWANI, MD
Mendik Foundation Professor and Chair, Department of Otolaryngology; Professor of Physiology and Neuroscience, New York University School of Medicine, New York [12]

H. CLIFFORD LANE, MD
Head, Clinical and Molecular Retrovirology Section, Laboratory of Immunoregulation; Clinical Director, National Institute of Allergy and Infectious Diseases, National Institutes of Health, Bethesda [31]

KENT B. LEWANDROWSKI, MD
Associate Chief of Pathology, Director, Core Laboratory, Massachusetts General Hospital; Associate Professor, Harvard Medical School, Boston [Appendix]

PHILLIP A. LOW, MD
Professor of Neurology, Mayo Medical School; Chairman, Division of Clinical Neurophysiology; Consultant in Neurology, Mayo Clinic, Rochester [22]

DANIEL H. LOWENSTEIN, MD
Professor of Neurology, Vice Chairman, Department of Neurology; Director, Physician-Scientist Education and Training Program; Director UCSF Epilepsy Center, University of California, San Francisco, San Francisco [2, 14]

JOSEPH B. MARTIN, MD, PhD, MA(Hon)
Dean of the Faculty of Medicine; Caroline Shields Walker Professor of Neurobiology and Clinical Neuroscience, Harvard Medical School, Boston [2, 4]

NANCY K. MELLO, PhD
Professor of Psychology, Harvard Medical School, Boston [43]

SHLOMO MELMED, MD
Professor and Associate Dean; David Geffen School of Medicine at University of California, Los Angeles; Senior Vice President and Chief Academic Officer at Cedars-Sinai Medical Center, Los Angeles [26]

JERRY R. MENDELL, MD
Helen C. Kurtz Professor and Chairman of Neurology, Ohio State University, Columbus [37, 38]

JACK H. MENDELSON, MD
Professor of Psychiatry (Neuroscience), Harvard Medical School, Belmont [43]

M.-MARSEL MESUAM, MD
Ruth and Evelyn Dunbar Professor of Neurology and Psychiatry; Director, Center for Behavioral and Cognitive Neurology; Director, Alzheimer's Program, Northwestern University Feinberg School of Medicine, Chicago [7]

BRUCE L. MILLER, MD
AW and Mary Margaret Clausen Distinguished Chair, Professor of Neurology, University of California, San Francisco, San Francisco [18, 32]

PHILIP J. NIVATPUMIN, MD
Department of Internal Medicine
The Johns Hopkins University School of Medicine
Baltimore (Review and Self-Assessment)

RICHARD K. OLNEY, MD
Professor of Neurology, University of California, San Francisco, San Francisco [10]

STANLEY B. PRUSINER, MD
Director, Institute for Neurodegenerative Diseases; Professor, Departments of Neurology, Biochemistry and Biophysics, University of California, San Francisco, San Francisco [32]

NEIL H. RASKIN, MD
Professor of Neurology, University of California, San Francisco, San Francisco [5]

VICTOR I. REUS, MD
Professor of Psychiatry, University of California, San Francisco; Medical Director, Langley Porter Hospital, San Francisco [41]

GARY S. RICHARDSON, MD
Assistant Professor of Psychiatry, Case Western Reserve University, Cleveland; Senior Research Scientist, Sleep Disorders and Research Center, Henry Ford Hospital, Detroit [13]

GARY L. ROBERTSON, MD
Professor of Medicine and Neurology, Northwestern University Feinberg School of Medicine, Chicago [26]

KAREN L. ROOS, MD
John and Nancy Nelson Professor of Neurology, Indiana University School of Medicine, Indianapolis [29]

ALLAN H. ROPPER, MD
Professor and Chairman of Neurology, Tufts University School of Medicine; Chief, Department of Neurology, St. Elizabeth's Medical Center, Boston [8, 16, 24]

ROGER N. ROSENBERG, MD
Zale Distinguished Chair and Professor of Neurology, University of Texas Southwestern Medical Center at Dallas; Attending Neurologist, Parkland Memorial Hospital and Zale-Lipsky University Hospital, Dallas [20]

MYRNA R. ROSENFELD, MD, PhD
Associate Professor of Neurology, Department of Neurology, University of Pennsylvania, Philadelphia [27]

STEPHEN M. SAGAR, MD
Professor of Neurology, Case Western Reserve School of Medicine; Director of Neuro-Oncology, Ireland Cancer Center, University Hospitals of Cleveland, Cleveland [25]

MARC A. SCHUCKIT, MD
Professor of Psychiatry, University of California, San Diego; Director, Alcohol Research Center, Director, Alcohol and Drug Treatment Program, Veterans Affairs San Diego Healthcare System, San Diego [42, 43]

DAVID S. SEGAL, PhD
Professor of Psychiatry, University of California, San Diego, La Jolla [43]

PATRICK M. SLUSS, PhD
Director, Immunodiagnostics Laboratory, Department of Pathology, Massachusetts General Hospital; Assistant Professor, Harvard Medical School, Boston [Appendix]

WADE S. SMITH, MD
Associate Professor of Neurology; Director, Neurointensive Care Service, University of California, San Francisco, San Francisco [17]

JAMES B. SNOW, JR., MD
Professor Emeritus, Department of Otorhinolaryngology, University of Pennsylvania; former Director, National Institute on Deafness and Other Communication Disorders, National Institutes of Health, Bethesda [12]

STEPHEN E. STRAUS, MD
Senior Investigator, Laboratory of Clinical Investigation, National Institute of Allergy and Infectious Diseases; Director, National Center for Complementary and Alternative Medicine, National Institutes of Health, Bethesda [40]

MORTON N. SWARTZ, MD
Professor, Department of Medicine, Harvard Medical School; Chief Emeritus, Infectious Disease, Chief, James Jackson Firm Medical Services, Massachusetts General Hospital, Boston [30]

KENNETH L. TYLER, MD
Roulor-Lewin Family Professor of Neurology; Professor of Medicine, Microbiology and Immunology, University of Colorado Health Sciences Center Chief, Neurology Service, Denver VA Medical Center, Denver [29]

CHARLES WIENER, MD
Vice-Chair, Department of Medicine
The Johns Hopkins University School of Medicine
Baltimore (Review and Self-Assessment)

JOHN W. WINKELMAN, MD, PhD
Assistant Professor of Psychiatry, Harvard Medical School; Medical Director, Sleep Health Center, Brigham and Women's Hospital, Boston [13]

PREFACE

Neurologic problems are often challenging. Acquisition of the requisite clinical skills may appear to be time-consuming, difficult to master, and dependent on a working knowledge of obscure anatomic facts and laundry lists of diagnostic possibilities. The patients themselves may be difficult, as neurologic disorders often alter an individual's capacity to recount the history of an illness or to even recognize that something is wrong. An additional obstacle is the development of independent neurology services, departments, and training programs at many medical centers, reducing the exposure of current internal medicine trainees to neurologic problems. All of these forces, acting within the fast-paced environment of modern medical practice, can lead to an overreliance on unfocused neuroimaging tests, suboptimal patient care, and unfortunate outcomes. Because neurologists represent only 1% of physicians, the vast majority of neurologic care must be delivered by nonspecialists who are often generalists and usually internists.

The old adage that neurologists "know everything but do nothing" has been rendered obsolete by advances in molecular medicine, imaging, bioengineering, and clinical research. Examples of new therapies include: thrombolytic therapy for acute ischemic stroke; endovascular recanalization for cerebrovascular disorders; intensive monitoring of brain pressure and cerebral blood flow for brain injury; effective therapies for immune-mediated neurologic disorders such as multiple sclerosis, immune neuropathies, myasthenia gravis, and myositis; new designer drugs for migraine; the first generation of rational therapies for neurodegenerative diseases; neural stimulators for Parkinson's disease; drugs for narcolepsy and other sleep disorders; and control of epilepsy by surgical resection of small seizure foci precisely localized by functional imaging and electrophysiology. Treatment breakthroughs continue, stimulated by a quickening tempo of discoveries generating opportunities for rational design of new diagnostics, interventions, and drugs.

The founding editors of *Harrison's Principles of Internal Medicine* acknowledged the importance of neurology but were uncertain as to its proper role in a textbook of internal medicine. An initial plan to exclude neurology from the first edition (1950) was reversed at the eleventh hour, and a neurology section was hastily prepared by Houston Merritt. By the second edition, the section was considerably enlarged by Raymond D. Adams, whose influence on the textbook was profound. The third neurology editor, Joseph B. Martin, brilliantly led the book during the 1980s and 1990s as neurology was transformed from a largely descriptive discipline to one of the most dynamic and rapidly evolving areas of medicine.

Our goal in publishing *Harrison's Neurology in Clinical Medicine* as a stand-alone volume is to provide expanded coverage of clinically important topics geared to the needs of the practicing internist, while retaining the focus on pathophysiology and therapy that has always been characteristic of *Harrison's*. New tables have been added, many illustrations have been redrawn using state-of-the-art graphics, and the catalog of neuroimaging findings has been enlarged. Questions and answers have been placed at the end of the book to provide important teaching points.

The Editors are indebted to our authors, a group of internationally recognized authorities who have magnificently distilled a daunting body of information into the essential principles required to understand and manage commonly encountered neurological problems. We are also grateful to Dr. Elizabeth Robbins, who has served for more than a decade as managing editor of the neurology section of *Harrison's* textbook; she has overseen the complex logistics required to produce a multiauthored textbook and has promoted exceptional standards for clarity, language, and style. This new product was championed by Jim Shanahan and Marty Wonsiewicz and impeccably managed in production by Mariapaz Ramos Englis, Catherine Saggese, and Charissa Baker.

It is our sincere hope that you will enjoy using *Harrison's Neurology in Clinical Medicine* as an authoritative source for the most up-to-date information in clinical neurology.

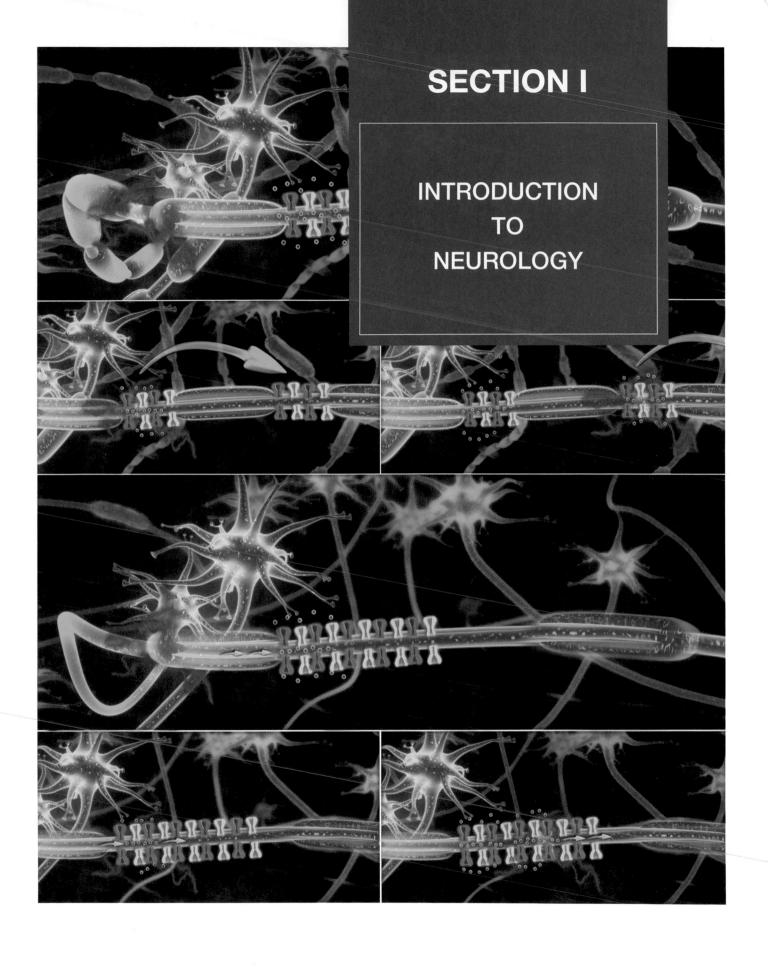

SECTION I

INTRODUCTION TO NEUROLOGY

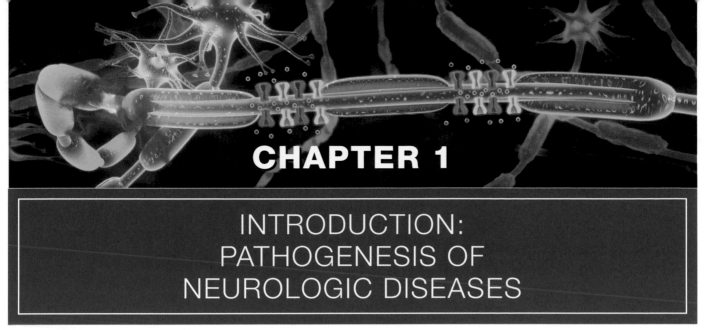

CHAPTER 1

INTRODUCTION: PATHOGENESIS OF NEUROLOGIC DISEASES

Stephen L. Hauser
M. Flint Beal

Neurologic diseases are common and costly. According to one estimate, 180 million Americans suffer from a nervous system disorder, resulting in an annual cost of $634 billion (**Table 1-1**). This aggregate cost is even greater than that for cardiovascular disorders. Globally, neurologic disorders are responsible for 28% of all years lived with a disability.

The human nervous system is the organ of consciousness, cognition, ethics, and behavior; as such, it is the most intricate structure known to exist. One-third of the 35,000 genes encoded in the human genome are expressed in the nervous system. Each mature brain is composed of 100 billion neurons, several million miles of axons and dendrites, and $>10^{15}$ synapses. Neurons exist within a dense parenchyma of multifunctional glial cells that synthesize myelin, preserve homeostasis, and regulate immune responses. Measured against this background of complexity, the achievements of molecular neuroscience have been extraordinary. This chapter reviews selected themes in neuroscience that provide a context for understanding fundamental mechanisms underlying neurologic disorders.

ION CHANNELS AND CHANNELOPATHIES

The resting potential of neurons and the action potentials responsible for impulse conduction are generated by ion currents and ion channels. Most ion channels are gated, meaning that they can transition between conformations that are open or closed to ion conductance. Individual ion channels are distinguished by the specific ions they conduct; by their kinetics; and by whether they directly sense voltage, are linked to receptors for neurotransmitters or other ligands such as neurotrophins, or are activated by second messengers. The diverse characteristics of different ion channels provide a means by which neuronal excitability can be exquisitely modulated at both the cellular and the subcellular levels. Mutations in ion channels—*channelopathies*—are responsible for a growing list of human neurologic disorders (**Table 1-2**). One example is epilepsy, a syndrome of diverse causes characterized by repetitive, synchronous firing of neuronal action potentials. Action potentials are normally generated by the opening of sodium channels and the inward movement of sodium ions down the intracellular concentration gradient. Depolarization of the neuronal membrane opens potassium channels, resulting in outward movement of potassium ions, repolarization, closure of the sodium channel, and hyperpolarization. Sodium or potassium channel subunit genes have long been considered candidate disease genes in inherited epilepsy syndromes, and recently such mutations have been identified. These mutations appear to alter the normal gating function of these channels, increasing the inherent excitability of neuronal membranes in regions where the abnormal channels are expressed.

TABLE 1-1

IMPACT OF NEUROLOGIC AND PSYCHIATRIC DISEASES IN THE U.S.

DISORDER	PATIENTS, MILLIONS	COST, BILLION $
Addiction	17.5	160
Alzheimer's disease	4	100
Blindness/vision loss	13	38.4
Deafness/hearing loss	28	56
Depression/manic depressive illness	17.5	47.3
Developmental disorders	8.6	30
Epilepsy	2.5	3.5
Head injury	2	25
Huntington's disease	0.03	—
Multiple sclerosis	0.3	2.5
Pain	80	100
Parkinson's disease	1	6
Schizophrenia	2	30
Spinal cord injury	0.25	5
Stroke	3	30
Total	180	634

Source: Modified from Dana Alliance for Brain Initiatives: *Delivery Results: A Progress Report on Brain Research*. New York, Dana Press, 1996.

Whereas the specific clinical manifestations of channelopathies are quite variable, one common feature is that manifestations tend to be intermittent or paroxysmal, such as occurs in epilepsy, migraine, ataxia, myotonia, or periodic paralysis. Exceptions are clinically progressive channel disorders such as autosomal dominant hearing impairment. The neurologic channelopathies identified to date are all uncommon disorders caused by obvious mutations in channel genes. As the full repertoire of human ion channels and related proteins are identified, it is likely that additional channelopathies will be discovered. In addition to rare disorders that result from obvious

TABLE 1-2

EXAMPLES OF NEUROLOGIC CHANNELOPATHIES

CATEGORY	DISORDER	CHANNEL TYPE	GENE	CHAP. REF.
Ataxias	Episodic ataxia-1	K	*KCNAI*	20
	Episodic ataxia-2	Ca	*CACNLIAd*	
	Spinocerebellar ataxia-6	Ca	*CACNLIAd*	
Migraine	Familial hemiplegic migraine	Ca	*CACNLIAd*	5
Epilepsy	Benign neonatal familial convulsions	K	*KCNQ2, KCNQ3*	14
	Generalized epilepsy with febrile convulsions plus	Na	*SCNIβ*	
Periodic paralysis	Hyperkalemic periodic paralysis	Na	*SCN4A*	38
	Hypokalemic periodic paralysis	Ca	*CACNLIA3*	
Myotonia	Myotonia congenita	C1	*CLCN1*	38
	Paramyotonia congenita	Na	*SCN4A*	
Deafness	Jorvell and Lange-Nielsen syndrome (deafness, prolonged QT interval, and arrythmia)	K	*KCNQ1, KCNE1*	12
	Autosomal dominant progressive deafness	K	*KCNQ4*	

mutations, it is possible that subtle allelic variations in channel genes or in their pattern of expression might underlie susceptibility to some common forms of epilepsy, migraine, or other disorders.

NEUROTRANSMITTERS AND NEUROTRANSMITTER RECEPTORS

Synaptic neurotransmission is the predominant means by which neurons communicate with each other. Classic neurotransmitters are synthesized in the presynaptic region of the nerve terminal; stored in vesicles; and released into the synaptic cleft, where they bind to receptors on the postsynaptic cell. Secreted neurotransmitters are eliminated by reuptake into the presynaptic neuron (or glia), by diffusion away from the synaptic cleft, and/or by specific inactivation. In addition to the classic neurotransmitters, many neuropeptides have been identified as definite or probable neurotransmitters; these include substance P, neurotensin, enkephalins, β-endorphin, histamine, vasoactive intestinal polypeptide, cholecystokinin, neuropeptide Y, and somatostatin. Peptide neurotransmitters are synthesized in the cell body rather than the nerve terminal and may colocalize with classic neurotransmitters in single neurons. Nitric oxide and carbon monoxide are gases that appear also to function as neurotransmitters, in part by signaling in a retrograde fashion from the postsynaptic to the presynaptic cell.

Neurotransmitters modulate the function of postsynaptic cells by binding to specific neurotransmitter receptors, of which there are two major types. *Ionotropic receptors* are direct ion channels that open after engagement by the neurotransmitter. *Metabotropic receptors* interact with G proteins, stimulating production of second messengers and activating protein kinases, which modulate a variety of cellular events. Ionotropic receptors are multiple subunit structures, whereas metabotropic receptors are composed of single subunits only. One important difference between ionotropic and metabotropic receptors is that the kinetics of ionotropic receptor effects are fast (generally <1 ms) because neurotransmitter binding directly alters the electrical properties of the postsynaptic cell, whereas metabotropic receptors function over longer time periods. These different properties contribute to the potential for selective and finely modulated signaling by neurotransmitters.

Neurotransmitter systems are perturbed in a large number of clinical disorders, examples of which are highlighted in **Table 1-3**. One example is the involvement of dopaminergic neurons originating in the substantia nigra of the midbrain and projecting to the striatum (nigrostriatal pathway) in Parkinson's disease and in heroin addicts after the ingestion of the toxin MPTP (1-methyl-4-phenyl-1,2,5,6-tetrahydropyridine).

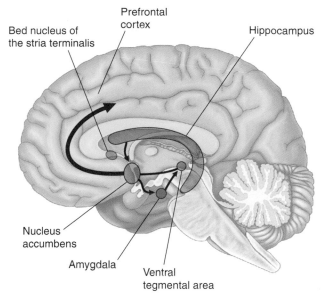

FIGURE 1-1

Mid-sagittal section of the human brain demonstrating limbic structures involved in brain reward pathways.

A second important dopaminergic system arising in the midbrain is the mediocorticolimbic pathway, which is implicated in the pathogenesis of addictive behaviors including drug reward. Its key components include the midbrain ventral tegmental area (VTA), median forebrain bundle, and nucleus accumbens (**Fig. 1-1**). *Addictive drugs share the property of increasing dopamine release in the nucleus accumbens.* Amphetamine increases intracellular release of dopamine from vesicles and reverses transport of dopamine through the dopamine transporters. Patients prone to addiction show increased activation of the nucleus accumbens following administration of amphetamine. Cocaine binds to dopamine transporters and inhibits dopamine reuptake. Ethanol inhibits inhibitory neurons in the VTA, leading to increased dopamine release in the nucleus accumbens. Opioids also disinhibit these dopaminergic neurons by binding to μ receptors expressed by GABA-containing interneurons in the VTA. Nicotine increases dopamine release by activating nicotinic acetylcholine receptors on cell bodies and nerve terminals of dopaminergic VTA neurons. Tetrahydrocannabinol, the active ingredient of cannabis, also increases dopamine levels in the nucleus accumbens. Blockade of dopamine in the nucleus accumbens can terminate the rewarding effects of addictive drugs.

Not all cell-to-cell communication in the nervous system occurs via neurotransmission. Gap junctions provide for direct neuron-neuron electrical conduction and also create openings for the diffusion of ions and metabolites between cells. In addition to neurons, gap

TABLE 1-3

PRINCIPAL CLASSIC NEUROTRANSMITTERS

NEUROTRANSMITTER	ANATOMY	CLINICAL ASPECTS
Acetylcholine (ACh) $CH_3-\overset{\overset{\textstyle O}{\|\|}}{C}-O-CH_2-CH_2-N-(CH_3)_3$	Motor neurons in spinal cord → neuromuscular junction	Acetylcholinesterases (nerve gases) Myasthenia gravis (antibodies to ACh receptor) Congenital myasthenic syndromes (mutations in ACh receptor subunits) Lambert-Eaton syndrome (antibodies to Ca channels impair ACh release) Botulism (toxin disrupts ACh release by exocytosis)
	Basal forebrain → widespread cortex	Alzheimer's disease (selective cell death) Autosomal dominant frontal lobe epilepsy (mutations in CNS ACh receptor)
	Interneurons in striatum Autonomic nervous system (preganglionic and postganglionic sympathetic)	Parkinson's disease (tremor)
Dopamine	Substantia nigra → striatum (nigrostriatal pathway)	Parkinson's disease (selective cell death) MPTP parkinsonism (toxin transported into neurons)
$HO-\text{(benzene ring)}-CH_2-CH_2-NH_3$ with HO	Substantia nigra → limbic system and widespread cortex	Addiction, behavioral disorders
	Arcuate nucleus of hypothalamus → anterior pituitary (via portal veins)	Inhibits prolactin secretion
Norepinephrine (NE)	Locus coeruleus (pons) → limbic system, hypothalamus, cortex	Mood disorders (MAOA inhibitors and tricyclics increase NE and improve depression)
$HO-\text{(benzene ring)}-CH(OH)-CH_2-NH_2$ with HO	Medulla → locus coeruleus, spinal cord	Anxiety
	Postganglionic neurons of sympathetic nervous system	Orthostatic tachycardia syndrome (mutations in NE transporter)
Serotonin $HO-\text{(indole ring)}-CH_2-CH_2-NH_2$	Pontine raphe nuclei → widespread projections Medulla/pons → dorsal horn of spinal cord	Mood disorders (SSRIs improve depression) Migraine pain pathway Pain pathway
γ-Aminobutyric acid (GABA) $H_2N-CH_2-CH_2-CH_2-COOH$	Major inhibitory neurotransmitter in brain; widespread cortical interneurons and long projection pathways	Stiff person syndrome (antibodies to glutamic acid decarboxylase, the biosynthetic enzyme for GABA) Epilepsy (gabapentin and valproic acid increase GABA)
Glycine $H_2N-CH-COOH$	Major inhibitory neurotransmitter in spinal cord	Spasticity Hyperekplexia (myoclonic startle syndrome) due to mutations in glycine receptor
Glutamate $H_2N-\underset{\underset{\textstyle COOH}{\|}}{CH}-CH_2-CH_2-COOH$	Major excitatory neurotransmitter; located throughout CNS, including cortical pyramidal cells	Seizures due to ingestion of domoic acid (a glutamate analogue) Rasmussen's encephalitis (antibody against glutamate receptor 3) Excitotoxic cell death

Note: CNS, central nervous system; MPTP, 1-methyl-4-phenyl-1,2,3,6-tetrahydropyridine; MAOA, monoamine oxidase A; SSRI, selective serotonin reuptake inhibitor.

junctions are also widespread in glia, creating a syncytium that protects neurons by removing glutamate and potassium from the extracellular environment. Gap junctions consist of membrane-spanning proteins, termed *connexins*, that pair across adjacent cells. Mechanisms that involve gap junctions have been related to a variety of neurologic disorders. Mutations in connexin 32, a gap junction protein expressed by Schwann cells, are responsible for the X-linked form of Charcot-Marie-Tooth disease (Chap. 34). Mutations in either of two gap junction proteins expressed in the inner ear—connexin 26 and connexin 31—result in autosomal dominant progressive hearing loss (Chap. 12). Glial calcium waves mediated through gap junctions also appear to explain the phenomenon of spreading depression associated with migraine auras and the march of epileptic discharges. Spreading depression is a neural response that follows a variety of different stimuli and is characterized by a circumferentially expanding negative potential that propagates at a characteristic speed of 20 m/s and is associated with an increase in extracellular potassium.

SIGNALING PATHWAYS AND GENE TRANSCRIPTION

The fundamental issue of how memory, learning, and thinking are encoded in the nervous system is likely to be clarified by identifying the signaling pathways involved in neuronal differentiation, axon guidance, and synapse formation, and by understanding how these pathways are modulated by experience. Many families of transcription factors, each comprising multiple individual components, are expressed in the nervous system. Elucidation of these signaling pathways has already begun to provide insights into the cause of a variety of neurologic disorders, including inherited disorders of cognition such as X-linked mental retardation. This problem affects approximately 1 in 500 males, and linkage studies in different families suggest that as many as 60 different X-chromosome encoded genes may be responsible. Rett syndrome, a common cause of (dominant) X-linked progressive mental retardation in females, is due to a mutation in a gene (*MECP2*) encoding a DNA-binding protein involved in transcriptional repression. As the X chromosome comprises only ~3% of germline DNA, then by extrapolation the number of genes that potentially contribute to clinical disorders affecting intelligence in humans must be potentially very large. As discussed below, there is increasing evidence that abnormal gene transcription may play a role in neurodegenerative diseases such as Huntington's disease in which proteins with polyglutamine expansions bind to and sequester transcription factors. A critical transcription factor for neu-

ronal survival is CREB (cyclic adenosine monophosphate responsive element-binding) protein, which also plays an important role in memory in the hippocampus.

MYELIN

Myelin is the multilayered insulating substance that surrounds axons and speeds impulse conduction by permitting action potentials to jump between naked regions of axons (nodes of Ranvier) and across myelinated segments. A single oligodendrocyte usually ensheaths multiple axons in the central nervous system (CNS), whereas in the peripheral nervous system (PNS) each Schwann cell typically myelinates a single axon. Myelin is a lipid-rich material formed by a spiraling process of the membrane of the myelinating cell around the axon, creating multiple membrane bilayers that are tightly apposed (compact myelin) by charged protein interactions. A number of clinically important neurologic disorders are caused by inherited mutations in myelin proteins of the CNS or PNS. Constituents of myelin also have a propensity to be targeted as autoantigens in autoimmune demyelinating disorders (**Fig. 1-2**).

NEUROTROPHIC FACTORS

Neurotrophic factors (**Table 1-4**) are secreted proteins that modulate neuronal growth, differentiation, repair, and survival; some have additional functions, including roles in neurotransmission and in the synaptic reorganization involved in learning and memory. The neurotrophin (NT) family contains nerve growth factor (NGF), brain-derived neurotrophic factor (BDNF), NT3, and NT4/5. The neurotrophins act at TrK and p75 receptors to promote survival of neurons. Because of their survival-promoting and antiapoptotic effects, neu-

TABLE 1-4

NEUROTROPHIC FACTORS	
Neurotrophin family	Transforming growth factor β family
Nerve growth factor	
Brain-derived neurotrophic factor	Glial-derived neurotrophic family
Neurotrophin-3	Neurturin
Neurotrophin-4	Persephin
Neurotrophin-6	Fibroblast growth factor family
Cytokine family	Hepatocyte growth factor
Ciliary neurotrophic factor	Insulin-like growth factor (IGF) family
Leukemia inhibitory factor	IGF-1
Interleukin-6	IGF-2
Cardiotrophin-1	

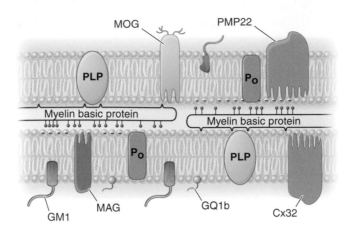

FIGURE 1-2

The molecular architecture of the myelin sheath illustrating the most important disease-related proteins. The illustration represents a composite of CNS and PNS myelin. Proteins restricted to CNS myelin are shown in green, proteins of PNS myelin are lavender, and proteins present in both CNS and PNS are red. In the CNS, the X-linked allelic disorders, Pelizaeus-Merzbacher disease and one variant of familial spastic paraplegia, are caused by mutations in the gene for proteolipid protein (PLP) that normally promotes extracellular compaction between adjacent myelin lamellae. The homologue of PLP in the PNS is the P_0 protein, mutations in which cause the neuropathy Charcot-Marie-Tooth disease (CMT) type 1B. The most common form of CMT is the 1A subtype caused by a duplication of the *PMP22* gene; deletions in *PMP22* are responsible for another inherited neuropathy termed *hereditary liability to pressure palsies* (Chap. 34).

In multiple sclerosis (MS), myelin basic protein (MBP) and the quantitatively minor CNS protein, myelin oligodendrocyte glycoprotein (MOG), are likely T cell and B cell antigens, respectively (Chap. 28). The location of MOG at the outermost lamella of the CNS myelin membrane may facilitate its targeting by autoantibodies. In the PNS, autoantibodies against myelin gangliosides are implicated in a variety of disorders, including GQ1b in the Fisher variant of Guillain-Barré syndrome, GM1 in multifocal motor neuropathy, and sulfatide constituents of myelin-associated glycoprotein (MAG) in peripheral neuropathies associated with monoclonal gammopathies (Chap. 35).

rotrophic factors are in theory outstanding candidates for therapy of disorders characterized by premature death of neurons such as occurs in amyotrophic lateral sclerosis (ALS) and other degenerative motor neuron disorders. Knockout mice lacking receptors for ciliary neurotrophic factor (CNTF) or BDNF show loss of motor neurons, and experimental motor neuron death can be rescued by treatment with various neurotrophic factors including CNTF and BDNF. However, in phase 3 clinical trials, growth factors were ineffective in human ALS. The growth factor glial-derived neurotrophic factor (GDNF) is important for survival of dopaminergic neurons. It has shown promising neurorestorative effects in experimental models of Parkinson's disease and in early-stage human clinical trials.

STEM CELLS AND TRANSPLANTATION

The nervous system is traditionally considered to be a nonmitotic organ, in particular with respect to neurons. These concepts have been challenged by the finding that neural progenitor or stem cells exist in the adult CNS that are capable of differentiation, migration over long distances, and extensive axonal arborization and synapse formation with appropriate targets. These capabilities also indicate that the repertoire of factors required for growth, survival, differentiation, and migration of these cells exists in the mature nervous system. In rodents, neural stem cells, defined as progenitor cells capable of differentiating into mature cells of neural or glial lineage, have been experimentally propagated from fetal CNS and neuroectodermal tissues and also from adult germinal matrix and ependyma regions. Human fetal CNS tissue is also capable of differentiation into cells with neuronal, astrocyte, and oligodendrocyte morphology when cultured in the presence of growth factors. Impressively, such cells could be stably engrafted into mouse CNS tissue, creating neural chimeras. Human adult neural stem cells have been identified in an astrocyte layer adjacent to the lateral ventricles; however, these neurons appeared to be unable to migrate or form connections. Once the repertoire of signals required for cell type specification is better understood, differentiation into specific neural or glial subpopulations can be directed in vitro; such cells could also be engineered to express therapeutic molecules. Another promising approach is to utilize growth factors, such as BDNF, to stimulate endogenous stem cells to proliferate and migrate to areas of neuronal damage. Administration of epidermal growth factor with fibroblast growth factor replenished up to 50% of hippocampal CA1 neurons a month after global ischemia in rats. The new neurons made connections and improved performance in a memory task.

Experimental transplantation of human fetal dopaminergic neurons in patients with Parkinson's disease has shown that these transplanted cells can survive within the host striatum; however, some patients developed disabling dyskinesias, and this approach is no longer in clinical development. Studies of transplantation for patients with Huntington's disease have also reported encouraging, although very preliminary, results. Oligodendrocyte precursor cells transplanted into mice with a dysmyelinating disorder effectively migrated in the new environment, interacted with axons, and mediated myelination; such experiments raise hope that similar transplantation strategies may be feasible in human disorders of myelin such as multiple sclerosis. The promise of stem cells for treatment of both neurodegenerative diseases and neural injury is great, but development has been slowed by unresolved concerns over safety (including the theoretical risk of malignant transformation of transplanted cells), ethics (particularly with respect to use of fetal tissue), and efficacy.

In developing brain, the extracellular matrix provides stimulatory and inhibitory signals that promote neuronal migration, neurite outgrowth, and axonal extension. After neuronal damage, reexpression of inhibitory molecules such as chondroitin sulfate proteoglycans may prevent tissue regeneration. Chondroitinase degraded these inhibitory molecules and enhanced axonal regeneration and motor recovery in a rat model of spinal cord injury. Several myelin proteins, specifically Nogo, oligodendrocyte myelin glycoprotein (OMGP), and myelin-associated glycoprotein (MAG), may also interfere with axon regeneration. Antibodies against Nogo promote regeneration after experimental focal ischemia. Nogo, OMGP, and MAG all bind to the same neural receptor, the Nogo receptor, which mediates its inhibitory function via the p75 neurotrophin receptor signaling.

CELL DEATH—EXCITOTOXICITY AND APOPTOSIS

Excitotoxicity refers to neuronal cell death caused by activation of excitatory amino acid receptors (**Fig. 1-3**). Compelling evidence for a role of excitotoxicity, especially in ischemic neuronal injury, is derived from experiments in animal models. Experimental models of stroke are associated with increased extracellular concentrations of the excitatory amino acid neurotransmitter glutamate, and neuronal damage is attenuated by denervation of glutamate-containing neurons or the administration of glutamate receptor antagonists. The distribution of cells sensitive to ischemia corresponds closely with that of N-methyl-D-aspartate (NMDA) receptors (except for cerebellar Purkinje cells, which are vulnerable to hypoxia-ischemia but lack NMDA receptors); and competitive and noncompetitive NMDA antagonists are effective in preventing focal ischemia. In global cerebral ischemia, non-NMDA receptors (kainic acid and AMPA) are activated, and antagonists to these receptors are protective. Experimental brain damage induced by hypoglycemia is also attenuated by NMDA antagonists.

Excitotoxicity is not a single event but rather a cascade of cell injury. Excitotoxicity causes influx of calcium into cells, and much of the calcium is sequestered in mitochondria rather than in the cytoplasm. Increased cytoplasmic calcium causes metabolic dysfunction and free radical generation; activates protein kinases, phospholipases, nitric oxide synthase, proteases, and endonucleases; and inhibits protein synthesis. Activation of nitric oxide synthase generates nitric oxide ($NO^{\bullet}$), which can react with superoxide ($O_2^{\bullet}$) to generate peroxynitrite ($ONOO^-$), which may play a direct role in neuronal injury. Another critical pathway is activation of poly-ADP-ribose polymerase, which occurs in response to free radical–mediated DNA damage. Experimentally, mice with knockout mutations of neuronal nitric oxide synthase or poly-ADP-ribose polymerase, or those that overexpress superoxide dismutase, are resistant to focal ischemia.

Apoptosis, or programmed cell death, plays an important role in both physiologic and pathologic conditions. During embryogenesis, apoptotic pathways operate to destroy neurons that fail to differentiate appropriately or reach their intended targets. There is mounting evidence for an increased rate of apoptotic cell death in a variety of acute and chronic neurologic diseases. Apoptosis is characterized by neuronal shrinkage, chromatin condensation, and DNA fragmentation, whereas necrotic cell death is associated with cytoplasmic and mitochondrial swelling followed by dissolution of the cell membrane. Apoptotic and necrotic cell death can coexist or be sequential events, depending on the severity of the initiating insult. Cellular energy reserves appear to have an important role in these two forms of cell death, with apoptosis favored under conditions in which ATP levels are preserved. Evidence of DNA fragmentation has been found in a number of degenerative neurologic disorders, including

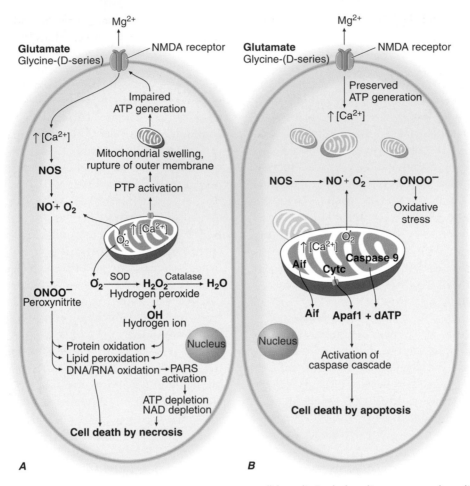

FIGURE 1-3

Involvement of mitochondria in cell death. A severe excitotoxic insult (*A*) results in cell death by necrosis, whereas a mild excitotoxic insult (*B*) results in apoptosis. After a severe insult (such as ischemia), there is a large increase in glutamate activation of NMDA receptors, an increase in intracellular Ca^{2+} concentrations, activation of nitric oxide synthase (NOS), and increased mitochondrial Ca^{2+} and superoxide generation followed by the formation of $ONOO^-$. This sequence results in damage to cellular macromolecules including DNA, leading to activation of poly-ADP-ribose polymerase (PARS). Both mitochondrial accumulation of Ca^{2+} and oxidative damage lead to activation of the permeability transition pore (PTP) that is linked to excitotoxic cell death. A mild excitotoxic insult can occur due either to an abnormality in an excitotoxicity amino acid receptor, allowing more Ca^{2+} flux, or to impaired functioning of other ionic channels or of energy production, which may allow the voltage-dependent NMDA receptor to be activated by ambient concentrations of glutamate. This event can then lead to increased mitochondrial Ca^{2+} and free radical production, yet relatively preserved ATP generation. The mitochondria may then release cytochrome c (Cytc), caspase 9, apoptosis-inducing factor (Aif), and perhaps other mediators that lead to apoptosis. The precise role of the PTP in this mode of cell death is still being clarified, but there does appear to be involvement of the adenine nucleotide transporter that is a key component of the PTP.

Alzheimer's disease, Huntington's disease, and ALS. The best characterized genetic neurologic disorder related to apoptosis is infantile spinal muscular atrophy (Werdnig-Hoffmann disease), in which two genes thought to be involved in the apoptosis pathways are causative.

Mitochondria are essential in controlling specific apoptosis pathways. The redistribution of cytochrome c, as well as apoptosis-inducing factor (AIF), from mitochondria during apoptosis leads to the activation of a cascade of intracellular proteases known as *caspases*. Caspase-independent apoptosis occurs after DNA damage, activation of poly-ADP-ribose polymerase, and translocation of AIF into the nucleus. Redistribution of cytochrome c is prevented by overproduction of the apoptotic protein BCL2 and is promoted by the proapoptotic protein BAX. These pathways may be triggered by activation of a large pore in the mitochondrial inner membrane known as the *permeability transition pore*, although in other circumstances they occur independently. Recent studies suggest that blocking the mitochondrial pore reduces both hypoglycemic and ischemic cell death.

PROTEIN AGGREGATION AND NEURODEGENERATION

The possibility that protein aggregation plays a role in the pathogenesis of neurodegenerative diseases is a major focus of current research. Protein aggregation is a major histopathologic hallmark of neurodegenerative diseases. Deposition of β-amyloid is strongly implicated in the pathogenesis of Alzheimer's disease. Genetic mutations in familial Alzheimer's disease produce increased amounts of β-amyloid with 42 amino acids, which has an increased propensity to aggregate, as compared to β-amyloid with 40 amino acids. Mutations in genes encoding the microtubule-associated protein tau lead to altered splicing of tau and the production of neurofibrillary tangles in frontotemporal dementia and progressive supranuclear palsy. Familial Parkinson's disease is associated with mutations in α-synuclein, parkin, and the ubiquitin carboxy-terminal hydrolase. Parkin, which causes autosomal recessive early-onset Parkinson's disease, is a ubiquitin ligase. The characteristic histopathologic feature of Parkinson's disease is the Lewy body, an eosinophilic cytoplasmic inclusion that contains both neurofilaments and α-synuclein. Huntington's disease and cerebellar degenerations are associated with expansions of polyglutamine repeats in proteins, which aggregate to produce neuronal intranuclear inclusions. Familial ALS is associated with superoxide dismutase mutations and cytoplasmic inclusions containing superoxide dismutase. In autosomal dominant neurohypophyseal diabetes insipidus, mutations in vasopressin result in abnormal protein processing, accumulation in the endoplasmic reticulum, and cell death.

The current major scientific question is whether protein aggregates contribute to neuronal death or whether they are merely secondary bystanders. Protein aggregates are usually ubiquinated, which targets them for degradation by the 26S component of the proteosome. An inability to degrade protein aggregates could lead to cellular dysfunction, impaired axonal transport, and cell death by apoptotic mechanisms.

In experimental models of Huntington's disease and cerebellar degeneration, protein aggregates are not well correlated with neuronal death. A substantial body of evidence suggests that the mutant proteins with polyglutamine expansions in these diseases bind to transcription factors and that this contributes to disease pathogenesis. Agents that upregulate gene transcription are neuroprotective in animal models of these diseases. A number of compounds have been developed to block β-amyloid production and/or aggregation, and these agents are being studied in early clinical trials in humans.

NEUROIMMUNOLOGY

The nervous system is traditionally considered to be an immunologically privileged organ, a concept originally derived from observations that tissue grafts implanted in the brain were not rejected efficiently. In this context, immune privilege of the CNS may be maintained by a variety of mechanisms, including the lack of an efficient surveillance function by T cells; the absence of a traditional lymphoid system; limited expression of major histocompatibility complex (MHC) molecules required for T cell recognition of antigen; effects of regulatory cytokines secreted spontaneously or in response to mediators such as NGF, creating an immunosuppressive milieu; and also from expression of fas ligand that can induce apoptosis of fas-expressing immune cells that enter the brain. The blood-brain barrier (BBB) partially isolates the brain from the peripheral environment and contributes to immune privilege. Anatomically, the barrier is created by the presence of impermeable tight junctions between endothelial cells and by a relative absence of transendothelial conduits for the passive diffusion of soluble molecules. The BBB serves to preserve CNS homeostasis by excluding neuroactive substances present in the serum, such as neurotransmitters and neurotrophic factors. Because of the BBB, lipid-insoluble molecules must utilize either ion channels or specific transport systems (for glucose or various amino acids) to gain entry to the CNS. Astrocyte foot processes that encircle the subendothelial basal surface of small blood vessels in the brain contribute to development and maintenance of the BBB.

The concept of immune privilege is at odds with clinical experience that vigorous immune reactions readily occur in the nervous system in response to infections and that autoimmune diseases of the nervous system are relatively common. Although primary (sensitizing) immune responses are not easily generated in the CNS for the reasons outlined above, this is not the case for secondary immune responses. When sensitization to nervous system antigens occurs *outside* the nervous system (e.g., in a regional lymph node), activated autoreactive T lymphocytes are easily generated, and these cells readily cross the BBB and induce immune-mediated injury. The paradigm for this mechanism of T cell–mediated CNS disease is experimental allergic encephalomyelitis (EAE), a laboratory model for the human autoimmune demyelinating disorders multiple sclerosis and acute disseminated encephalomyelitis; the sequence of events in EAE is illustrated in **Fig. 1–4.**

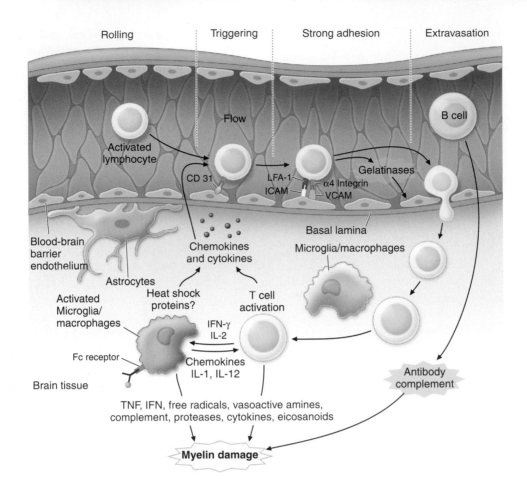

FIGURE 1-4

A model for experimental allergic encephalomyelitis (EAE). Crucial steps for disease initiation and progression include peripheral activation of preexisting autoreactive T cells; homing to the CNS and extravasation across the blood-brain barrier; reactivation of T cells by exposed autoantigens; secretion of cytokines; activation of microglia and astrocytes and recruitment of a secondary inflammatory wave; and immune-mediated myelin destruction. ICAM, intercellular adhesion molecule; LFA-1, leukocyte function-associated antigen-1; VCAM, vascular cell adhesion molecule; IFN, interferon; IL, interleukin; TNF, tumor necrosis factor.

Under normal circumstances the BBB is impermeable to antibodies. For autoantibodies to reach the CNS, the BBB must first be disrupted. In inflammatory conditions it is thought that this disruption most often occurs via actions of proinflammatory cytokines elaborated within the brain consequent to interactions between pathogenic T cells and antigen-presenting cells (APCs). In contrast to the BBB, in the PNS the blood–nerve barrier is incomplete. Endothelial tight junctions are lacking, and the capacity of charged molecules, including antibodies, to cross the barrier appears to be greatest in two regions of the PNS: proximally in the spinal roots and distally at neuromuscular junctions. This anatomical feature is likely to contribute to the propensity of antibody-mediated autoimmune disorders of the PNS to target proximal nerves (Guillain-Barré syndrome) or the neuromuscular junction (myasthenia gravis, Eaton-Lambert syndrome).

The major APCs in the CNS are microglial cells and macrophages; both cell types express MHC class 2 molecules as well as co-stimulatory molecules required for antigen presentation. Neurons do not express MHC class 2 molecules; however, some neurons express MHC class 1 proteins, which may be further increased in response to neuronal activity. Neuronal MHC class 1 molecules may function as retrograde postsynaptic signaling molecules that interact with presynaptic CD3 molecules to stabilize active synapses and transynaptically modulate neuronal function. A role of microglial activation as a contributor to cell death in neurodegenerative and chronic neuroinflammatory diseases is likely and is being actively investigated.

FURTHER READINGS

DAWSON TM, DAWSON VL: Rare genetic mutations shed light on the pathogenesis of Parkinson's disease. J Clin Invest 111:145, 2003

GAGE FH: Neurogenesis in the adult brain. J Neurosci 22:612, 2002

HADLEY EC et al: The future of aging therapies. Cell 120:557, 2005

☑ SANAI N et al: Unique astrocyte ribbon in adult human brain contains neural stem cells but lacks chain migration. Nature 427:740, 2004

Identification of multipotent neural stem cells in sub-ventricular zone of adult human brain.

SOTO C: Unfolding the role of protein misfolding in neurodegenerative diseases. Nature Rev Neurosci 4:49, 2003

☑ WATKINS TA, BARRES BA: Nerve regeneration: Regrowth stumped by shared receptor. Curr Biol 12:654, 2002

Review of myelin proteins Nogo, MAG, and OMGP that inhibit regeneration of CNS axons.

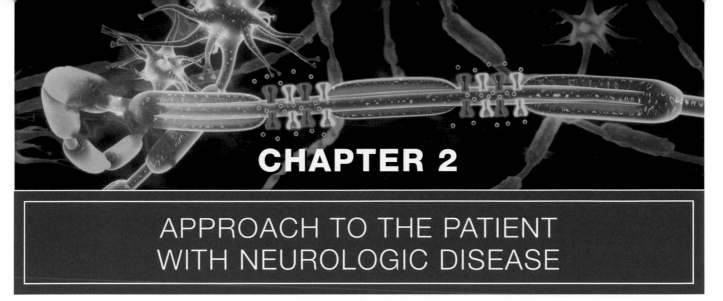

CHAPTER 2

APPROACH TO THE PATIENT WITH NEUROLOGIC DISEASE

Joseph B. Martin
Daniel H. Lowenstein
Stephen L. Hauser

Most patients with neurologic symptoms seek care from internists and other generalists rather than from neurologists, and this situation is likely to continue as primary care–based health care systems become increasingly prevalent. Because useful therapies now exist for these disorders, a skillful approach to diagnosis is essential. Many errors result from an overreliance on costly neuroimaging procedures and laboratory tests, which, while useful, do not substitute for an adequate history and examination. The proper approach to the patient with a neurologic illness begins with the patient and focuses the clinical problem first in anatomical and then in pathophysiologic terms; only then should a specific diagnosis be entertained. The direct evaluation of the patient also informs the subsequent workup and ensures that technology is judiciously applied, a correct diagnosis is established in an efficient manner, and treatment is promptly initiated.

THE NEUROLOGIC METHOD

LOCATE THE LESION(S)

The first priority is to identify the region of the nervous system that is likely to be responsible for the symptoms.

Can the disorder be mapped to one specific location, is it multifocal, or is a diffuse process present? Are the symptoms restricted to the nervous system, or do they arise in the context of a systemic illness? Is the problem in the central nervous system (CNS), the peripheral nervous system (PNS), or both? If in the CNS, is the cerebral cortex, basal ganglia, brainstem, cerebellum, or spinal cord responsible? Are the pain-sensitive meninges involved? If in the PNS, could the disorder be located in peripheral nerves and, if so, are motor or sensory nerves primarily affected, or is a lesion in the neuromuscular junction or muscle more likely?

The first clues to defining the anatomical area of involvement appear in the history, and the examination is then directed to confirm or rule out these impressions and to clarify uncertainties suggested by the history. A more detailed examination of a particular region of the CNS or PNS is often indicated. For example, the examination of a patient who presents with a history of ascending paresthesias and weakness should be directed toward deciding, among other things, if the location of the lesion is in the spinal cord or peripheral nerves. Focal back pain, a spinal cord sensory level, and incontinence suggest a spinal cord origin, whereas a stocking-glove pattern of sensory loss suggests peripheral nerve disease; areflexia usually indicates peripheral neuropathy but may also be present with spinal shock in acute spinal cord disorders.

Deciding "where the lesion is" accomplishes the task of limiting the possible etiologies to a manageable, finite number. In addition, this strategy safeguards against making tragic errors. Symptoms of recurrent vertigo, diplopia, and nystagmus should not trigger "multiple sclerosis" as an answer (etiology) but "brainstem" or "pons" (location); then a diagnosis of brainstem arteriovenous malformation will not be missed for lack of consideration. Similarly, the combination of optic neuritis and spastic ataxic paraparesis should initially suggest optic nerve and spinal cord disease; multiple sclerosis, CNS syphilis, and vitamin B_{12} deficiency are treatable disorders that can produce this syndrome. Once the question, "Where is the lesion?" is answered, then the question, "What is the lesion?" can be addressed.

DEFINE THE PATHOPHYSIOLOGY

Clues to the pathophysiology of the disease process may also be present in the history. Primary neuronal (gray matter) disorders may present as early cognitive disturbances, movement disorders, or seizures, whereas white matter involvement produces predominantly "long tract" disorders of motor, sensory, visual, and cerebellar pathways. Progressive and symmetric symptoms often have a metabolic or degenerative origin; in such cases lesions are usually not sharply circumscribed. Thus, a patient with paraparesis and a clear spinal cord sensory level is unlikely to have vitamin B_{12} deficiency as the explanation. A Lhermitte symptom (electric shock–like sensations evoked by neck flexion) is due to ectopic impulse generation in white matter pathways and occurs with demyelination in the cervical spinal cord. Symptoms that worsen after exposure to heat or exercise may indicate conduction block in demyelinated axons, as occurs in multiple sclerosis. A patient with recurrent episodes of diplopia and dysarthria associated with exercise or fatigue may have a disorder of neuromuscular transmission such as myasthenia gravis. Slowly advancing visual scotoma with luminous edges, termed *fortification spectra,* indicates spreading cortical depression, typically with migraine.

THE NEUROLOGIC HISTORY

As in all other aspects of clinical medicine, attention to the description of the symptoms experienced by the patient and substantiated by family members and others often permits an accurate localization and determination of the probable cause of the complaints, even before the neurologic examination is performed. Furthermore, a careful analysis of the history is a necessary prerequisite for bringing a focus to the neurologic examination that follows. Each complaint should be pursued as far as possible to elucidate the location of the lesion, the likely underlying pathophysiology, and potential etiologies. For example, a patient complains of weakness of the right arm. What are the associated features? Does the patient have difficulty with brushing hair or reaching upward (proximal) or buttoning buttons or opening a twist-top bottle (distal)? Also, negative associations may also be crucial. A patient with a right hemiparesis without a language deficit likely has a lesion (internal capsule, brainstem, or spinal cord) different from that of a patient with a right hemiparesis and aphasia (left hemisphere). Additional features of the history include the following:

1. ***Temporal course of the illness.*** It is important to determine the precise time of appearance and rate of progression of the symptoms experienced by the patient. The rapid onset of a neurologic complaint, occurring within seconds or minutes, usually indicates a vascular event, a seizure, or migraine. The onset of sensory symptoms located in one extremity that spread over a few seconds to adjacent portions of that extremity and then to the other regions of the body suggests a seizure. A more gradual onset and less well localized symptoms point to the possibility of a transient ischemic attack (TIA). A similar but slower temporal march of symptoms accompanied by headache, nausea, or visual disturbance suggests migraine. The presence of "positive" sensory symptoms (e.g., tingling or sensations that are difficult to describe) or involuntary motor movements suggests a seizure; in contrast, transient loss of function (negative symptoms) suggests a TIA. A stuttering onset where symptoms appear, stabilize, and then progress over hours or days also suggests cerebrovascular disease; an additional history of transient remission or regression indicates that the process is more likely due to ischemia rather than hemorrhage. A gradual evolution of symptoms over hours or days suggests a toxic, metabolic, infectious, or inflammatory process. Progressing symptoms associated with the systemic manifestations of fever, stiff neck, and altered level of consciousness imply an infectious process. Relapsing and remitting symptoms involving different levels of the nervous system suggest multiple sclerosis or other inflammatory processes; these disorders can occasionally produce new symptoms that are rapidly progressive over hours. Slowly progressive symptoms without remissions are characteristic of neurodegenerative disorders, chronic infections, gradual intoxications, and neoplasms.

2. ***Patients' descriptions of the complaint.*** The same words often mean different things to different patients. "Dizziness" may imply impending syncope, a sense of disequilibrium, or true spinning vertigo. "Numbness" may mean a complete loss of feeling, a positive sensation such as tingling, or paralysis. "Blurred vision" may be used to describe unilateral visual loss, as in transient monocular blindness, or diplopia. The interpretation of the true meaning of the words used by patients to describe symptoms becomes even more complex when there are differences in primary languages and cultures.

3. ***Corroboration of the history by others.*** It is almost always helpful to obtain additional information from family, friends, or other observers to corroborate or expand the patient's description. Memory loss, aphasia, loss of insight, intoxication, and other factors may impair the patient's capacity to communicate normally with the

examiner or prevent openness about factors that have contributed to the illness. Episodes of loss of consciousness necessitate that details be sought from observers to ascertain precisely what has happened during the event.

4. Family history. Many neurologic disorders have an underlying genetic component. The presence of a Mendelian disorder, such as Huntington's disease or Charcot-Marie-Tooth neuropathy, is often obvious if family data are available. More detailed questions about family history are often necessary in polygenic disorders such as multiple sclerosis, migraine, and many types of epilepsy. It is important to elicit family history about all illnesses, in addition to neurologic and psychiatric disorders. A familial propensity to hypertension or heart disease is relevant in a patient who presents with a stroke. There are numerous inherited neurologic diseases that are associated with multisystem manifestations that may provide clues to the correct diagnosis (e.g., neurofibromatosis, Wilson's disease, neuro-ophthalmic syndromes).

5. Medical illnesses. Many neurologic diseases occur in the context of systemic disorders. Diabetes mellitus, hypertension, and abnormalities of blood lipids predispose to cerebrovascular disease. A solitary mass lesion in the brain may be an abscess in a patient with valvular heart disease, a primary hemorrhage in a patient with a coagulopathy, a lymphoma or toxoplasmosis in a patient with AIDS, or a metastasis in a patient with underlying cancer. Patients with malignancy may also present with a neurologic paraneoplastic syndrome (Chap. 27) or complications from chemotherapy or radiotherapy. Marfan's syndrome and related collagen disorders predispose to dissection of the cranial arteries and aneurysmal subarachnoid hemorrhage; the latter may also occur with polycystic kidney disease. Various neurologic disorders occur with dysthyroid states or other endocrinopathies. It is especially important to look for the presence of systemic diseases in patients with peripheral neuropathy. Most patients with coma in a hospital setting have a metabolic, toxic, or infectious cause.

6. Drug use and abuse and toxin exposure. It is essential to inquire about the history of drug use, both prescribed and illicit. Aminoglycoside antibiotics may exacerbate symptoms of weakness in patients with disorders of neuromuscular transmission, such as myasthenia gravis, and may cause dizziness secondary to ototoxicity. Vincristine and other antineoplastic drugs can cause peripheral neuropathy, and immunosuppressive agents such as cyclosporine can produce encephalopathy. Excessive vitamin ingestion can lead to disease; for example vitamin A and pseudotumor cerebri, or pyridoxine and peripheral neuropathy. Many patients are unaware that over-the-counter sleeping pills, cold preparations, and diet pills are actually drugs. Alcohol, the most prevalent neurotoxin, is often not recognized as such by patients,

and other drugs of abuse such as cocaine and heroin can cause a wide range of neurologic abnormalities. A history of environmental or industrial exposure to neurotoxins may provide an essential clue; consultation with the patient's co-workers or employer may be required.

7. Formulating an impression of the patient. Use the opportunity while taking the history to form an impression of the patient. Is the information forthcoming, or does it take a circuitous course? Is there evidence of anxiety, depression, hypochondriasis? Are there any clues to defects in language, memory, insight, or inappropriate behavior? The neurologic assessment begins as soon as the patient comes into the room and the first introduction is made.

THE NEUROLOGIC EXAMINATION

The neurologic examination is challenging and complex; it has many components and includes a number of skills that can be mastered only through repeated use of the same techniques on a large number of individuals with and without neurologic disease. Mastery of the complete neurologic examination is usually important only for physicians in neurology and associated specialties. However, knowledge of the basics of the examination, especially those components that are effective in screening for neurologic dysfunction, is essential for all clinicians, especially generalists.

There is no single, universally accepted sequence of the examination that must be followed, but most clinicians begin with assessment of mental status followed by the cranial nerves, motor system, sensory system, coordination, and gait. Whether the examination is basic or comprehensive, it is essential that it be performed in an orderly and systematic fashion to avoid errors and serious omissions. Thus, the best way to learn and gain expertise in the examination is to choose one's own approach and practice it frequently and do it in the same exact sequence each time.

The detailed description of the neurologic examination that follows describes the more commonly used parts of the examination, with a particular emphasis on the components that are considered most helpful for the assessment of common neurologic problems. Each section also includes a brief description of the minimal examination necessary for adequate screening for abnormalities in a patient who has no symptoms suggesting neurologic dysfunction. A screening examination done in this way can be completed in 3 to 5 min.

Several additional points about the examination are worth noting. First, in recording observations, it is important to describe what is found rather than to apply a poorly defined medical term (e.g., "patient groans to sternal rub" rather than "obtunded"). Second, subtle CNS abnormalities are best detected by carefully comparing a patient's performance on tasks that require simultaneous activation of both cerebral hemispheres (e.g., eliciting a pronator drift of an outstretched arm with the eyes closed; extinction on one side of bilaterally applied light touch, also with eyes closed; or decreased arm swing or a slight asymmetry when walking). Third, if the patient's complaint is brought on by some activity, reproduce the activity in the office. If the complaint is of dizziness when the head is turned in one direction, have the patient do this and look for associated signs on examination (e.g., nystagmus or dysmetria). If pain occurs after walking two blocks, have the patient leave the office and walk this distance and immediately return, and repeat the relevant parts of the examination. Finally, the use of tests that are individually tailored to the patient's problem can be of value in assessing changes over time. Tests of walking a 7.5-m (25-ft) distance (normal, 5 to 6 s; note assistance, if any), repetitive finger or toe tapping (normal, 20 to 25 taps in 5 s), or handwriting are examples.

MENTAL STATUS EXAMINATION

- *The bare minimum: During the interview, look for difficulties with communication and determine whether the patient has recall and insight into recent and past events.*

The mental status examination is underway as soon as the physician begins observing and talking with the patient. If the history raises any concern for abnormalities of higher cortical function or if cognitive problems are observed during the interview, then detailed testing of the mental status is indicated. The patient's ability to understand the language used for the examination, cultural background, educational experience, sensory or motor problems, or comorbid conditions need to be factored into the applicability of the tests and interpretation of results.

The Folstein mini-mental status examination (MMSE) (Table 18-4) is a standardized screening examination of cognitive function that is extremely easy to administer and takes <10 min to complete. Using age-adjusted values for defining normal performance, the test is ~85% sensitive and 85% specific for making the diagnosis of dementia that is moderate or severe, especially in educated patients. When there is sufficient time available, the MMSE is one of the best methods for documenting the current mental status of the patient, and this is especially useful as a baseline assessment to which future scores of the MMSE can be compared.

Individual elements of the mental status examination can be subdivided into level of consciousness, orientation, speech and language, memory, fund of information, insight and judgment, abstract thought, and calculations.

Level of consciousness is the patient's relative state of awareness of the self and the environment, and ranges from fully awake to comatose. When the patient is not fully awake, the examiner should describe the responses to the minimum stimulus necessary to elicit a reaction, ranging from verbal commands to a brief, painful stimulus such as a squeeze of the trapezius muscle. Responses that are directed toward the stimulus and signify some degree of intact cerebral function (e.g., opening the eyes and looking at the examiner or reaching to push away a painful stimulus) must be distinguished from reflex responses of a spinal origin (e.g., triple flexion response—flexion at the ankle, knee, and hip in response to a painful stimulus to the foot).

Orientation is tested by asking the person to state his or her name, location, and time (day of the week and date); time is usually the first to be affected in a variety of conditions.

Speech is assessed by observing articulation, rate, rhythm, and prosody (i.e., the changes in pitch and accentuation of syllable and words).

Language is assessed by observing the content of the patient's verbal and written output, response to spoken commands, and ability to read. A typical testing sequence is to ask the patient to name successively more detailed components of clothing, a watch or a pen; repeat the phrase "No ifs, ands, or buts"; follow a three-step, verbal command; write a sentence; and read and respond to a written command.

Memory should be analyzed according to three main time scales: (1) immediate memory can be tested by saying a list of three items and having the patient repeat the list immediately, (2) short-term memory is assessed by asking the patient to recall the same three items 5 and 15 min later, and (3) long-term memory is evaluated by determining how well the patient is able to provide a coherent chronologic history of his or her illness or personal events.

Fund of information is assessed by asking questions about major historic or current events, with special attention to educational level and life experiences.

Insight and judgment abnormalities are usually detected during the patient interview; a more detailed assessment can be elicited by asking the patient to describe how he or she would respond to situations having a variety of potential outcomes (e.g., "What would you do if you found a wallet on the sidewalk?").

Abstract thought can be tested by asking the patient to describe similarities between various objects or concepts (e.g., apple and orange, desk and chair, poetry and sculpture) or to list items having the same attributes (e.g., a list of four-legged animals).

Calculation ability is assessed by having the patient carry out a computation that is appropriate to the patient's age and education (e.g., serial subtraction of 7 from 100 or 3 from 20; or word problems involving simple arithmetic).

CRANIAL NERVE EXAMINATION

- *The bare minimum: Check the fundi, visual fields, pupil size and reactivity, extraocular movements, and facial movements.*

The cranial nerves (CN) are best examined in numerical order, except for grouping together CN III, IV, and VI because of their similar function.

CN I (Olfactory)

Testing is usually omitted unless there is suspicion for inferior frontal lobe disease (e.g., meningioma). With eyes closed, ask the patient to sniff a mild stimulus such as toothpaste or coffee and identify the odorant.

CN II (Optic)

Check visual acuity (with eyeglasses or contact lens correction) using a Snellen chart or similar tool. Test the visual fields by confrontation, i.e., by comparing the patient's visual fields to your own. As a screening test, it is usually sufficient to examine the visual fields of both eyes simultaneously; individual eye fields should be tested if there is any reason to suspect a problem of vision by the history or other elements of the examination, or if the screening test reveals an abnormality. Face the patient at a distance of approximately 0.6 to 1.0 m (2 to 3 ft) and place your hands at the periphery of your visual fields in the plane that is equidistant between you and the patient. Instruct the patient to look directly at the center of your face and to indicate when and where he or she sees one of your fingers moving. Beginning with the two inferior quadrants and then the two superior quadrants, move your index finger of the right hand, left hand, or both hands simultaneously and observe whether the patient detects the movements. A single small-amplitude movement of the finger is sufficient for a normal response. Focal perimetry and tangent screen examinations should be used to map out visual field defects fully or to search for subtle abnormalities. Optic fundi should be examined with an ophthalmoscope, and the color, size, and degree of swelling or elevation of the optic disc noted, as well as the color and texture of the retina. The retinal vessels should be checked for size, regularity, arterial-venous nicking at crossing points, hemorrhage, exudates, etc.

CN III, IV, VI (Oculomotor, Trochlear, Abducens)

Describe the size and shape of pupils and reaction to light and accommodation (i.e., as the eyes converge while following your finger as it moves toward the bridge of the nose). To check extraocular movements, ask the patient to keep his or her head still while tracking the movement of the tip of your finger. Move the target slowly in the horizontal and vertical planes; observe any paresis, nystagmus, or abnormalities of smooth pursuit (saccades, oculomotor ataxia, etc.). If necessary, the relative position of the two eyes, both in primary and multidirectional gaze, can be assessed by comparing the reflections of a bright light off both pupils. However, in practice it is typically more useful to determine whether the patient describes diplopia in any direction of gaze; true diplopia should almost always resolve with one eye closed. Horizontal nystagmus is best assessed at 45° and not at extreme lateral gaze (which is uncomfortable for the patient); the target must often be held at the lateral position for at least a few seconds to detect an abnormality.

CN V (Trigeminal)

Examine sensation within the three territories of the branches of the trigeminal nerve (ophthalmic, maxillary, and mandibular) on each side of the face. As with other parts of the sensory examination, testing of two sensory modalities derived from different anatomical pathways (e.g., light touch and temperature) is sufficient for a screening examination. Testing of other modalities, the corneal reflex, and the motor component of CN V (jaw clench—masseter muscle) is indicated when suggested by the history.

CN VII (Facial)

Look for facial asymmetry at rest and with spontaneous movements. Test eyebrow elevation, forehead wrinkling, eye closure, smiling, and cheek puff. Look in particular for differences in the lower versus upper facial muscles; weakness of the lower two-thirds of the face with preservation of the upper third suggests an upper motor neuron lesion, whereas weakness of an entire side suggests a lower motor neuron lesion.

CN VIII (Vestibulocochlear)

Check the patient's ability to hear a finger rub or whispered voice with each ear. Further testing for air versus mastoid bone conduction (Rinne) and lateralization of a 512-Hz tuning fork placed at the center of the forehead (Weber) should be done if an abnormality is detected by history or examination. Any suspected problem should be followed up with formal audiometry. For further discussion of assessing vestibular nerve function in the setting of dizziness or coma, see Chaps. 9 and 8, respectively.

CN IX, X (Glossopharyngeal, Vagus)

Observe the position and symmetry of the palate and uvula at rest and with phonation ("aah"). The pharyngeal ("gag") reflex is evaluated by stimulating the posterior pharyngeal wall on each side with a sterile, blunt object (e.g., tongue blade), but the reflex is often absent in normal individuals.

CN XI (Spinal Accessory)

Check shoulder shrug (trapezius muscle) and head rotation to each side (sternocleidomastoid) against resistance.

CN XII (Hypoglossal)

Inspect the tongue for atrophy or fasciculations, position with protrusion, and strength when extended against the inner surface of the cheeks on each side.

MOTOR EXAMINATION

• *The bare minimum: Look for muscle atrophy and check extremity tone. Assess upper extremity strength by checking for pronator drift and strength of wrist or finger extensors. Tap the biceps, patellar, and Achilles reflexes. Test for lower extremity strength by having the patient walk normally and on heels and toes.*

The motor examination includes observations of muscle appearance, tone, strength, and reflexes. Although gait is in part a test of motor function, it is usually evaluated separately at the end of the examination.

Appearance

Inspect and palpate muscle groups under good light and with the patient in a comfortable and symmetric position. Check for muscle fasciculations, tenderness, and atrophy or hypertrophy. Involuntary movements may be present at rest (e.g., tics, myoclonus, choreoathetosis), during maintained posture (pill-rolling tremor of Parkinson's disease), or with voluntary movements (intention tremor of cerebellar disease or familial tremor).

Tone

Muscle tone is tested by measuring the resistance to passive movement of a relaxed limb. Patients often have difficulty relaxing during this procedure, so it is useful to

distract the patient to minimize active movements. In the upper limbs, tone is assessed by rapid pronation and supination of the forearm and flexion and extension at the wrist. In the lower limbs, while the patient is supine the examiner's hands are placed behind the knees and rapidly raised; with normal tone the ankles drag along the table surface for a variable distance before rising, whereas increased tone results in an immediate lift of the heel off the surface. Decreased tone is most commonly due to lower motor neuron or peripheral nerve disorders. Increased tone may be evident as spasticity (resistance determined by the angle and velocity of motion; corticospinal tract disease), rigidity (similar resistance in all angles of motion; extrapyramidal disease), or paratonia (fluctuating changes in resistance; frontal lobe pathways or normal difficulty in relaxing). Cogwheel rigidity, in which passive motion elicits jerky interruptions in resistance, is seen in parkinsonism.

Strength

Testing for pronator drift is an extremely useful method for screening upper limb weakness. The patient is asked to hold both arms fully extended and parallel to the ground with eyes closed. This position should be maintained for ~10 s; any flexion at the elbow or fingers or pronation of the forearm, especially if asymmetric, is a sign of potential weakness. Muscle strength is further assessed by having the patient exert maximal effort for the particular muscle or muscle group being tested. It is important to isolate the muscles as much as possible, i.e., hold the limb so that only the muscles of interest are active. It is also helpful to palpate accessible muscles as they contract. Grading muscle strength and evaluating the patient's effort is an art that takes time and practice. Muscle strength is traditionally graded using the following scale:

0 = no movement
1 = flicker or trace of contraction but no associated movement at a joint
2 = movement with gravity eliminated
3 = movement against gravity but not against resistance
$4-$ = movement against a mild degree of resistance
4 = movement against moderate resistance
$4+$ = movement against strong resistance
5 = full power

However, in many cases it is more practical to use the following terms:

Paralysis = no movement
Severe weakness = movement with gravity eliminated
Moderate weakness = movement against gravity but not against mild resistance

Mild weakness = movement against moderate
resistance

Full strength

Noting the pattern of weakness is as important as assessing the magnitude of weakness. Unilateral or bilateral weakness of the upper limb extensors and lower limb flexors ("pyramidal weakness") suggests a lesion of the pyramidal tract, bilateral proximal weakness suggests myopathy, and bilateral distal weakness suggests peripheral neuropathy.

Reflexes

Muscle Stretch Reflexes   Those that are typically assessed include the biceps (**C5**, C6), brachioradialis (C5, **C6**), and triceps (**C7**, C8) reflexes in the upper limbs and the patellar or quadriceps (**L3**, L4) and Achilles (**S1**, S2) reflexes in the lower limbs. The patient should be relaxed and the muscle positioned midway between full contraction and extension. Reflexes may be enhanced by asking the patient to voluntarily contract other, distant muscle groups (Jendrassik maneuver). For example, upper limb reflexes may be reinforced by voluntary teeth-clenching, and the Achilles reflex by hooking the flexed fingers of the two hands together and attempting to pull them apart. For each reflex tested, the two sides should be tested sequentially, and it is important to determine the smallest stimulus required to elicit a reflex rather than the maximum response. Reflexes are graded according to the following scale:

0 = absent
1 = present but diminished
2 = normoactive
3 = exaggerated
4 = clonus

Cutaneous Reflexes   The plantar reflex is elicited by stroking, with a noxious stimulus such as a tongue blade, the lateral surface of the sole of the foot beginning near the heel and moving across the ball of the foot to the great toe. The normal reflex consists of plantar flexion of the toes. With upper motor neuron lesions above the S1 level of the spinal cord, a paradoxical extension of the toe is observed, associated with fanning and extension of the other toes (termed an *extensor plantar response,* or *Babinski sign*). Superficial abdominal reflexes are elicited by gently stroking the abdominal surface near the umbilicus in a diagonal fashion with a sharp object (e.g., the wooden end of a cotton-tipped swab) and observing the movement of the umbilicus. Normally, the umbilicus will pull toward the stimulated quadrant. With upper motor neuron lesions, these reflexes are absent. They are most helpful when there is preservation of the upper (spinal cord level T9) but not lower (T12) abdominal reflexes, indicating a spinal lesion between T9 and T12, or when the response is asymmetric. Other useful cutaneous reflexes include the cremasteric (ipsilateral elevation of the testicle following stroking of the medial thigh; mediated by L1 and L2) and anal (contraction of the anal sphincter when the perianal skin is scratched; mediated by S2, S3, S4) reflexes. It is particularly important to test for these reflexes in any patient with suspected injury to the spinal cord or lumbosacral roots.

Primitive Reflexes   With disease of the frontal lobe pathways, several primitive reflexes not normally present in the adult may appear. The suck response is elicited by lightly touching the center of the lips, and the root response the corner of the lips, with a tongue blade; the patient will move the lips to suck or root in the direction of the stimulus. The grasp reflex is elicited by touching the palm between the thumb and index finger with the examiner's fingers; a positive response is a forced grasp of the examiner's hand. In many instances stroking the back of the hand will lead to its release. The palmomental response is contraction of the mentalis muscle (chin) ipsilateral to a scratch stimulus diagonally applied to the palm.

SENSORY EXAMINATION

- *The bare minimum: Ask whether the patient can feel light touch and the temperature of a cool object in each distal extremity. Check double simultaneous stimulation using light touch on the hands.*

Evaluating sensation is usually the most unreliable part of the examination, because it is subjective and is difficult to quantify. In the compliant and discerning patient, the sensory examination can be extremely helpful for the precise localization of a lesion. With patients who are uncooperative or lack an understanding of the tests, it may be useless. The examination should be focused on the suspected lesion. For example, in spinal cord, spinal root, or peripheral nerve abnormalities, all major sensory modalities should be tested while looking for a pattern consistent with a spinal level and dermatomal or nerve distribution. In patients with lesions at or above the brainstem, screening the primary sensory modalities in the distal extremities along with tests of "cortical" sensation is usually sufficient.

The five primary sensory modalities—light touch, pain, temperature, vibration, and joint position—are tested in each limb. Light touch is assessed by stimulating the skin with single, very gentle touches of the examiner's finger or a wisp of cotton. Pain is tested using a new pin, and temperature is assessed using a metal object (e.g., tuning fork) that has been immersed in cold and warm water. Vibration is tested using a 128-Hz tuning fork applied to the distal phalanx of the great toe or index finger just below the nailbed. By placing a finger on the opposite side of the joint being tested, the examiner compares the patient's threshold of vibration perception with his or her own. For joint position testing, the examiner grasps the digit or limb laterally and distal to the joint being assessed; small 1- to 2-mm excursions can usually be sensed. The Romberg maneuver is primarily a test of proprioception. The patient is asked to stand with the feet as close together as necessary to maintain balance while the eyes are open, and the eyes are then closed. A loss of balance with the eyes closed is an abnormal response.

"Cortical" sensation is mediated by the parietal lobes and represents an integration of the primary sensory modalities; testing cortical sensation is only meaningful when primary sensation is intact. Double simultaneous stimulation is especially useful as a screening test for cortical function; with the patient's eyes closed, the examiner lightly touches one or both hands and asks the patient to identify the stimuli. With a parietal lobe lesion, the patient may be unable to identify the stimulus on the contralateral side when both hands are touched. Other modalities relying on the parietal cortex include the discrimination of two closely placed stimuli as separate (two-point discrimination), identification of an object by touch and manipulation alone (stereognosis), and the identification of numbers or letters written on the skin surface (graphesthesia).

COORDINATION EXAMINATION

- *The bare minimum: Test rapid alternating movements of the fingers and feet, and the finger-to-nose maneuver.*

Coordination refers to the orchestration and fluidity of movements. Even simple acts require cooperation of agonist and antagonist muscles, maintenance of posture, and complex servomechanisms to control the rate and range of movements. Part of this integration relies on normal function of the cerebellar and basal ganglia systems. However, coordination also requires intact muscle strength and kinesthetic and proprioceptive information. Thus, if the examination has disclosed abnormalities of the motor or sensory systems, the patient's coordination should be assessed with these limitations in mind.

Rapid alternating movements in the upper limbs are tested separately on each side by having the patient make a fist, partially extend the index finger, and then tap the index finger on the distal thumb as quickly as possible. In the lower limb, the patient rapidly taps the

foot against the floor or the examiner's hand. Finger-to-nose testing is primarily a test of cerebellar function; the patient is asked to touch his or her index finger repetitively to the nose and then to the examiner's outstretched finger, which moves with each repetition. A similar test in the lower extremity is to have the patient raise the leg and touch the examiner's finger with the great toe. Another cerebellar test in the lower limbs is the heel-knee-shin maneuver; in the supine position the patient is asked to slide the heel of each foot from the knee down the shin of the other leg. For all these movements, the accuracy, speed, and rhythm are noted.

GAIT EXAMINATION

- *The bare minimum: Observe the patient while walking normally, on the heels and toes, and along a straight line.*

Watching the patient walk is the most important part of the neurologic examination. Normal gait requires that multiple systems—including strength, sensation, and coordination—function in a highly integrated fashion. Unexpected abnormalities may be detected that prompt the examiner to return, in more detail, to other aspects of the examination. The patient should be observed while walking and turning normally, walking on the heels, walking on the toes, and walking heel-to-toe along a straight line. The examination may reveal decreased arm swing on one side (corticospinal tract disease), a stooped posture and short-stepped gait (parkinsonism), a broad-based unstable gait (ataxia), scissoring (spasticity), or a high-stepped, slapping gait (posterior column or peripheral nerve disease), or the patient may appear to be stuck in place (apraxia with frontal lobe disease).

NEUROLOGIC DIAGNOSIS

The clinical data obtained from the history and the examination are interpreted in terms of neuroanatomy and neurophysiology and assembled into one of the known syndromes. From the syndrome the physician should be able to determine the anatomical localization that best explains the clinical findings, to narrow the list of diagnostic possibilities, and to select the laboratory tests most likely to be informative. The laboratory assessment may include (1) serum electrolytes; complete blood count; and renal, hepatic, endocrine, and immune studies; (2) cerebrospinal fluid examination; (3) focused neuroimaging studies (Chap. 3); or (4) electrophysiologic studies (Chap. 33). The anatomical localization, mode of onset and course of illness, other medical data, and laboratory findings are then integrated to establish an etiologic diagnosis.

It should be emphasized that the neurologic examination may be normal even in patients with a serious neurologic disease, such as seizures, chronic meningitis, or a TIA. A comatose patient may arrive with no available history, and in such cases the approach is as described in Chap. 8. In other patients, an inadequate history may be overcome by a succession of examinations from which the course of the illness can be inferred. In perplexing cases it is useful to remember that uncommon presentations of common diseases are more likely than rare etiologies. Thus, even in tertiary care settings, multiple strokes are usually due to emboli and not vasculitis, and dementia with myoclonus is usually Alzheimer's disease and not a prionopathy or a paraneoplastic disorder. Finally, the most important task of a primary care physician faced with a patient who has a new neurologic complaint is to assess the urgency of referral to a specialist. Here, the imperative is to rapidly identify patients likely to have nervous system infections, acute strokes, and spinal cord compression or other treatable mass lesions and arrange for immediate care.

FURTHER READINGS

▨ BLUMENFELD H: *Neuroanatomy Through Clinical Cases*. Sinauer Associates, Sunderland, MA, 2002

A simple, clinically based review of neuroanatomy and the neurologic examination.

ROPPER AH AND BROWN RH: *Principles of Neurology,* 8th ed. New York, McGraw-Hill, 2005

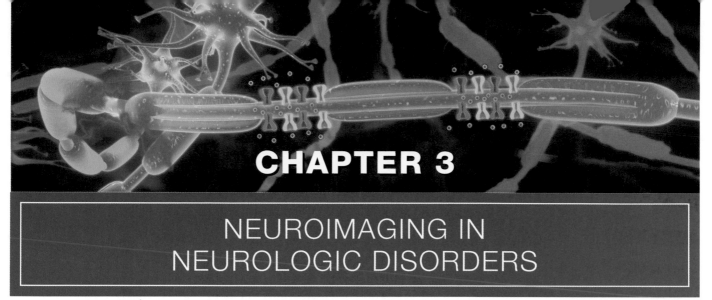

CHAPTER 3

NEUROIMAGING IN NEUROLOGIC DISORDERS

William P. Dillon

The clinician caring for patients with neurologic symptoms is faced with an expanding number of imaging options, including computed tomography (CT), CT angiography (CTA), perfusion CT (pCT), magnetic resonance imaging (MRI), MR angiography (MRA), functional MRI (fMRI), MR spectroscopy (MRS), MR neurography, and perfusion MRI (pMRI). In addition, an increasing number of interventional neuroradiologic techniques are available including angiography; embolization and stenting of vascular structures; and spine interventions such as discography, selective nerve root injection, and epidural injections. Recent developments, such as multidetector CT angiography and gadolinium-enhanced MRA, have narrowed the indications for conventional angiography, which is now reserved for patients in whom small-vessel detail is essential for diagnosis or for whom interventional therapies are planned (**Table 3-1**).

In general, MRI is more sensitive than CT for the detection of lesions affecting the central nervous system (CNS), particularly those of the spinal cord, cranial nerves, and posterior fossa structures. Diffusion MR, a sequence that detects reduction of microscopic motion of water, is the most sensitive technique for detecting acute ischemic stroke and is useful in the detection of encephalitis, abscesses, and prion diseases. CT, however, can be quickly obtained and is widely available, making it a pragmatic choice for the initial evaluation of patients with suspected acute stroke, hemorrhage, and intracranial or spinal trauma. CT is also more sensitive than MRI for visualizing fine osseous detail and is indicated in the initial evaluation of conductive hearing loss as well as lesions affecting the skull base and calvarium.

COMPUTED TOMOGRAPHY

TECHNIQUE

The CT image is a cross-sectional representation of anatomy created by a computer-generated analysis of the attenuation of x-ray beams passed through a section of the body. As the x-ray beam, collimated to the desired slice width, rotates around the patient, it passes through selected regions in the body. X-rays that are not attenuated by the body are detected by sensitive x-ray detectors aligned 180° from the x-ray tube. A computer calculates a "back projection" image from the 360° x-ray attenuation profile. Greater x-ray attenuation, e.g., as caused by bone, results in areas of high "density," while soft tissue structures, which have poor attenuation of x-rays, are lower in density. The resolution of an image depends on the radiation dose, the collimation (slice thickness), the field of view, and the matrix size of the

TABLE 3-1

GUIDELINES FOR THE USE OF CT, ULTRASOUND, AND MRI

CONDITION	RECOMMENDED TECHNIQUE
Hemorrhage	
Acute parenchymal	CT, MR
Subacute/chronic	MRI
Subarachnoid hemorrhage	CT, CTA, lumbar puncture → angiography
Aneurysm	Angiography > CTA, MRA
Ischemic infarction	
Hemorrhagic infarction	CT or MRI
Bland infarction	MRI > CT
Carotid or vertebral dissection	MRI/MRA, CTA, angiography
Vertebral basilar insufficiency	CTA, MRI/MRA
Carotid stenosis	CTA > Doppler ultrasound, MRA
Suspected mass lesion	
Neoplasm, primary or metastatic	MRI + contrast
Infection/abscess	MRI + contrast
Immunosuppressed with focal findings	MRI + contrast
Vascular malformation	MRI +/− angiography
White matter disorders	MRI
Demyelinating disease	MRI +/− contrast
Dementia	MRI > CT
Trauma	
Acute trauma	CT (noncontrast)
Shear injury/chronic hemorrhage	MRI
Headache/migraine	CT (noncontrast) / MRI
Seizure	
First time, no focal neurologic deficits	?CT as screen +/− contrast
Partial complex/refractory	MRI with coronal T2W imaging
Cranial neuropathy	MRI with contrast
Meningeal disease	MRI with contrast
SPINE	
Low back pain	
No neurologic deficits	MRI or CT after 4 weeks
With focal deficits	MRI > CT
Spinal stenosis	MRI or CT
Cervical spondylosis	MRI or CT myelography
Infection	MRI + contrast, CT
Myelopathy	MRI + contrast > myelography
Arteriovenous malformation	MRI, myelography/angiography

Note: CT, computed tomography; MRI, magnetic resonance imaging; MRA, MR angiography; CTA, CT angiography; T2W, T2-weighted.

display. A modern CT scanner is capable of obtaining sections as thin as 0.5 to 1 mm with submillimeter resolution at a speed of 0.5 to 1 s per section; complete studies of the brain can be completed in 20 to 60 s.

Helical CT is a type of scanner in which continuous CT information is obtained while the patient moves through the x-ray beam. In the helical scan mode, the table moves continuously through the rotating x-ray beam, generating a "helix" of information that can be reformatted into various slice thicknesses. Single or multiple (from 4 to 64) detectors positioned 180 degrees to the x-ray source may result in multiple slices per revolu-

tion of the beam around the patient. These "multidetector" scanners have further decreased the time per examination and permit rapid assessment of vascular anatomy as well as perfusion characteristics of brain parenchyma (**Figs. 3–1 and 3–2**). Advantages of multidetector scanning include shorter scan times, reduced patient and organ motion, and the ability to acquire images dynamically during the infusion of intravenous contrast that can be used to construct CT angiograms of vascular structures and CT perfusion images (Figs. 3–1*B* and 3–2). CTA images may be processed later for display in three dimensions to yield angiogram-like images (Fig. 3–1*C*).

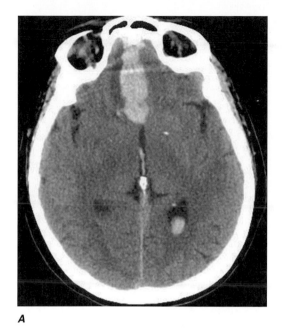

A

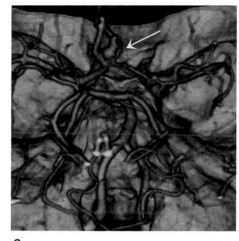

C

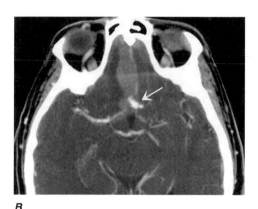

B

FIGURE 3-1

CT angiography (CTA) of ruptured anterior cerebral artery aneurysm. A 45-year-old man presents with acute headache. ***A***. Noncontrast CT demonstrates intraventricular, subarachnoid, and frontal lobe hemorrhage. ***B***. A partition from CT angiography demonstrates a suspicious enlargement of the anterior cerebral artery (*arrow*). ***C***. 3D surface reconstruction using a workstation confirms the anterior cerebral aneurysm and demonstrates its orientation and relationship to nearby vessels (*arrow*). CTA image is produced by 1-mm helical CT scans performed during a rapid bolus infusion of intravenous contrast medium.

CTA has proved useful in assessing the carotid bifurcation and intracranial arterial and venous anatomy.

Intravenous contrast is often administered prior to or during a CT study to identify vascular structures and to detect defects in the blood-brain barrier (BBB), which are associated with disorders such as tumors, infarcts, and infections. In the normal CNS, only vessels and structures lacking a BBB (e.g., the pituitary gland, choroid plexus, and dura) enhance after contrast administration. The use of iodinated contrast agents carries a risk of allergic reaction and adds additional expense and radiation dose. While helpful in characterizing mass lesions as well as essential for the acquisition of CTA studies, the decision to use contrast material should always be considered carefully.

INDICATIONS

CT is the primary study of choice in the evaluation of acute trauma to the brain and spine, suspected subarach-noid hemorrhage, and conductive hearing loss (Table 3-1). CT is complementary to MR in the evaluation of the skull base, orbit, and osseous structures of the spine. In the spine, CT is useful in evaluating patients with osseous spinal stenosis and spondylosis, but MRI is often preferred in those with neurologic deficits. CT can also be obtained following intrathecal contrast injection to evaluate the intracranial cisterns (*CT cisternography*) for cerebrospinal fluid (CSF) fistula, as well as the spinal subarachnoid space (*CT myelography*).

COMPLICATIONS

CT is safe, fast, and reliable. Radiation exposure is between 3 and 5 cGy per study. Care must be taken to reduce exposure when imaging children. The most frequent complications are associated with use of intravenous contrast agents. Two broad categories of contrast media, ionic and nonionic, are in use. Although ionic agents are relatively safe and inexpensive, they are

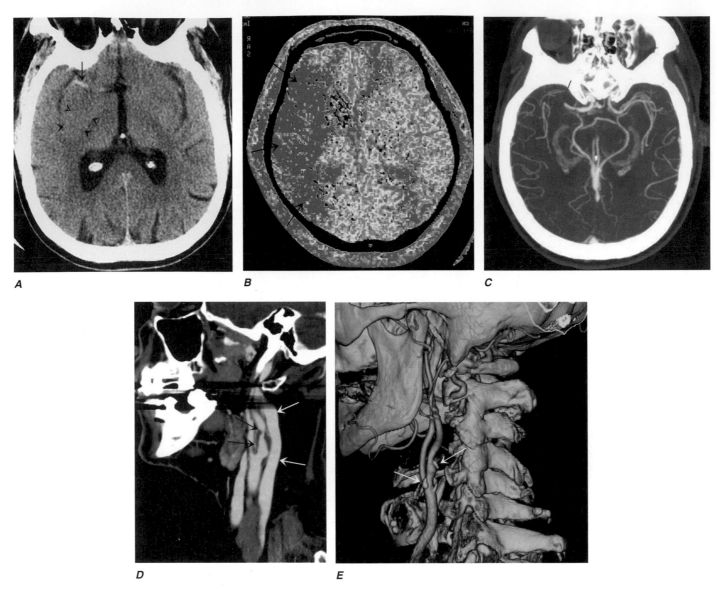

FIGURE 3-2

A 49-year-old man with acute neck pain and left hemiparesis. **A**. Axial noncontrast CT scan demonstrates high density within the right middle cerebral artery (*arrow*) associated with subtle low density involving the right putamen (*arrowheads*). **B**. Mean transit time map calculated from a CT perfusion study obtained with a 40-mL contrast injection during which 45 images were obtained at the same slice location. Prolongation of the mean transit time is visible throughout the right hemisphere (*arrows*). **C**. Axial maximum intensity projection from CTA study through the circle of Willis demonstrates an abrupt occlusion of the proximal right middle cerebral artery (*arrow*). Reconstitution of flow via collaterals is seen distal to the occlusion; however, the patient sustained a right basal ganglia infarction. **D**. Sagittal re-formation through the right internal carotid artery. Low-density lipid–laden plaque (*arrows*) narrows the lumen of the internal carotid artery (*black arrows*). The internal jugular vein is shown (*white arrows*). **E**. 3D surface CTA images (different patient) demonstrate calcification and narrowing of the right internal carotid artery, consistent with atherosclerotic disease.

associated with a higher incidence of reactions and side effects. As a result, ionic agents have been largely replaced by safer nonionic compounds (**Table 3–2**).

Contrast nephropathy may result from hemodynamic changes, renal tubular obstruction and cell damage, or immunologic reactions to contrast agents. A rise in serum creatinine of at least 85 μmol/L (1 mg/dL) within 48 h of contrast administration is often used as a definition of contrast nephropathy, although other causes of acute renal failure must be excluded. The prognosis is usually favorable, with serum creatinine levels returning to baseline within 1 to 2 weeks. Risk factors for contrast nephropathy include advanced age, preexisting renal disease, diabetes, dehydration, and high contrast dose. Patients with diabetes and those with mild renal failure should be well hydrated prior to the administration of contrast agents,

TABLE 3-2

GUIDELINES FOR USE OF INTRAVENOUS CONTRAST IN PATIENTS WITH IMPAIRED RENAL FUNCTION

SERUM CREATININE, μmol/L (mg/dL)[a]	RECOMMENDATION
<133 (<1.5)	Use either ionic or nonionic at 2 mL/kg to 150 mL total
133–177 (1.5–2.0)	Nonionic; hydrate diabetics 1 mL/kg per hour × 10 h
>177 (>2.0)	Consider noncontrast CT or MRI; nonionic contrast if required
177–221 (2.0–2.5)	Nonionic only if required (as above); contraindicated in diabetics
>265 (>3.0)	Nonionic IV contrast given only to patients undergoing dialysis within 24 h

[a]Risk is greatest in patients with rising creatinine levels.
Note: CT, computed tomography; MRI, magnetic resonance imaging.

TABLE 3-3

INDICATIONS FOR USE OF NONIONIC CONTRAST MEDIA

- Prior adverse reaction to contrast media, with the exception of heat, flushing, or an episode of nausea or vomiting
- Asthma or other serious lung disease
- History of atopic allergies (pretreatment with steroid/antihistamines recommended)
- Children under the age of 2 years
- Renal failure or creatinine >177 μmol/L (>2.0 mg/dL)
- Cardiac dysfunction, including recent or imminent cardiac decompensation, severe arrhythmias, unstable angina pectoris, recent myocardial infarction, and pulmonary hypertension
- Diabetes
- Severe debilitation

although careful consideration should be given to alternative imaging techniques, such as MR imaging. In addition, several agents including sodium bicarbonate and N-acetylcysteine have been shown to decrease the risk of contrast nephropathy when used prior to administration of contrast. Nonionic, low-osmolar media produce fewer abnormalities in renal blood flow and less endothelial cell damage but should still be used carefully in patients at risk (**Table 3-3**).

Other side effects are rare but include a sensation of warmth throughout the body and a metallic taste during intravenous administration of iodinated contrast media. Anaphylactic reactions to intravenous contrast media, while rare, are the most serious side effects and range from mild hives to bronchospasm, acute anaphylaxis, and death. The pathogenesis of these allergic reactions is not fully understood, but it is thought to include the release of mediators such as histamine, antibody-antigen reactions, and complement activation. Severe allergic reactions occur in ~0.04% of patients receiving nonionic media, sixfold fewer than with ionic media. Risk factors include a history of prior contrast reaction, food allergies to shellfish, and atopy (asthma and hay fever). In such patients, a noncontrast CT or MRI procedure should be considered as an alternative to contrast administration. If iodinated contrast is absolutely required, a nonionic agent should be used in conjunction with pretreatment with glucocorticoids and antihistamines (**Table 3-4**). Patients with allergic reactions to iodinated contrast material do not usually react to gadolinium-based MR contrast material, although it would be wise

to pretreat patients with a prior allergic history to contrast administration in a similar fashion.

MAGNETIC RESONANCE IMAGING

TECHNIQUE

Magnetic resonance is a complex interaction between hydrogen protons in biologic tissues, a static magnetic field (the magnet), and energy in the form of radiofrequency (Rf) waves of a specific frequency introduced by coils placed next to the body part of interest. Spatial localization is achieved by magnetic gradients surrounding the main magnet, which impart slight changes in magnetic field throughout the imaging volume. The energy state of the hydrogen protons is transiently excited by the Rf, which is administered at a frequency specific for the field strength of the magnet. The subsequent return to equilibrium energy state (*relaxation*) of the protons results in a release of Rf energy (the *echo*), which is

TABLE 3-4

GUIDELINES FOR PREMEDICATION OF PATIENTS WITH PRIOR CONTRAST ALLERGY

12 h prior to examination:
Prednisone, 40 mg PO *or* methylprednisolone, 32 mg PO
2 h prior to examination:
Prednisone, 40 mg PO *or* methylprednisolone, 32 mg PO *and*
Cimetidine, 300 mg PO *or* ranitidine, 150 mg PO
Immediately prior to examination:
Benadryl, 50 mg IV (alternatively, can be given PO 2 h prior to exam)

detected by the coils that delivered the Rf pulses. The echo is transformed by Fourier analysis into the information used to form an MR image. The MR image thus consists of a map of the distribution of hydrogen protons, with signal intensity imparted by both density of hydrogen protons as well as differences in the relaxation time (see below) of hydrogen protons on different molecules.

T1 and T2 Relaxation Times

The rate of return to equilibrium of perturbed protons is called the *relaxation rate*. The relaxation rate varies among normal and pathologic tissues. The relaxation rate of a hydrogen proton in a tissue is influenced by local interactions with surrounding molecules and atomic neighbors. Two relaxation rates, T1 and T2, influence the signal intensity of the image. The T1 relaxation time is the time, measured in milliseconds, for 63% of the hydrogen protons to return to their normal equilibrium state, while the T2 relaxation is the time for 63% of the protons to become dephased owing to interactions among nearby protons. The intensity of the signal within various tissues and image contrast can be modulated by altering acquisition parameters, such as the interval between Rf pulses (TR) and the time between the Rf pulse and the signal reception (TE). So-called T1-weighted (T1W) images are produced by keeping the TR and TE relatively short. T2-weighted (T2W) images are produced by using longer TR and TE times. Fat and subacute hemorrhage have short T1 relaxation rates and a high signal intensity on T1W images. Structures containing more water, such as CSF and edema, have long T1 and T2 relaxation rates, a low signal intensity on T1W images, and a high signal intensity on T2W images (**Table 3–5**). Gray matter contains 10 to 15% more water than white matter, which accounts for much of its contrast on MRI (**Fig. 3–3**). T2W images are more sensitive than T1W images to edema, demyelination,

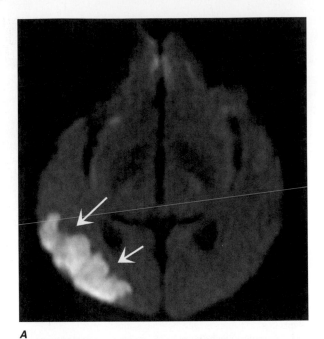

A

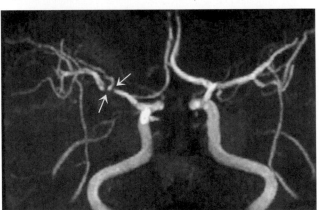

B

FIGURE 3-3

A. Axial echo-planar diffusion-weighted MR image demonstrates a large area of reduced diffusion consistent with acute cerebral ischemia (*arrows*) located in the right posterior frontotemporal lobe. Reduced diffusion is consistent with cytotoxic edema and is most commonly associated with acute cerebral infarction. *B*. Time-of-flight MR angiography through the circle of Willis demonstrates a high-grade stenosis at the left middle cerebral artery bifurcation (*arrows*).

TABLE 3-5

SOME COMMON INTENSITIES ON T1- AND T2-WEIGHTED MRI SEQUENCES						
			SIGNAL INTENSITY			
IMAGE	TR	TE	CSF	FAT	BRAIN	EDEMA
T1W	Short	Short	Low	High	Low	Low
T2W	Long	Long	High	Low	High	High

Note: TR, interval between radiofrequency (Rf) pulses; TE, interval between Rf pulse and signal reception; CSF, cerebrospinal fluid; T1W and T2W, T1- and T2-weighted.

infarction, and chronic hemorrhage, while T1-weighted imaging is more sensitive to subacute hemorrhage and fat-containing structures.

Many different MR pulse sequences exist, and each can be obtained in various planes (**Figs. 3–3, –4, –5**). The selection of a proper protocol that will best answer a clinical question depends on an accurate clinical history and indication for the examination. Fluid-attenuated inversion recovery (FLAIR) is a useful pulse sequence that pro-

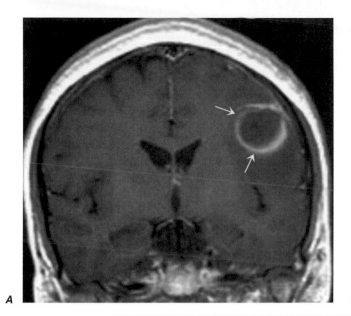

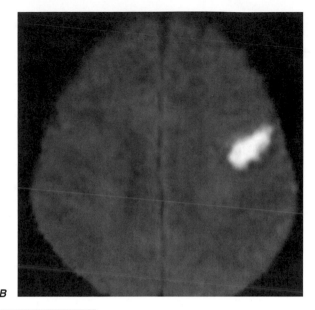

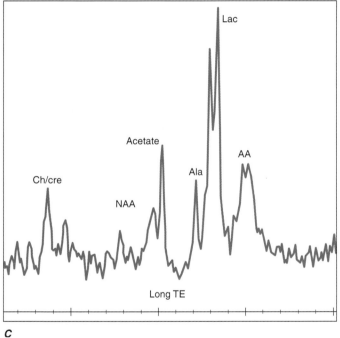

FIGURE 3-4

Middle-aged woman with fever and right hemiparesis. **A.** Coronal postcontrast T1-weighted image demonstrates a ring-enhancing mass in the left frontal lobe (*arrows*). **B.** Axial diffusion-weighted image demonstrates restricted diffusion (high signal intensity) within the lesion. Restricted diffusion in such a setting is highly suggestive of cerebral abscess.

C. Single-voxel proton spectroscopy obtained with a TE of 288 ms. In addition to the reduced *N*-acetylaspartate (NAA) peak, abnormal peaks including acetate, alanine (Ala), lactate (Lac), and amino acids (AA) are visualized. These are highly suggestive of cerebral abscess. At biopsy a streptococcal abscess was identified.

duces T2W images in which the normally high signal intensity of CSF is suppressed (Fig. 3-5*A*). FLAIR images are more sensitive than standard spine echo images for the detection of lesions within or adjacent to CSF. Gradient echo imaging is most sensitive to magnetic susceptibility as seen with blood, calcium, and air, and is indicated in patients with traumatic brain injury. MR images can be generated in sagittal, coronal, axial, or oblique planes without changing the patient's position. Each plane obtained requires a separate sequence lasting 1 to 10 min. Three-dimensional volumetric imaging is also possible with MRI, resulting in a volume of data that can be reformatted in any orientation on a workstation to highlight certain disease processes.

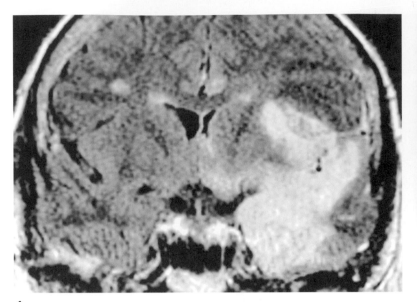

A

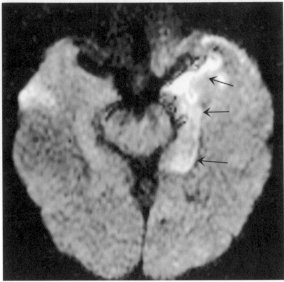

B

FIGURE 3-5

Herpes encephalitis. A 40-year-old man presents with altered mental status and fever. *A*. Coronal T2-weighted FLAIR image demonstrates expansion and high signal intensity involving the left medial temporal lobe, insular cortex, and left cingulate gyrus. *B*. Diffusion-weighted image demonstrates high signal intensity indicative of restricted diffusion involving the left medial temporal lobe and hippocampus (*arrows*). This is most consistent with neuronal destruction and can be seen in acute infarction as well as infectious and inflammatory encephalitis. Polymerase chain reaction evaluation of the CSF confirmed herpes encephalitis. (*Case courtesy of Howard Rowley, MD, University of Wisconsin.*)

MR Contrast Material

The heavy-metal element gadolinium forms the basis of all currently approved intravenous MR contrast agents. Gadolinium is a paramagnetic substance, which means that it reduces the T1 and T2 relaxation times of nearby water protons, resulting in a high signal on T1W images and a low signal on T2W images (the latter requires a sufficient local concentration, usually in the form of a bolus). Unlike iodinated contrast agents, the effect of MR contrast agents depends on the presence of local hydrogen protons on which it must act to achieve the desired effect. Gadolinium is chelated to DTPA (diethyl-enetriaminepentaacetic acid), which allows safe renal excretion. Approximately 0.2 mL/kg body weight is administered intravenously; the cost is ~$60 per dose. Gadolinium-DTPA does not cross the intact BBB but will enhance lesions lacking a BBB (Fig. 3-4*A*) and areas of the brain that normally are devoid of the BBB. The agent is well tolerated, and severe allergic reactions to gadolinium are rare but have been reported. The adverse reaction rate in patients with a prior history of atopy or asthma is 3.7%; however, the reaction rate increases to 6.3% in those patients with a prior history of unspecified allergic reaction to iodinated contrast. These agents can be administered safely to children as well as adults. Renal failure does not occur.

COMPLICATIONS AND CONTRAINDICATIONS

From the patient's perspective, an MRI examination can be intimidating, and a higher level of cooperation is required than with CT. The patient lies on a table that is moved into a long, narrow gap within the magnet. Approximately 5% of the population experiences severe claustrophobia in the MR environment. This can be reduced by mild sedation but remains a problem for some. Unlike CT, movement of the patient during an MR sequence distorts all the images; therefore, uncooperative patients should either be sedated for the MR study or scanned with CT. Generally, children under the age of 10 years usually require conscious sedation in order to complete the MR examination without motion degradation.

MRI is considered safe for patients, even at very high field strengths (>3 to 4 T). Serious injuries have been caused, however, by attraction of ferromagnetic objects into the magnet, which act as missiles if brought too close to the magnet. Likewise, ferromagnetic implants, such as aneurysm clips, may torque within the magnet, causing damage to vessels and even death. Metallic foreign bodies in the eye have moved and caused intraocular hemorrhage; screening for ocular metallic fragments is indicated in those with a history of metal work or ocular metallic foreign bodies. Implanted cardiac pacemakers are a contraindication to MRI owing to the risk of induced arrhythmias. All health care personnel and patients must be screened and educated thoroughly to prevent such disasters as the magnet is always "on." **Table 3-6** lists common contraindications for MRI.

MAGNETIC RESONANCE ANGIOGRAPHY

On routine spin echo MR sequences, moving protons (e.g., flowing blood, CSF) exhibit complex MR signals that range from high to low signal intensity relative to background stationary tissue. Fast-flowing blood returns no signal (flow void) on routine T1W or T2W spin echo MR images. Slower flowing blood, as occurs in veins or distal to arterial stenoses, may appear high in signal. However, using special pulse sequences called *gradient echo sequences,* it is possible to increase the signal intensity of moving protons in contrast to the low signal background intensity of stationary tissue. This creates angiography-like images, which can be manipulated in three dimensions to highlight vascular anatomy and relationships.

Two MRA techniques, time-of-flight (TOF) and phase-contrast, are routinely used. TOF, currently the technique used most frequently, relies on the suppression of nonmoving tissue to provide a low-intensity background for the high signal intensity of flowing blood entering the section; arterial or venous structures may be highlighted. A typical TOF angiography sequence

TABLE 3-6

COMMON CONTRAINDICATIONS TO MR IMAGING

Cardiac pacemaker or permanent pacemaker leads
Internal defibrillatory device
Cochlear prostheses
Bone growth stimulators
Spinal cord stimulators
Electronic infusion devices
Intracranial aneurysm clips (some but not all)
Ocular implants (some) or ocular metallic foreign body
McGee stapedectomy piston prosthesis
Omniphase penile implant
Swan-Ganz catheter
Magnetic stoma plugs
Magnetic dental implants
Magnetic sphincters
Ferromagnetic IVC filters, coils, stents — safe 6 weeks after implantation
Tattooed eyeliner (contains ferromagnetic material and may irritate eyes)

results in a series of contiguous thin MR sections (0.9 mm thick), which can be viewed as a stack and manipulated to create an angiographic image data set that can be reformatted and viewed in various planes and angles, much like that seen with conventional angiography (Fig. 3-3B). Noncontrast-enhanced MRA provides a vascular flow map rather than the anatomical map shown by conventional angiography.

Phase-contrast MRA has a longer acquisition time than TOF MRA, but in addition to providing anatomical information similar to that of TOF imaging, it can be used to reveal the velocity and direction of blood flow in a given vessel. Through the selection of different imaging parameters, differing blood velocities can be highlighted; selective venous and arterial MRA images can thus be obtained. One advantage of phase-contrast MRA is the excellent suppression of high-signal-intensity background structures.

MRA can also be acquired during infusion of contrast material. Recently, contrast-enhanced MRA has become the standard for extracranial vascular MRA. This technique entails rapid imaging using coronal three-dimensional TOF sequences during a bolus infusion of 15 to 20 mL of gadolinium-DTPA. Proper technique and timing of acquisition relative to bolus arrival are critical for success. Advantages include a reduction in the time of acquisition (1 to 2 min vs. 10 min) and flow-related artifacts.

MRA is lower in spatial resolution compared with conventional film-based angiography, and therefore the detection of small-vessel detail, such as is required in the workup of vasculitis, is problematic. MRA is also less sensitive to slowly flowing blood and thus may not reliably differentiate complete from near-complete occlusions. Motion, either by the patient or by anatomical structures, may distort the MRA images, creating artifacts. These limitations notwithstanding, MRA has proved useful in evaluation of the extracranial carotid and vertebral circulation as well as of larger-caliber intracranial arteries and dural sinuses. It has also proved useful in the noninvasive detection of intracranial aneurysms and vascular malformations.

ECHO-PLANAR MR IMAGING

Recent improvements in gradients, software, and high-speed computer processors now permit extremely rapid MRI of the brain. With echo-planar MRI (EPI), fast gradients are switched on and off at high speeds to create the information used to form an image. In routine spin echo imaging, images of the brain can be obtained in 5 to 10 min. With EPI, all of the information required for processing an image is accumulated in 50 to 150 ms, and the information for the entire brain is obtained in 1 to 2 min, depending on the degree of resolution required or desired. Fast MRI reduces patient and organ motion, permitting diffusion imaging (Figs. 3-3 to 3-5 and Fig. 17-12), perfusion imaging during contrast infusion fMRI, and kinematic motion studies.

Perfusion and diffusion imaging are EPI techniques that are useful in early detection of ischemic injury of the brain and may be useful together to demonstrate infarcted tissue as well as ischemic but potentially viable tissue at risk of infarction (e.g., the ischemic penumbra). Diffusion-weighted imaging (DWI) assesses microscopic motion of water; restriction of motion appears as relative high signal intensity on diffusion-weighted images. DWI is the most sensitive technique for detection of acute cerebral infarction of <7 days' duration and is also sensitive to encephalitis and abscess formation, all of which demonstrate reduced diffusion or high signal.

Perfusion MRI involves the acquisition of EPI images during a rapid bolus of contrast material. Relative perfusion abnormalities can be identified. The relative cerebral blood volume, mean transit time, and cerebral blood flow throughout the image can be calculated within regions of interest. Delay in mean transit time and reduction in cerebral blood volume and cerebral blood flow are typically seen in infarction. Elevated or normal cerebral blood volume in a setting of reduced blood flow may indicate tissue that is at risk of infarction. pMRI imaging can also be used in the assessment of brain tumors, where it has been shown to be helpful in differentiating intraaxial primary tumors from extraaxial tumors or metastasis.

Diffusion tract imaging (DTI) is a special diffusion technique that is capable of demonstrating white matter tracts and their relationship to lesions of the brain. Preferential microscopic motion of water along white matter tracts is detected by diffusion MR, which can also indicate the direction of white matter fiber tracts. This new technique has great potential in the assessment of brain maturation as well as disease entities that undermine the integrity of the white matter architecture.

fMRI of the brain is an EPI technique that localizes regions of activity in the brain following task activation. Neuronal activity elicits an increase in the delivery of oxygenated blood flow to a specific region of the brain, resulting in a slight alteration in the balance of oxyhemoglobin and deoxyhemoglobin, which yields a 2 to 3% increase in signal intensity within draining veins. Further work will determine whether these techniques are cost-effective or clinically useful, but currently preoperative somatosensory and auditory cortex localization is possible. This technique has proved useful to neuroscientists interested in interrogating the localization of certain brain functions.

MAGNETIC RESONANCE NEUROGRAPHY

MR neurography is an MR technique that shows promise in detecting increased signal in irritated, inflamed, or infiltrated nerves. These images are obtained with fat-suppressed fast spin echo imaging or short inversion recovery sequences, and they may indicate nerves that are responsible for pain syndromes more precisely. Irritated or infiltrated nerves will demonstrate high signal on T2W imaging.

POSITRON EMISSION TOMOGRAPHY (PET)

PET relies on the detection of positrons emitted during the decay of a radionuclide that has been injected into a patient. The most frequently used moiety is 2-[^{18}F]fluoro-2-deoxy-D-glucose (FDG), which is an analogue of glucose and is taken up by cells competitively with 2-deoxyglucose. Multiple images of glucose uptake activity are formed after 45 to 60 min. Images reveal differences in regional glucose activity among normal and pathologic brain structures. A lower activity of FDG in the parietal lobes has been associated with Alzheimer's disease (AD) and can be used to differentiate AD from other forms of dementia. FDG PET is used primarily for the detection of extracranial metastatic disease. PET is no longer used primarily for differentiation of tumor from radiation necrosis.

MYELOGRAPHY

TECHNIQUE

Myelography involves the intrathecal instillation of specially formulated water-soluble iodinated contrast medium into the lumbar or cervical subarachnoid space. CT scanning is usually performed after myelography (*CT myelography*) to better demonstrate the spinal cord and roots, which appear as filling defects in the opacified subarachnoid space. *Low-dose CT myelography,* in which CT is performed after the subarachnoid injection of a small amount of relatively dilute contrast material, has replaced conventional myelography for many indications, thereby reducing exposure to radiation and contrast media. Newer multidetector scanners now obtain CT studies quickly so that reformations in sagittal and coronal planes, equivalent to traditional myelography projections, are now routine.

INDICATIONS

Myelography has been largely replaced by CT myelography and MRI for diagnosis of diseases of the spinal canal and cord (Table 3-1). Remaining indications for conventional plain film myelography include the evaluation of suspected meningeal or arachnoid cysts and the localization of spinal dural arteriovenous or CSF fistulas. Conventional myelography and CT myelography provide the most precise information in patients with prior spinal fusion and spinal fixation hardware.

CONTRAINDICATIONS

Myelography is relatively safe; however, it should be performed with caution in any patient with elevated intracranial pressure or a history of allergic reaction to intrathecal contrast media. In patients with a suspected spinal block, MR is the preferred technique. If myelography is necessary, only a small amount of contrast medium should be instilled below the lesion in order to minimize the risk of neurologic deterioration. Lumbar puncture is to be avoided in patients with bleeding disorders, including patients receiving anticoagulant therapy, as well as in those with infections of the soft tissues.

COMPLICATIONS

Headache, nausea, and vomiting are the most frequent complications of myelography, occurring in up to 38% of patients. These symptoms are thought to result from neurotoxic effects of the contrast agent, persistent leakage of CSF at the puncture site, or psychological reactions to the procedure. Vasovagal syncope may occur during lumbar puncture; it is accentuated by the upright position used during lumbar myelography. Adequate hydration before and after myelography will reduce the incidence of this complication. Postural headache (post–lumbar puncture headache) is generally due to leakage of CSF from the puncture site, resulting in CSF hypotension; management is discussed in Chap. 5. Hearing loss is a rare complication of myelography. It may result from a direct toxic effect of the contrast medium or from an alteration of the pressure equilibrium between CSF and perilymph in the inner ear. Puncture of the spinal cord is a rare but serious complication of cervical (C1-2) and high lumbar puncture. The risk of cord puncture is greatest in patients with spinal stenosis or conditions that reduce CSF volume. In these settings, a low-dose lumbar injection followed by thin-section CT or MRI is a safer alternative to cervical puncture. Intrathecal contrast reactions are rare, but aseptic meningitis and encephalopathy may occur. The latter is usually dose-related and associated with contrast entering the intracranial subarachnoid space. Seizures occur following myelography in 0.1 to 0.3% of patients. Risk factors include a preexisting seizure disorder and the use of a total iodine dose of >4500 mg. Other reported symptoms include hyperthermia, hallucinations, depression, and anxiety states. These side effects have been reduced by the development of nonionic, water-soluble contrast agents, as well as by head elevation and generous hydration following myelography.

SPINE INTERVENTIONS

DISCOGRAPHY

The evaluation of back pain and radiculopathy may require diagnostic procedures that attempt either to reproduce the patient's pain or to relieve it, indicating its correct source. Discography is performed by fluoroscopic placement of a 22- to 25-gauge needle into the intervertebral disc and subsequent injection of 1 to 3 mL of contrast media. The intradiscal pressure is recorded, as is an assessment of the patient's response to the injection of contrast material. Typically little or no pain is felt during injection of a normal disc, which does not accept much more than 1 mL of contrast material, even at pressures as high as 415 to 690 kPa (60 to 100 lb/in^2). CT and plain films are obtained following the procedure.

SELECTIVE NERVE ROOT AND EPIDURAL SPINAL INJECTIONS

Percutaneous selective nerve root and epidural blocks with glucocorticoid and anesthetic mixtures may be both therapeutic and diagnostic, especially if a patient's pain is relieved. Typically 1 to 2 mL of an equal mixture of a long-acting glucocorticoid such as betamethasone and a long-acting anesthetic such as bupivacaine 0.75% is instilled under CT or fluoroscopic guidance in the intraspinal epidural space or adjacent to an existing nerve root.

ANGIOGRAPHY

TECHNIQUE

Catheter angiography is indicated in the evaluation of patients with vascular pathology, particularly of smaller intracranial vessels. However, it carries the greatest risk of morbidity of all diagnostic imaging procedures, owing to the necessity of inserting a catheter into a blood vessel, directing the catheter to the required location, injecting contrast material to visualize the vessel, and removing the catheter while maintaining hemostasis. Therapeutic transcatheter procedures (see below) have become important options for the treatment of some cerebrovascular diseases. The decision to undertake a diagnostic or therapeutic angiographic procedure requires careful assessment of the goals of the investigation and its attendant risks.

To improve tolerance to contrast agents, patients undergoing angiography should be well hydrated before and after the procedure. Since the femoral route is used most commonly, the femoral artery must be compressed after the procedure to prevent a hematoma from developing. The puncture site and distal pulses should be evaluated carefully after the procedure; complications can include thigh hematoma or lower extremity emboli.

INDICATIONS

Table 3-1 lists some of the indications for conventional angiography. Angiography has been replaced for many indications by CT/CTA or MRI/MRA; however, angiography is still used for evaluating intracranial small-vessel pathology (such as vasculitis), for assessing vascular malformations and aneurysms, and in endovascular therapeutic procedures.

COMPLICATIONS

A common femoral arterial puncture provides retrograde access via the aorta to the aortic arch and great vessels. The most feared complication of cerebral angiography is stroke. Thrombus can form on or inside the tip of the catheter, and atherosclerotic thrombus or plaque can be dislodged by the catheter or guidewire or by the force of injection and can embolize distally in the cerebral circulation. Risk factors for ischemic complications include limited experience on the part of the angiographer, atherosclerosis, vasospasm, low cardiac output, decreased oxygen-carrying capacity, advanced age, and possibly migraine. The risk of a neurologic complication varies but is ~4% for transient ischemic attack and stroke, 1% for permanent deficit, and <0.1% for death.

Ionic contrast material injected into the cerebral vasculature can be neurotoxic if the BBB is breached, either by an underlying disease or by the injection of hyperosmolar contrast agent. Ionic contrast media are less well tolerated than nonionic media, probably because they can induce changes in cell membrane electrical potentials. Patients with dolichoectasia of the basilar artery can suffer reversible brainstem dysfunction and acute short-term memory loss during angiography, owing to the slow percolation of the contrast material and the consequent prolonged exposure of the brain. Rarely, an intracranial aneurysm ruptures during an angiographic contrast injection, causing subarachnoid hemorrhage, perhaps as a result of injection under high pressure.

SPINAL ANGIOGRAPHY

Spinal angiography may be indicated to evaluate vascular malformations and tumors and to identify the artery of Adamkiewicz (Chap. 24) prior to aortic aneurysm repair. The procedure is lengthy and requires the use of relatively large volumes of contrast; the incidence of serious complications, including paraparesis, subjective visual blurring, and altered speech, is ~2%. Gadolinium-enhanced MRA has been used successfully in this setting and has promise for replacing diagnostic spinal angiography for some indications.

INTERVENTIONAL NEURORADIOLOGY

This rapidly developing field is providing new therapeutic options for patients with difficult neurovascular problems. Available procedures include detachable coil therapy for aneurysms, particulate or liquid adhesive embolization of arteriovenous malformations, balloon angioplasty and stenting of arterial stenosis or vasospasm, transarterial or transvenous embolization of dural arteriovenous fistulas, balloon occlusion of carotid-cavernous and vertebral fistulas, endovascular treatment of vein-of-Galen malformations, preoperative embolization of tumors, stenting of diseased extracranial carotid arteries, and thrombolysis or mechanical retrieval of acute arterial or venous thrombosis. Many of these disorders place the patient at high risk of cerebral hemorrhage, stroke, or death.

The highest complication rates are found with the therapies designed to treat the highest-risk diseases. In a large series of surgically difficult intracranial aneurysms treated with detachable balloons, Higashida and colleagues reported a 7.4% incidence of stroke and a 9.8% death rate. These figures must be considered in light of the high morbidity and mortality associated with untreated and surgically unapproachable aneurysms (Chap. 17). The advent of the electrolytically detachable coil has reduced these rates and ushered in a new era in the treatment of cerebral aneurysms. One recent double-blind trial (ISAT) found a 28% reduction of morbidity and mortality at 1 year among those treated for anterior circulation aneurysm with detachable coils versus neurosurgical clipping. It remains to be determined what the role of coils will be relative to surgical options, but in many centers, coiling of aneurysms has become standard therapy for many aneurysms.

FURTHER READINGS

CHA S et al: Intracranial mass lesions: Dynamic contrast-enhanced susceptibility-weighted echoplanar perfusion MR imaging. Radiology 223:11, 2002

JANKOWITZ B et al: Indications for catheter-based angiography of the cerebrovasculature. Neurosurg Clin N Am 16:241, 2005

LAW M: MR spectroscopy of brain tumors. Top Magn Reson Imaging. 15:291, 2004

MOLYNEUX AJ et al: International subarachnoid aneurysm trial (ISAT) of neurosurgical clipping versus endovascular coiling in 2143 patients with ruptured intracranial aneurysms: a randomised comparison of effects on survival, dependency, seizures, rebleeding, subgroups, and aneurysm occlusion. Lancet 366:809, 2005

A 7-year follow-up on patients randomized to surgery versus endovascular treatment of ruptured aneurysms.

MULLER M et al: Ischemia after carotid endarterectomy: Comparison between transcranial Doppler sonography and diffusion-weighted MR imaging (see comments). Am J Neuroradiol 21:47, 2000

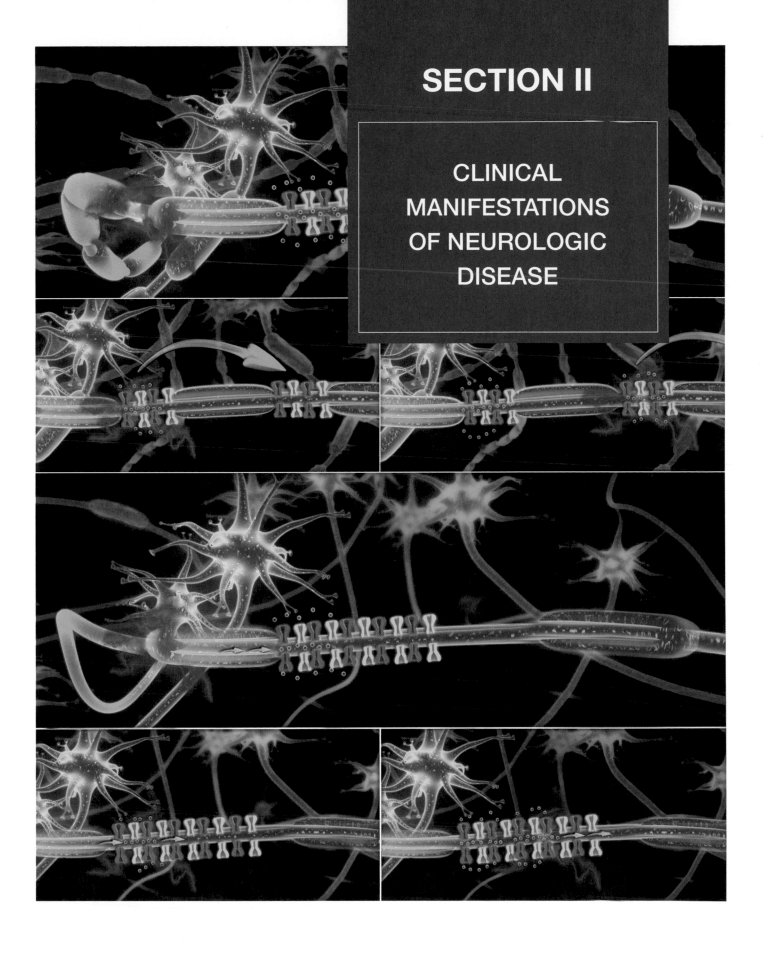

SECTION II

CLINICAL MANIFESTATIONS OF NEUROLOGIC DISEASE

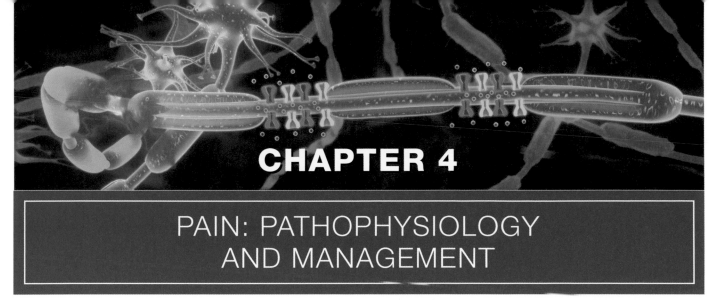

CHAPTER 4

PAIN: PATHOPHYSIOLOGY AND MANAGEMENT

Howard L. Fields
Joseph B. Martin

The task of medicine is to preserve and restore health and to relieve suffering. Understanding pain is essential to both these goals. Because pain is universally understood as a signal of disease, it is the most common symptom that brings a patient to a physician's attention. The function of the pain sensory system is to protect the body and maintain homeostasis. It does this by detecting, localizing, and identifying tissue-damaging processes. Since different diseases produce characteristic patterns of tissue damage, the quality, time course, and location of a patient's pain complaint and the location of tenderness provide important diagnostic clues and are used to evaluate the response to treatment. Once this information is obtained, it is the obligation of the physician to provide rapid and effective pain relief.

THE PAIN SENSORY SYSTEM

Pain is an unpleasant sensation localized to a part of the body. It is often described in terms of a penetrating or tissue-destructive process (e.g., stabbing, burning, twisting, tearing, squeezing) and/or of a bodily or emotional reaction (e.g., terrifying, nauseating, sickening). Furthermore, any pain of moderate or higher intensity is accompanied by anxiety and the urge to escape or terminate the feeling. These properties illustrate the duality of pain: it is both sensation and emotion. When acute, pain is characteristically associated with behavioral arousal and a stress response consisting of increased blood pressure, heart rate, pupil diameter, and plasma cortisol levels. In addition, local muscle contraction (e.g., limb flexion, abdominal wall rigidity) is often present.

PERIPHERAL MECHANISMS

The Primary Afferent Nociceptor

A peripheral nerve consists of the axons of three different types of neurons: primary sensory afferents, motor neurons, and sympathetic postganglionic neurons (**Fig. 4-1**). The cell bodies of primary afferents are located in the dorsal root ganglia in the vertebral foramina. The primary afferent axon bifurcates to send one process into the spinal cord and the other to innervate tissues. Primary afferents are classified by their diameter, degree of myelination, and conduction velocity. The largest-diameter fibers, A-beta (Aβ), respond maximally to light touch and/or moving stimuli; they are present primarily in nerves that innervate the skin. In normal individuals, the activity of these fibers does not produce pain. There are two other classes of primary afferents: the small-diameter myelinated A-delta (Aδ) and the unmyelinated (C fiber) axons (Fig. 4-1). These fibers are present in nerves to the skin and to deep somatic and visceral structures. Some tissues, such as the cornea, are innervated only by Aδ and C afferents. Most Aδ and C afferents respond maximally only to intense (painful) stimuli and produce the subjective experience of pain when they are electrically stimulated; this defines them as *primary afferent nociceptors (pain receptors)*. The ability to detect painful stimuli is completely abolished when Aδ and C axons are blocked.

Individual primary afferent nociceptors can respond to several different types of noxious stimuli. For example, most nociceptors respond to heating, intense mechanical stimuli such as a pinch, and application of irritating chemicals.

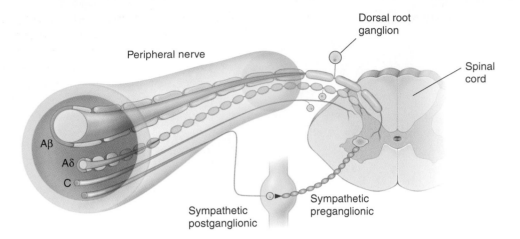

FIGURE 4-1

Components of a typical cutaneous nerve. There are two distinct functional categories of axons: primary afferents with cell bodies in the dorsal root ganglion, and sympathetic postganglionic fibers with cell bodies in the sympathetic ganglion. Primary afferents include those with large-diameter myelinated (Aβ), small-diameter myelinated (Aδ), and unmyelinated (C) axons. All sympathetic postganglionic fibers are unmyelinated.

Sensitization

When intense, repeated, or prolonged stimuli are applied to damaged or inflamed tissues the threshold for activating primary afferent nociceptors is lowered and the frequency of firing is higher for all stimulus intensities. Inflammatory mediators such as bradykinin, some prostaglandins, and leukotrienes contribute to this process, which is called *sensitization*. In sensitized tissues normally innocuous stimuli can produce pain. Sensitization is a clinically important process that contributes to tenderness, soreness, and hyperalgesia. A striking example of sensitization is sunburned skin, in which severe pain can be produced by a gentle slap on the back or a warm shower.

Sensitization is of particular importance for pain and tenderness in deep tissues. Viscera are normally relatively insensitive to noxious mechanical and thermal stimuli, although hollow viscera do generate significant discomfort when distended. In contrast, when affected by a disease process with an inflammatory component, deep structures such as joints or hollow viscera characteristically become exquisitely sensitive to mechanical stimulation.

A large proportion of Aδ and C afferents innervating viscera are completely insensitive in normal noninjured, noninflamed tissue. That is, they cannot be activated by known mechanical or thermal stimuli and are not spontaneously active. However, in the presence of inflammatory mediators, these afferents become sensitive to mechanical stimuli. Such afferents have been termed *silent nociceptors,* and their characteristic properties may explain how under pathologic conditions the relatively insensitive deep structures can become the source of severe and debilitating pain and tenderness. Low pH, prostaglandins, leukotrienes, and other inflammatory mediators such as bradykinin play a significant role in sensitization.

Nociceptor-Induced Inflammation

One important concept to emerge in recent years is that afferent nociceptors also have a neuroeffector function. Most nociceptors contain polypeptide mediators that are released from their peripheral terminals when they are activated (**Fig. 4-2**). An example is substance P, an 11-amino-acid peptide. Substance P is released from primary afferent nociceptors and has multiple biologic activities. It is a potent vasodilator, degranulates mast cells, is a chemoattractant for leukocytes, and increases the production and release of inflammatory mediators. Interestingly, depletion of substance P from joints reduces the severity of experimental arthritis. Primary afferent nociceptors are not simply passive messengers of threats to tissue injury but also play an active role in tissue protection through these neuroeffector functions.

CENTRAL MECHANISMS

The Spinal Cord and Referred Pain

The axons of primary afferent nociceptors enter the spinal cord via the dorsal root. They terminate in the dorsal horn of the spinal gray matter (**Fig. 4-3**). The terminals of primary afferent axons contact spinal neurons that transmit the pain signal to brain sites involved in pain perception. The axon of each primary afferent contacts many spinal neurons, and each spinal neuron receives convergent inputs from many primary afferents.

A

Primary activation

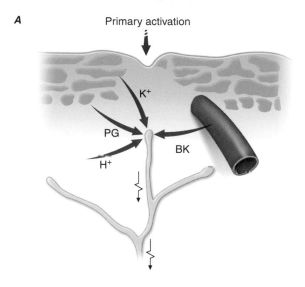

B

Secondary activation

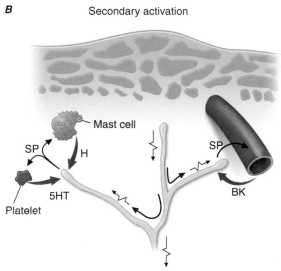

FIGURE 4-2

Events leading to activation, sensitization, and spread of sensitization of primary afferent nociceptor terminals. **A.** Direct activation by intense pressure and consequent cell damage. Cell damage induces lower pH (H⁺) and leads to release of potassium (K⁺) and to synthesis of prostaglandins (PG) and bradykinin (BK). Prostaglandins increase the sensitivity of the terminal to bradykinin and other pain-producing substances. **B.** Secondary activation. Impulses generated in the stimulated terminal propagate not only to the spinal cord but also into other terminal branches where they induce the release of peptides, including substance P (SP). Substance P causes vasodilation and neurogenic edema with further accumulation of bradykinin. Substance P also causes the release of histamine (H) from mast cells and serotonin (5HT) from platelets.

The convergence of sensory inputs to a single spinal pain-transmission neuron is of great importance because it underlies the phenomenon of referred pain. All spinal neurons that receive input from the viscera and deep musculoskeletal structures also receive input from the skin. The convergence patterns are determined by the spinal segment of the dorsal root ganglion that supplies the afferent innervation of a structure. For example, the afferents that supply the central diaphragm are derived from the third and fourth cervical dorsal root ganglia. Primary afferents with cell bodies in these same ganglia supply the skin of the shoulder and lower neck. Thus sensory inputs from both the shoulder skin and the central diaphragm converge on pain-transmission neurons in the third and fourth cervical spinal segments. *Because of this convergence and the fact that the spinal neurons are most often activated by inputs from the skin, activity evoked in spinal neurons by input from deep structures is mislocalized by the patient to a place that is roughly coextensive with the region of skin innervated by the same spinal segment.* Thus inflammation near the central diaphragm is usually reported as discomfort near the shoulder. This spatial displacement of pain sensation from the site of the injury that produces it is known as *referred pain.*

Ascending Pathways for Pain

A majority of spinal neurons contacted by primary afferent nociceptors send their axons to the contralateral thalamus. These axons form the contralateral spinothalamic tract, which lies in the anterolateral white matter of the spinal cord, the lateral edge of the medulla, and the lateral pons and midbrain. The spinothalamic pathway is crucial for pain sensation in humans. Interruption of this pathway produces permanent deficits in pain and temperature discrimination.

Spinothalamic tract axons ascend to several regions of the thalamus. There is tremendous divergence of the

Skin

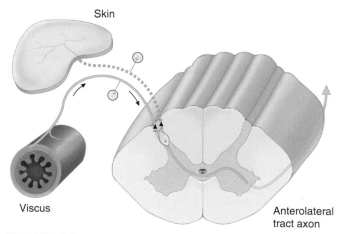

Viscus

Anterolateral tract axon

FIGURE 4-3

The convergence-projection hypothesis of referred pain. According to this hypothesis, visceral afferent nociceptors converge on the same pain-projection neurons as the afferents from the somatic structures in which the pain is perceived. The brain has no way of knowing the actual source of input and mistakenly "projects" the sensation to the somatic structure.

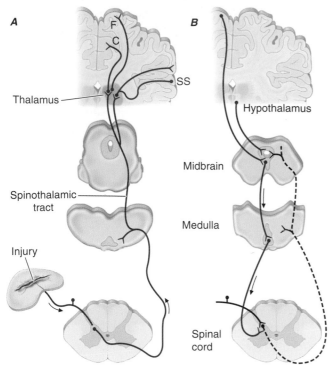

FIGURE 4-4

A. Transmission system for nociceptive messages. Noxious stimuli activate the sensitive peripheral ending of the primary afferent nociceptor by the process of transduction. The message is then transmitted over the peripheral nerve to the spinal cord, where it synapses with cells of origin of the major ascending pain pathway, the spinothalamic tract. The message is relayed in the thalamus to the anterior cingulate (C), frontal insular (F), and somatosensory cortex (SS). **B**. Pain-modulation network. Inputs from frontal cortex and hypothalamus (Hyp.) activate cells in the midbrain that control spinal pain-transmission cells via cells in the medulla.

pain signal from these thalamic sites to broad areas of the cerebral cortex that subserve different aspects of the pain experience (**Fig. 4-4**). One of the thalamic projections is to the somatosensory cortex. This projection mediates the purely sensory aspects of pain, i.e., its location, intensity, and quality. Other thalamic neurons project to cortical regions that are linked to emotional responses, such as the cingulate gyrus and other areas of the frontal lobes. These pathways to the frontal cortex subserve the affective or unpleasant emotional dimension of pain. This affective dimension of pain produces suffering and exerts potent control of behavior. Because of this dimension, fear is a constant companion of pain.

PAIN MODULATION

The pain produced by similar injuries is remarkably variable in different situations and in different individuals. For example, athletes have been known to sustain serious

fractures with only minor pain, and Beecher's classic World War II survey revealed that many soldiers in battle were unbothered by injuries that would have produced agonizing pain in civilian patients. Furthermore, even the suggestion of relief can have a significant analgesic effect (placebo). On the other hand, many patients find even minor injuries (such as venipuncture) frightening and unbearable, and the expectation of pain has been demonstrated to induce pain without a noxious stimulus.

The powerful effect of expectation and other psychological variables on the perceived intensity of pain implies the existence of brain circuits that can modulate the activity of the pain-transmission pathways. One of these circuits has links in the hypothalamus, midbrain, and medulla, and it selectively controls spinal pain-transmission neurons through a descending pathway (Fig. 4-4).

Human brain imaging studies have implicated this pain-modulating circuit in the pain-relieving effect of attention, suggestion, and opioid analgesic medications. Furthermore, each of the component structures of the pathway contains opioid receptors and is sensitive to the direct application of opioid drugs. In animals, lesions of the system reduce the analgesic effect of systemically administered opioids such as morphine. Along with the opioid receptor, the component nuclei of this pain-modulating circuit contain endogenous opioid peptides such as the enkephalins and β-endorphin.

The most reliable way to activate this endogenous opioid-mediated modulating system is by prolonged pain and/or fear. There is evidence that pain-relieving endogenous opioids are released following surgical procedures and in patients given a placebo for pain relief.

Pain-modulating circuits can enhance as well as suppress pain. Both pain-inhibiting and pain-facilitating neurons in the medulla project to and control spinal pain-transmission neurons. Since pain-transmission neurons can be activated by modulatory neurons, it is theoretically possible to generate a pain signal with no peripheral noxious stimulus. In fact, functional imaging studies have demonstrated increased activity in this circuit during migraine headache. A central circuit that facilitates pain could account for the finding that pain can be induced by suggestion and could provide a framework for understanding how psychological factors can contribute to chronic pain.

NEUROPATHIC PAIN

Lesions of the peripheral or central nervous pathways for pain typically result in a loss or impairment of pain sensation. Paradoxically, damage or dysfunction of these pathways can produce pain. For example, damage to peripheral nerves, as occurs in diabetic neuropathy, or to primary afferents, as in herpes zoster, can result in pain that is referred to the body region innervated by the damaged nerves. Though rare, pain may also be produced by damage to the central nervous system, particularly the spinothalamic pathway or thalamus. Such neuropathic pains are often severe and are notoriously intractable to standard treatments for pain.

Neuropathic pains typically have an unusual burning, tingling, or electric shock–like quality and may be triggered by very light touch. These features are rare in other types of pain. On examination, a sensory deficit is characteristically present in the area of the patient's pain. Hyperpathia is also characteristic of neuropathic pain; patients often complain that the very lightest moving stimuli evoke exquisite pain (allodynia). In this regard it is of clinical interest that a topical preparation of 5% lidocaine in patch form is effective for patients with posttherpetic neuralgia who have prominent allodynia.

A variety of mechanisms contribute to neuropathic pain. As with sensitized primary afferent nociceptors, damaged primary afferents, including nociceptors, become highly sensitive to mechanical stimulation and begin to generate impulses in the absence of stimulation. There is evidence that this increased sensitivity and spontaneous activity is due to an increased concentration of sodium channels. Damaged primary afferents may also develop sensitivity to norepinephrine. Interestingly, spinal cord pain-transmission neurons cut off from their normal input may also become spontaneously active. Thus both central and peripheral nervous system hyperactivity contribute to neuropathic pain.

Sympathetically Maintained Pain

Patients with peripheral nerve injury can develop a severe burning pain (causalgia) in the region innervated by the nerve. The pain typically begins after a delay of hours to days or even weeks. The pain is accompanied by swelling of the extremity, periarticular osteoporosis, and arthritic changes in the distal joints. The pain is dramatically and immediately relieved by blocking the sympathetic innervation of the affected extremity. Damaged primary afferent nociceptors acquire adrenergic sensitivity and can be activated by stimulation of the sympathetic outflow. A similar syndrome called *reflex sympathetic dystrophy* can be produced without obvious nerve damage by a variety of injuries, including fractures of bone, soft tissue trauma, myocardial infarction, and stroke (Chap. 22). Although the pathophysiology of this condition is poorly understood, the pain and the signs of inflammation are rapidly relieved by blocking the sympathetic nervous system. This implies that sympathetic activity can activate undamaged nociceptors when inflammation is present. Signs of sympathetic hyperactivity

should be sought in patients with posttraumatic pain and inflammation and no other obvious explanation.

TREATMENT FOR ACUTE PAIN

The ideal treatment for any pain is to remove the cause; thus diagnosis should always precede treatment planning. Sometimes treating the underlying condition does not immediately relieve pain. Furthermore, some conditions are so painful that rapid and effective analgesia is essential (e.g., the postoperative state, burns, trauma, cancer, sickle cell crisis). Analgesic medications are a first line of treatment in these cases, and all practitioners should be familiar with their use.

Aspirin, Acetaminophen, and Nonsteroidal Anti-Inflammatory Agents (NSAIDS)

These drugs are considered together because they are used for similar problems and may have a similar mechanism of action (**Table 4–1**). All these compounds inhibit cyclooxygenase (COX), and, except for acetaminophen, all have anti-inflammatory actions, especially at higher dosages. They are particularly effective for mild to moderate headache and for pain of musculoskeletal origin.

Since they are effective for these common types of pain and are available without prescription, COX inhibitors are by far the most commonly used analgesics. They are absorbed well from the gastrointestinal tract and, with occasional use, side effects are minimal. With chronic use, gastric irritation is a common side effect of aspirin and NSAIDs and is the problem that most frequently limits the dose that can be given. Gastric irritation is most severe with aspirin, which may cause erosion of the gastric mucosa, and because aspirin irreversibly acetylates platelets and thereby interferes with coagulation of the blood, gastrointestinal bleeding is a risk. The NSAIDs are less problematic, but their risk in this regard is still significant. In addition to their well-known gastrointestinal toxicity, nephrotoxicity is a significant problem for patients using NSAIDs on a chronic basis, and patients at risk for renal insufficiency should be monitored closely. NSAIDs also cause an increase in blood pressure in a significant number of individuals. Long-term treatment with NSAIDs requires regular blood pressure monitoring and treatment if necessary. Although toxic to the liver when taken in a high dose, acetaminophen rarely

TABLE 4-1

DRUGS FOR RELIEF OF PAIN

GENERIC NAME	DOSE, MG	INTERVAL	COMMENTS
Nonnarcotic Analgesics: Usual Doses and Intervals			
Acetylsalicylic acid	650 PO	q4h	Enteric-coated preparations available
Acetaminophen	650 PO	q4h	Side effects uncommon
Ibuprofen	400 PO	q4–6h	Available without prescription
Naproxen	250–500 PO	q12h	Delayed effects may be due to long half-life
Fenoprofen	200 PO	q4–6h	Contraindicated in renal disease
Indomethacin	25–50 PO	q8h	Gastrointestinal side effects common
Ketorolac	15–60 IM	q4–6h	Available for parenteral use (IM/IV)
Celecoxib	100–200 PO	q12–24h	Increased risk of MI in some patients; black box warning.

GENERIC NAME	PARENTERAL DOSE, MG	PO DOSE, MG	COMMENTS
Narcotic Analgesics: Usual Doses and Intervals			
Codeine	30–60 q4h	30–60 q4h	Nausea common
Oxycodone	—	5–10 q4–6h	Usually available with acetaminophen or aspirin
Morphine	10 q4h	60 q4h	
Morphine sustained release	—	30–200 bid to tid	Oral slow-release preparation
Hydromorphone	1–2 q4h	2–4 q4h	Shorter acting than morphine sulfate
Levorphanol	2 q6–8h	4 q6–8h	Longer acting than morphine sulfate; absorbed well PO
Methadone	10 q6–8h	20 q6–8h	Delayed sedation due to long half-life
Meperidine	75–100 q3–4h	300 q4h	Poorly absorbed PO; normeperidine a toxic metabolite
Butorphanol	—	1–2 q4h	Intranasal spray
Fentanyl	25–100 μg/h	—	72 h transdermal patch
Tramadol	—	50–100 q4–6h	Mixed opioid/adrenergic action

GENERIC NAME	UPTAKE BLOCKADE 5-HT	5-NE	SEDATIVE POTENCY	ANTICHOLINERGIC POTENCY	ORTHOSTATIC HYPOTENSION	CARDIAC ARRHYTHMIA	AVE. DOSE, MG/D	RANGE, MG/D
Antidepressants[a]								
Doxepin	++	+	High	Moderate	Moderate	Less	200	75–400
Amitriptyline	++++	++	High	Highest	Moderate	Yes	150	25–300
Imipramine	++++	++	Moderate	Moderate	High	Yes	200	75–400
Nortriptyline	+++	++	Moderate	Moderate	Low	Yes	100	40–150
Desipramine	+++	++++	Low	Low	Low	Yes	150	50–300
Venlafaxine	+++	++	Low	None	None	No	150	75–400

GENERIC NAME	PO DOSE, MG	INTERVAL
Anticonvulsants and Antiarrhythmics[a]		
Phenytoin	300	daily/qhs
Carbamazepine	200–300	q6h
Oxcarbazine	300	bid
Clonazepam	1	q6h
Mexiletine	150–300	q6–12h
Gabapentin[b]	600–1200	q8h

[a] Antidepressants, anticonvulsants, and antiarrhythmics have not been approved by the U.S. Food and Drug Administration (FDA) for the treatment of pain.
[b] Gabapentin in doses up to 1800 mg/d is FDA approved for postherpetic neuralgia.
Note: 5-HT, serotonin; NE, norepinephrine.

produces gastric irritation and does not interfere with platelet function.

The introduction of a parenteral form of NSAID, ketorolac, extends the usefulness of this class of compounds in the management of acute severe pain. Ketorolac is sufficiently potent and rapid in onset to supplant opioids for many patients with acute severe headache and musculoskeletal pain.

There are two major classes of COX: COX-1 is constitutively expressed, and COX-2 is induced in the inflammatory state. COX-2-selective drugs have moderate analgesic potency and may produce less gastric irritation than the nonselective COX inhibitors. It is not yet clear whether the use of COX-2-selective drugs is associated with a lower risk of nephrotoxicity compared to nonselective NSAIDs. On the other hand, COX-2-selective drugs offer a significant benefit in the management of acute postoperative pain because they do not affect platelet function. This is a situation in which the nonselective COX inhibitors would be contraindicated because they impair platelet-mediated blood clotting and are thus associated with increased bleeding at the operative site. A corollary of this is that COX-2 drugs do not provide the same degree of protection from thromboembolic cardiovascular adverse events such as myocardial infarction. Recent studies in patients with colon cancer and other conditions showed an increased risk of myocardial infarction and, in one case, stroke with COX-2 inhibitors, prompting the United States Food and Drug Administration to suspend sales or mandate black box warnings on all members of this class of drugs.

Opioid Analgesics

Opioids are the most potent pain-relieving drugs currently available. Furthermore, of all analgesics, they have the broadest range of efficacy, providing the most reliable and effective method for rapid pain relief. Although side effects are common, they are usually not serious except for respiratory depression and can be reversed rapidly with the narcotic antagonist naloxone. The physician should not hesitate to use opioid analgesics in patients with acute severe pain. Table 4-1 lists the most commonly used opioid analgesics.

Opioids produce analgesia by actions in the central nervous system. They activate pain-inhibitory neurons and directly inhibit pain-transmission neurons. Most of the commercially available opioid analgesics act at the same opioid receptor (mu receptor), differing mainly in potency, speed of onset, duration of action, and optimal route of administration. Although the dose-related side effects (sedation, respiratory depression, pruritus, constipation) are similar among the different opioids, some side effects are due to accumulation of nonopioid metabolites that are unique to individual drugs. One striking example of this is normeperidine, a metabolite of meperidine. Normeperidine produces hyperexcitability and seizures that are not reversible with naloxone. Normeperidine accumulation is increased in patients with renal failure.

The most rapid relief with opioids is obtained by intravenous administration; relief with oral administration is significantly slower. Common acute side effects include nausea, vomiting, and sedation. The most serious side effect is respiratory depression. Patients with any form of respiratory compromise must be kept under close observation following opioid administration; an oxygen saturation monitor may be useful. The opioid antagonist, naloxone, should be readily available. Opioid effects are dose-related, and there is great variability among patients in the doses that relieve pain and produce side effects. Because of this, initiation of therapy requires titration to optimal dose and interval. The most important principle is to provide adequate pain relief. This requires determining whether the drug has adequately relieved the pain and the duration of the relief. *The most common error made by physicians in managing severe pain with opioids is to prescribe an inadequate dose. Since many patients are reluctant to complain, this practice leads to needless suffering.* In the absence of sedation at the expected time of peak effect, a physician should not hesitate to repeat the initial dose to achieve satisfactory pain relief.

An innovative approach to the problem of achieving adequate pain relief is the use of patient-controlled analgesia (PCA). PCA requires a device that delivers a baseline continuous dose of an opioid drug, and preprogrammed additional doses whenever the patient pushes a button. The device can be programmed to limit the total hourly dose so that overdosing is impossible. The patient can then titrate the dose to the optimal level. This approach is used most extensively for the management of postoperative pain, but there is no reason why it should not be used for any hospitalized patient with persistent severe pain. PCA is also used for short-term home care of patients with intractable pain, such as is caused by metastatic cancer.

Many physicians, nurses, and patients have a certain trepidation about using opioids that is based on an exaggerated fear of addiction. In fact, there is a vanishingly small chance of patients becoming addicted to narcotics as a result of their appropriate medical use.

The availability of new routes of administration has extended the usefulness of opioid analgesics. Most important is the availability of spinal administration. Opioids can be infused through a spinal catheter placed either intrathecally or epidurally. By applying opioids directly to the spinal cord, regional analgesia can be obtained using a relatively low total dose. In this way, such side effects as sedation, nausea, and respiratory depression can be minimized. This approach has been used extensively in obstetric procedures and for lower-body postoperative pain. Opioids can also be given intranasally (butorphanol), rectally, and transdermally (fentanyl), thus avoiding the discomfort of frequent injections in patients who cannot be given oral medication. The fentanyl transdermal patch has the advantage of providing fairly steady plasma levels, which maximizes patient comfort.

Opioid and Cyclooxygenase Inhibitor Combinations

When used in combination, opioids and COX inhibitors have additive effects. Because a lower dose of each can be used to achieve the same degree of pain relief and their side effects are nonadditive, such combinations can be used to lower the severity of dose-related side effects. Fixed-ratio combinations of an opioid with acetaminophen carry a special risk. Dose escalation as a result of increased severity of pain or decreased opioid effect as a result of tolerance may lead to levels of acetaminophen that are toxic to the liver.

CHRONIC PAIN

Managing patients with chronic pain is intellectually and emotionally challenging. The patient's problem is often difficult to diagnose; such patients are demanding of the physician's time and often appear emotionally distraught. The traditional medical approach of seeking an obscure organic pathology is usually unhelpful. On the other hand, psychological evaluation and behaviorally based treatment paradigms are frequently helpful, particularly in the setting of a multidisciplinary pain-management center.

There are several factors that can cause, perpetuate, or exacerbate chronic pain. First, of course, the patient may simply have a disease that is characteristically painful for which there is presently no cure. Arthritis, cancer, migraine headaches, fibromyalgia, and diabetic neuropathy are examples of this. Second, there may be secondary perpetuating factors that are initiated by disease and persist after that disease has resolved. Examples include damaged sensory nerves, sympathetic efferent activity, and painful reflex muscle contraction. Finally, a variety of psychological conditions can exacerbate or even cause pain.

There are certain areas to which special attention should be paid in the medical history. Because depression is the most common emotional disturbance in patients with chronic pain, patients should be questioned about their mood, appetite, sleep patterns, and daily activity. A simple standardized questionnaire, such as the Beck Depression Inventory, can be a useful screening device. It is important to remember that major depression is a common, treatable, and potentially fatal illness.

Other clues that a significant emotional disturbance is contributing to a patient's chronic pain complaint include: pain that occurs in multiple unrelated sites; a pattern of recurrent, but separate, pain problems beginning in childhood or adolescence; pain beginning at a time of emotional trauma, such as the loss of a parent or spouse; a history of physical or sexual abuse; and past or present substance abuse.

On examination, special attention should be paid to whether the patient guards the painful area and whether certain movements or postures are avoided because of pain. Discovering a mechanical component to the pain can be useful both diagnostically and therapeutically. Painful areas should be examined for deep tenderness, noting whether this is localized to muscle, ligamentous structures, or joints. Chronic myofascial pain is very common, and in these patients deep palpation may reveal highly localized trigger points that are firm bands or knots in muscle. Relief of the pain following injection of local anesthetic into these trigger points supports the diagnosis. A neuropathic component to the pain is indicated by evidence of nerve damage, such as sensory impairment, exquisitely sensitive skin, weakness and muscle atrophy, or loss of deep tendon reflexes. Evidence suggesting sympathetic nervous system involvement includes the presence of diffuse swelling, changes in skin color and temperature, and hypersensitive skin and joint tenderness compared with the normal side. Relief of the pain with a sympathetic block is diagnostic.

A guiding principle in evaluating patients with chronic pain is to assess both emotional and organic factors before initiating therapy. Addressing these issues together, rather than waiting to address emotional issues after organic causes of pain have been ruled out, improves compliance in part because it assures patients that a psychological evaluation does not mean that the physician is questioning the validity of their complaint. Even when an organic cause for a patient's pain can be found, it is still wise to look for other factors. For example, a cancer patient with painful bony metastases may have additional pain due to nerve damage and may also be depressed. Optimal therapy requires that each of these factors be looked for and treated.

TREATMENT FOR CHRONIC PAIN

Once the evaluation process has been completed and the likely causative and exacerbating factors identified, an explicit treatment plan should be developed. An important part of this process is to identify specific and realistic functional goals for therapy, such as getting a good night's sleep, being able to go shopping, or returning to work. A multidisciplinary approach that utilizes medications, counseling, physical therapy, nerve blocks, and even surgery may be required to improve the patient's quality of life. There are also some newer, relatively invasive procedures that can be helpful for some patients with intractable pain. These procedures include implanting intraspinal electrodes for spinal stimulation. Intrathecal administration of opiates, baclofen, or other medications may be useful in refractory conditions. Ziconotide, a novel agent that blocks N-type voltage-sensitive calcium channels, was recently approved for use in the United States. This compound is administered intrathecally and was found to be useful in a multicenter trial for patients with cancer or AIDS who had pain refractory to opiates. There are no set criteria for predicting which patients will respond to these procedures. They are generally reserved for patients who have not responded to conventional pharmacologic approaches. Referral to a multidisciplinary pain clinic for a full evaluation should precede any of these procedures. Such referrals are clearly not necessary for all chronic pain patients. For some, pharmacologic management alone can often provide adequate relief.

Antidepressant Medications

The tricyclic antidepressants (TCAs; Table 4–1) are extremely useful for the management of patients with chronic pain. Although developed for the treatment of depression, the tricyclics have a spectrum of dose-related biologic activities that include the production of analgesia in a variety of clinical conditions. Although the mechanism is unknown, the analgesic effect of TCAs has a more rapid onset and occurs at a lower dose than is typically required for the treatment of depression. Furthermore, patients with chronic pain who are not depressed obtain pain relief with antidepressants. There is evidence that tricyclic drugs potentiate opioid analgesia, so they are useful adjuncts for the treatment of severe persistent pain such as occurs with malignant tumors. **Table 4–2** lists some of the painful conditions that respond to tricyclics. TCAs are of particular value in the management of neuropathic pain such as occurs in diabetic neuropathy and postherpetic neuralgia, for which there are few other therapeutic options.

The TCAs that have been shown to relieve pain have significant side effects (Table 4–1; Chap. 41). Some of these side effects, such as orthostatic hypotension, cardiac conduction delay, memory impairment, constipation, and urinary retention, are particularly problematic in elderly patients, and several are additive to the side effects of opioid analgesics. The selective serotonin reuptake inhibitors such as fluoxetine (Prozac) have fewer and less serious side effects than TCAs, but they are much less effective for relieving pain. It is of interest that venlafaxine (Effexor), a nontricyclic antidepressant that blocks both serotonin and norepinephrine reuptake, appears to retain most of the pain-relieving effect of TCAs with a side-effect profile more like that of the selective serotonin reuptake inhibitors. The drug may be particularly useful in patients who cannot tolerate the side effects of tricyclics.

TABLE 4-2

PAINFUL CONDITIONS THAT RESPOND TO TRICYCLIC ANTIDEPRESSANTS

Postherpetic neuralgia[a]
Diabetic neuropathy[a]
Tension headache[a]
Migraine headache[a]
Rheumatoid arthritis[a, b]
Chronic low back pain[b]
Cancer
Central post-stroke pain

[a] Controlled trials demonstrate analgesia.
[b] Controlled studies indicate benefit but not analgesia.

Anticonvulsants and Antiarrhythmics
(Table 4-1)

These drugs are useful primarily for patients with neuropathic pain. Phenytoin (Dilantin) and carbamazepine (Tegretol) were first shown to relieve the pain of trigeminal neuralgia. This pain has a characteristic brief, shooting, electric shock—like quality. In fact, anticonvulsants seem to be helpful largely for pains that have such a lancinating quality. A new-generation anticonvulsant, gabapentin (Neurontin), is effective for a broad range of neuropathic pains.

Antiarrhythmic drugs such as low-dose lidocaine and mexiletine (Mexitil) can also be effective for neuropathic pain. These drugs block the spontaneous activity of damaged primary afferent nociceptors.

Chronic Opioid Medication

The long-term use of opioids is accepted for patients with pain due to malignant disease. Although opioid use for chronic pain of nonmalignant origin is controversial, it is clear that for many such patients opioid analgesics are the best available option. This is understandable since opioids are the most potent and have the broadest range of efficacy of any analgesic medications. Although addiction is rare in patients who first use opioids for pain relief, some degree of tolerance and physical dependence are likely with long-term use. Therefore, before embarking on opioid therapy, other options should be explored, and the limitations and risks of opioids should be explained to the patient. It is also important to point out that some opioid analgesic medications have mixed agonist-antagonist properties (e.g., pentazocine and butorphanol). From a practical standpoint, this means that they may worsen pain by inducing an abstinence syndrome in patients who are physically dependent on other opioid analgesics.

With long-term outpatient use of orally administered opioids, it is desirable to use long-acting compounds such as levorphanol, methadone, or sustained-release morphine (Table 4-1). Transdermal fentanyl is another excellent option. The pharmacokinetic profile of these drug preparations enables prolonged pain relief, minimizes side effects such as sedation that are associated with high peak plasma levels, and reduces the likelihood of rebound pain associated with a rapid fall in plasma opioid concentration. Constipation is a virtually universal side effect of opioid use and should be treated expectantly. For some patients with neuropathic pain, the combination of gabapentin plus sustained-relief morphine may be more effective than either drug alone.

It is worth emphasizing that many patients, especially those with chronic pain, seek medical attention primarily because they are suffering and because only physicians can provide the medications required for their relief. A primary responsibility of all physicians is to minimize the physical and emotional discomfort of their patients. Familiarity with pain mechanisms and analgesic medications is an important step toward accomplishing this aim.

Adjuncts to Pain Management

Other nonpharmacologic methods may be useful for patients with refractory chronic pain. These can include acupuncture, biofeedback, and transcutaneous electrical nerve stimulation (TENS) devices. Randomized trials are needed in order to evaluate to efficacy of these approaches as adjuncts to current chronic pain management.

FURTHER READINGS

BRESALIER RS et al: Cardiovascular events associated with rofecoxib in a colorectal adenoma chemoprevention trial. N Engl J Med 352:1092, 2005

☑ CHEN H: Contemporary management of neuropathic pain for the primary care physician. Mayo Clin Proc 79:1533, 2004

A review of multiple pharmacologic and nonpharmacologic approaches to the management of neuropathic pain.

CRAIG AD: How do you feel? Interoception: The sense of the physiological condition of the body. Nat Rev Neurosci 8:655, 2002

☑ GILRON I et al: Morphine, gabapentin, or their combination for neuropathic pain. N Engl J Med 352:1324, 2005

Randomized double-blind trial showing that a combination of low doses of morphine and gabapentin is more effective than either alone as a single agent.

HARDEN RN: Chronic neuropathic pain: Mechanisms, diagnosis and treatment. Neurologist 11:111, 2005

PETROVIC P et al: Placebo and opioid analgesia—imaging a shared neuronal network. Science 5560:1737, 2002

STAATS PS: Intrathecal ziconotide in the treatment of refractory pain in patients with cancer or AIDS. JAMA 291:63, 2004

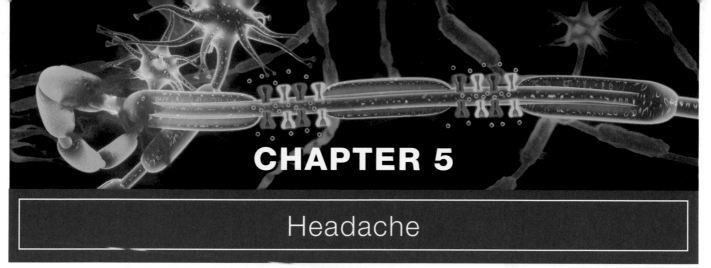

CHAPTER 5

Headache

Neil H. Raskin

Few of us are spared the experience of head pain. As many as 90% of individuals have at least one headache per year. Severe, disabling headache is reported to occur at least annually by 40% of individuals worldwide. A useful classification of the many causes of headache is shown in **Table 5-1**. Headache is usually a benign symptom, but occasionally it is the manifestation of a serious illness such as brain tumor, subarachnoid hemorrhage, meningitis, or giant cell arteritis. In emergency settings, approximately 5% of patients with headache are found to have a serious underlying neurologic disorder. Therefore, it is imperative that the serious causes of headache be diagnosed rapidly and accurately.

PAIN-SENSITIVE STRUCTURES OF THE HEAD

Pain usually occurs when peripheral nociceptors are stimulated in response to tissue injury, visceral distention, or other factors (Chap. 4). In such situations, pain perception is a normal physiologic response mediated by a healthy nervous system. Pain can also result when pain-sensitive pathways of the peripheral or central nervous system are damaged or activated inappropriately. Headache may originate from either or both mechanisms. Relatively few cranial structures are pain-sensitive: the scalp, middle meningeal artery, dural sinuses, falx cerebri, and the proximal segments of the large pial arteries. The ventricular ependyma, choroid plexus, pial veins, and much of the brain parenchyma are pain-insensitive. Electrical stimulation of the midbrain in the region of the dorsal raphe has resulted in migraine-like headaches. Thus, whereas most of the brain is insensitive to electrode probing, a site in the midbrain represents a possible source of headache generation. Sensory stimuli from the head are conveyed to the central nervous system via the trigeminal nerves for structures above the tentorium in the anterior and middle fossae of the skull, and via the first three cervical nerves for those in the posterior fossa and the inferior surface of the tentorium.

Headache can occur as the result of (1) distention, traction, or dilation of intracranial or extracranial arteries; (2) traction or displacement of large intracranial veins or their dural envelope; (3) compression, traction, or inflammation of cranial and spinal nerves; (4) spasm, inflammation, or trauma to cranial and cervical muscles; (5) meningeal irritation and raised intracranial pressure; or (6) other possible mechanisms such as activation of brainstem structures.

GENERAL CLINICAL CONSIDERATIONS

The quality, location, duration, and time course of the headache and the conditions that produce, exacerbate, or relieve it should be carefully reviewed. Ascertaining the *quality* of cephalic pain is occasionally helpful for diagnosis. Most tension-type headaches are described as tight "bandlike" pain or as dull, deeply located, and aching pain. Jabbing, brief, sharp cephalic pain, often occurring multifocally (ice pick–like pain), is usually benign. A throbbing quality and tight muscles about the head,

TABLE 5-1

INTERNATIONAL HEADACHE SOCIETY CLASSIFICATION OF HEADACHE

1. **Migraine**
   Migraine without aura
   Migraine with aura
   Retinal migraine
   Complications of migraine
   Childhood periodic syndromes that may be precursors to or associated with migraine
   Migraine-triggered seizure
2. **Tension-type headache**
   Episodic tension-type headache
   Chronic tension-type headache
3. **Cluster headache and trigeminal autonomic cephalgias**
   Cluster headache
   Chronic paroxysmal hemicrania
   Short-lasting unilateral neuralgiform headache attacks with conjunctival injection and tearing (SUNCT)
4. **Other primary headaches**
   Primary stabbing headache
   Primary cough headache
   Primary exertional headache
   Primary headache associated with sexual activity
   Hypnic headache (sleep associated)
   Primary thunderclap headache
   Hemicrania continua
   New daily-persistent headache (NDPH)
5. **Headache associated with head and/or neck trauma**
   Acute posttraumatic headache
   Chronic posttraumatic headache
   Acute headache attributed to whiplash injury
   Chronic headache attributed to whiplash injury
   Headache attributed to traumatic intracranial hematoma
   Headache attributed to other head and/or neck trauma
   Post-craniotomy headache
6. **Headache attributed to cranial or cervical vascular disorder**
   Acute ischemic stroke or transient ischemic attack
   Nontraumatic intracranial hematoma
   Unruptured vascular malformation
   Arteritis
   Carotid or vertebral artery pain
   Venous thrombosis
   Other vascular disorder
7. **Headache associated with nonvascular intracranial disorder**
   High CSF pressure
   Low CSF pressure
   Noninfectious inflammatory disease
   Related to intrathecal injections
   Intracranial neoplasm
   Epileptic seizure
   Chiari I malformation
   Syndrome of transient headache and neurologic deficits with CSF lymphocytosis (HaNDL)
   Associated with other nonvascular intracranial disorder
8. **Headache associated with substances or their withdrawal**
   Headache induced by acute substance use or exposure
   Medication-overuse headache (MOH)
   Attributed to chronic medication
   Headache from substance withdrawal
9. **Headache attributed to infection**
   Intracranial infection
   Systemic infection
   HIV/AIDS
   Chronic postinfection headache
10. **Headache attributed to disorder of homeostasis**
    Hypoxia and/or hypercapnia
    Arterial hypertension
    Hypothyroidism
    Fasting
    Cardiac
    Other metabolic abnormality
11. **Headache or facial pain attributed to disorder of cranium, neck, eyes, ears, nose, sinuses, teeth, mouth, or other facial or cranial structures**
    Cranial bone
    Neck
    Eyes
    Ears
    Rhinosinusitis
    Teeth, jaws, and related structures
    Temporomandibular joint disease
12. **Headache attributed to psychiatric disorder**
    Somatisation
    Psychotic disorder
13. **Cranial neuralgias and central causes of face pain**
    Trigeminal neuralgia
    Glossopharyngeal neuralgia
    Nervus intermedius neuralgia
    Superior laryngeal neuralgia
    Nasociliary neuralgia
    Supraorbital neuralgia
    Other terminal branch neuralgia
    Occipital neuralgia
    Neck-tongue syndrome
    External compression
    Cold-stimulus
    Constant pain caused by compression, irritation, or distortion of cranial nerves or upper cervical roots by structural lesions
    Optic neuritis
    Ocular diabetic neuropathy
    Herpes zoster
    Tolosa-Hunt
    Ophthalmoplegic "migraine"
    Central causes of face pain
    Other cranial neuralgia or other centrally mediated facial pain
14. **Other headache, cranial neuralgia, central or primary facial pain**
    Headache not elsewhere classified
    Headache unspecified

Note: CSF, cerebrospinal fluid.
Source: Cephalalgia 24 (Suppl 1):9, 2004. Reprinted by permission of Blackwell Publishing.

neck, and shoulder girdle are common nonspecific accompaniments of migraine headaches.

Pain *intensity* rarely has diagnostic value, although from the patient's perspective, it is the single aspect of pain that is most important. Although meningitis, subarachnoid hemorrhage, and cluster headache produce intense cranial pain, most patients entering emergency departments with the most severe headache of their lives usually have migraine. Contrary to common belief, the headache produced by a brain tumor is not usually distinctive or severe.

Data regarding *location* of headache may be informative. If the source is an extracranial structure, as in giant cell arteritis, the correspondence with the site of pain is fairly precise. Inflammation of an extracranial artery causes pain and exquisite tenderness localized to the site of the vessel. Lesions of paranasal sinuses, teeth, eyes, and upper cervical vertebrae induce less sharply localized pain, but pain that is still referred in a regional distribution. Intracranial lesions in the posterior fossa cause pain that is usually occipitonuchal, and supratentorial lesions most often induce frontotemporal pain.

Duration and *time-intensity* curves of headaches are diagnostically useful. A ruptured aneurysm results in head pain that peaks in an instant, thunderclap-like; much less often, unruptured aneurysms may signal their presence in the same way. Cluster headache attacks reach their peak over 3 to 5 min, remain at maximal levels for about 45 min, and then taper off. Migraine attacks build up over hours, are maintained for several hours to days, and are characteristically relieved by sleep. Sleep disruption and early morning headaches that improve during the day are characteristics of headaches produced by brain tumors or other disorders that produce increased intracranial pressure.

Facial pain must be distinguished from headache. Trigeminal and, less commonly, glossopharyngeal neuralgia are frequent causes of facial pain (Chap. 23). *Neuralgias* are painful disorders characterized by paroxysmal, fleeting, often electric shock–like episodes that are frequently caused by demyelinating lesions of nerves (the trigeminal or glossopharyngeal nerves in cranial neuralgias). Certain maneuvers characteristically trigger paroxysms of pain. However, the most common cause of facial pain by far is dental; provocation by hot, cold, or sweet foods is typical. The application of a cold stimulus will repeatedly induce dental pain, whereas in neuralgic disorders, a refractory period usually occurs after the initial response so that pain cannot be repeatedly induced.

The effect of eating on facial pain may provide insight into its cause. Is it the chewing, swallowing, or taste of the food that elicits pain? Chewing suggests trigeminal neuralgia, temporomandibular joint dysfunction, or giant cell arteritis ("jaw claudication"), whereas swallowing *and* taste provocation suggest glossopharyngeal neuralgia. Pain with swallowing is common in patients with caroti-

dynia (see below) because the inflamed, tender carotid artery abuts the esophagus during deglutition.

Many patients with facial pain do not experience stereotypic neuralgias; the term *atypical facial pain* has been used in this setting. Vague, poorly localized, continuous facial pain is characteristic of nasopharyngeal carcinoma; a burning pain often develops as deafferentation occurs and evidence of cranial neuropathy appears. Burning facial pain may also occur with tumors of the fifth cranial nerve (meningioma or schwannoma) or with lesions of the pons that interrupt the dorsal root entry zone of the nerve (multiple sclerosis). In patients with facial pain, the finding of objective sensory loss is an important clue to a serious underlying disorder. Occasionally, the cause of a pain problem cannot be resolved promptly, necessitating periodic follow-up until further signs appear.

CLINICAL EVALUATION OF ACUTE, NEW-ONSET HEADACHE

Patients who present with their first severe headache raise entirely different diagnostic possibilities than those with recurrent headaches over many years. In new-onset and severe headaches, the probability of finding a potentially serious cause is considerably greater than in recurrent headache. When a patient complains of an acute, new-onset headache, a number of causes should be considered including meningitis, subarachnoid hemorrhage, epidural or subdural hematoma, glaucoma, and purulent sinusitis. Clinical features of acute, new-onset headache caused by serious underlying conditions are summarized in **Table 5-2**.

A complete neurologic examination is an essential first step in the evaluation. In most cases, an abnormal examination should be followed by a computed tomography (CT) or a magnetic resonance imaging (MRI) study. As a screening procedure for intracranial pathology in this setting, CT and MRI methods appear to be equally sensitive. A general evaluation of acute headache might include the investigation of cardiovascular and renal status by blood

TABLE 5-2

HEADACHE SYMPTOMS THAT SUGGEST A SERIOUS UNDERLYING DISORDER

"Worst" headache ever
First severe headache
Subacute worsening over days or weeks
Abnormal neurologic examination
Fever or unexplained systemic signs
Vomiting precedes headache
Induced by bending, lifting, cough
Disturbs sleep or presents immediately upon awakening
Known systemic illness
Onset after age 55

pressure monitoring and urine examination; eyes by fundoscopy, intraocular pressure measurement, and refraction; cranial arteries by palpation; and cervical spine by the effect of passive movement of the head and imaging.

The psychological state of the patient should also be evaluated since a relationship exists between head pain and depression. Many patients in chronic daily pain cycles become depressed; moreover, there is a greater-than-chance coincidence of migraine with both bipolar (manic-depressive) and unipolar major depressive disorders. Drugs with antidepressant actions are also effective in the prophylactic treatment of both tension-type headache and migraine.

Underlying recurrent headache disorders may be activated by pain that follows otologic or endodontic surgical procedures. Thus, pain about the head as the result of diseased tissue or trauma may reawaken an otherwise quiescent migrainous syndrome. Treatment of the headache is largely ineffective until the cause of the primary problem is addressed.

Serious underlying conditions that are associated with headache are described below and in **Table 5–3**.

MENINGITIS

In general, acute, severe headache with stiff neck and fever suggests meningitis. Lumbar puncture is mandatory.

Often there is striking accentuation of pain with eye movement. Meningitis is particularly easy to mistake for migraine in that the cardinal symptoms of pounding headache, photophobia, nausea, and vomiting are present. A detailed discussion of meningitis can be found in Chaps. 29 and 30.

INTRACRANIAL HEMORRHAGE

In general, acute, severe headache with stiff neck but without fever suggests subarachnoid hemorrhage. A ruptured aneurysm, arteriovenous malformation, or intraparenchymal hemorrhage may also present with headache alone. Rarely, if the hemorrhage is small or below the foramen magnum, the head CT scan can be normal. Therefore, a lumbar puncture may be required to make the definitive diagnosis of a subarachnoid hemorrhage. A detailed discussion of intracranial hemorrhage can be found in Chap. 17.

BRAIN TUMOR

Approximately 30% of patients with brain tumors consider headache to be their chief complaint. The head pain is usually nondescript—an intermittent deep, dull aching of moderate intensity, which may worsen with

TABLE 5-3

SYMPTOMS OF SERIOUS UNDERLYING CAUSES OF HEADACHE	
CAUSE	**SYMPTOMS**
Meningitis	Nuchal rigidity, headache, photophobia, and prostration; may not be febrile. Lumbar puncture is diagnostic.
Intracranial hemorrhage	Nuchal rigidity and headache; may not have clouded consciousness or seizures. Hemorrhage may not be seen on CT scan. Lumbar puncture shows "bloody tap" that does not clear by the last tube. A fresh hemorrhage may not be xanthochromic.
Brain tumor	May present with prostrating pounding headaches that are associated with nausea and vomiting. Should be suspected in progressively severe new "migraine" that is invariably unilateral.
Temporal arteritis	May present with a unilateral pounding headache. Onset generally in older patients (>50 years) and frequently associated with visual changes. The erythrocyte sedimentation rate is the best screening test and is usually markedly elevated (i.e., >50). Definitive diagnosis can be made by arterial biopsy.
Glaucoma	Usually consists of severe eye pain. May have nausea and vomiting. The eye is usually painful and red. The pupil may be partially dilated.

Note: CT, computed tomography.

exertion or change in position and may be associated with nausea and vomiting. This pattern of symptoms results from migraine far more often than from brain tumor. Headache of brain tumor disturbs sleep in about 10% of patients. Vomiting that precedes the appearance of headache by weeks is highly characteristic of posterior fossa brain tumors. A history of amenorrhea or galactorrhea should lead one to question whether a prolactin-secreting pituitary adenoma (or the polycystic ovary syndrome) is the source of headache. Headache arising de novo in a patient with known malignancy suggests either cerebral metastases and/or carcinomatous meningitis. Head pain appearing abruptly after bending, lifting, or coughing can be due to a posterior fossa mass (or a Chiari malformation). A detailed discussion of brain tumors can be found in Chap. 25.

TEMPORAL ARTERITIS

Temporal (giant cell) arteritis is an inflammatory disorder of arteries that frequently involves the extracranial carotid circulation. This is a common disorder of the elderly; its annual incidence is 77:100,000 in individuals aged 50 and older. The average age of onset is 70 years, and women account for 65% of cases. About half of patients with untreated temporal arteritis develop blindness due to involvement of the ophthalmic artery and its branches; indeed, the ischemic optic neuropathy induced by giant cell arteritis is the major cause of rapidly developing bilateral blindness in patients >60 years. Because treatment with glucocorticoids is effective in preventing this complication, prompt recognition of this disorder is important.

Typical presenting symptoms include headache, polymyalgia rheumatica, jaw claudication, fever, and weight loss. Headache is the dominant symptom and often appears in association with malaise and muscle aches. Head pain may be unilateral or bilateral and is located temporally in 50% of patients but may involve any and all aspects of the cranium. Pain usually appears gradually over a few hours before peak intensity is reached; occasionally, it is explosive in onset. The quality of pain is only seldom throbbing; it is almost invariably described as dull and boring with superimposed episodic ice pick–like lancinating pains similar to the sharp pains that appear in migraine. Most patients can recognize that the origin of their head pain is superficial, external to the skull, rather than originating deep within the cranium (the pain site for migraineurs). Scalp tenderness is present, often to a marked degree; brushing the hair or resting the head on a pillow may be impossible because of pain. Headache is usually worse at night and is often aggravated by exposure to cold. Reddened, tender nodules or red streaking of the skin overlying the temporal arteries may be found in patients with headache, as is tenderness of the temporal or, less commonly, the occipital arteries.

The erythrocyte sedimentation rate (ESR) is often, though not always, elevated; a normal ESR does not exclude giant cell arteritis. A temporal artery biopsy and treatment with prednisone at 80 mg daily for the first 4 to 6 weeks should be initiated when clinical suspicion is high. The prevalence of migraine among the elderly is substantial, considerably higher than that of giant cell arteritis. Migraineurs often report amelioration of their headaches with prednisone, so that one must be cautious about interpreting the therapeutic response.

GLAUCOMA

Glaucoma may present with a prostrating headache associated with nausea and vomiting. The history will usually reveal that the headache started with severe eye pain. On physical examination, the eye is often red with a fixed, moderately dilated pupil. A discussion of glaucoma can be found in Chap. 11.

OTHER CAUSES OF HEADACHE
Systemic Illness

There is hardly any illness that is never manifested by headache; however, some illnesses are frequently associated with headache. These include infectious mononucleosis, systemic lupus erythematosus, chronic pulmonary failure with hypercapnia (early morning headaches), Hashimoto's thyroiditis, inflammatory bowel disease, many of the illnesses associated with HIV, and the acute blood pressure elevations that occur in pheochromocytoma and in malignant hypertension. The last two examples are the exceptions to the generalization that hypertension per se is a very uncommon cause of headache; diastolic pressures of at least 120 mmHg are requisite for hypertension to cause headache. Persistent headache and fever are often the manifestations of an acute systemic viral infection; if the neck is supple in such a patient, lumbar puncture may be deferred. Some drugs and drug-withdrawal states, e.g., oral contraceptives, ovulation-promoting medications, and glucocorticoid withdrawal, are also associated with headache in some individuals.

Idiopathic Intracranial Hypertension (Pseudotumor Cerebri)

Headache, clinically resembling that of brain tumor, is a common presenting symptom of pseudotumor cerebri, a disorder of raised intracranial pressure probably resulting from impaired cerebrospinal fluid (CSF) absorption by the arachnoid villi. Morning headaches that are worsened by coughing and straining are typical. The pain is sometimes retroocular and worsened by eye movements. Transient visual obscurations and papilledema with enlarged blind spots and loss of peripheral visual fields are additional manifestations. Most patients are young, female, and obese. They often have a history of exposure to provoking agents such as vitamin A and glucocorticoids. Treatment of idiopathic intracranial hypertension is discussed in Chap. 11.

Cough

A male-dominated (4:1) syndrome, cough headache is characterized by transient, severe head pain upon coughing, bending, lifting, sneezing, or stooping. Head pain persists for seconds to a few minutes. Many patients date the origins of the syndrome to a lower respiratory infection accompanied by severe coughing or to strenuous weight-lifting programs. Headache is usually diffuse but is lateralized in about one-third of patients. The incidence of serious intracranial structural anomalies causing this condition is about 25%; the Chiari malformation (Chap. 24) is a common cause. Thus, MRI is indicated for most patients with cough headache. The benign disorder may persist for a few years; it responds dramatically to indomethacin at doses ranging from 50 to 200 mg daily. Approximately half of patients will also show a response to therapeutic lumbar puncture with removal of 40 mL of CSF.

Many patients with migraine note that attacks of headache may be provoked by *sustained* physical exertion, such as during the third mile of a 5-mile run. Such headaches build up over hours, in contrast to cough headache. The term *effort migraine* has been used for this syndrome to avoid the ambiguous term *exertional headache*.

Lumbar Puncture

Headache following lumbar puncture usually begins within 48 h but may be delayed for up to 12 days. Its incidence is between 10 and 30%. Head pain is dramatically positional; it begins when the patient sits or stands upright; there is relief upon reclining or with abdominal compression. The longer the patient is upright, the longer the latency before head pain subsides. It is worsened by head shaking and jugular vein compression. The pain is usually a dull ache but may be throbbing; its location is occipitofrontal. Nausea and stiff neck often accompany headache, and occasional patients report blurred vision, photophobia, tinnitus, and vertigo. The symptoms resolve over a few days but may on occasion persist for weeks to months.

Loss of CSF volume decreases the brain's supportive cushion, so that when a patient is upright there is probably dilation and tension placed on the brain's anchoring structures, the pain-sensitive dural sinuses, resulting in pain. Intracranial hypotension often occurs, but severe lumbar puncture headache may be present even in patients who have normal CSF pressure.

Treatment with intravenous caffeine sodium benzoate given over a few minutes as a 500-mg dose will promptly terminate headache in 75% of patients; a second dose given in 1 h brings the total success rate to 85%. An epidural blood patch accomplished by injection of 15 mL of autologous whole blood rarely fails for those who do not respond to caffeine. The mechanism for these treatment effects is not straightforward. The blood patch has an *immediate* effect, making it unlikely that sealing off a dural hole with blood clot is its mechanism of action.

Postconcussion

Following seemingly trivial head injuries and particularly after rear-end motor vehicle collisions, many patients report varying combinations of headache, dizziness, vertigo, and impaired memory. Anxiety, irritability, and difficulty with concentration are other hallmarks of this syndrome. Symptoms may remit after several weeks or persist for months and even years after the injury. Postconcussion headaches may occur whether or not a person was rendered unconscious by head trauma. Typically, the neurologic examination is normal with the exception of the behavioral abnormalities, and CT or MRI studies are unrevealing. Chronic subdural hematoma may on occasion mimic this disorder. Although the cause of postconcussive headache disorder is not known, it should not in general be viewed as a primary psychological disturbance. It often persists long after the settlement of pending lawsuits. The treatment is symptomatic support. Repeated encouragement that the syndrome eventually remits is important.

Coital Headache

This is another male-dominated (4:1) syndrome. Attacks occur periorgasmically, are very abrupt in onset, and subside in a few minutes if coitus is interrupted. These are nearly always benign events and usually occur sporadically; if they persist for hours or are accompanied by vomiting, subarachnoid hemorrhage must be excluded (Chap. 17).

PRINCIPAL CLINICAL VARIETIES OF RECURRENT HEADACHE

There is usually little difficulty in diagnosing the serious types of headaches listed above because of the clues provided by the associated symptoms and signs. It is when headache is chronic, recurrent, and unattended by other important signs of disease that the physician faces a challenging and unique medical problem. The following sections describe a variety of headache types, ranging from the most common (e.g., migraine) to rare causes of recurrent headache.

TENSION-TYPE HEADACHE

The term *tension-type headache* is still commonly used to describe a chronic head pain syndrome characterized by bilateral tight, bandlike discomfort. Patients may report that the head feels as if it is in a vise or that the posterior neck muscles are tight. The pain typically builds slowly, fluctuates in severity, and may persist more or less continuously for many days. Exertion does not usually worsen the headache. The headache may be episodic or chronic (i.e., present >15 days per month). Tension-type headache is common in all age groups, and females tend to predominate. In some patients, anxiety or depression coexist with tension headache.

The pathophysiologic basis of tension-type headache remains unknown. Many investigators believe that periodic tension headache is biologically indistinguishable from migraine, whereas others believe that tension-type headache and migraine are two distinct clinical entities.

Abnormalities of cervical and temporal muscle contraction are likely to exist, but the exact nature of the dysfunction has not yet been elucidated.

Relaxation almost always relieves tension-type headaches. Patients should be encouraged to find a means of relaxation, which, for a given individual, could include bed rest, massage, and/or formal biofeedback training. Pharmacologic treatment consists of either simple analgesics and/or muscle relaxants. Ibuprofen and naproxen sodium are useful treatments for most individuals. When simple over-the-counter analgesics such as acetaminophen, aspirin, ibuprofen, and/or other nonsteroidal anti-inflammatory drugs (NSAIDs) alone fail, the addition of butalbital and caffeine (in a combination compound such as Fiorinal, Fioricet) to these analgesics may be effective. A list of commonly used analgesics for tension-type headaches is presented in **Table 5-4**. For chronic tension-type headache, prophylactic therapy is recommended. Low doses of amitriptyline (10 to 50 mg at bedtime) can provide effective prophylaxis.

MIGRAINE

Migraine, the most common cause of headache, afflicts approximately 15% of women and 6% of men. A useful definition of migraine is a benign and recurring syndrome of headache, nausea, vomiting, and/or other

TABLE 5-4

DRUGS EFFECTIVE IN THE TREATMENT OF TENSION-TYPE HEADACHE		
DRUG	**TRADE NAME**	**DOSAGE**
NONSTEROIDAL ANTI-INFLAMMATORY AGENTS		
Acetaminophen	Tylenol, generic	650 mg PO q4–6h
Aspirin	Generic	650 mg PO q4–6h
Diclofenac	Cataflam, generic	50–100 mg q4–6h (max 200 mg/d)
Ibuprofen	Advil, Motrin, Nuprin, generic	400 mg PO q3–4h
Naproxen sodium	Aleve, Anaprox, generic	220–550 mg bid
COMBINATION ANALGESICS		
Acetaminophen, 325 mg, *plus* butalbital, 50 mg	Phrenilin, generic	1–2 tablets; max 6 per day
Acetaminophen, 650 mg, *plus* butalbital, 50 mg	Phrenilin Forte	1 tablet; max 6 per day
Acetaminophen, 325 mg, *plus* butalbital, 50 mg, *plus* caffeine, 40 mg	Fioricet; Esgic, generic	1–2 tablets; max 6 per day
Acetaminophen, 500 mg, *plus* butalbital, 50 mg, *plus* caffeine, 40 mg	Esgic-plus	1–2 tablets; max 6 per day
Aspirin, 325 mg, *plus* butalbital, 50 mg, *plus* caffeine, 40 mg	Fiorinal	1–2 tablets; max 6 per day
Aspirin, 650 mg, *plus* butalbital, 50 mg	Axotal	1 tablet q4h; max 6 per day
PROPHYLACTIC MEDICATIONS		
Amitriptyline	Elavil, generic	10–50 mg at bedtime
Doxepin	Sinequan, generic	10–75 mg at bedtime
Nortriptyline	Pamelor, generic	25–75 mg at bedtime

TABLE 5-5

SYMPTOMS ACCOMPANYING SEVERE MIGRAINE ATTACKS IN 500 PATIENTS

SYMPTOM	PATIENTS AFFECTED, %
Nausea	87
Photophobia	82
Lightheadedness	72
Scalp tenderness	65
Vomiting	56
Visual disturbances	36
Photopsia	26
Fortification spectra	10
Paresthesias	33
Vertigo	33
Alteration of consciousness	18
Syncope	10
Seizure	4
Confusional state	4
Diarrhea	16

Source: From NH Raskin, *Headache,* 2d ed. New York, Churchill Livingston, 1998; with permission.

symptoms of neurologic dysfunction in varying admixtures (**Table 5-5**). Migraine can often be recognized by its activators (red wine, menses, hunger, lack of sleep, glare, estrogen, worry, perfumes, let-down periods) and its deactivators (sleep, pregnancy, exhilaration, triptans). A classification of the many subtypes of migraine, as defined by the International Headache Society, is shown in Table 5-1.

Severe headache attacks, regardless of cause, are more likely to be described as throbbing and associated with vomiting and scalp tenderness. Milder headaches tend to be nondescript—tight, bandlike discomfort often involving the entire head—the profile of tension-type headache.

Pathogenesis

Genetic Basis of Migraine   Migraine has a definite genetic predisposition. Specific mutations leading to *rare* causes of vascular headache have been identified (**Table 5-6**). For example, the MELAS syndrome consists of a *m*itochondrial *e*ncephalomyopathy, *l*actic *a*cidosis, and *s*troke-like episodes and is caused by an A → G point mutation in the mitochondrial gene encoding for tRNA$^{Leu(UUR)}$ at nucleotide position 3243. Episodic migraine-like headaches are another common clinical feature of this syndrome, especially early in the course of the disease. The genetic pattern of mitochondrial disorders is unique, since only mothers transmit mitochondrial DNA. Thus, all children of mothers with MELAS syndrome are affected with the disorder.

Familial hemiplegic migraine (FHM) is characterized by episodes of recurrent hemiparesis or hemiplegia during the aura phase of a migraine headache. Other associated symptoms may include hemianesthesia or paresthesias; hemianopic visual field disturbances; dysphasia; and variable degrees of drowsiness, confusion, and/or coma. In severe attacks, these symptoms can be quite prolonged and persist for days or weeks, but characteristically they last for only 30 to 60 min and are followed by a unilateral throbbing headache.

Approximately 50% of cases of FHM appear to be caused by mutations within the CACNL1A4 gene on chromosome 19, which encodes a P/Q type calcium channel subunit expressed only in the central nervous system. The gene is very large (>300 kb in length) and consists of 47 exons. Four distinct point mutations have been identified within the gene (in five different families) that cosegregate with the clinical diagnosis of FHM. Analysis of haplotypes in the two families with the same mutation suggest that each mutation arose independently rather than representing a founder effect. CACNL1A4 is likely to play a role in calcium-induced

TABLE 5-6

MIGRAINE GENETICS

GENE (LOCUS)	FUNCTION OF GENE	CLINICAL SYNDROME	COMMENT
tRNA$^{Leu(UUR)}$ (mitochondrial)	Unknown	MELAS syndrome	Extremely rare syndrome
CACNL1A4 (19p13)	P/Q calcium channel regulating neurotransmitter release	Familial hemiplegic migraine (FHM)	Mutations account for ~50% of FHM cases
DRD2 (11q23)	G protein–coupled D$_2$ receptor for dopamine	Migraine	Positive association reported in two independent laboratories
Notch3	Unknown	Cerebral autosomal dominant arteriopathy with subcortical infarcts and leukoencephalopathy (CADASIL)	

Note: MELAS, mitochondrial encephalomyopathy, lactic acidosis, and stroke-like episodes.

neurotransmitter release and/or contraction of smooth muscle. Different mutations within this gene are the cause of two other neurogenetic disorders, spinocerebellar ataxia type 6 and episodic ataxia type 2 (Chap. 20).

In a genetic association study, a *Nco*I polymorphism in the gene encoding the D_2 dopamine receptor (DRD2) was overrepresented in a population of patients with migraine with aura compared to a control group of nonmigraineurs, suggesting that susceptibility to migraine with aura is modified by certain DRD2 alleles. In a Sardinian population, an association between different DRD2 alleles and migraine has also been demonstrated. These initial studies suggest that variations in dopamine receptor regulation and/or function may alter susceptibility to migraine since molecular variations within the DRD2 gene have been associated with variations in dopaminergic function. However, since not all individuals with the implicated DRD2 genotypes suffer from migraine with aura, additional genes or factors must also be involved. Migraine is likely to be a complex disorder with polygenic inheritance and a strong environmental component.

The Vascular Theory of Migraine It was widely held for many years that the headache phase of migrainous attacks was caused by extracranial vasodilatation and that the neurologic symptoms were produced by intracranial vasoconstriction (i.e., the "vascular" hypothesis of migraine). Regional cerebral blood flow studies have shown that in patients with classic migraine there is, during attacks, a modest cortical hypoperfusion that begins in the visual cortex and spreads forward at a rate of 2 to 3 mm/min. The decrease in blood flow averages 25 to 30% (insufficient to explain symptoms on the basis of ischemia) and progresses anteriorly in a wavelike fashion independent of the topography of cerebral arteries. The wave of hypoperfusion persists for 4 to 6 h, appears to follow the convolutions of the cortex, and does not cross the central or lateral sulcus, progressing to the frontal lobe via the insula. Perfusion of subcortical structures is normal. Contralateral neurologic symptoms appear during temporoparietal hypoperfusion; at times, hypoperfusion persists in these regions after symptoms cease. More often, frontal spread continues as the headache phase begins. A few patients with classic migraine show no flow abnormalities; an occasional patient has developed focal ischemia sufficient to cause symptoms. However, focal ischemia does not appear to be *necessary* for focal symptoms to occur.

The ability of these changes to induce the symptoms of migraine has been questioned. Specifically, the decrease in blood flow that is observed does not appear to be significant enough to cause focal neurologic symptoms. Second, the increase in blood flow per se is not painful, and vasodilatation alone cannot account for the

local edema and focal tenderness often observed in migraineurs. Moreover, in migraine without aura, no flow abnormalities are usually seen. Thus, it is unlikely that simple vasoconstriction and vasodilatation are the fundamental pathophysiologic abnormalities in migraine. However, it is clear that cerebral blood flow is altered during certain migraine attacks, and these changes may explain some, but clearly not all, of the clinical syndrome of migraine.

The Neuronal Theory of Migraine *Fortification spectrum* is a migraine aura characterized by a slowly enlarging visual scotoma with luminous edges (see below). It is believed to result from *spreading depression,* a slowly moving (2 to 3 mm/min), potassium-liberating depression of cortical activity, preceded by a wavefront of increased metabolic activity. Spreading depression can be produced by a variety of experimental stimuli, including hypoxia, mechanical trauma, and the topical application of potassium. These observations suggest that neuronal abnormalities could be the cause of a migraine attack.

Physiologically, electrical stimulation near dorsal raphe neurons in the upper brainstem can result in migraine-like headaches. Blood flow in the pons and midbrain increases focally during migraine headache episodes; this alteration probably results from increased activity of cells in the dorsal raphe and locus coeruleus. There are projections from the dorsal raphe that terminate on cerebral arteries and alter cerebral blood flow. There are also major projections from the dorsal raphe to important visual centers, including the lateral geniculate body, superior colliculus, retina, and visual cortex. These various serotonergic projections may represent the neural substrate for the circulatory and visual characteristics of migraine. The dorsal raphe cells stop firing during deep sleep, and sleep is known to ameliorate migraine; the antimigraine prophylactic drugs also inhibit activity of the dorsal raphe cells through a direct or indirect agonist effect.

Positron emission tomography (PET) scan studies have demonstrated that midbrain structures near the dorsal raphe are activated during a migraine attack. In one study of acute migraine, an injection of sumatriptan relieved the headache but did not alter the brainstem changes noted on the PET scan. These data suggest that a "brainstem generator" may be the cause of migraine and that certain antimigraine medications may not interfere with the underlying pathologic process in migraine.

The Trigeminovascular System in Migraine Activation of cells in the trigeminal nucleus caudalis in the medulla (a pain-processing center for the head and face region) results in the release of vasoactive neuropeptides, including substance P and calcitonin gene–related peptide, at vascular terminations of the trigeminal nerve. These peptide neurotransmitters have been proposed to induce a sterile inflammation that activates trigeminal nociceptive afferents originating on the vessel wall, further contributing to the production of pain. This provides a potential mechanism for the soft tissue swelling and tenderness of blood vessels that accompany migraine attacks. However, numerous pharmacologic agents that are effective in preventing or reducing inflammation in this animal model (e.g., selective $5HT_{1D}$ agonists, NK-1 antagonists, endothelin antagonists) have failed to demonstrate any clinical efficacy in migraine trials.

5-Hydroxytryptamine in Migraine Pharmacologic and other data point to the involvement of the neurotransmitter 5-hydroxytryptamine (5HT; also known as serotonin) in migraine. Approximately 40 years ago, methysergide was found to antagonize certain peripheral actions of 5HT and was introduced as the first drug capable of preventing migraine attacks. Subsequently, it was found that platelet levels of 5HT fall consistently at the onset of headache and that drugs that cause 5HT to be released may trigger migrainous episodes. Such changes in circulating 5HT levels proved to be pharmacologically trivial, however, and interest in the humoral role of 5HT in migraine declined.

More recently, interest in the role of 5HT in migraine has been renewed due to the introduction of the triptan class of antimigraine drugs. The triptans are designed to stimulate selectively a particular subpopulation of 5HT receptors. At least 14 specific 5HT receptors exist in humans. The triptans (e.g., naratriptan, rizatriptan, sumatriptan, and zolmitriptan) are potent agonists of $5HT_{1B}$, $5HT_{1D}$, and $5HT_{1F}$ receptors and are less potent at $5HT_{1A}$ and $5HT_{1E}$ receptors. A growing body of data indicates that the antimigraine efficacy of the triptans relates to their ability to stimulate $5HT_{1B}$ receptors, which are located on both blood vessels and nerve terminals. Selective $5HT_{1D}$ receptor agonists have, thus far, failed to demonstrate clinical efficacy in migraine. Triptans that are weak $5HT_{1F}$ agonists are also effective in migraine; however, only $5HT_{1B}$ efficacy is currently thought to be essential for antimigraine efficacy.

Dopamine in Migraine A growing body of biologic, pharmacologic, and genetic data supports a role for dopamine in the pathophysiology of certain subtypes of migraine. Most migraine symptoms can be induced by dopaminergic stimulation. Moreover, there is dopamine receptor hypersensitivity in migraineurs, as demonstrated by the induction of yawning, nausea, vomiting, hypotension, and other symptoms of a migraine attack by dopaminergic agonists at doses that do not affect nonmigraineurs. Conversely, dopamine receptor antagonists are effective therapeutic agents in migraine, especially when given parenterally or concurrently with other antimigraine agents. As noted above, genetic data also suggest that molecular variations within dopamine receptor genes play a modifying role in the pathophysiology of migraine with aura. Therefore, modulation of dopaminergic neurotransmission should be considered in the therapeutic management of migraine.

The Sympathetic Nervous System in Migraine Alterations occur within the sympathetic nervous system (SNS) of migraineurs before, during, and between migraine attacks. Factors that activate the SNS are all triggers for migraine. Specific examples include environmental changes (e.g., stress, sleep patterns, hormonal shifts, hypoglycemia) and agents that cause release and a secondary depletion of peripheral catecholamines (e.g., tyramine, phenylethylamine, fenfluramine, m-chlorophenylpiperazine, and reserpine). By contrast, effective therapeutic approaches to migraine share an ability to mimic and/or enhance the effects of norepinephrine in the peripheral SNS. For example, norepinephrine itself, sympathomimetics (e.g., isometheptene), monoamine oxidase inhibitors (MAOIs), and reuptake blockers alleviate migraine. Dopamine antagonists, prostaglandin synthesis inhibitors, and adenosine antagonists are pharmacologic agents effective in the acute treatment of migraine. These drugs block the negative feedback inhibition or norepinephrine release induced by endogenous dopamine, prostaglandins, and adenosine. Therefore, migraine susceptibility may relate to genetically based variations in the ability to maintain adequate concentrations of certain neurotransmitters within postganglionic sympathetic nerve terminals. This hypothesis has been called the *empty neuron theory* of migraine.

Clinical Features

Migraine without Aura (Common Migraine) In this syndrome no focal neurologic disturbance precedes the recurrent headaches. Migraine without aura is by far the more frequent type of vascular headache. The International Headache Society criteria for migraine include moderate to severe head pain, pulsating quality, unilateral location, aggravation by walking stairs or similar routine activity, attendant nausea and/or vomiting, photophobia and phonophobia, and multiple attacks, each lasting 4 to 72 h.

Migraine with Aura (Classic Migraine) In this syndrome headache is associated with characteristic premonitory sensory, motor, or visual symptoms. Focal neurologic disturbances are more common during headache attacks than as prodromal symptoms. Focal neurologic disturbances without headache or vomiting have come to be known as *migraine equivalents* or *migraine accompaniments* and appear to occur more commonly in patients between the ages of 40 and 70 years. The term *complicated migraine* has generally been used to describe migraine with dramatic transient focal neurologic features or a migraine attack that leaves a persisting residual neurologic deficit.

The most common premonitory symptoms reported by migraineurs are visual, arising from dysfunction of occipital lobe neurons. Scotomas and/or hallucinations occur in about one-third of migraineurs and usually appear in the central portions of the visual fields. A highly characteristic syndrome occurs in about 10% of patients; it usually begins as a small paracentral scotoma, which slowly expands into a "C" shape. Luminous angles appear at the enlarging outer edge, becoming colored as the scintillating scotoma expands and moves toward the periphery of the involved half of the visual field, eventually disappearing over the horizon of peripheral vision. The entire process lasts 20 to 25 min. This phenomenon is pathognomonic for migraine and has never been described in association with a cerebral structural anomaly. It is commonly referred to as a *fortification spectrum* because the serrated edges of the hallucinated "C" seemed to resemble a fortified town with bastions around it; spectrum is used in the sense of an apparition or specter.

Basilar Migraine Symptoms referable to a disturbance in brainstem function, such as vertigo, dysarthria, or diplopia, occur as the only neurologic symptoms of the attack in about 25% of patients. A dramatic form of basilar migraine (Bickerstaff's migraine) occurs primarily in adolescent females. Episodes begin with total blindness accompanied or followed by admixtures of vertigo, ataxia, dysarthria, tinnitus, and distal and perioral paresthesias. In about one-quarter of patients, a confusional state supervenes. The neurologic symptoms usually persist for 20 to 30 min and are generally followed by a throbbing occipital headache. This basilar migraine syndrome is now known also to occur in children and in adults over age 50. An altered sensorium may persist for as long as 5 days and may take the form of confusional states superficially resembling psychotic reactions. Full recovery after the episode is the rule.

Carotidynia The carotidynia syndrome, sometimes called *lower-half headache* or *facial migraine,* is most common among older patients, with the incidence peaking in the fourth through sixth decades. Pain is usually located at the jaw or neck, although sometimes periorbital or maxillary pain occurs; it may be continuous,

deep, dull, and aching, and it becomes pounding or throbbing episodically. There are often superimposed sharp, ice pick–like jabs. Attacks occur one to several times per week, each lasting several minutes to hours. Tenderness and prominent pulsations of the cervical carotid artery and soft tissue swelling overlying the carotid are usually present ipsilateral to the pain; many patients also report throbbing ipsilateral headache concurrent with carotidynia attacks as well as between attacks. Dental trauma is a common precipitant of this syndrome. Carotid artery involvement also appears to be common in the more traditional forms of migraine; over 50% of patients with frequent migraine attacks are found to have carotid tenderness at several points on the side most often involved during hemicranial migraine attacks.

TREATMENT FOR MIGRAINE

Nonpharmacologic Approaches for All Migraineurs

Migraine can often be managed to some degree by a variety of nonpharmacologic approaches (**Table 5–7**). The measures that apply to a given individual should be used routinely since they provide a simple, cost-effective approach to migraine management. Patients with migraine do not encounter more stress than headache-free individuals; overresponsiveness to stress appears to be the issue. Since the stresses of everyday living cannot be eliminated, lessening one's response to stress by

TABLE 5-7

NONPHARMACOLOGIC APPROACHES TO MIGRAINE

Identify and then avoid trigger factors such as:
 Alcohol (e.g., red wine)
 Foods (e.g., chocolate, certain cheeses, monosodium glutamate, nitrate-containing foods)
 Hunger (avoid missing meals)
 Irregular sleep patterns (both lack of sleep and excessive sleep)
 Organic odors
 Sustained exertion
 Acute changes in stress levels
 Miscellaneous (glare, flashing lights)
Attempt to manage environmental shifts such as:
 Time zone shifts
 High altitude
 Barometric pressure changes
 Weather changes
 Assess menstrual cycle relationship

various techniques is helpful for many patients. These include yoga, transcendental meditation, hypnosis, and conditioning techniques such as biofeedback. For most patients, this approach is, at best, an adjunct to pharmacotherapy. Avoidance of migraine trigger factors may also provide significant prophylactic benefits. Unfortunately, these measures are unlikely to prevent all migraine attacks. When these measures fail to prevent an attack, pharmacologic approaches are then needed to abort an attack.

Pharmacologic Treatment of Acute Migraine

The mainstay of pharmacologic therapy is the judicious use of one or more of the many drugs that are effective in migraine. The selection of the optimal regimen for a given patient depends on a number of factors, the most important of which is the severity of the attack (**Table 5-8**). Mild migraine attacks can usually be managed by oral agents; the average efficacy rate is 50 to 70%. Severe migraine attacks may require parenteral therapy. Most drugs effective in the treatment of migraine are members of one of three major pharmacologic classes: anti-inflammatory agents, $5HT_1$ agonists, and dopamine antagonists.

Table 5-9 lists specific drugs effective in migraine. In general, an adequate dose of whichever agent is chosen should be used as soon as possible after the onset of an attack. If additional medication is required within 60 min because symptoms return or have not abated, the initial dose should be increased for subsequent attacks. Migraine therapy must be individualized for each patient; a standard approach for all patients is not possible. A therapeutic regimen may need to be constantly refined and personalized until one is identified that provides the patient with rapid, complete, and consistent relief with minimal side effects.

NONSTEROIDAL ANTI-INFLAMMATORY AGENTS

Both the severity and duration of a migraine attack can be reduced significantly by anti-inflammatory agents. Indeed, many undiagnosed migraineurs are self-treated with nonprescription anti-inflammatory agents (Table 5-4). A general consensus is that NSAIDs are most effective when taken early in the migraine attack. However, the effectiveness of anti-inflammatory agents in migraine is usually less than optimal in moderate or severe migraine attacks. The combination of acetaminophen, aspirin, and caffeine (Excedrin Migraine) has been approved for use by the U.S. Food and Drug Administration (FDA) for the treatment of mild to moderate migraine. The combination of aspirin and metoclopramide has been shown to be equivalent to a single dose of sumatriptan. Major side effects of NSAIDs include dyspepsia and gastrointestinal irritation.

TABLE 5-8

A STAGED APPROACH TO MIGRAINE PHARMACOTHERAPY		
STAGE	**DIAGNOSIS**	**THERAPIES**
Mild migraine	Occasional throbbing headaches	NSAIDs
		Combination analgesics
	No major impairment of functioning	Oral $5HT_1$ agonists
Moderate migraine	Moderate or severe headaches	Oral, nasal, or SC $5HT_1$ agonists
	Nausea common	Oral dopamine antagonists
	Some impairment of functioning	
Severe migraine	Severe headaches >3 times per month	SC, IM, or IV $5HT_1$ agonists
	Significant functional impairment	IM or IV dopamine antagonists
	Marked nausea and/or vomiting	Prophylactic medications

Note: NSAIDs, nonsteroidal anti-inflammatory drugs; 5HT, 5-hydroxytryptamine.

TABLE 5-9

TREATMENT OF ACUTE MIGRAINE

DRUG	TRADE NAME	DOSAGE
NSAIDS		
Acetaminophen, aspirin, caffeine	Excedrin Migraine	Two tablets or caplets q6h (max 8 per day)
5HT₁ AGONISTS		
Oral		
Ergotamine	Ergomar	One 2-mg sublingual tablet at onset and q1/2h (max 3 per day, 5 per week)
Ergotamine 1 mg, caffeine 100 mg	Ercaf, Wigraine	One or two tablets at onset, then one tablet q1/2h (max 6 per day, 10 per week)
Naratriptan	Amerge	2.5-mg tablet at onset; may repeat once after 4 h
Rizatriptan	Maxalt Maxalt-MLT	5- to 10-mg tablet at onset; may repeat after 2 h (max 30 mg/d)
Sumatriptan	Imitrex	50- to 100-mg tablet at onset; may repeat after 2 h (max 200 mg/d)
Zolmitriptan	Zomig	2.5-mg tablet at onset; may repeat after 2 h (max 10 mg/d)
Under oral 5HT agonists	Zomig Rapimelt	
Nasal		
Dihydroergotamine	Migranal Nasal Spray	Prior to nasal spray, the pump must be primed 4 times; one spray (0.5 mg) is administered followed, in 15 min, by a second spray
Sumatriptan	Imitrex Nasal Spray	5 to 20 mg intranasal spray as 4 sprays of 5 mg or a single 20-mg spray (may repeat once after 2 h, not to exceed a dose of 40 mg/d)
Frovatriptan	Frova	2.5-mg tablet at onset, may repeat after 2 h (max 5 mg/d)
Almotriptan	Axert	12.5-mg tablet at onset, may repeat after 2 h (max 25 mg/d)
Zolmitriptan	Zomig Nasal Spray	2.5 mg intranasal spray as one spray, may repeat after 2 h (max 5 mg/d)
Parenteral		
Dihydroergotamine	DHE-45	1 mg IV, IM, or SC at onset and q1h (max 3 mg/d, 6 mg per week)
Sumatriptan	Imitrex Injection	6 mg SC at onset (may repeat once after 1 h for max of two doses in 24 h)
DOPAMINE ANTAGONISTS		
Oral		
Metoclopramide	Reglan,[a] generic[a]	5–10 mg/d
Prochlorperazine	Compazine,[a] generic[a]	1–25 mg/d
Parenteral		
Chlorpromazine	Generic[a]	0.1 mg/kg IV at 2 mg/min; max 35 mg/d
Metoclopramide	Reglan,[a] generic	10 mg IV
Prochlorperazine	Compazine,[a] generic[a]	10 mg IV
OTHER		
Oral		
Acetaminophen, 325 mg, *plus* dichloralphenazone, 100 mg, *plus* isometheptene, 65 mg	Midrin, Duradrin, generic	Two capsules at onset followed by 1 capsule q1h (max 5 capsules)
Nasal		
Butorphanol	Stadol[a]	1 mg (1 spray in 1 nostril), may repeat if necessary in 1–2 h
Parenteral		
Narcotics	Generic[a]	Multiple preparations and dosages; see Table 4-1.

[a]Not specifically indicated by the U.S. Food and Drug Administration for migraine.
Note: NSAIDs, nonsteroidal anti-inflammatory drugs; 5HT, 5-hydroxytryptamine.

5HT₁ AGONISTS

Oral   Stimulation of $5HT_1$ receptors can stop an acute migraine attack. Ergotamine and dihydroergotamine are nonselective receptor agonists, while the series of drugs known as triptans are selective $5HT_1$ receptor agonists. A variety of triptans (e.g., naratriptan, rizatriptan, sumatriptan, zolmitriptan, almotriptan, frovatriptan) are now available for the treatment of migraine (Table 5-9).

Each of the triptan class of drugs has similar pharmacologic properties but varies slightly in terms of clinical efficacy. Rizatriptan and almotriptan are the fastest acting and most efficacious of the triptans currently available in the United States. Sumatriptan and zolmitriptan have similar rates of efficacy as well as time to onset, whereas naratriptan and frovatriptan are the slowest acting and the least efficacious. Clinical efficacy appears to be related more to the t_{max} (time to peak plasma level) than to the potency, half-life, or bioavailability (**Table 5-10**). This observation is in keeping with a significant body of data indicating that faster-acting analgesics are more efficacious than slower-acting agents.

Unfortunately, monotherapy with a selective oral $5HT_1$ agonist does not result in rapid, consistent, and complete relief of migraine in all patients. Triptans are not effective in migraine with aura unless given after the aura is completed and the headache initiated. Side effects, although often mild and transient, occur in up to 89% of patients. Moreover, $5HT_1$ agonists are contraindicated in individuals with a history of cardiovascular disease. Recurrence of headache is a major limitation of triptan use, and occurs at least occasionally in 40 to 78% of patients.

Ergotamine preparations offer a nonselective means of stimulating $5HT_1$ receptors. A nonnauseating dose of ergotamine should be sought since a dose that provokes nausea is too high and may intensify head pain. Except for a sublingual formulation of ergotamine (Ergomar), oral formulations of ergotamine also contain 100 mg caffeine (theoretically to enhance ergotamine absorption and possibly to add additional vasoconstrictor activity). The average oral ergotamine dose for a migraine attack is 2 mg. Since the clinical studies demonstrating the efficacy of ergotamine in migraine predated the clinical trial methodologies used with the triptans, it is difficult to assess the clinical efficacy of ergotamine versus the triptans. In general, ergotamine appears to have a much higher incidence of nausea than triptans, but less headache recurrence.

Nasal   The fastest acting nonparenteral antimigraine therapies that can be self-administered include nasal formulations of dihydroergotamine (Migranal), *zolmitriptan (Zomig nasal),* or sumatriptan (Imitrex Nasal). The nasal sprays result in substantial blood levels within 30 to 60 min. However, the nasal formulations suffer from inconsistent dosing, poor taste, and variable efficacy. Although in theory the nasal sprays might provide faster and more effective relief of a migraine attack than oral formulations, their reported efficacy is only approximately 50 to 60%.

Parenteral   Parenteral administration of drugs such as dihydroergotamine (DHE-45 Injectable) and sumatriptan (Imitrex SC) is approved by the FDA for the rapid relief of a migraine attack. Peak plasma levels of dihydroergotamine are achieved 3 min after intravenous dosing, 30 min after intramuscular dosing, and 45 min after subcutaneous dosing. If an attack has not already peaked, subcutaneous or intramuscular administration of 1 mg dihydroergotamine suffices for about 80 to 90% of patients. Sumatriptan, 6 mg subcutaneously, is effective in approximately 70 to 80% of patients.

TABLE 5-10

COMPARATIVE PHARMACOLOGY OF ORAL TRIPTANS[a]				
DRUG AND DOSE, MG	T_{MAX}, H	$T_{1/2}$, H	ORAL BIOAVAILABILITY, %	CLINICAL EFFICACY AT 2 H, %
Rizatriptan, 10	1–2	2–3	45	71
Zolmitriptan, 2.5	2	2.5–3	44	65
Sumatriptan, 50	2–3	2	14	61
Naratriptan, 2.5	2–4	5–6	68	45
Frovatriptan, 2.5	2–3	26	25	43
Almotriptan, 12.5	2–3	3	70	58

[a]Data adapted from package inserts approved by the U.S. Food and Drug Administration.

DOPAMINE ANTAGONISTS

Oral   Oral dopamine antagonists should be considered as adjunctive therapy in migraine. Drug absorption is impaired during migrainous attacks because of reduced gastrointestinal motility. Delayed absorption occurs in the absence of nausea and is related to the severity of the attack and not its duration. Therefore, when oral NSAIDs and/or triptan agents fail, the addition of a dopamine antagonist such as metoclopramide, 10 mg, should be considered to enhance gastric absorption. In addition, dopamine antagonists decrease nausea/vomiting and restore normal gastric motility.

Parenteral   Parenteral dopamine antagonists (e.g., chlorpromazine, prochlorperazine, metoclopramide) can also provide significant acute relief of migraine; they can be used in combination with parenteral 5HT$_1$ agonists. A common intravenous protocol used for the treatment of severe migraine is the administration over 2 min of a mixture of 5 mg of prochlorperazine and 0.5 mg of dihydroergotamine.

OTHER MEDICATIONS FOR ACUTE MIGRAINE

Oral   The combination of acetaminophen, dichloralphenazone, and isometheptene (i.e., Midrin, Duradrin, generic), one to two capsules, has been classified by the FDA as "possibly" effective in the treatment of migraine. Since the clinical studies demonstrating the efficacy of this combination analgesic in migraine predated the clinical trial methodologies used with the triptans, it is difficult to assess the clinical efficacy of this sympathomimetic compound in comparison to other agents.

Nasal   A nasal preparation of butorphanol is available for the treatment of acute pain. As with all narcotics, the use of nasal butorphanol should be limited to a select group of migraineurs, as described below.

Parenteral   Narcotics are effective in the acute treatment of migraine. For example, intravenous meperidine (Demerol), 50 to 100 mg, is given frequently in the emergency room. This regimen "works" in the sense that the pain of migraine is eliminated. However, this regimen is clearly suboptimal in patients with recurrent headache for two major reasons. First, narcotics do not treat the underlying headache mechanism; rather, they act at the thalamic level to alter pain sensation. Second, the recurrent use of narcotics can lead to significant problems. In patients taking oral narcotics such as oxycodone (Percodan) or hydrocodone (Vicodin), narcotic addiction can greatly confuse the treatment of migraine. The headache that results from narcotic craving and/or withdrawal can be difficult to distinguish from chronic migraine. Therefore, it is recommended that narcotic use in migraine be limited to patients with severe, but infrequent, headaches that are unresponsive to other pharmacologic approaches.

Prophylactic Treatment for Migraine

A substantial number of drugs are now available that have the capacity to stabilize migraine (**Table 5-11**). The decision of whether to use this approach depends on the frequency of attacks and on how well acute treatment is working. The occurrence of at least three attacks per month could be an indication for this approach. Drugs must be taken daily, and there is usually a lag of at least 2 to 6 weeks before an effect is seen. The drugs that have been approved by the FDA for the prophylactic treatment of migraine include propranolol, timolol, sodium valproate, and methysergide. In addition, a number of other drugs appear to display prophylactic efficacy. This group of drugs includes amitriptyline, nortriptyline, verapamil, phenelzine, gabapentin, and cyproheptadine. Phenelzine and methysergide are usually reserved for recalcitrant cases because of their serious potential side effects. Phenelzine is an MAOI; therefore, tyramine-containing foods, decongestants, and meperidine are contraindicated. Methysergide may cause retroperitoneal or cardiac valvular fibrosis when it is used for >8 months, thus monitoring is required for patients using this drug; the risk of the fibrotic complication is about 1:1500 and is likely to reverse after the drug is stopped.

The probability of success with any one of the antimigraine drugs is 50 to 75%; thus, if one drug is assessed each month, there is a good chance that effective stabilization will be achieved within a few months. Many patients are managed adequately with low-dose amitriptyline, propranolol, or valproate. If these agents fail or lead to unacceptable side effects, then methysergide or phenelzine can be used. Once effective stabilization is achieved, the drug is continued for 5 to 6 months and then slowly tapered to assess the continued need. Many patients are able to discontinue medication and

TABLE 5-11

DRUGS EFFECTIVE IN THE PROPHYLACTIC TREATMENT OF MIGRAINE

DRUG	TRADE NAME	DOSAGE
β-Adrenergic agents		
Propranolol	Inderal, Inderal LA	80–320 mg qd
Timolol	Blocadren	20–60 mg qd
Anticonvulsants		
Sodium valproate	Depakote	250 mg bid (max 1000 mg/d)
Topirimate	Topamax	25–50 mg bid
Tricyclic antidepressants		
Amitriptyline	Elavil,[a] generic	10–50 mg qhs
Nortriptyline	Pamelor,[a] generic	25–75 mg qhs
Monoamine oxidase inhibitors		
Phenelzine	Nardil[a]	15 mg tid
Serotonergic drugs		
Methysergide	Sansert	4–8 mg qd
Cyproheptadine	Periactin[a]	4–16 mg qd
Other		
Verapamil	Calan,[a] Isoptin[a]	80–480 mg qd

[a]Not specifically indicated for migraine by the U.S. Food and Drug Administration.

experience fewer and milder attacks for long periods, suggesting that these drugs may alter the natural history of migraine.

CLUSTER HEADACHE

A variety of names have been used for this condition, including *Raeder's syndrome, histamine cephalalgia,* and *sphenopalatine neuralgia. Cluster headache* is a distinctive and treatable vascular headache syndrome. The episodic type is most common and is characterized by one to three short-lived attacks of periorbital pain per day over a 4- to 8-week period, followed by a pain-free interval that averages 1 year. The chronic form, which may begin de novo or several years after an episodic pattern has become established, is characterized by the absence of sustained periods of remission. Each type may transform into the other. Men are affected seven to eight times more often than women; hereditary factors are usually absent. Although the onset is generally between ages 20 and 50, it may occur as early as the first decade of life. Propranolol and amitriptyline are largely ineffective. Lithium is beneficial for cluster headache and ineffective in migraine. The cluster syndrome is thus clinically, genetically, and therapeutically different from migraine. Nevertheless, mixed features of the two disorders are occasionally present, suggesting some common elements to their pathogenesis.

Clinical Features

Periorbital or, less commonly, temporal pain begins without warning and reaches a crescendo within 5 min. It is often excruciating in intensity and is deep, nonfluctuating, and explosive in quality; only rarely is it pulsatile. Pain is strictly unilateral and usually affects the same side in subsequent months. Attacks last from 30 min to 2 h; there are often associated symptoms of homolateral lacrimation, reddening of the eye, nasal stuffiness, lid ptosis, and nausea. Alcohol provokes attacks in about 70% of patients but ceases to be provocative when the bout remits; this on-off vulnerability to alcohol is pathognomonic of cluster headache. Only rarely do foods or emotional factors precipitate pain, in contrast to migraine.

There is a striking periodicity of attacks in at least 85% of patients. At least one of the daily attacks of pain recurs at about the same hour each day for the duration of a cluster bout. Onset is nocturnal in about 50% of the cases, and then the pain usually awakens the patient within 2 h of falling asleep.

Pathogenesis

No consistent cerebral blood flow changes accompany attacks of pain. Perhaps the strongest evidence for a central mechanism is the periodicity of attacks; the existence of a central mechanism is also suggested by the observation that autonomic symptoms that accompany the pain are bilateral and are more severe on the painful side. The hypothalamus is probably the site of activation in this disorder. The posterior hypothalamus contains cells that regulate autonomic functions, and the anterior hypothalamus contains cells (in the suprachiasmatic nuclei) that constitute the principal circadian pacemaker in mammals. Activation of both is necessary to explain the symptoms of cluster headache. The pacemaker is modulated via serotonergic dorsal raphe projections. It can be concluded tentatively that both migraine and cluster headache result from abnormal serotonergic neurotransmission, albeit at different loci.

TREATMENT FOR CLUSTER EADACHE

The most satisfactory treatment is the administration of drugs to prevent cluster attacks until the bout is over. Effective prophylactic drugs are prednisone, lithium, methysergide, ergotamine, sodium valproate, and verapamil. Lithium (600 to 900 mg daily) appears to be particularly useful for the chronic form of the disorder. A 10-day course of prednisone, beginning at 60 mg daily for 7 days followed by a rapid taper, may interrupt the pain bout for many patients. When ergotamine is used, it is most effective when given 1 to 2 h before an expected attack. Patients who use ergotamine daily must be educated regarding the early symptoms of ergotism, which may include vomiting, numbness, tingling, pain, and cyanosis of the limbs; a weekly limit of 14 mg should be adhered to.

For the attacks themselves, oxygen inhalation (9 L/min via a loose mask) is the most effective modality; 15 min of inhalation of 100% oxygen is often necessary. Sumatriptan, 6 mg subcutaneously, will usually shorten an attack to 10 to 15 min.

CLINICAL TREATMENT PEARL
Indomethacin-Reponsive Headaches

Over the past decades, there have emerged rare headache syndromes that respond selectively to indomethacin. These include chronic paroxysmal hemicrania, cough headache, and the icepick headache syndrome. There are other headaches such as coital headache, hemicrania continua, and post-craniotomy headache, that respond well to both indomethacin and other agents. A trial of indomethacin should be given to patients suspected of having these headache syndromes.

FURTHER READINGS

BIONDI DM: Physical treatments for headache: A structured review. Headache 45:738, 2005

Review of some nonpharmacologic treatments for headache.

FERRARI MD et al: Oral triptans in acute migraine treatment: A meta-analysis of 53 trials. Lancet 358:1668, 2001

LODER E: Safety of sumatriptan in pregnancy. CNS Drugs 17:1, 2003

NARBONE MC: Acute drug treatment of migraine attack. Neurol Sci 25:S113, 2004

SILBERSTEIN SD: Migraine pathophysiology and its clinical implications. Cephalalgia 24(Suppl 2):2, 2004

Further review of possible mechanisms involved in the pathogenesis of migraine.

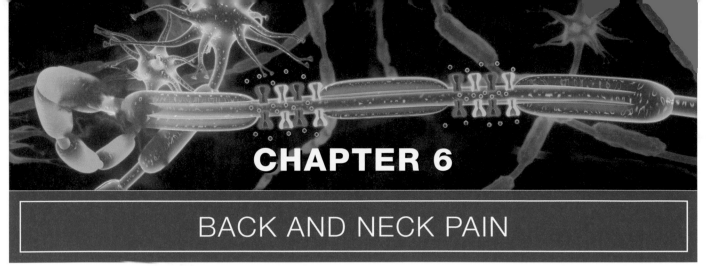

CHAPTER 6

BACK AND NECK PAIN

John W. Engstrom

The importance of back and neck pain in our society is underscored by the following: (1) the cost of back pain in the United States is between $20 and $50 billion annually, (2) back symptoms are the most common cause of disability in patients under 45 years of age, (3) low back pain is the second most common reason for visiting a physician in the United States, and (4) approximately 1% of the U.S. population is chronically disabled because of back pain.

ANATOMY OF THE SPINE

The anterior portion of the spine consists of cylindrical vertebral bodies separated by intervertebral disks and held together by the anterior and posterior longitudinal ligaments. The intervertebral disks are composed of a central gelatinous nucleus pulposus surrounded by a tough cartilagenous ring, the annulus fibrosis; disks are responsible for 25% of spinal column length (**Figs. 6-1**

and **6-2**). The disks are largest in the cervical and lumbar regions where movements of the spine are greatest. The disks are elastic in youth and allow the bony vertebrae to move easily upon each other. Elasticity is lost with age. The function of the anterior spine is to absorb the shock of body movements such as walking and running.

The posterior portion of the spine consists of the vertebral arches and seven processes. Each arch consists of paired cylindrical pedicles anteriorly and paired laminae posteriorly. The vertebral arch gives rise to two transverse processes laterally, one spinous process posteriorly, plus two superior and two inferior articular facets. The functions of the posterior spine are to protect the spinal cord and nerves within the spinal canal and to stabilize the spine by providing sites for the attachment of muscles and ligaments. The contraction of muscles attached to the spinous and transverse processes produces a system of pulleys and levers that results in flexion, extension, and lateral bending movements of the spine.

Nerve root injury (*radiculopathy*) is a common cause of neck, arm, low back, and leg pain (**Figs. 6-3** and **6-4**). The nerve roots exit at a level above their respective vertebral bodies in the cervical region (the C7 nerve root exits at the C6-C7 level) and below their respective vertebral bodies in the thoracic and lumbar regions (the T1 nerve root exits at the T1-T2 level). The cervical nerve roots follow a relatively short intraspinal course before exiting. By contrast, because the spinal cord ends at the vertebral L1 or L2 level, the lumbar nerve roots follow a long intraspinal course and can be injured anywhere from the upper lumbar spine to their exit at the intervertebral foramen. For example, it is common for disk herniation at the L4-L5 level to produce compression of the S1 nerve root (**Fig. 6-5**).

Pain-sensitive structures in the spine include the periosteum of the vertebrae, dura, facet joints, annulus fibrosus of the intervertebral disk, epidural veins, and the posterior longitudinal ligament. The nucleus pulposus of the intervertebral disk is not pain-sensitive under normal

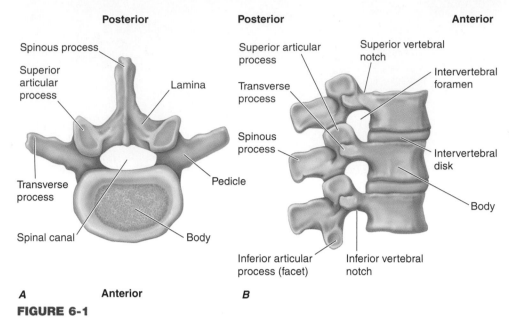

FIGURE 6-1

Vertebral anatomy. (*From A Gauthier Cornuelle, DH Gronefeld: Radiographic Anatomy Positioning. New York, McGraw-Hill, 1998, with permission.*)

circumstances. Pain sensation is conveyed partially by the sinuvertebral nerve that arises from the spinal nerve at each spine segment and reenters the spinal canal through the intervertebral foramen at the same level. Disease of these diverse pain-sensitive spine structures may explain many cases of back pain without nerve root compression. The lumbar and cervical spine possess the greatest potential for movement and injury.

APPROACH TO THE PATIENT WITH BACK PAIN

Types of Back Pain

Understanding the type of pain experienced by the patient is the essential first step. Attention is also focused on identification of risk factors for serious underlying diseases; the majority of these are due to tumor, fracture, radiculopathy or infection (**Table 6-1**).

Local pain is caused by stretching of pain-sensitive structures that compress or irritate sensory nerve endings. The site of the pain is near the affected part of the back.

Pain referred to the back may arise from abdominal or pelvic viscera. The pain is usually described as primarily abdominal or pelvic but is accompanied by back pain and usually unaffected by posture. The patient may occasionally complain of back pain only.

Pain of spine origin may be located in the back or referred to the buttocks or legs. Diseases affecting the upper lumbar spine tend to refer pain to the lumbar region, groin, or anterior thighs. Diseases affecting the lower lumbar spine tend to produce pain referred to the buttocks, posterior thighs, or rarely the calves or feet. Provocative injections into pain-sensitive structures of the spine may produce leg pain that does not follow a dermatomal distribution. This "sclerotomal" pain may explain instances in which back and leg pain is unaccompanied by evidence of nerve root compression.

Radicular back pain is typically sharp and radiates from the spine to the leg within the territory of a nerve root (see "Lumbar Disk Disease," below). Coughing, sneezing, or voluntary contraction of abdominal muscles (lifting heavy objects or straining at stool) may elicit the radiating pain. The pain may increase in postures that stretch the nerves and nerve roots. Sitting stretches the sciatic nerve (L5 and S1 roots) because the nerve passes posterior to the hip. The femoral nerve (L2, L3, and L4 roots) passes anterior to the hip and is not stretched by sitting. The description of the pain alone often fails to distinguish clearly between sclerotomal pain and radiculopathy.

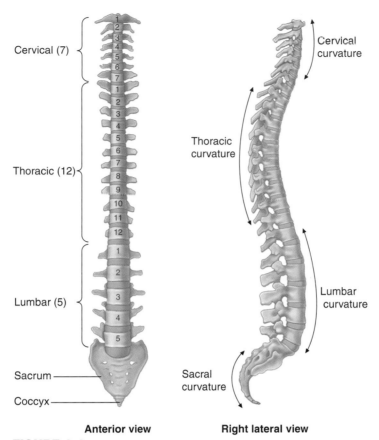

Cervical (7)

Thoracic (12)

Lumbar (5)

Sacrum

Coccyx

Cervical curvature

Thoracic curvature

Lumbar curvature

Sacral curvature

Anterior view   **Right lateral view**

FIGURE 6-2

Spinal column. (*From A Gauthier Cornuelle, DH Gronefeld: Radiographic Anatomy Positioning. New York, McGraw-Hill, 1998, with permission.*)

Pain associated with muscle spasm, although of obscure origin, is commonly associated with many spine disorders. The spasms are accompanied by abnormal posture, taut paraspinal muscles, and dull pain.

Knowledge of the circumstances associated with the onset of back pain is important when weighing possible serious underlying causes for the pain. Some patients involved in accidents or work-related injuries may exaggerate their pain for the purpose of compensation or for psychological reasons.

Examination of the Back

A physical examination that includes the abdomen and rectum is advisable. Back pain referred from visceral organs may be reproduced during palpation of the abdomen [pancreatitis, abdominal aortic aneurysm (AAA)] or percussion over the costovertebral angles (pyelonephritis, adrenal disease).

The normal spine has a thoracic kyphosis, lumbar lordosis, and cervical lordosis. Exaggeration of these normal alignments may result in hyperkyphosis (lameback) of the thoracic spine or hyperlordosis (swayback) of the lumbar spine. Spasm of lumbar paraspinal muscles results in flattening of the usual lumbar lordosis. Inspection may reveal lateral curvature of the spine (scoliosis) or an asymmetry in the paraspinal muscles, suggesting muscle spasm. Taut paraspinal muscles limit motion of the lumbar spine. Back pain of bony spine origin is often reproduced by palpation or percussion over the spinous process of the affected vertebrae.

Forward bending is frequently limited by paraspinal muscle spasm. Flexion of the hips is

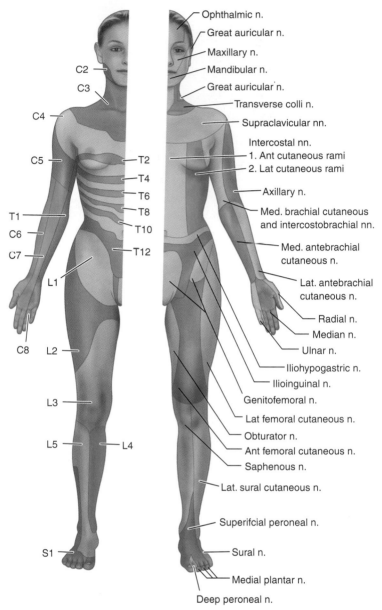

FIGURE 6-3

Anterior view of dermatomes (*left*) and cutaneous areas (*right*) supplied by individual nerves. (*Modified from MB Carpenter and J Sutin, in Human Neuroanatomy, 8th ed, Baltimore, Williams & Wilkins, 1983.*)

normal in patients with lumbar spine disease, but flexion of the lumbar spine is limited and sometimes painful. Lateral bending to the side opposite the injured spinal element may stretch the damaged tissues, worsen pain, and limit motion. Hyperextension of the spine (with the patient prone or standing) is limited when nerve root compression or bony spine disease is present.

Pain from hip disease may resemble the pain of lumbar spine disease. Hip pain can be reproduced by internal and external rotation at the hip, with the knee and hip in flexion (Patrick sign), and by percussion of the heel with the examiner's palm while the leg is extended.

With the patient lying flat, passive flexion of the extended leg at the hip stretches the L5 and S1 nerve roots and the sciatic nerve. Passive dorsiflexion of the foot during the maneuver adds to the stretch. While flexion to at least 80° is normally possible without causing pain, tight hamstring

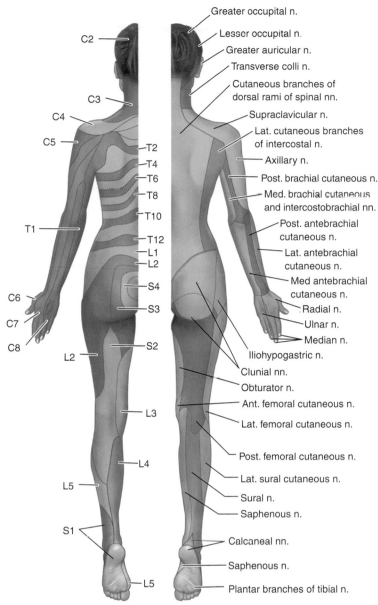

FIGURE 6-4

Posterior view of dermatomes (*left*) and cutaneous areas (*right*) supplied by individual peripheral nerves. (*Modified from MB Carpenter and J Sutin, in Human Neuroanatomy, 8th ed, Baltimore, Williams & Wilkins, 1983.*)

muscles are a source of pain in many patients. The *straight leg–raising* (SLR) test is positive if the maneuver reproduces the patient's usual back or limb pain, not the discomfort associated with tight hamstring muscles. Eliciting the SLR sign in the sitting position may help determine if the finding is reproducible. The patient may describe pain in the low back, buttocks, posterior thigh, or lower leg, but the key feature is reproduction of the pa-

tient's usual pain. The *crossed SLR sign* is positive when flexion of one leg reproduces the pain in the opposite leg or buttocks. The crossed SLR sign is less sensitive but more specific for disk herniation than the SLR sign. The nerve or nerve root lesion is always on the side of the pain. The *reverse SLR sign* is elicited by standing the patient next to the examination table and passively extending each leg with the knee fully extended. This ma-

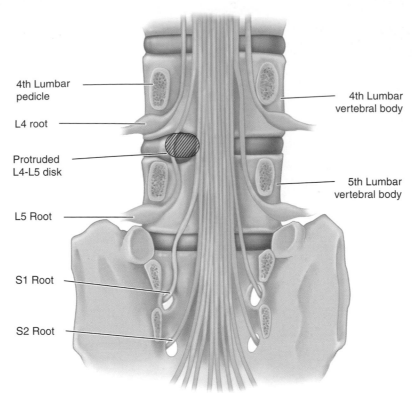

4th Lumbar pedicle

L4 root

Protruded L4-L5 disk

L5 Root

S1 Root

S2 Root

4th Lumbar vertebral body

5th Lumbar vertebral body

FIGURE 6-5

Compression of L5 and S1 roots by herniated disk. (*Modified from AH Ropper, RH Brown: Adams and Victor's Principles of Neurology, 8th ed. New York, McGraw-Hill, 2005, with permission.*)

neuver, which stretches the L2-L4 nerve roots and the femoral nerve, is considered positive if the patient's usual back or limb pain is reproduced.

The neurologic examination includes a search for weakness, muscle atrophy, focal reflex changes, diminished sensation in the legs, and signs of spinal cord injury. The examiner should be alert to the possibility of breakaway weakness, defined as fluctuating strength during the examination of one or more muscles. The weakness may be due to pain or a combination of pain and underlying true weakness. Breakaway weakness without pain is due to lack of effort. In uncertain cases, electromyography (EMG) can determine whether or not true weakness is present. Findings with specific nerve root lesions are shown in **Table 6-2** and are discussed below.

Laboratory, Imaging, and EMG Studies

Routine laboratory studies such as a complete blood count, erythrocyte sedimentation rate, chemistry panel, and urinalysis are rarely needed for the initial evaluation of nonspecific, acute (<3 months' duration) low back pain (ALBP). If risk factors for a serious underlying disease are present,

then laboratory studies (guided by the history and examination) are indicated.

Plain films of the lumbar or cervical spine are helpful when risk factors for vertebral fracture (history of trauma, chronic steroid use, malignancy, osteoporosis, or focal tenderness to palpation over the spinous process of the affected segment) are present. In the absence of risk factors, routine x-rays of the lumbar spine in nonspecific ALBP are expensive and rarely helpful. Magnetic resonance imaging (MRI) and computed tomography (CT)-myelography are the radiologic tests of choice for evaluation of most serious diseases involving the spine. MRI is superior for the definition of soft tissue structures, whereas CT-myelography provides optimal imaging of bony lesions and is tolerated by claustrophobic patients. With rare exceptions, conventional myelography and bone scan are inferior to MRI and CT-myelography.

EMG can be used to assess the functional integrity of the peripheral nervous system. Sensory nerve conduction studies are normal when focal sensory loss is due to nerve root damage because the nerve roots are proximal to the nerve cell

TABLE 6-1

ACUTE LOW BACK PAIN: RISK FACTORS FOR AN IMPORTANT STRUCTURAL CAUSE

History
- Pain worse at rest or at night
- Prior history of cancer
- History of chronic infection (esp. lung, urinary tract, skin)
- History of trauma
- Age >50 years
- Intravenous drug use
- Glucocorticoid use
- History of a rapidly progressive neurologic deficit

Examination
- Unexplained fever
- Unexplained weight loss
- Percussion tenderness over the spine
- Abdominal, rectal, or pelvic mass
- Patrick's sign or heel percussion sign
- Straight leg or reverse straight–leg raising signs
- Progressive focal neurologic deficit

bodies in the dorsal root ganglia. The diagnostic yield of needle EMG is higher than that of nerve conduction studies for radiculopathy. Denervation changes in a myotomal (segmental) distribution are detected by sampling multiple muscles supplied by different nerve roots and nerves; the pattern of muscle involvement indicates the nerve root(s) responsible for the injury. Needle EMG provides objective information about motor nerve fiber injury when the clinical evaluation of weakness is limited by pain or poor effort. EMG and nerve conduction studies will be normal when only limb pain or sensory nerve root injury or irritation is present. Mixed nerve somatosensory evoked potentials and F-wave studies are of little value in the evaluation of radiculopathy.

CAUSES OF BACK PAIN (See Table 6-3)

CONGENITAL ANOMALIES OF THE LUMBAR SPINE

Spondylolysis is a bony defect in the pars interarticularis (a segment near the junction of the pedicle with the lamina) of the vertebra; the etiology may be a stress fracture in a congenitally abnormal segment. The defect (usually bilateral) is best visualized on oblique projections in plain x-rays or by CT scan and occurs in the setting of a single injury, repeated minor injuries, or growth.

TABLE 6-2

LUMBOSACRAL RADICULOPATHY — NEUROLOGIC FEATURES

LUMBOSACRAL NERVE ROOTS	EXAMINATION FINDINGS			
	REFLEX	SENSORY	MOTOR	PAIN DISTRIBUTION
L2[a]	—	Upper anterior thigh	Psoas (hip flexion)	Anterior thigh
L3[a]	—	Lower anterior thigh Anterior knee	Psoas (hip flexion) Quadriceps (knee extension) Thigh adduction	Anterior thigh, knee
L4[a]	Quadriceps (knee)	Medial calf	Quadriceps (knee extension)[b] Thigh adduction Tibialis anterior (foot dorsiflexion)	Knee, medial calf Anterolateral thigh
L5[c]	—	Dorsal surface — foot Lateral calf	Peroneii (foot eversion)[b] Tibialis anterior (foot dorsiflexion) Gluteus medius (hip abduction) Toe dorsiflexors	Lateral calf, dorsal foot, posterolateral thigh, buttocks
S1[c]	Gastrocnemius/ soleus (ankle)	Plantar surface — foot Lateral aspect — foot	Gastrocnemius/soleus (foot plantar flexion)[b] Abductor hallucis (toe flexors)[b] Gluteus maximus (hip extension)	Bottom foot, posterior calf, posterior thigh, buttocks

[a]Reverse straight leg — raising sign present — see "Examination of the Back."
[b]These muscles receive the majority of innervation from this root.
[c]Straight leg — raising sign present — see "Examination of the Back."

TABLE 6-3

CAUSES OF LOW BACK AND NECK PAIN

Congenital/developmental
    Spondylolysis and spondylolisthesis[a]
    Kyphoscoliosis[a]
    Spina bifida occulta[a]
    Tethered spinal cord[a]
Minor trauma
    Strain or sprain
    Whiplash injury[b]
Fractures
    Traumatic — falls, motor vehicle accidents
    Atraumatic — osteoporosis, neoplastic infiltration,
        exogenous steroids
Intervertebral disk herniation
Degenerative
    Disk-osteophyte complex
    Internal disk disruption
    Spinal stenosis with neurogenic claudication[a]
    Uncovertebral joint disease[b]
    Atlantoaxial joint disease (e.g., rheumatoid arthritis)[a]
Arthritis
    Spondylosis
    Facet or sacroiliac arthropathy
    Autoimmune (e.g., anklyosing spondylitis, Reiter's
        syndrome)
Neoplasms — metastatic, hematologic, primary bone
tumors
Infection/inflammation
    Vertebral osteomyelitis
    Spinal epidural abscess
    Septic disk
    Meningitis
    Lumbar arachnoiditis[a]
Metabolic
    Osteoporosis — hyperparathyroidism, immobility
    Osteosclerosis (e.g., Paget's disease)
Other
    Referred pain from visceral disease
    Postural
    Psychiatric, malingering, chronic pain syndromes
    Vertebral artery dissection[a]

[a]Low back pain only.
[b]Neck pain only.

Spondylolisthesis is the anterior slippage of the vertebral body, pedicles, and superior articular facets, leaving the posterior elements behind. Spondylolisthesis is associated with spondylolysis and degenerative spine disease and occurs more frequently in women. The slippage may be asymptomatic but may also cause low back pain, nerve root injury (the L5 root most frequently), or symptomatic spinal stenosis. Tenderness may be elicited near the segment that has "slipped" forward (most often L4 on L5 or occasionally L5 on S1). A "step" may be present on deep palpation of the posterior elements of the segment above the spondylolisthetic joint. The trunk may be shortened and the abdomen protuberant as a result of extreme forward displacement of L4 on L5; in severe cases, cauda equina syndrome (CES) may occur (see below).

Spina bifida occulta is a failure of closure of one or several vertebral arches posteriorly; the meninges and spinal cord are normal. A dimple or small lipoma may overlie the defect. Most cases are asymptomatic and discovered incidentally during evaluation for back pain.

Tethered cord syndrome usually presents as a progressive cauda equina disorder (see below), although myelopathy may also be the initial manifestation. The patient is often a young adult who complains of perineal or perianal pain, sometimes following minor trauma. Neuroimaging studies reveal a low-lying conus (below L1-L2) and a short and thickened filum terminale.

TRAUMA

A patient complaining of back pain and inability to move the legs may have a spinal fracture or dislocation and, with fractures above L1, spinal cord compression. Care must be taken to avoid further damage to the spinal cord or nerve roots by immobilizing the back pending results of x-rays.

Sprains and Strains

The terms *low back sprain, strain,* or *mechanically induced muscle spasm* refer to minor, self-limited injuries associated with lifting a heavy object, a fall, or a sudden deceleration such as in an automobile accident. These terms are used loosely and do not clearly describe a specific anatomical lesion. The pain is usually confined to the lower back, and there is no radiation to the buttocks or legs. Patients with paraspinal muscle spasm often assume unusual postures.

Traumatic Vertebral Fractures

Most traumatic fractures of the lumbar vertebral bodies result from injuries producing anterior wedging or compression. With severe trauma, the patient may sustain a fracture-dislocation or a "burst" fracture involving the vertebral body and posterior elements. Traumatic vertebral fractures are caused by falls from a height (a pars interarticularis fracture of the L5 vertebra is common), sudden deceleration in an automobile accident, or direct injury. Neurologic impairment is common, and early surgical treatment is indicated.

LUMBAR DISK DISEASE

This is a common cause of chronic or recurrent low back and leg pain (**Fig. 6-6**). Disk disease is most likely

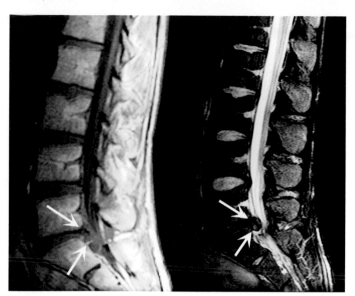

FIGURE 6-6

MRI of lumbar herniated disk; left S1 radiculopathy. Sagittal T1-weighted image on the left with arrows outlining disk margins. Sagittal T2 image on the right reveals a protruding disk at the L5-S1 level (*arrows*), which displaces the central thecal sac.

to occur at the L4-L5 and L5-S1 levels, but upper lumbar levels are involved occasionally. The cause is often unknown; the risk is increased in overweight individuals. Disk herniation is unusual prior to age 20 and is rare in the fibrotic disks of the elderly. Degeneration of the nucleus pulposus and the annulus fibrosus increases with age and may be asymptomatic or painful. The pain may be located in the low back only or referred to the leg, buttock, or hip. A sneeze, cough, or trivial movement may cause the nucleus pulposus to prolapse, pushing the frayed and weakened annulus posteriorly. With severe disk disease, the nucleus may protrude through the annulus (herniation) or become extruded to lie as a free fragment in the spinal canal.

The mechanism by which intervertebral disk injury causes back pain is controversial. The inner annulus fibrosus and nucleus pulposus are normally devoid of innervation. Inflammation and production of proinflammatory cytokines within the protruding or ruptured disk may trigger or perpetuate back pain. Ingrowth of nociceptive (pain) nerve fibers into inner portions of a diseased disk may be responsible for chronic "diskogenic" pain. Nerve root injury (radiculopathy) from disk herniation may be due to compression, inflammation, or both; pathologically, demyelination and axonal loss are usually present.

Symptoms of a ruptured disk include back pain, abnormal posture, limitation of spine motion (particularly flexion), or radicular pain. A dermatomal pattern of sensory loss or a reduced or absent deep tendon reflex is more suggestive of a specific root lesion than the pattern of pain. Motor findings (focal weakness, muscle atrophy, or fasciculations) occur less frequently than sensory or reflex changes. Symptoms and signs are usually unilateral, but bilateral involvement does occur with large central disk herniations that compress several nerve roots at the same level. Clinical manifestations of specific nerve root lesions are summarized in Table 6-3. There is evidence to suggest that lumbar disk herniation with a nonprogressive nerve root deficit can be managed conservatively without surgery. Large disk herniations that rupture through the annulus are naturally more likely to decrease in size over time than small protrusions that are contained within the annulus.

The differential diagnosis includes a variety of serious and treatable conditions that include epidural abscess, hematoma, or tumor. Fever, constant pain uninfluenced by position, sphincter abnormalities, or signs of spinal cord disease suggest an etiology other than lumbar disk disease. Bilateral absence of ankle reflexes can be a normal finding in old age, a sign of bilateral S1 radiculopathy, or a polyneuropathy. While an absent deep tendon reflex or focal sensory loss may reflect injury to a nerve root, other sites of injury along the nerve must also be considered. For example, an absent knee reflex may be due to a femoral neuropathy rather than an L4 nerve root injury. A loss of sensation over the foot and distal lateral calf may result from a peroneal or lateral sciatic neuropathy rather than an L5 nerve root injury. Focal muscle atrophy may reflect a nerve root or peripheral nerve injury, an anterior horn cell disease, or disuse.

An MRI scan or CT-myelogram is necessary to establish the location and type of pathology. Simple MRI yields exquisite views of intraspinal and adjacent soft tissue anatomy. Bony lesions of the lateral recess or intervertebral foramen may be seen with optimal clarity on CT-myelographic studies. The correlation of neuroradiologic findings to symptoms, particularly pain, is not simple. Contrast-enhancing tears in the annulus fibrosus or disk protrusions are widely accepted as common sources of back pain; however, one study found that over half of asymptomatic adults have similar findings. Asymptomatic disk protrusions are also common, and these abnormalities may enhance with contrast. Furthermore, in patients with known disk herniation treated either medically or surgically, persistence of the herniation 10 years later had no relationship to the clinical outcome. MRI findings of disk protrusion, tears in the annulus fibrosus, or contrast enhancement are common incidental findings that by themselves should not dictate management decisions for patients with back pain.

There are four indications for intervertebral disk surgery: (1) progressive motor weakness from nerve root injury demonstrated on clinical examination or EMG; (2) bowel or bladder disturbance or other signs of spinal cord compression; (3) incapacitating pain of nerve root origin, despite conservative treatment for at least 4 weeks; and (4) recurrent incapacitating pain despite conservative treatment. The latter two criteria are more subjective and less well established than the first two criteria. Surgical treatment may be considered if the pain and/or neurologic findings do not substantially improve over the first 12 weeks.

The usual surgical procedure is a partial hemilaminectomy with excision of the prolapsed disk. Fusion of the involved lumbar segments is considered only if significant spinal instability is present (i.e., degenerative spondylolisthesis or isthmic spondylolysis).

CES is an injury of multiple lumbosacral nerve roots within the spinal canal. Low back pain, weakness and areflexia in the lower extremities, saddle anesthesia, and loss of bladder function may occur. The problem must be distinguished from disorders of the lower spinal cord (conus medullaris syndrome), acute transverse myelitis (Chap. 24), and Guillain-Barré syndrome (Chap. 35). Combined involvement of the conus medullaris and cauda equina can occur. CES is commonly due to a ruptured lumbosacral intervertebral disk, lumbosacral spine fracture, hematoma within the spinal canal (e.g., following lumbar puncture in patients with coagulopathy), compressive tumors, or other mass lesions. Treatment options include surgical decompression, sometimes urgently in an attempt to restore or preserve motor or sphincter function, or palliative radiotherapy or chemotherapy for metastatic tumors.

DEGENERATIVE CONDITIONS

Lumbar spinal stenosis describes a narrowed lumbar spinal canal. When severe, neurogenic claudication, consisting of back and buttock or leg pain induced by walking or standing and relieved by sitting, can occur. Symptoms in the legs are usually bilateral. Unlike vascular claudication, symptoms are often provoked by standing without walking. Unlike lumbar disk disease, symptoms are usually relieved by sitting. Focal weakness, sensory loss, or reflex changes may occur when spinal stenosis is associated with radiculopathy. Severe neurologic deficits, including paralysis and urinary incontinence, occur rarely. Spinal stenosis can be acquired (75%), congenital, or due to a combination of both causes. Congenital forms (achondroplasia, idiopathic) are characterized by short, thick pedicles that produce both spinal canal and lateral recess stenosis. Acquired factors that may contribute to spinal stenosis include degenerative diseases (spondylosis,

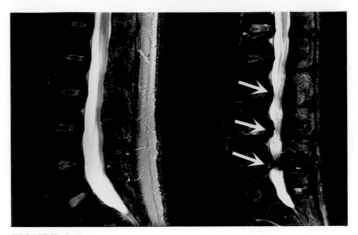

FIGURE 6-7

Spinal stenosis. Sagittal T2 fast spin echo magnetic resonance imaging of a normal (*left*) and (*right*) lumbar spine, revealing multifocal narrowing (*arrows*) of the cerebrospinal fluid spaces surrounding the nerve roots within the thecal sac.

spondylolisthesis, scoliosis), trauma, spine surgery (postlaminectomy, fusion), metabolic or endocrine disorders (epidural lipomatosis, osteoporosis, acromegaly, renal osteodystrophy, hypoparathyroidism), and Paget's disease. MRI or CT-myelography provides the best definition of the abnormal anatomy (**Fig. 6-7**).

Conservative treatment of symptomatic spinal stenosis includes nonsteroidal anti-inflammatory drugs (NSAIDs), exercise programs, and symptomatic treatment of acute pain exacerbations. Surgical therapy is considered when medical therapy does not relieve pain sufficiently to allow for activities of daily living or when significant focal neurologic signs are present. Between 65 and 80% of properly selected patients treated surgically experience 75% relief of back and leg pain. Up to 25% develop recurrent stenosis at the same spinal level or an adjacent level 5 years after the initial surgery; recurrent symptoms usually respond to a second surgical decompression.

Facet joint hypertrophy can produce unilateral radicular symptoms or signs due to bony compression of a nerve root that are indistinguishable from disk-related radiculopathy. Patients may exhibit stretch signs, focal motor weakness, hyporeflexia, or dermatomal sensory loss. Hypertrophic superior or inferior facets can often be visualized radiologically. Foraminotomy results in long-term relief of leg and back pain in 80 to 90% of patients.

ARTHRITIS

Spondylosis, or osteoarthritic spine disease, typically occurs in later life and primarily involves the cervical and lumbosacral spine. Patients often complain of back pain that is increased by motion and associated with stiffness or limitation of motion. The relationship between clinical symptoms and radiologic findings is usually not straightforward. Pain may be prominent when x-ray findings are minimal; alternatively, large osteophytes can be seen in asymptomatic patients in middle and later life. Hypertrophied facets and osteophytes may compress nerve roots in the lateral recess or intervertebral foramen. Osteophytes arising from the vertebral body may cause or contribute to central spinal canal stenosis. Loss of intervertebral disk height reduces the cross-sectional area of the intervertebral foramen; the descending pedicle may compress the nerve root exiting at that level. Rarely, osteoarthritic changes in the lumbar spine compress the cauda equina.

Ankylosing Spondylitis

This distinctive arthritic spine disease typically presents with the insidious onset of low back and buttock pain. Patients are often males below age 40. Associated features include morning back stiffness, nocturnal pain, pain unrelieved by rest, an elevated sedimentation rate, and the histocompatibility antigen HLA-B27. Onset at a young age and back pain improving with exercise is characteristic. Loss of the normal lumbar lordosis and exaggeration of thoracic kyphosis are seen as the disease progresses. Inflammation and erosion of the outer fibers of the annulus fibrosus at the point of contact with the vertebral body are followed by ossification and bony growth that bridges adjacent vertebral bodies and reduces spine mobility in all planes. Radiologic hallmarks are periarticular destructive changes, sclerosis of the sacroiliac joints, and bridging of vertebral bodies to produce the fused "bamboo spine." Similar restricted movements may accompany Reiter's syndrome, psoriatic arthritis, and chronic inflammatory bowel disease. Stress fractures through the spontaneously ankylosed posterior bony elements of the rigid, osteoporotic spine may produce focal pain, spinal cord compression, or CES. Atlantoaxial subluxation with spinal cord compression occasionally occurs. Ankylosis of the ribs to the spine and a decrease in the height of the thoracic spine may compromise respiratory function.

NEOPLASMS (See Also Chap. 25)

Back pain is the most common neurologic symptom in patients with systemic cancer and is usually due to vertebral metastases. Metastatic carcinoma (breast, lung, prostate, thyroid, kidney, gastrointestinal tract), multiple myeloma, and non-Hodgkin's and Hodgkin's lymphomas frequently involve the spine. Back pain may be the presenting symptom. The pain tends to be constant, dull, unrelieved by rest, and worse at night. In contrast, mechanical low back pain usually improves with rest. Plain x-rays usually, but not always, show destructive lesions in one or several vertebral bodies without disk space involvement. MRI or CT-myelography are the studies of choice when spinal metastasis is suspected. MRI is usually preferred, but the procedure of choice is the study most rapidly available because the patient's condition may worsen quickly.

INFECTIONS/INFLAMMATION

Vertebral osteomyelitis is usually caused by staphylococci, but other bacteria or the tubercle bacillus (Pott's disease) may be responsible. A primary source of infection, most often the urinary tract, skin, or lungs, can be identified in 40% of patients. Intravenous drug use is a well-recognized risk factor. Back pain exacerbated by motion and unrelieved by rest, spine tenderness over the involved spine segment, and an elevated erythrocyte sedimentation rate are the most common findings. Fever or an elevated white blood cell count are found in a minority of patients. Plain radiographs may show a narrowed disk space with erosion of adjacent vertebrae; however, these diagnostic changes may take weeks or months to appear. MRI and CT are sensitive and specific for osteomyelitis; CT may be more readily available in emergency settings and better tolerated by some patients with severe back pain.

Spinal epidural abscess (Chap. 24) presents with back pain (aggravated by movement or palpation) and fever. Signs of nerve root injury or spinal cord compression may be present. The abscess may track over multiple spinal levels and is best delineated by spine MRI.

Lumbar adhesive arachnoiditis with radiculopathy is due to fibrosis following inflammation within the subarachnoid space. The fibrosis results in nerve root adhesions, producing back and leg pain associated with motor, sensory, or reflex changes. Myelography-induced arachnoiditis has become rare with the abandonment of oil-based contrast. Other causes of arachnoiditis include multiple lumbar operations, chronic spinal infections, spinal cord injury, intrathecal hemorrhage, intrathecal injection of glucocorticoids or anesthetics, and foreign bodies. The MRI may show nerve roots that clump together centrally and adhere to the dura peripherally, or loculations of cerebrospinal fluid within the thecal sac. Treatment is often unsatisfactory. Microsurgical lysis of adhesions, dorsal rhizotomy, and dorsal root ganglionectomy have resulted in poor outcomes. Dorsal column stimulation for pain relief has produced varying results. Epidural injections of glucocorticoids have been of limited value.

METABOLIC CAUSES
Osteoporosis and Osteosclerosis

Immobilization or underlying systemic disorders such as osteomalacia, hyperparathyroidism, hyperthyroidism, multiple myeloma, metastatic carcinoma, or glucocorticoid use may accelerate osteoporosis and weaken the vertebral body. The most common causes of atraumatic vertebral body fractures are postmenopausal (type 1) or senile (type 2) osteoporosis. Compression fractures occur in up to half of patients with severe osteoporosis, and those who sustain a fracture have a 4.5-fold increased risk for recurrent fracture. The sole manifestation of a compression fracture may be localized aching (often after a trivial injury) that is exacerbated by movement. Other patients experience radicular pain only. Focal tenderness to palpation is common. The clinical context, neurologic signs, and x-ray appearance of the spine establish the diagnosis. When compression fractures are found, treatable risk factors should be sought. Antiresorptive drugs including bisphosphonates (e.g., alendronate), transdermal estrogen, and tamoxifen have been shown to reduce the risk of osteoporotic fractures. Compression fractures above the midthoracic region suggest malignancy; if tumor is suspected, a bone biopsy or diagnostic search for a primary tumor is indicated.

Interventions [percutaneous vertebroplasty (PVP), kyphoplasty] exist for osteoporotic compression fractures associated with debilitating pain. Candidates for PVP should have midline pain, focal tenderness over the spinous process of the affected vertebral body, <80% loss of vertebral body height, and onset of symptoms within the prior 4 months. The technique consists of injection of polymethylmethacrylate, under fluoroscopic guidance, into the affected vertebral body. Rare major complications include extravasation of cement into the epidural space (resulting in myelopathy) or fatal pulmonary embolism from migration of cement into paraspinal veins. Approximately three-quarters of patients who meet selection criteria have reported enhanced quality of life. Relief of pain following PVP has also been reported in patients with vertebral metastases, myeloma, or hemangiomas.

Osteosclerosis (abnormally increased bone density) is readily identifiable on routine x-ray studies (e.g., Paget's disease) and may or may not produce back pain. Spinal cord or nerve root compression may result from bony encroachment on the spinal canal or intervertebral foramina. Single dual-beam photon absorptiometry or quantitative CT can be used to detect small changes in bone mineral density.

REFERRED PAIN FROM VISCERAL DISEASE

Diseases of the thorax, abdomen, or pelvis may refer pain to the posterior portion of the spinal segment that innervates the diseased organ. Occasionally, back pain may be the first and only sign. Upper abdominal diseases generally refer pain to the lower thoracic or upper lumbar region (eighth thoracic to the first and second lumbar vertebrae), lower abdominal diseases to the lumbar region (second to fourth lumbar vertebrae), and pelvic diseases to the sacral region. Local signs (pain with spine palpation, paraspinal muscle spasm) are absent, and minimal or no pain accompanies normal spine movements.

Low Thoracic or Lumbar Pain with Abdominal Disease

Peptic ulcers or tumors of the posterior wall of the stomach or duodenum typically produce epigastric pain, but midline back or paraspinal pain may occur if retroperitoneal extension is present. Back pain due to peptic ulcer may be precipitated by ingestion of an orange, alcohol, or coffee and relieved by food or antacids. Fatty foods are more likely to induce back pain associated with biliary disease. Diseases of the pancreas produce back pain to the right of the spine (head of the pancreas involved) or to the left (body or tail involved). Pathology in retroperitoneal structures (hemorrhage, tumors, pyelonephritis) produces paraspinal pain that radiates to the lower abdomen, groin, or anterior thighs. A mass in the iliopsoas region often produces unilateral lumbar pain with radiation toward the groin, labia, or testicles. The sudden appearance of lumbar pain in a patient receiving anticoagulants suggests retroperitoneal hemorrhage.

Isolated low back pain occurs in 6 to 20% of patients with a contained rupture of an abdominal aortic aneurysm (AAA). The classic clinical triad of abdominal pain, shock, and back pain in an elderly man occurs in <20% of patients. Two of these three features are present in two-thirds of patients, and hypotension is present in half. The typical patient is an elderly male smoker with back pain. The diagnosis is initially missed in at least one-third of patients because the symptoms and signs can be nonspecific. Common misdiagnoses include nonspecific back pain, diverticulitis, renal colic, sepsis, and myocardial infarction. A careful abdominal examination revealing a pulsatile mass (present in 50 to 75% of patients) is an important physical finding. Patients with suspected AAA should be evaluated with ultrasound, CT, or MRI.

Inflammatory bowel disorders (colitis, diverticulitis) or cancers of the colon may produce lower abdominal pain, midlumbar back pain, or both. The pain may have a beltlike distribution around the body. A lesion in the transverse or proximal descending colon may refer pain to the middle or left back at the L2–L3 level. Lesions of the sigmoid colon may refer pain to the upper sacral or midline suprapubic regions or left lower quadrant of the abdomen.

Sacral Pain with Gynecologic and Urologic Disease

Pelvic organs rarely cause low back pain, except for gynecologic disorders involving the uterosacral ligaments. The pain is referred to the sacral region. Endometriosis or cancers of the uterus may invade the uterosacral ligaments; malposition of the uterus may cause uterosacral ligament traction. Pain associated with endometriosis is typically premenstrual and often continues until it merges with menstrual pain. Malposition of the uterus (retroversion, descensus, and prolapse) may produce sacral pain after prolonged standing. Menstrual pain may be felt in the sacral region. The poorly localized, cramping pain can radiate down the legs. Pain due to neoplastic infiltration of nerves is typically continuous, progressive in severity, and unrelieved by rest at night. Less commonly, radiation therapy of pelvic tumors may produce sacral pain from late radiation necrosis of tissue or nerves. Low back pain that radiates into one or both thighs is common in the last weeks of pregnancy.

Urologic sources of lumbosacral back pain include chronic prostatitis, prostate cancer with spinal metastasis, and diseases of the kidney and ureter. Lesions of the bladder and testes do not usually produce back pain. The diagnosis of metastatic prostate carcinoma is established by rectal examination, spine imaging studies (MRI or CT), and measurement of prostate-specific antigen. Infectious, inflammatory, or neoplastic renal diseases may produce ipsilateral lumbosacral pain, as can renal artery or vein thrombosis. Paraspinal lumbar pain may be a symptom of ureteral obstruction due to nephrolithiasis.

OTHER CAUSES OF BACK PAIN

Postural Back Pain

There is a group of patients with nonspecific chronic low back pain (CLBP) in whom no anatomical or pathologic lesion can be found despite exhaustive investigation. These individuals complain of vague, diffuse back pain with prolonged sitting or standing that is relieved by rest. The physical examination is unrevealing except for "poor posture." Imaging studies and laboratory evaluations are normal. Exercises to strengthen the paraspinal and abdominal muscles are sometimes therapeutic.

Psychiatric Disease

CLBP may be encountered in patients who seek financial compensation, in malingerers, or in those with concurrent substance abuse, chronic anxiety states, or depression. Many patients with CLBP have a history of psychiatric illness (depression, anxiety, substance abuse) or childhood trauma (physical or sexual abuse) that antedates the onset

of back pain. Preoperative psychological assessment has been used to exclude patients with marked psychological impairments; these patients are likely to have a poor surgical outcome.

Unidentified

The cause of low back pain occasionally remains unclear. Some patients have had multiple operations for disk disease but have persistent pain and disability. The original indications for surgery may have been questionable, with back pain only, no definite neurologic signs, or a minor disk bulge noted on CT or MRI. Scoring systems based upon neurologic signs, psychological factors, physiologic studies, and imaging studies have been devised to minimize the likelihood of unsuccessful surgical explorations.

TREATMENT FOR BACK PAIN

Acute Low Back Pain (ALBP)

A practical approach to the management of low back pain is to consider acute and chronic presentations separately. ALBP is defined as pain of <3 months' duration. Full recovery can be expected in 85% of adults with ALBP unaccompanied by leg pain. Most have purely "mechanical" symptoms—i.e., pain that is aggravated by motion and relieved by rest.

Observational studies have been used to justify a minimalist approach to this problem. These studies share a number of limitations: (1) a true placebo control group is often lacking; (2) patients who consult different provider groups (generalists, orthopedists, neurologists) are assumed to have similar etiologies for their back pain; (3) no information is provided about the details of treatment; and (4) there is no attempt to tabulate serious causes of ALBP.

The algorithms (clinical practice guidelines or CPGs) for the treatment of back pain (**Fig. 6-8**) draw from published guidelines. However, since CPGs are based on incomplete evidence, guidelines should not substitute for clinical judgment.

The initial assessment excludes clinically important underlying causes of back pain that require urgent intervention including infection, cancer, and trauma (Table 6-1). Pain increasing with standing and relieved by sitting, percussion tenderness over the costovertebral angle, an abdominal mass (pulsatile or nonpulsatile), or a rectal mass are addi-

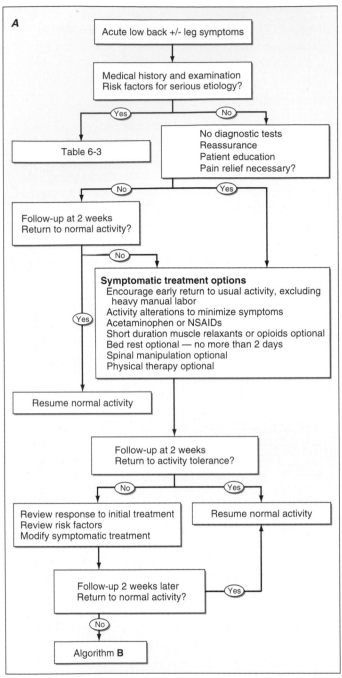

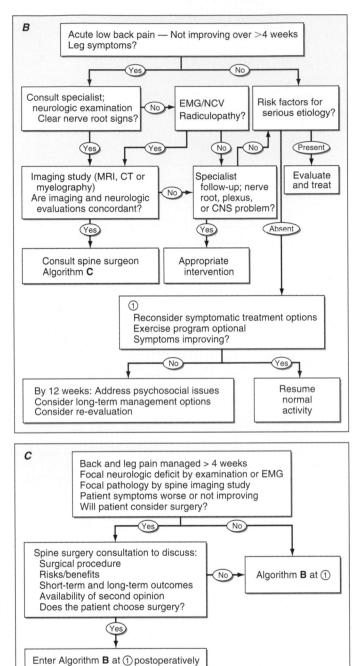

FIGURE 6-8

Algorithms for management of acute low back pain, age ≥18 years. **A**. Symptoms <3 months, first 4 weeks. **B**. Management weeks 4–12. **C**. Surgical options.①, entry point from Algorithm C postoperatively or if patient declines surgery. (NSAIDs, nonsteroidal anti-inflammatory drugs; CBC, com-

plete blood count; ESR, erythrocyte sedimentation rate; UA, urinalysis; EMG, electromyography; NCV, nerve conduction velocity studies; MRI, magnetic resonance imaging; CT, computed tomography; CNS, central nervous system.)

tional findings that trigger concern. Worrisome focal neurologic signs include sensory loss (saddle anesthesia or focal limb sensory loss), leg weakness, spasticity, or reflex asymmetry. Laboratory studies are unnecessary unless a clinically important underlying

cause is suspected. Plain spine films are rarely indicated in the first month of symptoms unless a spine fracture is suspected.

Clinical trials have shown no benefit of prolonged (>2 days) bed rest for uncomplicated ALBP.

There is evidence that bed rest is also ineffective for patients with sciatica or for acute back pain with findings of nerve root injury. Theoretical advantages of early ambulation for ALBP include maintenance of cardiovascular conditioning, improved disk and cartilage nutrition, improved bone and muscle strength, and increased endorphin levels. A trial examining the effects of a program of early vigorous exercise was negative, but the benefits of less vigorous exercise or other exercise programs are unknown. The early resumption of normal physical activity (without heavy manual labor) is likely to be beneficial. Traction for ALBP is not effective, as shown in well-designed clinical trials that include a "sham" traction control group. Despite this knowledge, physicians in one survey identified strict bed rest for 3 days, trigger point injections (see below), and physical therapy (PT) as beneficial for ALBP. In many instances, the behavior of treating physicians does not reflect the current medical literature.

Proof is lacking to support the treatment of acute back and neck pain with acupuncture, transcutaneous electrical nerve stimulation, massage, ultrasound, diathermy, or electrical stimulation. Cervical collars can be modestly helpful by limiting spontaneous and reflex neck movements that exacerbate pain. Evidence regarding the efficacy of ice or heat is lacking, but these interventions are optional given the lack of negative evidence, low cost, and low risk. Biofeedback has not been studied rigorously. Facet joint, trigger point, and ligament injections are not recommended for ALBP.

A role for modification of posture has not been validated by rigorous clinical studies. As a practical matter, temporary suspension of activity known to increase mechanical stress on the spine (heavy lifting, prolonged sitting, bending or twisting, straining at stool) may be helpful.

Education is an important part of treatment. Satisfaction and the likelihood of follow-up increase when patients are educated about prognosis, treatment methods, activity modifications, and strategies to prevent future exacerbations. In one study, patients who felt they did not receive an adequate explanation for their symptoms wanted further diagnostic tests. Evidence for the efficacy of structured education programs ("back school") is inconclusive; in one study, patients attending back school had a shorter duration of sick leave during the initial episode but not during subsequent episodes. Randomized studies of back school for primary prevention of low back

injury and pain have failed to demonstrate any benefit.

NSAIDs and acetaminophen are effective over-the-counter agents for ALBP. Muscle relaxants (cyclobenzaprine, methocarbamol) provide short-term (4 to 7 days) benefit, but drowsiness limits daytime use. Opioid analgesics are no more effective than NSAIDs or acetaminophen for initial treatment of ALBP, nor do they increase the likelihood of return to work. Short-term use of opioids in patients unresponsive to or intolerant of acetaminophen or NSAIDs may be helpful. There is no evidence to support the use of oral glucocorticoids or tricyclic antidepressants for ALBP.

Epidural glucocorticoids may occasionally produce short-term pain relief in ALBP and radiculopathy, but proof is lacking for pain relief beyond 1 month. Epidural anesthetics, glucocorticoids, or opioids are not indicated in the initial treatment of ALBP without radiculopathy. Diagnostic nerve root blocks have been advocated to determine if pain originates from a specific nerve root. However, improvement may result even when the nerve root is not responsible for the pain syndrome; this may occur with placebo effects, painful lesions located distally along the peripheral nerve, or anesthesia of the sinuvertebral nerve. Therapeutic nerve root blocks with injection of glucocorticoids and a local anesthetic is an option after conservative measures fail, particularly when temporary relief of pain is necessary.

A short course of spinal manipulation or PT for symptomatic relief of uncomplicated ALBP is an option. A prospective, randomized study comparing PT, chiropractic manipulation, and education interventions for patients with ALBP found modest trends toward benefit with both PT and chiropractic manipulation at 1 year. Costs per year were equivalent in the PT/chiropractic group and ~$280 less for the group treated with the education booklet alone. The value of such treatment beyond 1 year is unknown. Similarly, specific PT or chiropractic protocols that may provide benefit have not been fully defined.

Chronic Low Back Pain

CLBP, defined as pain lasting >12 weeks, accounts for 50% of total back pain costs. Overweight individuals appear to be at particular risk. Other risk factors include: female gender, older age, prior history of back pain, restricted spinal mobility, pain radiating into a leg, high levels of psychological distress, poor self-rated health, minimal physical activity, smoking, job dissatisfaction, and widespread pain. Combinations of these premorbid factors have been used to predict which individuals with ALBP are likely to develop CLBP. The initial approach to these patients is similar to that for ALBP, and the differential diagnosis is similar. Treatment of this heterogeneous group of patients is directed toward the underlying cause when known; the ultimate goal is to restore function to the greatest extent possible.

Many conditions that produce CLBP can be identified by a combination of neuroimaging and electrophysiologic studies. Spine MRI or CT-myelography are the techniques of choice but are generally not indicated within the first month after initial evaluation in the absence of risk factors for a serious underlying cause. Imaging studies should be performed only in circumstances where the results are likely to influence surgical or medical treatment.

Diskography provides no additional anatomical information beyond what is available by MRI. Reproduction of the patient's typical pain with the injection is often used as evidence that a specific disk is the pain generator, but it is not known whether this information has any value in selecting candidates for surgery. A recent study concluded that there is no proof that diskography improves surgical outcome. There is no proven role for thermography in the assessment of radiculopathy.

The diagnosis of nerve root injury is most secure when the history, examination, results of imaging studies, and the EMG are concordant. The correlation between CT and EMG for localization of nerve root injury is between 65 and 73%. Up to one-third of asymptomatic adults have a disk protrusion detected by CT or MRI scans. Thus, surgical intervention based solely upon radiologic findings increases the likelihood of an unsuccessful outcome.

CLBP can be treated with a variety of conservative measures. Acute and subacute exacerbations are managed with NSAIDs and comfort measures. There is no good evidence to suggest that one NSAID is more effective than another. Bed rest should not exceed 2 days. Activity tolerance is the primary goal, while pain relief is secondary. Exercise programs can reverse atrophy in paraspinal muscles and strengthen extensors of the trunk. Intensive physical exercise or "work hardening" regimens (under the guidance of a physical therapist)

have been effective in returning some patients to work, improving walking distances, and diminishing pain. The benefit can be sustained with home exercise regimens; compliance with the exercise regimen strongly influences outcome. The role of manipulation, back school, or epidural steroid injections in the treatment of CLBP is unclear. Up to 30% of epidural steroid injections performed without fluoroscopic guidance miss the epidural space even when performed by an experienced anesthesiologist. There is no strong evidence to support the use of acupuncture or traction. A reduction in sick leave days, long-term health care utilization, and pension expenditures may offset the initial expense of multidisciplinary treatment programs. In one study comparing 3 weeks of hydrotherapy versus routine ambulatory care, hydrotherapy reduced the duration and intensity of back pain, reduced analgesic drug consumption, improved spine mobility, and improved function. Function returned to baseline at the 9-month follow-up, but all other beneficial effects were sustained. Percutaneous electrical nerve stimulation (PENS) has been shown to provide significant short-term relief of CLBP, but additional studies regarding its long-term efficacy and cost are needed.

PAIN IN THE NECK AND SHOULDER

Neck pain, which usually arises from diseases of the cervical spine and soft tissues of the neck, is common (4.6% of adults in one study). Neck pain arising from the cervical spine is typically precipitated by movements and may be accompanied by focal tenderness and limitation of motion. Pain arising from the brachial plexus, shoulder, or peripheral nerves can be confused with cervical spine disease, but the history and examination usually identify a more distal origin for the pain. When the distinction between nerve root and brachial plexus tissue involvement is unclear on clinical grounds alone, then magnetic resonance neurography is sometimes helpful to directly visualize both the plexus and nerve roots simultaneously. Cervical spine trauma, disk disease, or spondylosis may be asymptomatic or painful and can produce a myelopathy, radiculopathy, or both. The nerve roots most commonly affected are C7 and C6.

TRAUMA TO THE CERVICAL SPINE

Trauma to the cervical spine (fractures, subluxation) places the spinal cord at risk for compression. Motor vehicle accidents, violent crimes, or falls account for 87% of spinal cord injuries (Chap. 24). Immediate immobilization of the neck is essential to minimize further spinal cord injury from movement of unstable cervical spine segments.

Whiplash injury is due to trauma (usually automobile accidents) causing cervical musculoligamental sprain or strain due to hyperflexion or hyperextension of the neck. This diagnosis should not be applied to patients with fractures, disk herniation, head injury, or altered consciousness. One prospective study found that 18% of patients with whiplash injury had persistent injury-related symptoms 2 years after the car accident. These patients were older, had a higher incidence of inclined or rotated head position at impact, greater intensity of initial neck and head pain, greater number of initial symptoms, and more osteoarthritic changes on cervical spine x-rays at baseline compared to patients who ultimately recovered. Severe initial symptoms are associated with a poor long-term outcome.

CERVICAL DISK DISEASE

Herniation of a lower cervical disk is a common cause of neck, shoulder, arm, or hand pain. Neck pain (worse with movement), stiffness, and a limited range of motion are the usual manifestations. With nerve root compression, pain may radiate into a shoulder or arm. Extension and lateral rotation of the neck narrows the intervertebral foramen and may reproduce radicular symptoms (Spurling's sign). In young individuals, acute nerve root compression from a ruptured cervical disk is often due to trauma. Subacute radiculopathy is less likely to be related to a specific traumatic incident and is usually due to a combination of disk disease and spondylosis. Cervical disk herniations are usually posterolateral near the lateral recess and intervertebral foramen. Typical patterns of reflex, sensory, and motor changes that accompany specific cervical nerve root lesions are summarized in **Table 6-4**; however it is helpful to remember that (1) overlap in function between adjacent nerve roots is common, (2) symptoms and signs may be evident in only part of the

TABLE 6-4

CERVICAL RADICULOPATHY — NEUROLOGIC FEATURES

CERVICAL NERVE ROOTS	EXAMINATION FINDINGS			PAIN DISTRIBUTION
	REFLEX	SENSORY	MOTOR	
C5	Biceps	Over lateral deltoid	Supraspinatus[a] (initial arm abduction) Infraspinatus[a] (arm external rotation) Deltoid[a] (arm abduction) Biceps (arm flexion)	Lateral arm, medial scapula
C6	Biceps	Thumb, index fingers Radial hand/forearm	Biceps (arm flexion) Pronator teres (internal forearm rotation)	Lateral forearm, thumb, index finger
C7	Triceps	Middle fingers Dorsum forearm	Triceps[a] (arm extension) Wrist extensors[a] Extensor digitorum[a] (finger extension)	Posterior arm, dorsal forearm, lateral hand
C8	Finger flexors	Little finger Medial hand and forearm	Abductor pollicis brevis (abduction D1) First dorsal interosseous (abduction D2) Abductor digiti minimi (abduction D5)	4th and 5th fingers, medial forearm
T1	Finger flexors	Axilla and medial arm	Abductor pollicis brevis (abduction D1) First dorsal interosseous (abduction D2) Abductor digiti minimi (abduction D5)	Medial arm, axilla

[a]These muscles receive the majority of innervation from this root.

injured nerve root territory, and (3) the location of pain is the most variable of the clinical features.

CERVICAL SPONDYLOSIS

Osteoarthritis of the cervical spine may produce neck pain that radiates into the back of the head, shoulders, or arms, or may be the source of headaches in the posterior occipital region (supplied by the C2-C4 nerve roots). Osteophyte formation in the lateral recess or hypertrophic facet joints may produce a monoradiculopathy (**Fig. 6-9**). Narrowing of the spinal canal by osteophytes, ossification of the posterior longitudinal ligament, or a large central disk may compress the cervical spinal cord. Combinations of radiculopathy and myelopathy also occur. An electrical sensation elicited by neck flexion and radiating down the spine from the neck (Lhermitte's symptom) usually indicates involvement of the cervical or upper thoracic (T1-T2) spinal cord. When little or no neck pain accompanies the cord compression, the diagnosis may be confused with amyotrophic lateral sclerosis (Chap. 21), multiple sclerosis (Chap. 28), spinal cord tumors, or syringomyelia (Chap. 24). The possibility of treatable cervical spondylosis must be considered even when the patient presents with leg complaints only. In other cases, an unrelated lumbar radiculopathy or polyneuropathy may mask signs of an associated cervical myelopathy. MRI or CT-myelography can define the anatomical abnormalities, and EMG and nerve conduction studies can localize and assess the severity of the motor nerve root injury.

OTHER CAUSES OF NECK PAIN

Rheumatoid arthritis (RA) of the cervical apophyseal joints produces neck pain, stiffness, and limitation of motion. In typical cases with symmetric inflammatory polyarthritis, the diagnosis of RA is straightforward. In advanced RA, synovitis of the atlantoaxial joint (C1-2; Fig. 6-4) may damage the transverse ligament of the atlas, producing forward displacement of the atlas on the axis (atlantoaxial subluxation). Radiologic evidence of atlantoaxial subluxation occurs in 30% of patients with RA. Not surprisingly, the degree of subluxation correlates with the severity of erosive disease. When subluxation is present, careful neurologic assessment is important to identify early signs of myelopathy. Occasional patients develop high spinal cord compression leading to quadriparesis, respiratory insufficiency, and death. Low back pain is common in RA; however, the frequency of facet disease, fracture, and spondylolisthesis is no greater than in controls with mechanical low back pain.

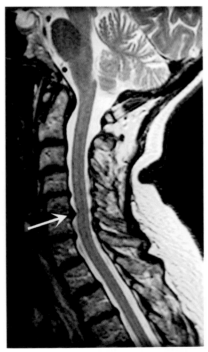

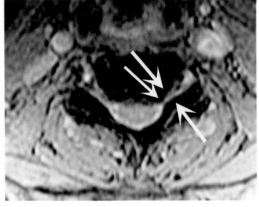

B

A

FIGURE 6-9

Cervical spondylosis; left C6 radiculopathy. **A**. Sagittal T2 fast spin echo magnetic resonance imaging reveals a hypointense osteophyte that protrudes from the C5-C6 level into the thecal sac, displacing the spinal cord posteriorly (*white arrows*). **B**. Axial 2-mm section from a 3-D volume gradient echo sequence of the cervical spine. The high signal of the right C5-C6 intervertebral foramen contrasts with the narrow high signal of the left C5-C6 intervertebral foramen produced by osteophytic spurring (*arrows*).

Ankylosing spondylitis can cause neck pain and on occasion atlantoaxial subluxation; when spinal cord compression is present or threatened, surgical intervention is indicated. *Herpes zoster* produces acute posterior occipital or neck pain prior to the outbreak of vesicles. *Neoplasms* metastatic to the cervical spine, *infections* (osteomyelitis and epidural abscess), and *metabolic bone diseases* may also be the cause of neck pain. Neck pain may also be referred from the heart with coronary artery ischemia (cervical angina syndrome).

THORACIC OUTLET

The thoracic outlet contains the first rib, the subclavian artery and vein, the brachial plexus, the clavicle, and the lung apex. Injury to these structures may result in postural or movement-induced pain around the shoulder and supraclavicular region. *True neurogenic thoracic outlet syndrome* (TOS) results from compression of the lower trunk of the brachial plexus or ventral rami of the C8 or T1 nerve roots by an anomalous band of tissue connecting an elongate transverse process at C7 with the first rib. Weakness and numbness of the hand are the most common symptoms; in general, pain is not prominent. Signs include weakness of intrinsic muscles of the hand and diminished sensation on the palmar aspect of the fourth and fifth digits. EMG and nerve conduction studies confirm the diagnosis. Treatment consists of surgical division of the anomalous band. The weakness and wasting of intrinsic hand muscles typically does not improve, but surgery halts the insidious progression of weakness. *Arterial TOS* results from compression of the subclavian artery by a cervical rib; the compression results in poststenotic dilatation of the artery and thrombus formation. Blood pressure is reduced in the affected limb, and signs of emboli may be present in the hand; neurologic signs are absent. Ultrasound can confirm the diagnosis noninvasively. Treatment is with thrombolysis or anticoagulation (with or without embolectomy) and surgical excision of the cervical rib compressing the subclavian artery or vein. *Disputed TOS* includes a large number of patients with chronic arm and shoulder pain of unclear cause. The lack of sensitive and specific findings on physical examination or laboratory markers for this condition frequently results in diagnostic uncertainty. The role of surgery in disputed TOS is controversial. Multidisciplinary pain management is a conservative approach, although treatment is often unsuccessful.

BRACHIAL PLEXUS AND NERVES

Pain from injury to the brachial plexus or peripheral nerves of the arm can occasionally mimic pain of cervical spine origin. Neoplastic infiltration of the lower trunk of the brachial plexus may produce shoulder pain radiating down the arm, numbness of the fourth and fifth fingers, and weakness of intrinsic hand muscles innervated by the ulnar and median nerves. Postradiation fibrosis (breast carcinoma is the most common setting) may produce similar findings, although pain is less often present. A Pancoast tumor of the lung is another cause and should be considered, especially when a Horner's syndrome is present. *Suprascapular neuropathy* may produce severe shoulder pain, wasting of the supraspinatous and infraspinatous muscles, and weakness in external rotation of the arm at the shoulder and the first 6° of arm abduction laterally. *Acute brachial neuritis* is often confused with radiculopathy. It consists of the acute onset of severe shoulder or scapular pain followed over days to weeks by weakness of the proximal arm and shoulder girdle muscles innervated by the upper brachial plexus. The onset is often preceeded by an infection or immunization. Complete recovery occurs in 75% of patients after 2 years and in 89% after 3 years. Occasional cases of carpal tunnel syndrome produce pain and paresthesias extending into the forearm, arm, and shoulder resembling a C5 or C6 root lesion. Lesions of the radial or ulnar nerve can mimic a radiculopathy at C7 or C8, respectively. EMG and nerve conduction studies can accurately localize lesions to the nerve roots, brachial plexus, or peripheral nerves. ***For further discussion of peripheral nerve disorders, see Chap. 33.***

SHOULDER

Pain from the shoulder can be difficult to distinguish from neck pain. If symptoms and signs of radiculopathy are absent, then the differential diagnosis includes mechanical shoulder pain (tendonitis, bursitis, rotator cuff tear, dislocation, adhesive capsulitis, and cuff impingement under the acromion) and referred pain (subdiaphragmatic irritation, angina, Pancoast tumor). Mechanical pain is often worse at night, associated with local shoulder tenderness and aggravated by abduction, internal rotation, or extension of the arm. Pain from shoulder disease may on occasion radiate into the arm or hand, but sensory, motor, and reflex changes are absent.

TREATMENT FOR NECK PAIN

There are few well-designed clinical trials that address optimal treatment of neck pain. Symptomatic treatment can include the use of analgesic medications and/or a soft cervical collar. Current indications for cervical disk surgery are similar to those for lumbar disk surgery; because of the risk of spinal cord injury with cervical spine disease, an aggressive approach is generally indicated whenever spinal cord injury is threatened. Surgical management of cervical herniated disks usually consists of an anterior approach with diskectomy followed by anterior interbody fusion. A simple posterior partial laminectomy with diskectomy is an acceptable alternative approach. The risk of subsequent radiculopathy or myelopathy at cervical segments adjacent to the fusion is ~3% per year and 26% per decade. Although this risk is sometimes portrayed as a late complication of surgery, it may also reflect the natural history of degenerative cervical spine disease in patients selected for surgery. Nonprogressive cervical radiculopathy (associated with a focal neurologic deficit) due to a herniated cervical disk may be treated conservatively with a high rate of success. Cervical spondylosis with bony, compressive cervical radiculopathy is generally treated with surgical decompression to forstall the progression of neurologic signs. Cervical spondylotic myelopathy is typically managed with either anterior decompression and fusion or laminectomy. Outcomes in both surgical groups vary, but late functional deterioration occurs in 20 to 30% of patients; a prospective, controlled study comparing different surgical interventions is needed.

FURTHER READINGS

☑ ATLAS SJ, NARDIN RA: Evaluation and treatment of low back pain: An evidence-based approach to clinical care. Muscle Nerve 27:265, 2003.

Updated Clinical Guidelines for the management of low back pain.

☑ CASSIDY JD et al: Effect of eliminating compensation for pain and suffering on the outcome of insurance claims for whiplash injury. N Engl J Med 342:1179, 2000.

Decreased incidence and improved prognosis for whiplash injury.

CHERKIN DC et al: Randomized trial comparing traditional Chinese medical acupuncture, therapeutic massage, and self-care education for chronic low back pain. Arch Intern Med 161:1081, 2001.

☑ COHEN SP et al: Lumbar discography: A comprehensive review of outcome studies, diagnostic accuracy, and principles. Reg Anesth Pain Med 30(2):163, 2005.

Role of lumber discography in establishing "discogenic" low back pain.

☑ GIBSON JN, WADDELL G: Surgery for degenerative lumbar spondylosis. Cochrane Database Syst Rev 2:CD001352, 2000.

Literature-based review of indications for surgery.

☑ NG PP et al: Percutaneous vertebroplasty: An emerging therapy for vertebral compression fractures. Semin Neurol 22(2):149, 2002.

Review of vertebroplasty for treatment of incapacitating pain.

POHJOLAINEN T et al: Treatment of acute low back pain with the COX-2-selective anti-inflammatory drug nimesulide. Results of a randomized, double-blind comparative trial. Spine 25:1579, 2000

☑ RIEW KD et al: The effect of nerve root injections on the need for operative treatment of lumbar radicular pain. J Bone Joint Surg 82A:689, 2000.

Role of selective nerve root blocks in selecting patients for surgery.

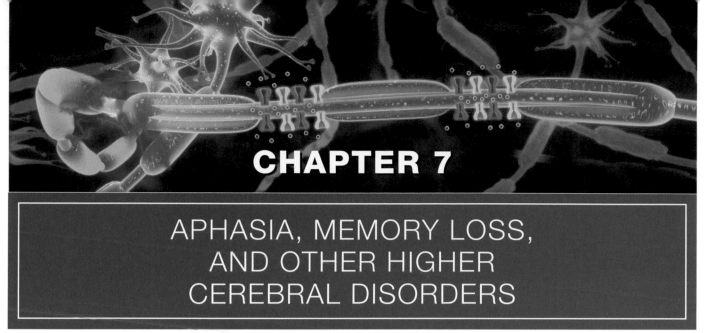

CHAPTER 7

APHASIA, MEMORY LOSS, AND OTHER HIGHER CEREBRAL DISORDERS

M.-Marsel Mesulam

The cerebral cortex of the human brain contains approximately 20 billion neurons spread over an area of 2.5 m². The *primary sensory* areas provide an obligatory portal for the entry of sensory information into cortical circuitry, whereas the *primary motor* areas provide a final common pathway for coordinating complex motor acts. The primary sensory and motor areas constitute 10% of the cerebral cortex. The rest is subsumed by unimodal, heteromodal, paralimbic, and limbic areas, collectively known as the *association cortex* (Fig. 7-1). The association cortex mediates the integrative processes that subserve cognition, emotion, and behavior. A systematic testing of these mental functions is necessary for the effective clinical assessment of the association cortex and its diseases.

According to current thinking, there are no centers for "hearing words," "perceiving space," or "storing memories." Cognitive and behavioral functions (domains) are coordinated by intersecting *large-scale neural networks* that contain interconnected cortical and subcortical components. The network approach to higher cerebral function has at least four implications of clinical relevance: (1) a single domain such as language or memory can be disrupted by damage to any one of several areas, as long as these areas belong to the same network; (2) damage confined to a single area can give rise to multiple deficits, involving the functions of all networks that intersect in that region; (3) damage to a network component may give rise to minimal or transient deficits if other parts of the network undergo compensatory reorganization; and (4) individual anatomical sites within a network display a relative (but not absolute) specialization for different behavioral aspects of the relevant function. Five anatomically defined large-scale networks are most relevant to clinical practice: a perisylvian network for language; a parietofrontal network for spatial cognition; an occipitotemporal network for face and object recognition; a limbic network for retentive memory; and a prefrontal network for attention and behavior.

THE LEFT PERISYLVIAN NETWORK FOR LANGUAGE: APHASIAS AND RELATED CONDITIONS

Language allows the communication and elaboration of thoughts and experiences by linking them to arbitrary symbols known as words. The neural substrate of language is composed of a distributed network centered in the perisylvian region of the *left* hemisphere. The posterior pole of this network is known as *Wernicke's area* and includes the posterior third of the superior temporal gyrus and a surrounding rim of inferior parietal and midtemporal cortex (see **Fig. 7-1**). An essential function of Wernicke's area is to transform sensory inputs into

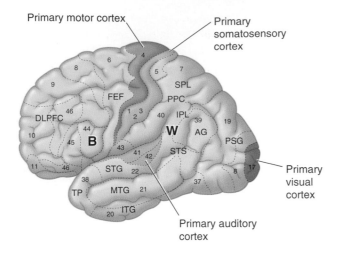

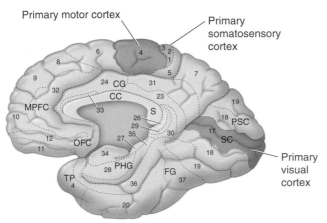

FIGURE 7-1

Lateral (*top*) and medial (*bottom*) views of the cerebral hemispheres. The numbers refer to the Brodmann cytoarchitectonic designations. Area 17 corresponds to primary visual cortex, 41–42 to primary auditory cortex, 1–3 to primary somatosensory cortex, and 4 to primary motor cortex. The rest of the cerebral cortex contains association areas. AG, angular gyrus; B, Broca's area; CC, corpus callosum; CG, cingulate cortex; DLPFC, dorsolateral prefrontal cortex; FEF, frontal eye fields (premotor cortex); FG, fusiform gyrus; IPL, inferior parietal lobule; ITG, inferior temporal gyrus; LG, lingual gyrus; MPFC, medial prefrontal cortex; MTG, middle temporal gyrus; OFC, orbitofrontal cortex; PHG, parahippocampal gyrus; PPC, posterior parietal cortex; PSC, peristriate cortex; SC, striate cortex; SMG, supramarginal gyrus; SPL, superior parietal lobule; STG, superior temporal gyrus; STS, superior temporal sulcus; TP, temporopolar cortex; W, Wernicke's area.

their neural word representations so that these can establish the distributed associations that give the word its meaning. The anterior pole of the language network, known as *Broca's area,* includes the posterior part of the inferior frontal gyrus and a surrounding rim of prefrontal heteromodal cortex. An essential function of this area is to transform neural word representations into

their articulatory sequences so that the words can be uttered in the form of spoken language. The sequencing function of Broca's area also appears to involve the ordering of words into sentences that contain a meaning-appropriate *syntax* (grammar). Wernicke's and Broca's areas are interconnected with each other and with additional perisylvian, temporal, prefrontal, and posterior parietal regions, making up a neural network subserving the various aspects of language function. Damage to any one of these components or to their interconnections can give rise to language disturbances (*aphasia*). Aphasia should be diagnosed only when there are deficits in the formal aspects of language such as naming, word choice, comprehension, spelling, and syntax. Dysarthria and mutism do not, by themselves, lead to a diagnosis of aphasia. The language network shows a left hemisphere dominance pattern in the vast majority of the population. In ~90% of right handers and 60% of left handers, aphasia occurs only after lesions of the left hemisphere. In some individuals no hemispheric dominance for language can be discerned, and in some others (including a small minority of right handers) there is a right hemisphere dominance for language. A language disturbance occurring after a right hemisphere lesion in a right hander is called *crossed aphasia.*

CLINICAL EXAMINATION

The clinical examination of language should include the assessment of naming, spontaneous speech, comprehension, repetition, reading, and writing. A deficit of naming (*anomia*) is the single most common finding in aphasic patients. When asked to name common objects (pencil or wristwatch), the patient may fail to come up with the appropriate word, may provide a circumlocutious description of the object ("the thing for writing"), or may come up with the wrong word (*paraphasia*). If the patient offers an incorrect but legitimate word ("pen" for "pencil"), the naming error is known as a *semantic paraphasia*; if the word approximates the correct answer but is phonetically inaccurate ("plentil" for "pencil"), it is known as a *phonemic paraphasia*. Asking the patient to name body parts, geometric shapes, and component parts of objects (lapel of coat, cap of pen) can elicit mild forms of anomia in patients who can otherwise name common objects. In most anomias, the patient cannot retrieve the appropriate name when shown an object but can point to the appropriate object when the name is provided by the examiner. This is known as a one-way (or retrieval-based) naming deficit. A two-way naming deficit exists if the patient can neither provide nor recognize the correct name, indicating the presence of a language comprehension impairment. *Spontaneous speech* is described as "fluent" if it maintains appropriate output volume, phrase length, and melody or as "nonfluent" if it is sparse, halting, and average utterance length is below four words. The examiner should also note if the speech is paraphasic or circumlocutious; if it shows a relative paucity of substantive nouns and action verbs versus function words (prepositions, conjunctions); and if word order, tenses, suffixes, prefixes, plurals, and possessives are appropriate. *Comprehension* can be tested by assessing the patient's ability to follow conversation, by asking yes-no questions ("Can a dog fly?", "Does it snow in summer?") or asking the patient to point to appropriate objects ("Where is the source of illumination in this room?"). Statements with embedded clauses or passive voice construction ("If a tiger is eaten by a lion, which animal stays alive?") help to assess the ability to comprehend complex syntactic structure. Commands to close or open the eyes, stand up, sit down, or roll over should not be used to assess overall comprehension since appropriate responses aimed at such axial movements can be preserved in patients who otherwise have profound comprehension deficits.

Repetition is assessed by asking the patient to repeat single words, short sentences, or strings of words such as "No ifs, ands, or buts." The testing of repetition with tongue-twisters such as "hippopotamus" or "Irish constabulary" provides a better assessment of dysarthria and pallilalia than aphasia. Aphasic patients may have little difficulty with tongue-twisters but have a particularly hard time repeating a string of function words. It is important to make sure that the number of words does not exceed the patient's attention span. Otherwise, the failure of repetition becomes a reflection of the narrowed attention span rather than an indication of an aphasic deficit. *Reading* should be assessed for deficits in reading aloud as well as comprehension. *Writing* is assessed for spelling errors, word order, and grammar. *Alexia* describes an inability to either read aloud or comprehend single words and simple sentences; *agraphia* (or dysgraphia) is used to describe an acquired deficit in the spelling or grammar of written language.

The correspondence between individual deficits of language function and lesion location does not display a rigid one-to-one relationship and should be conceptualized within the context of the distributed network model. Nonetheless, the classification of aphasic patients into specific clinical syndromes helps to determine the most likely anatomical distribution of the underlying neurologic disease and has implications for etiology and prognosis (Fig. 7-1). Aphasic syndromes can be divided into "central" syndromes, which result from damage to the two epicenters of the language network (Broca's and Wernicke's areas), and "disconnection" syndromes, which arise from lesions that interrupt the functional connectivity of these centers with each other and with the other components of the language network. The syndromes outlined below are idealizations; pure syndromes occur rarely.

Wernicke's Aphasia

Comprehension is impaired for spoken and written language. Language output is fluent but is highly paraphasic and circumlocutious. The tendency for paraphasic errors may be so pronounced that it leads to strings of neologisms, which form the basis of what is known as "jargon aphasia." Speech contains large numbers of function words (e.g., prepositions, conjunctions) but few substantive nouns or verbs that refer to specific actions. The output is therefore voluminous but uninformative. For example, a patient attempts to describe how his wife accidentally threw away something important, perhaps his dentures: "We don't need it anymore, she says. And with it when that was downstairs was my teeth-tick...a...den...dentith...my dentist. And they happened to be in that bag...see? How could this have happened? How could a thing like this happen...So she says we won't need it anymore...I didn't think we'd use it. And now if I have any problems anybody coming a month from now, 4 months from now, or 6 months from now, I have a new dentist. Where my two . . . two little pieces of dentist that I use . . . that I . . . all gone. If she throws the whole thing away . . . visit some friends of hers and she can't throw them away."

Gestures and pantomime do not improve communication. The patient does not seem to realize that his or her language is incomprehensible and may appear angry and impatient when the examiner fails to decipher the meaning of a severely paraphasic statement. In some patients this type of aphasia can be associated with severe agitation and paranoid behaviors. One area of comprehension that may be preserved is the ability to follow commands aimed at axial musculature. The dissociation between the failure to understand simple questions ("What is your name") in a patient who rapidly closes his or her eyes, sits up, or rolls over when asked to do so is characteristic of Wernicke's aphasia and helps to differentiate it from deafness, psychiatric disease, or malingering. Patients with Wernicke's aphasia cannot express their thoughts in meaning-appropriate words and cannot decode the meaning of words in any modality of input. This aphasia therefore has expressive as well as receptive components. Repetition, naming, reading, and writing are also impaired.

The lesion site most commonly associated with Wernicke's aphasia is the posterior portion of the language network and tends to involve at least parts of Wernicke's area. An embolus to the inferior division of the middle cerebral artery, and to the posterior temporal or angular branches in particular, is the most common etiology

(Chap. 17). Intracerebral hemorrhage, severe head trauma, or neoplasm are other causes. A coexisting right hemi- or superior quadrantanopia is common, and mild right nasolabial flattening may be found, but otherwise the examination is often unrevealing. The paraphasic, neologistic speech in an agitated patient with an otherwise unremarkable neurologic examination may lead to the suspicion of a primary psychiatric disorder such as schizophrenia or mania, but the other components characteristic of acquired aphasia and the absence of prior psychiatric disease usually settle the issue. Some patients with Wernicke's aphasia due to intracerebral hemorrhage or head trauma may improve as the hemorrhage or the injury heals. In most other patients, prognosis for recovery is guarded. Fluent transcortical aphasia (transcortical sensory aphasia) is similar to Wernicke's aphasia, but repetition is intact.

Broca's Aphasia

Speech is nonfluent, labored, interrupted by many word-finding pauses, and usually dysarthric. It is impoverished in function words but enriched in meaning-appropriate nouns and verbs. Abnormal word order and the inappropriate deployment of *bound morphemes* (word endings used to denote tenses, possessives, or plurals) lead to a characteristic agrammatism. Speech is telegraphic and pithy but quite informative. In the following passage, a patient with Broca's aphasia describes his medical history: "I see . . .   the dotor, dotor sent me . . . Bosson. Go to hospital. Dotor . . .   kept me beside. Two, tee days, doctor send me home."

   Output may be reduced to a grunt or single word ("yes" or "no"), which is emitted with different intonations in an attempt to express approval or disapproval. In addition to fluency, naming and repetition are also impaired. Comprehension of spoken language is intact, except for syntactically difficult sentences with passive voice structure or embedded clauses. Reading comprehension is also preserved, with the occasional exception of a specific inability to read small grammatical words such as conjunctions and pronouns. The last two features indicate that Broca's aphasia is not just an "expressive" or "motor" disorder and that it may also involve a comprehension deficit for function words and syntax. Patients with Broca's aphasia can be tearful, easily frustrated, and profoundly depressed. Insight into their condition is preserved, in contrast to Wernicke's aphasia. Even when spontaneous speech is severely dysarthric, the patient may be able to display a relatively normal articulation of words when singing. This dissociation has been used to develop specific therapeutic approaches (melodic intonation therapy) for Broca's aphasia. Additional neurologic deficits usually include right facial weakness, hemiparesis or hemiplegia, and a buccofacial apraxia

characterized by an inability to carry out motor commands involving oropharyngeal and facial musculature (e.g., patients are unable to demonstrate how to blow out a match or suck through a straw). Visual fields are intact. The cause is most often infarction of Broca's area (the inferior frontal convolution; Fig. 7-1) and surrounding anterior perisylvian and insular cortex, due to occlusion of the superior division of the middle cerebral artery (Chap. 17). Mass lesions including tumor, intracerebral hemorrhage, or abscess may also be responsible. Small lesions confined to the posterior part of Broca's area may lead to a nonaphasic and often reversible deficit of speech articulation, usually accompanied by mild right facial weakness. When the cause of Broca's aphasia is stroke, recovery of language function generally peaks within 2 to 6 months, after which time further progress is limited. Nonfluent transcortical aphasia (transcortical motor aphasia) is similar to Broca's aphasia, but repetition is intact and agrammatism may be less pronounced.

Global Aphasia

Speech output is nonfluent, and comprehension of spoken language is severely impaired. Naming, repetition, reading, and writing are also impaired. This syndrome represents the combined dysfunction of Broca's and Wernicke's areas and usually results from strokes that involve the entire middle cerebral artery distribution in the left hemisphere. Most patients are initially mute or say a few words, such as "hi" or "yes." Related signs include right hemiplegia, hemisensory loss, and homonymous hemianopia. Occasionally, a patient with a lesion in Wernicke's area will present with a global aphasia that soon resolves into Wernicke's aphasia.

Conduction Aphasia

Speech output is fluent but paraphasic, comprehension of spoken language is intact, and repetition is severely impaired. Naming and writing are also impaired. Reading aloud is impaired, but reading comprehension is preserved. The lesion sites spare Broca's and Wernicke's areas but may induce a functional disconnection between the two so that neural word representations formed in Wernicke's area and adjacent regions cannot be conveyed to Broca's area for assembly into corresponding articulatory patterns. Occasionally, a Wernicke's area lesion gives rise to a transient Wernicke's aphasia that rapidly resolves into a conduction aphasia. The paraphasic output in conduction aphasia interferes with the ability to express meaning, but this deficit is not nearly as severe as the one displayed by patients with Wernicke's aphasia. Associated neurologic signs in conduction aphasia vary according to the primary lesion site.

Anomic Aphasia

This form of aphasia may be considered the "minimal dysfunction" syndrome of the language network. Articulation, comprehension, and repetition are intact, but confrontation naming, word finding, and spelling are impaired. Speech is enriched in function words but impoverished in substantive nouns and verbs denoting specific actions. Language output is fluent but paraphasic, circumlocutious, and uninformative. The lesion sites can be anywhere within the left hemisphere language network, including the middle and inferior temporal gyri. *Anomic aphasia is the single most common language disturbance seen in head trauma, metabolic encephalopathy, and Alzheimer's disease.* The language impairment of Alzheimer's disease almost always leads to fluent aphasias (e.g., anomic, Wernicke's, conduction, or fluent transcortical aphasia). The insidious onset and relentless progression of nonfluent language disturbances (Broca's or nonfluent transcortical aphasia) can be seen in *primary progressive aphasia,* a degenerative syndrome most commonly associated with focal nonspecific neuronal loss or Pick's disease.

Pure Word Deafness

This is not a true aphasic syndrome because the language deficit is modality-specific. The most common lesions are either bilateral or left-sided in the superior temporal gyrus. The net effect of the underlying lesion is to interrupt the flow of information from the unimodal auditory association cortex to Wernicke's area. Patients have no difficulty understanding written language and can express themselves well in spoken or written language. They have no difficulty interpreting and reacting to environmental sounds since primary auditory cortex and subcortical auditory relays are intact. Since auditory information cannot be conveyed to the language network, however, it cannot be decoded into neural word representations and the patient reacts to speech as if it were in an alien tongue that cannot be deciphered. Patients cannot repeat spoken language but have no difficulty naming objects. In time, patients with pure word deafness teach themselves lip reading and may appear to have improved. There may be no additional neurologic findings, but agitated paranoid reactions are frequent in the acute stages. Cerebrovascular lesions are the most frequent cause.

Pure Alexia without Agraphia

This is the visual equivalent of pure word deafness. The lesions (usually a combination of damage to the left occipital cortex and to a posterior sector of the corpus callosum—the splenium) interrupt the flow of visual input into the language network. There is usually a right hemianopia, but the core language network remains unaffected. The patient can understand and produce spoken language, name objects in the left visual hemifield, repeat, and write. However, the patient acts as if illiterate when asked to read even the simplest sentence because the visual information from the written words (presented to the intact left visual hemifield) cannot reach the language network. Objects in the left hemifield may be named accurately because they activate nonvisual associations in the right hemisphere, which, in turn, can access the language network through transcallosal pathways anterior to the splenium. Patients with this syndrome may also lose the ability to name colors, although they can match colors. This is known as a *color anomia.* The most common etiology of pure alexia is a vascular lesion in the territory of the posterior cerebral artery or an infiltrating neoplasm in the left occipital cortex that involves the optic radiations as well as the crossing fibers of the splenium. Since the posterior cerebral artery also supplies medial temporal components of the limbic system, the patient with pure alexia may also experience an amnesia, but this is usually transient because the limbic lesion is unilateral.

Apraxia

This generic term designates a complex motor deficit that cannot be attributed to pyramidal, extrapyramidal, cerebellar, or sensory dysfunction and that does not arise from the patient's failure to understand the nature of the task. The form that is most frequently encountered in clinical practice is known as *ideomotor apraxia.* Commands to perform a specific motor act ("cough," "blow out a match") or to pantomime the use of a common tool (a comb, hammer, straw, or toothbrush) in the absence of the real object cannot be followed. The patient's ability to comprehend the command is ascertained by demonstrating multiple movements and establishing that the correct one can be recognized. Some patients with this type of apraxia can imitate the appropriate movement (when it is demonstrated by the examiner) and show no impairment when handed the real object, indicating that the sensorimotor mechanisms necessary for the movement are intact. Some forms of ideomotor apraxia represent a disconnection of the language network from pyramidal motor systems: commands to execute complex movements are understood but cannot be conveyed to the appropriate motor areas, even though the relevant motor mechanisms are intact. *Buccofacial apraxia* involves apraxic deficits in movements of the face and mouth. *Limb apraxia* encompasses apraxic deficits in movements of the arms and legs. Ideomotor apraxia is almost always caused by lesions in the left hemisphere and is commonly associated with aphasic syndromes, especially Broca's aphasia and conduction aphasia. Its presence cannot be ascertained in patients with language comprehension deficits. The ability to follow commands aimed at axial musculature ("close the eyes," "stand up") is subserved by different pathways and may be intact in otherwise severely aphasic and apraxic patients. Patients with lesions of the anterior corpus callosum can display a special type of ideomotor apraxia confined to the left side of the body. Since the handling of real objects is not impaired, ideomotor apraxia, by itself, causes no major limitation of daily living activities.

Ideational apraxia refers to a deficit in the execution of a goal-directed sequence of movements in patients who have no difficulty executing the individual components of the sequence. For example, when asked to pick up a pen and write, the sequence of uncapping the pen, placing the cap at the opposite end, turning the point towards the writing surface, and writing may be disrupted, and the patient may be seen trying to write with the wrong end of the pen or even with the removed cap. These motor sequencing problems are usually seen in the context of confusional states and dementias rather than focal lesions associated with aphasic conditions. *Limb-kinetic apraxia* involves a clumsiness in the actual use of tools that cannot be attributed to sensory, pyramidal, extrapyramidal, or cerebellar dysfunction. This condition can emerge in the context of focal premotor cortex lesions or *corticobasal ganglionic degeneration.*

Gerstmann's Syndrome

The combination of *acalculia* (impairment of simple arithmetic), *dysgraphia* (impaired writing), *finger anomia* (an inability to name individual fingers such as the index or thumb), and *right-left confusion* (an inability to tell whether a hand, foot, or arm of the patient or examiner is on the right or left side of the body) is known as Gerstmann's syndrome. In making this diagnosis it is important to establish that the finger and left-right naming deficits are not part of a more generalized anomia and that the patient is not otherwise aphasic. When Gerstmann's syndrome is seen in isolation, it is commonly associated with damage to the inferior parietal lobule (especially the angular gyrus) in the left hemisphere.

THE PARIETOFRONTAL NETWORK FOR SPATIAL ORIENTATION: NEGLECT

HEMISPATIAL NEGLECT

Adaptive orientation to significant events within the extrapersonal space is subserved by a large-scale network containing three major cortical components. The *cingu-late cortex* provides access to a limbic-motivational mapping of the extrapersonal space, the *posterior parietal cortex* to a sensorimotor representation of salient extrapersonal events, and the *frontal eye fields* to motor strategies for attentional behaviors (**Fig. 7–2**). Subcortical components of this network include the striatum and the thalamus. Contralesional hemispatial neglect represents one outcome of damage to any of the cortical or subcortical components of this network. *The traditional view that hemispatial neglect always denotes a parietal lobe lesion is inaccurate.* In keeping with this anatomical organization, the clinical manifestations of neglect display three behavioral components: sensory events (or their mental representations) within the neglected hemispace have a lesser impact on overall awareness; there is a paucity of exploratory and orienting acts directed toward the

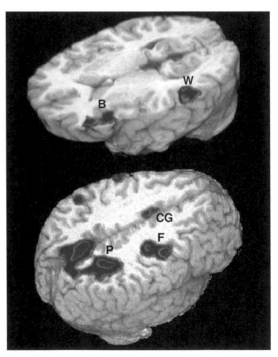

FIGURE 7-2

Functional magnetic resonance imaging of language and spatial attention in neurologically intact subjects. The dark areas show regions of task-related significant activation. (*Top*) The subjects were asked to determine if two words were synonymous. This language task led to the simultaneous activation of the two epicenters of the language network, Broca's area (B) and Wernicke's area (W). The activations are exclusively in the left hemisphere. (*Bottom*) The subjects were asked to shift spatial attention to a peripheral target. This task led to the simultaneous activation of the three epicenters of the attentional network, the posterior parietal cortex (P), the frontal eye fields (F), and the cingulate gyrus (CG). The activations are predominantly in the right hemisphere. (*Courtesy of Darren Gitelman, MD.*)

neglected hemispace; and the patient behaves as if the neglected hemispace was motivationally devalued.

According to one model of spatial cognition, the right hemisphere directs attention within the *entire* extrapersonal space, whereas the left hemisphere directs attention mostly within the contralateral right hemispace. Consequently, unilateral left hemisphere lesions do not give rise to much contralesional neglect since the ipsilateral attentional mechanisms of the right hemisphere can compensate for the loss of the *contralaterally* directed attentional functions of the left hemisphere. Unilateral right hemisphere lesions, however, give rise to severe contralesional left hemispatial neglect because the unaffected left hemisphere does not contain ipsilateral attentional mechanisms. This model is consistent with clinical experience, which shows that contralesional neglect is more common, severe, and lasting after damage to the right hemisphere than after damage to the left hemisphere. Severe neglect for the right hemispace is rare, even in left handers with left hemisphere lesions.

Patients with severe neglect may fail to dress, shave, or groom the left side of the body; may fail to eat food placed on the left side of the tray; and may fail to read the left half of sentences. When the examiner draws a large circle [12 to 15 cm (5 to 6 in.) in diameter] and asks the patient to place the numbers 1 to 12 as if the circle represented the face of a clock, there is a tendency to crowd the numbers on the right side and leave the left side empty. When asked to copy a simple line drawing, the patient fails to copy detail on the left; and when asked to write, there is a tendency to leave an unusually wide margin on the left.

Two bedside tests that are useful in assessing neglect are *simultaneous bilateral stimulation* and *visual target cancellation*. In the former, the examiner provides either unilateral or simultaneous bilateral stimulation in the visual, auditory, and tactile modalities. Following right hemisphere injury, patients who have no difficulty detecting unilateral stimuli on either side experience the bilaterally presented stimulus as coming only from the right. This phenomenon is known as *extinction* and is a manifestation of the sensory-representational aspect of hemispatial neglect. In the target detection task, targets (e.g., As) are interspersed with foils (e.g., other letters of the alphabet) on a 21.5 by 28.0 cm (8.5 by 11 in.) sheet of paper and the patient is asked to circle all the targets. A failure to detect targets on the left is a manifestation of the exploratory deficit in hemispatial neglect (**Fig. 7-3A**). Hemianopia, by itself, does not interfere with performance in this task since the patient is free to turn the head and eyes to the left. The normal tendency in target detection tasks is to start from the left upper quadrant and move systematically in horizontal or vertical sweeps. Some patients show a tendency to start

the process from the right and proceed in a haphazard fashion. This represents a subtle manifestation of left neglect, even if the patient eventually manages to detect all the appropriate targets. Some patients with neglect may also deny the existence of hemiparesis and may even deny ownership of the paralyzed limb, a condition known as *anosognosia*.

Cerebrovascular lesions and neoplasms in the right hemisphere are the most common causes of hemispatial neglect. Depending on the site of the lesion, the patient with neglect may also have hemiparesis, hemihypesthesia, and hemianopia on the left, but these are not invariant findings. The majority of patients display considerable improvement of hemispatial neglect, usually within the first several weeks.

BALINT'S SYNDROME, SIMULTANAGNOSIA, DRESSING APRAXIA, AND CONSTRUCTION APRAXIA

Bilateral involvement of the network for spatial attention, especially its parietal components, leads to a state of severe spatial disorientation known as *Bálint's syndrome*. Bálint's syndrome involves deficits in the orderly visuomotor scanning of the environment (*oculomotor apraxia*) and in accurate manual reaching toward visual targets (*optic ataxia*). The third and most dramatic component of Bálint's syndrome is known as *simultanagnosia* and reflects an inability to integrate visual information in the center of gaze with more peripheral information. The patient gets stuck on the detail that falls in the center of gaze without attempting to scan the visual environment for additional information. The patient with simultanagnosia "misses the forest for the trees." Complex visual scenes cannot be grasped in their entirety, leading to severe limitations in the visual identification of objects and scenes. For example, a patient who is shown a table lamp and asked to name the object may look at its circular base and call it an ash tray. Some patients with simultanagnosia report that objects they look at may suddenly vanish, probably indicating an inability to look back at the original point of gaze after brief saccadic displacements. Movement and distracting stimuli greatly exacerbate the difficulties of visual perception. Simultanagnosia can sometimes occur without the other two components of Bálint's syndrome.

A modification of the letter cancellation task described above can be used for the bedside diagnosis of simultanagnosia. In this modification, some of the targets (e.g., As) are made to be much larger than the others [7.5 to 10 cm vs 2.5 cm (3 to 4 in. vs 1 in.) in height], and all targets are embedded among foils. Patients with simultanagnosia display a counterintuitive but character-

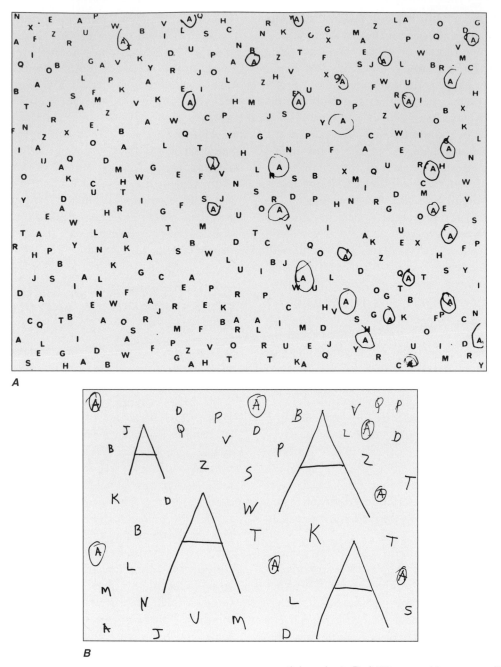

A

B

FIGURE 7-3

A. A 47-year-old man with a large frontoparietal lesion in the right hemisphere was asked to circle all the As. Only targets on the right are circled. This is a manifestation of left hemi-spatial neglect. *B.* A 70-year-old woman with a 2-year history of degenerative dementia was able to circle most of the small targets but ignored the larger ones. This is a manifestation of simultanagnosia.

istic tendency to miss the larger targets (Fig. 7-3B). This occurs because the information needed for the identification of the larger targets cannot be confined to the immediate line of gaze and requires the integration of visual information across a more extensive field of view. The greater difficulty in the detection of the larger targets also indicates that poor acuity is not responsible for the impairment of visual function and that the problem is central rather than peripheral. Bálint's syndrome results from bilateral dorsal parietal lesions; common settings include watershed infarction between the middle and posterior cerebral artery territories, hypoglycemia, sagittal sinus thrombosis, or atypical forms of Alzheimer's disease. In patients with Bálint's syndrome due to stroke, bilateral visual field defects (usually inferior quadrantanopias) are common.

Another manifestation of bilateral (or right-sided) dorsal parietal lobe lesions is *dressing apraxia*. The patient with this condition is unable to align the body axis with the axis of the garment and can be seen struggling as he or she holds a coat from its bottom or extends his or her arm into a fold of the garment rather than into its sleeve. Lesions that involve the posterior parietal cortex also lead to severe difficulties in copying simple line drawings. This is known as a *construction apraxia* and is much more severe if the lesion is in the right hemisphere. In some patients with right hemisphere lesions, the drawing difficulties are confined to the left side of the figure and represent a manifestation of hemispatial neglect; in others, there is a more universal deficit in reproducing contours and three-dimensional perspective. Dressing apraxia and construction apraxia represent special instances of a more general disturbance in spatial orientation.

THE OCCIPITOTEMPORAL NETWORK FOR FACE AND OBJECT RECOGNITION: PROSOPAGNOSIA AND OBJECT AGNOSIA

Perceptual information about faces and objects is initially encoded in primary (striate) visual cortex and adjacent (upstream) peristriate visual association areas. This information is subsequently relayed first to the downstream visual association areas of occipitotemporal cortex and then to other heteromodal and paralimbic areas of the cerebral cortex. Bilateral lesions in the fusiform and lingual gyri of occipitotemporal cortex disrupt this process and interfere with the ability of otherwise intact perceptual information to activate the distributed multimodal associations that lead to the recognition of faces and objects. The resultant face and object recognition deficits are known as *prosopagnosia* and *visual object agnosia*.

The patient with prosopagnosia cannot recognize familiar faces, including, sometimes, the reflection of his or her own face in the mirror. This is not a perceptual deficit since prosopagnosic patients can easily tell if two faces are identical or not. Furthermore, a prosopagnosic patient who cannot recognize a familiar face by visual inspection alone can use auditory cues to reach appropriate recognition if allowed to listen to the person's voice. The deficit in prosopagnosia is therefore modality-specific and reflects the existence of a lesion that prevents the activation of otherwise intact multimodal templates by relevant visual input. Damasio has pointed out that the deficit in prosopagnosia is not limited to the recognition of faces but that it can also extend to the recognition of individual members of larger generic object groups. For example, prosopagnosic patients characteristically have no difficulty with the generic identification of a face as a face or of a car as a car, but they cannot recognize the identity of an individual face or the make of an individual car. This reflects a visual recognition deficit for proprietary features that characterize individual members of an object class. When recognition problems become more generalized and extend to the generic identification of common objects, the condition is known as *visual object agnosia*. In contrast to prosopagnosic patients, those with object agnosia cannot recognize a face as a face or a car as a car.

It is important to distinguish visual object agnosia from anomia. The patient with anomia cannot name the object but can describe its use. In contrast, the patient with visual agnosia is unable either to name a visually presented object or to describe its use. The characteristic lesions in prosopagnosia and visual object agnosia consist of bilateral infarctions in the territory of the posterior cerebral arteries. Associated deficits can include visual field defects (especially superior quadrantanopias) or a centrally based color blindness known as achromatopsia. Rarely, the responsible lesion is unilateral. In such cases, prosopagnosia is associated with lesions in the right hemisphere and object agnosia with lesions in the left.

THE LIMBIC NETWORK FOR MEMORY: AMNESIAS

Limbic and paralimbic areas (such as the hippocampus, amygdala, and entorhinal cortex), the anterior and medial nuclei of the thalamus, the medial and basal parts of the striatum, and the hypothalamus collectively constitute a distributed network known as the *limbic system*. The behavioral affiliations of this network include the coordination of emotion, motivation, autonomic tone, and endocrine function. An additional area of specialization for the limbic network, and the one which is of most relevance to clinical practice, is that of declarative (conscious) memory for recent episodes and experiences. A disturbance in this function is known as an *amnestic state*. In the absence of deficits in motivation, attention, language, or visuospatial function, the clinical diagnosis of a persistent global amnestic state is always associated with bilateral damage to the limbic network, usually within the hippocampo-entorhinal complex or the thalamus.

Although the limbic network is the site of damage for amnestic states, it is almost certainly not the storage site for memories. Memories are stored in widely distributed form throughout the cerebral cortex. The role attributed to the limbic network is to bind these distributed fragments into coherent events and experiences that can sustain conscious recall. Damage to the limbic network does not necessarily destroy memories but interferes with their conscious (declarative) recall in coherent form. The individual fragments of information remain preserved despite the limbic lesions and can sustain what is known as *implicit memory*. For example, patients with amnestic states can acquire new motor or perceptual skills, even though they may have no conscious knowledge of the experiences that led to the acquisition of these skills.

The memory disturbance in the amnestic state is multimodal and includes retrograde and anterograde components. The *retrograde amnesia* involves an inability to recall experiences that occurred before the onset of the amnestic state. Relatively recent events are more vulnerable to retrograde amnesia than more remote and more extensively consolidated events. A patient who comes to the emergency room complaining that he cannot remember his identity but who can remember the events of the previous day is almost certainly not suffering from a neurologic cause of memory disturbance. The second and most important component of the amnestic state is the *anterograde amnesia,* which indicates an inability to store, retain, and recall new knowledge. Patients with amnestic states cannot remember what they ate a few minutes ago or the details of an important event they may have experienced a few hours ago. In the acute stages, there may also be a tendency to fill in memory gaps with inaccurate, fabricated, and often implausible information. This is known as *confabulation*. Patients with the amnestic syndrome forget that they forget and tend to deny the existence of a memory problem when questioned.

The patient with an amnestic state is almost always disoriented, especially to time. Accurate temporal orientation and accurate knowledge of current news rule out a major amnestic state. The anterograde component of an amnestic state can be tested with a list of four to five words read aloud by the examiner up to five times or until the patient can immediately repeat the entire list without intervening delay. In the next phase of testing, the patient is allowed to concentrate on the words and to rehearse them internally for 1 min before being asked to recall them. Accurate performance in this phase indicates that the patient is motivated and sufficiently attentive to hold the words online for at least 1 min. The final phase of the testing involves a retention period of 5 to 10 min, during which the patient is engaged in other tasks. Adequate recall at the end of this interval requires offline storage, retention, and retrieval. Amnestic patients fail this phase of the task and may even forget that they were given a list of words to remember. Accurate recognition of the words by multiple choice in a patient who cannot recall them indicates a less severe memory disturbance that affects mostly the retrieval stage of memory. The retrograde component of an amnesia can be assessed with questions related to autobiographical or historical events. The anterograde component of amnes-

tic states is usually much more prominent than the retrograde component. In rare instances, usually associated with temporal lobe epilepsy or benzodiazepine intake, the retrograde component may dominate.

The assessment of memory can be quite challenging. Bedside evaluations may only detect the most severe impairments. Less severe memory impairments, as in the case of patients with temporal lobe epilepsy, mild head injury, or early dementia, require quantitative evaluations by neuropsychologists. Confusional states caused by toxic-metabolic encephalopathies and some types of frontal lobe damage interfere with attentional capacity and lead to secondary memory impairments, even in the absence of any limbic lesions. This sort of memory impairment can be differentiated from the amnestic state by the presence of additional impairments in the attention-related tasks described below in the section on the frontal lobes.

Many neurologic diseases can give rise to an amnestic state. These include tumors (of the sphenoid wing, posterior corpus callosum, thalamus, or medial temporal lobe), infarctions (in the territories of the anterior or posterior cerebral arteries), head trauma, herpes simplex encephalitis, Wernicke-Korsakoff encephalopathy, paraneoplastic limbic encephalitis, and degenerative dementias such as Alzheimer's or Pick's disease. The one common denominator of all these diseases is that they lead to the bilateral lesions within one or more components in the limbic network, most commonly the hippocampus, entorhinal cortex, the mammillary bodies of the hypothalamus, and the limbic thalamus. Occasionally, unilateral left-sided lesions can give rise to an amnestic state, but the memory disorder tends to be transient. Depending on the nature and distribution of the underlying neurologic disease, the patient may also have visual field deficits, eye movement limitations, or cerebellar findings.

Transient global amnesia (TGA) is a distinctive syndrome usually seen in late middle age. Patients become acutely disoriented and repeatedly ask who they are, where they are, what they are doing. The spell is characterized by anterograde amnesia (inability to retain new information) and a retrograde amnesia for relatively recent events that occurred before the onset. The syndrome usually resolves within 24 to 48 h and is followed by the filling-in of the period affected by the retrograde amnesia, although there is persistent loss of memory for the events that occurred during the ictus. Recurrences are noted in ~20% of patients. Migraine, temporal lobe seizures, and transient ischemic events in the posterior cerebral territory have been postulated as causes of transient global amnesia. Recent studies of diffusion-weighted imaging of the hippocampus in TGA patients support a vascular etiology, at least in some patients. The absence of associated neurologic findings may occasionally lead to the incorrect diagnosis of a psychiatric disorder.

THE PREFRONTAL NETWORK FOR ATTENTION AND BEHAVIOR

Approximately one-third of all the cerebral cortex in the human brain is located in the frontal lobes. The frontal lobes can be subdivided into motor-premotor, dorsolateral prefrontal, medial prefrontal, and orbitofrontal components. The terms *frontal lobe syndrome* and *prefrontal cortex* refer only to the last three of these four components. These are the parts of the cerebral cortex that show the greatest phylogenetic expansion in primates and especially in humans. The dorsolateral prefrontal, medial prefrontal, and orbitofrontal areas, and the subcortical structures with which they are interconnected (i.e., the head of the caudate and the dorsomedial nucleus of the thalamus), collectively make up a large-scale network that coordinates exceedingly complex aspects of human cognition and behavior.

The prefrontal network plays an important role in behaviors that require an integration of thought with emotion and motivation. There is no simple formula for summarizing the diverse functional affiliations of the prefrontal network. Its integrity appears important for the simultaneous awareness of context, options, consequences, relevance, and emotional impact so as to allow the formulation of adaptive inferences, decisions, and actions. Damage to this part of the brain impairs mental flexibility, reasoning, hypothesis formation, abstract thinking, foresight, judgment, the online (attentive) holding of information, and the ability to inhibit inappropriate responses. Behaviors impaired by prefrontal cortex lesions, especially those related to the manipulation of mental content, are often referred to as "executive functions."

Even very large bilateral prefrontal lesions may leave all sensory, motor, and basic cognitive functions intact while leading to isolated but dramatic alterations of personality and behavior. The most common clinical manifestations of damage to the prefrontal network take the form of two relatively distinct syndromes. In the *frontal abulic syndrome,* the patient shows a loss of initiative, creativity, and curiosity and displays a pervasive emotional blandness and apathy. In the *frontal disinhibition syndrome,* the patient becomes socially disinhibited and shows severe impairments of judgment, insight, and foresight. The dissociation between intact intellectual function and a total lack of even rudimentary common sense is striking. Despite the preservation of all essential memory functions, the patient cannot learn from experience and continues to display inappropriate behaviors without appearing to feel emotional pain, guilt, or regret when such behaviors repeatedly lead to disastrous consequences. The impairments may emerge only in real-life situations when behavior is under minimal external control and may not be apparent within the structured environment of the medical office. Testing judgment by asking patients what they would do if they detected a fire in a theater or found a stamped and addressed envelope on the road is not very informative since patients who answer these questions wisely in the office may still act very foolishly in the more complex real-life setting. The physician must therefore be prepared to make a diagnosis of frontal lobe disease on the basis of historic information alone even when the office examination of mental state may be quite intact.

The abulic syndrome tends to be associated with damage to the dorsolateral prefrontal cortex, and the disinhibition syndrome with the medial prefrontal or orbitofrontal cortex. These syndromes tend to arise almost exclusively after bilateral lesions, most frequently in the setting of head trauma, stroke, ruptured aneurysms, hydrocephalus, tumors (including metastases, glioblastoma, and falx or olfactory groove meningiomas), or focal degenerative diseases. Unilateral lesions confined to the prefrontal cortex may remain silent until the pathology spreads to the other side. The emergence of developmentally primitive reflexes, also known as frontal release signs, such as grasping (elicited by stroking the palm) and sucking (elicited by stroking the lips) are seen primarily in patients with large structural lesions that extend into the premotor components of the frontal lobes or in the context of metabolic encephalopathies. The vast majority of patients with prefrontal lesions and frontal lobe behavioral syndromes do not display these reflexes.

Damage to the frontal lobe disrupts a variety of attention-related functions including working memory (the transient online holding of information), concentration span, the scanning and retrieval of stored information, the inhibition of immediate but inappropriate responses, and mental flexibility. The capacity for focusing on a trend of thought and the ability to voluntarily shift the focus of attention from one thought or stimulus to another can become impaired. Digit span (which should be seven forward and five reverse) is decreased; the recitation of the months of the year in reverse order (which should take less than 15 s) is slowed; and the fluency in producing words starting with a, f, or s that can be generated in 1 min (normally 12 or more per letter) is diminished even in nonaphasic patients. Characteristically, there is a progressive slowing of performance as the task proceeds; e.g., the patient asked to count backwards by 3s may say "100, 97, 94, . . 91, ... 88," etc., and may not complete the task. In "go–no-go" tasks (where the instruction is to raise the finger upon hearing one tap but to keep it still upon hearing two taps), the patient shows a characteristic inability to keep still in response to the "no go" stimulus; mental flexibility (tested by the ability to shift from one criterion to another in sorting or matching tasks) is impoverished; distractibility by irrelevant stimuli is increased; and there is a pronounced tendency for impersistence and perseveration.

These attentional deficits disrupt the orderly registration and retrieval of new information and lead to *secondary* memory deficits. Such memory deficits can be differentiated from the *primary* memory impairments of the amnestic state by showing that they improve when the attentional load of the task is decreased. Working memory (also known as immediate memory) is an attentional function based on the temporary online holding of information. It is closely associated with the integrity of the prefrontal network and the ascending reticular activating system. Retentive memory, on the other hand, depends on the stable (offline) storage of information and is associated with the integrity of the limbic network. The distinction of the underlying neural mechanisms is illustrated by the observation that severely amnestic patients who cannot remember events that occurred a few minutes ago may have intact if not superior working memory capacity as shown in tests of digit span.

Lesions in the caudate nucleus or in the dorsomedial nucleus of the thalamus (subcortical components of the prefrontal network) can also produce a frontal lobe syndrome. This is one reason why the mental state changes associated with degenerative basal ganglia diseases, such as Parkinson's or Huntington's disease, may take the form of a frontal lobe syndrome. Because of its widespread connections with other regions of association cortex, one essential computational role of the prefrontal network is to function as an integrator, or "orchestrator," for other networks. Bilateral multifocal lesions of the cerebral hemispheres, none of which are individually large enough to cause specific cognitive deficits such as aphasia or neglect, can collectively interfere with the connectivity and integrating function of prefrontal cortex. A frontal lobe syndrome is the single most common behavioral profile associated with a variety of bilateral multifocal brain diseases including metabolic encephalopathy, multiple sclerosis, vitamin B_{12} deficiency, and others. In fact, the vast majority of patients with the clinical diagnosis of a frontal lobe syndrome tend to have lesions that do not involve prefrontal cortex but involve either the subcortical components of the prefrontal network or its connections with other parts of the brain. In order to avoid making a diagnosis of "frontal lobe syndrome" in a patient with no evidence of frontal cortex disease, it is advisable to use the diagnostic term *frontal network syndrome,* with

the understanding that the responsible lesions can lie anywhere within this distributed network.

The patient with frontal lobe disease raises potential dilemmas in differential diagnosis: the abulia and blandness may be misinterpreted as depression, and the disinhibition as idiopathic mania or acting-out. Appropriate intervention may be delayed while a treatable tumor keeps expanding. An informed approach to frontal lobe disease and its behavioral manifestations may help to avoid such errors.

CARING FOR THE PATIENT WITH DEFICITS OF HIGHER CEREBRAL FUNCTION

Some of the deficits described in this chapter are so complex that they may bewilder not only the patient and family but also the physician. It is imperative to carry out a systematic clinical evaluation in order to characterize the nature of the deficits and explain them in lay terms to the patient and family. Such an explanation can allay at least some of the anxieties, address the mistaken impression that the deficit (e.g., social disinhibition or inability to recognize family members) is psychologically motivated, and lead to practical suggestions for daily living activities. The consultation of a skilled neuropsychologist may aid in the formulation of diagnosis and management. Patients with simultanagnosia, for example, may benefit from the counterintuitive instruction to stand back when they cannot find an item so that a greater search area falls within the immediate field of gaze. Some patients with frontal lobe disease can be extremely irritable and abusive to spouses and yet display all the appropriate social graces during the visit to the medical office. In such cases, the history may be more important than the bedside examination in charting a course of treatment.

Reactive depression is common in patients with higher cerebral dysfunction and should be treated. These patients may be sensitive to the usual doses of antidepressants or anxiolytics and deserve a careful titration of dosage. Brain damage may cause a dissociation between feeling states and their expression, so that a patient who may superficially appear jocular could still be suffering from an underlying depression that deserves to be treated. In many cases, agitation may be controlled with reassurance. In other cases, treatment with benzodiazepines or sedating antidepressants may become necessary. The use of neuroleptics for the control of agitation should be reserved for refractory cases since extrapyramidal side effects are frequent in patients with coexisting brain damage.

Spontaneous improvement of cognitive deficits due to acute neurologic lesions is common. It is most rapid in the first few weeks but may continue for up to 2 years, especially in young individuals with single brain lesions. The mechanisms for this recovery are incompletely understood. Some of the initial deficits appear to arise from remote dysfunction (diaschisis) in parts of the brain that are interconnected with the site of initial injury. Improvement in these patients may reflect, at least in part, a normalization of the remote dysfunction. Other mechanisms may involve functional reorganization in surviving neurons adjacent to the injury or the compensatory use of homologous structures, e.g., the right superior temporal gyrus with recovery from Wernicke's aphasia. In some patients with large lesions involving Broca's and Wernicke's areas, only Wernicke's area may show contralateral compensatory reorganization (or bilateral functionality), giving rise to a situation where a lesion that should have caused a global aphasia becomes associated with a residual Broca's aphasia. Prognosis for recovery from aphasia is best when Wernicke's area is spared. Cognitive rehabilitation procedures have been used in the treatment of higher cortical deficits. There are few controlled studies, but some do show a benefit of rehabilitation in the recovery from hemispatial neglect and aphasia. Some types of deficits may be more prone to recovery than others. For example, patients with nonfluent aphasias are more likely to benefit from speech therapy than patients with fluent aphasias and comprehension deficits. In general, lesions that lead to a denial of illness (e.g., anosognosia) are associated with cognitive deficits that are more resistant to rehabilitation. The recovery of higher cortical dysfunction is rarely complete. Periodic neuropsychological assessment is necessary for quantifying the pace of the improvement and for generating specific recommendations for cognitive rehabilitation, modifications in the home environment, and the timetable for returning to school or work.

In general medical practice, most patients with deficits in higher cognitive functions will be suffering from dementia. There is a mistaken belief that dementias are anatomically diffuse and that they cause global cognitive impairments. This is only true at the terminal stages. During most of the clinical course, dementias are exquisitely selective with respect to anatomy and cognitive pattern. Alzheimer's disease, for example, causes the greatest destruction in medial temporal areas belonging to the memory network and is clinically characterized by a correspondingly severe amnesia. There are other dementias where memory is intact. Frontal lobe dementia results from a selective degeneration of the frontal lobe and leads to a gradual dissolution of behavior and complex attention. Primary progressive aphasia is characterized by a gradual atrophy of the left perisylvian language network and leads to a progressive dissolution of language that can remain isolated for up to 10 years. An enlightened approach to the differential diagnosis and treatment of these patients requires an understanding of the principles that link neural networks to higher cerebral functions.

FURTHER READINGS

DAMASIO AR, DAMASIO H: Aphasia and the neural basis of language, in *Principles of Behavioral and Cognitive Neurology,* 2d ed, M-M Mesulam (ed). New York, Oxford University Press, 2000

LEIGUARDA RC, MARSDEN CD: Limb apraxias. Higher-order disorders of sensorimotor integration. Brain 123:860, 2000

☑ MEINZER M et al: Long-term stability of improved language functions in chronic aphasia after constraint-induced aphasia therapy. Stroke 36:1462,2005

Trial of short-term intense aphasia rehabilitation showed promising results.

MESULAM M-M: Behavioral neuroanatomy: Large-scale networks, association cortex, frontal syndromes, the limbic system and hemispheric specializations, in *Principles of Behavioral and Cognitive Neurology,* 2d ed, M-M Mesulam (ed). New York, Oxford University Press, 2000

———: The human frontal lobes: Transcending the default mode through contingent encoding, in *Principles of Frontal Lobe Function,* DT Stuss, RT Knight (eds). New York, Oxford University Press, 2002

SEDLACZEK O et al: Detection of delayed focal MR changes in the lateral hippocampus in transient global amnesia. Neurology 62:2165, 2004

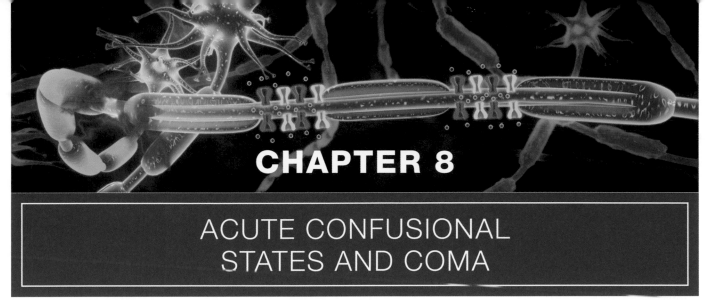

CHAPTER 8

ACUTE CONFUSIONAL STATES AND COMA

Allan H. Ropper

Confusional states and coma are among the most common problems in general medicine. They account for a substantial portion of admissions to emergency wards and occur frequently on all hospital services. Because confusion and a diminished level of consciousness frequently coexist and are caused by many of the same diseases, they are presented together here, but from a medical perspective they have different clinical characteristics and physiologic explanations.

Almost all instances of diminished alertness can be traced to widespread abnormalities of the cerebral hemispheres or to reduced activity of a special thalamocortical alerting system termed the *reticular activating system* (RAS). The proper functioning of this system, its ascending projections to the cortex, and the cortex itself are required to maintain alertness and coherence of thought.

THE CONFUSIONAL STATE

Confusion is a mental and behavioral state of reduced comprehension, coherence, and capacity to reason. Inattention, as defined by the inability to sustain uninterrupted thought and actions, and disorientation are its earliest outward signs. As the state of confusion worsens, there are more global mental failings, including impairments of memory, perception, comprehension, problem solving, language, praxis, visuospatial function, and various aspects of emotional behavior that are attributable to particular regions of the brain. In some instances an apparent confusional state may be due to an isolated deficit in mental function such as an impairment of language (*aphasia*), loss of memory (*amnesia*), or lack of appreciation of spatial relations of self or the external environment (*agnosia*) (Chap. 7). Confusion is also a feature of dementia (Chap. 18), in which case the chronicity of the process distinguishes it from an acute encephalopathy.

The confused patient is usually subdued, not inclined to speak, and is physically inactive. A state of confusion that is accompanied by agitation, hallucinations, tremor, and illusions (misperceptions of environmental sight, sound, or touch) is termed *delirium,* as typified by delirium tremens from alcohol or drug withdrawal.

APPROACH TO THE PATIENT WITH A CONFUSIONAL STATE

Confusion and delirium always signify a disorder of the nervous system. They may be the major manifestations of a head injury; a seizure; drug toxicity (or drug withdrawal); a metabolic disorder resulting from hepatic, renal, pulmonary or cardiac failure; a systemic infection; meningitis or encephalitis; or a chronic dementing disease.

Evaluation begins with a careful history emphasizing the patient's condition before the onset of confusion. The clinical examination should focus on signs of diminished attentiveness, disorientation, and drowsiness and on the presence of localizing neurologic signs. From the clinical data the clinician is directed to the appropriate laboratory tests (see below). Often, even after all diagnostic tests are completed, one may still not know the cause of a confusional state. The patient should then be observed in the hospital for a number of days under stable conditions. New clues may appear or confusion caused by a medication may resolve.

Orientation and memory are tested by asking the patient the date, inclusive of month, day, year, and day of week; the precise place; and some items of universally known information (the names of the President and Vice President, a recent national event, the state capital). Further probing may be necessary to reveal a defect in clarity—why is the patient in the hospital; what is his or her address, zip code, telephone number, social security number? Problems of increasing complexity may be pursued, but they usually provide little additional information. Attention and coherence of thought can be gauged by the accuracy and speed of responses but are examined more explicitly by having the patient repeat strings of numbers (most adults easily retain seven digits forward and four backward), spell a word such as "world" backwards, and perform serial calculations—tests of serial subtraction of 3 from 30 or 7 from 100 are useful. It is the inability to sustain coherent mental activity in performing tasks such as these that exposes the most subtle confusional states.

Other salient findings are the level of alertness, which fluctuates if there is drowsiness; indications of focal damage of the cerebrum such as hemiparesis, hemianopia, and aphasia; or adventitious movements of myoclonus or partial convulsions. The language of the confused patient may be disorganized and rambling, even to the extent of incorporating paraphasic words. These features, along with impaired comprehension that is due mainly to inattention, may be mistaken for aphasia.

One of the most specific signs of a metabolic encephalopathy is *asterixis,* which is an arrhythmic flapping tremor that is typically elicited by asking the patient to hold the arms outstretched with the wrists and hands fully extended. After a few seconds, there is a large jerking lapse in the posture of the hand and then a rapid return to the original position. The same movements can be found in any tonically held posture, even of the protruded tongue. Bilateral asterixis always signifies a metabolic encephalopathy, e.g., from hepatic failure, hypercapnia, or drug intoxication, especially with anticonvulsant medications. Myoclonic jerking and tremor are typical of uremic encephalopathy or

exposure to antipsychotic drugs such as lithium, phenothiazines, or butyrophenones; myoclonus is also common with severe anoxic cerebral damage.

Confusion in the postoperative period, particularly after cardiac and extensive orthopedic procedures, is common but at times so subtle as to escape attention. Often a careful history will reveal that a mild but compensated dementia existed prior to the operation. Medications, particularly those with anticholinergic activity (including meperidine), inadvertent withdrawal from sleeping pills or alcohol, fever, and any of the endogenous metabolic derangements listed above may be responsible, or a stroke may have occurred. In many cases, particularly in the elderly, transient confusion and drowsiness arise with a febrile infection of the urinary tract, lungs, blood, or peritoneum. The term *septic encephalopathy* is used to describe this association, but the mechanism by which systemic infection leads to cerebral dysfunction is unknown.

Distinguishing dementia from an acute confusional state is a problem in the elderly. The two may coexist if an acute medical problem or a poorly tolerated medication supervenes in a mildly demented patient, producing a so-called beclouded dementia. The memory loss of dementia brings about a confusional state that varies little in severity from day to day. Poor mental performance in dementia is manifested primarily as incomplete recollection; inadequate access to names and words, and ideas; and the inability to retain new information, thus affecting orientation and factual knowledge. In contrast to the acute confusional states, attention, alertness, and coherence are preserved until the most advanced stages. Dementia in its advanced stages produces a chronic confusion with breakdown of all types of mental performance; the distinction from an acute encephalopathy then depends mainly on the longstanding nature of the condition.

Treatment of the confused patient requires that all unnecessary medication be stopped, metabolic alterations be rectified, and infection be treated. Skilled nursing and a quiet room with a window are important. Careful explanations should be given at regular intervals to the family. In the elderly, regular reorientation and active measures to lessen risk factors (sleep deprivation, immobility, and vision and hearing impairments) have been shown to reduce the number and severity of episodes of delirium in hospitalized patients.

COMA AND RELATED DISORDERS OF CONSCIOUSNESS

States of reduced alertness and responsiveness represent a continuum that in its severest form is called *coma,* a deep sleeplike state from which the patient cannot be aroused. *Stupor* refers to lesser degrees of unarousability in which the patient can be awakened only by vigorous stimuli, accompanied by motor behavior that leads to avoidance of uncomfortable or aggravating stimuli. *Drowsiness,* which is familiar to all persons, simulates light sleep and is characterized by easy arousal and the persistence of alertness for brief periods. Drowsiness and stupor are usually attended by some degree of confusion. A narrative description of the level of arousal and of the type of responses evoked by various stimuli precisely as observed at the bedside is preferable to ambiguous terms such as semicoma or obtundation.

Several other neurologic conditions render patients apparently unresponsive and simulate coma, and certain subsyndromes of coma must be considered separately because of their special significance. Among the latter, the *vegetative state* signifies an awake but unresponsive state. These patients have emerged from coma after a period of days or weeks to an unresponsive state in which the eyelids are open, giving the appearance of wakefulness. Yawning, coughing, swallowing, as well as limb and head movements persist, but there are few, if any, meaningful responses to the external and internal environment—in essence, an "awake coma." Respiratory and autonomic functions are retained. The term "vegetative" is unfortunate as it is subject to misinterpretation by lay persons. There are always accompanying signs that indicate extensive damage in both cerebral hemispheres, e.g., decerebrate or decorticate limb posturing and absent responses to visual stimuli (see below). In the closely related *minimally conscious state* the patient may make intermittent rudimentary vocal or motor responses. Cardiac arrest and head injuries are the most common causes of the vegetative state (Chaps. 15 and 16). The prognosis for regaining mental faculties once the vegetative state has supervened for several months is almost nil, hence the term *persistent vegetative state.* Most reports of dramatic recovery, when investigated carefully, are found to yield to the usual rules for prognosis, but there have been rare instances of awakening to a demented condition.

Certain clinical states are prone to be misinterpreted as stupor or coma. *Akinetic mutism* refers to a partially or fully awake patient who is able to form impressions and think but remains immobile and mute, particularly when unstimulated. The condition results from damage in the regions of the medial thalamic nuclei, the frontal lobes (particularly situated deeply or on the orbitofrontal

surfaces), or from hydrocephalus. The term *abulia* is used to describe a mental and physical slowness and diminished ability to initiate activity that is in essence a mild form of akinetic mutism, with the same anatomical origins. *Catatonia* is a curious hypomobile and mute syndrome associated with a major psychosis. In the typical form patients appear awake with eyes open but make no voluntary or responsive movements, although they blink spontaneously, swallow, and may not appear distressed. Often, the eyes are half-open as if the patient is in a fog or light sleep. There are signs that indicate the patient is responsive, though it may take some ingenuity on the part of the examiner to demonstrate these. For example, eyelid elevation is actively resisted, blinking occurs in response to a visual threat, and the eyes move concomitantly with head rotation, all of which are inconsistent with a brain lesion. It is characteristic but not invariable in catatonia for the limbs to retain the posture, no matter how bizarre, in which they have been placed by the examiner ("waxy flexibility," or catalepsy.) Upon recovery, such patients have some memory of events that occurred during their catatonic stupor. The appearance is superficially similar to akinetic mutism, but clinical evidence of cerebral damage is lacking.

The *locked-in state* describes a pseudocoma in which an awake patient has no means of producing speech or volitional movement in order to indicate that he is awake, but vertical eye movements and lid elevation remain unimpaired, thus allowing the patient to signal. Such individuals have written entire treatises using Morse code. Infarction or hemorrhage of the ventral pons, which transects all descending corticospinal and corticobulbar pathways, is the usual cause. A similar awake but de-efferented state occurs as a result of total paralysis of the musculature in severe cases of Guillain-Barré syndrome (Chap. 35), critical illness neuropathy (Chap. 15), and pharmacologic neuromuscular blockade.

THE ANATOMY AND PHYSIOLOGY OF UNCONSCIOUSNESS

To the extent that all complex waking behaviors require the widespread participation of the cerebral cortex, consciousness cannot exist without the activity of this structure. The RAS, a loosely grouped aggregation of neurons located in the upper brainstem and medial thalamus, maintains the cerebral cortex in a state of wakeful consciousness. It follows that the principal causes of coma are (1) lesions that damage the RAS or its projections; (2) destruction of large portions of both cerebral hemispheres; and (3) suppression of reticulo-cerebral function by drugs, toxins, or metabolic derangements such as hypoglycemia, anoxia, azotemia, or hepatic failure.

The regions of the reticular formation that are critical to the maintenance of wakefulness extend from the caudal midbrain to the lower thalamus. The neurons of the RAS project rostrally to the cortex primarily via thalamic relay nuclei that in turn exert a tonic influence on the activity of the entire cerebral cortex. The behavioral arousal effected by somesthetic, auditory, and visual stimuli depends upon the rich reciprocal innervation that the RAS receives from these sensory systems. A most important practical consideration derives from the anatomical proximity of the RAS to structures that control pupillary function and eye movements. Pupillary enlargement and loss of vertical and adduction movements of the globes suggest that upper brainstem damage may be the source of coma.

Coma due to Cerebral Mass Lesions and Herniations

The cranial cavity is separated into compartments by infoldings of the dura—the two cerebral hemispheres are separated by the falx, and the anterior and posterior fossae by the tentorium. *Herniation* refers to displacement of brain tissue into a compartment that it normally does not occupy. Many of the signs associated with coma, and indeed coma itself, can be attributed to these tissue shifts (**Fig. 8–1**).

Uncal transtentorial herniation refers to impaction of the anterior medial temporal gyrus (the uncus) into the an-

terior portion of the tentorial opening. The displaced tissue compresses the third nerve as it traverses the subarachnoid space and results in enlargement of the ipsilateral pupil (putatively because the fibers subserving parasympathetic pupillary function are located peripherally in the nerve). The coma that follows may be due to lateral compression of the midbrain against the opposite tentorial edge by the displaced parahippocampal gyrus (**Fig. 8–2**). In some cases the lateral displacement causes compression of the opposite cerebral peduncle, producing a Babinski response and hemiparesis contralateral to the original hemiparesis (the Kernohan–Woltman sign). In addition to compressing the upper brainstem, tissue shifts, including herniations, may compress major blood vessels, particularly the anterior and posterior cerebral arteries as they pass over the tentorial reflections, thus producing brain infarctions. The distortions may also entrap portions of the ventricular system, resulting in regional hydrocephalus.

Central transtentorial herniation denotes a symmetric downward movement of the upper thalamic region through the tentorial opening. Miotic pupils and drowsiness are the heralding signs. Both temporal and central herniations are thought to cause progressive compression of the brainstem from above: first the midbrain, then the pons, and finally the medulla. The result is a sequential appearance of neurologic signs that correspond to the affected level. Other forms of herniation are *transfalcial herniation* (displacement of the cingulate gyrus under the falx and across the midline), and *foraminal herniation* (downward forcing of the cerebellar tonsils into the foramen magnum).

A direct relationship between the various configurations of transtentorial herniations and coma is not always found. Displacement of deep brain structures by a mass in any direction, with or without herniation, is adequate to compress the region of the RAS and result in coma. Furthermore, drowsiness and stupor typically occur with moderate horizontal shifts at the level of the diencephalon (thalami) well before transtentorial or other herniations are evident. Lateral shift is easily quantified on axial images of computed tomography (CT) and magnetic resonance imaging (MRI) scans (Fig. 8–2). In cases of *acutely appearing masses,* a fairly consistent relationship exists between the degree of horizontal displacement of midline structures and the level of consciousness. Specifically, horizontal displacement of the pineal calcification of 3 to 5 mm is generally associated with drowsiness, 6 to 8 mm with stupor, and >9 mm with coma. At the same time, intrusion of the medial temporal lobe into the tentorial opening may be apparent on MRI and CT scan by an obliteration of the cisterns that surround the upper brainstem.

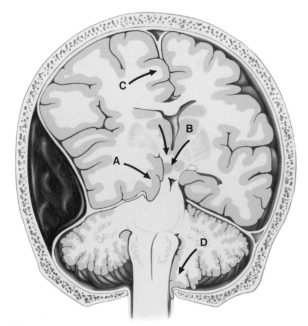

FIGURE 8-1

Types of cerebral herniation; (A) uncal; (B) central; (C) transfalcial; (D) foraminal

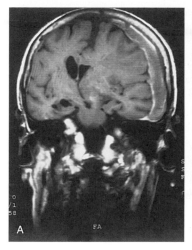
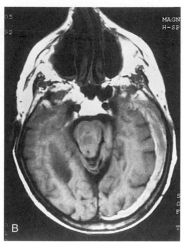

FIGURE 8-2

Coronal (*A*) and axial (*B*) magnetic resonance images from a stuporous patient with a left third nerve palsy as a result of a large left-sided subdural hematoma (seen as a gray-white rim). The upper midbrain and lower thalamic regions are compressed and displaced horizontally away from the mass, and there is transtentorial herniation of the medial temporal lobe structures, including the uncus anteriorly. The lateral ventricle opposite to the hematoma has become enlarged as a result of compression of the third ventricle.

Coma and Confusional States due to Metabolic Disorders

Many systemic metabolic abnormalities cause coma by interrupting the delivery of energy substrates (hypoxia, ischemia, hypoglycemia) or by altering neuronal excitability (drug and alcohol intoxication, anesthesia, and epilepsy). The same metabolic abnormalities that produce coma may in milder form induce widespread cortical dysfunction and an acute confusional state. Thus, in metabolic encephalopathies, clouded consciousness and coma are in a continuum. Neuropathologic changes are variable—prominent in hypoxia-ischemia, evident as astrocytic changes in hepatic coma, and negligible in renal and other metabolic encephalopathies.

Cerebral neurons are fully dependent on cerebral blood flow (CBF) and the related delivery of oxygen and glucose. CBF approximates 75 mL per 100 g/min in gray matter and 30 mL per 100 g/min in white matter (mean = 55 mL per 100 g/min); oxygen consumption is 3.5 mL per 100 g/min, and glucose utilization is 5 mg per 100 g/min. Brain stores of glucose provide energy for ~2 min after blood flow is interrupted, and oxygen stores last 8 to 10 s after the cessation of blood flow. Simultaneous hypoxia and ischemia exhaust glucose more rapidly. The electroencephalogram (EEG) rhythm in these circumstances becomes diffusely slowed, typical of metabolic encephalopathies, and as conditions of substrate delivery worsen, eventually all recordable brain electrical activity ceases. In almost all instances of metabolic encephalopathy, the global metabolic activity of the brain is reduced in proportion to the degree of unconsciousness.

Conditions such as hypoglycemia, hyponatremia, hyperosmolarity, hypercapnia, hypercalcemia, and he-

patic and renal failure are associated with a variety of alterations in neurons and astrocytes. The reversible effects of these conditions on the brain are not understood, but may result from impaired energy supplies, changes in ion fluxes across neuronal membranes, and neurotransmitter abnormalities. For example, the high brain ammonia concentration of hepatic coma interferes with cerebral energy metabolism and with the Na^+, K^+-ATPase pump, increases the number and size of astrocytes, alters nerve cell function, and causes increased concentrations of potentially toxic products of ammonia metabolism; it may also result in abnormalities of neurotransmitters, including putative "false" neurotransmitters that are active at receptor sites. Apart from hyperammonemia, which of these mechanisms is of critical importance is not clear. The mechanism of the encephalopathy of renal failure is also not known. Unlike ammonia, urea itself does not produce central nervous system (CNS) toxicity. A multifactorial causation has been proposed, including increased permeability of the blood-brain barrier to toxic substances such as organic acids and an increase in brain calcium or cerebrospinal fluid (CSF) phosphate content.

Coma and seizures are a common accompaniment of any large shifts in sodium and water balance. These changes in osmolarity arise from systemic medical disorders including diabetic ketoacidosis, the nonketotic hyperosmolar state, and hyponatremia from any cause (e.g., water intoxication, excessive secretion of antidiuretic hormone or atrial natriuretic peptides). The volume of brain water correlates with the level of consciousness in these states, but other factors also play a role. Sodium levels <125 mmol/L induce confusion and <115 mmol/L are associated with coma and convulsions. In hyperosmolar coma the serum osmolarity generally exceeds 350 mosmol/L. *As in most other metabolic encephalopathies, the severity of neurologic change depends to a large degree on the rapidity with which the serum changes occur.* Hypercapnia depresses the level of consciousness in proportion to the rise in CO_2 tension in the blood; the level of consciousness also depends on the rapidity of change. The pathophysiology of other metabolic encephalopathies such as hypercalcemia, hypothyroidism, vitamin B_{12} deficiency, and hypothermia are incompletely understood but must also reflect derangements of CNS biochemistry and membrane function.

Epileptic Coma

Continuous, generalized electrical discharges of the cortex (*seizures*) are associated with coma even in the absence of epileptic motor activity (*convulsions*). The self-limited coma that follows seizures, termed the *postictal state,* may be due to exhaustion of energy reserves or effects of locally toxic molecules that are the byproduct of seizures. The postictal state produces a pattern of continuous, generalized slowing of the background EEG activity similar to that of other metabolic encephalopathies.

Pharmacologic Coma

This class of encephalopathy is in large measure reversible and leaves no residual damage providing hypoxia does not supervene. Many drugs and toxins are capable of depressing nervous system function. Some produce coma by affecting both the brainstem nuclei, including the RAS, and the cerebral cortex. The combination of cortical and brainstem signs, which occurs in certain drug overdoses, may lead to an incorrect diagnosis of structural brainstem disease.

APPROACH TO THE PATIENT IN A COMA

Acute respiratory and cardiovascular problems should be attended to prior to neurologic assessment. In most instances, a complete medical evaluation, except for vital signs, funduscopy, and examination for nuchal rigidity, may be deferred until the neurologic evaluation has established the severity and nature of coma. *The approach to the patient with trauma is discussed in Chap. 16.*

History

In many cases, the cause of coma is immediately evident (e.g., trauma, cardiac arrest, or known drug ingestion). In the remainder, certain points are especially useful: (1) the circumstances and rapidity with which neurologic symptoms developed; (2) the antecedent symptoms (confusion, weakness, headache, fever, seizures, dizziness, double vision, or vomiting); (3) the use of medications, illicit drugs, or alcohol; and (4) chronic liver, kidney, lung, heart, or other medical disease. Direct interrogation or telephone calls to family and observers on the scene are an important part of the initial evaluation. Ambulance technicians often provide the most useful information.

General Physical Examination

The temperature, pulse, respiratory rate and pattern, and blood pressure should be measured quickly. Fever suggests a systemic infection, bacterial meningitis, or encephalitis; only rarely is it attributable to a brain lesion that has disturbed temperature-regulating centers. A slight elevation in temperature may follow vigorous convulsions. High body temperature, 42 to 44°C, associated with dry skin should arouse the suspicion of heat stroke or anticholinergic drug intoxication. Hypothermia is observed with alcoholic, barbiturate, sedative, or phenothiazine intoxication; hypoglycemia; peripheral circulatory failure; or hypothyroidism. Hypothermia itself causes coma only when the temperature is <31°C. Tachypnea may indicate acidosis or pneumonia. Aberrant respiratory patterns that reflect brainstem disorders are discussed below. Marked hypertension indicates hypertensive encephalopathy or a rapid rise in intracranial pressure (ICP) and may occur acutely after head injury. Hypotension is characteristic of coma from alcohol or barbiturate intoxication, internal hemorrhage, myocardial infarction, sepsis, profound hypothyroidism, or Addisonian crisis. The funduscopic examination can detect subarachnoid hemorrhage (subhyaloid hemorrhages), hypertensive encephalopathy (exudates, hemorrhages, vessel-crossing changes, papilledema), and increased ICP (papilledema). Petechiae suggest thrombotic thrombocytopenic purpura, meningococcemia, or a bleeding diathesis from which an intracerebral hemorrhage arises.

Neurologic Assessment

First, the patient should be observed without intervention by the examiner. Patients who toss about, reach up toward the face, cross their legs, yawn, swallow, cough, or moan are close to being awake. Lack of restless movements on one side or an outturned leg suggests a hemiplegia. Intermittent twitching movements of a foot, finger, or facial muscle may be the only sign of seizures. Multifocal myoclonus almost always indicates a metabolic disorder, particularly uremia, anoxia, or drug intoxication (lithium and haloperidol are particularly likely to cause this sign), or the rarer conditions of spongiform encephalopathy and Hashimoto disease. In a drowsy and confused patient bilateral asterixis is a certain sign of metabolic encephalopathy or drug intoxication.

The terms *decorticate rigidity* and *decerebrate rigidity,* or "posturing," describe stereotyped arm and leg movements occurring spontaneously or elicited by sensory stimulation. Flexion of the elbows and wrists and supination of the arm (decortication) suggests bilateral damage rostral to the midbrain, whereas extension of the elbows and wrists with pronation (decerebration) indicates damage to motor tracts in the midbrain or caudal diencephalon. The less frequent combination of arm extension with leg flexion or flaccid legs is associated with lesions in the pons. These concepts have been adapted from animal work and cannot be applied with the same precision to coma in humans. In fact, acute and widespread cerebral disorders of any type, regardless of location, frequently cause limb extension, and almost all such extensor posturing becomes predominantly flexor as time passes. Posturing may also be unilateral and may coexist with purposeful limb movements, usually reflecting incomplete damage to the motor system.

Level of Arousal and Elicited Movements

If the patient is not aroused by a conversational volume of voice, a sequence of increasingly intense stimuli is used to determine the threshold for arousal and the optimal motor response of each side of the body. The results of testing may vary from minute to minute and serial examinations are most useful. Tickling the nostrils with a cotton wisp is a moderate stimulus to arousal—all but deeply stuporous and comatose patients will move the head away and rouse to some degree. Using the hand to remove the offending stimulus represents an even greater degree of responsiveness.

Responses to noxious stimuli should be appraised critically. Stereotyped posturing indicates severe dysfunction of the corticospinal system. Abduction-avoidance movement of a limb is usually purposeful and denotes an intact corticospinal system. Pressure

on the knuckles or bony prominences and pinprick are humane forms of noxious stimuli; pinching the skin causes unsightly ecchymoses and is generally not necessary but may be useful in eliciting abduction withdrawal movements of the limbs.

Brainstem Reflexes

Assessment of brainstem function is essential to localization of the lesion in coma (**Fig. 8-3**). The brainstem reflexes that are conveniently examined are pupillary responses to light, spontaneous and

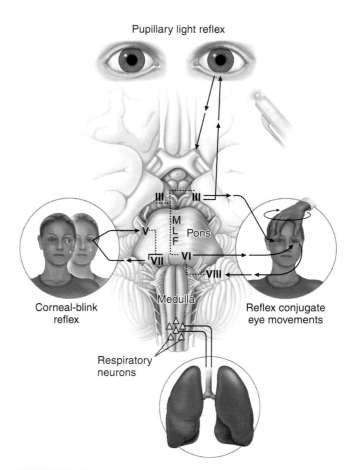

FIGURE 8-3

Examination of brainstem reflexes in coma. Midbrain and third nerve function are tested by pupillary reaction to light, pontine function by spontaneous and reflex eye movements and corneal responses, and medullary function by respiratory and pharyngeal responses. Reflex conjugate, horizontal eye movements are dependent on the medial longitudinal fasciculus (MLF) interconnecting the sixth and contralateral third nerve nuclei. Head rotation (oculocephalic reflex) or caloric stimulation of the labyrinths (oculovestibular reflex) elicits contraversive eye movements (for details see text).

elicited eye movements, corneal responses, and the respiratory pattern. As a rule, when these brainstem activities are preserved, particularly the pupil reactions and eye movements, coma must be ascribed to bilateral hemispheral disease. The converse, however, is not always true as a mass in the hemispheres may be the underlying cause of coma but nonetheless produce brainstem signs.

PUPILS

Pupillary reactions are examined with a bright, diffuse light (not an ophthalmoscope); if the response is absent, this should be confirmed by observation through a magnifying lens. Normally reactive and round pupils of midsize (2.5 to 5 mm) essentially exclude midbrain damage, either primary or secondary to compression. Reaction to light is often difficult to appreciate in pupils <2 mm in diameter, and bright room lighting mutes pupillary reactivity. One unreactive and enlarged pupil (>6 mm) or one that is poorly reactive signifies a compression or stretching of the third nerve from the effects of a mass above. Enlargement of the pupil contralateral to a mass may occur first but is infrequent. An oval and slightly eccentric pupil is a transitional sign that accompanies early midbrain–third nerve compression. The most extreme pupillary sign, bilaterally dilated and unreactive pupils, indicates severe midbrain damage, usually from compression by a mass. Ingestion of drugs with anticholinergic activity, the use of mydriatic eye drops, and direct ocular trauma are among the causes of misleading pupillary enlargement.

Unilateral miosis in coma has been attributed to dysfunction of sympathetic efferents originating in the posterior hypothalamus and descending in the tegmentum of the brainstem to the cervical cord. It is an occasional finding with a large cerebral hemorrhage that affects the thalamus. Reactive and bilaterally small (1 to 2.5 mm) but not pinpoint pupils are seen in metabolic encephalopathies or in deep bilateral hemispheral lesions such as hydrocephalus or thalamic hemorrhage. Very small but reactive pupils (<1 mm) characterize narcotic or barbiturate overdoses but also occur with extensive pontine hemorrhage. The response to naloxone and the presence of reflex eye movements (see below) distinguish these.

OCULAR MOVEMENTS

The eyes are first observed by elevating the lids and noting the resting position and spontaneous movements of the globes. Lid tone, tested by lifting the eyelids and noting their resistance to opening and the speed of closure, is reduced progressively as coma deepens. Horizontal divergence of the eyes at rest is normal in drowsiness. As coma deepens, the ocular axes may become parallel again.

Spontaneous eye movements in coma often take the form of conjugate horizontal roving. This finding alone exonerates the midbrain and pons and has the same significance as normal reflex eye movements (see below). Conjugate horizontal ocular deviation to one side indicates damage to the pons on the opposite side or a lesion in the frontal lobe on the same side. This phenomenon may be summarized by the following maxim: *The eyes look toward a hemispheral lesion and away from a brainstem lesion*. Seizures also drive the eyes to one side. On rare occasions, the eyes may turn paradoxically away from the side of a deep hemispheral lesion ("wrong-way eyes"). The eyes turn down and inward as a result of thalamic and upper midbrain lesions, typically with thalamic hemorrhage. "Ocular bobbing" describes a brisk downward and slow upward movement of the eyes associated with loss of horizontal eye movements and is diagnostic of bilateral pontine damage, usually from thrombosis of the basilar artery. "Ocular dipping" is a slower, arrhythmic downward movement followed by a faster upward movement in patients with normal reflex horizontal gaze; it indicates diffuse cortical anoxic damage. Many other complex eye movements are known but do not have the same significance as the ones already mentioned.

The oculocephalic reflexes depend on the integrity of the ocular motor nuclei and their interconnecting tracts that extend from the midbrain to the pons and medulla. These reflexes are elicited by moving the head from side to side or vertically and observing evoked eye movements in the direction opposite to the head movement (Fig. 8–3). These movements, called somewhat inappropriately "doll's eyes" (which refers more accurately to the reflex elevation of the eyelids with flexion of the neck), are normally suppressed in the awake patient by visual fixation. Their presence therefore indicates a reduced cortical influence on the brainstem. Furthermore, preservation of evoked reflex eye movements signifies the integrity of the brainstem and, by implication, that the origin of unconsciousness lies in the cerebral hemispheres.

The opposite—the absence of reflex eye movements—signifies damage within the brainstem but can be produced infrequently by profound overdoses of certain drugs. Normal pupillary size and light reaction distinguishes most drug-induced comas from structural brainstem damage.

Thermal, or "caloric," stimulation of the vestibular apparatus (oculovestibular response) provides a more intense stimulus for the oculocephalic reflex but gives fundamentally the same information. The test is performed by irrigating the external auditory canal with cool water in order to induce convection currents in the labyrinths. After a brief latency, the result is tonic deviation of both eyes to the side of cool-water irrigation and nystagmus in the opposite direction. (The acronym "COWS" has been used to remind generations of medical students of the direction of nystagmus—"cold water opposite, warm water same"). The absence of nystagmus despite conjugate deviation of the globes signifies that the cerebral hemispheres are damaged or suppressed. The loss of conjugate ocular movements indicates brainstem damage.

By touching the cornea with a wisp of cotton, a response consisting of brief bilateral lid closure is normally observed. The corneal reflexes depend on the integrity of pontine pathways between the fifth (afferent) and both seventh (efferent) cranial nerves; although rarely useful alone, in conjunction with reflex eye movements they are important clinical tests of pontine function. CNS depressant drugs diminish or eliminate the corneal responses soon after reflex eye movements are paralyzed but before the pupils become unreactive to light. The corneal (and pharyngeal) response may be lost for a time on the side of an acute hemiplegia.

RESPIRATION

Respiratory patterns are of less localizing value in comparison to other brainstem signs. Shallow, slow, but regular breathing suggests metabolic or drug depression. Cheyne-Stokes respiration in its classic cyclic form, ending with a brief apneic period, signifies bihemispheral damage or metabolic suppression and commonly accompanies light coma. Rapid, deep (Kussmaul) breathing usually implies metabolic acidosis but may also occur with pontomesencephalic lesions. Agonal gasps reflect bilateral lower brainstem damage and are well known as the terminal respiratory pattern of severe brain damage. A number of other cyclic breathing variations are of lesser significance.

LABORATORY STUDIES AND IMAGING

The studies that are most useful in the diagnosis of confusional states and coma are: chemical-toxicologic analysis of blood and urine, cranial CT or MRI, EEG, and CSF examination. Arterial blood-gas analysis is helpful in patients with lung disease and acid-base disorders. The metabolic aberrations commonly encountered in clinical practice require measurements of electrolytes, glucose, calcium, osmolarity, and renal (blood urea nitrogen) and hepatic (NH_3) function. Toxicologic analysis is necessary in any case of coma where the diagnosis is not immediately clear. However, the presence of exogenous drugs or toxins, especially alcohol, does not exclude the possibility that other factors, particularly head trauma, are also contributing to the clinical state. An ethanol level of 43 mmol/L (200 mg/dL) in nonhabituated patients generally causes impaired mental activity and of >65 mmol/L (300 mg/dL) is associated with stupor. The development of tolerance may allow the chronic alcoholic to remain awake at levels >87 mmol/L (400 mg/dL).

The availability of CT and MRI has focused attention on causes of coma that are radiologically detectable (e.g., hemorrhages, tumors, or hydrocephalus). Resorting primarily to this approach, although at times expedient, is imprudent because most cases of coma (and confusion) are metabolic or toxic in origin. The notion that a normal CT scan excludes anatomical lesions as the cause of coma is also erroneous. Bilateral hemisphere infarction, small brainstem lesions, encephalitis, meningitis, mechanical shearing of axons as a result of closed head trauma, sagittal sinus thrombosis, and subdural hematomas that are isodense to adjacent brain are some of the disorders that may not be detected. Nevertheless, if the source of coma remains unknown, a scan should be obtained.

The EEG is useful in metabolic or drug-induced confusional states but is rarely diagnostic, except when coma is due to clinically unrecognized seizures, to herpesvirus encephalitis, or to Creutzfeldt-Jakob disease. The amount of background slowing of the EEG is a reflection of the severity of any diffuse encephalopathy. Predominant high-voltage slowing (δ or triphasic waves) in the frontal regions is typical of metabolic coma, as from hepatic failure, and widespread fast (β) activity implicates sedative drugs (e.g., diazepines, barbiturates). A special pattern of "α coma," defined by widespread, variable 8- to 12-Hz activity, superficially resembles the normal α rhythm of waking but is unresponsive to environmental stimuli. It results from pontine or diffuse cortical damage and is associated with a poor prognosis. Most importantly, EEG recordings may reveal clinically inapparent epileptic discharges in a patient with coma. Normal α activity on the EEG also alerts the clinician to the locked-in syndrome or to hysteria or catatonia.

Lumbar puncture is performed less frequently than in the past because neuroimaging scans effectively exclude intracerebral and subarachnoid hemorrhages that are severe enough to cause coma. However, examination of the CSF is indispensable in the diagnosis of meningitis and encephalitis. Lumbar puncture should therefore not be deferred if meningitis is a possibility.

DIFFERENTIAL DIAGNOSIS OF COMA
(Table 8-1)

The causes of coma can be conceptualized in three broad categories: those without focal neurologic signs (e.g., metabolic encephalopathies); meningitis syndromes, characterized by fever or stiff neck and an excess of cells in the spinal fluid (e.g., bacterial meningitis, subarachnoid hemorrhage); and those with prominent focal signs (e.g., stroke, cerebral hemorrhage). In most instances confusion and coma are part of an obvious medical problem such as drug ingestion, hypoxia, stroke, trauma, or liver or kidney failure. Conditions that cause sudden coma include drug ingestion, cerebral hemorrhage, trauma, cardiac arrest, epilepsy, or basilar artery embolism. Coma that appears subacutely is usually related to a preceding medical or neurologic problem, including the secondary brain swelling of a mass lesion such as tumor or cerebral infarction.

Cerebrovascular diseases cause the greatest difficulty in coma diagnosis (Chap. 17). These may be summarized as follows: (1) basal ganglia and thalamic hemorrhage (acute but not instantaneous onset, vomiting, headache, hemiplegia, and characteristic eye signs); (2) pontine hemorrhage (sudden onset, pinpoint pupils, loss of reflex eye movements and corneal responses, ocular bobbing, posturing, hyperventilation, and excessive sweating); (3) cerebellar hemorrhage (occipital headache, vomiting, gaze paresis, and inability to stand); (4) basilar artery thrombosis (neurologic prodrome or warning spells, diplopia, dysarthria, vomiting, eye movement and corneal response abnormalities, and asymmetric limb paresis); and (5) subarachnoid hemorrhage (precipitous coma after headache and vomiting). The most common stroke, infarction in the territory of the middle cerebral artery, does not cause coma, but edema surrounding large infarcts may expand during the first few days and act as a mass. The syndrome of acute hydrocephalus accompanies many intracranial diseases, particularly subarachnoid hemorrhage. It is characterized by headache and sometimes vomiting that may progress quickly to coma, with extensor posturing of the limbs, bilateral Babinski signs, small nonreactive pupils, and impaired oculocephalic movements in the vertical direction.

If the history and examination do not indicate the cause of coma, then information obtained from CT or

---

TABLE 8-1

DIFFERENTIAL DIAGNOSIS OF COMA

1. Diseases that cause no focal or lateralizing neurologic signs, usually with normal brainstem functions; CT scan and cellular content of the CSF are normal
   a. Intoxications: alcohol, sedative drugs, opiates, etc.
   b. Metabolic disturbances: anoxia, hyponatremia, hypernatremia, hypercalcemia, diabetic acidosis, nonketotic hyperosmolar hyperglycemia, hypoglycemia, uremia, hepatic coma, hypercarbia, addisonian crisis, hypo- and hyperthyroid states, profound nutritional deficiency
   c. Severe systemic infections: pneumonia, septicemia, typhoid fever, malaria, Waterhouse-Friderichsen syndrome
   d. Shock from any cause
   e. Postseizure states, status epilepticus, subclinical epilepsy
   f. Hypertensive encephalopathy, eclampsia
   g. Severe hyperthermia, hypothermia
   h. Concussion
   i. Acute hydrocephalus

2. Diseases that cause meningeal irritation with or without fever, and with an excess of WBCs or RBCs in the CSF, usually without focal or lateralizing cerebral or brainstem signs; CT or MRI shows no mass lesion
   a. Subarachnoid hemorrhage from ruptured aneurysm, arteriovenous malformation, trauma
   b. Acute bacterial meningitis
   c. Viral encephalitis
   d. Miscellaneous: Fat embolism, cholesterol embolism, carcinomatous and lymphomatous meningitis, etc.

3. Diseases that cause focal brainstem or lateralizing cerebral signs, with or without changes in the CSF; CT and MRI are abnormal
   a. Hemispheral hemorrhage (basal ganglionic, thalamic) or infarction (large middle cerebral artery territory) with secondary brainstem compression
   b. Brainstem infarction due to basilar artery thrombosis or embolism
   c. Brain abscess, subdural empyema
   d. Epidural and subdural hemorrhage, brain contusion
   e. Brain tumor with surrounding edema
   f. Cerebellar and pontine hemorrhage and infarction
   g. Widespread traumatic brain injury
   h. Metabolic coma (see above) with preexisting focal damage
   i. Miscellaneous: cortical vein thrombosis, herpes simplex encephalitis, multiple cerebral emboli due to bacterial endocarditis, acute hemorrhagic leukoencephalitis, acute disseminated (postinfectious) encephalomyelitis, thrombotic thrombocytopenic purpura, cerebral vasculitis, gliomatosis cerebri, pituitary apoplexy, intravascular lymphoma, etc.

Note: CT, computed tomography; CSF, cerebrospinal fluid; WBC, white blood cells; RBCs, red blood cells; MRI, magnetic resonance imaging.

MRI may be needed. As mentioned earlier, the majority of medical causes of coma can be established without a neuroimaging study.

BRAIN DEATH

This is a state in which there has been cessation of cerebral blood flow; as a result there is global loss of brain function while respiration is maintained by artificial means and the heart continues to pump. It is the only type of brain damage that is recognized as equivalent to death. Many roughly equivalent criteria have been advanced for the diagnosis of brain death, and it is essential to adhere to those standards endorsed by the local medical community. Ideal criteria are simple, can be conducted at the bedside, and allow no chance of diagnostic error. They contain three essential elements: (1) widespread cortical destruction shown by deep coma—unresponsiveness to all forms of stimulation; (2) global brainstem damage demonstrated by absent pupillary light reaction and the loss of oculovestibular and corneal reflexes; and (3) destruction of the medulla manifested by complete apnea. The pulse rate is invariant and unresponsive to atropine. Diabetes insipidus is often present, but may develop hours or days after the other clinical signs of brain death. The pupils are often enlarged but may be mid-sized; they should not be constricted. The absence of deep tendon reflexes is not required because the spinal cord remains functional.

Demonstration that apnea is due to irreversible medullary damage requires that the P_{CO_2} be high enough to stimulate respiration during a test of spontaneous breathing (apnea test). This can be done safely by the use, prior to removing the ventilator, of diffusion oxygenation. This is accomplished by preoxygenation with 100% oxygen, which is then sustained during the test by oxygen administered through a tracheal cannula. CO_2 tension increases approximately 0.3 to 0.4 kPa/min (2 to 3 mmHg/min) during apnea. At the end of the period of observation, typically several minutes in duration, arterial P_{CO_2} should be at least >6.6 to 8.0 kPa (50 to 60 mmHg) for the test to be valid. Complete apnea is considered to be present if no respiratory effort is observed in the presence of a sufficiently elevated P_{CO_2}.

The possibility of profound drug-induced or hypothermic depression of the nervous system should be excluded, and some period of observation, usually 6 to 24 h, is desirable during which this state is shown to be sustained. It is particularly advisable to delay clinical testing for at least 24 h if a cardiac arrest has caused brain death or if the inciting disease is not known. An isoelectric EEG may be used as a confirmatory test for total cerebral damage but is not absolutely necessary. Radionuclide brain scanning, cerebral angiography, or transcranial Doppler measurements may also be used to demonstrate the absence of cerebral blood flow but they have not been extensively correlated with pathologic changes.

There is no compelling reason to embark on the demonstration of brain death except when organ transplantation is involved. Although it is largely accepted in western society that the respirator can be disconnected from a brain-dead patient, problems frequently arise because of poor communication and inadequate preparation of the family by the physician. Reasonable medical practice allows the removal of support or transfer out of an intensive care unit of patients who are not brain dead but whose condition is nonetheless hopeless and are likely to live for only a brief time.

TREATMENT FOR NERVOUS SYSTEM DAMAGE

The immediate goal is prevention of further nervous system damage. Hypotension, hypoglycemia, hypercalcemia, hypoxia, hypercapnia, and hyperthermia should be corrected rapidly. An oropharyngeal airway is adequate to keep the pharynx open in drowsy patients who are breathing normally. Tracheal intubation is indicated if there is apnea, upper airway obstruction, hypoventilation, or emesis, or if the patient is liable to aspirate because of coma. Mechanical ventilation is required if there is hypoventilation or a need to induce hypocapnia in order to lower ICP as described below. Intravenous access is established, and naloxone and dextrose are administered if narcotic overdose or hypoglycemia are even remote possibilities; thiamine is given along with glucose to avoid provoking Wernicke disease in malnourished patients. In cases of suspected basilar thrombosis with brainstem ischemia, intravenous heparin or a thrombolytic agent is often utilized, after cerebral hemorrhage is excluded by a neuroimaging study. Physostigmine may awaken patients with anticholinergic-type drug overdose, but must be used only by experienced physicians and with careful monitoring; many physicians believe that it should only be used to treat anticholinergic overdose–associated cardiac arrhythmias. The use of benzodiazepine antagonists offers some prospect of improvement after overdoses of soporific drugs and has transient benefit in hepatic encephalopathy. Intravenous administration of hypotonic solutions should be monitored carefully in any serious acute brain illness because of the potential for exacerbating brain swelling. Cervical spine injuries must not be overlooked, particularly prior to attempting intubation or evaluating of oculocephalic responses. Headache accompanied by fever and meningismus indicates an urgent need for examination of the CSF to diagnose meningitis. If the lumbar puncture in a case of suspected meningitis is delayed for any reason, an antibiotic such as a third-generation cephalosporin should be administered as soon as possible, preferably after obtaining blood cultures. The management of raised ICP is discussed in Chap. 15.

PROGNOSIS

The prediction of the outcome of coma must be considered in reference to long-term care and medical resources. One hopes to avoid the emotionally painful, hopeless outcome of a patient who is left severely disabled or vegetative. The uniformly pessimistic outcome of the persistent vegetative state has already been mentioned. Children and young adults may have ominous early clinical findings such as abnormal brainstem reflexes and yet recover, so that temporization in offering a prognosis in this group of patients is wise. Metabolic comas have a far better prognosis than traumatic comas. All schemes for prognosis in adults should be taken as approximations, and medical judgments must be tempered by factors such as age, underlying systemic disease, and general medical condition. In an attempt to collect prognostic information from large numbers of patients

with head injury, the Glasgow Coma Scale was devised; empirically it has predictive value in cases of brain trauma (Chap. 16). For anoxic and metabolic coma, clinical signs such as the pupillary and motor responses after 1 day, 3 days, and 1 week have been shown to have predictive value (Chap. 15). The absence of the cortical waves of the somatosensory evoked potentials has also proved a strong indicator of poor outcome in coma from any cause.

FURTHER READINGS

☑ LAUREYS S et al: Brain function in coma, vegetative state, and related disorders. Lancet Neurol 3:537, 2004

Excellent overview of the spectrum of abnormal states of consciousness and their respective neuroanatomic localizations.

☑ PANDHARIPANDE P et al: Delirium: Acute cognitive dysfunction in the critically ill. Curr Opin Crit Care 11: 360, 2005

Approach to delirium in medical and surgical intensive care units.

PARVIZI J, DAMASIO AR: Neuroanatomical correlates of brainstem coma. Brain 126:1524, 2003

ROPPER AH: *Neurological and Neurosurgical Intensive Care,* 4th ed. New York, Lippincott Williams & Wilkins, 2004

WIJDICKS EFM: Current concepts: The diagnosis of brain death. N Engl J Med 344:1215, 2001

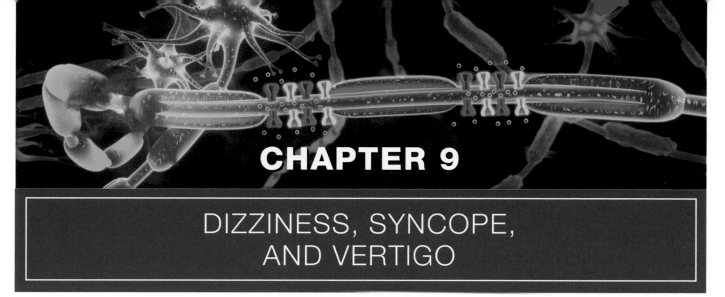

CHAPTER 9

DIZZINESS, SYNCOPE, AND VERTIGO

Robert B. Daroff
Mark D. Carlson

DIZZINESS

Dizziness is a common and often vexing symptom. Patients use the term to encompass a variety of sensations, including those that seem semantically appropriate (e.g., lightheadedness, faintness, spinning, giddiness) and those that are misleadingly inappropriate, such as mental confusion, blurred vision, headache, or tingling. Moreover, some individuals with gait disorders caused by peripheral neuropathy, myelopathy, spasticity, parkinsonism, or cerebellar ataxia complain of "dizziness" despite the absence of vertigo or other abnormal cephalic sensations. In this context, the term *dizziness* is being used to describe disturbed ambulation. There may be mild associated lightheadedness, particularly with impaired sensation from the feet or poor vision; this is known as *multiple-sensory-defect dizziness* and occurs in elderly individuals who complain of dizziness only when walking. Decreased position sense (secondary to neuropathy or myelopathy) and poor vision (from cataracts or retinal degeneration) create an overreliance on the aging vestibular apparatus. A less precise but sometimes comforting designation to patients is *benign dysequilibrium of aging*. Thus, a careful history is necessary to determine exactly what a patient who states, "Doctor, I'm dizzy," is experiencing. After eliminating the misleading symptoms or gait disturbance, "dizziness" usually means either

faintness (presyncope) or *vertigo* (an illusory or hallucinatory sense of movement of the body or environment, most often a feeling of spinning). Operationally, after obtaining the history, dizziness may be classified into three categories: (1) faintness/presyncope, (2) vertigo, and (3) miscellaneous head sensations.

FAINTNESS AND SYNCOPE

Syncope is defined as transient loss of consciousness due to reduced cerebral blood flow. Syncope is associated with postural collapse and spontaneous recovery. It may occur suddenly, without warning, or may be preceded by prodromal symptoms of faintness ("presyncope"). These include lightheadedness, "dizziness" without true vertigo, a feeling of warmth, diaphoresis, nausea, and visual blurring occasionally proceeding to blindness. Presyncopal symptoms vary in duration and may increase in severity until loss of consciousness occurs or may resolve prior to loss of consciousness if the cerebral ischemia is corrected. The differentiation of syncope from seizure is an important, sometimes difficult, diagnostic problem.

Syncope may be benign when it occurs as a result of normal cardiovascular reflex effects on heart rate and vascular tone, or serious when due to a life-threatening arrhythmia. Syncope may occur as a single event or may be recurrent. Recurrent, unexplained syncope, particularly in an individual with structural heart disease, is associated with a high risk of death (40% mortality within 2 years).

PATHOPHYSIOLOGY

Syncope results from a sudden impairment of brain metabolism, usually brought about by hypotension with reduction of cerebral blood flow. Several mechanisms subserve circulatory adjustments to the upright posture. Approximately three-fourths of the systemic blood volume is contained in the venous bed, and any interference in venous return may lead to a reduction in cardiac output. Cerebral blood flow may still be maintained as long as systemic arterial vasoconstriction occurs, but when this adjustment fails, serious hypotension, with resultant cerebral underperfusion to less than half of normal, results in syncope. Normally, the pooling of blood in the lower parts of the body is prevented by (1) pressor reflexes that induce constriction of peripheral arterioles and venules, (2) reflex acceleration of the heart by means of aortic and carotid reflexes, and (3) improvement of venous return to the heart by activity of the muscles of the limbs. Tilting a normal person upright on a tilt table causes some blood to accumulate in the lower limbs and diminishes cardiac output slightly; this may be followed by a slight transitory fall in systolic blood pressure. In a patient with defective

vasomotor reflexes, however, tilt table testing may produce an abrupt and sustained fall in blood pressure, precipitating a faint.

CAUSES OF SYNCOPE

Transiently decreased cerebral blood flow is usually due to one of three general mechanisms: disorders of vascular tone or blood volume, cardiovascular disorders including cardiac arrhythmias, or cerebrovascular disease (**Table 9–1**). Not infrequently, however, the cause of syncope is multifactorial.

Disorders of Vascular Tone or Blood Volume

Disorders of autonomic control of the heart and circulation share common pathophysiologic mechanisms: a cardioinhibitory component (e.g., bradycardia due to increased vagal activity), a vasodepressor component

TABLE 9–1

CAUSES OF SYNCOPE

I. **Disorders of vascular tone or blood volume**
A. Vasovagal (vasodepressor, neurocardiogenic)
B. Postural (orthostatic) hypotension
1. Drug induced (especially antihypertensive or vasodilator drugs)
2. Peripheral neuropathy (diabetic, alcoholic, nutritional, amyloid)
3. Idiopathic postural hypotension
4. Multisystem atrophies
5. Physical deconditioning
6. Sympathectomy
7. Acute dysautonomia (Guillain-Barré syndrome variant)
8. Decreased blood volume (adrenal insufficiency, acute blood loss, etc.)
C. Carotid sinus hypersensitivity
D. Situational
1. Cough
2. Micturition
3. Defecation
4. Valsalva
5. Deglutition
E. Glossopharyngeal neuralgia
II. **Cardiovascular disorders**
A. Cardiac arrhythmias
1. Bradyarrhythmias
a. Sinus bradycardia, sinoatrial block, sinus arrest, sick-sinus syndrome
b. Atrioventricular block
2. Tachyarrhythmias
a. Supraventricular tachycardia with structural cardiac disease

b. Atrial fibrillation associated with the Wolff-Parkinson-White syndrome
c. Atrial flutter with 1:1 atrioventricular conduction
d. Ventricular tachycardia
B. Other cardiopulmonary etiologies
1. Pulmonary embolism
2. Pulmonary hypertension
3. Atrial myxoma
4. Myocardial disease (massive myocardial infarction)
5. Left ventricular myocardial restriction or constriction
6. Pericardial constriction or tamponade
7. Aortic outflow tract obstruction
8. Aortic valvular stenosis
9. Hypertrophic obstructive cardiomyopathy
III. **Cerebrovascular disease (Chap. 17)**
A. Vertebrobasilar insufficiency
B. Basilar artery migraine
IV. **Other disorders that may resemble syncope**
A. Metabolic
1. Hypoxia
2. Anemia
3. Diminished carbon dioxide due to hyperventilation
4. Hypoglycemia
B. Psychogenic
1. Anxiety attacks
2. Hysterical fainting
C. Seizures

(e.g., inappropriate vasodilatation due to sympathetic withdrawal), or both.

Neurocardiogenic (Vasovagal and Vasodepressor) Syncope

The term *neurocardiogenic* is generally used to encompass both vasovagal and vasodepressor syncope. Strictly speaking, vasovagal syncope is associated with both sympathetic withdrawal (vasodilatation) and increased parasympathetic activity (bradycardia), whereas vasodepressor syncope is associated with sympathetic withdrawal alone.

These forms of syncope are the common faint that may be experienced by normal persons and account for approximately half of all episodes of syncope. Neurocardiogenic syncope is frequently recurrent and commonly precipitated by a hot or crowded environment, alcohol, extreme fatigue, severe pain, hunger, prolonged standing, and emotional or stressful situations. Episodes are often preceded by a presyncopal prodrome lasting seconds to minutes, and rarely occur in the supine position. The individual is usually sitting or standing and experiences weakness, nausea, diaphoresis, lightheadedness, blurred vision, and often a forceful heart beat with tachycardia followed by cardiac slowing and decreasing blood pressure prior to loss of consciousness. The individual appears pale or ashen; in dark-skinned individuals, the pallor may only be notable in the conjunctivae and lips. Patients with a gradual onset of presyncopal symptoms have time to protect themselves against injury; in others, syncope occurs suddenly, without warning.

The depth and duration of unconsciousness vary. Sometimes the patient remains partly aware of the surroundings, or there may be complete unresponsiveness. The unconscious patient usually lies motionless with skeletal muscles relaxed, but a few clonic jerks of the limbs and face may occur. Sphincter control is usually maintained, in contrast to a seizure. The pulse may be feeble or apparently absent, the blood pressure low or undetectable, and breathing may be almost imperceptible. The duration of unconsciousness is rarely longer than a few minutes if the conditions that provoke the episode are reversed. Once the patient is placed in a horizontal position, the strength of the pulse improves, color begins to return to the face, breathing becomes quicker and deeper, and consciousness is restored. Some patients may experience a sense of residual weakness after regaining consciousness, and rising too soon may precipitate another faint. Unconsciousness may be prolonged if an individual remains upright, thus it is essential that individuals with vasovagal syncope assume a recumbent position as soon as possible. Although commonly benign, neurocardiogenic syncope can be associated with prolonged asystole and hypotension, resulting in injury.

The syncope often occurs in the setting of increased peripheral sympathetic activity and venous pooling. Under these conditions, vigorous myocardial contraction of a relatively empty left ventricle activates myocardial mechanoreceptors and vagal afferent nerve fibers that inhibit sympathetic activity and increase parasympathetic activity. The resultant vasodilatation and bradycardia induce hypotension and syncope. Although the reflex involving myocardial mechanoreceptors is the mechanism usually accepted as responsible for neurocardiogenic syncope, other reflexes may also be operative. Patients with transplanted (denervated) hearts have experienced cardiovascular responses identical to those present during neurocardiogenic syncope. This should not be possible if the response depends solely on the reflex mechanisms described above, unless the transplanted heart has become reinnervated. Moreover, neurocardiogenic syncope often occurs in response to stimuli (fear, emotional stress, or pain) that may not be associated with venous pooling in the lower extremities, which suggests a cortical component to the reflex. Thus, a variety of afferent and efferent responses may cause neurocardiogenic syncope.

As distinct from the peripheral mechanisms, the central nervous system (CNS) mechanisms responsible for neurocardiogenic syncope are uncertain, but a sudden surge in central serotonin levels may contribute to the sympathetic withdrawal. Endogenous opiates (endorphins) and adenosine are also putative participants in the pathogenesis.

Postural (Orthostatic) Hypotension

This occurs in patients who have a chronic defect in, or variable instability of, vasomotor reflexes. Systemic arterial blood pressure falls on assumption of upright posture due to loss of vasoconstriction reflexes in resistance and capacitance vessels of the lower extremities. Although the syncopal attack differs little from vasodepressor syncope, the effect of posture is critical. Sudden rising from a recumbent position or standing quietly are precipitating circumstances. *Orthostatic hypotension may be the cause of syncope in up to 30% of the elderly; polypharmacy with antihypertensive or antidepressant drugs is often a contributor in these patients.*

Postural syncope may occur in otherwise normal persons with defective postural reflexes. Patients with *idiopathic postural hypotension* may be identified by a characteristic response to upright tilt on a table. Initially, the blood pressure diminishes slightly before stabilizing at a lower level. Shortly thereafter, the compensatory reflexes fail and the arterial pressure falls precipitously. The condition is often familial.

Orthostatic hypotension, often accompanied by disturbances in sweating, impotence, and sphincter difficulties, is also a primary feature of autonomic nervous system disorders (Chap. 22). The most common causes of neurogenic orthostatic hypotension are chronic diseases of the peripheral nervous system that involve postganglionic unmyelinated fibers (e.g., diabetic, nutritional, and amyloid polyneuropathy). Much less common are the multiple system atrophies; these are CNS disorders in which orthostatic hypotension is associated with (1) parkinsonism (Shy-Drager syndrome), (2) progressive cerebellar degeneration, or (3) a more variable parkinsonian and cerebellar syndrome (striatonigral degeneration) (Chap. 19). A rare, acute postganglionic dysautonomia may represent a variant of Guillain-Barré syndrome (Chap. 35).

There are several additional causes of postural syncope: (1) After physical deconditioning (such as after prolonged illness with recumbency, especially in elderly individuals with reduced muscle tone) or after prolonged weightlessness, as in space flight; (2) after sympathectomy that has abolished vasopressor reflexes; and (3) in patients receiving antihypertensive or vasodilator drugs and those who are hypovolemic because of diuretics, excessive sweating, diarrhea, vomiting, hemorrhage, or adrenal insufficiency.

■ Carotid Sinus Hypersensitivity   Syncope due to carotid sinus hypersensitivity is precipitated by pressure on the carotid sinus baroreceptors, which are located just cephalad to the bifurcation of the common carotid artery. This typically occurs in the setting of shaving, a tight collar, or turning the head to one side. Carotid sinus hypersensitivity occurs predominantly in men ≥50 years old. Activation of carotid sinus baroreceptors gives rise to impulses carried via the nerve of Hering, a branch of the glossopharyngeal nerve, to the medulla oblongata. These afferent impulses activate efferent sympathetic nerve fibers to the heart and blood vessels, cardiac vagal efferent nerve fibers, or both. In patients with carotid sinus hypersensitivity, these responses may cause sinus arrest or atrioventricular (AV) block (a cardioinhibitory response), vasodilatation (a vasodepressor response), or both (a mixed response). The mechanisms responsible for the syndrome are not clear, and validated diagnostic criteria do not exist; some authorities have questioned its very existence.

■ Situational Syncope   A variety of activities, including cough, deglutition, micturition, and defecation, are associated with syncope in susceptible individuals. These syndromes are caused, at least in part, by abnormal autonomic control and may involve a cardioinhibitory response, a vasodepressor response, or both. Cough, micturition, and defecation are associated with maneuvers (such as Valsalva, straining, and coughing) that may con-

tribute to hypotension and syncope by decreasing venous return. Increased intracranial pressure secondary to the increased intrathoracic pressure may also contribute by decreasing cerebral blood flow.

Cough syncope typically occurs in men with chronic bronchitis or chronic obstructive lung disease during or after prolonged coughing fits. Micturition syncope occurs predominantly in middle-aged and older men, particularly those with prostatic hypertrophy and obstruction of the bladder neck; loss of consciousness usually occurs at night during or immediately after voiding. Deglutition syncope and defecation syncope occur in men and women. Deglutition syncope may be associated with esophageal disorders, particularly esophageal spasm. In some individuals, particular foods and carbonated or cold beverages initiate episodes by activating esophageal sensory receptors that trigger reflex sinus bradycardia or AV block. Defecation syncope is probably secondary to a Valsalva maneuver in older individuals with constipation.

■ Glossopharyngeal Neuralgia   Syncope due to glossopharyngeal neuralgia (Chap. 23) is preceded by pain in the oropharynx, tonsillar fossa, or tongue. Loss of consciousness is usually associated with asystole rather than vasodilatation. The mechanism is thought to involve activation of afferent impulses in the glossopharyngeal nerve that terminate in the nucleus solitarius of the medulla and, via collaterals, activate the dorsal motor nucleus of the vagus nerve.

CARDIOVASCULAR DISORDERS

Cardiac syncope results from a sudden reduction in cardiac output, caused most commonly by a cardiac arrhythmia. In normal individuals, heart rates between 30 and 180 beats/min do not reduce cerebral blood flow, especially if the person is in the supine position. As the heart rate decreases, ventricular filling time and stroke volume increase to maintain normal cardiac output. At rates <30 beats/min, stroke volume can no longer increase to compensate adequately for the decreased heart rate. At rates greater than ~180 beats/min, ventricular filling time is inadequate to maintain adequate stroke volume. In either case, cerebral hypoperfusion and syncope may occur. Upright posture; cerebrovascular disease; anemia; loss of atrioventricular synchrony; and coronary, myocardial, or valvular disease all reduce the tolerance to alterations in rate.

Bradyarrhythmias may occur as a result of an abnormality of impulse generation (e.g., sinoatrial arrest) or impulse conduction (e.g., AV block). Either may cause syncope if the escape pacemaker rate is insufficient to maintain cardiac output. Syncope due to bradyarrhythmias may occur abruptly, without presyncopal symptoms, and recur several times daily. Patients with *sick-sinus syndrome* may have sinus pauses (>3 s), and those with syncope due to high-degree AV block (*Stokes-Adams-Morgagni syndrome*) may have evidence of conduction system disease (e.g., prolonged PR interval, bundle branch block). However, the arrhythmia is often transitory, and the surface electrocardiogram or continuous electrocardiographic monitor (Holter monitor) taken later may not reveal the abnormality. The *bradycardia-tachycardia syndrome* is a common form of sinus node dysfunction in which syncope generally occurs as a result of marked sinus pauses, some following termination of paroxysms of atrial tachyarrhythmias. Drugs are a common cause for bradyarrhythmias, particularly in patients with underlying structural heart disease. Digoxin, α-adrenergic receptor antagonists, calcium channel blockers, and many antiarrhythmic drugs may suppress sinoatrial node impulse generation or slow AV nodal conduction.

Syncope due to a *tachyarrhythmia* is usually preceded by palpitation or lightheadedness but may occur abruptly with no warning symptoms. *Supraventricular tachyarrhythmias* are unlikely to cause syncope in individuals with structurally normal hearts but may if they occur in patients with (1) heart disease that also compromises cardiac output, (2) cerebrovascular disease, (3) a disorder of vascular tone or blood volume, or (4) a rapid ventricular rate. These tachycardias result most commonly from paroxysmal atrial flutter, atrial fibrillation, or reentry involving the AV node or accessory pathways that bypass part or all of the AV conduction system. Patients with the *Wolff-Parkinson-White syndrome* may experience syncope when a very rapid ventricular rate occurs due to reentry across an accessory AV connection.

In patients with structural heart disease, ventricular tachycardia is a common cause of syncope, particularly in patients with a prior myocardial infarction. Patients with aortic valvular stenosis and hypertrophic obstructive cardiomyopathy are also at risk for ventricular tachycardia. Individuals with abnormalities of ventricular repolarization (prolongation of the QT interval) are at risk to develop polymorphic ventricular tachycardia (*torsades de pointes*). Those with the inherited form of this syndrome often have a family history of sudden death in young individuals. Genetic markers can identify some patients with familial long-QT syndrome, but the clinical utility of these markers remains unproven. Drugs (i.e., certain antiarrhythmics and erythromycin) and electrolyte disorders (i.e., hypokalemia, hypocalcemia, hypomagnesemia) can prolong the QT interval and predispose to torsades de pointes. Antiarrhythmic medications may precipitate ventricular tachycardia, particularly in patients with structural heart disease.

In addition to arrhythmias, syncope may also occur with a variety of structural cardiovascular disorders.

Episodes are usually precipitated when the cardiac output cannot increase to compensate adequately for peripheral vasodilatation. Peripheral vasodilatation may be appropriate, such as following exercise, or may occur due to inappropriate activation of left ventricular mechanoreceptor reflexes, as occurs in aortic outflow tract obstruction (aortic valvular stenosis or hypertrophic obstructive cardiomyopathy). Obstruction to forward flow is the most common reason that cardiac output cannot increase. Pericardial tamponade is a rare cause of syncope. Syncope occurs in up to 10% of patients with massive pulmonary embolism and may occur with exertion in patients with severe primary pulmonary hypertension. The cause is an inability of the right ventricle to provide appropriate cardiac output in the presence of obstruction or increased pulmonary vascular resistance. Loss of consciousness is usually accompanied by other symptoms such as chest pain and dyspnea. Atrial myxoma, a prosthetic valve thrombus, and, rarely, mitral stenosis may impair left ventricular filling, decrease cardiac output, and cause syncope.

Cerebrovascular Disease

Cerebrovascular disease alone rarely causes syncope but may lower the threshold for syncope in patients with other causes. The vertebrobasilar arteries, which supply brainstem structures responsible for maintaining consciousness, are usually involved when cerebrovascular disease causes or contributes to syncope. An exception is the rare patient with tight bilateral carotid stenosis and recurrent syncope, often precipitated by standing or walking. Most patients who experience lightheadedness or syncope due to cerebrovascular disease also have symptoms of focal neurologic ischemia, such as arm or leg weakness, diplopia, ataxia, dysarthria, or sensory disturbances. Basilar artery migraine is a rare disorder that causes syncope in adolescents.

DIFFERENTIAL DIAGNOSIS OF SYNCOPE

Anxiety Attacks and the Hyperventilation Syndrome

Anxiety, such as occurs in panic attacks, is frequently interpreted as a feeling of faintness or dizziness resembling presyncope. The symptoms are not accompanied by facial pallor and are not relieved by recumbency. The diagnosis is made on the basis of the associated symptoms such as a feeling of impending doom, air hunger, palpitations, and tingling of the fingers and perioral region. Attacks can often be reproduced by hyperventilation, resulting in hypocapnia, alkalosis, increased cerebrovascular resistance, and decreased cerebral blood flow. The release of epinephrine also contributes to the symptoms.

Seizures

A seizure may be heralded by an aura, which is caused by a focal seizure discharge and hence has localizing significance (Chap. 14). The aura is usually followed by a rapid return to normal or by a loss of consciousness. Injury from falling is frequent in a seizure and rare in syncope, since only in generalized seizures are protective reflexes abolished instantaneously. Sustained tonic-clonic movements are characteristic of convulsive seizures but brief clonic, or tonic-clonic, seizure-like activity can accompany fainting episodes. The period of unconsciousness tends to be longer in seizures than in syncope. Urinary incontinence is frequent in seizures and rare in syncope. The return of consciousness is prompt in syncope, slow after a seizure. Mental confusion, headache, and drowsiness are common sequelae of seizures, whereas physical weakness with a clear sensorium characterizes the postsyncopal state. Repeated spells of unconsciousness in a young person at a rate of several per day or month are more suggestive of epilepsy than syncope. See Table 14-7 for a comparison of seizures and syncope.

Hypoglycemia

Severe hypoglycemia is usually due to a serious disease such as a tumor of the islets of Langerhans; advanced adrenal, pituitary, or hepatic disease; or to excessive administration of insulin.

Acute Hemorrhage

Hemorrhage, usually within the gastrointestinal tract, is an occasional cause of syncope. In the absence of pain and hematemesis, the cause of the weakness, faintness, or even unconsciousness may remain obscure until the passage of a black stool.

Hysterical Fainting

The attack is usually unattended by an outward display of anxiety. Lack of change in pulse and blood pressure or color of the skin and mucous membranes distinguish it from the vasodepressor faint.

APPROACH TO THE PATIENT WITH SYNCOPE

The diagnosis of syncope is often challenging. The cause may only be apparent at the time of the event, leaving few, if any, clues when the patient is seen later by the physician. The physician should think first of those causes that constitute a therapeutic

emergency. Among them are massive internal hemorrhage or myocardial infarction, which may be painless, and cardiac arrhythmias. In elderly persons, a sudden faint, without obvious cause, should arouse the suspicion of complete heart block or a tachyarrhythmia, even though all findings are negative when the patient is seen.

Figure 9-1 depicts an algorithmic approach to syncope. A careful history is the most important diagnostic tool, both to suggest the correct cause and to exclude important potential causes (Table 9-1). The nature of the events and their time course immediately prior to, during, and after an episode of syncope often provide valuable etiologic clues. Loss of consciousness in particular situations, such as during venipuncture, micturition, or with volume depletion, suggests an abnormality of vascular tone. The position of the patient at the time of the syncopal episode is important; syncope in the supine position is unlikely to be vasovagal and suggests an arrhythmia or a seizure. Syncope due to carotid sinus syndrome may occur when

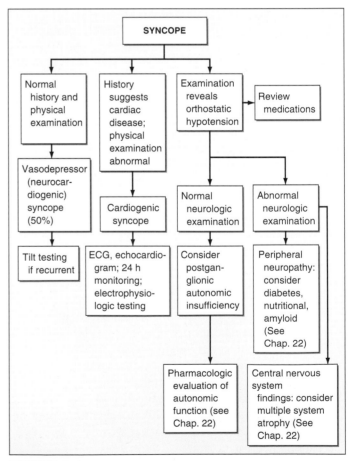

FIGURE 9-1

Approach to the patient with syncope.

the individual is wearing a shirt with a tight collar, turning the head (turning to look while driving in reverse), or manipulating the neck (as in shaving). The patient's medications must be noted, including nonprescription drugs or health store supplements, with particular attention to recent changes.

The physical examination should include evaluation of heart rate and blood pressure in the supine, sitting, and standing positions. In patients with unexplained recurrent syncope, an attempt to reproduce an attack may assist in diagnosis. Anxiety attacks induced by hyperventilation can be reproduced readily by having the patient breathe rapidly and deeply for 2 to 3 min. Cough syncope may be reproduced by inducing the Valsalva maneuver. Carotid sinus massage should generally be avoided, even in patients with suspected carotid sinus hypersensitivity; it is a risky procedure that can cause a transient ischemic attack (TIA) or stroke in individuals with carotid atheromas.

Diagnostic Tests

The choice of diagnostic tests should be guided by the history and the physical examination. Measurements of serum electrolytes, glucose, and the hematocrit are usually indicated. Cardiac enzymes should be evaluated if myocardial ischemia is suspected. Blood and urine toxicology screens may reveal the presence of alcohol or other drugs. In patients with possible adrenocortical insufficiency, plasma aldosterone and mineralocorticoid levels should be obtained.

Although the surface electrocardiogram is unlikely to provide a definitive diagnosis, it may provide clues to the cause of syncope *and should be performed in almost all patients*. The presence of conduction abnormalities (PR prolongation and bundle branch block) suggests a bradyarrhythmia, whereas pathologic Q waves or prolongation of the QT interval suggests a ventricular tachyarrhythmia. Inpatients should undergo continuous electrocardiographic monitoring; outpatients should wear a Holter monitor for 24 to 48 h. Whenever possible, symptoms should be correlated with the occurrence of arrhythmias. Continuous electrocardiographic monitoring may establish the cause of syncope in as many as 15% of patients. Cardiac event monitors may be useful in patients with infrequent symptoms, particularly in patients with presyncope. The presence of a late potential on a signal-averaged electrocardiogram is associated with increased risk for ventricular tacharrhythmias in patients with a prior myocardial infarction. Low-voltage (visually inapparent) T wave alternans is also associated with development of sustained ventricular arrhythmias.

Invasive cardiac electrophysiologic testing provides diagnostic and prognostic information regarding sinus node function, AV conduction, and supraventricular and ventricular arrhythmias. Prolongation of the sinus node recovery time (>1500 ms) is a specific finding (85 to 100%) for diagnosis of sinus node dysfunction but has a low sensitivity; continuous electrocardiographic monitoring is usually more effective for diagnosing this abnormality. Prolongation of the HV interval and conduction block below the His bundle indicate that His-Purkinje disease may be responsible for syncope. Programmed stimulation for ventricular arrhythmias is most useful in patients who have experienced a myocardial infarction; the sensitivity and specificity of this technique is lower in patients with normal hearts or those with heart disease other than coronary artery disease.

Upright tilt table testing is indicated for recurrent syncope, a single syncopal episode that caused injury, or a single syncopal event in a "high-risk" setting (pilot, commercial vehicle driver, etc.), whether or not there is a history of preexisting heart disease or prior vasovagal episodes. In susceptible patients, upright tilt at an angle between 60 and 80° for 30 to 60 min induces a vasovagal episode. The protocol can be shortened if upright tilt is combined with administration of drugs that cause venous pooling or increase adrenergic stimulation (isoproterenol, nitroglycerin, edrophonium, or adenosine). The sensitivity and specificity of tilt table testing is difficult to ascertain because of the lack of validated criteria. Moreover, the reflexes responsible for vasovagal syncope can be elicited in most, if not all, individuals given the appropriate stimulus. The reported accuracy of the test ranges from 30 to 80%, depending on the population studied and the techniques used. Whereas the reproducibility of a negative test is 85 to 100%, the reproducibility of a positive tilt table test is only between 62 and 88%.

A variety of other tests may be useful to determine the presence of structural heart disease that may cause syncope. The echocardiogram with Doppler examination detects valvular, myocardial, and pericardial abnormalities. The echocardiogram is the "gold standard" for the diagnosis of hypertrophic cardiomyopathy and atrial myxoma. Cardiac cine magnetic resonance (MR) imaging provides an alternative noninvasive modality that may be useful for patients in whom diagnostic-quality echocardiographic images cannot be obtained. This test is also indicated for patients suspected of having arrhythmogenic right ventricular dysplasia or right ventricular outflow tract ventricular tachycardia. Both are associated with right ventricular structural abnormalities that are better visualized on MR imaging than by echocardiogram. Exercise testing may detect ischemia or exercise-induced arrhythmias. In some patients, cardiac catheterization may be necessary to diagnose the presence or severity of coronary artery disease or valvular abnormalities. Ultrafast computed tomographic scan, ventilation-perfusion scan, or pulmonary angiography is indicated in patients in whom syncope may be due to pulmonary embolus.

In possible cases of cerebrovascular syncope neuroimaging tests may be indicated, including Doppler ultrasound studies of the carotid and vertebrobasilar systems, MR imaging, MR angiography, and x-ray angiography of the cerebral vasculature (Chap. 17). Electroencephalography is indicated if seizures are suspected.

TREATMENT FOR SYNCOPE

The treatment is directed toward the underlying cause. This discussion will focus on disorders of autonomic control. Cerebrovascular disorders are discussed in Chap. 17.

Certain precautions should be taken regardless of the cause of syncope. At the first sign of symptoms, patients should make every effort to avoid injury should they lose consciousness. Patients with frequent episodes, or those who have experienced syncope without warning symptoms, should avoid situations in which sudden loss of consciousness might result in injury (e.g., climbing ladders, swimming alone, operating heavy machinery, driving). Patients should lower their head to the extent possible and preferably should lie down. Lowering the head by bending at the waist should be avoided because it may further compromise venous return to the heart. When appropriate, family members or other close contacts should be educated as to the problem. This will ensure appropriate therapy and may prevent delivery of inappropriate therapy

(chest compressions associated with cardiopulmonary resuscitation) that may inflict trauma.

Patients who have lost consciousness should be placed in a position that maximizes cerebral blood flow, offers protection from trauma, and secures the airway. Whenever possible, the patient should be placed supine with the head turned to the side to prevent aspiration and the tongue from blocking the airway. Assessment of the pulse and direct cardiac auscultation may assist in determining if the episode is associated with a bradyarrhythmia or tachyarrhythmia. Clothing that fits tightly around the neck or waist should be loosened. Peripheral stimulation, such as by sprinkling cold water on the face, may be helpful. Patients should not be given anything by mouth or be permitted to rise until the sense of physical weakness has passed.

Patients with vasovagal syncope should be instructed to avoid situations or stimuli that have caused them to lose consciousness and to assume a recumbent position when premonitory symptoms occur. These behavioral modifications alone may be sufficient for patients with infrequent and relatively benign episodes of vasovagal syncope, particularly when loss of consciousness occurs in response to a specific stimulus. Tilt training (standing and leaning against a wall for progressively longer periods each day) has been used with limited success, particularly for those patients who have profound orthostatic intolerance. Episodes associated with intravascular volume depletion may be prevented by salt and fluid loading prior to provocative events.

Prescription drug therapy may be necessary when vasovagal syncope is resistant to these measures, when episodes occur frequently, or when syncope is associated with a significant risk for injury. β-Adrenergic receptor antagonists (metoprolol, 25 to 50 mg bid; atenolol, 25 to 50 mg qd; or nadolol, 10 to 20 mg bid; all starting doses), the most widely used agents, mitigate the increase in myocardial contractility that stimulates left ventricular mechanoreceptors and also block central serotonin receptors. Serotonin reuptake inhibitors (paroxetine, 20 to 40 mg qd; or sertraline, 25 to 50 mg qd), appear to be effective for some patients. Bupropion SR (150 mg qd), another antidepressant, has also been used with success. β-Adrenergic receptor antagonists and serotonin reuptake inhibitors are well tolerated and are often used as first-line agents for younger patients. Hydrofludrocortisone (0.1 to 0.2 mg qd), a mineralocorticoid, promotes sodium retention, volume expansion, and peripheral vasoconstriction by increasing β-receptor sensitivity to endogenous catecholamines. Hydrofludrocortisone is useful for patients with intravascular volume depletion and those who also have postural hypotension. Proamatine (2.5 to 10 mg bid or tid), an α-agonist, has been used as a first-line agent for some patients. In a recent randomized controlled trial, proamatine was more effective than placebo in preventing syncope during an upright tilt-test. However, in some patients, proamatine and hydrofludrocortisone may increase resting supine systemic blood pressure, a property that may be problematic for those with hypertension.

Disopyramide (150 mg bid), a vagolytic antiarrhythmic drug with negative inotropic properties, and another vagolytic, transdermal scopolamine, have been used to treat vasovagal syncope, as have theophylline and ephedrine. Side effects associated with these drugs have limited their use for this indication. Disopyramide is a type 1A antiarrhythmic drug and should be used with great caution, if at all, in patients who are at risk for ventricular arrhythmias. Although several clinical trials have suggested that pharmacologic therapy for vasovagal syncope is effective, long-term prospective randomized controlled trials have yet to be completed.

Permanent dual-chamber cardiac pacing is effective for patients with frequent episodes of vasovagal syncope and is indicated for those with prolonged asystole associated with vasovagal episodes. Patients in whom vasodilatation contributes to loss of consciousness may also experience symptomatic benefit from permanent pacing. Pacemakers that can be programmed to transiently pace at a high rate (90 to 100 beats/min) after a profound drop in the patient's intrinsic heart rate are most effective.

Patients with orthostatic hypotension should be instructed to rise slowly and systematically (supine to seated, seated to standing) from the bed or a chair. Movement of the legs prior to rising facilitates venous return from the lower extremities. Whenever possible, medications that aggravate the problem (vasodilators, diuretics, etc.) should be discontinued. Elevation of the head of the bed [20 to 30 cm (8 to 12 in.)] and use of compression stockings may help.

Additional therapeutic modalities include an antigravity or g suit or compression stockings to prevent lower limb blood pooling; salt loading; and a variety of pharmacologic agents including sympathomimetic amines, monamine oxidase inhibitors, beta blockers, and levodopa. The treatment of orthostatic hypotension secondary to central or peripheral disorders of the autonomic nervous system is discussed in Chap. 22.

Glossopharyngeal neuralgia is treated with carbamazepine, which is effective for the syncope as well as for the pain. Patients with carotid sinus syndrome should be instructed to avoid clothing and situations that stimulate carotid sinus baroreceptors. They should turn their entire body, rather than just their head, when looking to the side. Those with intractable syncope due to the cardioinhibitory response to carotid sinus stimulation should undergo permanent pacemaker implantation.

Patients with syncope should be hospitalized when the episode may have resulted from a life-threatening abnormality or if recurrence with significant injury seems likely. These individuals should be admitted to a bed with continuous electrocardiographic monitoring. Patients who are known to have a normal heart and for whom the history strongly suggests vasovagal or situational syncope may be treated as outpatients if the episodes are neither frequent nor severe.

VERTIGO

Vertigo is usually due to a disturbance in the vestibular system. The end organs of this system, situated in the bony labyrinths of the inner ears, consist of the three semicircular canals and the otolithic apparatus (utricle and saccule) on each side. The canals transduce angular acceleration, while the otoliths transduce linear acceleration and the static gravitational forces that provide a sense of head position in space. The neural output of the end organs is conveyed to the vestibular nuclei in the brainstem via the eighth cranial nerves. The principal projections from the vestibular nuclei are to the nuclei of cranial nerves III, IV, and VI; spinal cord; cerebral cortex; and cerebellum. The vestibuloocular reflex (VOR) serves to maintain visual stability during head movement and depends on direct projections from the vestibular nuclei to the sixth cranial nerve (abducens) nuclei in the pons and, via the medial longitudinal fasciculus, to the third (oculomotor) and fourth (trochlear) cranial nerve nuclei in the midbrain. These connections account for the nystagmus (to-and-fro oscillation of the eyes) that is an almost invariable accompaniment of vestibular dysfunction. The vestibular nerves and nuclei project to areas of the cerebellum (primarily the flocculus and nodulus) that modulate the VOR. The vestibulospinal pathways assist in the maintenance of postural stability. Projections to the cerebral cortex, via the thalamus, provide conscious awareness of head position and movement.

The vestibular system is one of three sensory systems subserving spatial orientation and posture; the other two are the visual system (retina to occipital cortex) and the somatosensory system that conveys peripheral information from skin, joint, and muscle receptors. The three stabilizing systems overlap sufficiently to compensate (partially or completely) for each other's deficiencies. Vertigo may represent either physiologic stimulation or pathologic dysfunction in any of the three systems.

Physiologic Vertigo

This occurs in normal individuals when (1) the brain is confronted with a mismatch among the three stabilizing sensory systems; (2) the vestibular system is subjected to unfamiliar head movements to which it is unadapted, such as in seasickness; (3) unusual head/neck positions, such as the extreme extension when painting a ceiling; or (4) following a spin. Intersensory mismatch explains carsickness, height vertigo, and the visual vertigo most commonly experienced during motion picture chase scenes; in the latter, the visual sensation of environmental movement is unaccompanied by concomitant vestibular and somatosensory movement cues. Space sickness, a frequent transient effect of active head movement in the weightless zero-gravity environment, is another example of physiologic vertigo.

Pathologic Vertigo

This results from lesions of the visual, somatosensory, or vestibular systems. Visual vertigo is caused by new or incorrect spectacles or by the sudden onset of an extraocular muscle paresis with diplopia; in either instance, CNS compensation rapidly counteracts the vertigo. Somatosensory vertigo, rare in isolation, is usually due to a peripheral neuropathy or myelopathy that reduces the sensory input necessary for central compensation when there is dysfunction of the vestibular or visual systems.

The most common cause of pathologic vertigo is vestibular dysfunction involving either its end organ (labyrinth), nerve, or central connections. The vertigo is frequently accompanied by nausea, jerk nystagmus, postural unsteadiness, and gait ataxia. Since vertigo increases with rapid head movements, patients tend to hold their heads still.

Labyrinthine Dysfunction   This causes severe rotational or linear vertigo. When rotational, the hallucination

of movement, whether of environment or self, is directed away from the side of the lesion. The fast phases of nystagmus beat away from the lesion side, and the tendency to fall is toward the side of the lesion, particularly in darkness or with the eyes closed.

Under normal circumstances, when the head is straight and immobile, the vestibular end organs generate a tonic resting firing frequency that is equal from the two sides. With any rotational acceleration, the anatomical positions of the semicircular canals on each side necessitate an increased firing rate from one and a commensurate decrease from the other. This change in neural activity is ultimately projected to the cerebral cortex, where it is summed with inputs from the visual and somatosensory systems to produce the appropriate conscious sense of rotational movement. After cessation of movement, the firing frequencies of the two end organs reverse; the side with the initially increased rate decreases, and the other side increases. A sense of rotation in the opposite direction is experienced; since there is no actual head movement, this hallucinatory sensation is physiologic postrotational vertigo.

Any disease state that changes the firing frequency of an end organ, producing unequal neural input to the brainstem and ultimately the cerebral cortex, causes vertigo. The symptom can be conceptualized as the cortex inappropriately interpreting the abnormal neural input as indicating actual head rotation. Transient abnormalities produce short-lived symptoms. With a fixed unilateral deficit, central compensatory mechanisms ultimately diminish the vertigo. Since compensation depends on the plasticity of connections between the vestibular nuclei and the cerebellum, patients with brainstem or cerebellar disease have diminished adaptive capacity, and symptoms may persist indefinitely. Compensation is always inadequate for severe fixed bilateral lesions despite normal cerebellar connections: these patients are permanently symptomatic.

Acute unilateral labyrinthine dysfunction is caused by infection, trauma, and ischemia. Often, no specific etiology is uncovered, and the nonspecific terms acute labyrinthitis, acute peripheral vestibulopathy, or vestibular neuritis are used to describe the event. The vertiginous attacks are brief and leave the patient with mild vertigo for several days. Infection with herpes simplex virus type 1 has been implicated. It is impossible to predict whether a patient recovering from the first bout of vertigo will have recurrent episodes.

Labyrinthine ischemia, presumably due to occlusion of the labyrinthine branch of the internal auditory artery, may be the sole manifestation of vertebrobasilar insufficiency (Chap. 17); patients with this syndrome present with the abrupt onset of severe vertigo, nausea, and vomiting, but without tinnitus or hearing loss.

Acute bilateral labyrinthine dysfunction is usually the result of toxins such as drugs or alcohol. The most common offending drugs are the aminoglycoside antibiotics that damage the hair cells of the vestibular end organs and may cause a permanent disorder of equilibrium.

Recurrent unilateral labyrinthine dysfunction, in association with signs and symptoms of cochlear disease (progressive hearing loss and tinnitus), is usually due to Ménière's disease (Chap. 12). When auditory manifestations are absent, the term *vestibular neuronitis* denotes recurrent monosymptomatic vertigo. TIAs of the posterior cerebral circulation (vertebrobasilar insufficiency) only infrequently cause recurrent vertigo without concomitant motor, sensory, visual, cranial nerve, or cerebellar signs (Chap. 17).

Positional vertigo is precipitated by a recumbent head position, either to the right or to the left. Benign paroxysmal positional (or positioning) vertigo (BPPV) of the posterior semicircular canal is particularly common. Although the condition may be due to head trauma, usually no precipitating factors are identified. It generally abates spontaneously after weeks or months. The vertigo and accompanying nystagmus have a distinct pattern of latency, fatigability, and habituation that differs from the less common central positional vertigo (**Table 9-2**) due to lesions in and around the fourth ventricle. Moreover, the pattern of nystagmus in posterior canal BPPV is distinctive. When supine, with the head turned to the side of the offending ear (bad ear down), the lower eye displays a large-amplitude torsional nystagmus, and the upper eye has a lesser degree of torsion combined with upbeating nystagmus. If the eyes are directed to the upper ear, the vertical nystagmus in the upper eye increases in amplitude. Mild dysequilibrium when upright may also be present.

A *perilymphatic fistula* should be suspected when episodic vertigo is precipitated by Valsalva or exertion, particularly upon a background of a stepwise progressive sensory-neural hearing loss. The condition is usually caused by head trauma or barotrauma or occurs after middle ear surgery.

■ **Vertigo of Vestibular Nerve Origin** This occurs with diseases that involve the nerve in the petrous bone or the cerebellopontine angle. Although less severe and less frequently paroxysmal, it has many of the characteristics of labyrinthine vertigo. The adjacent auditory division of the eighth cranial nerve is usually affected, which

TABLE 9-2

CLINICAL PEARLS: DISTINGUISHING PERIPHERAL VS. CENTRAL CAUSES OF VERTIGO.		
Feature	Peripheral (Labyrinth or Nerve)	Central (Brainstem or Cerebellum)
Latency[a]	3–40 s	None: immediate vertigo and nystagmus
Fatigability[b]	Yes	No
Habituation[c]	Yes	No
Direction of associated nystagmus	Unidirectional; fast phase opposite lesion[d]	Bidirectional or unidirectional
Vertical or purely torsional nystagmus	Never present	May be present
Visual fixation	Inhibits nystagmus and vertigo	No inhibition
Intensity of vertigo	Severe	Mild
Tinnitus and/or deafness	Often present	Usually absent
Associated CNS abnormalities	None	Extremely common (e.g., diplopia, hiccups, cranial neuropathies, dysarthria)
Common causes	BPPV, infection (labyrinthitis), Ménière's, ischemia, trauma, toxin	Vascular, demyelinating, neoplasm

[a]Time between attaining head position and onset of symptoms.
[b]Disappearance of symptoms with maintenance of offending position.
[c]Lessening of symptoms with repeated trials.
[d]In Ménière's disease, the direction of the fast phase is variable.
Note: BPPV, benign paroxysmal positional vertigo.

explains the frequent association of vertigo with unilateral tinnitus and hearing loss. The most common cause of eighth cranial nerve dysfunction is a tumor, usually a schwannoma (*acoustic neuroma*) or a meningioma. These tumors grow slowly and produce such a gradual reduction of labyrinthine output that central compensatory mechanisms can prevent or minimize the vertigo; auditory symptoms of hearing loss and tinnitus are the most common manifestations.

Central Vertigo Lesions of the brainstem or cerebellum can cause acute vertigo, but associated signs and symptoms usually permit distinction from a labyrinthine etiology (Table 9-2). Occasionally, an acute lesion of the vestibulocerebellum may present with monosymptomatic vertigo indistinguishable from a labyrinthopathy.

Vertigo may be a manifestation of a migraine aura (Chap. 5), but some patients with migraine have episodes of vertigo unassociated with their headaches. Antimigrainous treatment should be considered in such patients with otherwise enigmatic vertiginous episodes.

Vestibular epilepsy, vertigo secondary to temporal lobe epileptic activity, is rare and almost always intermixed with other epileptic manifestations.

Psychogenic Vertigo This is usually a concomitant of panic attacks (Chap. 41) or agoraphobia (fear of large open spaces, crowds, or leaving the safety of home) and should be suspected in patients so "incapacitated" by their symptoms that they adopt a prolonged housebound status. Most patients with organic vertigo attempt to function despite their discomfort. Organic vertigo is accompanied by nystagmus; a psychogenic etiology is almost certain when nystagmus is absent during a vertiginous episode.

Miscellaneous Head Sensations

This designation is used, primarily for purposes of initial classification, to describe dizziness that is neither faintness nor vertigo. Cephalic ischemia or vestibular dysfunction may be of such low intensity that the usual symptomatology is not clearly identified. For example, a small decrease in blood pressure or a slight vestibular imbalance may cause sensations different from distinct faintness or vertigo but that may be identified properly during provocative testing techniques (see below). Other causes of dizziness in this category are hyperventilation syndrome, hypoglycemia, and the somatic symptoms of a clinical depression; these patients should all have normal neurologic examinations and vestibular function tests. Depressed patients often insist that the depression is "secondary" to the dizziness.

APPROACH TO THE PATIENT WITH VERTIGO

The most important diagnostic tool is a detailed history focused on the meaning of "dizziness" to the patient. Is it faintness (presyncope)? Is there a sensation of spinning? If either of these is affirmed and the neurologic examination is normal, appropriate investigations for the multiple causes of cephalic ischemia or vestibular dysfunction are undertaken.

When the meaning of "dizziness" is uncertain, provocative tests may be helpful. These office procedures simulate either cephalic ischemia or vestibular dysfunction. Cephalic ischemia is obvious if the dizziness is duplicated during maneuvers that produce orthostatic hypotension. Further provocation involves the Valsalva maneuver, which decreases cerebral blood flow and should reproduce ischemic symptoms.

Hyperventilation is the cause of dizziness in many anxious individuals; tingling of the hands and face may be absent. Forced hyperventilation for 1 min is indicated for patients with enigmatic dizziness and normal neurologic examinations.

The simplest provocative test for vestibular dysfunction is rapid rotation and abrupt cessation of movement in a swivel chair. This always induces vertigo that the patients can compare with their symptomatic dizziness. The intense induced vertigo may be unlike the spontaneous symptoms, but shortly thereafter, when the vertigo has all but subsided, a lightheadedness supervenes that may be identified as "my dizziness." When this occurs, the dizzy patient, originally classified as suffering from "miscellaneous head sensations," is now properly diagnosed as having mild vertigo secondary to a vestibulopathy.

Patients with symptoms of positional vertigo should be appropriately tested (Table 9-2). A final provocative and diagnostic vestibular test, requiring the use of Frenzel eyeglasses (self-illuminated goggles with convex lenses that blur out the patient's vision, but allow the examiner to see the eyes greatly magnified), is vigorous head shaking in the horizontal plane for about 10 s. If nystagmus develops after the shaking stops, even in the absence of vertigo, vestibular dysfunction is demonstrated. The maneuver can then be repeated in the vertical plane. If the provocative tests establish the dizziness as a vestibular symptom, an evaluation of vestibular vertigo is undertaken.

Evaluation of Patients with Pathologic Vestibular Vertigo

The evaluation depends on whether a central etiology is suspected (Table 9–2). If so, MR imaging of the head is mandatory. Such an examination is rarely helpful in cases of recurrent monosymptomatic vertigo with a normal neurologic examination. Typical BPPV requires no investigation after the diagnosis is made.

Vestibular function tests serve to (1) demonstrate an abnormality when the distinction between organic and psychogenic is uncertain, (2) establish the side of the abnormality, and (3) distinguish between peripheral and central etiologies. The standard test is electronystagmography (calorics), where warm and cold water (or air) are applied, in a prescribed fashion, to the tympanic membranes, and the slow-phase velocities of the resultant nystagmus from the two are compared. A velocity decrease from one side indicates hypofunction ("canal paresis"). An inability to induce nystagmus with ice water denotes a "dead labyrinth." Some institutions have the capability of quantitatively determining various aspects of the VOR using computer-driven rotational chairs and precise oculographic recording of the eye movements.

CNS disease can produce dizzy sensations of all types. Consequently, a neurologic examination is always required even if the history or provocative tests suggest a cardiac, peripheral vestibular, or psychogenic etiology. Any abnormality on the neurologic examination should prompt appropriate neurodiagnostic studies.

TABLE 9–3

TREATMENT OF VERTIGO

AGENT[a]	DOSE[b]
Antihistamines	
Meclizine	25–50 mg 3 times/day
Dimenhydrinate	50 mg 1–2 times/day
Promethazine[c]	25–50-mg suppository or IM
Benzodiazepines	
Diazepam	2.5 mg 1–3 times/day
Clonazepam	0.25 mg 1–3 times/day
Phenothiazines	
Prochlorperazine[c]	5 mg IM or 25-mg suppository
Anticholinergic[d]	
Scopolamine transdermal	Patch
Sympathomimetics[d]	
Ephedrine	25 mg/d
Combination preparations[d]	
Ephedrine and promethazine	25 mg/d of each
Exercise therapy	
Repositioning maneuvers[e]	
Vestibular rehabilitation[f]	
Other	
Diuretics or low-salt (1 g/d) diet[g]	
Antimigrainous drugs[h]	
Inner ear surgery[i]	
Glucocorticoids[c]	

[a]All listed drugs are U.S. Food and Drug Administration approved, but most are not approved for the treatment of vertigo.
[b]Usual oral (unless otherwise stated) starting dose in adults; maintenance dose can be reached by a gradual increase.
[c]For acute vertigo only.
[d]For motion sickness only.
[e]For benign paroxysmal positional vertigo.
[f]For vertigo other than Ménière's and positional.
[g]For Ménière's disease.
[h]For migraine-associated vertigo (see Chap. 5 for a listing of prophylactic antimigrainous drugs).
[i]For perilymphatic fistula and refractory cases of Ménière's disease.

TREATMENT FOR VERTIGO

Treatment for acute vertigo consists of bed rest (1 to 2 days maximum) and vestibular suppressant drugs such as antihistaminics (meclizine, dimenhydrinate, promethazine), tranquilizers with GABA-ergic effects (diazepam, clonazepam), phenothiazines (prochlorperazine), or glucocorticoids (**Table 9-3**). If the vertigo persists beyond a few days, most authorities advise ambulation in an attempt to induce central compensatory mechanisms, despite the short-term discomfort to the patient. Chronic vertigo of labyrinthine origin may be treated with a systematized vestibular rehabilitation program to facilitate central compensation.

BPPV is often self-limited but, when persistent, may respond dramatically to specific repositioning exercise programs designed to empty particulate debris from the posterior semicircular canal. One of these exercises, the Epley procedure, is graphically demonstrated, in four languages, on a website for use in both physician's offices and self-treatment (*www.charite.de/ch/neuro/vertigo.html*).

Prophylactic measures to prevent recurrent vertigo are variably effective. Antihistamines are commonly utilized but are of limited value. Ménière's disease may respond to a diuretic or, more effectively, to a very low salt diet (1 g/d). Recurrent episodes of migraine-associated vertigo should be treated with antimigrainous therapy (Chap. 5). There are a variety of inner ear surgical procedures for refractory Ménière's disease, but these are only rarely necessary.

Helpful websites for both physicians and vertigo patients are: *www.iVertigo.net* and *www.tchain.com*.

FURTHER READINGS

Baloh RW, Honrubia V: *Clinical Neurophysiology of the Vestibular System*, 3d ed. New York, Oxford University, 2001

☑ Grubb BP: Neurocardiogenic syncope. N Engl J Med 352:1004, 2005

A concise review of one of the most common causes of syncope.

Kapoor WN: Current evaluation in management of syncope. Circulation 106:1606, 2002

Kaufman H et al: Midodrine in neurally mediated syncope: A double-blind, randomized, crossover study. Ann Neurol 52:342, 2002

Kaufman NH, Bhattacharya K: Diagnosis and treatment of neurally mediated syncope. The Neurologist 8:175, 2002

☑ Lempert T, von Brevern M: Episodic vertigo. Curr Opin Neurol 18:5, 2005

A focused discussion of common peripheral causes of episodic vertigo and their specific treatments.

Soteriades E et al: Incidence and prognosis of syncope. N Engl J Med 347:878, 2002

Strupp M, Arbusow V: Acute vestibulopathy. Curr Opin Neurol 14:11, 2001

Woodworth BA et al: The canalith repositioning procedure for benign positional vertigo: A meta-analysis. Laryngoscope 114:1143, 2004

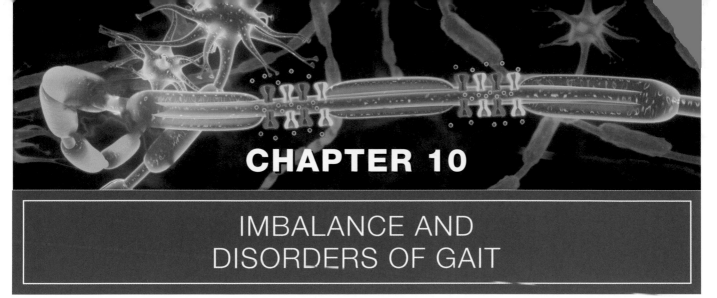

CHAPTER 10

IMBALANCE AND DISORDERS OF GAIT

Richard K. Olney

Imbalance is the impaired ability to maintain the intended orientation of the body in space. It is generally manifest as difficulty in maintaining an upright posture while standing or walking; a severe imbalance may also affect the ability to maintain posture while seated. Patients with imbalance commonly complain of a feeling of unsteadiness or dysequilibrium. Whereas imbalance and unsteadiness are synonymous, *dysequilibrium* implies the additional component of impaired spatial orientation even while lying down. Patients with dysequilibrium commonly also experience *vertigo*, defined as an hallucination of rotatory movement.

PATHOGENESIS

IMBALANCE AND LIMB ATAXIA

Imbalance results from disorders of the vestibular, sensory, or cerebellar systems, whereas limb ataxia is produced by disorders of the sensory or cerebellar systems. Asymmetric vestibular sensory input to the brainstem and cerebellum produces asymmetric imbalance, but not limb ataxia. Sensory ataxia is caused by lesions that affect the peripheral sensory fibers; dorsal root ganglia cells; posterior columns of the spinal cord; or lemniscal system in the brainstem, thalamus, or parietal cortex. Impairment of the proprioceptive sensory feedback to the cerebellum, basal ganglia, and cortex produces sensory ataxia. Sensory ataxia results

in imbalance and disturbs the fluency and integration of limb movements that can be partially alleviated by visual feedback. Imbalance with cerebellar ataxia results from disorders of proprioceptive, spinocerebellar, or vestibular sensory input; the integration of these inputs in the brainstem or midline cerebellar vermis or flocculonodular lobe; or the motor output to the spinal neurons that control muscles of the proximal limbs and trunk. Cerebellar limb ataxia results from disorders of the spinocerebellar and corticopontocerebellar inputs, the integration of these inputs in the intermediate and lateral cerebellum, or the output to the spinal neurons (via the red nucleus and rubrospinal tract) or to the cortex. These pathways ensure adequate speed, fluency, and integration of limb movements. The lateral cerebellar hemispheres coordinate a polysynaptic feedback circuit that modulates cortically initiated limb movement.

DISORDERS OF GAIT

Walking is one of the most complicated motor activities. Cyclical stepping movements produced by the lumbosacral spinal cord centers are modified by cortical, basal ganglionic, brainstem, and cerebellar influences based on proprioceptive, vestibular, and visual feedback.

IMBALANCE

A guide to interpretation of imbalance without weakness is presented in **Fig. 10-1**.

Imbalance with cerebellar ataxia typically produces truncal ataxia, which is usually revealed during the process of rising from a chair, assuming the upright stance with the feet together, or performing some other activity while standing. Once a desired position is reached, imbalance may be surprisingly mild. As walking begins, the imbalance recurs. Patients usually learn to lessen the imbal-

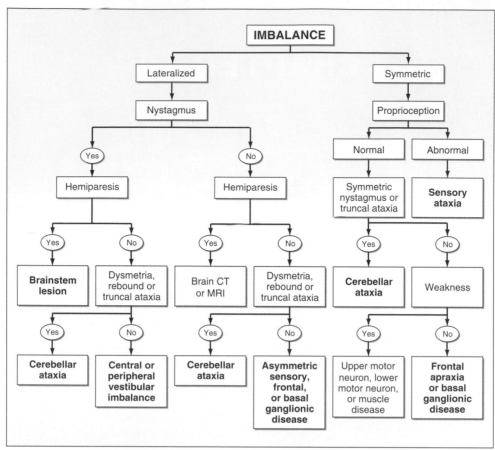

Figure 10-1

An algorithm for evaluation of imbalance without weakness.

ance by walking with the legs widely separated. The imbalance is usually not lateralized; may be accompanied by symmetric nystagmus; and is caused by toxic, metabolic, inflammatory, or neurodegenerative diseases. Asymmetric cerebellar ataxia suggests structural disease from ischemia, tumor, or other mass lesion.

Cerebellar limb ataxia is characterized by dysmetria (irregular errors in amplitude and force of movements); intention tremor (accentuation as the target is approached); dysdiadochokinesia (errors in rhythm, velocity, or force); and excessive rebound of outstretched arms against a resistance that is suddenly removed. Muscle tone is often modestly reduced; this contributes to the abnormal rebound due to decreased activation of segmental spinal cord reflexes and also to pendular reflexes, i.e., a tendency for a tendon reflex to produce multiple swings to and fro after a single tap. If involvement is asymmetric, lateralized imbalance is common and usually associated with asymmetric nystagmus. For further discussion of cerebellar diseases, see Chap. 20.

Imbalance with vestibular dysfunction is characterized by a consistent tendency to fall to one side. The patient commonly complains of vertigo rather than imbalance,

especially if the onset is acute. Acute vertigo associated with lateralized imbalance but no other neurologic signs is often due to disorders of the semicircular canal; the presence of other neurologic signs suggests brainstem ischemia (Chap. 17) or multiple sclerosis (Chap. 28). When the vestibular dysfunction is peripheral, positional nystagmus and vertigo tend to resolve if a provocative position is maintained (extinction) or repeated (habituation). Lateralized imbalance of gradual onset or persisting for >2 weeks, accompanied by nystagmus, may result from lesions of the semicircular canal or vestibular nerve, brainstem, or cerebellum.

Imbalance with sensory ataxia is characterized by marked worsening when visual feedback is removed. The patient can often assume the upright stance with feet together cautiously with eyes open. With eye closure, balance is rapidly lost (positive Romberg sign) in various directions at random. Sensory examination reveals impairment of proprioception at the toes and ankles, usually associated with an even more prominent abnormality of vibratory perception. Prompt evaluation for vitamin B_{12} deficiency is important, as this disorder is reversible if recognized early. Depression or absence of reflexes points to peripheral nerve disorders. Spasticity with extensor plantar responses suggests posterior column and spinal cord disorders. Rarely, sensory ataxia produces lateralized imbalance. In these cases, the disorder is usually in the parietal lobe or thalamus, but may also be due to an asymmetric sensory neuropathy or posterior column disease.

Sensory limb ataxia is similar to cerebellar limb ataxia but is markedly worse when the eyes are closed. Examination also reveals abnormal proprioception and vibratory perception. The approach focuses on localizing the proprioceptive impairment to the peripheral nerves, the posterior columns of the spinal cord, or rarely the parietal lobe.

Other forms of imbalance occur, but the fundamental problem is usually a primary disorder of strength, extrapyramidal function, or cortical initiation of movement, as indicated in Fig. 10-1.

ABNORMAL GAIT

Each of the disorders discussed in this chapter produces a characteristic gait disturbance. If the neurologic examination is normal except for an abnormal gait, diagnosis may be difficult even for the experienced clinician.

Hemiparetic gait characterizes spastic hemiparesis. In its most severe form, an abnormal posture of the limbs is produced by spasticity. The arm is adducted and internally rotated, with flexion of the elbow, wrist, and fingers and with extension of the hip, knee, and ankle. Forward swing of the spastic leg during walking requires abduction and circumduction at the hip, often with contralateral tilt of the trunk to prevent the toes catching on the floor as the leg is advanced. In its mildest form, the affected arm is held in a normal position, but swings less than the normal arm. The affected leg is flexed less than the normal leg during its forward swing and is more externally rotated. A hemiparetic gait is a common residual sign of a stroke.

Paraparetic gait is a walking pattern in which both legs are moved in a slow, stiff manner with circumduction, similar to the leg movement in a hemiparetic gait. In many patients, the legs tend to cross with each forward swing ("scissoring"). A paraparetic gait is a common sign of spinal cord disease and also occurs in cerebral palsy.

Steppage gait is produced by weakness of ankle dorsiflexion. Because of the partial or complete foot drop, the leg must be lifted higher than usual to avoid catching the toe on the floor during the forward swing of the leg. If unilateral, steppage gait is usually due to L5 radiculopathy, sciatic neuropathy, or peroneal neuropathy. If bilateral, it is the common result of a distal polyneuropathy or lumbosacral polyradiculopathy.

Waddling gait results from proximal lower limb weakness, most often from myopathy but occasionally from neuromuscular junction disease or a proximal symmetric spinal muscular atrophy. With weakness of hip flexion, the trunk is tilted away from the leg that is being moved to lift the hip and provide extra distance between the foot and the floor, and the pelvis is rotated forward to assist with forward motion of the leg. Because pelvic girdle weakness is customarily bilateral, the pelvic lift and rotation alternate from side to side, giving the waddling appearance to the gait.

Parkinsonian gait is characterized by a forward stoop, with modest flexion at the hips and knees. The arms are flexed at the elbows and adducted at the shoulders, often with a 4- to 6-Hz resting pronation-supination tremor but little other movement, even during walking. Walking is initiated slowly by leaning forward and maintained with short rapid steps, during which the feet shuffle along the floor. The pace tends to accelerate (festination) as the upper body gradually leans further ahead of the feet, whether movement is forward (propulsion) or backward (retropulsion). The postural instability leads to falls (Chap. 19).

Apraxic gait results from bilateral frontal lobe disease with impaired ability to plan and execute sequential movements. This gait superficially resembles that of parkinsonism, in that the posture is stooped and any steps taken are short and shuffling. However, initiation and maintenance of walking are impaired in a different manner. Each movement that is required for walking can usually be performed, if tested in isolation while sitting or lying. However, when asked to step forward while standing, a long pause often occurs before any attempt is made to flex at the hip and advance, as if the patient is "glued to the ground." Once walking is initiated, it is not maintained, even in an abnormal festinating manner. Rather, after one or several steps are taken, walking is stopped for several seconds or longer. The process is then repeated. Dementia and incontinence may coexist.

Choreoathetotic gait is characterized by an intermittent, irregular movement that disrupts the smooth flow of a normal gait. Flexion or extension movements at the hip are common and unpredictable but readily observed as a pelvic lurch.

Cerebellar ataxic gait is a broad-based gait disorder in which the speed and length of stride vary irregularly from step to step. With midline cerebellar disease, as in alcoholics, posture is erect but the feet are separated; lower limb ataxia is commonly present as well. With disease of the cerebellar hemispheres, limb ataxia and nystagmus are commonly present as well.

Sensory ataxic gait may resemble a cerebellar gait, with its broad-based stance and difficulty with change in position. However, although balance may be maintained with the eyes open, loss of visual input through eye closure results in rapid loss of balance with a fall (positive Romberg sign), unless the physician assists the patient.

Vestibular gait is one in which the patient consistently tends to fall to one side, whether walking or standing. Cranial nerve examination usually demonstrates an asymmetric nystagmus. The possibilities of unilateral sensory ataxia and hemiparesis are excluded by the findings of normal proprioception and strength.

Astasia-abasia is a typical hysterical gait disorder. Although the patient usually has normal coordination of leg movements in bed or while sitting, the patient is unable to stand or walk without assistance. If distracted, stationary balance is sometimes maintained and several steps are taken normally, followed by a dramatic demonstration of imbalance with a lunge toward the examiner's arms or a nearby bed.

FURTHER READINGS

CAPADAY C: The special nature of human walking and its neural control. Trends Neurosci 25:370, 2002

An excellent overview of neural pathways that control ambulation; rehabilitation strategies for stroke and spinal cord patients.

DIETZ V: Proprioception and locomotor disorders. Nat Rev Neurosci 3:781, 2002

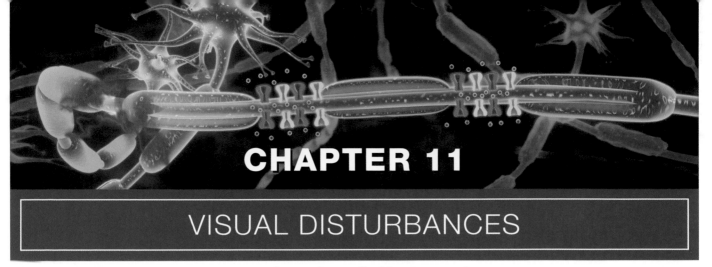

CHAPTER 11

VISUAL DISTURBANCES

Jonathan C. Horton

THE HUMAN VISUAL SYSTEM

The visual system provides a supremely efficient means for the rapid assimilation of information from the environment to aid in the guidance of behavior. The act of seeing begins with the capture of images focused by the cornea and lens upon a light-sensitive membrane in the back of the eye, called the *retina*. The retina is actually part of the brain, banished to the periphery to serve as a transducer for the conversion of patterns of light energy into neuronal signals. Light is absorbed by photopigment in two types of receptors: rods and cones. In the human retina there are 100 million rods and 5 million cones. The rods operate in dim (scotopic) illumination. The cones function under daylight (photopic) conditions. The cone system is specialized for color perception and high spatial resolution. The majority of cones are located within the macula, the portion of the retina serving the central 10° of vision. In the middle of the macula a small pit termed the *fovea,* packed exclusively with cones, provides best visual acuity.

Photoreceptors hyperpolarize in response to light, activating bipolar, amacrine, and horizontal cells in the inner nuclear layer. After processing of photoreceptor re-

sponses by this complex retinal circuit, the flow of sensory information ultimately converges upon a final common pathway: the ganglion cells. These cells translate the visual image impinging upon the retina into a continuously varying barrage of action potentials that propagate along the primary optic pathway to visual centers within the brain. There are a million ganglion cells in each retina, and hence a million fibers in each optic nerve.

Ganglion cell axons sweep along the inner surface of the retina in the nerve fiber layer, exit the eye at the optic disc, and travel through the optic nerve, optic chiasm, and optic tract to reach targets in the brain. The majority of fibers synapse upon cells in the lateral geniculate body, a thalamic relay station. Cells in the lateral geniculate body project in turn to the primary visual cortex. This massive afferent retinogeniculocortical sensory pathway provides the neural substrate for visual perception. Although the lateral geniculate body is the main target of the retina, separate classes of ganglion cells project to other subcortical visual nuclei involved in different functions. Ganglion cells that mediate pupillary constriction and circadian rhythms are light sensitive, owing to a novel visual pigment, melanopsin. Pupil responses are mediated by input to the pretectal olivary nuclei in the midbrain. The pretectal nuclei send their output to the Edinger-Westphal nuclei, which in turn provide parasympathetic innervation to the iris sphincter via an interneuron in the ciliary ganglion. Circadian rhythms are timed by a retinal projection to the suprachiasmatic nucleus. Visual orientation and eye movements are served by retinal input to the superior colliculus. Gaze stabilization and optokinetic reflexes are governed by a group of small retinal targets known collectively as the *brainstem accessory optic system.*

The eyes must be rotated constantly within their orbits to place and maintain targets of visual interest upon the fovea. This activity, called *foveation,* or looking, is governed by an elaborate efferent motor system. Each eye is moved by six extraocular muscles, supplied by cranial nerves from the oculomotor (III), trochlear (IV), and abducens (VI) nuclei. Activity in these ocular motor nuclei is coordinated by pontine and midbrain mechanisms for smooth pursuit, saccades, and gaze stabilization during head and body movements. Large regions of the frontal and parietooccipital cortex control these brainstem eye movement centers by providing descending supranuclear input.

CLINICAL ASSESSMENT OF VISUAL FUNCTION

REFRACTIVE STATE

In approaching the patient with reduced vision, the first step is to decide whether refractive error is responsible. In *emmetropia,* parallel rays from infinity are focused perfectly upon the retina. Sadly, this condition is enjoyed by only a minority of the population. In *myopia,* the globe is too long, and light rays come to a focal point in front of the retina. Near objects can be seen clearly, but distant objects require a diverging lens in front of the eye. In *hyperopia,* the globe is too short, and hence a converging lens is used to supplement the refractive power of the eye. In *astigmatism,* the corneal surface is not perfectly spherical, necessitating a cylindrical corrective lens. In recent years it has become possible to correct refractive error with the excimer laser by performing LASIK (laser in situ keratomileusis) to alter the curvature of the cornea.

With the onset of middle age, *presbyopia* develops as the lens within the eye becomes unable to increase its refractive power to accommodate upon near objects. To compensate for presbyopia, the emmetropic patient must use reading glasses. The patient already wearing glasses for distance correction usually switches to bifocals. The only exception is the myopic patient, who may achieve clear vision at near simply by removing glasses containing the distance prescription.

Refractive errors usually develop slowly and remain stable after adolescence, except in unusual circumstances. For example, the acute onset of diabetes mellitus can produce sudden myopia because of lens edema induced by hyperglycemia. Testing vision through a pinhole aperture is a useful way to screen quickly for refractive error. If the visual acuity is better through a pinhole than with the unaided eye, the patient needs a refraction to obtain best corrected visual acuity.

VISUAL ACUITY

The Snellen chart is used to test acuity at a distance of 6 m (20 ft). For convenience, a scale version of the Snellen chart, called the Rosenbaum card, is held at 36 cm (14 in) from the patient (**Fig. 11–1**). All subjects should be able to read the 6/6 m (20/20 ft) line with each eye using their refractive correction, if any. Patients who need reading glasses because of presbyopia must wear them for ac-

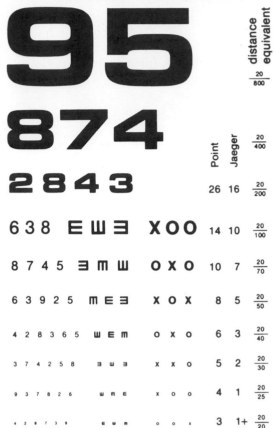

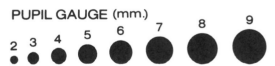

FIGURE 11–1

The Rosenbaum card is a miniature, scale version of the Snellen chart for testing visual acuity at near. When the visual acuity is recorded, the Snellen distance equivalent should bear a notation indicating that vision was tested at near, not at 6 m (20 ft), or else the Jaeger number system should be used to report the acuity.

curate testing with the Rosenbaum card. If 6/6 (20/20) acuity is not present in each eye, the deficiency in vision must be explained. If worse than 6/240 (20/800), acuity should be recorded in terms of counting fingers, hand motions, light perception, or no light perception. Legal blindness is defined by the Internal Revenue Service as a best corrected acuity of 6/60 (20/200) or less in the better eye, or a binocular visual field subtending 20° or less. For driving the laws vary by state, but most require a corrected acuity of 6/12 (20/40) in at least one eye. Patients with a homonymous hemianopia should not drive.

PUPILS

The pupils should be tested individually in dim light with the patient fixating on a distant target. If they respond briskly to light, there is no need to check the near response, because isolated loss of constriction (miosis) to accommodation does not occur. For this reason, the ubiquitous abbreviation PERRLA (pupils equal, round, and reactive to light and accommodation) implies a wasted effort with the last step. However, it is important to test the near response if the light response is poor or absent. Light-near dissociation occurs with neurosyphilis (Argyll Robertson pupil), lesions of the dorsal midbrain (obstructive hydrocephalus, pineal region tumors), and after aberrant regeneration (oculomotor nerve palsy, Adie's tonic pupil).

An eye with no light perception has no pupillary response to direct light stimulation. If the retina or optic nerve is only partially injured, the direct pupillary response will be weaker than the consensual pupillary response evoked by shining a light into the other eye. This *relative afferent pupillary defect* (Marcus Gunn pupil) can be elicited with the swinging flashlight test (**Fig. 11–2**). It is an extremely useful sign in retrobulbar optic neuritis and other optic nerve diseases, where it may be the sole objective evidence for disease.

Subtle inequality in pupil size, up to 0.5 mm, is a fairly common finding in normal persons. The diagnosis of essential or physiologic anisocoria is secure as long as the relative pupil asymmetry remains constant as ambient lighting varies. Anisocoria that increases in dim light indicates a sympathetic paresis of the iris dilator muscle. The triad of miosis with ipsilateral ptosis and anhidrosis constitutes Horner's syndrome, although anhidrosis is an inconstant feature. Brainstem stroke, carotid dissection, or neoplasm impinging upon the sympathetic chain are occasionally identified as the cause of Horner's syndrome, but most cases are idiopathic.

Anisocoria that increases in bright light suggests a parasympathetic palsy. The first concern is an oculomotor nerve paresis. This possibility is excluded if the eye movements are full and the patient has no ptosis or diplopia. Acute pupillary dilation (mydriasis) can occur from damage to the ciliary ganglion in the orbit. Common mechanisms are infection (herpes zoster, influenza), trauma (blunt, penetrating, surgical), or ischemia (diabetes, temporal arteritis). After denervation of the iris sphincter the pupil does not respond well to light, but the response to near is often relatively intact. When the near stimulus is removed, the pupil redilates very slowly compared with the normal pupil, hence the term *tonic pupil*. In Adie's syndrome, a tonic pupil occurs in conjunction with weak or absent tendon reflexes in the lower extremities. This benign disorder, which occurs predominantly in healthy young women, is assumed to represent a mild dysautono-

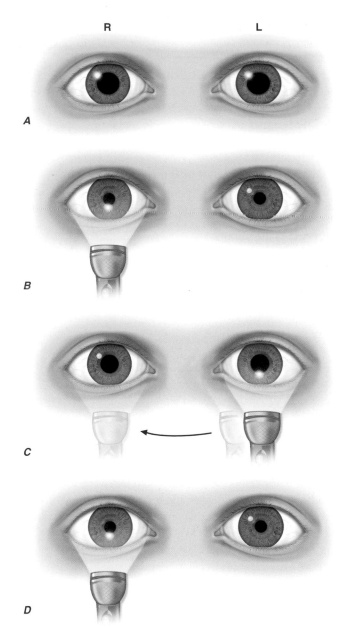

R   L

FIGURE 11-2

The swinging flashlight test shows a relative afferent pupil defect (Marcus Gunn pupil) in the left eye. **A.** With the patient fixating on a distant target and background lighting dim, the pupils are equal and relatively large. **B.** Shining a flashlight into the right eye evokes equal, strong constriction of both pupils. **C.** Swinging the flashlight over to the damaged left eye causes dilation of both pupils, although they remain smaller than in **A. D.** Swinging the flashlight back over to the healthy right eye results in symmetric constriction back to the appearance shown in **B.** Note that the pupils always remain equal; the damage to the left retina/optic nerve is revealed by weaker bilateral pupil constriction to a flashlight in the left eye compared with the right eye. (*Legend adapted from P Levatin, Arch Ophthalmol 62:768, 1959.*)

mia. Tonic pupils are also associated with Shy-Drager syndrome, segmental hypohidrosis, diabetes, and amyloidosis. Occasionally, a tonic pupil is discovered incidentally in an otherwise completely normal, asymptomatic individual. The diagnosis is confirmed by placing a drop of dilute (0.125%) pilocarpine into each eye. Denervation hypersensitivity produces pupillary constriction in a tonic pupil, whereas the normal pupil shows no response. Pharmacologic dilation from accidental or deliberate instillation of anticholinergic agents (atropine, scopolamine) into the eye can also produce pupillary mydriasis. In this situation, normal strength (1%) pilocarpine causes no constriction.

Both pupils are affected equally by systemic medications. They are small with narcotic use (morphine, heroin) and large with anticholinergics (scopolamine). Parasympathetic agents (pilocarpine, demecarium bromide) used to treat glaucoma produce miosis. In any patient with an unexplained pupillary abnormality, a slit-lamp examination is helpful to exclude surgical trauma to the iris, an occult foreign body, perforating injury, intraocular inflammation, adhesions (synechia), angle-closure glaucoma, and iris sphincter rupture from blunt trauma.

EYE MOVEMENTS AND ALIGNMENT

Eye movements are tested by asking the patient with both eyes open to pursue a small target such as a penlight into the cardinal fields of gaze. Normal ocular versions are smooth, symmetric, full, and maintained in all directions without nystagmus. Saccades, or quick refixation eye movements, are assessed by having the patient look back and forth between two stationary targets. The eyes should move rapidly and accurately in a single jump to their target. Ocular alignment can be judged by holding a penlight directly in front of the patient at about 1 m. If the eyes are straight, the corneal light reflex will be centered in the middle of each pupil. To test eye alignment more precisely, the cover test is useful. The patient is instructed to gaze upon a small fixation target in the distance. One eye is covered suddenly while observing the second eye. If the second eye shifts to fixate upon the target, it was misaligned. If it does not move, the first eye is uncovered and the test is repeated on the second eye. If neither eye moves, the eyes are aligned orthotropically. If the eyes are orthotropic in primary gaze but the patient complains of diplopia, the cover test should be performed with the head tilted or turned in whatever direction elicits diplopia. With practice the examiner can detect an ocular deviation (heterotropia) as small as 1 to 2° with the cover test. Deviations can be measured by placing prisms in front of the misaligned eye to determine the power required to neutralize the fixation shift evoked by covering the other eye.

STEREOPSIS

Stereoacuity is determined by presenting targets with retinal disparity separately to each eye using polarized images. The most popular office tests measure a range of thresholds from 800 to 40 seconds of arc. Normal stereoacuity is 40 seconds of arc. If a patient achieves this level of stereoacuity, one is assured that the eyes are aligned orthotropically and that vision is intact in each eye. Random dot stereograms have no monocular depth cues and provide an excellent screening test for strabismus and amblyopia in children.

COLOR VISION

The retina contains three classes of cones, with visual pigments of differing peak spectral sensitivity: red (560 nm), green (530 nm), and blue (430 nm). The red and green cone pigments are encoded on the X chromosome; the blue cone pigment on chromosome 7. Mutations of the blue cone pigment are exceedingly rare. Mutations of the red and green pigments cause congenital X-linked color blindness in 8% of males. Affected individuals are not truly color blind; rather, they differ from normal subjects in how they perceive color and how they combine primary monochromatic lights to match a given color. Anomalous trichromats have three cone types, but a mutation in one cone pigment (usually red or green) causes a shift in peak spectral sensitivity, altering the proportion of primary colors required to achieve a color match. Dichromats have only two cone types and will therefore accept a color match based upon only two primary colors. Anomalous trichromats and dichromats have 6/6 (20/20) visual acuity, but their hue discrimination is impaired. Ishihara color plates can be used to detect red-green color blindness. The test plates contain a hidden number, visible only to subjects with color confusion from red-green color blindness. Because color blindness is almost exclusively X-linked, it is worth screening only male children.

The Ishihara plates are often used to detect acquired defects in color vision, although they are intended as a screening test for congenital color blindness. Acquired defects in color vision frequently result from disease of the macula or optic nerve. For example, patients with a history of optic neuritis often complain of color desaturation long after their visual acuity has returned to normal. Color blindness can also occur from bilateral strokes involving the ventral portion of the occipital lobe (cerebral achromatopsia). Such patients can perceive only shades of gray and may also have difficulty recognizing faces (prosopagnosia). Infarcts of the dominant occipital lobe sometimes give rise to color anomia. Affected patients can discriminate colors, but they cannot name them.

VISUAL FIELDS

Vision can be impaired by damage to the visual system anywhere from the eyes to the occipital lobes. One can localize the site of the lesion with considerable accuracy by mapping the visual field deficit by finger confrontation and then correlating it with the topographic anatomy of the visual pathway (**Fig. 11–3**). Quantitative visual field mapping is performed by computer-driven perimeters (Humphrey, Octopus) that present a target of variable intensity at fixed positions in the visual field (Fig. 11–3*A*). By generating an automated printout of light thresholds, these static perimeters provide a sensitive means of detecting scotomas in the visual field. They are exceedingly useful for serial assessment of visual function in chronic diseases such as glaucoma or pseudotumor cerebri.

The crux of visual field analysis is to decide whether a lesion is before, at, or behind the optic chiasm. If a scotoma is confined to one eye, it must be due to a lesion anterior to the chiasm, involving either the optic nerve or retina. Retinal lesions produce scotomas that correspond optically to their location in the fundus. For example, a superior-nasal retinal detachment results in an inferior-temporal field cut.

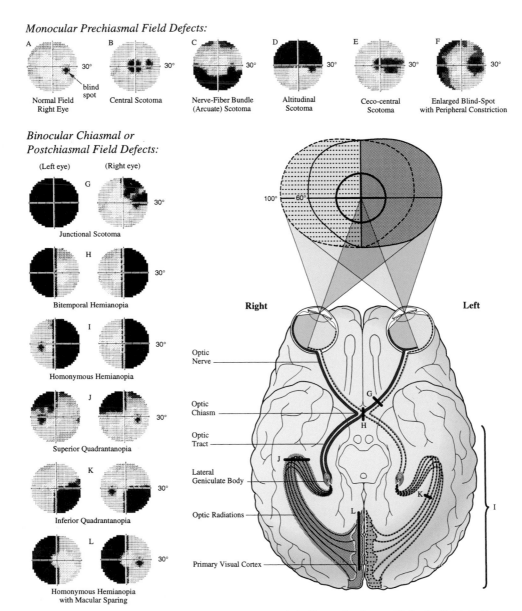

FIGURE 11-3

Ventral view of the brain, correlating patterns of visual field loss with the sites of lesions in the visual pathway. The visual fields overlap partially, creating 120° of central binocular field flanked by a 40° monocular crescent on either side. The visual field maps in this figure were done with a computer-driven perimeter (Humphrey Instruments, Carl Zeiss, Inc.). It plots the retinal sensitivity to light in the central 30° using a gray scale format. Areas of visual field loss are shown in black. The examples of common monocular, prechiasmal field defects are all shown for the right eye. By convention, the visual fields are always recorded with the left eye's field on the left, and the right eye's field on the right, just as the patient sees the world.

Damage to the macula causes a central scotoma (Fig. 11-3*B*).

Optic nerve disease produces characteristic patterns of visual field loss. Glaucoma selectively destroys axons that enter the superotemporal or inferotemporal poles of the optic disc, resulting in arcuate scotomas shaped like a Turkish scimitar, which emanate from the blind spot and curve around fixation to end flat against the horizontal meridian (Fig. 11-3*C*). This type of field defect mirrors the arrangement of the nerve fiber layer in the temporal retina. Arcuate or nerve fiber layer scotomas also occur from optic neuritis, ischemic optic neuropathy, optic disc drusen, and branch retinal artery or vein occlusion.

Damage to the entire upper or lower pole of the optic disc causes an altitudinal field cut that follows the horizontal meridian (Fig. 11-3*D*). This pattern of visual field loss is typical of ischemic optic neuropathy but also occurs from retinal vascular occlusion, advanced glaucoma, and optic neuritis.

About half the fibers in the optic nerve originate from ganglion cells serving the macula. Damage to papillomacular fibers causes a cecocentral scotoma encompassing the blind spot and macula (Fig. 11-3*E*). If the damage is irreversible, pallor eventually appears in the temporal portion of the optic disc. Temporal pallor from a cecocentral scotoma may develop in optic neuritis, nutritional optic neuropathy, toxic optic neuropathy, Leber's hereditary optic neuropathy, and compressive optic neuropathy. It is worth mentioning that the temporal side of the optic disc is slightly more pale than the nasal side in most normal individuals. Therefore, it can sometimes be difficult to decide whether the temporal pallor visible on fundus examination represents a pathologic change. Pallor of the nasal rim of the optic disc is a less equivocal sign of optic atrophy.

At the optic chiasm, fibers from nasal ganglion cells decussate into the contralateral optic tract. Crossed fibers are damaged more by compression than uncrossed fibers. As a result, mass lesions of the sellar region cause a temporal hemianopia in each eye. Tumors anterior to the optic chiasm, such as meningiomas of the tuberculum sella, produce a junctional scotoma characterized by an optic neuropathy in one eye and a superior temporal field cut in the other eye (Fig. 11-3*G*). More symmetric compression of the optic chiasm by a pituitary adenoma (Fig. 26-4), meningioma, craniopharyngioma, glioma, or aneurysm results in a bitemporal hemianopia (Fig. 11-3*H*). The insidious development of a bitemporal hemianopia often goes unnoticed by the patient and will escape detection by the physician unless each eye is tested separately.

It is difficult to localize a postchiasmal lesion accurately, because injury anywhere in the optic tract, lateral geniculate body, optic radiations, or visual cortex can produce a homonymous hemianopia, i.e., a temporal hemifield defect in the contralateral eye and a matching nasal hemifield defect in the ipsilateral eye (Fig. 11-3*I*). A unilateral postchiasmal lesion leaves the visual acuity in each eye unaffected, although the patient may read the letters on only the left or right half of the eye chart. Lesions of the optic radiations tend to cause poorly matched or incongruous field defects in each eye. Damage to the optic radiations in the temporal lobe (Meyer's loop) produces a superior quadrantic homonymous hemianopia (Fig. 11-3*J*), whereas injury to the optic radiations in the parietal lobe results in an inferior quadrantic homonymous hemianopia (Fig. 11-3*K*). Lesions of the primary visual cortex give rise to dense, congruous hemianopic field defects. Occlusion of the posterior cerebral artery supplying the occipital lobe is a frequent cause of total homonymous hemianopia. Some patients with hemianopia after occipital stroke have macular sparing, because the macular representation at the tip of the occipital lobe is supplied by collaterals from the middle cerebral artery (Fig. 11-3*L*). Destruction of both occipital lobes produces cortical blindness. This condition can be distinguished from bilateral prechiasmal visual loss by noting that the pupil responses and optic fundi remain normal.

TRANSIENT OR SUDDEN VISUAL LOSS

Amaurosis Fugax

This term refers to a transient ischemic attack of the retina (Chap. 17). Because neural tissue has a high rate of metabolism, interruption of blood flow to the retina for more than a few seconds results in *transient monocular blindness,* a term used interchangeably with amaurosis fugax. Patients describe a rapid fading of vision like a curtain descending, sometimes affecting only a portion of the visual field. Amaurosis fugax usually occurs from an embolus that becomes stuck within a retinal arteriole (**Fig. 11-4**). If the embolus breaks up or passes, flow is

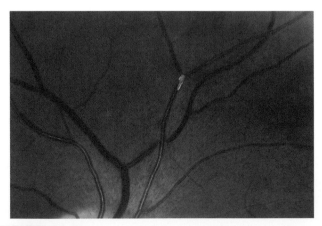

FIGURE 11-4
Hollenhorst plaque lodged at the bifurcation of a retinal arteriole proves that a patient is shedding emboli from either the carotid artery, great vessels, or heart.

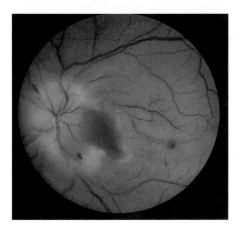

FIGURE 11-5

Central retinal artery occlusion combined with ischemic optic neuropathy in a 19-year-old woman with an elevated titer of anticardiolipin antibodies. Note the orange dot (rather than cherry red) corresponding to the fovea and the spared patch of retina just temporal to the optic disc.

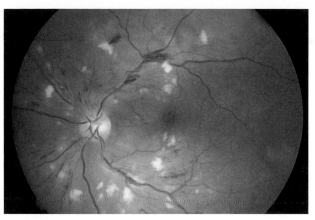

FIGURE 11-6

Hypertensive retinopathy with scattered flame (splinter) hemorrhages and cotton wool spots (nerve fiber layer infarcts) in a patient with headache and a blood pressure of 234/120.

restored and vision returns quickly to normal without permanent damage. With prolonged interruption of blood flow, the inner retina suffers infarction. Ophthalmoscopy reveals zones of whitened, edematous retina following the distribution of branch retinal arterioles. Complete occlusion of the central retinal artery produces arrest of blood flow and a milky retina with a cherry-red fovea (**Fig. 11-5**). Emboli are composed of either cholesterol (Hollenhorst plaque), calcium, or platelet-fibrin debris. The most common source is an atherosclerotic plaque in the carotid artery or aorta, although emboli can also arise from the heart, especially in patients with diseased valves, atrial fibrillation, or wall motion abnormalities.

In rare instances, amaurosis fugax occurs from low central retinal artery perfusion pressure in a patient with a critical stenosis of the ipsilateral carotid artery and poor collateral flow via the circle of Willis. In this situation, amaurosis fugax develops when there is a dip in systemic blood pressure or a slight worsening of the carotid stenosis. Sometimes there is contralateral motor or sensory loss, indicating concomitant hemispheric cerebral ischemia.

Retinal arterial occlusion also occurs rarely in association with retinal migraine, lupus erythematosus, anticardiolipin antibodies (Fig. 11-5), anticoagulant deficiency states (protein S, protein C, and antithrombin III deficiency), pregnancy, intravenous drug abuse, blood dyscrasias, dysproteinemias, and temporal arteritis.

Marked *systemic hypertension* causes sclerosis of retinal arterioles, splinter hemorrhages, focal infarcts of the nerve fiber layer (cotton-wool spots), and leakage of lipid and fluid (hard exudate) into the macula (**Fig. 11-6**). In hypertensive crisis, sudden visual loss can result from

vasospasm of retinal arterioles and retinal ischemia. In addition, acute hypertension may produce visual loss from ischemic swelling of the optic disc. Patients with acute hypertensive retinopathy should be treated by lowering the blood pressure. However, the blood pressure should not be reduced precipitously, because there is a danger of optic disc infarction from sudden hypoperfusion.

Impending *branch* or *central retinal vein occlusion* can produce prolonged visual obscurations that resemble those described by patients with amaurosis fugax. The veins appear engorged and phlebitic, with numerous retinal hemorrhages (**Fig. 11-7**). In some patients, venous blood flow recovers spontaneously, while others evolve a frank obstruction with extensive retinal bleeding ("blood and thunder" appearance), infarction, and visual loss.

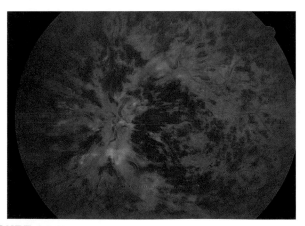

FIGURE 11-7

Central retinal vein occlusion can produce massive retinal hemorrhage ("blood and thunder"), ischemia, and vision loss.

Venous occlusion of the retina is often idiopathic, but hypertension, diabetes, and glaucoma are prominent risk factors. Polycythemia, thrombocythemia, or other factors leading to an underlying hypercoagulable state should be corrected; aspirin treatment may be beneficial.

Anterior Ischemic Optic Neuropathy (AION)

This is caused by insufficient blood flow through the posterior ciliary arteries supplying the optic disc. It produces painless, monocular visual loss that is usually sudden, although some patients have progressive worsening. The optic disc appears swollen and surrounded by nerve fiber layer splinter hemorrhages (**Fig. 11–8**). AION is divided into two forms: arteritic and nonarteritic. The nonarteritic form of AION is most common. No specific cause can be identified, although diabetes and hypertension are frequent risk factors. No treatment is available. About 5% of patients, especially those over age 60, develop the arteritic form of AION in conjunction with giant cell (temporal) arteritis. It is urgent to recognize arteritic AION so that high doses of glucocorticoids can be instituted immediately to prevent blindness in the second eye. Symptoms of polymyalgia rheumatica may be present; the sedimentation rate and C-reactive protein level are usually elevated. In a patient with visual loss from suspected arteritic AION, temporal artery biopsy is mandatory to confirm the diagnosis. Glucocorticoids should be started immediately, without waiting for the biopsy to be completed. The diagnosis of arteritic AION is difficult to sustain in the face of a negative temporal artery biopsy, but such cases do occur.

Posterior Ischemic Optic Neuropathy

This is an infrequent cause of acute visual loss, induced by the combination of severe anemia and hypotension. Cases have been reported after major blood loss during surgery, exsanguinating trauma, gastrointestinal bleeding, and renal dialysis. The fundus usually appears normal, although optic disc swelling develops if the process extends far enough anteriorly. Vision can be salvaged in some patients by prompt blood transfusion and reversal of hypotension.

Optic Neuritis

This is a common inflammatory disease of the optic nerve. In the Optic Neuritis Treatment Trial (ONTT), the mean age of patients was 32 years, 77% were female, 92% had ocular pain (especially with eye movements), and 35% had optic disc swelling. In most patients, the demyelinating event was retrobulbar and the ocular fundus appeared normal on initial examination (**Fig. 11–9**), although optic disc pallor slowly developed over subsequent months.

Virtually all patients experience a gradual recovery of vision after a single episode of optic neuritis, even without treatment. This rule is so reliable that failure of vision to improve after a first attack of optic neuritis casts doubt upon the original diagnosis. Treatment with high-dose intravenous methylprednisolone (250 mg every 6 h for 3 days) followed by oral prednisone (1 mg/kg per day for 11 days) makes no difference in final acuity (measured 6 months after the attack), but the recovery of visual function occurs more rapidly.

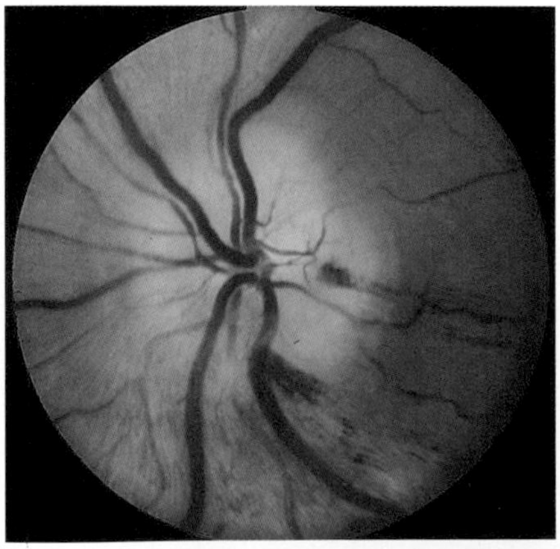

FIGURE 11-8
Anterior ischemic optic neuropathy from temporal arteritis in a 78-year-old woman with pallid disc swelling, hemorrhage, visual loss, myalgia, and an erythrocyte sedimentation rate of 86 mm/h.

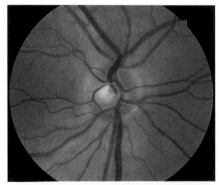

FIGURE 11-9
Retrobulbar optic neuritis is characterized by a normal fundus examination initially, hence the rubric, "the doctor sees nothing, and the patient sees nothing." Optic atrophy develops after severe or repeated attacks.

For some patients, optic neuritis remains an isolated event. However, the ONTT showed that the 5-year cumulative probability of developing clinically definite multiple sclerosis (MS) following optic neuritis is 30%. In patients with two or more demyelinating plaques on brain magnetic resonance (MR) imaging, the 5-year risk for MS increases to 45%, and treatment with interferon (IFN) β-1a has been shown to retard the development of additional lesions and protect against evolution to MS. An MR scan is recommended in every patient with a first attack of optic neuritis (Chap. 28). When visual loss is severe (worse than 20/100), treatment with intravenous followed by oral glucocorticoids hastens recovery. If multiple lesions are present on the MR scan, treatment with IFN-β-1a should be broached with the patient.

Leber's Hereditary Optic Neuropathy

This is a disease of young men, characterized by gradual painless, severe, central visual loss in one eye, followed weeks or months later by the same process in the other eye. Acutely, the optic disc appears mildly plethoric with surface capillary telangiectases, but no vascular leakage on fluorescein angiography. Eventually optic atrophy ensues. Leber's optic neuropathy is caused by a point mutation at codon 11778 in the mitochondrial gene encoding nicotinamide adenine dinucleotide dehydrogenase (NADH) subunit 4. Additional mutations responsible for the disease have been identified, most in mitochondrial genes encoding proteins involved in electron transport. Mitochondrial mutations causing Leber's neuropathy are inherited from the mother by all her children, but usually only sons develop symptoms. There is no treatment.

Toxic Optic Neuropathy

This can result in acute visual loss with bilateral optic disc swelling and central or cecocentral scotomas. Such cases have been reported to result from exposure to ethambutol, methyl alcohol (moonshine), ethylene glycol (antifreeze), or carbon monoxide. In toxic optic neuropathy, visual loss can also develop gradually and produce optic atrophy (**Fig. 11-10**) without a phase of acute optic disc edema. Many agents have been implicated as a cause of toxic optic neuropathy, but the evidence supporting the association for many is weak. The following is a partial list of potential offending drugs or toxins: disulfiram, ethchlorvynol, chloramphenicol, amiodarone, monoclonal anti-CD3 antibody, ciprofloxacin, digitalis, streptomycin, lead, arsenic, thallium, D-penicillamine, isoniazid, emetine, and sulfonamides. Deficiency states, induced either by starvation, malabsorption, or alcoholism, can lead to insidious visual loss. Thiamine, vitamin B_{12}, and folate levels should be checked in any patient with unexplained, bilateral central scotomas and optic pallor.

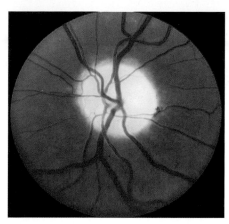

FIGURE 11-10

Optic atrophy is not a specific diagnosis, but refers to the combination of optic disc pallor, arteriolar narrowing, and nerve fiber layer destruction produced by a host of eye diseases, especially optic neuropathies.

Papilledema

This connotes bilateral optic disc swelling from raised intracranial pressure (**Fig. 11-11**). Headache is a frequent, but not invariable, accompaniment. All other forms of optic disc swelling, e.g., from optic neuritis or ischemic optic neuropathy, should be called "optic disc edema." This convention is arbitrary but serves to avoid confusion. Often it is difficult to differentiate papilledema from other forms of optic disc edema by fundus examination alone. Transient visual obscurations are a classic symptom of papilledema. They can occur in only one eye or simultaneously in both eyes. They usually last seconds but can persist longer if the papilledema is fulminant. Obscurations follow abrupt shifts in posture or happen sponta-

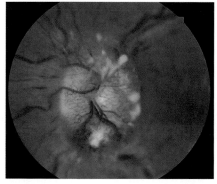

FIGURE 11-11

Papilledema means optic disc edema from raised intracranial pressure. This obese young woman with pseudotumor cerebri was misdiagnosed as a migraineur until fundus examination was performed, showing optic disc elevation, hemorrhages, and cotton wool spots.

neously. When obscurations are prolonged or sponta-neous, the papilledema is more threatening. Visual acuity is not affected by papilledema unless the papilledema is severe, long-standing, or accompanied by macular edema and hemorrhage. Visual field testing shows enlarged blind spots and peripheral constriction (Fig. 11-3F). With un-remitting papilledema, peripheral visual field loss pro-gresses in an insidious fashion while the optic nerve de-velops atrophy. In this setting, reduction of optic disc swelling is an ominous sign of a dying nerve rather than an encouraging indication of resolving papilledema.

Evaluation of papilledema requires neuroimaging to exclude an intracranial lesion. MR angiography is appropriate in selected cases to search for a dural venous sinus occlusion or an arteriovenous shunt. If neuroradio-logic studies are negative, the subarachnoid opening pressure should be measured by lumbar puncture. An elevated pressure, with normal cerebrospinal fluid, points by exclusion to the diagnosis of *pseudotumor cerebri* (idio-pathic intracranial hypertension). The majority of patients are young, female, and obese. Treatment with a carbonic anhydrase inhibitor such as acetazolamide low-ers intracranial pressure by reducing the production of cerebrospinal fluid. Weight reduction is vital but often unsuccessful. If acetazolamide and weight loss fail, and visual field loss is progressive, a shunt should be per-formed without delay to prevent blindness. Occasionally, emergency surgery is required for sudden blindness caused by fulminant papilledema.

Optic Disc Drusen

These are refractile deposits within the substance of the op-tic nerve head (**Fig. 11-12**). They are unrelated to drusen of the retina, which occur in age-related macular degenera-tion. Optic disc drusen are most common in people of northern European descent. Their diagnosis is obvious when they are visible as glittering particles upon the surface of the optic disc. However, in many patients they are hidden beneath the surface, producing pseudo-papilledema. It is im-portant to recognize optic disc drusen to avoid an unnec-essary evaluation for papilledema. Ultrasound or computed tomography (CT) scanning is sensitive for detection of buried optic disc drusen because they contain calcium. In most patients, optic disc drusen are an incidental, innocuous finding, but they can produce visual obscurations. On perimetry they give rise to enlarged blind spots and arcuate scotomas from damage to the optic disc. With increasing age, drusen tend to become more exposed on the disc sur-face as optic atrophy develops. Hemorrhage, choroidal neo-vascular membrane, and AION are more likely to occur in patients with optic disc drusen. No treatment is available.

Vitreous Degeneration

This occurs in all individuals with advancing age, leading to visual symptoms. Opacities develop in the vitreous, casting annoying shadows upon the retina. As the eye moves, these distracting "floaters" move synchronously, with a slight lag caused by inertia of the vitreous gel. Vit-reous traction upon the retina causes mechanical stimula-tion, resulting in perception of flashing lights. This pho-topsia is brief and confined to one eye, in contrast to the bilateral, prolonged scintillations of cortical migraine. Contraction of the vitreous can result in sudden separa-tion from the retina, heralded by an alarming shower of floaters and photopsia. This process, known as *vitreous de-tachment,* is a frequent involutional event in the elderly. It is not harmful unless it damages the retina. A careful ex-amination of the dilated fundus is important in any pa-tient complaining of floaters or photopsia to search for peripheral tears or holes. If such a lesion is found, laser application or cryotherapy can forestall a retinal detach-ment. Occasionally a tear ruptures a retinal blood vessel, causing vitreous hemorrhage and sudden loss of vision. On attempted ophthalmoscopy the fundus is hidden by a dark red haze of blood. Ultrasound is required to exam-ine the interior of the eye for a retinal tear or detach-ment. If the hemorrhage does not resolve spontaneously, the vitreous can be removed surgically. Vitreous hemor-rhage also occurs from the fragile neovascular vessels that proliferate on the surface of the retina in diabetes, sickle cell anemia, and other ischemic ocular diseases.

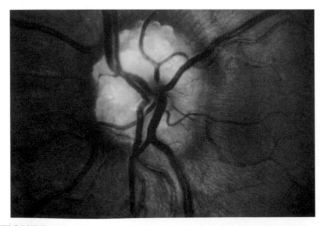

FIGURE 11-12
Optic disc drusen are calcified deposits of unknown etiology within the optic disc. They are sometimes confused with pa-pilledema.

Retinal Detachment

This produces symptoms of floaters, flashing lights, and a scotoma in the peripheral visual field corresponding to the detachment (**Fig. 11-13**). If the detachment includes

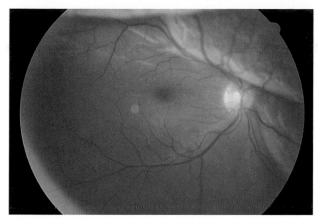

FIGURE 11-13

Retinal detachment appears as an elevated sheet of retinal tissue with folds. In this patient the fovea was spared, so acuity was normal, but a superior detachment produced an inferior scotoma.

the fovea, there is an afferent pupil defect and the visual acuity is reduced. In most eyes, retinal detachment starts with a hole, flap, or tear in the peripheral retina (rhegmatogenous retinal detachment). Patients with peripheral retinal thinning (lattice degeneration) are particularly vulnerable to this process. Once a break has developed in the retina, liquified vitreous is free to enter the subretinal space, separating the retina from the pigment epithelium. The combination of vitreous traction upon the retinal surface and passage of fluid behind the retina leads inexorably to detachment. Patients with a history of myopia, trauma, or prior cataract extraction are at greatest risk for retinal detachment. The diagnosis is confirmed by ophthalmoscopic examination of the dilated eye.

Classic Migraine (See also Chap. 5)

This usually occurs with a visual aura lasting about 20 min. In a typical attack, a small central disturbance in the field of vision marches toward the periphery, leaving a transient scotoma in its wake. The expanding border of migraine scotoma has a scintillating, dancing, or zig-zag edge, resembling the bastions of a fortified city, hence the term *fortification spectra*. Patients' descriptions of fortification spectra vary widely and can be confused with amaurosis fugax. Migraine patterns usually last longer and are perceived in both eyes, whereas amaurosis fugax is briefer and occurs in only one eye. Migraine phenomena also remain visible in the dark or with the eyes closed. Generally they are confined to either the right or left visual hemifield, but sometimes both fields are involved simultaneously. Patients often have a long history of stereotypic attacks. After the visual symptoms recede, headache develops in most patients.

Transient Ischemic Attacks

Vertebrobasilar insufficiency may result in acute homonymous visual symptoms. Many patients mistakenly describe symptoms in their left or right eye, when in fact they are occurring in the left or right hemifield of both eyes. Interruption of blood supply to the visual cortex causes a sudden fogging or graying of vision, occasionally with flashing lights or other positive phenomena that mimic migraine. Cortical ischemic attacks are briefer in duration than migraine, occur in older patients, and are not followed by headache. There may be associated signs of brainstem ischemia, such as diplopia, vertigo, numbness, weakness, or dysarthria.

Stroke

This occurs when interruption of blood supply from the posterior cerebral artery to the visual cortex is prolonged. The only finding on examination is a homonymous visual field defect that stops abruptly at the vertical meridian. Occipital lobe stroke is usually due to thrombotic occlusion of the vertebrobasilar system, embolus, or dissection. Lobar hemorrhage, tumor, abscess, and arteriovenous malformation are other common causes of hemianopic cortical visual loss.

Factitious (Functional, Nonorganic) Visual Loss

This is claimed by hysterics or malingerers. The latter comprise the vast majority, seeking sympathy, special treatment, or financial gain by feigning loss of sight. The diagnosis is suspected when the history is atypical, physical findings are lacking or contradictory, inconsistencies emerge on testing, and a secondary motive can be identified. In our litigious society, the fraudulent pursuit of recompense has spawned an epidemic of factitious visual loss.

CHRONIC VISUAL LOSS

Cataract

This is a clouding of the lens sufficient to reduce vision. Most cataracts develop slowly as a result of aging, leading to gradual impairment of vision. The formation of cataract occurs more rapidly in patients with a history of ocular trauma, uveitis, or diabetes mellitus. Cataracts are acquired in a variety of genetic diseases, such as myotonic dystrophy, neurofibromatosis type 2, and galactosemia. Radiation therapy and glucocorticoid treatment can induce cataract as a side effect. The cataracts associated with radiation or glucocorticoids have a typical posterior subcapsular location. Cataract can be detected by noting an impaired red reflex when viewing light reflected from the fundus with an ophthalmoscope or by examining the dilated eye using the slit lamp.

The only treatment for cataract is surgical extraction of the opacified lens. Over a million cataract operations are performed each year in the United States. The operation is generally done under local anesthesia on an outpatient basis. A plastic or silicone intraocular lens is placed within the empty lens capsule in the posterior chamber, substituting for the natural lens and leading to rapid recovery of sight. More than 95% of patients who undergo cataract extraction can expect an improvement in vision. In many patients, the lens capsule remaining in the eye after cataract extraction eventually turns cloudy, causing a secondary loss of vision. A small opening is made in the lens capsule with a laser to restore clarity.

Glaucoma

This is a slowly progressive, insidious optic neuropathy, usually associated with chronic elevation of intraocular pressure. In Americans of African descent it is the leading cause of blindness. The mechanism whereby raised intraocular pressure injures the optic nerve is not understood. Axons entering the inferotemporal and superotemporal aspects of the optic disc are damaged first, producing typical nerve fiber bundle or arcuate scotomas on perimetric testing. As fibers are destroyed, the neural rim of the optic disc shrinks and the physiologic cup within the optic disc enlarges (**Fig. 11–14**). This process is referred to as pathologic "cupping." The cup-to-disc diameter is expressed as a ratio, e.g., 0.2/1. The cup-to-disc ratio ranges widely in normal individuals, making it difficult to diagnose glaucoma reliably simply by observing an unusually large or deep optic cup. Careful documentation of serial examinations is helpful. In the patient with physiologic cupping, the large cup remains stable, whereas in the patient with glaucoma it expands relentlessly over the years. Detection of visual field loss by

computerized perimetry also contributes to the diagnosis. Finally, most patients with glaucoma have raised intraocular pressure. However, many patients with typical glaucomatous cupping and visual field loss have intraocular pressures that apparently never exceed the normal limit of 20 mmHg (so-called low-tension glaucoma).

In acute angle-closure glaucoma, the eye is red and painful due to abrupt, severe elevation of intraocular pressure. Such cases account for only a handful of patients with glaucoma. Most patients with glaucoma have open anterior chamber angles. The cause of raised intraocular pressure in open angle glaucoma is unknown but is associated with gene mutations in the heritable forms.

Glaucoma is usually painless (except in angle-closure glaucoma). Foveal acuity is spared until end-stage disease is reached. For these reasons, severe and irreversible damage can occur before either the patient or physician recognizes the diagnosis. Screening of patients for glaucoma by noting the cup-to-disc ratio on ophthalmoscopy and by measuring intraocular pressure is vital. Glaucoma is treated with topical adrenergic agonists, cholinergic agonists, beta blockers, and prostaglandin analogues. Occasionally, systemic absorption of beta blocker from eye drops can be sufficient to cause side effects of bradycardia, hypotension, heart block, bronchospasm, or depression. Topical or oral carbonic anhydrase inhibitors are used to lower intraocular pressure by reducing aqueous production. Laser treatment of the trabecular meshwork in the anterior chamber angle improves aqueous outflow from the eye. If medical or laser treatments fail to halt optic nerve damage from glaucoma, a filter must be constructed surgically (trabeculectomy) to release aqueous from the eye in a controlled fashion.

Macular Degeneration

This is a major cause of gradual, painless, bilateral central visual loss in the elderly. The old term, "senile macular degeneration," misinterpreted by many patients as an unflattering reference, has been replaced with "age-related macular degeneration." It occurs in a nonexudative (dry) form and an exudative (wet) form. The nonexudative process begins with the accumulation of extracellular deposits, called drusen, underneath the retinal pigment epithelium. On ophthalmoscopy, they are pleomorphic but generally appear as small discrete yellow lesions clustered in the macula (**Fig. 11–15**). With time they become larger, more numerous, and confluent. The retinal pigment epithelium becomes focally detached and atrophic, causing visual loss by interfering with photoreceptor function. Treatment with vitamins C and E, beta carotene, and zinc may retard dry macular degeneration.

Exudative macular degeneration, which develops in only a minority of patients, occurs when neovascular

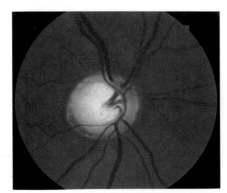

FIGURE 11-14

Glaucoma results in "cupping" as the neural rim is destroyed and the central cup becomes enlarged and excavated. The cup-to-disc ratio is about 0.7/1.0 in this patient.

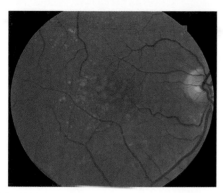

FIGURE 11-15
Age-related macular degeneration begins with the accumulation of drusen within the macula. They appear as scattered yellow subretinal deposits.

vessels from the choroid grow through defects in Bruch's membrane into the potential space beneath the retinal pigment epithelium. Leakage from these vessels produces elevation of the retina and pigment epithelium, with distortion (metamorphopsia) and blurring of vision. Although onset of these symptoms is usually gradual, bleeding from subretinal choroidal neovascular membranes sometimes causes acute visual loss. The neovascular membranes can be difficult to see on fundus examination because they are beneath the retina. Fluorescein or indocyanine green angiography is extremely useful for their detection. In some patients, prompt laser ablation of choroidal neovascular membranes seen on fluorescein angiography can halt the exudative process. However, the neovascular membranes frequently recur, requiring constant vigilance and repeated photocoagulation.

Major or repeated hemorrhage under the retina from neovascular membranes results in fibrosis, development of a round (disciform) macular scar, and permanent loss of central vision. Surgical attempts to remove subretinal membranes in age-related macular degeneration have not improved vision in most patients. However, outcomes have been more encouraging for patients with choroidal neovascular membranes from ocular histoplasmosis syndrome.

Central Serous Chorioretinopathy

This primarily affects males between the ages of 20 and 50. Leakage of serous fluid from the choroid causes small, localized detachment of the retinal pigment epithelium and the neurosensory retina. These detachments produce acute or chronic symptoms of metamorphopsia and blurred vision when the macula is involved. They are difficult to visualize with a direct ophthalmoscope because the detached retina is transparent and only slightly elevated. Diagnosis of central serous chorioretinopathy is

made easily by fluorescein angiography, which shows dye streaming into the subretinal space. The cause of central serous chorioretinopathy is unknown. Symptoms may resolve spontaneously if the retina reattaches, but recurrent detachment is common. Laser photocoagulation has benefited some patients with this condition.

Diabetic Retinopathy

A rare disease until 1921, when the discovery of insulin resulted in a dramatic improvement in life expectancy for patients with diabetes mellitus, it is now a leading cause of blindness in the United States. The retinopathy of diabetes takes years to develop but eventually appears in nearly all cases. Regular surveillance of the dilated fundus is crucial for any patient with diabetes. In advanced diabetic retinopathy, the proliferation of neovascular vessels leads to blindness from vitreous hemorrhage, retinal detachment, and glaucoma. These complications can be avoided in most patients by administration of panretinal laser photocoagulation at the appropriate point in the evolution of the disease.

Retinitis Pigmentosa

This is a general term for a disparate group of rod and cone dystrophies characterized by progressive night blindness, visual field constriction with a ring scotoma, loss of acuity, and an abnormal electroretinogram (ERG). It occurs sporadically or in an autosomal recessive, dominant, or X-linked pattern. Irregular black deposits of clumped pigment in the peripheral retina, called *bone spicules* because of their vague resemblance to the spicules of cancellous bone, give the disease its name (**Fig. 11-16**). The name is actually a

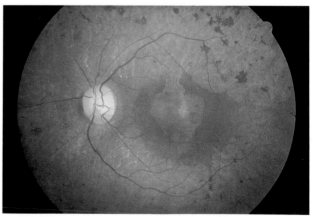

FIGURE 11-16
Retinitis pigmentosa with black clumps of pigment in the retinal periphery known as "bone spicules." There is also atrophy of the retinal pigment epithelium, making the vasculature of the choroid easily visible.

misnomer because retinitis pigmentosa is not an inflammatory process. Most cases are due to a mutation in the gene for rhodopsin, the rod photopigment, or in the gene for peripherin, a glycoprotein located in photoreceptor outer segments. Vitamin A (15,000 IU/day) slightly retards the deterioration of the ERG in patients with retinitis pigmentosa but has no beneficial effect on visual acuity or fields. Some forms of retinitis pigmentosa occur in association with rare, hereditary systemic diseases (olivopontocerebellar degeneration, Bassen-Kornzweig disease, Kearns-Sayre syndrome, Refsum's disease). Chronic treatment with chloroquine, hydroxychloroquine, and phenothiazines (especially thioridazine) can produce visual loss from a toxic retinopathy that resembles retinitis pigmentosa.

Epiretinal Membrane

This is a fibrocellular tissue that grows across the inner surface of the retina, causing metamorphopsia and reduced visual acuity from distortion of the macula. A crinkled, cellophane-like membrane is visible on the retinal examination. Epiretinal membrane is most common in patients over 50 years of age and is usually unilateral. Most cases are idiopathic, but some occur as a result of hypertensive retinopathy, diabetes, retinal detachment, or trauma. When visual acuity is reduced to the level of about 6/24 (20/80), vitrectomy and surgical peeling of the membrane to relieve macular puckering are recommended. Contraction of an epiretinal membrane sometimes gives rise to a *macular hole*. Most macular holes, however, are caused by local vitreous traction within the fovea. Vitrectomy can improve acuity in selected cases.

Melanoma and Other Tumors

Melanoma is the most common primary tumor of the eye (**Fig. 11-17**). It causes photopsia, an enlarging scotoma, and loss of vision. A small melanoma is often difficult to differentiate from a benign choroidal nevus. Serial examinations are required to document a malignant pattern of growth. Treatment of melanoma is controversial. Options include enucleation, local resection, and irradiation. *Metastatic tumors* to the eye outnumber primary tumors. Breast and lung carcinoma have a special propensity to spread to the choroid or iris. Leukemia and lymphoma also commonly invade ocular tissues. Sometimes their only sign on eye examination is cellular debris in the vitreous, which can masquerade as a chronic posterior uveitis. *Retrobulbar tumor* of the optic nerve (meningioma, glioma) or *chiasmal tumor* (pituitary adenoma, meningioma) produces gradual visual loss with few objective findings, except for optic disc pallor. Rarely, sudden expansion of a pituitary adenoma from infarction and bleeding (*pituitary apoplexy*) causes acute

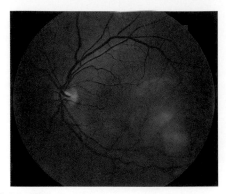

FIGURE 11-17
Melanoma of the choroid, appearing as an elevated dark mass in the inferior temporal fundus, just encroaching upon the fovea.

retrobulbar visual loss, with headache, nausea, and ocular motor nerve palsies. In any patient with visual field loss or optic atrophy, CT or MR scanning should be considered if the cause remains unknown after careful review of the history and thorough examination of the eye.

PROPTOSIS

When the globes appear asymmetric, the clinician must first decide which eye is abnormal. Is one eye recessed within the orbit (*enophthalmos*) or is the other eye protuberant (*exophthalmos,* or *proptosis*)? A small globe or a Horner's syndrome can give the appearance of enophthalmos. True enophthalmos occurs commonly after trauma, from atrophy of retrobulbar fat, or fracture of the orbital floor. The position of the eyes within the orbits is measured using a Hertel exophthalmometer, a hand-held instrument that records the position of the anterior corneal surface relative to the lateral orbital rim. If this instrument is not available, relative eye position can be judged by bending the patient's head forward and looking down upon the orbits. A proptosis of only 2 mm in one eye is detectable from this perspective. The development of proptosis implies a space-occupying lesion in the orbit, and usually warrants CT or MR imaging.

Graves' Ophthalmopathy

This is the leading cause of proptosis in adults. The proptosis is often asymmetric and can even appear to be unilateral. Orbital inflammation and engorgement of the extraocular muscles, particularly the medial rectus and the inferior rectus, account for the protrusion of the globe. Corneal exposure, lid retraction, conjunctival injection, restriction of gaze, diplopia, and visual loss from optic nerve compression are cardinal symptoms. Graves' ophthalmopathy is treated with oral prednisone (60 mg/d) for 1 month, followed by a taper over several months, topical lubricants, eyelid surgery, eye muscle surgery, or orbital decompression. Radiation therapy is not effective.

Orbital Pseudotumor

This is an idiopathic, inflammatory orbital syndrome, frequently confused with Graves' ophthalmopathy. Symptoms are pain, limited eye movements, proptosis, and congestion. Evaluation for sarcoidosis, Wegener's granulomatosis, and other types of orbital vasculitis or collagen-vascular disease is negative. Imaging often shows swollen eye muscles (orbital myositis) with enlarged tendons. By contrast, in Graves' ophthalmopathy the tendons of the eye muscles are usually spared. The Tolosa-Hunt syndrome may be regarded as an extension of orbital pseudotumor through the superior orbital fissure into the cavernous sinus. The diagnosis of orbital pseudotumor is difficult. Biopsy of the orbit frequently yields nonspecific evidence of fat infiltration by lymphocytes, plasma cells, and eosinophils. A dramatic response to a therapeutic trial of systemic glucocorticoids indirectly provides the best confirmation of the diagnosis.

Orbital Cellulitis

This causes pain, lid erythema, proptosis, conjunctival chemosis, restricted motility, decreased acuity, afferent pupillary defect, fever, and leukocytosis. It often arises from the paranasal sinuses, especially by contiguous spread of infection from the ethmoid sinus through the lamina papyracea of the medial orbit. A history of recent upper respiratory tract infection, chronic sinusitis, thick mucous secretions, or dental disease is significant in any patient with suspected orbital cellulitis. Blood cultures should be obtained, but they are usually negative. Most patients respond to empirical therapy with broad-spectrum intravenous antibiotics. Occasionally, orbital cellulitis follows an overwhelming course, with massive proptosis, blindness, septic cavernous sinus thrombosis, and meningitis. To avert this disaster, orbital cellulitis should be managed aggressively in the early stages, with immediate antibiotic therapy and imaging of the orbits. Prompt surgical drainage of an orbital abscess or paranasal sinusitis is indicated if optic nerve function deteriorates despite antibiotics.

Tumors

Tumors of the orbit cause painless, progressive proptosis. The most common primary tumors are hemangioma, lymphangioma, neurofibroma, dermoid cyst, adenoid cystic carcinoma, optic nerve glioma, optic nerve meningioma, and benign mixed tumor of the lacrimal gland. Metastatic tumor to the orbit occurs frequently in breast carcinoma, lung carcinoma, and lymphoma. Diagnosis by fine-needle aspiration followed by urgent radiation therapy can sometimes preserve vision.

Carotid Cavernous Fistulas

With anterior drainage through the orbit these produce proptosis, diplopia, glaucoma, and corkscrew, arterialized conjunctival vessels. Direct fistulas usually result from trauma. They are easily diagnosed because of the prominent signs produced by high-flow, high-pressure shunting. Indirect fistulas, or dural arteriovenous malformations, are more likely to occur spontaneously, especially in older women. The signs are more subtle and the diagnosis is frequently missed. The combination of slight proptosis, diplopia, enlarged muscles, and an injected eye is often mistaken for thyroid ophthalmopathy. A bruit heard upon auscultation of the head, or reported by the patient, is a valuable diagnostic clue. Imaging shows an enlarged superior ophthalmic vein in the orbits. Carotid cavernous shunts can be eliminated by intravascular embolization.

PTOSIS

Blepharoptosis

This is an abnormal drooping of the eyelid. Unilateral or bilateral ptosis can be congenital, from dysgenesis of the levator palpebrae superioris, or from abnormal insertion of its aponeurosis into the eyelid. Acquired ptosis can develop so gradually that the patient is unaware of the problem. Inspection of old photographs is helpful in dating the onset. A history of prior trauma, eye surgery, contact lens use, diplopia, systemic symptoms (e.g., dysphagia or peripheral muscle weakness), or a family history of ptosis should be sought. Fluctuating ptosis that worsens late in the day is typical of myasthenia gravis. Examination should focus upon evidence for proptosis, eyelid masses or deformities, inflammation, pupil inequality, or limitation of motility. The width of the palpebral fissures is measured in primary gaze to quantitate the degree of ptosis. The ptosis will be underestimated if the patient compensates by lifting the brow with the frontalis muscle.

Mechanical Ptosis

This occurs in many elderly patients from stretching and redundancy of eyelid skin and subcutaneous fat (dermatochalasis). The extra weight of these sagging tissues causes the lid to droop. Enlargement or deformation of the eyelid from infection, tumor, trauma, or inflammation also results in ptosis on a purely mechanical basis.

Aponeurotic Ptosis

This is an acquired dehiscence or stretching of the aponeurotic tendon, which connects the levator muscle to the tarsal plate of the eyelid. It occurs commonly in older patients, presumably from loss of connective tissue elasticity. Aponeurotic ptosis is also a frequent sequela of eyelid swelling from infection or blunt trauma to the orbit, cataract surgery, or hard contact lens usage.

Myogenic Ptosis

The causes of *myogenic ptosis* include myasthenia gravis (Chap. 36) and a number of rare *myopathies* that manifest with ptosis. The term *chronic progressive external ophthalmoplegia* refers to a spectrum of systemic diseases caused by mutations of mitochondrial DNA. As the name implies, the most prominent findings are symmetric, slowly progressive ptosis and limitation of eye movements. In general, diplopia is a late symptom because all eye movements are reduced equally. In the *Kearns-Sayre* variant, retinal pigmentary changes and abnormalities of cardiac conduction develop. Peripheral muscle biopsy shows characteristic "ragged-red fibers." *Oculopharyngeal dystrophy* is a distinct autosomal dominant disease with onset in middle age, characterized by ptosis, limited eye movements, and trouble swallowing. *Myotonic dystrophy,* another autosomal dominant disorder, causes ptosis, ophthalmoparesis, cataract, and pigmentary retinopathy. Patients have muscle wasting, myotonia, frontal balding, and cardiac abnormalities.

Neurogenic Ptosis

This results from a lesion affecting the innervation to either of the two muscles that open the eyelid: Müller's muscle or the levator palpebrae superioris. Examination of the pupil helps to distinguish between these two possibilities. In Horner's syndrome, the eye with ptosis has a smaller pupil and the eye movements are full. In an oculomotor nerve palsy, the eye with the ptosis has a larger, or a normal, pupil. If the pupil is normal but there is limitation of adduction, elevation, and depression, a pupil-sparing oculomotor nerve palsy is likely (see next section). Rarely, a lesion affecting the small, central subnucleus of the oculomotor complex will cause bilateral ptosis with normal eye movements and pupils.

DOUBLE VISION

The first point to clarify is whether diplopia persists in either eye after covering the fellow eye. If it does, the diagnosis is monocular diplopia. The cause is usually intrinsic to the eye and therefore has no dire implications for the patient. Corneal aberrations (e.g., keratoconus, pterygium), uncorrected refractive error, cataract, or foveal traction may give rise to monocular diplopia. Occasionally it is a symptom of malingering or psychiatric disease. Diplopia alleviated by covering one eye is binocular diplopia and is caused by disruption of ocular alignment. Inquiry should be made into the nature of the double vision (purely side-by-side versus partial vertical displacement of images), mode of onset, duration, intermittency, diurnal variation, and associated neurologic or systemic symptoms. If the patient has diplopia while being examined, motility testing should reveal a deficiency corresponding to the patient's symptoms. However, subtle limitation of ocular excursions is often difficult to detect. For example, a patient with a slight left abducens nerve paresis may appear to have full eye movements, despite a complaint of horizontal diplopia upon looking to the left. In this situation, the cover test provides a more sensitive method for demonstrating the ocular misalignment. It should be conducted in primary gaze, and then with the head turned and tilted in each direction. In the above example, a cover test with the head turned to the right will maximize the fixation shift evoked by the cover test.

Occasionally, a cover test performed in an asymptomatic patient during a routine examination will reveal an ocular deviation. If the eye movements are full and the ocular misalignment is equal in all directions of gaze (concomitant deviation), the diagnosis is strabismus. In this condition, which affects about 1% of the population, fusion is disrupted in infancy or early childhood. To avoid diplopia, vision is suppressed from the nonfixating eye. In some children, this leads to impaired vision (amblyopia, or "lazy" eye) in the deviated eye.

Binocular diplopia occurs from a wide range of processes: infectious, neoplastic, metabolic, degenerative, inflammatory, and vascular. One must decide if the diplopia is neurogenic in origin or due to restriction of globe rotation by local disease in the orbit. Orbital pseudotumor, myositis, infection, tumor, thyroid disease, and muscle entrapment (e.g., from a blowout fracture) cause restrictive diplopia. The diagnosis of restriction is usually made by recognizing other associated signs and symptoms of local orbital disease in conjunction with imaging.

Myasthenia Gravis (See also Chap. 36)

This is a major cause of diplopia. The diplopia is often intermittent, variable, and not confined to any single ocular motor nerve distribution. The pupils are always normal. Fluctuating ptosis may be present. Many patients have a purely ocular form of the disease, with no evidence of systemic muscular weakness. The diagnosis can be confirmed by an intravenous edrophonium injection or by an assay for antiacetylcholine receptor antibodies. Negative results from these tests do not exclude the diagnosis. *Botulism* from food or wound poisoning can mimic ocular myasthenia.

After restrictive orbital disease and myasthenia gravis are excluded, a lesion of a cranial nerve supplying innervation to the extraocular muscles is the most likely cause of binocular diplopia.

Oculomotor Nerve

The third cranial nerve innervates the medial, inferior, and superior recti; inferior oblique; levator palpebrae superioris; and the iris sphincter. Total palsy of the oculomotor nerve causes ptosis, a dilated pupil, and leaves the eye "down and out" because of the unopposed action of the lateral rectus and superior oblique. This combination of findings is obvious. More challenging is the diagnosis of an early or partial oculomotor nerve palsy. In this setting, any combination of ptosis, pupil dilation, and weakness of the eye muscles supplied by the oculomotor nerve may be encountered. Frequent serial examinations during the evolving phase of the palsy and a high index of suspicion help ensure that the diagnosis is not missed. The advent of an oculomotor nerve palsy with any degree of pupil involvement in an otherwise healthy patient, especially when accompanied by pain, raises the specter of a circle of Willis aneurysm. If an MR imaging shows no compressive lesion, an arteriogram must be considered to rule out an aneurysm of either the posterior communicating artery or the basilar artery. If the pupil is entirely normal, with all other components of an oculomotor palsy present, aneurysm is so rare that an angiogram is seldom indicated.

A lesion of the oculomotor nucleus in the rostral midbrain produces signs that differ from those caused by a lesion of the nerve itself. There is bilateral ptosis because the levator muscle is innervated by a single central subnucleus. There is also weakness of the contralateral superior rectus, because it is supplied by the oculomotor nucleus on the other side. Occasionally both superior recti are weak. Isolated nuclear oculomotor palsy is rare. Usually neurologic examination reveals additional signs to suggest brainstem damage from infarction, hemorrhage, tumor, or infection.

Injury to structures surrounding fascicles of the oculomotor nerve descending through the midbrain has given rise to a number of classic eponymic designations. In *Nothnagel's syndrome,* injury to the superior cerebellar peduncle causes ipsilateral oculomotor palsy

and contralateral cerebellar ataxia. In *Benedikt's syndrome,* injury to the red nucleus results in ipsilateral oculomotor palsy and contralateral tremor, chorea, and athetosis. *Claude's syndrome* incorporates features of both the aforementioned syndromes, by injury to both the red nucleus and the superior cerebellar peduncle. Finally, in *Weber's syndrome,* injury to the cerebral peduncle causes ipsilateral oculomotor palsy with contralateral hemiparesis.

In the subarachnoid space the oculomotor nerve is vulnerable to aneurysm, meningitis, tumor, infarction, and compression. In cerebral herniation the nerve becomes trapped between the edge of the tentorium and the uncus of the temporal lobe. Oculomotor palsy can also occur from midbrain torsion and hemorrhages during herniation. In the cavernous sinus, oculomotor palsy arises from carotid aneurysm, carotid cavernous fistula, cavernous sinus thrombosis, tumor (pituitary adenoma, meningioma, metastasis), herpes zoster infection, and the Tolosa-Hunt syndrome.

The etiology of an isolated, pupil-sparing oculomotor palsy often remains an enigma, even after neuroimaging and extensive laboratory testing. Most cases are thought to result from microvascular infarction of the nerve, somewhere along its course from the brainstem to the orbit. Usually the patient complains of pain. Diabetes, hypertension, and vascular disease are major risk factors. Spontaneous recovery over a period of months is the rule. If this fails to occur, or if new findings develop, the diagnosis of microvascular oculomotor nerve palsy should be reconsidered. Aberrant regeneration is common when the oculomotor nerve is injured by trauma or compression (tumor, aneurysm). Miswiring of sprouting fibers to the levator muscle and the rectus muscles results in elevation of the eyelid upon downgaze or adduction. The pupil also constricts upon attempted adduction, elevation, or depression of the globe. Aberrant regeneration is not seen after oculomotor palsy from microvascular infarct and hence vitiates that diagnosis.

Trochlear Nerve

The fourth cranial nerve originates in the midbrain, just caudal to the oculomotor nerve complex. Fibers exit the brainstem dorsally and cross to innervate the contralateral superior oblique. The principal actions of this muscle are to depress and to intort the globe. A palsy therefore results in hypertropia and excyclotorsion. The cyclotorsion is seldom noticed by patients. Instead, they complain of vertical diplopia, especially upon reading or looking down. The vertical diplopia is also exacerbated by tilting the head toward the side with the muscle palsy, and alleviated by tilting it away. This "head tilt test" is a cardinal diagnostic feature.

Isolated trochlear nerve palsy occurs from all the causes listed above for the oculomotor nerve, except aneurysm. The trochlear nerve is particularly apt to suffer injury after closed head trauma. The free edge of the tentorium is thought to impinge upon the nerve during a concussive blow. Most isolated trochlear nerve palsies are idiopathic and hence diagnosed by exclusion as "microvascular." Spontaneous improvement occurs over a period of months in most patients. A base-down prism (conveniently applied to the patient's glasses as a stick-on Fresnel lens) may serve as a temporary measure to alleviate diplopia. If the palsy does not resolve, the eyes can be realigned by weakening the inferior oblique muscle.

Abducens Nerve

The sixth cranial nerve innervates the lateral rectus muscle. A palsy produces horizontal diplopia, worse on gaze to the side of the lesion. A nuclear lesion has different consequences, because the abducens nucleus contains interneurons that project via the medial longitudinal fasciculus to the medial rectus subnucleus of the contralateral oculomotor complex. Therefore, an abducens nuclear lesion produces a complete lateral gaze palsy, from weakness of both the ipsilateral lateral rectus and the contralateral medial rectus. *Foville's syndrome* following dorsal pontine injury includes lateral gaze palsy, ipsilateral facial palsy, and contralateral hemiparesis incurred by damage to descending corticospinal fibers. *Millard-Gubler syndrome* from ventral pontine injury is similar, except for the eye findings. There is lateral rectus weakness only, instead of gaze palsy, because the abducens fascicle is injured rather than the nucleus. Infarct, tumor, hemorrhage, vascular malformation, and multiple sclerosis are the most common etiologies of brainstem abducens palsy.

After leaving the ventral pons, the abducens nerve runs forward along the clivus to pierce the dura at the petrous apex, where it enters the cavernous sinus. Along its subarachnoid course it is susceptible to meningitis, tumor (meningioma, chordoma, carcinomatous meningitis), subarachnoid hemorrhage, trauma, and compression by aneurysm or dolichoectatic vessels. At the petrous apex, mastoiditis can produce deafness, pain, and ipsilateral abducens palsy (*Gradenigo's syndrome*). In the cavernous sinus, the nerve can be affected by carotid aneurysm, carotid cavernous fistula, tumor (pituitary adenoma, meningioma, nasopharyngeal carcinoma), herpes infection, and Tolosa-Hunt syndrome.

Unilateral or bilateral abducens palsy is a classic sign of raised intracranial pressure. The diagnosis can be confirmed if papilledema is observed on fundus examination. The mechanism is still debated but is probably related to rostral-caudal displacement of the brainstem. The same phenomenon accounts for abducens palsy from low intracranial pressure (e.g., after lumbar puncture, spinal anesthesia, or spontaneous dural cerebrospinal fluid leak).

Treatment of abducens palsy is aimed at prompt correction of the underlying cause. However, the cause remains obscure in many instances, despite diligent evaluation. As mentioned above for isolated trochlear or oculomotor palsy, most cases are assumed to represent microvascular infarcts because they often occur in the setting of diabetes or other vascular risk factors. Some cases may develop as a postinfectious mononeuritis (e.g., following a viral flu). Patching one eye or applying a temporary prism will provide relief of diplopia until the palsy resolves. If recovery is incomplete, eye muscle surgery can nearly always realign the eyes, at least in primary position. A patient with an abducens palsy that fails to improve should be reevaluated for an occult etiology (e.g., chordoma, carcinomatous meningitis, carotid cavernous fistula, myasthenia gravis).

Multiple Ocular Motor Nerve Palsies

These should not be attributed to spontaneous microvascular events affecting more than one cranial nerve at a time. This remarkable coincidence does occur, especially in diabetic patients, but the diagnosis is made only in retrospect after exhausting all other diagnostic alternatives. Neuroimaging should focus on the cavernous sinus, superior orbital fissure, and orbital apex, where all three ocular motor nerves are in close proximity. In the diabetic or compromised host, fungal infection (*Aspergillus,* Mucorales, *Cryptococcus*) is a frequent cause of multiple nerve palsies. In the patient with systemic malignancy, carcinomatous meningitis is a likely diagnosis. Cytologic examination may be negative despite repeated sampling of the cerebrospinal fluid. The cancer-associated Lambert-Eaton myasthenic syndrome can also produce ophthalmoplegia. Giant cell (temporal) arteritis occasionally manifests as diplopia from ischemic palsies of extraocular muscles. Fisher syndrome, an ocular variant of Guillain-Barré, can produce ophthalmoplegia with areflexia and ataxia. Often the ataxia is mild, and the areflexia is overlooked because the physician's attention is focused upon the eyes. Antiganglioside antibodies (GQ1b) can be detected in about 50% of cases.

Supranuclear Disorders of Gaze

These are often mistaken for multiple ocular motor nerve palsies. For example, Wernicke's encephalopathy can produce nystagmus and a partial deficit of horizontal and vertical gaze that mimics a combined abducens and oculomotor nerve palsy. The disorder occurs in malnourished or alcoholic patients and can be reversed by thiamine. Infarct, hemorrhage, tumor, multiple sclerosis, encephalitis, vasculitis, and Whipple's disease are other important causes of supranuclear gaze palsy. Disorders of vertical gaze, especially downwards saccades, are an early feature of progressive supranuclear palsy. Smooth pursuit is affected later in the course of the disease. Parkinson's disease, Huntington's chorea, and olivopontocerebellar degeneration can also affect vertical gaze.

The *frontal eye field* of the cerebral cortex is involved in generation of saccades to the contralateral side. After hemispheric stroke, the eyes usually deviate towards the lesioned side because of the unopposed action of the frontal eye field in the normal hemisphere. With time, this deficit resolves. Seizures generally have the opposite effect: the eyes deviate conjugately away from the irritative focus. *Parietal lesions* disrupt smooth pursuit of targets moving toward the side of the lesion. Bilateral parietal lesions produce *Balint's syndrome,* characterized by impaired eye-hand coordination (optic ataxia), difficulty initiating voluntary eye movements (ocular apraxia), and visuospatial disorientation (simultanagnosia).

Horizontal Gaze

Descending cortical inputs mediating horizontal gaze ultimately converge at the level of the pons. Neurons in the paramedian pontine reticular formation are responsible for controlling conjugate gaze toward the same side. They project directly to the ipsilateral abducens nucleus. A lesion of either the paramedian pontine reticular formation or the abducens nucleus causes an ipsilateral conjugate gaze palsy. Lesions at either locus produce nearly identical clinical syndromes, with the following exception: vestibular stimulation (oculocephalic maneuver or caloric irrigation) will succeed in driving the eyes conjugately to the side in a patient with a lesion of the paramedian pontine reticular formation, but not in a patient with a lesion of the abducens nucleus.

■ **Internuclear Ophthalmoplegia** This results from damage to the medial longitudinal fasciculus ascending from the abducens nucleus in the pons to the oculomotor nucleus in the midbrain (hence, "internuclear"). Damage to fibers carrying the conjugate signal from abducens interneurons to the contralateral medial rectus motoneurons results in a failure of adduction on attempted lateral gaze. For example, a patient with a left internuclear ophthalmoplegia will have slowed or absent adducting movements of the left eye. A patient with bilateral injury to the medial longitudinal fasciculus will have bilateral internuclear ophthalmoplegia. Multiple sclerosis is the most common cause, although tumor, stroke, trauma, or any brainstem process may be responsible. *One-and-a-half syndrome* is due to a combined lesion of the medial longitudinal fasciculus and the abducens nucleus on the same side. The patient's only horizontal eye movement is abduction of the eye on the other side **(Fig. 11-18)**.

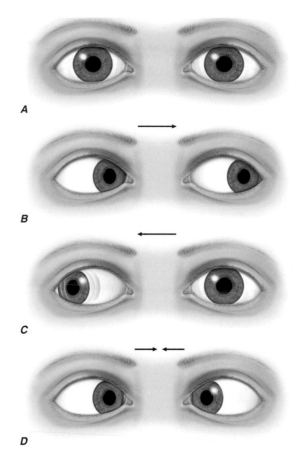

FIGURE 11-18

Left internuclear ophthalmoplegia (INO). *A.* In the primary position of gaze the eyes appear normal. *B.* Similarly, horizontal gaze to the left is intact. *C.* On attempted horizontal gaze to the right, there is a delay or complete loss of adduction on attempted horizontal gaze to one side accompanied by nystagmus in the abducting eye. *D.* Convergence is preserved, distinguishing INO from medial rectus palsy.

Vertical Gaze

This is controlled at the level of the midbrain. The neuronal circuits affected in disorders of vertical gaze are not fully elucidated, but lesions of the rostral interstitial nucleus of the medial longitudinal fasciculus and the interstitial nucleus of Cajal cause supranuclear paresis of upgaze, downgaze, or all vertical eye movements. Distal basilar artery ischemia is the most common etiology. *Skew deviation* refers to a vertical misalignment of the eyes, usually constant in all positions of gaze. The finding has poor localizing value because skew deviation has been reported after lesions in widespread regions of the brainstem and cerebellum.

■ **Parinaud's Syndrome** Also known as *dorsal midbrain syndrome,* this is a distinct supranuclear vertical gaze disorder from damage to the posterior commissure. It is a classic sign of hydrocephalus from aqueductal stenosis.

Pineal region tumors, cysticercosis, and stroke also cause Parinaud's syndrome. Features include loss of upgaze (and sometimes downgaze), convergence-retraction nystagmus on attempted upgaze, downwards ocular deviation ("setting sun" sign), lid retraction (Collier's sign), skew deviation, pseudoabducens palsy, and light-near dissociation of the pupils.

Nystagmus

This is a rhythmical oscillation of the eyes, occurring physiologically from vestibular and optokinetic stimulation or pathologically in a wide variety of diseases (Chap. 9). Abnormalities of the eyes or optic nerves, present at birth or acquired in childhood, can produce a complex, searching nystagmus with irregular pendular (sinusoidal) and jerk features. This nystagmus is commonly referred to as *congenital sensory nystagmus*. It is a poor term, because even in children with congenital lesions, the nystagmus does not appear until several months of age. *Congenital motor nystagmus,* which looks similar to congenital sensory nystagmus, develops in the absence of any abnormality of the sensory visual system. Visual acuity is also reduced in congenital motor nystagmus, probably by the nystagmus itself, but seldom below a level of 20/200.

Jerk Nystagmus This is characterized by a slow drift off the target, followed by a fast corrective saccade. By convention, the nystagmus is named after the quick phase. Jerk nystagmus can be downbeat, upbeat, horizontal (left or right), and torsional. The pattern of nystagmus may vary with gaze position. Some patients will be oblivious to their nystagmus. Others will complain of blurred vision, or a subjective, to-and-fro movement of the environment (oscillopsia) corresponding to their nystagmus. Fine nystagmus may be difficult to see upon gross examination of the eyes. Observation of nystagmoid movements of the optic disc on ophthalmoscopy is a sensitive way to detect subtle nystagmus.

Gaze-evoked Nystagmus This is the most common form of jerk nystagmus. When the eyes are held eccentrically in the orbits, they have a natural tendency to drift back to primary position. The subject compensates by making a corrective saccade to maintain the deviated eye position. Many normal patients have mild gaze-evoked nystagmus. Exaggerated gaze-evoked nystagmus can be induced by drugs (sedatives, anticonvulsants, alcohol); muscle paresis; myasthenia gravis; demyelinating disease; and cerebellopontine angle, brainstem, and cerebellar lesions.

Vestibular Nystagmus *Vestibular nystagmus* results from dysfunction of the labyrinth (Ménière's disease),

vestibular nerve, or vestibular nucleus in the brainstem. Peripheral vestibular nystagmus often occurs in discrete attacks, with symptoms of nausea and vertigo. There may be associated tinnitus and hearing loss. Sudden shifts in head position may provoke or exacerbate symptoms.

Downbeat Nystagmus *Downbeat nystagmus* occurs from lesions near the craniocervical junction (Chiari malformation, basilar invagination). It has also been reported in brainstem or cerebellar stroke, lithium or anticonvulsant intoxication, alcoholism, and multiple sclerosis. *Upbeat nystagmus* is associated with damage to the pontine tegmentum, from stroke, demyelination, or tumor.

Opsoclonus

This rare, dramatic disorder of eye movements consists of bursts of consecutive saccades (saccadomania). When the saccades are confined to the horizontal plane, the term *ocular flutter* is preferred. It can occur from viral encephalitis, trauma, or a paraneoplastic effect of neuroblastoma, breast carcinoma, and other malignancies. It has also been reported as a benign, transient phenomenon in otherwise healthy patients.

FURTHER READINGS

ALBERT DM, JAKOBIEC FA (eds): *Principles and Practice of Ophthalmology,* 2d ed. Philadelphia, Saunders, 2000

BENAVENTE O et al: Prognosis after transient monocular blindness associated with carotid artery stenosis. N Engl J Med 345:1084, 2001

☑ KEANE JR: Internuclear ophthalmoplegia: Unusual causes in 114 of 410 patients. Arch Neurol 62:714, 2005

Excellent case series report of common and unusual causes of internuclear ophthalmoplegia.

NEGI A, VERNON SA: An overview of the eye in diabetes. J R Soc Med 96:266, 2003

PAMBAKIAN A et al: Rehabilitation strategies for patients with homonymous visual field defects. J Neuroophthalmol 25:136, 2005

PIERROT-DESEILLIGNY C, MILEA D: Vertical nystagmus: Clinical facts and hypotheses. Brain 128:1237, 2005

RUCKER JC, TOMSAK RL: Binocular diplopia. A practical approach. Neurologist 11:98, 2005

SOLOMON R, DONNENFELD ED: Recent advances and future frontiers in treating age-related cataracts. JAMA 290:248, 2003

TROBE JD: *The Neurology of Vision,* (Contemporary Neurology Series 60), Oxford University Press, New York, New York 2001

☑ VAN WIJNGAARDEN P et al: Inhibitors of ocular neovascularization: Promises and potential problems. JAMA 293:1509, 2005

Update on evolving therapies for macular degeneration.

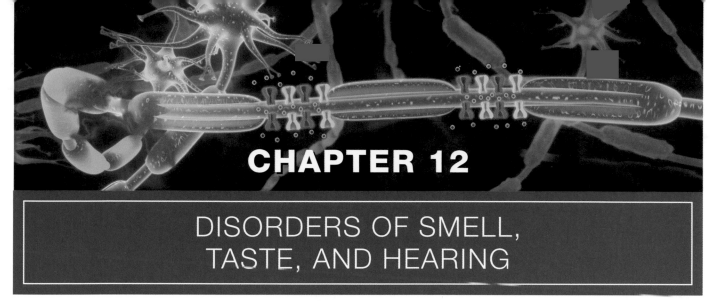

CHAPTER 12

DISORDERS OF SMELL, TASTE, AND HEARING

Anil K. Lalwani

James B. Snow, Jr.

SMELL

The sense of smell determines the flavor and palatability of food and drink. It serves, along with the trigeminal system, as a monitor of inhaled chemicals, including dangerous substances such as natural gas, smoke, and air pollutants. Olfactory dysfunction affects ~1% of people under age 60 and more than half of the population beyond this age.

DEFINITIONS

Smell is the perception of odor by the nose. *Taste* is the perception of salty, sweet, sour, or bitter by the tongue. Related sensations during eating such as somatic sensations of coolness, warmth, and irritation are mediated through the trigeminal, glossopharyngeal, and vagal afferents in the nose, oral cavity, tongue, pharynx, and larynx. *Flavor* is the complex interaction of taste, smell, and somatic sensation. Terms relating to disorders of smell include *anosmia,* an absence of the ability to smell; *hypos-*

mia, a decreased ability to smell; *hyperosmia,* an increased sensitivity to an odorant; *dysosmia,* distortion in the perception of an odor; *phantosmia,* perception of an odorant where none is present; and *agnosia,* inability to classify, contrast, or identify odor sensations verbally, even though the ability to distinguish between odorants or to recognize them may be normal. An odor stimulus is referred to as an *odorant.* Each category of smell dysfunction can be further subclassified as total (applying to all odorants) or partial (dysfunction of only select odorants).

PHYSIOLOGY OF SMELL

The *olfactory neuroepithelium* is located in the superior part of the nasal cavities. It contains an orderly arrangement of bipolar olfactory receptor cells, microvillar cells, sustentacular cells, and basal cells. The dendritic process of the bipolar cell has a bulb-shaped vesicle that projects into the mucous layer and bears six to eight cilia containing the odorant. Each bipolar cell contains 56 cm^2 (9 in.^{2}) of surface area to receive olfactory stimuli.

Microvillar cells are located adjacent to the receptor cells on the surface of the neuroepithelium. Sustentacular cells, unlike their counterparts in the respiratory epithelium, are not specialized to secrete mucus. Although they form a tight barrier separating neurons from the outside environment, their complete function is unknown. The basal cells are progenitors of other cell types in the olfactory neuroepithelium, including the bipolar receptor cells. There is a regular turnover of bipolar receptor cells, which function as the primary sensory neurons. In addition, with injury to the cell body or its axon, the receptor cell is replaced by a differentiated basal cell, which reestablishes a central neural connection. These primary sensory neurons are unique among sensory systems in that they are regularly replaced and regenerate after injury.

153

The unmyelinated axons of receptor cells form the fila of the olfactory nerve, pass through the cribriform plate, and terminate within spherical masses of neuropil, termed *glomeruli*, in the olfactory bulb. The glomeruli are the focus of a high degree of convergence of information, since many more fibers enter than leave them. The main second-order neurons are mitral cells. The primary dendrite of each mitral cell extends into a single glomerulus. Axons of the mitral cells project along with the axons of adjacent tufted cells to the limbic system, including the anterior olfactory nucleus and the amygdala. Cognitive awareness of smell requires stimulation of the prepiriform cortex or amygdaloid nuclei.

A secondary site of olfactory chemosensation is located in the epithelium of the vomeronasal organ, a tubular structure that opens on the ventral aspect of the nasal septum. Sensory neurons located in the vomeronasal organ detect pheromones, nonvolatile chemical signals that in lower mammals trigger innate and stereotyped reproductive and social behaviors, as well as neuroendocrine changes. Neurons from the organ project to the accessory olfactory bulbs and not the main olfactory bulb, as does the olfactory neuroepithelium. Whether humans use the vomeronasal organ to detect and respond to chemical signals from others remains controversial. Development of the olfactory and vomeronasal system appears to be required for normal sexual maturation.

The sensation of smell begins with introduction of an odorant to the cilia of the bipolar neuron. Most odorants are hydrophobic; as they move from the air phase of the nasal cavity to the aqueous phase of the olfactory mucous, they are transported toward the cilia by small water-soluble proteins called *odorant-binding proteins* and reversibly bind to receptors on the cilia surface. Binding leads to confor-mational changes in the receptor protein, activation of G protein–coupled second messengers, and generation of action potentials in the primary neurons. Intensity appears to be coded by the amount of firing in the afferent neurons.

Olfactory receptor proteins belong to the large family of G protein–coupled receptors that also includes rhodopsins; α- and β-adrenergic receptors; muscarinic acetylcholine receptors; and neurotransmitter receptors for dopamine, serotonin, and substance P. In humans, there are 300 to 1000 olfactory receptor genes belonging to 20 different families located in clusters at more than 25 different chromosomal locations. Each olfactory neuron seems to express only one or, at most, a few receptor genes, thus providing the molecular basis of odor discrimination. Bipolar cells that express similar receptors appear to be scattered across discrete spatial zones. These similar cells converge on a select few glomeruli in the olfactory bulb. The result is a potential spatial map of how we receive odor stimului, much like the tonotopic organization of how we perceive sound.

DISORDERS OF THE SENSE OF SMELL

These are caused by conditions that interfere with the access of the odorant to the olfactory neuroepithelium (transport loss), injure the receptor region (sensory loss), or damage central olfactory pathways (neural loss). Currently no clinical tests exist to differentiate these different types of olfactory losses. Fortunately, the history of the disease provides important clues to the cause. The leading causes of olfactory disorders are summarized in **Table 12-1;** the most common etiologies are head trauma in children and young adults, and viral infections in older adults.

TABLE 12-1

CAUSES OF OLFACTORY DYSFUNCTION	
Transport Losses	**Neural Losses**
Allergic rhinitis	AIDS
Bacterial rhinitis and sinusitis	Alcoholism
Congenital abnormalities	Alzheimer's disease
Nasal neoplasms	Cigarette smoke
Nasal polyps	Depression
Nasal septal deviation	Diabetes mellitus
Nasal surgery	Drugs/toxins
Viral infections	Huntington's chorea
Sensory Losses	Hypothyroidism
Drugs	Kallmann syndrome
Neoplasms	Malnutrition
Radiation therapy	Neoplasms
Toxin exposure	Neurosurgery
Viral infections	Parkinson's disease
	Trauma
	Vitamin B_{12} deficiency
	Zinc deficiency

Head trauma is followed by unilateral or bilateral impairment of smell in up to 15% of cases; anosmia is more common than hyposmia. Olfactory dysfunction is more common when trauma is associated with loss of consciousness, moderately severe head injury and skull fracture. Frontal injuries and fractures disrupt the cribriform plate and olfactory axons that perforate it. Sometimes there is an associated cerebrospinal fluid (CSF) rhinorrhea resulting from a tearing of the dura overlying the cribriform plate and paranasal sinuses. Anosmia may also follow blows to the occiput. Once traumatic anosmia develops, it is usually permanent; only 10% of patients ever improve or recover. Perversion of the sense of smell may occur as a transient phase in the recovery process.

Viral infections destroy the olfactory neuroepithelium, which is replaced by respiratory epithelium. Parainfluenza virus type 3 appears to be especially detrimental to human olfaction. HIV infection is associated with subjective distortion of taste and smell, which may become more severe as the disease progresses. The loss of taste and smell may play an important role in the development and progression of HIV-associated wasting. Congenital anosmias are rare but important. Kallmann syndrome is an X-linked disorder characterized by congenital anosmia and hypogonadotropic hypogonadism resulting from a failure of migration from the olfactory placode of olfactory receptor neurons and neurons synthesizing gonadotropin-releasing hormone. Anosmia can also occur in albinos. The receptor cells are present but are hypoplastic, lack cilia, and do not project above the surrounding supporting cells.

Meningiomas of the inferior frontal region are the most frequent neoplastic cause of anosmia; loss of smell may be the only neurologic abnormality. Rarely, anosmia can occur with gliomas of the frontal lobe. Occasionally, pituitary adenomas, craniopharyngiomas, suprasellar meningiomas, and aneurysms of the anterior part of the circle of Willis extend forward and damage olfactory structures. These tumors and hamartomas may also induce seizures with olfactory hallucinations, indicating involvement of the uncus of the temporal lobe.

Dysosmia, subjective distortions of olfactory perception, may occur with intranasal diseases that partially impair smell or may represent a phase in the recovery from a neurogenic anosmia. Most dysosmic disorders consist of disagreeable odors, sometimes accompanied by distortions of taste. Dysosmia also can occur with depression.

APPROACH TO THE PATIENT WITH ANOSMIA

Unilateral anosmia is rarely a complaint and is only recognized by separate testing of smell in each nasal cavity. Bilateral anosmia, on the other hand, brings patients to medical attention. Anosmic patients usually complain of a loss of the sense of taste even though their taste thresholds may be within normal limits. In actuality, they are complaining of a loss of flavor detection, which is mainly an olfactory function. The physical examination should include a thorough inspection of the ears, upper respiratory tract, and head and neck. A neurologic examination emphasizing the cranial nerves and cerebellar and sensorimotor function is essential. Any signs of depression should be noted.

Sensory olfactory function can be assessed by any of several methods. The Odor Stix test uses a commercially available odor-producing magic marker–like pen held approximately 8 to 15 cm (3 to 6 in.) from the patient's nose. The 30-cm alcohol test uses a freshly opened isopropyl alcohol packet held ~30 cm (12 in.) from the patient's nose. There is a commercially available scratch-and-sniff card containing three odors available for testing olfaction grossly. A superior test is the University of Pennsylvania Smell Identification Test (UPSIT). This consists of a 40-item, forced choice, microencapsulated odor, scratch-and-sniff paradigm. For example, one of the items reads, "This odor smells most like (a) chocolate, (b) banana, (c) onion, or (d) fruit punch." The test is highly reliable, is sensitive to age and sex differences, and provides an accurate quantitative determination of the olfactory deficit. The average score for total anosmics is slightly higher than that expected on the basis of chance because of the inclusion of some odorants that act by trigeminal stimulation.

Following assessment of sensory olfactory function, the detection threshold for the odorant phenyl ethyl alcohol should be established using a graduated stimulus. Sensitivity for each side of the nose is determined with a detection threshold for phenyl ethyl methyl ethyl carbinol. Nasal resistance can also be measured with anterior rhinomanometry for each side of the nose.

Computed tomography (CT) or magnetic resonance imaging (MRI) of the head is required to rule out paranasal sinusitis; neoplasms of the anterior cranial fossa, nasal cavity, or paranasal sinuses; or unsuspected fractures of the anterior cranial fossa. Bone abnormalities are best seen with CT. MRI is useful in evaluating olfactory bulbs, ventricles, and other soft tissue of the brain. Coronal CT is optimal for assessing cribriform plate, anterior cranial fossa, and sinus anatomy.

Techniques have been developed to biopsy the olfactory neuroepithelium, but in view of the widespread degeneration of the olfactory neuroepithelium and intercalation of respiratory epithelium in the olfactory area of adults with no apparent olfactory dysfunction, biopsy material must be interpreted cautiously.

TREATMENT FOR OLFACTORY LOSSES

Therapy for patients with transport olfactory losses due to allergic rhinitis, bacterial rhinitis and sinusitis, polyps, neoplasms, and structural abnormalities of the nasal cavities can be undertaken with a high likelihood for improvement. Allergy management; antibiotic therapy; topical and systemic glucocorticoid therapy; and surgery for nasal polyps, deviation of the nasal septum, and chronic hyperplastic sinusitis are frequently effective in restoring the sense of smell.

There is no proven treatment for sensorineural olfactory losses. Fortunately, spontaneous recovery often occurs. Zinc and vitamin therapy (especially with vitamin A) are advocated by some. Profound zinc deficiency can produce loss and distortion of the sense of smell but is not a clinically important problem except in very limited geographic areas. The epithelial degeneration associated with vitamin A deficiency can cause anosmia, but in western societies the prevalence of vitamin A deficiency is low. Exposure to cigarette smoke and other airborne toxic chemicals can cause metaplasia of the olfactory epithelium. Spontaneous recovery can occur if the insult is discontinued. Counseling of patients is therefore helpful in these cases.

More than half of people over age 60 suffer from olfactory dysfunction. No effective treatment exists for presbyosmia, but patients are often reassured to learn that this problem is common in their age group. In addition, early recognition and counseling can help patients to compensate for the loss of smell. The incidence of natural gas–related accidents is disproportionately high in the elderly, perhaps due in part to the gradual loss of smell. Mercaptan, the pungent odor in natural gas, is an olfactory stimulant and does not activate taste receptors. Many elderly with olfactory dysfunction experience a decrease in flavor sensation and find it necessary to hyperflavor food, usually by increasing the amount of salt in their diet.

TASTE

Compared with disorders of smell, gustatory disorders are uncommon. Loss of olfactory sensitivity is often accompanied by complaints of loss of the sense of taste, usually with normal detection thresholds for taste.

DEFINITIONS

Disturbances of the sense of taste may be categorized as *total ageusia,* total absence of gustatory function or inability to detect the qualities of sweet, salt, bitter, or sour; *partial ageusia,* ability to detect some of but not all the qualitative gustatory sensations; *specific ageusia,* inability to detect the taste quality of certain substances; *total hypogeusia,* decreased sensitivity to all tastants; *partial hypogeusia,* decreased sensitivity to some tastants; and *dysgeusia* or *phantogeusia,* distortion in the perception of a tastant, i.e., the perception of the wrong quality when a tastant is presented or the perception of a taste when there has been no tastant ingested. Confusions between sour and bitter, and less commonly between salty and bitter, may represent semantic misunderstandings or have true pathophysiologic bases. It may be possible to differentiate between the loss of flavor recognition in patients with olfactory losses who complain of a loss of taste as well as smell by asking if they are able to taste sweetness in sodas, saltiness in potato chips, etc.

PHYSIOLOGY OF TASTE

The taste receptor cells are located in the taste buds, spherical groups of cells arranged in a pattern resembling the segments of a citrus fruit. At the surface, the taste bud has a pore into which microvilli of the receptor cells project. Unlike the olfactory system, the receptor cell is not the primary neuron. Instead, gustatory afferent nerve fibers contact individual taste receptor cells. There are at least five receptor populations. Taste buds are located in the papillae along the lateral margin and dorsum of the tongue; at the junction of the dorsum and the base of the tongue; and in the palate, epiglottis, larynx, and esophagus.

The sense of taste is mediated through the facial, glossopharyngeal, and vagal nerves. The chorda tympani branch of the facial nerve subserves taste from the anterior two-thirds of the tongue. The posterior third of the tongue is supplied by the lingual branch of the glossopharyngeal nerve. Afferents from the palate travel with the greater superficial petrosal nerve to the geniculate ganglion and then via the facial nerve to the brainstem. The internal branch of the superior laryngeal nerve of the vagus nerve contains the taste afferents from the larynx, including the epiglottis and esophagus.

The central connections of the nerves terminate in the brainstem in the nucleus of the tractus solitarius. The central pathway from the nucleus of the tractus solitarius projects to the ipsilateral parabrachial nuclei of the pons. Two divergent pathways project from the parabrachial nuclei. One ascends to the gustatory relay in the dorsal thalamus, synapses, and continues to the cortex of the insula. There is also evidence for a direct pathway from the parabrachial nuclei to the cortex. (Olfaction and gustation appear to be unique among sensory systems in that at least some fibers bypass the thalamus.) The other pathway from the parabrachial nuclei goes to the ventral forebrain, including the lateral hypothalamus, substantia innominata, central nucleus of the amygdala, and the stria terminalis.

Tastants gain access to the receptor cells through the taste pore. Four classes of taste are recognized: sweet, salt, sour, and bitter. Individual gustatory afferent fibers almost always respond to a number of different chemicals. Response patterns of gustatory afferent axons can be grouped into classes based on the stimulus chemical that produces the largest response. For example, for sucrose-best response neurons, the second-best stimulus is almost always sodium chloride. The fact that individual gustatory afferent fibers respond to a large number of different chemicals led to the *across-fiber-pattern* theory of gustatory coding, while the best-stimulus analysis led to the concept of *labeled* afferents. It appears that labeled fibers are important for establishing gross quality, but the across-fiber pattern within a best-stimulus category, and perhaps among categories, is needed for discriminating

chemicals within qualities. For example, sweetness may be carried by sucrose-best neurons, but the differentiation of sucrose and fructose may require a comparison of the relative activity among sucrose-best, salt-best, and quinine-best neurons. As with olfaction and other sensory systems, intensity appears to be encoded by the quantity of neural activity.

DISORDERS OF THE SENSE OF TASTE

Disorders of the sense of taste are caused by conditions that interfere with the access of the tastant to the receptor cells in the taste bud (transport loss), injure receptor cells (sensory loss), or damage gustatory afferent nerves and central gustatory pathways (neural loss) (**Table 12–2**). *Transport gustatory losses* result from xerostomia due to many causes, including Sjögren's syndrome, radiation therapy, heavy-metal intoxication, and bacterial colonization of the taste pore. *Sensory gustatory losses* are caused by inflammatory and degenerative diseases in the oral cavity; a vast number of drugs, particularly those that interfere with cell turnover such as antithyroid and antineoplastic agents; radiation therapy to the oral cavity and pharynx; viral infections; endocrine disorders; neoplasms; and aging. *Neural gustatory losses* occur with neoplasms, trauma, and surgical procedures in which the gustatory afferents are injured. Taste buds degenerate when their gustatory afferents are transected but remain when their somatosensory afferents are severed. Patients with renal disease have increased thresholds for sweet and sour tastes, which resolves with dialysis.

A side effect of medication is the single most common cause of taste dysfunction in clinical practice. Xerostomia, regardless of the etiology, can be associated

TABLE 12-2

CAUSES OF GUSTATORY DYSFUNCTION	
Transport Gustatory Losses	**Neural Gustatory Losses**
Drugs	Diabetes mellitus
Heavy-metal intoxication	Hypothyroidism
Radiation therapy	Neuropathies of the facial nerve (e.g.,
Sjögren's syndrome	Bell's palsy and the Miller-Fisher
Xerostomia	variant of Guillain-Barré syndrome)
Sensory Gustatory Losses	Oral neoplasms
Aging	Oral surgery
Candidiasis	Radiation therapy
Drugs (antithyroid and antineoplastic)	Renal disease
Endocrine disorders	Stroke and other CNS disorders
Oral neoplasms	Trauma
Pemphigus	Upper respiratory tract infections
Radiation therapy	
Viral infections (especially with herpes viruses)	

with taste dysfunction. It is associated with poor oral clearance and poor dental hygeine, and can adversely affect the oral mucosa, all leading to dysgeusia. However, severe salivary gland failure does not necessarily lead to taste complaints. Xerostomia, the use of antibiotics or glucocorticoids, or immunodeficiency can lead to overgrowth of *Candida*; overgrowth alone, without thrush or overt signs of infection, can be associated with bad taste or hypogeusia. When taste dysfunction occurs in a patient at risk for fungal overgrowth, a trial of nystatin or other antifungal medication is warranted.

Upper respiratory infections and head trauma can lead to both smell and taste dysfunction; taste is more likely to improve than smell. The mechanism of taste disturbance in these situations is not well understood. Trauma to the chorda tympani branch of the facial nerve during middle ear surgery or third molar extractions is relatively common and can cause dysgeusia. Peripheral neuropathies involving the facial nerve proximal to the stylomastoid foramen (thus involving the chorda tympani) are associated with impairment of taste. Unilateral Bell's palsy often produces only limited symptoms detectable by detailed testing (Chap. 23). Bilateral facial nerve palsies (such as can be seen in the Fisher variant of the Guillain-Barré syndrome and sarcoidosis) can be associated with either hypogeusia or total ageusia (Chap. 35). Finally, aging itself may be associated with reduced taste sensitivity. The taste dysfunction may be limited to a single compound and may be mild.

APPROACH TO THE PATIENT WITH TASTE DISORDERS

Patients who complain of loss of taste should be evaluated for both gustatory and olfactory function. Clinical assessment of taste is not as well developed or standardized as that of smell. The first step is to perform suprathreshold whole-mouth taste testing for quality, intensity, and pleasantness perception of four taste qualities: sweet, salty, sour, and bitter. Most commonly used reagents for taste testing are sucrose, citric acid or hydrochloric acid, caffeine or quinine (sulfate or hydrochloride), and sodium chloride. The taste stimuli should be freshly prepared. For quantification, detection thresholds are obtained by applying graduated dilutions to the tongue quandrants or by whole-mouth sips. Electric taste testing (*electrogustometry*) is used clinically to identify taste deficits in specific quandrants of the tongue. Regional gustatory testing may also be performed to assess for the possibility of loss localized to one or more receptor fields as a result of a peripheral or central lesion.

The history of the disease and localization studies provide important clues to the reason for taste disturbance. For example, absence of taste on the anterior two-thirds of the tongue associated with a facial paralysis indicates that the lesion is proximal to the juncture of the chorda tympani branch with the facial nerve in the mastoid.

TREATMENT FOR TASTE DISORDERS

Treatment of gustatory disorders is limited. No effective therapies exist for the sensorineural disorders of taste. Altered taste due to surgical stretch injury of chorda tympani nerve usually improves within 3 to 4 months, while dysfunction is usually permanent with transection of the nerve. Taste dysfunction following trauma may resolve spontaneously without intervention and is more likely to do so than posttraumatic smell dysfunction. Idiopathic alterations of taste sensitivity usually remain stable or worsen; zinc and vitamin therapy are of unproven value. Directed therapy to address factors that affect taste perception can be of value. Xerostomia can be treated with artificial saliva, providing some benefits to patients with a disturbed salivary milieu. Oral pilocarpine may be beneficial for a variety of forms of xerostomia. Appropriate treatment of bacterial and fungal infections of the oral cavity can be of great help in improving taste function. Taste disturbance related to drugs can often be resolved by changing the prescribed medication.

HEARING

Hearing loss is one of the most common sensory disorders in humans and can present at any age. Nearly 10% of the adult population has some hearing loss, and one-third of individuals over the age of 65 have a hearing loss of sufficient magnitude to require a hearing aid.

PHYSIOLOGY OF HEARING (Fig. 12-1)

The function of the external and middle ear is to amplify sound to facilitate mechanotransduction by hair cells in the inner ear. Sound waves enter the external auditory canal and set the tympanic membrane in motion, which in turn moves the malleus, incus, and stapes of the middle ear. Movement of the footplate of the stapes causes pressure changes in the fluid-filled inner

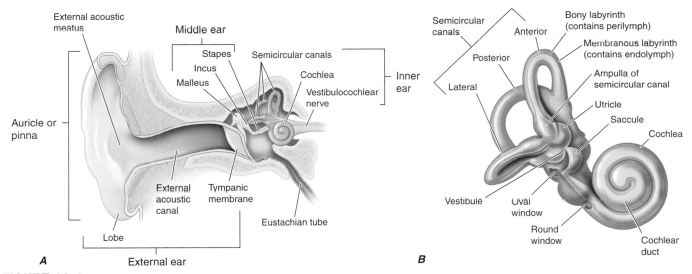

FIGURE 12-1
A. Drawing of modified coronal section through external ear and temporal bone, with structures of the middle and inner ear demonstrated. *B*. High-resolution view of inner ear.

ear eliciting a traveling wave in the basilar membrane of the cochlea. The tympanic membrane and the ossicular chain in the middle ear serve as an impedence-matching mechanism, improving the efficiency of energy transfer from air to the fluid-filled inner ear.

Stereocilia of the hair cells of the organ of Corti, which rests on the basilar membrane, are in contact with the tectorial membrane and are deformed by the traveling wave. A point of maximal displacement of the basilar membrane is determined by the frequency of the stimulating tone. High-frequency tones cause maximal displacement of the basilar membrane near the base of the cochlea. As the frequency of the stimulating tone decreases, the point of maximal displacement moves toward the apex of the cochlea.

The inner and outer hair cells of the organ of Corti have different innervation patterns, but both are mechanoreceptors. The afferent innervation relates principally to the inner hair cells, and the efferent innervation relates principally to outer hair cells. The motility of the outer hair cells alters the micromechanics of the inner hair cells creating a cochlear amplifier, which explains the exquisite sensitivity and frequency selectivity of the cochlea.

The current concept of cochlear transduction is that displacement of the tips of the stereocilia allows potassium to flow into the cell, resulting in its depolarization. The potassium influx opens calcium channels near the base of the cell, stimulating transmitter release. The neurotransmitter at the hair cell and cochlear nerve dendrite interface is thought to be glutamate. Each of the cochlear nerve neurons can be activated at a frequency and intensity specific for that cell. This specificity is maintained at

each point of the central auditory pathway: dorsal and ventral cochlear nuclei, trapezoid body, superior olivary complex, lateral lemniscus, inferior colliculus, medial geniculate body, and auditory cortex. At low frequencies, individual auditory nerve fibers can respond more or less synchronously with the stimulating tone. At higher frequencies, phase-locking occurs so that neurons alternate in response to particular phases of the cycle of the sound wave. Intensity is encoded by the amount of neural activity in individual neurons, the number of neurons that are active, and the specific neurons that are activated.

GENETIC CAUSES OF HEARING LOSS

More than half of childhood hearing impairment is thought to be hereditary; hereditary hearing impairment (HHI) can also manifest later in life. HHI may be classified as either nonsyndromic, when hearing loss is the only clinical abnormality, or syndromic, when hearing loss is associated with anomalies in other organ systems. Nearly two-thirds of HHIs are nonsyndromic, and the remaining one-third are syndromic. Between 70 and 80% of nonsyndromic HHI is inherited in an autosomal recessive manner; another 15 to 20% is autosomal dominant. Less than 5% is X-linked or maternally inherited via the mitochondria.

Over 60 loci harboring genes for nonsyndromic HHI have been mapped, with equal numbers of dominant and recessive modes of inheritance; numerous genes have now been cloned (**Table 12–3**). The hearing genes fall into the categories of structural proteins (MYO7A, MYO15, TECTA, DIAPH1), transcription factors (POU3F4, POU4F3), ion channels (KCNQ4, PDS), and gap junc-

TABLE 12-3

NONSYNDROMIC GENES AND LOCI

LOCUS	GENE	FUNCTION	INHERITANCE
DFNB1	GBJ2 (Cx26)	Forms gap junctions, or plasma membrane channels, with connexins	AR
DFNB2	MYO7A	Moves different macromolecular structures relative to actin filaments	AR
DFNB3	MYO15	Organizes actin in hair cells	AR
DFNB4	PDS	Encodes highly hydrophobic proteins containing the sulphate transporter signature	AR
DFNB9	OTOF	Involved in trafficking of membrane vesicles	AR
DFNB21	TECTA	Includes an amino-terminal hydrophobic signal sequence for translocation across the membrane and a carboxy-terminal hydrophobic region characteristic of precursors of glycosylphosphatidyl-inositol-linked membrane-bound proteins	AR
DFNA1	DIAPH1	Involved in cytokinesis and establishment of cell polarity	AD
DFNA2	GJB3 (Cx31)	Forms gap junction protein	AD
	KCNQ4	Forms potassium channel	
DFNA3	GJB2 (Cx26)	Forms gap junctions, or plasma membrane channels, with connexins	AD
	GBJ6 (Cx30)		
DFNA5	DFNA5	Unknown; related to a gene that is upregulated in estrogen receptor-negative breast carcinomas	AD
DFNA8/12	TECTA	Includes an amino-terminal hydrophobic signal sequence for translocation across the membrane and a carboxy-terminal hydrophobic region characteristic of precursors of glycosylphosphatidylinositol-linked membrane-bound proteins	AD
DFNA9	COCH	Involved in hemostasis, complement system, immune system, and extracellular matrix assembly	AD
DFNA11	MYO7A	Moves different macromolecular structures relative to actin filaments	AD
DFNA15	POU4F3	Serves as a critical developmental regulator for the determination of cellular phenotypes	AD
DFN3	POU3F4	Serves as a critical developmental regulator for the determination of cellular phenotypes	X-linked

Note: AD, autosomal dominant; AR, autosomal recessive.

tion proteins (Cx26, Cx30, Cx31). Several of these genes, including connexin 26 (Cx26), TECTA, and MYO7A, cause both autosomal dominant and recessive forms of nonsyndromic HHI. In general, the hearing loss associated with dominant genes has its onset in adolescence or adulthood and varies in severity, whereas the hearing loss associated with recessive inheritance is congenital and profound. Connexin 26 is particularly important because it is associated with nearly 20% of cases of childhood deafness; in heterozygotes the onset of hearing loss may be in adolescence or adulthood. Two frame-shift mutations, 30delG and 167delT, account for >50% of the cases, making population screening feasible. The 167delT mutation is highly prevalent in Ashkenazi Jews; it is predicted that 1 in 1765 individuals in this population will be homozygous and affected. The hearing loss can also vary among the members of the same family, suggesting that other genes or factors likely influence the auditory phenotype.

The contribution of genetics to presbycusis (see below) is also becoming better understood. In addition to connexin 26, several other nonsyndromic genes are associated with hearing loss that progresses with age. Sensitivity to aminoglycoside ototoxicity can be maternally transmitted through a mitochondrial mutation. Susceptibility to noise-induced hearing loss may also be genetically determined.

There are over 200 syndromic forms of hearing loss. These include Usher syndrome (retinitis pigmentosa and hearing loss), Waardenburg syndrome (pigmentary abnormality and hearing loss), Pendred syndrome (thyroid organification defect and hearing loss), Alport syndrome (renal disease and hearing loss), Jervell and Lange-Nielsen syndrome (prolonged QT interval and hearing loss), neurofibromatosis type 2 (bilateral acoustic schwannoma), and mitochondrial disorders [mitochondrial encephalopathy, lactic acidosis, and stroke-like episodes (MELAS); myoclonic epilepsy and ragged red fibers (MERRF); progressive external ophthalmoplegia (PEO)].

DISORDERS OF THE SENSE OF HEARING

Hearing loss can result from disorders of the auricle, external auditory canal, middle ear, inner ear, or central auditory pathways (**Fig. 12-2**). *In general, lesions in the auricle, external auditory canal, or middle ear cause conductive hearing losses, whereas lesions in the inner ear or eighth nerve cause sensorineural hearing losses.*

Conductive Hearing Loss

This results from obstruction of the external auditory canal by cerumen, debris, and foreign bodies; swelling of

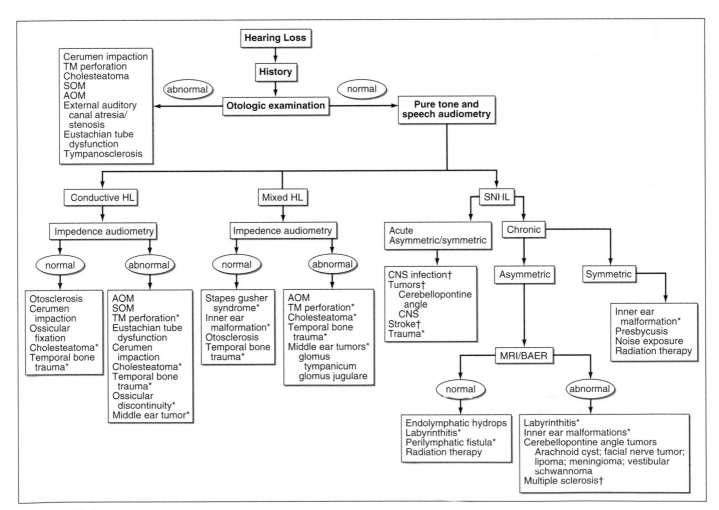

FIGURE 12-2

An algorithm for the approach to hearing loss. HL, hearing loss; SNHL, sensorineural hearing loss; TM, tympanic membrane; SOM, serous otitis media; AOM, acute otitis media; *, CT scan of temporal bone; †, MRI scan.

the lining of the canal; atresia or neoplasms of the canal; perforations of the tympanic membrane; disruption of the ossicular chain, as occurs with necrosis of the long process of the incus in trauma or infection; otosclerosis; or fluid, scarring, or neoplasms in the middle ear.

Cholesteatoma, stratified squamous epithelium in the middle ear or mastoid, occurs frequently in adults. This is a benign, slowly growing lesion that destroys bone and normal ear tissue. Theories of pathogenesis include traumatic implantation and invasion, immigration and invasion through a perforation, and metaplasia following chronic infection and irritation. On examination, there is often a perforation of the tympanic membrane filled with cheesy white squamous debris. A chronically draining ear that fails to respond to appropriate antibiotic therapy should raise suspicion of a cholesteatoma. Conductive hearing loss secondary to ossicular erosion is common. Surgery is required to remove this destructive process.

Conductive hearing loss with a normal ear canal and intact tympanic membrane suggests ossicular pathology. Fixation of the stapes from *otosclerosis* is a common cause of low-frequency conductive hearing loss. It occurs equally in men and women and has a simple autosomal dominant inheritance with incomplete penetrance. Hearing impairment usually presents between the late teens to the forties. In women, the hearing loss is often first noticeable during pregnancy, as the otosclerotic process is accelerated during pregnancy. A hearing aid or a simple outpatient surgical procedure (stapedectomy) can provide adequate auditory rehabilitation. Extension of otosclerosis beyond the stapes footplate to involve the cochlea (cochlear otosclerosis) can lead to mixed or sensorineural hearing loss. Fluoride therapy to prevent hearing loss associated with cochlear otosclerosis is of uncertain value.

Eustachian tube dysfunction is extremely common in adults and may predispose to acute otitis media (AOM) or serous otitis media (SOM). Trauma, AOM, or chronic otitis media are the usual factors responsible for tympanic membrane perforation. While small perforations often heal spontaneously, larger defects usually require surgical intervention. Tympanoplasty is highly effective (>90%) in the repair of tympanic membrane perforations. Otoscopy is usually sufficient to diagnose AOM, SOM, chronic otitis media, cerumen impaction, tympanic membrane perforation, and eustachian tube dysfunction.

Sensorineural Hearing Loss

Damage to the hair cells of the organ of Corti may be caused by intense noise, viral infections, ototoxic drugs (e.g., salicylates, quinine and its synthetic analogues, aminoglycoside antibiotics, loop diuretics such as furosemide and ethacrynic acid, and cancer chemotherapeutic agents such as cisplatin), fractures of the temporal bone, meningitis, cochlear otosclerosis (see above), Ménière's disease, and aging. Congenital malformations of the inner ear may be the cause of hearing loss in some adults. Genetic predisposition alone or in concert with environmental influences may also be responsible.

Presbycusis (age-associated hearing loss) is the most common cause of sensorineural hearing loss in adults. In the early stages, it is characterized by symmetric, gentle to sharply sloping high-frequency hearing loss. With progression, the hearing loss involves all frequencies. More importantly, the hearing impairment is associated with significant loss in clarity. There is a loss of discrimination for phonemes, recruitment (abnormal growth of loudness), and particular difficulty in understanding speech in noisy environments. Hearing aids may provide limited rehabilitation once the word recognition score deteriorates below 50%. Improvements in cochlear implants have made them the treatment of choice when hearing aids prove inadequate.

Ménière's disease is characterized by episodic vertigo, fluctuating sensorineural hearing loss, tinnitus, and aural fullness. Tinnitus and/or deafness may be absent during the initial attacks of vertigo, but they invariably appear as the disease progresses and are increased in severity during an acute attack. The annual incidence of Ménière's disease is 0.5 to 7.5 per 1000; onset is most frequently in the fifth decade of life but may also occur in young adults or the elderly. Histologically, there is distention of the endolymphatic system (endolymphatic hydrops) leading to degeneration of vestibular and cochlear hair cells. This may result from endolymphatic sac dysfunction secondary to infection, trauma, autoimmune disease, inflammatory causes, or tumor; an idiopathic etiology constitutes the largest category and is most accurately referred to as Ménière's disease. Although any pattern of hearing loss can be observed, typically, low-frequency, unilateral sensorineural hearing impairment is present. MRI should be obtained to exclude retrocochlear pathology such as cerebellopontine angle tumors or demyelinating disorders. Therapy is directed towards the control of vertigo. A low-salt diet is the mainstay of treatment of the control of rotatory vertigo. Diuretics, a short course of glucocorticoids, and intratympanic gentamicin may also be useful adjuncts in recalcitrant cases. Surgical therapy of vertigo is reserved for unresponsive cases and includes endolymphatic sac decompression, labyrinthectomy, and vestibular nerve section. Both labyrinthectomy and vestibular nerve section abolish rotatory vertigo in >90% of the cases. Unfortunately, there is no effective therapy for hearing loss, tinnitus, or aural fullness associated with Ménière's disease.

Sensorineural hearing loss may also result from any neoplastic, vascular, demyelinating, infectious, or degenerative disease or trauma affecting the central auditory pathways. HIV leads to both peripheral and central auditory system pathology and is associated with sensorineural hearing impairment.

A finding of conductive and sensory hearing loss in combination is termed *mixed hearing loss.* Mixed hearing losses are due to pathology that can affect the middle and inner ear simultaneously such as otosclerosis involving the ossicles and the cochlea, head trauma, chronic otitis media, cholesteatoma, middle ear tumors, and some inner ear malformations.

Trauma resulting in temporal bone fractures may be associated with conductive, sensorineural, and mixed hearing loss. If the fracture spares the inner ear, there may simply be conductive hearing loss due to rupture of the tympanic membrane or disruption of the ossicular chain. These abnormalities are amenable to surgical correction. Profound hearing loss and severe vertigo are associated with temporal bone fractures involving the inner ear. A perilymphatic fistula associated with leakage of inner-ear fluid into the middle ear can occur and may require surgical repair. An associated facial nerve injury is not uncommon. CT is best suited to assess fracture of the traumatized temporal bone, evaluate the ear canal, and determine the integrity of the ossicular chain and the involvement of the inner ear. CSF leaks that accompany temporal bone fractures are usually self-limited; the use of prophylactic antibiotics is controversial.

Tinnitus is defined as the perception of a sound when there is no sound in the environment. It may have a buzzing, roaring, or ringing quality and may be pulsatile (synchronous with the heartbeat). Tinnitus is often associated with either a conductive or sensorineural hearing loss. The pathophysiology of tinnitus is not well understood. The cause of the tinnitus can usually be determined by finding the cause of the associated hearing loss. Tinnitus may be the first symptom of a serious condition such as a vestibular schwannoma. Pulsatile tinnitus requires evaluation of the vascular system of the head to exclude vascular tumors such as glomus jugulare tumors, aneurysms, stenotic arterial lesions, and dural arteriovenous fistulas; it may also occur with SOM.

APPROACH TO THE PATIENT WITH HEARING DISORDERS

The goal in the evaluation of a patient with auditory complaints is to determine (1) the nature of the hearing impairment (conductive vs. sensorineural), (2) the severity of the impairment (mild, moderate, severe, profound), (3) the anatomy of the impairment (external ear, middle ear, inner ear, or central auditory pathway), and (4) the etiol-

ogy. The history should elicit characteristics of the hearing loss, including the duration of deafness, unilateral vs. bilateral involvement, nature of onset (sudden vs. insidious), and rate of progression (rapid vs. slow). The presence or absence of tinnitus, vertigo, imbalance, aural fullness, otorrhea, headache, facial nerve dysfunction, and head and neck paresthesias should be ascertained. Information regarding head trauma, exposure to ototoxins, occupational or recreational noise exposure, and family history of hearing impairment may also be important. A sudden onset of unilateral hearing loss, with or without tinnitus, may represent a viral infection of the inner ear or a stroke. Patients with unilateral hearing loss (sensory or conductive) usually complain of reduced hearing, poor sound localization, and difficulty hearing clearly with background noise. Gradual progression of a hearing deficit is common with otosclerosis, noise-induced hearing loss, vestibular schwannoma, or Ménière's disease. Small vestibular schwannomas typically present with asymmetric hearing impairment, tinnitus, and imbalance (rarely vertigo); cranial neuropathy, in particular of the trigeminal or facial nerve, may accompany larger tumors. In addition to hearing loss, Ménière's disease may be associated with episodic vertigo, tinnitus, and aural fullness. Hearing loss with otorrhea is most likely due to chronic otitis media or cholesteatoma.

Examination should include the auricle, external ear canal, and tympanic membrane. The external ear canal of the elderly is often dry and fragile; it is preferable to clean cerumen with wall-mounted suction and cerumen loops and to avoid irrigation. In examining the eardrum, the topography of the tympanic membrane is more important than presence or absence of the light reflex. In addition to the pars tensa (the lower two-thirds of the eardrum), the pars flaccida above the short process of the malleus should also be examined for retraction pockets that may be evidence of chronic eustachian tube dysfunction or cholesteatoma. Insufflation of the ear canal is necessary to assess tympanic membrane mobility and compliance. Careful inspection of the nose, nasopharynx, and upper respiratory tract is indicated. Unilateral serous effusion should prompt a fiberoptic examination of the nasopharynx to exclude neoplasms. Cranial nerves should be evaluated with special attention to facial and trigeminal nerves, which are commonly disturbed with tumors involving the cerebellopontine angle.

The Rinne and Weber tuning fork tests, with a 256- or 512-Hz tuning fork, are used to screen for hearing loss, differentiate conductive from sensorineural hearing losses, and to confirm the findings of audiologic evaluation. Rinne's test compares the ability to hear by air conduction with the ability to hear by bone conduction. The tines of a vibrating tuning fork are held near the opening of the external auditory canal, and then the stem is placed on the mastoid process; for direct contact, it may be placed on teeth or dentures. The patient is asked to indicate whether the tone is louder by air conduction or bone conduction. Normally, and in the presence of sensorineural hearing loss, a tone is heard louder by air conduction than by bone conduction; however, with conductive hearing loss of $\geqslant 30$ dB (see "Audiologic Assessment," below), the bone-conduction stimulus is perceived as louder than the air-conduction stimulus. For the Weber test, the stem of a vibrating tuning fork is placed on the head in the midline and the patient asked whether the tone is heard in both ears or better in one ear than in the other. With a unilateral conductive hearing loss, the tone is perceived in the affected ear. With a unilateral sensorineural hearing loss, the tone is perceived in the unaffected ear. A 5-dB difference in hearing between the two ears is required for lateralization.

LABORATORY ASSESSMENT OF HEARING

Audiologic Assessment

The minimum audiologic assessment for hearing loss should include the measurement of pure tone air-conduction and bone-conduction thresholds, speech reception threshold, discrimination score, tympanometry, acoustic reflexes, and acoustic-reflex decay. This test battery provides a comprehensive screening evaluation of the whole auditory system and allows one to determine whether further differentiation of a sensory (cochlear) from a neural (retrocochlear) hearing loss is indicated.

Pure tone audiometry assesses hearing acuity for pure tones. The test is administered by an audiologist and is performed in a sound-attenuated chamber. The pure tone stimulus is delivered with an audiometer, an electronic device that allows the presentation of specific frequencies (generally between 250 and 8000 Hz) at specific intensities. Air and bone conduction thresholds are established for each ear. Air conduction thresholds are established by presenting the stimulus in air with the use of headphones. Bone conduction thresholds are accomplished by placing the stem of a vibrating tuning fork or an oscillator of an audiometer in contact with the head. In the presence of a hearing loss, broad-spectrum noise is presented to the nontest ear for *masking* purposes so that responses are based on perception from the ear under test.

The responses are measured in decibels. An *audiogram* is a plot of intensity in decibels of hearing threshold versus frequency. A decibel (dB) is equal to 20 times the logarithm of the ratio of the sound pressure required to achieve threshold in the patient to the sound pressure required to achieve threshold in a normal hearing person. Therefore, a change of 6 dB represents doubling of sound pressure, and a change of 20 dB represents a tenfold change in sound pressure. Loudness, which depends on the frequency, intensity, and duration of a sound, doubles with approximately each 10-dB increase in sound pressure level. Pitch, on the other hand, does not directly correlate with frequency. The perception of pitch changes slowly in the low and high frequencies. In the middle tones, which are important for human speech, pitch varies more rapidly with changes in frequency.

Pure tone audiometry establishes the presence and severity of hearing impairment, unilateral vs. bilateral involvement, and the type of hearing loss. Conductive hearing losses with a large mass component, as is often seen in middle-ear effusions, produce elevation of thresholds that predominate in the higher frequencies. Conductive hearing losses with a large stiffness component, as in fixation of the footplate of the stapes in early otosclerosis, produce threshold elevations in the lower frequencies. Often, the conductive hearing loss involves all frequencies, suggesting involvement of both stiffness and mass. In general, sensorineural hearing losses such as presbycusis affect higher frequencies more than lower frequencies. An exception is Ménière's disease, which is characteristically associated with low-frequency sensorineural hearing loss. Noise-induced hearing loss has an unusual pattern of hearing impairment in which the loss at 4000 Hz is greater than at higher frequencies. Vestibular schwannomas characteristically affect the higher frequencies, but any pattern of hearing loss can be observed.

Speech recognition requires greater synchronous neural firing than is necessary for appreciation of pure tones. *Speech audiometry* tests the clarity with which one hears. The *speech reception threshold* (SRT) is defined as the intensity at which speech is recognized as a meaningful symbol and is obtained by presenting two-syllable words with an equal accent on each syllable. The intensity at which the patient can repeat 50% of the words correctly is the SRT. Once the SRT is determined, discrimination or word recognition ability is tested by presenting one-syllable words at 25 to 40 dB above the speech reception threshold. The words are phonetically balanced in that the phonemes (speech sounds) occur in the list of words at the same frequency that they occur in ordinary conversational English. An individual with normal hearing or conductive hearing loss can repeat 88 to 100% of the phonetically balanced words correctly. Patients with a sensorineural hearing loss have variable loss of discrimination. As a general rule, neural lesions are associated with more deterioration in discrimination ability than are lesions in the inner ear. For example, in a patient with mild asymmetric sensorineural hearing loss, a clue to the diagnosis of vestibular schwannoma is the presence of greater than expected deterioration in discrimination ability. Deterioration in discrimination ability at higher intensities above the SRT also suggests a lesion in the eighth nerve or central auditory pathways.

Tympanometry measures the impedance of the middle ear to sound and is useful in diagnosis of middle-ear effusions. A *tympanogram* is the graphic representation of change in impedance or compliance as the pressure in the ear canal is changed. Normally, the middle ear is most compliant at atmospheric pressure, and the compliance decreases as the pressure is increased or decreased; this pattern is seen with normal hearing or in the presence of sensorineural hearing loss. Compliance that does not change with change in pressure suggests middle-ear effusion. With a negative pressure in the middle ear, as with eustachian tube obstruction, the point of maximal compliance occurs with negative pressure in the ear canal. A tympanogram in which no point of maximal compliance can be obtained is most commonly seen with discontinuity of the ossicular chain. A reduction in the maximal compliance peak can be seen in otosclerosis.

During tympanometry, an intense tone elicits contraction of the stapedius muscle. The change in compliance of the middle ear with contraction of the stapedius muscle can be detected. The presence or absence of this *acoustic reflex* is important in the anatomical localization of facial nerve paralysis as well as hearing loss. Normal or elevated acoustic reflex thresholds in an individual with sensorineural hearing impairment suggests a cochlear hearing loss. Assessment of *acoustic reflex decay* helps differentiate sensory from neural hearing losses. In neural hearing loss, the reflex adapts or decays with time.

Otoacoustic emissions (OAE) can be measured with microphones inserted into the external auditory canal. The emissions may be spontaneous or evoked with sound stimulation. The presence of OAEs indicates that the outer hair cells of the organ of Corti are intact and can be used to assess auditory thresholds and to distinguish sensory from neural hearing losses.

Evoked Responses

Electrocochleography measures the earliest evoked potentials generated in the cochlea and the auditory nerve. Receptor potentials recorded include the cochlear microphonic, generated by the outer hair cells of the organ of Corti, and the summating potential, generated by the inner hair cells in response to sound. The whole nerve action potential representing the composite firing of the first-order neurons can also be recorded during electrocochleography. Clinically, the test is useful in the diagnosis of Ménière's disease, where an elevation of the ratio of summating potential to action potential is seen.

Brainstem auditory evoked responses (BAERs) are useful in differentiating the site of sensorineural hearing loss. In response to sound, five distinct electrical potentials arising from different stations along the peripheral and central auditory pathway can be identified using computer averaging from scalp surface electrodes. BAERs are valuable in situations in which patients cannot or will not give reliable voluntary thresholds. They are also used to assess the integrity of the auditory nerve and brainstem in various clinical situations, including intraoperative monitoring and in determination of brain death.

Imaging Studies

The choice of radiologic tests is largely determined by whether the goal is to evaluate the bony anatomy of the external, middle, and inner ear or to image the auditory nerve and brain. Axial and coronal CT of the temporal bone with fine 1-mm cuts is ideal for determining the caliber of the external auditory canal, integrity of the ossicular chain, and presence of middle-ear or mastoid disease; it can also detect inner-ear malformations. CT is also ideal for the detection of bone erosion often seen in the presence of chronic otitis media and cholesteatoma. MRI is superior to CT for imaging of retrocochlear pathology such as vestibular schwannoma, meningioma, other lesions of the cerebellopontine angle, demyelinating lesions of the brainstem, and brain tumors. Recent experience suggests that both CT and MRI are equally capable of identifying inner-ear malformations and assessing cochlear patency for preoperative evaluation of patients for cochlear implantation.

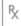

TREATMENT FOR HEARING DISORDERS

In general, conductive hearing losses are amenable to surgical intervention and correction, while sensorineural hearing losses are permanent. Atresia of the ear canal can be surgically repaired, often with significant improvement in hearing. Tympanic membrane perforations due to chronic otitis media or trauma can be repaired with an outpatient tympanoplasty. Likewise, conductive hearing loss associated with otosclerosis can be treated by stapedectomy, which is successful in 90 to 95% of cases. Tympanostomy tubes allow the prompt return of normal hearing in individuals with middle-ear effusions. Hearing aids are effective and well-tolerated in patients with conductive hearing losses.

Patients with mild, moderate, and severe sensorineural hearing losses are regularly rehabilitated with hearing aids of varying configuration and strength. Hearing aids have been improved to provide greater fidelity and have been miniaturized. The current generation of hearing aids can be placed entirely within the ear canal, thus reducing the stigma associated with their use. In general, the more severe the hearing impairment, the larger the hearing aid required for auditory rehabilitation. Digital hearing aids lend themselves to individual programming, and multiple and directional microphones at the ear level may be helpful in noisy surroundings. Since all hearing aids amplify noise as well as speech, the only absolute solution to the problem found thus far is to place the microphone closer to the speaker than the noise source. This arrangement is not possible with a self-contained, cosmetically acceptable device. It is cumbersome and requires a user-friendly environment.

In many situations, including lectures and the theater, hearing-impaired persons benefit from assistive devices that are based on the principle of having the speaker closer to the microphone than any source of noise. Assistive devices include infrared and frequency modulated (FM) transmission as well as an electromagnetic loop around the room for transmission to the individual's hearing aid. Hearing aids with telecoils can also be used with properly equipped telephones in the same way.

In the event that the hearing aid provides inadequate rehabilitation, cochlear implants may be appropriate. Criteria for implantation include severe to profound hearing loss with word recognition score ≤30% under best aided conditions. Worldwide, more than 20,000 deaf individuals (including 4000 children) have received cochlear implants. Cochlear implants are neural prostheses that convert sound energy to electrical energy and can be used to stimulate the auditory division of the eighth nerve directly. In most cases of profound hearing impairment, the auditory hair cells are lost but the ganglionic cells of the auditory division of the eighth nerve are preserved. Cochlear implants

consist of electrodes that are inserted into the cochlea through the round window, speech processors that extract acoustical elements of speech for conversion to electrical currents, and a means of transmitting the electrical energy through the skin. Patients with implants experience sound that helps with speech reading, allows open-set word recognition, and helps in modulating the person's own voice. Usually, within 3 months after implantation, adult patients can understand speech without visual cues. With the current generation of multichannel cochlear implants, nearly 75% of patients are able to converse on the telephone. It is anticipated that improvements in the electrode design and speech processors will permit further enhancement in understanding speech, especially in the presence of background noise.

For individuals who have had both eighth nerves destroyed by trauma or bilateral vestibular schwannomas (e.g., neurofibromatosis type 2), brainstem auditory implants placed near the cochlear nucleus may provide auditory rehabilitation. It is hoped that additional advances may provide benefits similar to those with the cochlear implant.

Tinnitus often accompanies hearing loss. Therapy for tinnitus is usually directed toward minimizing the appreciation of tinnitus. Relief of the tinnitus may be obtained by masking it with background music. Hearing aids are also helpful in tinnitus suppression, as are tinnitus maskers, devices that present a sound to the affected ear that is more pleasant to listen to than the tinnitus. The use of a tinnitus masker is often followed by several hours of inhibition of the tinnitus. Antidepressants have also shown beneficial effect in helping patients deal with tinnitus.

Tinnitus and background noise can significantly affect understanding of speech in individuals with hearing impairment. Hard-of-hearing individuals often benefit from a reduction in unnecessary noise (e.g., radio or television) to enhance the signal-to-noise ratio. Speech comprehension is aided by lip reading; therefore the impaired listener should be seated so that the face of the speaker is well-illuminated and easily seen. Speaking directly into the ear is occasionally helpful, but usually more is lost than gained because the speaker's face can no longer be seen. Speech should be slow enough to make each word distinct, but overly slow speech is distracting and loses contextual and speech-reading benefits. Although speech should be in a loud, clear voice, one should be aware that in sensorineural hearing losses in general and in elderly hard-of-hearing persons in particular, recruitment (abnormal perception of loud sounds) may be troublesome. Above all, optimal communication cannot take place without both parties giving it their full and undivided attention.

PREVENTION

Conductive hearing losses may be prevented by prompt antibiotic therapy of adequate duration for AOM and by ventilation of the middle ear with tympanostomy tubes in middle-ear effusions lasting ≤12 weeks. Loss of vestibular function and deafness due to aminoglycoside antibiotics can largely be prevented by careful monitoring of serum peak and trough levels.

Some 10 million Americans have noise-induced hearing loss, and 20 million are exposed to hazardous noise in their employment. Noise-induced hearing loss can be prevented by avoidance of exposure to loud noise or by regular use of ear plugs or fluid-filled ear muffs to attenuate intense sound. Noise-induced hearing loss results from recreational as well as occupational activities and begins in adolescence. High-risk activities for noise-induced hearing loss include wood and metal working with electrical equipment and target practice and hunting with small firearms. All internal-combustion and electric engines, including snow and leaf blow-

ers, snowmobiles, outboard motors, and chain saws, require protection of the user with hearing protectors. Virtually all noise-induced hearing loss is preventable through education, which should begin before the teenage years. Programs of industrial conservation of hearing are required when the exposure over an 8-h period averages 85 dB. Workers in such noisy environments can be protected with preemployment audiologic assessment, the mandatory use of hearing protectors, and annual audiologic assessments.

FURTHER READINGS

BALLENGER JJ, SNOW JB (eds): *Ballenger's Otorhinolaryngology Head and Neck Surgery,* 16th ed. Baltimore, BC Decker, 2002

EGGERMONT JJ, ROBERTS LE: The neuroscience of tinnitus. Trends Neurosci, 27:676, 2004

GURTLER N, LALWANI AK: Etiology of syndromic and nonsyndromic sensorineural hearing loss. Otolaryngol Clin North Am 35:891, 2002

KOVACS T: Mechanisms of olfactory dysfunction in aging and neurodegenerative disorders. Ageing Res Rev 3: 215, 2004

> ◪ SMITH RJH et al: Sensorineural hearing loss in children. Lancet 355:879, 2005
>
> *Excellent review of inherited causes of hearing loss.*

WROBEL BB, LEOPOLD DA: Clinical assessment of patients with smell and taste disorders. Otolaryngol Clin North Am 37: 1127, 2004

ZADEH MH et al: Diagnosis and treatment of sudden-onset sensorineural hearing loss: A study of 51 patients. Otolaryngol Head Neck Surg 128:92, 2003

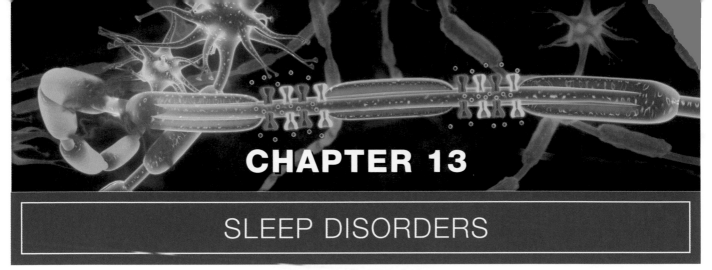

CHAPTER 13

SLEEP DISORDERS

Charles A. Czeisler
John W. Winkelman
Gary S. Richardson

Disturbed sleep is among the most frequent health complaints physicians encounter. More than one-half of adults in the United States experience at least intermittent sleep disturbances. For most, it is an occasional night of poor sleep or daytime sleepiness. However, at least 15 to 20% of adults report chronic sleep disturbance or misalignment of circadian timing, which can lead to serious impairment of daytime functioning. In addition, such problems may contribute to or exacerbate medical or psychiatric conditions. Thirty years ago, many such complaints were treated with hypnotic medications without further diagnostic evaluation. Since then, a distinct class of sleep and arousal disorders has been identified.

PHYSIOLOGY OF SLEEP AND WAKEFULNESS

Most adults sleep 7 to 8 h per night, although the timing, duration, and internal structure of sleep vary among healthy individuals and as a function of age. At the extremes, infants and the elderly have frequent interruptions of sleep. In the United States, adults of intermediate age tend to have one consolidated sleep episode per day, although in some cultures sleep may be divided into a midafternoon nap and a shortened night sleep. Two principal systems govern the sleep-wake cycle: one actively generates sleep and sleep-related processes and another times sleep within the 24-h day. Either intrinsic abnormalities in these systems or extrinsic disturbances (environmental, drug- or illness-related) can lead to sleep or circadian rhythm disorders.

STATES AND STAGES OF SLEEP

States and stages of human sleep are defined on the basis of characteristic patterns in the electroencephalogram (EEG), the electrooculogram (EOG—a measure of eye-movement activity), and the surface electromyogram (EMG) measured on the chin and neck. The continuous recording of this array of electrophysiologic parameters to define sleep and wakefulness is termed *polysomnography*.

Polysomnographic profiles define two states of sleep: (1) rapid-eye-movement (REM) sleep, and (2) non-rapid-eye-movement (NREM) sleep. NREM sleep is further subdivided into four stages, characterized by increasing arousal threshold and slowing of the cortical EEG. REM sleep is characterized by a low-amplitude, mixed-frequency EEG similar to that of NREM stage 1 sleep. The EOG shows bursts of REM similar to those seen during eyes-open wakefulness. Chin EMG activity is absent, reflecting the brainstem-mediated muscle atonia that is characteristic of that state.

ORGANIZATION OF HUMAN SLEEP

Normal nocturnal sleep in adults displays a consistent organization from night to night (**Fig. 13-1**). After sleep onset, sleep usually progresses through NREM stages 1 to 4 within 45 to 60 min. Slow-wave sleep (NREM stages 3 and 4) predominates in the first third of the night and comprises 15 to 25% of total nocturnal sleep time in young adults. The percentage of slow-wave sleep is influenced by several factors, most notably age (see below). Prior sleep deprivation increases the rapidity of sleep onset and both the intensity and amount of slow-wave sleep.

The first REM sleep episode usually occurs in the second hour of sleep. More rapid onset of REM sleep in a young adult (particularly if <30 min) may suggest pathology such as endogenous depression, narcolepsy, circadian rhythm disorders, or drug withdrawal. NREM and REM alternate through the night with an average period of 90 to 110 min (the "ultradian" sleep cycle). Overall, REM sleep constitutes 20 to 25% of total sleep, and NREM stages 1 and 2 are 50 to 60%.

Age has a profound impact on sleep state organization (Fig. 13-1). Slow-wave sleep is most intense and prominent during childhood, decreasing sharply at puberty and across the second and third decades of life. After age 30, there is a progressive decline in the amount of slow-wave sleep, and the amplitude of delta EEG activity comprising slow-wave sleep is profoundly reduced. The depth of slow-wave sleep, as measured by the arousal threshold to auditory stimulation, also decreases with age. In the oth-erwise healthy older person, slow-wave sleep may be completely absent, particularly in males.

A different age profile exists for REM sleep than for slow-wave sleep. In infancy, REM sleep may comprise 50% of total sleep time, and the percentage is inversely proportional to developmental age. The amount of REM sleep falls off sharply over the first postnatal year as a mature REM-NREM cycle develops; thereafter, REM sleep occupies a relatively constant percentage of total sleep time.

NEUROANATOMY OF SLEEP

Experimental studies in animals have variously implicated the medullary reticular formation, the thalamus, and the basal forebrain in the generation of sleep, while the brainstem reticular formation, the midbrain, the subthalamus, the thalamus, and the basal forebrain have all been suggested to play a role in the generation of wakefulness or EEG arousal.

Current hypotheses suggest that the capacity for sleep and wakefulness generation is distributed along an axial "core" of neurons extending from the brainstem rostrally to the basal forebrain. Complex commingling of neuronal groups occurs at many points along this brainstem-forebrain axis. A cluster of γ-aminobutyric acid (GABA) and galaninergic neurons in the ventrolateral preoptic (VLPO) hypothalamus is selectively activated coincident with sleep onset. These neurons project to and inhibit histaminergic cell groups in the tuberomammilary nucleus that are important to the ascending arousal system, suggesting that the hypothalamic VLPO neurons may play a key executive role in sleep regulation.

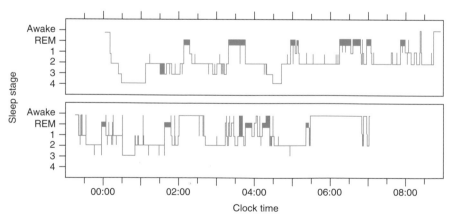

FIGURE 13-1

Stages of REM sleep (solid bars), the four stages of NREM sleep, and wakefulness over the course of the entire night for representative young and older adult men. Characteristic features of sleep in older people include reduction of slow-wave sleep, frequent spontaneous awakenings, early sleep onset, and early morning awakening. *(From the Division of Sleep Medicine, Brigham and Women's Hospital.)*

Specific regions in the pons are associated with the neurophysiologic correlates of REM sleep. Small lesions in the dorsal pons result in the loss of the descending muscle inhibition normally associated with REM sleep; microinjections of the cholinergic agonist carbachol into the pontine reticular formation appear to produce a state with all of the features of REM sleep. These experimental manipulations are mimicked by pathologic conditions in humans and animals. In narcolepsy, for example, abrupt, complete, or partial paralysis (cataplexy) occurs in response to a variety of stimuli. In dogs with this condition, physostigmine, a central cholinesterase inhibitor, increases the frequency of cataplectic attacks, while atropine decreases their frequency. Conversely, in REM sleep behavior disorder (see below), patients suffer from incomplete motor inhibition during REM sleep, resulting in involuntary, occasionally violent movement during REM sleep.

NEUROCHEMISTRY OF SLEEP

Early experimental studies that focused on the raphe nuclei of the brainstem appeared to implicate serotonin as the primary sleep-promoting neurotransmitter, while catecholamines were considered to be responsible for wakefulness. Subsequent work has demonstrated that the raphe-serotonin system may facilitate sleep but is not necessary for its expression. Pharmacologic studies of sleep and wakefulness suggest roles for other neurotransmitters as well. Pontine cholinergic neurotransmission is known to play a role in REM sleep generation. The alerting influence of caffeine implicates adenosine, whereas the hypnotic effect of benzodiazepines and barbiturates suggests a role for endogenous ligands of the $GABA_A$ receptor complex. A newly characterized neuropeptide, hypocretin (orexin), has recently been implicated in the pathophysiology of narcolepsy (see below), but its role in normal sleep regulation remains to be defined.

A variety of sleep-promoting substances have been identified, although it is not known whether or not they are involved in the endogenous sleep-wake regulatory process. These include prostaglandin D_2, delta sleep-inducing peptide, muramyl dipeptide, interleukin 1, fatty acid primary amides, and melatonin. The hypnotic effect of these substances is commonly limited to NREM or slow-wave sleep, although peptides that increase REM sleep have also been reported. Many putative "sleep factors," including interleukin 1 and prostaglandin D_2, are immunologically active as well, suggesting a link between immune function and sleep-wake states.

PHYSIOLOGY OF CIRCADIAN RHYTHMICITY

The sleep-wake cycle is the most evident of the many 24-h rhythms in humans. Prominent daily variations also occur in endocrine, thermoregulatory, cardiac, pulmonary, renal, gastrointestinal, and neurobehavioral functions. At the molecular level, endogenous circadian rhythmicity is driven by self-sustaining transcriptional/translational feedback loops (**Fig. 13-2**). In evaluating a daily variation in humans, it is important to distinguish between those rhythmic components passively evoked by periodic environmental or behavioral changes (e.g., the increase in blood pressure and heart rate upon assumption of the upright posture) and those actively driven by an endogenous oscillatory process (e.g., the circadian variation in plasma cortisol that persists under a variety of environmental and behavioral conditions).

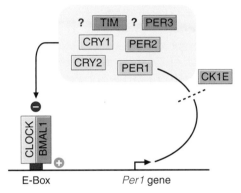

FIGURE 13-2

Model of the molecular feedback loop at the core of the mammalian circadian clock. The positive element of the feedback loop (+) is the transcriptional activation of the *Per1* gene (and probably other clock genes) by a heterodimer of the transcription factors CLOCK and BMAL1 (also called MOP3) bound to an E-box DNA regulatory element. The *Per1* transcript and its product, the clock component PER1 protein, accumulate in the cell cytoplasm. As it accumulates, the PER1 protein is recruited into a multiprotein complex thought to contain other circadian clock component proteins such as cryptochromes (CRYs), period proteins (PERs), and others. This complex is then transported into the cell nucleus (across the dotted line), where it functions as the negative element in the feedback loop (−) by inhibiting the activity of the CLOCK-BMAL1 transcription factor heterodimer. As a consequence of this action, the concentration of PER1 and other clock proteins in the inhibitory complex falls, allowing CLOCK-BMAL1 to activate transcription of *Per1* and other genes and begin another cycle. The dynamics of the 24-h molecular cycle are controlled at several levels, including regulation of the rate of PER protein degradation by casein kinase-1 epsilon (CK1E). Additional limbs of this genetic regulatory network, omitted for the sake of clarity, are thought to contribute stability. Question marks denote putative clock proteins, such as Timeless (TIM), as yet lacking genetic proof of a role in the mammalian clock mechanism. (*Copyright © Charles J. Weitz, Ph.D., Department of Neurobiology, Harvard Medical School.*)

While it is now recognized that many peripheral tissues in mammals have circadian clocks that regulate diverse physiologic processes, these independent tissue-specific oscillations are coordinated by a central neural pacemaker located in the suprachiasmatic nuclei (SCN) of the hypothalamus. Bilateral destruction of these nuclei results in a loss of the endogenous circadian rhythm of locomotor activity, which can be restored only by transplantation of the same structure from a donor animal. The genetically determined period of this endogenous neural oscillator, which averages ∼24.2 h in humans, is normally synchronized to the 24-h period of the environmental light-dark cycle. Small differences in circadian period underlie variations in diurnal preference, with the circadian period shorter in morning than in evening types. Entrainment of mammalian circadian rhythms by the light-dark cycle is mediated via the retinohypothalamic tract, a monosynaptic pathway that links specialized, photoreceptive retinal ganglion cells directly to the SCN. Humans are exquisitely sensitive to the resetting effects of light, particularly at the blue end (∼460 to 480 nm) of the visible spectrum.

The timing and internal architecture of sleep are directly coupled to the output of the endogenous circadian pacemaker. Paradoxically, the endogenous circadian rhythms of sleep tendency, sleepiness, and REM sleep propensity all peak near the habitual wake time, just after the nadir of the endogenous circadian temperature cycle, whereas the circadian wake propensity rhythm peaks 1 to 3 h before the habitual bedtime. These rhythms are thus timed to oppose the homeostatic decline of sleep tendency during the habitual sleep episode and the rise of sleep tendency throughout the usual waking day, respectively. Misalignment of the output of the endogenous circadian pacemaker with the desired sleep-wake cycle can, therefore, induce insomnia, decreased alertness, and impaired performance evident in night-shift workers and airline travelers.

BEHAVIORAL CORRELATES OF SLEEP STATES AND STAGES

Polysomnographic staging of sleep correlates with behavioral changes during specific states and stages. During the transitional state between wakefulness and sleep (stage 1 sleep), subjects may respond to faint auditory or visual signals without "awakening." Memory incorporation is inhibited at the onset of NREM stage 1 sleep, which may explain why individuals aroused from that transitional sleep stage frequently deny having been asleep. Such transitions may intrude upon behavioral wakefulness after sleep deprivation, notwithstanding attempts to remain continuously awake (see "Shift-Work Sleep Disorder," below).

Awakenings from REM sleep are associated with recall of vivid dream imagery >80% of the time. The reliability of dream recall increases with REM sleep episodes occurring later in the night. Imagery may also be reported after NREM sleep interruptions, though these typically lack the detail and vividness of REM sleep dreams. The incidence of NREM sleep dream recall can be increased by selective REM sleep deprivation, suggesting that REM sleep and dreaming per se are not inexorably linked.

PHYSIOLOGIC CORRELATES OF SLEEP STATES AND STAGES

All major physiologic systems are influenced by sleep. Changes in cardiovascular function include a decrease in blood pressure and heart rate during NREM and particularly during slow-wave sleep. During REM sleep, phasic activity (bursts of eye movements) is associated with variability in both blood pressure and heart rate mediated principally by the vagus. Cardiac dysrhythmias may occur selectively during REM sleep. Respiratory function also changes. In comparison to relaxed wakefulness, respiratory rate becomes more regular during NREM sleep (especially slow-wave sleep) and tonic REM sleep and becomes very irregular during phasic REM sleep. Minute ventilation decreases in NREM sleep out of proportion to the decrease in metabolic rate at sleep onset, resulting in a higher P_{CO_2}.

Endocrine function also varies with sleep. Slow-wave sleep is associated with secretion of growth hormone, while sleep in general is associated with augmented secretion of prolactin. Sleep has a complex effect on the secretion of luteinizing hormone (LH): during puberty, sleep is associated with increased LH secretion, whereas sleep in the mature woman inhibits LH secretion in the early follicular phase of the menstrual cycle. Sleep onset (and probably slow-wave sleep) is associated with inhibition of thyroid-stimulating hormone and of the adrenocorticotropic hormone–cortisol axis, an effect that is superimposed on the prominent circadian rhythms in the two systems.

The pineal hormone melatonin is secreted predominantly at night in both day- and night-active species, reflecting the direct modulation of pineal activity by the circadian pacemaker through a circuitous neural pathway from the SCN to the pineal gland. Melatonin secretion is not dependent upon the occurrence of sleep, persisting in individuals kept awake at night. In addition, exogenous melatonin increases sleepiness and may potentiate sleep when administered to good sleepers attempting to sleep during daylight hours at a time when endogenous melatonin levels are low. The efficacy of melatonin as a sleep-promoting therapy for patients with insomnia is currently not known.

Sleep is also accompanied by alterations of thermoregulatory function. NREM sleep is associated with an attenuation of thermoregulatory responses to either heat or cold stress, and animal studies of thermosensitive neurons in the hypothalamus document an NREM-sleep-dependent reduction of the thermoregulatory set-point. REM sleep is associated with complete absence of thermoregulatory responsiveness, effectively resulting in functional poikilothermy. However, the potential adverse impact of this failure of thermoregulation is blunted by inhibition of REM sleep by extreme ambient temperatures.

DISORDERS OF SLEEP AND WAKEFULNESS

APPROACH TO THE PATIENT WITH A SLEEP DISORDER

Patients may seek help from a physician because of one of several symptoms: (1) an acute or chronic inability to sleep adequately at night (insomnia); (2) chronic fatigue, sleepiness, or tiredness during the day; or (3) a behavioral manifestation associated with sleep itself. Complaints of insomnia or excessive daytime sleepiness should be viewed as symptoms (much like fever or pain) of underlying disorders. Knowledge of the differential diagnosis of these presenting complaints is essential to identify the underlying medical disorder. Only then can appropriate treatment, rather than nonspecific approaches (e.g., over-the-counter sleeping aids), be applied. Diagnoses of exclusion, such as primary insomnia, should be made only after other diagnoses have been ruled out **Table 13-1** outlines the diagnostic and therapeutic approach to the patient with a complaint of excessive daytime sleepiness.

A careful history is essential. In particular, the duration, severity, and consistency of the symptoms are important, along with the patient's estimate of the consequences of reported sleep loss on waking function. Information from a friend or family member can be invaluable; some patients may be unaware of, or will underreport, such potentially embarrassing symptoms as heavy snoring or falling asleep while driving.

TABLE 13-1

EVALUATION OF THE PATIENT WITH THE COMPLAINT OF EXCESSIVE DAYTIME SOMNOLENCE

FINDINGS ON HISTORY AND PHYSICAL EXAMINATION	DIAGNOSTIC EVALUATION	DIAGNOSIS	THERAPY
Obesity, snoring, hypertension	Polysomnography with respiratory monitoring	Obstructive sleep apnea	Continuous positive airway pressure; ENT surgery (e.g., uvulopalatopharyngoplasty); dental appliance; pharmacologic therapy (e.g., protriptyline); weight loss
Cataplexy, hypnogogic hallucinations, sleep paralysis, family history	Polysomnography with multiple sleep latency testing	Narcolepsy-cataplexy syndrome	Stimulants (e.g., modafinil, methylphenidate); REM-suppressant antidepressants (e.g., protriptyline); genetic counseling
Restless legs syndrome, disturbed sleep, predisposing medical condition (e.g., anemia or renal failure)	Polysomnography with bilateral anterior tibialis EMG monitoring	Periodic limb movements of sleep	Treatment of predisposing condition, if possible; dopamine agonists (e.g., pramipexole); benzodiazepines (e.g., clonazepam)
Disturbed sleep, predisposing medical conditions (e.g., asthma) and/or predisposing medical therapies (e.g., theophylline)	Sleep-wake diary recording	Insomnias (see text)	Treatment of predisposing condition and/or change in therapy, if possible; behavioral therapy; short-acting benzodiazepine receptor agonist (e.g., zolpidem)

Note: ENT, ears, nose, throat; REM, rapid eye movement; EMG, electromyogram.

Completion by the patient of a day-by-day sleep-work-drug log for at least 2 weeks can help the physician better understand the nature of the complaint. Work times and sleep times (including daytime naps and nocturnal awakenings) as well as drug and alcohol use, including caffeine and hypnotics, should be noted each day. In addition, the sleep times should be recorded.

Polysomnography is necessary for the diagnosis of specific disorders such as narcolepsy and sleep apnea and may be of utility in other settings as well. In addition to the three electrophysiologic variables used to define sleep states and stages, the standard clinical polysomnogram includes measures of respiration (respiratory effort, air flow, and oxygen saturation), anterior tibialis EMG, and electrocardiogram. Evaluation of penile tumescence during nocturnal sleep can also help determine whether the cause of erectile dysfunction in a patient is psychogenic or organic.

EVALUATION OF INSOMNIA

Insomnia is the complaint of inadequate sleep; it can be classified according to the nature of sleep disruption and the duration of the complaint. Insomnia is subdivided into difficulty falling asleep (*sleep onset insomnia*), frequent or sustained awakenings (*sleep maintenance insomnia*), early morning awakenings (*sleep offset insomnia*), or persistent sleepiness despite sleep of adequate duration (*nonrestorative sleep*). Similarly, the duration of the symptom influences diagnostic and therapeutic considerations. An insomnia complaint lasting one to several nights (within a single episode) is termed *transient insomnia* and is typically the result of situational stress or a change in sleep schedule or environment (e.g., jet lag). *Short-term insomnia* lasts from a few days to 3 weeks. Disruption of this duration is usually associated with more protracted stress, such as recovery from surgery or short-term illness. *Long-term insomnia*, or *chronic insomnia*, lasts for months or years and, in contrast with short-term insomnia, requires a thorough evaluation of underlying causes (see below). Chronic insomnia is often a waxing and waning disorder, with spontaneous or stressor-induced exacerbations.

An occasional night of poor sleep, typically in the setting of stress or excitement about external events, is both common and without lasting consequences. However, persistent insomnia can lead to impaired daytime function, injury due to accidents, and the development of major depression. In addition, there is emerging evidence that individuals with chronic insomnia have increased utilization of health care resources, even after controlling for co-morbid medical and psychiatric disorders.

All insomnias can be exacerbated and perpetuated by behaviors that are not conducive to initiating or maintaining sleep. *Inadequate sleep hygiene* is characterized by a behavior pattern prior to sleep or a bedroom environment that is not conducive to sleep. Noise or light in the bedroom can interfere with sleep, as can a bed partner with periodic limb movements during sleep or one who snores loudly. Clocks can heighten the anxiety about the time it has taken to fall asleep. Drugs that act on the central nervous system, large meals, vigorous exercise, or hot showers just before sleep may interfere with sleep onset. Many individuals participate in stressful work-related activities in the evening, producing a state incompatible with sleep onset. In preference to hypnotic medications, patients should be counseled to avoid stressful activities before bed, develop a soporific bedtime ritual, and to prepare and reserve the bedroom environment for sleeping. Consistent, regular rising times should be maintained daily, including weekends.

PRIMARY INSOMNIA

Insomnia without Identifiable Cause

Many patients with chronic insomnia have no clear, single identifiable underlying cause for their difficulties with sleep. Rather, such patients often have multiple etiologies for their insomnia, which may evolve over the years. Primary insomnia is thus a diagnosis of exclusion, often without a clear underlying single cause. In addition, the chief sleep complaint may change over time, with initial insomnia predominating at one point, and multiple awakenings or nonrestorative sleep occurring at other times. Subsyndromal psychiatric disorders (e.g., anxiety and mood complaints), negative conditioning to the sleep environment (psychophysiologic insomnia, see below), amplification of the time spent awake (sleep-state misperception), physiologic hyperarousal, and poor sleep hygiene (see above) may all be present. As these processes may be both causes and consequences of chronic insomnia, many individuals will have a progressive course to their symptoms in which the severity is proportional to the chronicity, and much of the complaint may persist even after effective treatment of the initial inciting etiology. Treatment of primary insomnia is often directed to each of the putative contributing factors: behavior therapies for anxiety and negative conditioning (see below), pharmacotherapy for mood/anxiety disorders, an emphasis on maintenance of good sleep hygiene, and intermittent hypnotics for exacerbations of the insomnia.

If insomnia persists after treatment of these contributing factors, empirical pharmacotherapy is often used on a nightly or intermittent basis. A variety of sedative compounds are used for this purpose. Alcohol and antihistamines are the most commonly used nonprescription sleep aids. The former may help with sleep onset, but is associated with sleep disruption during the night and can escalate into abuse, dependence, and withdrawal in the predisposed individual. Antihistamines may be of benefit when used intermittently, but produce rapid tolerance and have multiple side effects (especially anticholinergic), which limit their use. Benzodiazepine receptor agonists are the most effective and well-tolerated class of medications for insomnia. The broad range of half-lives allows flexibility in the duration of sedative action. Zaleplon (5 to 20 mg), with a half-life of 1 to 2 h, zolpidem (5 to 10 mg) and triazolam (0.125 to 0.25 mg), with half-lives of 2 to 3 h, and temazepam (15 to 30 mg) and lorazepam (0.5 to 2 mg), with half-lives of 6 to 12 h, are the most commonly prescribed agents in this family. Generally, side effects are minimal if the dose is kept low and the serum concentration is minimized during the waking hours (by using the shortest-acting, effective agent). However, with even brief continuous use, rebound insomnia can occur upon discontinuation. There are only limited data supporting sustained efficacy of benzodiazepine receptor agonists; caution should be exercised in long-term use. The likelihood of rebound insomnia and tolerance can be minimized by short durations of treatment, intermittent use, or gradual tapering of the dose. For acute insomnia, nightly use of a benzodiazepine receptor agonist for a maximum of 2 to 4 weeks is advisable. For chronic insomnia, intermittent use is recommended. Benzodiazepine receptor agonists should be avoided, or used very judiciously, in patients with a history of substance abuse. The heterocyclic antidepressants (trazodone, amitriptyline, and doxepin) are the most commonly prescribed alternatives to benzodiazepine receptor agonists due to their lack of abuse potential and lower cost. Trazodone (25 to 100 mg) is used more commonly than the tricyclic antidepressants as it has a much shorter half-life (5 to 9 h), has much less anticholinergic activity (sparing patients, particularly the elderly, constipation, urinary retention, and tachycardia), is associated with less weight gain, and is much safer in overdose. The risk of priapism is small (~1 in 10,000).

Psychophysiologic Insomnia

Persistent *psychophysiologic insomnia* is a behavioral disorder in which patients are preoccupied with a perceived inability to sleep adequately at night. The sleep disturbance is often triggered by an emotionally stressful event; however, the poor sleep habits and beliefs about sleep acquired during the stressful period persist long after the initial incident. Such patients become hyperaroused by their own persistent efforts to sleep or the sleep environment, and the insomnia is a conditioned or learned response. They may be able to fall asleep more easily at unscheduled times (when not trying) or outside the home environment. Polysomnographic recording in patients with psychophysiologic insomnia reveals an objective sleep disturbance, often with an abnormally long sleep latency; frequent nocturnal awakenings; and an increased amount of stage 1 transitional sleep. Rigorous attention should be paid to sleep hygiene and correction of counterproductive, arousing behaviors before bedtime. Behavioral therapies are the treatment modality of choice, with only intermittent use of medications. When patients are awake for >20 min, they should read or perform other relaxing activities to distract themselves from insomnia-related anxiety. In addition, bedtime and waketime should be scheduled to restrict time in bed to be equal to their perceived total sleep time. This will generally produce sleep deprivation, greater sleep drive, and, eventually, better sleep. Time in bed can then be gradually expanded.

SECONDARY INSOMNIA

Transient Situational Insomnia

This typically develops after a change in the sleeping environment (e.g., in an unfamiliar hotel or hospital bed) or before or after a significant life event, such as a change of occupation, loss of a loved one, illness, or anxiety over a deadline or examination. Increased sleep latency, frequent awakenings from sleep, and early morning awakening can all occur. Recovery is generally rapid, usually within a few weeks. Treatment is symptomatic, with intermittent use of hypnotics and resolution of the underlying stress. *Altitude insomnia* describes a sleep disturbance that is a common consequence of exposure to high altitude. Periodic breathing of the Cheyne-Stokes type occurs during NREM sleep about half the time at high altitude, with restoration of a regular breathing pattern during REM sleep. Both hypoxia and hypocapnia are thought to be involved in the development of periodic breathing. Frequent awakenings and poor quality sleep characterize altitude insomnia, which is generally worst on the first few nights at high altitude but may persist. Treatment with acetazolamide can decrease time spent in periodic breathing and substantially reduce hypoxia during sleep.

Insomnia Associated with Mental Disorders

Approximately 80% of patients with psychiatric disorders describe sleep complaints. There is considerable heterogeneity, however, in the nature of the sleep disturbance both between conditions and among patients with the same condition. *Depression* can be associated with sleep onset insomnia, sleep maintenance insomnia, or early morning wakefulness. However, hypersomnia occurs in some depressed patients, especially adolescents and those with either bipolar or seasonal (fall/winter) depression (Chap. 41). Indeed, sleep disturbance is an important vegetative sign of depression and may commence before any mood changes are perceived by the patient. Consistent polysomnographic findings in depression include decreased REM sleep latency, lengthened first REM sleep episode, and shortened first NREM sleep episode; however, these findings are not specific for depression, and the extent of these changes varies with age and symptomatology. Depressed patients also show decreased slow-wave sleep and reduced sleep continuity.

In *mania* and *hypomania*, sleep latency is increased and total sleep time can be reduced. Patients with *anxiety disorders* tend not to show the changes in REM sleep and slow-wave sleep seen in endogenously depressed patients. *Chronic alcoholics* lack slow-wave sleep, have decreased amounts of REM sleep (as an acute response to alcohol), and have frequent arousals throughout the night. This is associated with impaired daytime alertness. The sleep of chronic alcoholics may remain disturbed for years after discontinuance of alcohol usage. Sleep architecture and physiology are disturbed in *schizophrenia* (with a decreased amount of stage 4 sleep and a lack of augmentation of REM sleep following REM sleep deprivation); chronic schizophrenics often show day-night reversal, sleep fragmentation, and insomnia.

Insomnia Associated with Neurologic Disorders

A variety of neurologic diseases result in sleep disruption through both indirect, nonspecific mechanisms (e.g., pain in cervical spondylosis or low back pain) or by impairment of central neural structures involved in the generation and control of sleep itself. For example, *dementia* from any cause has long been associated with disturbances in the timing of the sleep-wake cycle, often characterized by nocturnal wandering and an exacerbation of symptomatology at night (so-called sundowning).

Epilepsy may rarely present as a sleep complaint (Chap. 14). Often the history is of abnormal behavior, at times with convulsive movements during sleep, and the differential diagnosis includes REM sleep behavior disorder, sleep apnea syndrome, and periodic movements of sleep (see above). Diagnosis requires nocturnal EEG recording. Other neurologic diseases associated with abnormal movements, such as *Parkinson's disease, hemiballismus,*

Huntington's chorea, and *Gilles de la Tourette syndrome* (Chap. 19), are also associated with disrupted sleep, presumably through secondary mechanisms. However, the abnormal movements themselves are greatly reduced during sleep. Headache syndromes (*migraine* or *cluster headache*) may show sleep-associated exacerbations (Chap. 5) by unknown mechanisms.

Fatal familial insomnia is a rare hereditary disorder caused by degeneration of anterior and dorsomedial nuclei of the thalamus. Insomnia is a prominent early symptom. Progressively, the syndrome produces autonomic dysfunction, dysarthria, myoclonus, coma, and death. The pathogenesis is a mutation in the prion gene (Chap. 32).

Insomnia Associated with Other Medical Disorders

A number of medical conditions are associated with disruptions of sleep. The association is frequently nonspecific, e.g., that between sleep disruption and chronic pain from rheumatologic disorders. Attention to this association is important in that sleep-associated symptoms are often the presenting complaint. Treatment of the underlying medical disorder or symptom is the most useful approach. Sleep disruption can also result from the appropriate use of drugs such as glucocorticoids (see below).

One prominent association is between sleep disruption and *asthma*. In many asthmatics there is a prominent daily variation in airway resistance that results in marked increases in asthmatic symptoms at night, especially during sleep. In addition, treatment of asthma with theophylline-based compounds, adrenergic agonists, or glucocorticoids can independently disrupt sleep. When sleep disruption is a side effect of asthma treatment, inhaled glucocorticoids (e.g., beclomethasone) that do not disrupt sleep may provide a useful alternative.

Cardiac ischemia may also be associated with sleep disruption. The ischemia itself may result from increases in sympathetic tone as a result of sleep apnea. Patients may present with complaints of nightmares or vivid, disturbing dreams, with or without awareness of the more classic symptoms of angina or of the sleep disordered breathing. Treatment of the sleep apnea may substantially improve the angina and the nocturnal sleep quality. *Paroxysmal nocturnal dyspnea* can also occur as a consequence of sleep-associated cardiac ischemia that causes pulmonary congestion exacerbated by the recumbent posture.

Chronic obstructive pulmonary disease is also associated with sleep disruption, as is *cystic fibrosis, menopause, hyperthyroidism, gastroesophageal reflux, chronic renal failure,* and *liver failure.*

Medication-, Drug-, or Alcohol-Dependent Insomnia

Disturbed sleep can result from ingestion of a wide variety of agents. Caffeine is perhaps the most common pharmacologic cause of insomnia. It produces increased latency to sleep onset, more frequent arousals during sleep, and a reduction in total sleep time for up to 8 to 14 h after ingestion. As few as three to five cups of coffee can significantly disturb sleep in some patients; therefore, a 1- to 2-month trial without caffeine should be attempted in patients with these symptoms. Similarly, alcohol and nicotine can interfere with sleep, despite the fact that many patients use them to relax and promote sleep. Although alcohol can increase drowsiness and shorten sleep latency, even moderate amounts of alcohol increase awakenings in the second half of the night. In addition, alcohol ingestion prior to sleep is contraindicated in patients with sleep apnea because of the inhibitory effects of alcohol on upper airway muscle tone. Acutely, amphetamines and cocaine suppress both REM sleep and total sleep time, which return to normal with chronic use. Withdrawal leads to a REM sleep rebound. A number of prescribed medications can produce insomnia. Antidepressants, sympathomimetics, and glucocorticoids are common causes. In addition, severe rebound insomnia can result from the acute withdrawal of hypnotics, especially following the use of high doses of benzodiazepines with a short half-life. For this reason, hypnotic doses should be low to moderate, the total duration of hypnotic therapy should usually be limited to 2 to 3 weeks, and prolonged drug tapering is encouraged.

RESTLESS LEGS SYNDROME (RLS)

Patients with this sensory-motor disorder report a creeping or crawling dysesthesia deep within the calves or feet, or sometimes even in the upper extemities, that is associated with an irresistible urge to move the affected limbs. For most patients with RLS, the dysesthesias and restlessness are much worse in the evening or night compared to the daytime and frequently interfere with the ability to fall asleep. The disorder is exacerbated by inactivity and temporarily relieved by movement. In contrast, paresthesias secondary to peripheral neuropathy persist with activity. The severity of this chronic disorder may wax and wane with time and can be exacerbated by sleep deprivation, caffeine, and pregnancy. The prevalence is 1 to 5% of young to middle-age adults and increases to 10 to 20% in those >60 years. There appear to be important differences in RLS prevalence among racial groups, with higher prevalence in those of Northern European ancestry. Roughly one-third of patients (particularly those with an early age of onset) will have multiple affected family members, possibly with an autosomal dominant pattern. Iron deficiency and renal failure may cause RLS, which is then considered secondary RLS. The symptoms of RLS are exquisitely sensitive to dopaminergic drugs (e.g., pramipexole 0.25 to 1.0 mg q8PM or ropinirole 0.5 to 4.0 mg q8PM), which are the treatment of choice. Narcotics, benzodiazepines, and certain anticonvulsants may also be of therapeutic value. Most patients with restless legs also experience periodic limb movements of sleep, although the reverse is not the case.

PERIODIC LIMB MOVEMENT DISORDER

Periodic limb movement disorder, previously known as *nocturnal myoclonus*, is the principal objective polysomnographic finding in 17% of patients with insomnia and 11% of those with excessive daytime somnolence (**Fig. 13-3**). It is often unclear whether it is an incidental finding or the cause of disturbed sleep. Stereotyped, 0.5- to 5.0-s extensions of the great toe and dorsiflexion of the foot recur every 20 to 40 s during NREM sleep, in episodes lasting from minutes to hours. Most such episodes occur during the first half of the night. The disorder occurs in a wide variety of sleep disorders (including narcolepsy, sleep apnea, REM sleep behavior disorder, and various forms of insomnia) and may be associated with frequent arousals and an increased number of sleep-stage transitions. The incidence increases with age: 44% of people over age 65 without a sleep complaint have more than five periodic leg movements per hour of sleep. The pathophysiology is not well understood, though individuals with high spinal transections can exhibit periodic leg movements during sleep, suggesting the existence of a spinal generator. Polysomnography with bilateral surface EMG recording of the anterior tibialis is used to establish the diagnosis. Treatment options include dopaminergic medications or benzodiazepines.

EVALUATION OF DAYTIME SLEEPINESS

Daytime impairment due to sleep loss may be difficult to quantify for several reasons. First, sleepiness is not necessarily proportional to subjectively assessed sleep deprivation. In obstructive sleep apnea, for example, the repeated brief interruptions of sleep associated with resumption of respiration at the end of apneic episodes result in daytime sleepiness, despite the fact that the patient may be unaware of the sleep fragmentation. Second, subjective descriptions of waking impairment vary from patient to patient. Patients may describe themselves as "sleepy," "fatigued," or "tired" and may

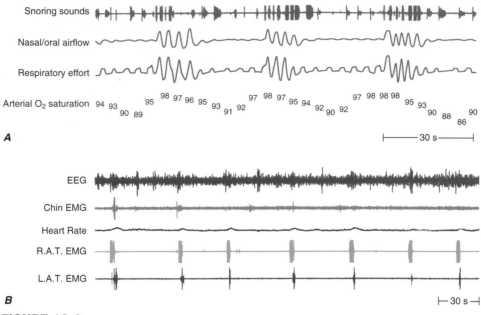

FIGURE 13-3

Polysomnographic recordings of (**A**) obstructive sleep apnea and (**B**) periodic limb movement of sleep. Note the snoring and reduction in air flow in the presence of continued respiratory effort, associated with the subsequent oxygen desaturation (upper panel). Periodic limb movements occur with a relatively constant intermovement interval and are associated with changes in the EEG and heart rates acceleration (lower panel). Abbreviations: R.A.T., right anterior tibialis; L.A.T., left anterior tibialis. (*From the Division of Sleep Medicine, Brigham and Women's Hospital.*)

have a clear sense of the meaning of those terms, while others may use the same terms to describe a completely different condition. Third, sleepiness, particularly when profound, may affect judgment in a manner analogous to ethanol, such that subjective awareness of the condition and the consequent cognitive and motor impairment is reduced. Finally, patients may be reluctant to admit that sleepiness is a problem, both because they are generally unaware of what constitutes normal alertness and because sleepiness is generally viewed pejoratively, ascribed more often to a deficit in motivation than to an inadequately addressed physiologic sleep need.

Specific questioning about the occurrence of sleep episodes during normal waking hours, both intentional and unintentional, can overcome the inconsistencies among subjective characterizations and help to interpret the adverse impact of sleepiness on daytime function. Specific areas to be addressed include the occurrence of inadvertent sleep episodes while driving or in other safety-related settings, sleepiness while at work or school (and the relationship of sleepiness to work and school performance), and the effect of sleepiness on social and family life. Evidence for significant daytime impairment [in association either with the diagnosis of a primary sleep disorder, such as narcolepsy or sleep apnea, or with

imposed or self-selected sleep-wake schedules (see "Shift-Work Sleep Disorder," below)] raises the question of the physician's responsibility to notify motor vehicle licensing authorities of the increased risk of sleepiness-related vehicle accidents. As with epilepsy, legal requirements vary from state to state, and existing legal precedents do not provide a consistent interpretation of the balance between the physician's responsibility and the patient's right to privacy. At a minimum, physicians should document discussions with the patient regarding the increased risk of operating a vehicle, as well as a recommendation that driving be suspended until successful treatment or schedule modification can be instituted.

The distinction between fatigue and sleepiness can be useful in the differentiation of patients with complaints of fatigue or tiredness in the setting of disorders such as fibromyalgia, chronic fatigue syndrome (Chap. 40), or endocrine deficiencies such as hypothyroidism or Addison's disease. While patients with these disorders can typically distinguish their daytime symptoms from the sleepiness that occurs with sleep deprivation, substantial overlap can occur. This is particularly true when the primary disorder also results in chronic sleep disruption (e.g., sleep apnea in hypothyroidism) or in abnormal sleep (e.g., fibromyalgia).

While clinical evaluation of the complaint of excessive sleepiness is usually adequate, objective quantification is sometimes necessary. Assessment of daytime functioning as an index of the adequacy of sleep can be made with the multiple sleep latency test (MSLT), which involves repeated measurement of sleep latency (time to onset of sleep) under standardized conditions during a day following quantified nocturnal sleep. The average latency across four to six tests (administered every 2 h across the waking day) provides an objective measure of daytime sleep tendency. Disorders of sleep that result in pathologic daytime somnolence can be reliably distinguished with the MSLT. In addition, the multiple measurements of sleep onset may identify direct transitions from wakefulness to REM sleep that are suggestive of specific pathologic conditions (e.g., narcolepsy).

NARCOLEPSY

Narcolepsy is both a disorder of the ability to sustain wakefulness voluntarily and a disorder of REM sleep regulation (**Table 13-2**). The classic "narcolepsy tetrad" consists of excessive daytime somnolence plus three specific symptoms related to an intrusion of REM sleep characteristics (e.g., muscle atonia, vivid dream imagery) into the transition between wakefulness and sleep: (1) sudden weakness or loss of muscle tone without loss of consciousness, often elicited by emotion (cataplexy); (2) hallucinations at sleep onset (hypnogogic hallucinations) or upon awakening (hypnopompic hallucinations); and (3) muscular paralysis upon awakening (sleep paralysis). The severity of cataplexy varies, as patients may have two to three attacks per day or per decade. Some patients with objectively confirmed narcolepsy (see below) may show no evidence of cataplexy. In those with cataplexy, the extent and duration of an attack may also vary, from a transient sagging of the jaw lasting a few seconds to rare cases of flaccid paralysis of the entire voluntary musculature

TABLE 13-2

PREVALENCE OF SYMPTOMS IN NARCOLEPSY	
SYMPTOM	PREVALENCE, %
Excessive daytime somnolence	100
Disturbed sleep	87
Cataplexy	76
Hypnogogic hallucinations	68
Sleep paralysis	64
Memory problems	50

Source: Modified from TA Roth, L Merlotti in SA Burton et al (eds), *Narcolepsy 3rd International Symposium: Selected Symposium Proceedings*, Chicago, Matrix Communications, 1989.

for up to 20 to 30 min. Symptoms of narcolepsy typically begin in the second decade, although the onset ranges from ages 5 to 50. Once established, the disease is chronic without remissions. Secondary forms of narcolepsy have been described (e.g., after head trauma).

Narcolepsy affects about 1 in 4000 people in the United States and appears to have a genetic basis. Recently, several convergent lines of evidence suggest that the hypothalamic neuropeptide hypocretin (orexin) is involved in the pathogenesis of narcolepsy: (1) a mutation in the hypocretin receptor 2 gene has been associated with canine narcolepsy; (2) hypocretin "knockout" mice that are genetically unable to produce this neuropeptide exhibit a phenotype, as assessed by behavioral and electrophysiologic criteria, that is similar to human narcolepsy; and (3) cerebrospinal fluid levels of hypocretin are reduced in most patients who have narcolepsy with cataplexy. The inheritance pattern of narcolepsy in humans is more complex than in the canine model. However, almost all narcoleptics with cataplexy are positive for HLA DQB1*0602, suggesting that an autoimmune process may be responsible.

Diagnosis

The diagnostic criteria continue to be a matter of debate. Certainly, objective verification of excessive daytime somnolence, typically with MSLT mean sleep latencies <8 min, is an essential if nonspecific diagnostic feature. Other conditions that cause excessive sleepiness, such as sleep apnea or chronic sleep restriction, must be rigorously excluded. The other objective diagnostic feature of narcolepsy is the presence of REM sleep in at least two of the naps during the MSLT. Abnormal regulation of REM sleep is also manifested by the appearance of REM sleep immediately or within minutes after sleep onset in 50% of narcoleptic patients, a rarity in unaffected individuals maintaining a conventional sleep-wake schedule. The REM-related symptoms of the classic narcolepsy tetrad are variably present. There is increasing evidence that narcoleptics with cataplexy (one-half to two-thirds of patients) may represent a more homogeneous group than those without this symptom. However, a history of cataplexy can be difficult to establish reliably. Hypnogogic and hypnopompic hallucinations and sleep paralysis are often found in nonnarcoleptic individuals and may be present in only one-half of narcoleptics. Nocturnal sleep disruption is commonly observed in narcolepsy but is also a nonspecific symptom. Similarly, a history of "automatic behavior" during wakefulness (a trancelike state during which simple motor behaviors persist) is not specific for narcolepsy and serves principally to corroborate the presence of daytime somnolence.

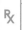

TREATMENT FOR NARCOLEPSY

The treatment of narcolepsy is symptomatic. Somnolence is treated with wake-promoting therapeutics. Modafinil is now the drug of choice, principally because it is associated with fewer side effects than older stimulants and has a long half-life; 200 to 400 mg is given as a single daily dose. Older drugs such as methylphenidate (10 mg bid to 20 mg qid or dextroamphetamine (10 mg bid) are still used as alternatives, particularly in refractory patients.

Many antidepressant medications are potent suppressors of REM sleep and thus useful in the treatment of the REM-related phenomena of cataplexy, hypnogogic hallucinations, and sleep paralysis. The tricyclic antidepressants [e.g., protriptyline (10 to 40 mg/d) and clomipramine (25 to 50 mg/d)], the selective serotonin reuptake inhibitors (SSRIs) [e.g., fluoxetine (10 to 20 mg/d)], and the monoamine oxidase inhibitors [e.g., selegiline (20 to 40 mg/d)] are commonly used for this purpose. Efficacy of the antidepressants is limited largely by anticholinergic side effects (tricyclics) and by sleep disturbance and sexual dysfunction (SSRIs); in addition, rebound cataplexy is a complication of abrupt discontinuation of these medications. Recently, two randomized double-blind placebo-controlled trials have demonstrated a significant reduction in cataleptic attacks with sodium oxybate (previously known as γ-hydroxybutyrate or GHB). This drug is now approved by the U.S. Food and Drug Administration (FDA) for treatment of cataplexy; given concern over its potential use as a drug of abuse, it is a Schedule III medication with strict regulations and a special risk management program (see also *http://xyrem.info* for details). Finally, adequate nocturnal sleep time and planned daytime naps (when possible) are important preventative measures for these REM-related phenomena.

SLEEP APNEA SYNDROMES

Respiratory dysfunction during sleep is a common, serious cause of excessive daytime somnolence as well as of disturbed nocturnal sleep. An estimated 2 to 5 million people in the United States have a reduction or cessation of breathing for 10 to 150 s, from thirty to several hundred times every night during sleep. These episodes may be due to either an occlusion of the airway (*obstructive sleep apnea*), absence of respiratory effort (*central sleep apnea*), or a combination of these factors (*mixed sleep apnea*) (Fig. 13-3). Failure to recognize and treat these conditions appropriately may lead to impairment of daytime alertness; increased risk of sleep-related motor vehicle accidents; hypertension and other serious cardiovascular and cerebrovascular complications; and increased mortality. Sleep apnea is particularly prevalent in overweight men and in the elderly, yet it is estimated to remain undiagnosed in 80 to 90% of affected individuals. This is unfortunate since effective treatments are available.

PARASOMNIAS

The term *parasomnia* refers to abnormal behaviors that arise from or occur during sleep. A continuum of parasomnias arise from NREM sleep, from brief confusional arousals to sleepwalking and night terrors. The presenting complaint is usually related to the behavior itself, but the parasomnias can disturb sleep continuity or lead to mild impairments in daytime alertness. Only one parasomnia is known to occur in REM sleep, i.e., REM sleep behavior disorder (RBD; see below).

Sleepwalking (Somnambulism)

Patients affected by this disorder carry out automatic motor activities that range from simple to complex. Individuals may leave the bed, walk, urinate inappropriately, eat, or exit from the house while remaining only partially aware. Full arousal may be difficult, and some patients may respond to attempted awakening with agitation or even violence. Sleepwalking arises from stage 3 or 4 NREM sleep and is most common in children and adolescents, when these sleep stages are most robust. Episodes are usually isolated but may be recurrent in 1 to 6% of patients. The cause is unknown, though it has a familial basis in roughly one-third of cases.

Sleep Terrors

This disorder, also called *pavor nocturnus*, occurs primarily in young children during the first several hours after sleep onset, in stages 3 and 4 of NREM sleep. The child suddenly screams, exhibiting autonomic arousal with sweating, tachycardia, and hyperventilation. The individual may be difficult to arouse and rarely recalls the episode on awakening in the morning. Recurrent attacks are rare. Parents are usually reassured to learn that the condition is self-limited and benign, and that no specific therapy is indicated. Both sleep terrors and sleepwalking represent abnormalities of arousal. In contrast, *nightmares* (dream anxiety attacks) occur during REM sleep and cause full arousal, with intact memory for the unpleasant episode.

REM Sleep Behavior Disorder

RBD is a rare condition that is distinct from other parasomnias in that it occurs during REM sleep. It primarily afflicts men of middle age or older, many of whom have a history of prior neurologic disease. In fact, over one-third of patients will go on to develop Parkinson's disease (Chap. 19) within 10 to 20 years. Presenting symptoms consist of agitated or violent behavior during sleep, reported by a bed partner. In contrast to typical somnambulism, injury to patient or bed partner is not uncommon, and, upon awakening, the patient reports vivid, often unpleasant, dream imagery. The principal differential diagnosis is that of nocturnal seizures, which can be excluded with polysomnography. In RBD, seizure activity is absent on the EEG, and disinhibition of the usual motor atonia is observed in the EMG during REM sleep, at times associated with complex motor behaviors. The pathogenesis is unclear, but damage to brainstem areas mediating descending motor inhibition during REM sleep may be responsible. In support of this hypothesis are the remarkable similarities between RBD and the sleep of animals with bilateral lesions of the pontine tegmentum in areas controlling REM sleep motor inhibition. Treatment with clonazepam (0.5 to 1.0 mg qhs) provides sustained improvement in almost all reported cases.

Sleep Bruxism

Bruxism is an involuntary, forceful grinding of teeth during sleep that affects 10 to 20% of the population. The patient is usually unaware of the problem. The typical age of onset is 17 to 20 years, and spontaneous remission usually occurs by age 40. Sex distribution appears to be equal. In many cases, the diagnosis is made during dental examination, damage is minor, and no treatment is indicated. In more severe cases, treatment with a rubber tooth guard is necessary to prevent disfiguring tooth injury. Stress management or, in some cases, biofeedback can be useful when bruxism is a manifestation of psychological stress. There are anecdotal reports of benefit using benzodiazepines.

Sleep Enuresis

Bedwetting, like sleepwalking and night terrors, is another parasomnia that occurs during sleep in the young. Before age 5 or 6, nocturnal enuresis should probably be considered a normal feature of development. The condition usually improves spontaneously at puberty, has a prevalence in late adolescence of 1 to 3%, and is rare in adulthood. In older patients with enuresis a distinction must be made between primary and secondary enuresis, the latter being defined as bedwetting in patients who have been fully continent for 6 to 12 months. Treatment of primary enuresis is reserved for patients of appropriate age (>5 or 6 years) and consists of bladder training exercises and behavioral therapy. Urologic abnormalities are more common in primary enuresis and must be assessed by urologic examination. Important causes of secondary enuresis include emotional disturbances, urinary tract infections or malformations, cauda equina lesions, epilepsy, sleep apnea, and certain medications. Symptomatic pharmacotherapy is usually accomplished with desmopressin (0.2 mg qhs), oxybutynin chloride (5 to 10 mg qhs) or imipramine (10 to 50 mg qhs).

Miscellaneous Parasomnias

Other clinical entities fulfill the definition of a parasomnia in that they occur selectively during sleep and are associated with some degree of sleep disruption. Examples include *jactatio capitis nocturna* (nocturnal headbanging), sleep talking, nocturnal paroxysmal dystonia, and nocturnal leg cramps.

CIRCADIAN RHYTHM SLEEP DISORDERS

A subset of patients presenting with either insomnia or hypersomnia may have a disorder of sleep *timing* rather than sleep *generation*. Disorders of sleep timing can be either organic (i.e., due to an intrinsic defect in the circadian pacemaker or its input from entraining stimuli) or environmental (i.e., due to a disruption of exposure to entraining stimuli from the environment). Regardless of etiology, the symptoms reflect the influence of the underlying circadian pacemaker on sleep-wake function. Thus, effective therapeutic approaches should aim to entrain the oscillator at an appropriate phase.

Rapid Time-Zone Change (Jet Lag) Syndrome

More than 60 million people experience transmeridian air travel annually, which is often associated with excessive daytime sleepiness, sleep onset insomnia, and frequent arousals from sleep, particularly in the latter half of the night. Gastrointestinal discomfort is common. The syndrome is transient, typically lasting 2 to 14 d depending on the number of time zones crossed, the direction of travel, and the traveler's age and phase-shifting capacity. Travelers who spend more time outdoors reportedly adapt more quickly than those who remain in hotel rooms, presumably due to bright (outdoor) light exposure. Avoidance of antecedent sleep loss and obtaining nap sleep on the afternoon prior to overnight travel greatly reduces the difficulty of extended wakefulness. Laboratory studies suggest that submilligram doses of the pineal hormone melatonin can enhance sleep efficiency, but only if taken when endogenous melatonin concentrations are low (i.e., during biologic daytime), and furthermore that melatonin may induce phase shifts in human rhythms. A large-scale clinical trial evaluating the safety and efficacy of melatonin as a treatment for jet lag and other circadian sleep disorders is needed.

Shift-Work Sleep Disorder

More than 7 million workers in the United States regularly work at night, either on a permanent or rotating schedule. In addition, each week millions elect to remain awake at night to meet deadlines, drive long distances, or participate in recreational activities, leading to both sleep loss and misalignment of their circadian rhythms with respect to their sleep-wake cycle. Chronic shift workers have higher rates of cardiac, gastrointestinal, and reproductive disorders. Studies of regular night-shift workers indicate that the circadian timing system usually fails to adapt successfully to such inverted schedules. This leads to a misalignment between the desired work-rest schedule and the output of the pacemaker and in disturbed daytime sleep. Sleep deprivation, increased length of time awake prior to work, and misalignment of circadian phase produce decreased alertness and performance, increased reaction time, and increased risk of performance lapses, thereby resulting in greater safety hazards among night workers and other sleep-deprived individuals. Sleep disturbance nearly doubles the risk of a fatal work accident. Recently, modafinil given as 200 mg prior to the shift was shown to be modestly useful as prophylaxis against excessive sleepiness.

Sleep onset is associated with marked attenuation in perception of both auditory and visual stimuli and lapses of consciousness. The sleepy individual may thus attempt to perform routine and familiar motor tasks during the transition state between wakefulness and sleep (stage 1 sleep) in the absence of adequate sensory input from the environment. Motor vehicle operators are especially vulnerable to sleep-related accidents since the sleep-deprived driver or operator often fails to heed the warning signs of fatigue. Such attempts to override the powerful biologic drive for sleep by the sheer force of will can yield a catastrophic outcome when sleep processes intrude involuntarily upon the waking brain. Such intrusions typically last only seconds but are known on occasion to persist for longer durations. These frequent brief intrusions of stage 1 sleep into behavioral wakefulness are a major component of the impaired psychomotor performance seen with sleepiness. There is a significant increase in the risk of sleep-related, fatal-to-the-driver highway crashes in the early morning and late afternoon hours, coincident with bimodal peaks in the daily rhythm of sleep tendency.

Safety programs should promote education about sleep and increase awareness of the hazards associated with night work and should be aimed at minimizing both circadian disruption and sleep deprivation. The work schedule should minimize: (1) exposure to night work, (2) the frequency of shift rotation so that shifts do not rotate more than once every 2 to 3 weeks, (3) the number of consecutive night shifts, and (4) the duration of night shifts. In fact, shift durations of >18 h should be universally recognized as increasing the risk of sleep-related errors and performance lapses. Caffeine is undoubtedly the most widely used wake-promoting drug, but it cannot forestall sleep indefinitely and does not shield users from sleep-related performance lapses. Postural changes, exercise, and strategic placement of nap opportunities can sometimes temporarily reduce the risk of fatigue-related performance lapses. Properly timed exposure to bright light can facilitate rapid adaptation to night-shift work. An adequate number of safe highway rest areas, shoulder rumble strips, and strict enforcement and compliance monitoring of hours-of-service policies are needed to reduce the risk of sleep-related transportation crashes.

Delayed Sleep Phase Syndrome

Delayed sleep phase syndrome is characterized by: (1) reported sleep onset and wake times intractably later than desired, (2) actual sleep times at nearly the same clock hours daily, and (3) essentially normal all-night polysomnography except for delayed sleep onset. Patients exhibit an abnormally delayed endogenous circadian phase, with the temperature minimum during the constant routine occurring later than normal. This delayed phase could be due to: (1) an abnormally long, genetically determined intrinsic period of the endogenous circadian pacemaker; (2) an abnormally reduced phase-advancing capacity of the pacemaker; or (3) an irregular prior sleep-wake schedule, characterized by frequent nights when the patient chooses to remain awake well past midnight (for social, school, or work reasons). In most cases, it is difficult to distinguish among these factors, since patients with an abnormally long intrinsic period are more likely to "choose" such late-night activities because they are unable to sleep at that time. Patients tend to be young adults. This self-perpetuating condition can persist for years and does not usually respond to attempts to reestablish normal bedtime hours. Treatment methods involving bright-light phototherapy during the morning hours or melatonin administration in the evening hours show promise in these patients, although the relapse rate is high.

Advanced Sleep Phase Syndrome

Advanced sleep phase syndrome (ASPS) is the converse of the delayed sleep phase syndrome. Most commonly, this syndrome occurs in older people, 15% of whom report that they cannot sleep past 5 A.M., with twice that number complaining that they wake up too early at least several times per week. Patients with ASPS experience excessive daytime sleepiness during the evening hours, when they have great difficulty remaining awake, even in social settings. Typically, patients awaken from 3 to 5 A.M. each day, often several hours before their desired wake times. In addition to age-related ASPS, an early-onset familial variant of this condition has also been reported. In one such family, autosomal dominant ASPS was due to a missense mutation in a circadian clock component (PER2, as shown in Fig. 13-2) that altered the circardian period. Patients with ASPS may benefit from bright-light phototherapy during the evening hours, designed to reset the circadian pacemaker to a later hour.

Non-24-H Sleep-Wake Disorder

This condition can occur when the maximal phase-advancing capacity of the circadian pacemaker is not adequate to accommodate the difference between the 24-h geophysical day and the intrinsic period of the pacemaker in the patient. Alternatively, patients' self-selected exposure to artificial light may drive the circadian pacemaker to a >24-h schedule. Affected patients are not able to maintain a stable phase relationship between the output of the pacemaker and the 24-h day. Such patients typically present with an incremental pattern of successive delays in sleep onsets and wake times, progressing in and out of phase with local time. When the patient's endogenous rhythms are out of phase with the local environment, insomnia coexists with excessive daytime sleepiness. Conversely, when the endogenous rhythms are in phase with the local environment, symptoms remit. The intervals between symptomatic periods may last several weeks to several months. Blind individuals unable to perceive light are particularly susceptible to this disorder. Nightly low-dose (0.5 mg) melatonin administration has been reported to improve sleep and, in some cases, even to induce synchronization of the circadian pacemaker.

MEDICAL IMPLICATIONS OF CIRCADIAN RHYTHMICITY

Prominent circadian variations have been reported in the incidence of acute myocardial infarction, sudden cardiac death, and stroke, the leading causes of death in the United States. Platelet aggregability is increased after arising in the early morning hours, coincident with the peak incidence of these cardiovascular events. A better understanding of the possible role of circadian rhythmicity in the acute destabilization of a chronic condition such as atherosclerotic disease could improve the understanding of the pathophysiology.

Diagnostic and therapeutic procedures may also be affected by the time of day at which data are collected. Examples include blood pressure, body temperature, the dexamethasone suppression test, and plasma cortisol levels. The timing of chemotherapy administration has been reported to have an effect on the outcome of treatment. Few physicians realize the extent to which routine measures are affected by the time (or sleep/wake state) when the measurement is made.

In addition, both the toxicity and effectiveness of drugs can vary during the day. For example, more than a fivefold difference has been observed in mortality rates following administration of toxic agents to experimental animals at different times of day. Anesthetic agents are particularly sensitive to time-of-day effects. Finally, the physician must be increasingly aware of the public health risks associated with the ever-increasing demands made by the duty-rest-recreation schedules in our round-the-clock society.

FURTHER READINGS

ANTLE MC, SILVER R: Orchestrating time: Arrangements of the brain circadian clock. Trends Neurosci 28:145, 2005

CAPLES SM et al: Obstructive sleep apnea. Ann Intern Med 142:187, 2005

CHOKROVERTY S et al: Sleep and Movement Disorders. Philadelphia, Butterworth-Heinemann, 2003

DAUVILLIERS Y et al: Genetics of normal and pathological sleep in humans. Sleep Med Rev 9:91, 2005

GIGLIO P et al: The primary parasomnias. A review for neurologists. Neurologist 11:90, 2005

Excellent approach to the diagnosis and treatment of common sleep disorders.

LESAGE S, HENING WA: The restless legs syndrome and periodic limb movement disorder: A review of management. Semin Neurol 24:249, 2004

NAU SD et al: Treatment of insomnia in older adults. Clin Psychol Rev 25:645, 2005

NISHINO S, KANBAYASHI T: Symptomatic narcolepsy, cataplexy and hypersomnia, and their implications in the hypothalamic hypocretin/orexin system. Sleep Med Rev 9:269, 2005

Sateia MJ, Nowell PD: Insomnia. Lancet 364:1959, 2004

Evaluation and treatment of insomnia, with a focus on both behavioral modification and pharmacologic therapies.

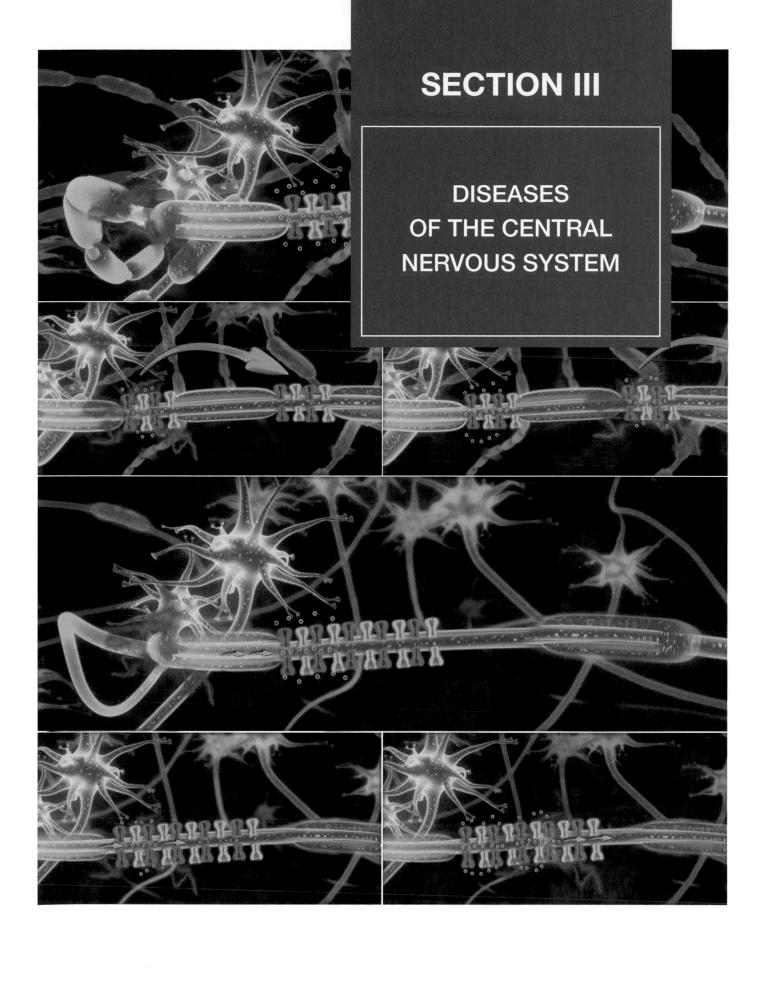

SECTION III

DISEASES
OF THE CENTRAL
NERVOUS SYSTEM

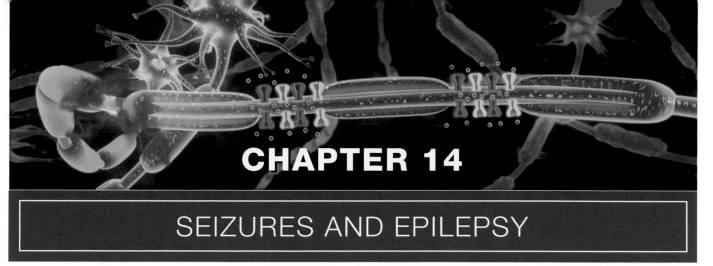

CHAPTER 14

SEIZURES AND EPILEPSY

Daniel H. Lowenstein

A *seizure* (from the Latin *sacire,* "to take possession of") is a paroxysmal event due to abnormal, excessive, hypersynchronous discharges from an aggregate of central nervous system (CNS) neurons. Depending on the distribution of discharges, this abnormal CNS activity can have various manifestations, ranging from dramatic convulsive activity to experiential phenomena not readily discernible by an observer. Although a variety of factors influence the incidence and prevalence of seizures, ~5 to 10% of the population will have at least one seizure, with the highest incidence occurring in early childhood and late adulthood.

The meaning of the term seizure needs to be carefully distinguished from that of epilepsy. *Epilepsy* describes a condition in which a person has *recurrent* seizures due to a chronic, underlying process. This defin-ition implies that a person with a single seizure, or recurrent seizures due to correctable or avoidable circumstances, does not necessarily have epilepsy. Epilepsy refers to a clinical phenomenon rather than a single disease entity, since there are many forms and causes of epilepsy. However, among the many causes of epilepsy there are various *epilepsy syndromes* in which the clinical and pathologic characteristics are distinctive and suggest a specific underlying etiology.

Using the definition of epilepsy as two or more unprovoked seizures, the incidence of epilepsy is ~0.3 to 0.5% in different populations throughout the world, and the prevalence of epilepsy has been estimated at 5 to 10 persons per 1000.

CLASSIFICATION OF SEIZURES

Determining the type of seizure that has occurred is essential for focusing the diagnostic approach on particular etiologies, selecting the appropriate therapy, and providing potentially vital information regarding prognosis. In 1981, the International League Against Epilepsy (ILAE) published a modified version of the International Classi-fication of Epileptic Seizures that has continued to be a useful classification system (**Table 14-1**). This system is based on the clinical features of seizures and associated electroencephalographic findings. Other potentially distinctive features such as etiology or cellular substrate are not considered in this classification system, although this will undoubtedly change in the future as more is learned about the pathophysiologic mechanisms that underlie specific seizure types.

A fundamental principle is that seizures may be either partial (synonymous with focal) or generalized. *Partial seizures* are those in which the seizure activity is restricted to discrete areas of the cerebral cortex. *Generalized seizures* involve diffuse regions of the brain simultaneously. Partial seizures are usually associated with structural abnormalities of the brain. In contrast,

TABLE 14-1

CLASSIFICATION OF SEIZURES

1. **Partial seizures**
   a. Simple partial seizures (with motor, sensory, autonomic, or psychic signs)
   b. Complex partial seizures
   c. Partial seizures with secondary generalization
2. **Primarily generalized seizures**
   a. Absence (petit mal)
   b. Tonic-clonic (grand mal)
   c. Tonic
   d. Atonic
   e. Myoclonic
3. **Unclassified seizures**
   a. Neonatal seizures
   b. Infantile spasms

generalized seizures may result from cellular, biochemical, or structural abnormalities that have a more widespread distribution.

PARTIAL SEIZURES

Partial seizures occur within discrete regions of the brain. If consciousness is fully preserved during the seizure, the clinical manifestations are considered relatively simple and the seizure is termed a *simple partial seizure.* If consciousness is impaired, the symptomatology is more complex and the seizure is termed a *complex partial seizure.* An important additional subgroup comprises those seizures that begin as partial seizures and then spread diffusely throughout the cortex, i.e., *partial seizures with secondary generalization.*

Simple Partial Seizures

Simple partial seizures cause motor, sensory, autonomic, or psychic symptoms without an obvious alteration in consciousness. For example, a patient having a partial motor seizure arising from the right primary motor cortex in the vicinity controlling hand movement will note the onset of involuntary movements of the contralateral, left hand. These movements are typically clonic (i.e., repetitive, flexion/extension movements) at a frequency of ~2 to 3 Hz; pure tonic posturing may be seen as well. Since the cortical region controlling hand movement is immediately adjacent to the region for facial expression, the seizure may also cause abnormal movements of the face synchronous with the movements of the hand. The electroencephalogram (EEG) recorded with scalp electrodes during the seizure (i.e., an ictal EEG) may show abnormal discharges in a very limited region over the appropriate area of cerebral cortex if the seizure focus involves the cerebral convexity. Seizure

activity occurring within deeper brain structures is often not recorded by the standard EEG, however, and may require intracranial electrodes for its detection.

Three additional features of partial motor seizures are worth noting. First, in some patients the abnormal motor movements may begin in a very restricted region such as the fingers and gradually progress (over seconds to minutes) to include a larger portion of the extremity. This phenomenon, described by Hughlings Jackson and known as a "Jacksonian march," represents the spread of seizure activity over a progressively larger region of motor cortex. Second, patients may experience a localized paresis (Todd's paralysis) for minutes to many hours in the involved region following the seizure. Third, in rare instances the seizure may continue for hours or days. This condition, termed *epilepsia partialis continua,* is often refractory to medical therapy.

Simple partial seizures may also manifest as changes in somatic sensation (e.g., paresthesias), vision (flashing lights or formed hallucinations), equilibrium (sensation of falling or vertigo), or autonomic function (flushing, sweating, piloerection). Simple partial seizures arising from the temporal or frontal cortex may also cause alterations in hearing, olfaction, or higher cortical function (psychic symptoms). This includes the sensation of unusual, intense odors (e.g., burning rubber or kerosene) or sounds (crude or highly complex sounds), or an epigastric sensation that rises from the stomach or chest to the head. Some patients describe odd, internal feelings such as fear, a sense of impending change, detachment, depersonalization, déjà vu, or illusions that objects are growing smaller (micropsia) or larger (macropsia). When such symptoms precede a complex partial or secondarily generalized seizure, these simple partial seizures serve as a warning, or *aura.*

Complex Partial Seizures

Complex partial seizures are characterized by focal seizure activity accompanied by a transient impairment of the patient's ability to maintain normal contact with the environment. The patient is unable to respond appropriately to visual or verbal commands during the seizure and has impaired recollection or awareness of the ictal phase. The seizures frequently begin with an aura (i.e., a simple partial seizure) that is stereotypic for the patient. The start of the ictal phase is often a sudden behavioral arrest or motionless stare, which marks the onset of the period of amnesia. The behavioral arrest is usually accompanied by *automatisms,* which are involuntary, automatic behaviors that have a wide range of manifestations. Automatisms may consist of very basic behaviors such as chewing, lip smacking, swallowing, or "picking" movements of the hands, or more elaborate behaviors such as a display of emotion or running. The patient is typically confused following the seizure, and the transition to full recovery of consciousness may range from seconds up to an hour. Examination immediately following the seizure may show an anterograde amnesia or, in cases involving the dominant hemisphere, a postictal aphasia.

The routine, interictal (i.e., between seizures) EEG in patients with complex partial seizures is often normal or may show brief discharges termed *epileptiform spikes,* or *sharp waves.* Since complex partial seizures can arise from the medial temporal lobe or inferior frontal lobe, i.e., regions distant from the scalp, the EEG recorded during the seizure may be nonlocalizing. However, the seizure focus is often detected using sphenoidal or surgically placed intracranial electrodes.

The range of potential clinical behaviors linked to complex partial seizures is so broad that extreme caution is advised before concluding that stereotypic episodes of bizarre or atypical behavior are not due to seizure activity. In such cases additional, detailed EEG studies may be helpful.

Partial Seizures with Secondary Generalization

Partial seizures can spread to involve both cerebral hemispheres and produce a generalized seizure, usually of the tonic-clonic variety (discussed below). Secondary generalization is observed frequently following simple partial seizures, especially those with a focus in the frontal lobe, but may also be associated with partial seizures occurring elsewhere in the brain. A partial seizure with secondary generalization is often difficult to distinguish from a primarily generalized tonic-clonic seizure, since bystanders tend to emphasize the more dramatic, generalized convulsive phase of the seizure and overlook the more subtle, focal symptoms present at onset. In some cases, the focal onset of the seizure becomes apparent only when a careful history identifies a preceding aura (i.e., simple partial seizure). Often, however, the focal onset is not clinically evident and may be established only through careful EEG analysis. Nonetheless, distinguishing between these two entities is extremely important, as there may be substantial differences in the evaluation and treatment of partial versus generalized seizure disorders.

GENERALIZED SEIZURES

By definition, generalized seizures arise from both cerebral hemispheres simultaneously. However, it is currently impossible to exclude entirely the existence of a focal region of abnormal activity that initiates the seizure prior to rapid secondary generalization. For this reason,

generalized seizures may be practically defined as bilateral clinical and electrographic events without any detectable focal onset. Fortunately, several types of generalized seizures have distinctive features that facilitate clinical diagnosis.

Absence Seizures (Petit Mal)

Absence seizures are characterized by sudden, brief lapses of consciousness without loss of postural control. The seizure typically lasts for only seconds, consciousness returns as suddenly as it was lost, and there is no postictal confusion. Although the brief loss of consciousness may be clinically inapparent or the sole manifestation of the seizure discharge, absence seizures are usually accompanied by subtle, bilateral motor signs such as rapid blinking of the eyelids, chewing movements, or small-amplitude, clonic movements of the hands.

Absence seizures usually begin in childhood (ages 4 to 8) or early adolescence and are the main seizure type in 15 to 20% of children with epilepsy. The seizures can occur hundreds of times per day, but the child may be unaware of or unable to convey their existence. The patient may be constantly piecing together experiences that have been interrupted by the seizures. Since the clinical signs of the seizures are subtle, especially to new parents, it is not surprising that the first clue to absence epilepsy is often unexplained "daydreaming" and a decline in school performance recognized by a teacher.

The electrophysiologic hallmark of typical absence seizures is a generalized, symmetric, 3-Hz spike-and-wave discharge that begins and ends suddenly, superimposed on a normal EEG background. Periods of spike-and-wave discharges lasting more than a few seconds usually correlate with clinical signs, but the EEG often shows many more brief bursts of abnormal cortical activity than were suspected clinically. Hyperventilation tends to provoke these electrographic discharges and even the seizures themselves and is routinely used when recording the EEG.

Typical absence seizures are often associated with generalized, tonic-clonic seizures, but patients usually have no other neurologic problems and respond well to treatment with specific anticonvulsants. Although estimates vary, ~60 to 70% of such patients will have a spontaneous remission during adolescence.

Atypical Absence Seizures

Atypical absence seizures have features that deviate both clinically and electrophysiologically from typical absence seizures. For example, the lapse of consciousness is usually of longer duration and less abrupt in onset and cessation, and the seizure is accompanied by more obvious motor signs that may include focal or lateralizing features. The EEG shows a generalized, slow spike-and-wave pattern with a frequency of ≤2.5/s, as well as other abnormal activity. Atypical absence seizures are usually associated with diffuse or multifocal structural abnormalities of the brain and therefore may accompany other signs of neurologic dysfunction such as mental retardation. Furthermore, the seizures are less responsive to anticonvulsants compared to typical absence seizures.

Generalized, Tonic-Clonic Seizures (Grand Mal)

Primarily generalized, tonic-clonic seizures are the main seizure type in ~10% of all persons with epilepsy. They are also the most common seizure type resulting from metabolic derangements and are therefore frequently encountered in many different clinical settings. The seizure usually begins abruptly without warning, although some patients describe vague premonitory symptoms in the hours leading up to the seizure. This prodrome is distinct from the stereotypic auras associated with focal seizures that secondarily generalize. The initial phase of the seizure is usually tonic contraction of muscles throughout the body, accounting for a number of the classic features of the event. Tonic contraction of the muscles of expiration and the larynx at the onset will produce a loud moan or "ictal cry." Respirations are impaired, secretions pool in the oropharynx, and cyanosis develops. Contraction of the jaw muscles may cause biting of the tongue. A marked enhancement of sympathetic tone leads to increases in heart rate, blood pressure, and pupillary size. After 10 to 20 s, the tonic phase of the seizure typically evolves into the clonic phase, produced by the superimposition of periods of muscle relaxation on the tonic muscle contraction. The periods of relaxation progressively increase until the end of the ictal phase, which usually lasts no more than 1 min. The postictal phase is characterized by unresponsiveness, muscular flaccidity, and excessive salivation that can cause stridorous breathing and partial airway obstruction. Bladder or bowel incontinence may occur at this point. Patients gradually regain consciousness over minutes to hours, and during this transition there is typically a period of postictal confusion. Patients subsequently complain of headache, fatigue, and muscle ache that can last for many hours. The duration of impaired consciousness in the postictal phase can be extremely long, i.e., many hours, in patients with prolonged seizures or underlying CNS diseases such as alcoholic cerebral atrophy.

The EEG during the tonic phase of the seizure shows a progressive increase in generalized low-voltage fast activity, followed by generalized high-amplitude, polyspike discharges. In the clonic phase, the high-amplitude activity is typically interrupted by slow waves to create a spike-and-wave pattern. The postictal EEG shows diffuse slowing that gradually recovers as the patient awakens.

There are many variants of the generalized tonic-clonic seizure, including pure tonic and pure clonic seizures. Brief tonic seizures lasting only a few seconds are especially noteworthy since they are usually associated with specific epileptic syndromes having mixed seizure phenotypes, such as the Lennox-Gastaut syndrome (discussed below).

Atonic Seizures

Atonic seizures are characterized by sudden loss of postural muscle tone lasting 1 to 2 s. Consciousness is briefly impaired, but there is usually no postictal confusion. A very brief seizure may cause only a quick head drop or nodding movement, while a longer seizure will cause the patient to collapse. This can be extremely dangerous, since there is a substantial risk of direct head injury with the fall. The EEG shows brief, generalized spike-and-wave discharges followed immediately by diffuse slow waves that correlate with the loss of muscle tone. Similar to pure tonic seizures, atonic seizures are usually seen in association with known epileptic syndromes.

Myoclonic Seizures

Myoclonus is a sudden and brief muscle contraction that may involve one part of the body or the entire body. A normal, common physiologic form of myoclonus is the sudden jerking movement observed while falling asleep. Pathologic myoclonus is most commonly seen in association with metabolic disorders, degenerative CNS diseases, or anoxic brain injury (Chap. 15). Although the distinction from other forms of myoclonus is imprecise, myoclonic seizures are considered to be true epileptic events since they are caused by cortical (versus subcortical or spinal) dysfunction. The EEG may show bilaterally synchronous spike-and-wave discharges synchronized with the myoclonus, although these can be obscured by movement artifact. Myoclonic seizures usually coexist with other forms of generalized seizure disorders but are the predominant feature of juvenile myoclonic epilepsy (discussed below).

UNCLASSIFIED SEIZURES

Not all seizure types can be classified as partial or generalized. This appears to be especially true of seizures that occur in neonates and infants. The distinctive phenotypes of seizures at these early ages likely result, in part, from differences in neuronal function and connectivity in the immature versus mature CNS.

EPILEPSY SYNDROMES

Epilepsy syndromes are disorders in which epilepsy is a predominant feature, and there is sufficient evidence (e.g., through clinical, EEG, radiologic, or genetic observations) to suggest a common underlying mechanism. Three important epilepsy syndromes are listed below; additional examples with a known genetic basis are shown in **Table 14-2.**

JUVENILE MYOCLONIC EPILEPSY

Juvenile myoclonic epilepsy (JME) is a generalized seizure disorder of unknown cause that appears in early adolescence and is usually characterized by bilateral myoclonic jerks that may be single or repetitive. The myoclonic seizures are most frequent in the morning after awakening and can be provoked by sleep deprivation. Consciousness is preserved unless the myoclonus is especially severe. Many patients also experience generalized tonic-clonic seizures, and up to one-third have absence seizures. The condition is otherwise benign, and although complete remission is uncommon, the seizures respond well to appropriate anticonvulsant medication. There is often a family history of epilepsy, and genetic linkage studies suggest a polygenic cause.

LENNOX-GASTAUT SYNDROME

Lennox-Gastaut syndrome occurs in children and is defined by the following triad: (1) multiple seizure types (usually including generalized tonic-clonic, atonic, and atypical absence seizures); (2) an EEG showing slow (<3 Hz) spike-and-wave discharges and a variety of other abnormalities; and (3) impaired cognitive function in most but not all cases. Lennox-Gastaut syndrome is associated with CNS disease or dysfunction from a variety of causes, including developmental abnormalities, perinatal hypoxia/ischemia, trauma, infection, and other acquired lesions. The multifactorial nature of this syndrome suggests that it is a nonspecific response of the brain to diffuse neural injury. Unfortunately, many patients have a poor prognosis due to the underlying CNS disease and the physical and psychosocial consequences of severe, poorly controlled epilepsy.

MESIAL TEMPORAL LOBE EPILEPSY SYNDROME

Mesial temporal lobe epilepsy (MTLE) is the most common syndrome associated with complex partial seizures and is an example of a symptomatic, partial epilepsy with distinctive clinical, electroencephalographic, and pathologic features (**Table 14-3**). High-resolution magnetic resonance imaging (MRI) can detect the characteristic hippocampal sclerosis that appears to be essential in the pathophysiology of MTLE for many patients (**Fig. 14-1**). Recognition of this syndrome is especially important because it tends to be refractory to treatment with anticonvulsants but responds extremely well to surgical intervention. Advances in the understanding of basic mechanisms of epilepsy have come through studies of experimental models of MTLE, discussed below.

THE CAUSES OF SEIZURES AND EPILEPSY

Seizures are a result of a shift in the normal balance of excitation and inhibition within the CNS. Given the numerous properties that control neuronal excitability, it is not surprising that there are many different ways to perturb this normal balance, and therefore many different causes of both seizures and epilepsy. Three clinical observations emphasize how a variety of factors determine why certain conditions may cause seizures or epilepsy in a given patient.

1. *The normal brain is capable of having a seizure under the appropriate circumstances, and there are differences between individuals in the susceptibility or threshold for seizures.* For example, seizures may be induced by high fevers in children who are otherwise normal and who never develop other neurologic problems, including epilepsy. However, febrile seizures occur only in a relatively small proportion of children. This implies there are various underlying, *endogenous factors* that influence the threshold for having a seizure. Some of these factors are clearly genetic, as it has been shown that a family history of epilepsy will influence the likelihood of seizures occurring in otherwise normal individuals. Normal development also plays an important role, since the brain appears to have different seizure thresholds at different maturational stages.

2. *There are a variety of conditions that have an extremely high likelihood of resulting in a chronic seizure disorder.* One of the best examples of this is severe, penetrating head trauma, which is associated with up to a 50% risk of subsequent epilepsy. The high propensity for severe traumatic brain injury to lead to epilepsy suggests that the injury results in a long-lasting, pathologic change in the CNS that transforms a presumably normal neural network into one that is abnormally hyperexcitable. This process is known as *epileptogenesis,* and the specific changes that result in a lowered seizure threshold can be considered *epileptogenic factors.* Other processes associated with epileptogenesis include stroke, infections, and abnormalities of CNS development. Likewise, the genetic

TABLE 14-2

EXAMPLES OF GENES ASSOCIATED WITH EPILEPSY SYNDROMES[a]

GENE (LOCUS)	FUNCTION OF GENE	CLINICAL SYNDROME	COMMENTS
KCNQ2 (20q13.3) KCNQ3 (8q24)	Voltage-gated potassium channel subunits; mutation in pore regions may cause a 20–40% reduction of potassium currents, which will lead to impaired repolarization	Benign familial neonatal convulsions (BFNC); autosomal dominant inheritance; onset in 1st week of life in infants who are otherwise normal; remission usually within weeks to months; long-term epilepsy in 10–15%	Rare; sequence and functional homology to KCNQ1, mutations of which cause long QT syndrome and a cardiac-auditory syndrome
SCN1B (19q12.1)	β-subunit of a voltage-gated sodium channel; mutation disrupts disulfide bridge that is crucial for structure of extracellular domain; mutated β-subunit leads to slower sodium channel inactivation	Generalized epilepsy with febrile seizures plus (GEFS+); autosomal dominant inheritance; presents with febrile seizures at median 1 year, which may persist >6 years, then variable seizure types not associated with fever	Incidence uncertain; GEFS+ identified in other families with mutations in other sodium channel subunits (SCN1A and SCN2A) and GABA$_A$ receptor subunit (GABRG2); significant phenotypic heterogeneity within same family, including members with febrile seizures only
LGI1 (10q24)	Leucine-rich glioma-inactivated gene; previous evidence for role in glial tumor progression; likely to be involved in nervous system development	Autosomal dominant partial epilepsy with auditory features (ADPEAF); temporal lobe epilepsy with wide range of auditory and other sensory symptoms as major manifestation; age of onset usually between 10 and 25 years	Rare; at least one family with similar syndrome has mutation(s) elsewhere; LGI1 mutation is the only known mutation identified in temporal lobe epilepsy and the only non-ion-channel gene mutation known in idiopathic epilepsy
EPM2A (6q24)	Laforin, a protein tyrosine phosphatase (PTP); may influence glycogen metabolism, which is known to be regulated by phosphatases	Progressive myoclonus epilepsy (Lafora's disease); autosomal recessive inheritance; onset age 6–19 years, death within 10 years; brain degeneration associated with polyglucosan intracellular inclusion bodies in numerous organs	Most common PME in Southern Europe, Middle East, Northern Africa, and Indian subcontinent; genetic heterogeneity; unknown whether seizure phenotype due to degeneration or direct effects of abnormal laforin expression.
Doublecortin (Xq21-24)	Doublecortin, expressed primarily in frontal lobes; function unknown; potentially an intracellular signalling molecule	Classic lissencephaly associated with severe mental retardation and seizures in males; subcortical band heterotopia with more subtle findings in females (presumably due to random X-inactivation); X-linked dominant	Relatively rare but of uncertain incidence, recent increased ascertainment due to improved imaging techniques; relationship between migration defect and seizure phenotype unknown

[a]The first three syndromes listed in the table (BFNC, GEFS+, and ADPEAF) are examples of idiopathic generalized epilepsies associated with identified gene mutations. The last two syndromes are examples of the numerous Mendelian disorders in which seizures are one part of the phenotype.
Note: GABA, γ-aminobutyric acid.

TABLE 14-3

CHARACTERISTICS OF THE MESIAL TEMPORAL LOBE EPILEPSY SYNDROME

History

History of febrile seizures

Family history of epilepsy

Early onset

Rare secondarily generalized seizures

Seizures may remit and reappear

Seizures often intractable

Clinical observations

Aura common

Behavioral arrest/stare

Complex automatisms

Unilateral posturing

Postictal disorientation, memory loss, dysphasia (with focus in dominant hemisphere)

Laboratory studies

Unilateral or bilateral anterior temporal spikes on EEG

Hypometabolism on interictal PET

Hypoperfusion on interictal SPECT

Material-specific memory deficits on intracranial amobarbital (Wada) test

MRI findings

Small hippocampus with increased signal on T2-weighted sequences

Small temporal lobe

Enlarged temporal horn

Pathologic findings

Highly selective loss of specific cell populations within hippocampus in most cases

Note: EEG, electroencephalogram; PET, positron emission tomography; SPECT, single photon emission computed tomography.

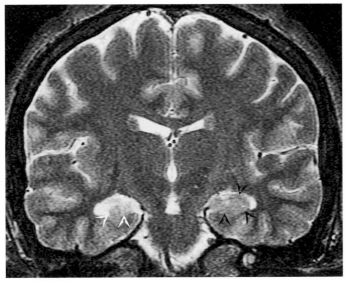

FIGURE 14-1

Mesial temporal lobe epilepsy. The EEG suggested a right temporal lobe focus. Coronal high-resolution T2-weighted fast spin echo magnetic resonance image obtained through the body of the hippocampus demonstrates abnormal high signal intensity in the right hippocampus (white arrows; compare with the normal hippocampus on the left, black arrows) consistent with mesial temporal sclerosis.

abnormalities associated with epilepsy likely involve processes that trigger the appearance of specific sets of epileptogenic factors.

3. Seizures are episodic. Patients with epilepsy have seizures intermittently and, depending on the underlying cause, many patients are completely normal for months or even years between seizures. This implies there are important provocative or *precipitating factors* that induce seizures in patients with epilepsy. Similarly, precipitating factors are responsible for causing the single seizure in someone without epilepsy. Precipitants include those due to intrinsic physiologic processes, such as psychological or physical stress, sleep deprivation, or hormonal changes associated with the menstrual cycle. They also include exogenous factors such as exposure to toxic substances and certain medications.

These observations emphasize the concept that the many causes of seizures and epilepsy result from a dynamic interplay between endogenous factors, epileptogenic factors, and precipitating factors. The potential role of each needs to be carefully considered when determining the appropriate management of a patient with seizures. For example, the identification of predisposing factors (e.g., family history of epilepsy) in a patient with febrile seizures may increase the necessity for closer follow-up and a more aggressive diagnostic evaluation. Finding an epileptogenic lesion may help in the estimation of seizure recurrence and duration of therapy. Finally, removal or modification of a precipitating factor may be an effective and safer method for preventing further seizures than the prophylactic use of anticonvulsant drugs.

CAUSES ACCORDING TO AGE

In practice, it is useful to consider the etiologies of seizures based on the age of the patient, as age is one of the most important factors determining both the incidence and likely causes of seizures or epilepsy (**Table 14-4**). During the *neonatal period* and *early infancy,* potential causes include hypoxic-ischemic encephalopathy, trauma, CNS infection, congenital CNS abnormalities, and metabolic disorders. Babies born to mothers using

neurotoxic drugs such as cocaine, heroin, or ethanol are susceptible to drug-withdrawal seizures in the first few days after delivery. Hypoglycemia and hypocalcemia, which can occur as secondary complications of perinatal injury, are also causes of seizures early after delivery. Seizures due to inborn errors of metabolism usually present once regular feeding begins, typically 2 to 3 days after birth. Pyridoxine (vitamin B_6) deficiency, an important cause of neonatal seizures, can be effectively treated with pyridoxine replacement. The idiopathic or inherited forms of benign neonatal convulsions are also seen during this time period.

The most common seizures arising in *late infancy and early childhood* are febrile seizures, which are seizures associated with fevers but without evidence of CNS infection or other defined causes. The overall prevalence is 3 to 5% and even higher in some parts of the world, such as Asia. Patients often have a family history of

TABLE 14-4

CAUSES OF SEIZURES

Neonates (<1 month)	Perinatal hypoxia and ischemia
	Intracranial hemorrhage and trauma
	Acute CNS infection
	Metabolic disturbances (hypoglycemia, hypocalcemia, hypomagnesemia, pyridoxine deficiency)
	Drug withdrawal
	Developmental disorders
	Genetic disorders
Infants and children (>1 mo and <12 years)	Febrile seizures
	Genetic disorders (metabolic, degenerative, primary epilepsy syndromes)
	CNS infection
	Developmental disorders
	Trauma
	Idiopathic
Adolescents (12–18 years)	Trauma
	Genetic disorders
	Infection
	Brain tumor
	Illicit drug use
	Idiopathic
Young adults (18–35 years)	Trauma
	Alcohol withdrawal
	Illicit drug use
	Brain tumor
	Idiopathic
Older adults (>35 years)	Cerebrovascular disease
	Brain tumor
	Alcohol withdrawal
	Metabolic disorders (uremia, hepatic failure, electrolyte abnormalities, hypoglycemia)
	Alzheimer's disease and other degenerative CNS diseases
	Idiopathic

Note: CNS, central nervous system.

febrile seizures or epilepsy. Febrile seizures usually occur between 3 months and 5 years of age and have a peak incidence between 18 and 24 months. The typical scenario is a child who has a generalized, tonic-clonic seizure during a febrile illness in the setting of a common childhood infection such as otitis media, respiratory infection, or gastroenteritis. The seizure is likely to occur during the rising phase of the temperature curve (i.e., during the first day) rather than well into the course of the illness. A *simple* febrile seizure is a single, isolated event, brief, and symmetric in appearance. *Complex* febrile seizures are characterized by repeated seizure activity, duration >15 min, or have focal features. Approximately one-third of patients with febrile seizures will have a recurrence, but <10% have three or more episodes. Recurrences are much more likely when the febrile seizure occurs in the first year of life. Simple febrile seizures are not associated with an increase in the risk of developing epilepsy, while complex febrile seizures have a risk of 2 to 5%; other risk factors include the presence of preexisting neurologic deficits and a family history of nonfebrile seizures.

Childhood marks the age at which many of the well-defined epilepsy syndromes present. Some children who are otherwise normal develop idiopathic, generalized tonic-clonic seizures without other features that fit into specific syndromes. Temporal lobe epilepsy usually presents in childhood and may be related to mesial temporal lobe sclerosis (as part of the MTLE syndrome) or other focal abnormalities such as cortical dysgenesis. Other types of partial seizures, including those with secondary generalization, may be the relatively late manifestation of a developmental disorder, an acquired lesion such as head trauma, CNS infection (especially viral encephalitis), or very rarely a CNS tumor.

The period of *adolescence and early adulthood* is one of transition during which the idiopathic or genetically based epilepsy syndromes, including JME and juvenile absence epilepsy, become less common, while epilepsies secondary to acquired CNS lesions begin to predominate. Seizures that begin in patients in this age range may be associated with head trauma, CNS infections (including parasitic infections such as cysticercosis), brain tumors, congenital CNS abnormalities, illicit drug use, or alcohol withdrawal.

Head trauma is a common cause of epilepsy in adolescents and adults. The head injury can be caused by a variety of mechanisms, and the likelihood of developing epilepsy is strongly correlated with the severity of the injury. A patient with a penetrating head wound, depressed skull fracture, intracranial hemorrhage, or prolonged posttraumatic coma or amnesia has a 40 to 50% risk of developing epilepsy, while a patient with a closed head injury and cerebral contusion has a 5 to 25% risk.

Recurrent seizures usually develop within 1 year after head trauma, although intervals of ≥10 years are well known. In controlled studies, mild head injury, defined as a concussion with amnesia or loss of consciousness of <30 min, was found to be associated with only a slightly increased likelihood of epilepsy. Nonetheless, most epileptologists know of patients who have partial seizures within hours or days of a mild head injury and subsequently develop chronic seizures of the same type; such cases may represent rare examples of chronic epilepsy resulting from mild head injury.

The causes of seizures in *older adults* include cerebrovascular disease, trauma (including subdural hematoma), CNS tumors, and degenerative diseases. Cerebrovascular disease may account for ~50% of new cases of epilepsy in patients older than 65. Acute seizures (i.e., occurring at the time of the stroke) are seen more often with embolic rather than hemorrhagic or thrombotic stroke. Chronic seizures typically appear months to years after the initial event and are associated with all forms of stroke.

Metabolic disturbances such as electrolyte imbalance, hypo- or hyperglycemia, renal failure, and hepatic failure may cause seizures at any age. Similarly, endocrine disorders, hematologic disorders, vasculitides, and many other systemic diseases may cause seizures over a broad age range. A wide variety of medications and abused substances are known to precipitate seizures as well (**Table 14-5**).

BASIC MECHANISMS

MECHANISMS OF SEIZURE INITIATION AND PROPAGATION

Partial seizure activity can begin in a very discrete region of cortex and then spread to neighboring regions, i.e., there is a *seizure initiation* phase and a *seizure propagation* phase. The initiation phase is characterized by two concurrent events in an aggregate of neurons: (1) high-frequency bursts of action potentials, and (2) hypersynchronization. The bursting activity is caused by a relatively long-lasting depolarization of the neuronal membrane due to influx of extracellular calcium (Ca^{2+}), which leads to the opening of voltage-dependent sodium (Na^+) channels, influx of Na^+, and generation of repetitive action potentials. This is followed by a hyperpolarizing afterpotential mediated by γ-aminobutyric acid (GABA) receptors or potassium (K^+) channels, depending on the cell type. The synchronized bursts from a sufficient number of neurons result in a so-called spike discharge on the EEG.

Normally, the spread of bursting activity is prevented by intact hyperpolarization and a region of surrounding inhi-

TABLE 14-5

DRUGS AND OTHER SUBSTANCES THAT CAN CAUSE SEIZURES

Antimicrobials/antivirals	Psychotropics
β-lactam and related compounds	Antidepressants
Quinolones	Antipsychotics
Acyclovir	Lithium
Isoniazid	Radiographic contrast agents
Ganciclovir	Theophylline
Anesthetics and analgesics	Sedative-hypnotic drug withdrawal
Meperidine	Alcohol
Tramadol	Barbiturates
Local anesthetics	Benzodiazepines
Immunomodulatory drugs	Drugs of abuse
Cyclosporine	Amphetamine
OKT3 (monoclonal antibodies to T cells)	Cocaine
Tacrolimus (FK-506)	Phencyclidine
Interferons	Methylphenidate
	Flumazenil[a]

[a]In benzodiazepine-dependent patients.

bition created by inhibitory neurons. With sufficient activation there is a recruitment of surrounding neurons via a number of mechanisms. Repetitive discharges lead to the following: (1) an increase in extracellular K^+, which blunts hyperpolarization and depolarizes neighboring neurons; (2) accumulation of Ca^{2+} in presynaptic terminals, leading to enhanced neurotransmitter release; and (3) depolarization-induced activation of the N-methyl-D-aspartate (NMDA) subtype of the excitatory amino acid receptor, which causes Ca^{2+} influx and neuronal activation. The recruitment of a sufficient number of neurons leads to a loss of the surrounding inhibition and propagation of seizure activity into contiguous areas via local cortical connections, and to more distant areas via long commissural pathways such as the corpus callosum.

Many factors control neuronal excitability, and thus there are many potential mechanisms for altering a neuron's propensity to have bursting activity. Mechanisms *intrinsic* to the neuron include changes in the conductance of ion channels, response characteristics of membrane receptors, cytoplasmic buffering, second-messenger systems, and protein expression as determined by gene transcription, translation, and posttranslational modification. Mechanisms *extrinsic* to the neuron include changes in the amount or type of neurotransmitters present at the synapse, modulation of receptors by extracellular ions and other molecules, and temporal and spatial properties of synaptic and nonsynaptic input. Nonneural cells, such as astrocytes and oligodendrocytes, have an important role in many of these mechanisms as well.

Certain recognized causes of seizures are explained by these mechanisms. For example, accidental ingestion of domoic acid, which is an analogue of glutamate (the principal excitatory neurotransmitter in the brain), causes profound seizures via direct activation of excitatory amino acid receptors throughout the CNS. Penicillin, which can lower the seizure threshold in humans and is a potent convulsant in experimental models, reduces inhibition by antagonizing the effects of GABA at its receptor. The basic mechanisms of other precipitating factors of seizures, such as sleep deprivation, fever, alcohol withdrawal, hypoxia, and infection, are not as well understood but presumably involve analogous perturbations in neuronal excitability. Similarly, the endogenous factors that determine an individual's seizure threshold may relate to these properties as well.

Knowledge of the mechanisms responsible for initiation and propagation of most generalized seizures (including tonic-clonic, myoclonic, and atonic types) remains rudimentary and reflects the limited understanding of the connectivity of the brain at a systems level. Much more is understood about the origin of generalized spike-and-wave discharges in absence seizures. These appear to be related to oscillatory rhythms normally generated during sleep by circuits connecting the thalamus and cortex. This oscillatory behavior involves an interaction between $GABA_B$ receptors, T-type Ca^{2+} channels, and K^+ channels located within the thalamus. Pharmacologic studies indicate that modulation of these receptors and channels can induce absence seizures, and there is speculation that the genetic forms of absence epilepsy may be associated with mutations of components of this system.

MECHANISMS OF EPILEPTOGENESIS

Epileptogenesis refers to the transformation of a normal neuronal network into one that is chronically hyperexcitable. There is often a delay of months to years between an initial CNS injury such as trauma, stroke, or infection and the first seizure. The injury appears to initiate a process that gradually lowers the seizure threshold in the affected region until a spontaneous seizure occurs. In many genetic and idiopathic forms of epilepsy, epileptogenesis is presumably determined by developmentally regulated events.

Pathologic studies of the hippocampus from patients with temporal lobe epilepsy have led to the suggestion that some forms of epileptogenesis are related to *structural changes in neuronal networks*. For example, many patients with MTLE have a highly selective loss of neurons that may contribute to inhibition of the main excitatory neurons within the dentate gyrus. There is also evidence that, in response to the loss of neurons, there is reorganization or "sprouting" of surviving neurons in a way that affects the excitability of the network. Some of these changes can be seen in experimental models of prolonged electrical seizures or traumatic brain injury. Thus, an initial injury such as head injury may lead to a very focal, confined region of structural change that causes local hyperexcitability. The local hyperexcitability leads to further structural changes that evolve over time until the focal lesion produces clinically evident seizures. Similar models have also provided strong evidence for long-term alterations in *intrinsic, biochemical properties of cells* within the network, such as chronic changes in glutamate receptor function.

GENETIC CAUSES OF EPILEPSY

The most important recent progress in epilepsy research has been the identification of genetic mutations associated with a variety of epilepsy syndromes (Table 14-2). Although all of the mutations identified to date cause rare forms of epilepsy, their discovery has led to extremely important conceptual advances. For example, it appears that many of the inherited, idiopathic epilepsies (i.e., the relatively "pure" forms of epilepsy in which seizures are the phenotypic abnormality and brain structure and function are otherwise normal) are due to mutations affecting ion channel function. These syndromes are therefore part of the larger group of channelopathies causing paroxysmal disorders such as cardiac arrhythmias, episodic ataxia, periodic weakness, and familial hemiplegic migraine. In contrast, gene mutations observed in symptomatic epilepsies (i.e., disorders in which other neurologic abnormalities, such as cognitive

impairment, coexist with seizures) are proving to be associated with pathways influencing CNS development or neuronal homeostasis. A current challenge is to identify the multiple susceptibility genes that underlie the more common forms of idiopathic epilepsies.

MECHANISMS OF ACTION OF ANTIEPILEPTIC DRUGS

Antiepileptic drugs appear to act primarily by blocking the initiation or spread of seizures. This occurs through a variety of mechanisms that modify the activity of ion channels or neurotransmitters, and in most cases the drugs have pleiotropic effects. The mechanisms include inhibition of Na^+-dependent action potentials in a frequency-dependent manner (e.g., phenytoin, carbamazepine, lamotrigine, topiramate, zonisamide), inhibition of voltage-gated Ca^{2+} channels (phenytoin), decrease of glutamate release (lamotrigine), potentiation of GABA receptor function (benzodiazepines and barbiturates), and increase in the availability of GABA (valproic acid, gabapentin, tiagabine). The two most effective drugs for absence seizures, ethosuximide and valproic acid, probably act by inhibiting T-type Ca^{2+} channels in thalamic neurons.

In contrast to the relatively large number of antiepileptic drugs that can attenuate seizure activity, there are currently no drugs known to prevent the formation of a seizure focus following CNS injury. The eventual development of such "antiepileptogenic" drugs will provide an important means of preventing the emergence of epilepsy following injuries such as head trauma, stroke, and CNS infection.

EVALUATION OF THE PATIENT WITH A SEIZURE

When a patient presents shortly after a seizure, the first priorities are attention to vital signs, respiratory and cardiovascular support, and treatment of seizures if they resume (see "Treatment"). Life-threatening conditions such as CNS infection, metabolic derangement, or drug toxicity must be recognized and managed appropriately.

When the patient is not acutely ill, the evaluation will initially focus on whether there is a history of earlier seizures (**Fig. 14-2**). If this is the first seizure, then the emphasis will be to (1) establish whether the reported episode was a seizure rather than another paroxysmal event, (2) determine the cause of the seizure by identifying risk factors and precipitating events, and (3) decide whether anticonvulsant therapy is required in addition to treatment for any underlying illness.

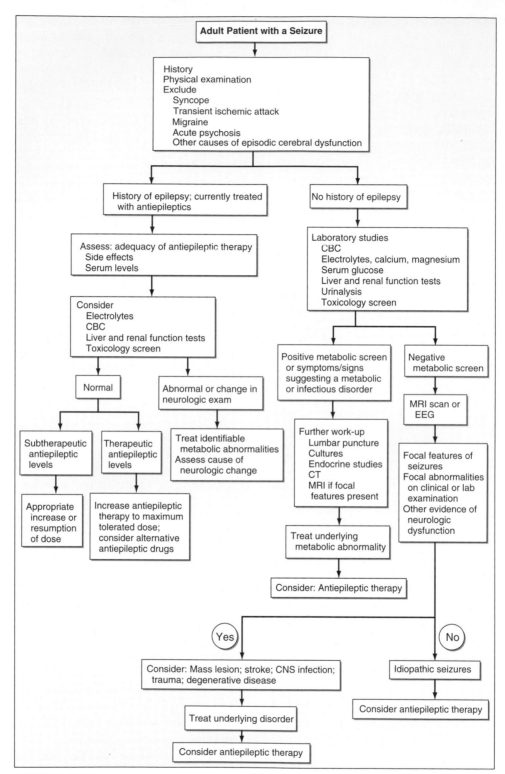

FIGURE 14-2

Evaluation of the adult patient with a seizure. CBC, complete blood count; CT, computed tomography; MRI, magnetic resonance imaging; EEG, electroencephalogram; CNS, central nervous system.

In the patient with prior seizures or a known history of epilepsy, the evaluation is directed toward (1) identification of the underlying cause and precipitating factors, and (2) determination of the adequacy of the patient's current therapy.

HISTORY AND EXAMINATION

The first goal is to determine whether the event was truly a seizure. An in-depth history is essential, for *in many cases the diagnosis of a seizure is based solely on clinical grounds—the examination and laboratory studies are often normal.* Questions should be focused on the symptoms before, during, and after the episode in order to discriminate a seizure from other paroxysmal events (see "Differential Diagnosis of Scizures"). Seizures frequently occur out-of-hospital, and the patient may be unaware of the ictal and immediate postictal phases; thus witnesses to the event should be interviewed carefully.

The history should also focus on risk factors and predisposing events. Clues for a predisposition to seizures include a history of febrile seizures, earlier auras or brief seizures not recognized as such, and a family history of seizures. Epileptogenic factors such as prior head trauma, stroke, tumor, or vascular malformation should be identified. In children, a careful assessment of developmental milestones may provide evidence for underlying CNS disease. Precipitating factors such as sleep deprivation, systemic diseases, electrolyte or metabolic derangements, acute infection, drugs that lower the seizure threshold (Table 14-5), or alcohol or illicit drug use should also be identified.

The general physical examination includes a search for signs of infection or systemic illness. Careful examination of the skin may reveal signs of neurocutaneous disorders, such as tuberous sclerosis or neurofibromatosis, or chronic liver or renal disease. A finding of organomegaly may indicate a metabolic storage disease, and limb asymmetry may provide a clue to brain injury early in development. Signs of head trauma and use of alcohol or illicit drugs should be sought. Auscultation of the heart and carotid arteries may identify an abnormality that predisposes to cerebrovascular disease.

All patients require a complete neurologic examination, with particular emphasis on eliciting signs of cerebral hemispheric disease (Chap. 2). Careful assessment of mental status (including memory, language function, and abstract thinking) may suggest lesions in the anterior frontal, parietal, or temporal lobes. Testing of visual fields will help screen for lesions in the optic pathways and occipital lobes. Screening tests of motor function such as pronator drift, deep tendon reflexes, gait, and coordination may suggest lesions in motor (frontal) cortex, and

cortical sensory testing (e.g., double simultaneous stimulation) may detect lesions in the parietal cortex.

LABORATORY STUDIES

Routine blood studies are indicated to identify the more common metabolic causes of seizures, such as abnormalities in electrolytes, glucose, calcium, or magnesium, and hepatic or renal disease. A screen for toxins in blood and urine should also be obtained from all patients in appropriate risk groups, especially when no clear precipitating factor has been identified. A lumbar puncture is indicated if there is any suspicion of meningitis or encephalitis and is mandatory in all patients infected with HIV, even in the absence of symptoms or signs suggesting infection.

Electroencephalography

All patients who have a possible seizure disorder should be evaluated with an EEG as soon as possible. The EEG measures electrical activity of the brain by recording from electrodes placed on the scalp. The potential difference between pairs of electrodes is amplified and displayed on a computer monitor, oscilloscope, or paper. The characteristics of the normal EEG depend on the patient's age and level of arousal. The recorded activity represents the postsynaptic potentials of vertically oriented pyramidal cells in the cerebral cortex and is characterized by its frequency. In normal awake adults lying quietly with the eyes closed, an 8- to 13-Hz alpha rhythm is seen posteriorly in the EEG, intermixed with a variable amount of generalized faster beta activity (>13 Hz); the alpha rhythm is attenuated when the eyes are opened (**Fig. 14-3**). During drowsiness, the alpha rhythm is also attenuated; with light sleep, slower activity in the theta (4 to 7 Hz) and delta (<4 Hz) ranges becomes more apparent.

The EEG is best recorded from several different electrode arrangements (montages) in turn, and activating procedures are usually performed in an attempt to provoke abnormalities. Such procedures commonly include hyperventilation (for 3 or 4 min), photic stimulation, sleep, and sleep deprivation on the night prior to the recording.

In the evaluation of a patient with suspected epilepsy, the presence of *electrographic seizure activity* during the clinically evident event, i.e., of abnormal, repetitive, rhythmic activity having an abrupt onset and termination, clearly establishes the diagnosis. The absence of electrographic seizure activity does not exclude a seizure disorder, however, because simple or complex seizures may originate from a region of cortex that is not within range of the scalp electrodes. The EEG is always abnormal during generalized tonic-clonic seizures. Since seizures are typically

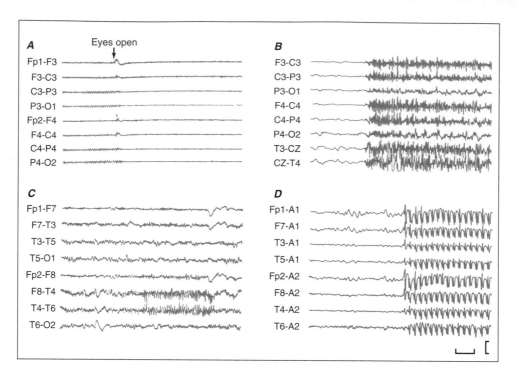

FIGURE 14-3

A. A normal EEG showing a posteriorly situated 9-Hz alpha rhythm that attenuates with eye opening. ***B***. Onset of a tonic seizure showing generalized repetitive sharp activity with synchronous onset over both hemispheres. ***C***. Burst of repetitive spikes in the right temporal region during a clinical spell suggestive of a complex partial seizure. ***D***. Generalized 3-Hz spike-wave activity occurring synchronously over both hemispheres during an absence seizure. Horizontal calibration: 1s; vertical calibration: 200 μV in ***A*** and ***C***, 400 μV in ***B***, and 750 μV in ***D***. Electrode placements are indicated at the left of each panel in accord with the international 10:20 system. A, earlobe; C, central; F, frontal; Fp, frontal polar; P, parietal; T, temporal; O, occipital. Right-sided placements are indicated by even numbers, left-sided placements by odd numbers, and midline placements by Z. [*From MJ Aminoff (ed): Electrodiagnosis in Clinical Neurology, 5th ed. New York, Churchill Livingstone, 2005. Reprinted with permission from Elsevier.*]

infrequent and unpredictable, it is often not possible to obtain the EEG during a clinical event. Continuous monitoring for prolonged periods in video-EEG telemetry units for hospitalized patients or the use of portable equipment to record the EEG continuously on cassettes for ≥24 h in ambulatory patients has made it easier to capture the electrophysiologic accompaniments of clinical events.

The EEG may also be helpful in the interictal period by showing certain abnormalities that are highly supportive of the diagnosis of epilepsy. Such *epileptiform activity* consists of bursts of abnormal discharges containing spikes or sharp waves. The presence of epileptiform activity is not specific for epilepsy, but it has a much greater prevalence in patients with epilepsy than in normal individuals. However, even in an individual who is known to have epilepsy, the initial routine interictal EEG may be normal up to 60% of the time. Thus, the EEG cannot establish the diagnosis of epilepsy in many cases.

The EEG is also used for classifying seizure disorders and aiding in the selection of anticonvulsant medications. For example, episodic generalized spike-wave activity is usually seen in patients with typical absence epilepsy and may be seen with other generalized epilepsy syndromes. Focal interictal epileptiform discharges would support the diagnosis of a partial seizure disorder such as temporal lobe epilepsy or frontal lobe seizures, depending on the location of the discharges.

The routine scalp-recorded EEG may also be used to assess the prognosis of seizure disorders; in general, a normal EEG implies a better prognosis, whereas an abnormal background or profuse epileptiform activity suggests a poor outlook. Unfortunately, the EEG has not proved to be useful in predicting which patients with predisposing conditions, such as head injury or brain tumor, will go on to develop epilepsy, because in such circumstances epileptiform activity is commonly encountered regardless of whether seizures occur.

Brain Imaging

Almost all patients with new-onset seizures should have a brain imaging study to determine whether there is an underlying structural abnormality that is responsible. The only potential exception to this rule is children who have an unambiguous history and examination suggestive of a benign, generalized seizure disorder such as absence epilepsy. MRI has been shown to be superior to computed tomography (CT) for the detection of cerebral lesions associated with epilepsy. In some cases MRI will identify lesions such as tumors, vascular malformations, or other pathologies that need immediate therapy. The use of newer MRI methods, such as fluid-attenuated inversion recovery (FLAIR), has increased the sensitivity for detection of abnormalities of cortical architecture, including hippocampal atrophy associated with mesial temporal sclerosis, and abnormalities of cortical neuronal migration. In such cases the findings may not lead to immediate therapy, but they do provide an explanation for the patient's seizures and point to the need for chronic anticonvulsant therapy or possible surgical resection.

In the patient with a suspected CNS infection or mass lesion, CT scanning should be performed emergently when MRI is not immediately available. Otherwise, it is usually appropriate to obtain an MRI study within a few days of the initial evaluation. Functional imaging procedures such as positron emission tomography (PET) and single photon emission computed tomography (SPECT) are also used to evaluate certain patients with medically refractory seizures (discussed below).

DIFFERENTIAL DIAGNOSIS OF SEIZURES

Disorders that may mimic seizures are listed in **Table 14-6**. In most cases seizures can be distinguished from other conditions by meticulous attention to the history and relevant laboratory studies. On occasion, additional studies, such as video-EEG monitoring, sleep studies, tilt table analysis, or cardiac electrophysiology, may be required to reach a correct diagnosis. Two of the more common nonepileptic syndromes in the differential diagnosis are detailed below.

Syncope (See also Chap. 9)

The diagnostic dilemma encountered most frequently is the distinction between a generalized seizure and syncope. Observations by the patient and bystanders that can help discriminate between the two are listed in **Table 14-7**. Characteristics of a seizure include the presence of an aura, cyanosis, unconsciousness, motor manifestations lasting >30 s, postictal disorientation, muscle soreness, and sleepiness. In contrast, a syncopal episode is more likely if the event was provoked by acute pain or anxiety or occurred immediately after arising from the lying or sitting position. Patients with syncope often describe a stereotyped transition from consciousness to unconsciousness that includes tiredness, sweating, nausea, and tunneling of vision, and they experience a relatively brief loss of

TABLE 14-6

DIFFERENTIAL DIAGNOSIS OF SEIZURES	
Syncope	Transient ischemic attack (TIA)
Vasovagal syncope	Basilar artery TIA
Cardiac arrhythmia	Sleep disorders
Valvular heart disease	Narcolepsy/cataplexy
Cardiac failure	Benign sleep myoclonus
Orthostatic hypotension	Movement disorders
Psychological disorders	Tics
Psychogenic seizure	Nonepileptic myoclonus
Hyperventilation	Paroxysmal choreoathetosis
Panic attack	Special considerations in children
Metabolic disturbances	Breath-holding spells
Alcoholic blackouts	Migraine with recurrent abdominal pain
Delirium tremens	and cyclic vomiting
Hypoglycemia	Benign paroxysmal vertigo
Hypoxia	Apnea
Psychoactive drugs (e.g., hallucinogens)	Night terrors
Migraine	Sleepwalking
Confusional migraine	
Basilar migraine	

TABLE 14-7

FEATURES THAT DISTINGUISH GENERALIZED TONIC-CLONIC SEIZURE FROM SYNCOPE

FEATURE	SEIZURE	SYNCOPE
Immediate precipitating factors	Usually none	Emotional stress, Valsalva, orthostatic hypotension, cardiac etiologies
Premonitory symptoms	None or aura (e.g., odd odor)	Tiredness, nausea, diaphoresis, tunneling of vision
Posture at onset	Variable	Usually erect
Transition to unconsciousness	Often immediate	Gradual over seconds[a]
Duration of unconsciousness	Minutes	Seconds
Duration of tonic or clonic movements	30–60 s	Never more than 15 s
Facial appearance during event	Cyanosis, frothing at mouth	Pallor
Disorientation and sleepiness after event	Many minutes to hours	<5 min
Aching of muscles after event	Often	Sometimes
Biting of tongue	Sometimes	Rarely
Incontinence	Sometimes	Sometimes
Headache	Sometimes	Rarely

[a]May be sudden with certain cardiac arrhythmias.

consciousness. Headache or incontinence usually suggests a seizure but may on occasion also occur with syncope. A brief period (i.e., 1 to 10 s) of convulsive motor activity is frequently seen immediately at the onset of a syncopal episode, especially if the patient remains in an upright posture after fainting (e.g., in a dentist's chair) and therefore has a sustained decrease in cerebral perfusion. Rarely, a syncopal episode can induce a full tonic-clonic seizure. In such cases the evaluation must focus on both the cause of the syncopal event as well as the possibility that the patient has a propensity for recurrent seizures.

Psychogenic Seizures

Psychogenic seizures are nonepileptic behaviors that resemble seizures. They are often part of a conversion reaction precipitated by underlying psychological distress. Certain behaviors, such as side-to-side turning of the head, asymmetric and large-amplitude shaking movements of the limbs, twitching of all four extremities without loss of consciousness, and pelvic thrusting are more commonly associated with psychogenic rather than epileptic seizures. Psychogenic seizures often last longer than epileptic seizures and may wax and wane over minutes to hours. However, the distinction is sometimes difficult on clinical grounds alone, and there are many examples of diagnostic errors made by experienced epileptologists. This is especially true for psychogenic seizures that resemble complex partial seizures, since the behavioral manifestations of complex partial seizures (especially of frontal lobe origin) can be extremely unusual, and in both cases the routine surface EEG may be normal. Video-EEG monitoring is often useful when historic features are nondiagnostic. Generalized tonic-clonic seizures always produce marked EEG abnormalities during and after the seizure. For suspected complex partial seizures of temporal lobe origin, the use of additional electrodes beyond the standard scalp locations (e.g., sphenoidal electrodes) may be required to localize a seizure focus. Measurement of serum prolactin levels may also help to discriminate between organic and psychogenic seizures, since most generalized seizures and many complex partial seizures are accompanied by rises in serum prolactin (during the immediate 30-min postictal period), whereas psychogenic seizures are not. The diagnosis of psychogenic seizures does not exclude a concurrent diagnosis of epilepsy, since the two often coexist.

TREATMENT FOR SEIZURE

Therapy for a patient with a seizure disorder is almost always multimodal and includes treatment of underlying conditions that cause or contribute to the seizures, avoidance of precipitating factors, suppression of recurrent seizures by prophylactic therapy with antiepileptic medications or surgery, and addressing a variety of psychological and social issues. Treatment plans must be individualized, given the many different types and causes of seizures as well as the differences in efficacy and toxicity of antiepileptic medications for each patient. In almost all cases a neurologist with experience in the treatment of epilepsy should design and oversee implementation of the treatment strategy. Furthermore, patients with refractory epilepsy or those who require polypharmacy with antiepileptic drugs should remain under the regular care of a neurologist.

Treatment of Underlying Conditions

If the sole cause of a seizure is a metabolic disturbance such as an abnormality of serum electrolytes or glucose, then treatment is aimed at reversing the metabolic problem and preventing its recurrence. Therapy with antiepileptic drugs is usually unnecessary unless the metabolic disorder cannot be corrected promptly and the patient is at risk of having further seizures. If the apparent cause of a seizure was a medication (e.g., theophylline) or illicit drug use (e.g., cocaine), then appropriate therapy is avoidance of the drug; there is usually no need for antiepileptic medications unless subsequent seizures occur in the absence of these precipitants.

Seizures caused by a structural CNS lesion such as a brain tumor, vascular malformation, or brain abscess may not recur after appropriate treatment of the underlying lesion. However, despite removal of the structural lesion, there is a risk that the seizure focus will remain in the surrounding tissue or develop de novo as a result of gliosis and other processes induced by surgery, radiation, or other therapies. Most patients are therefore maintained on an antiepileptic medication for at least 1 year, and an attempt is made to withdraw medications only if the patient has been completely seizure-free. If seizures are refractory to medication, the patient may benefit from surgical removal of the epileptic brain region (see below).

Avoidance of Precipitating Factors

Unfortunately, little is known about the specific factors that determine precisely when a seizure will occur in a patient with epilepsy. Some patients can identify particular situations that appear to lower their seizure threshold; these situations should be avoided. For example, a patient who has seizures in the setting of sleep deprivation should obviously be advised to maintain a normal sleep schedule. Many patients note an association between alcohol intake and seizures, and they should be encouraged to modify their drinking habits accordingly. There are also relatively rare cases of patients with seizures that are induced by highly specific stimuli such as a video game monitor, music, or an individual's voice ("reflex epilepsy"). If there is an association between stress and seizures, stress reduction techniques such as physical exercise, meditation, or counseling may be helpful.

Antiepileptic Drug Therapy

Antiepileptic drug therapy is the mainstay of treatment for most patients with epilepsy. The overall goal is to completely prevent seizures without causing any untoward side effects, preferably with a single medication and a dosing schedule that is easy for the patient to follow. Seizure classification is an important element in designing the treatment plan, since some antiepileptic drugs have different activities against various seizure types. However, there is considerable overlap between many antiepileptic drugs, such that the choice of therapy is often determined more by specific needs of the patient, especially the patient's assessment of side effects.

WHEN TO INITIATE ANTIEPILEPTIC DRUG THERAPY

Antiepileptic drug therapy should be started in any patient with recurrent seizures of unknown etiology or a known cause that cannot be reversed. Whether to initiate therapy in a patient with a single seizure is controversial. Patients with a single seizure due to an identified lesion such as a CNS tumor, infection, or trauma, in which there is strong evidence that the lesion is epileptogenic, should be treated. The risk of seizure recurrence in a patient with an apparently unprovoked or idiopathic seizure is uncertain, with estimates ranging from 31 to 71% in the first 12 months after the initial seizure. This uncertainty arises from differences in the underlying seizure types and etiologies in various published epidemiologic studies. Generally accepted risk factors associated with recurrent seizures include the following: (1) an abnormal neurologic examination, (2) seizures presenting as status epilepticus, (3) postictal Todd's paralysis, (4) a strong family history of seizures, or (5) an abnormal EEG. Most patients with one or more of these risk factors should be treated. Issues such as employment or driving may influence the decision whether or not to start medications as well. For example, a patient with a single, idiopathic seizure whose job depends on driving may prefer taking antiepileptic drugs rather than risk a seizure recurrence and the potential loss of driving privileges.

SELECTION OF ANTIEPILEPTIC DRUGS

Antiepileptic drugs available in the United States are shown in **Table 14-8**, and the main pharmacologic characteristics of commonly used drugs are listed in **Table 14-9**. Older medications such as phenytoin, valproic acid, carbamazepine, and ethosuximide are generally used as first-line therapy for most seizure disorders since, overall, they are as effective as recently marketed drugs and significantly less expensive. Most of the new drugs that have become available in the past decade are used as add-on or alternative therapy.

In addition to efficacy, factors influencing the choice of an initial medication include the convenience of dosing (e.g., once daily versus three or four times daily) and potential side effects. Almost all of the commonly used antiepileptic drugs can cause similar, dose-related side effects such as sedation, ataxia, and diplopia. Close follow-up is required to ensure these are promptly recognized and reversed. Most of the drugs can also cause

idiosyncratic toxicity such as rash, bone marrow suppression, or hepatotoxicity. Although rare, these side effects should be considered during drug selection, and patients require laboratory tests (e.g., complete blood count and liver function tests) prior to the institution of a drug (to establish baseline values) and during initial dosing and titration of the agent.

Antiepileptic Drug Selection for Partial Seizures

Carbamazepine, phenytoin, or lamotrigine is currently the initial drug of choice for the treatment of partial seizures, including those that secondarily generalize. Overall they have very similar efficacy, but differences in pharmacokinetics and toxicity are the main determinants for use in a given patient. Phenytoin has a relatively long half-life and offers the advantage of once or twice daily dosing compared to two or three times daily dosing for carbamazepine (although a more expensive, extended-release form of carbamazepine is now available) and lamotrigine. An advantage of carbamazepine is that its metabolism follows first-order pharmacokinetics, and the relationship between drug dose, serum levels, and toxicity is linear. By contrast, phenytoin shows properties of saturation kinetics, such that small increases in phenytoin doses above a standard maintenance dose can precipitate marked side effects. This is one of the main causes of acute phenytoin toxicity. Long-term use

TABLE 14-8

SELECTION OF ANTIEPILEPTIC DRUGS

	PRIMARY GENERALIZED TONIC-CLONIC	PARTIAL[a]	ABSENCE	ATYPICAL ABSENCE, MYOCLONIC, ATONIC
First-Line	Valproic acid Lamotrigine	Carbamazepine Phenytoin Lamotrigine Valproic acid	Valproic acid Ethosuximide	Valproic acid
Alternatives	Phenytoin Carbamazepine Topiramate[b] Zonisamide[b] Felbamate Primidone Phenobarbital	Topiramate[b] Levetiracetam[b] Tiagabine[b] Zonisamide[b] Gabapentin[b] Primidone Phenobarbital	Lamotrigine Clonazepam	Lamotrigine Topiramate[b] Clonazepam Felbamate

[a]Includes simple partial, complex partial, and secondarily generalized seizures.
[b]As adjunctive therapy.

TABLE 14-9

DOSAGE AND ADVERSE EFFECTS OF COMMONLY USED ANTIEPILEPTIC DRUGS

GENERIC NAME	TRADE NAME	PRINCIPAL USES	TYPICAL DOSE; DOSE INTERVAL	HALF-LIFE	THERAPEUTIC RANGE	ADVERSE EFFECTS		DRUG INTERACTIONS
						NEUROLOGIC	SYSTEMIC	
Phenytoin (diphenyl-hydantoin	Dilantin	Tonic-clonic (grand mal) Focal-onset	300–400 mg/d (3–6 mg/kg, adult; 4–8 mg/kg, child); qd-bid	24 h (wide variation, dose-dependent)	10–20 μg/mL	Dizziness Diplopia Ataxia Incoordi- nation Confusion	Gum hyperplasia Lymphade- nopathy Hirsutism Osteom- alacia Facial coarsening Skin rash	Level increased by isoniazid, sulfonamides, fluoxetine Level decreased by enzyme- inducing drugs[a] Altered folate metabolism
Carbamazepine	Tegretol Carbatrol	Tonic-clonic Focal-onset	600–1800 mg/d (15–35 mg/kg, child); bid-qid	10–17 h	6–12 μg/mL	Ataxia Dizziness Diplopia Vertigo	Aplastic anemia Leukopenia Gastroin- testinal irritation Hepatotoxicity Hyponatremia	Level decreased by enzyme- inducing drugs[a] Level increased by erythromycin, propoxyphene, isoniazid, cimetidine, fluoxetine
Valproic acid	Depakene Depakote	Tonic-clonic Absence Atypical absence Myoclonic Focal-onset	750–2000 mg/d (20–60 mg/kg); bid-qid	15 h	50–150 μg/mL	Ataxia Sedation Tremor	Hepatotoxicity Thrombocy- topenia Gastrointestinal irritation Weight gain Transient alopecia Hyperam- monemia	Level decreased by enzyme- inducing drugs[a]
Lamotrigine	Lamictal	Focal-onset Tonic-clonic Atypical absence Myoclonic Lennox- Gastaut syndrome	150–500 mg/d; bid	25 h 14 h (with enzyme- inducers) 59 h (with valproic acid)	Not established	Dizziness Diplopia Sedation Ataxia Headache	Skin rash Stevens- Johnson syndrome	Level decreased by enzyme- inducing drugs[a] Level increased by valproic acid
Ethosuximide	Zarontin	Absence (petit mal)	750–1250 mg/d (20-40 mg/kg); qd-bid	60 h, adult 30 h, child	40–100 μg/mL	Ataxia Lethargy Headache	Gastrointestinal irritation Skin rash Bone marrow suppression	
Gabapentin	Neurontin	Focal-onset	900–2400 mg/d; tid-qid	5–9 h	Not established	Sedation Dizziness Ataxia Fatigue	Gastrointestinal irritation Weight gain Edema	No known significant interactions
Topiramate	Topamax	Focal-onset Tonic-clonic Lennox- Gastaut syndrome	200–400 mg/d; bid	20–30 h	Not established	Psychomotor slowing Sedation Speech or language problems Fatigue Paresthesias	Renal stones (avoid use with other carbonic anhydrase inhibitors) Weight loss	Level decreased by enzyme- inducing drugs[a]

(continued)

TABLE 14-9 *(continued)*

DOSAGE AND ADVERSE EFFECTS OF COMMONLY USED ANTIEPILEPTIC DRUGS

GENERIC NAME	TRADE NAME	PRINCIPAL USES	TYPICAL DOSE; DOSE INTERVAL	HALF-LIFE	THERAPEUTIC RANGE	ADVERSE EFFECTS		DRUG INTERACTIONS
						NEUROLOGIC	SYSTEMIC	
Tiagabine	Gabitril	Focal-onset Tonic-clonic	32–56 mg/d; bid-qid	7–9 h	Not established	Confusion Sedation Depression Dizziness Speech or language problems Paresthesias Psychosis	Gastrointestinal irritation	Level decreased by enzyme-inducing drugs[a]
Phenobarbital	Luminol	Tonic-clonic Focal-onset	60–180 mg/d (1–4 mg/kg, adult); (3–6 mg/kg, child); qd	90 h (70 h in children)	10–40 μg/mL	Sedation Ataxia Confusion Dizziness Decreased libido Depression	Skin rash	Level increased by valproic acid, phenytoin
Primidone	Mysoline	Tonic-clonic Focal-onset	750–1000 mg/d (10–25 mg/kg); bid-tid	Primidone, 8–15 h Phenobarbital, 90 h	Primidone, 4–12 μg/mL Phenobarbital, 10–40 μg/mL	Same as phenobarbital		
Clonazepam	Klonopin	Absence Atypical absence Myoclonic	1–12 mg/d (0.1–0.2 mg/kg); qd-tid	24–48 h	10–70 ng/mL	Ataxia Sedation Lethargy	Anorexia	Level decreased by enzyme-inducing drugs[a]
Felbamate	Felbatol	Focal-onset Lennox-Gastaut syndrome	2400–3600 mg/d, (45 mg/kg, child); tid-qid	16–22 h	Not established	Insomnia Dizziness Sedation Headache	Aplastic anemia Hepatic failure Weight loss Gastrointestinal irritation	Increases phenytoin, valproic acid, active carbamazepine metabolite
Levetiracetam	Keppra	Focal-onset	1000–3000 mg/d; bid	6–8 h	Not established	Sedation Fatigue Incoordination Psychosis	Anemia Leukopenia	None known
Zonisamide	Zonegran	Focal-onset	200–400 mg/d;qd-bid	50–68 h	Not established	Sedation Dizziness Confusion Headache Psychosis	Anorexia Renal stones	Level decreased by enzyme-inducing drugs[a]
Oxcarbazepine	Trileptal	Focal-onset	900–2400 mg/d (30–45 mg/kg, child); bid	10–17 h (for active metabolite)	Not established	Fatigue Ataxia Dizziness Diplopia Vertigo Headache	See carbamaze-pine	Level decreased by enzyme-inducing drugs[a] May increase phenytoin

[a]Phenytoin, carbamazepine, phenobarbital.

of phenytoin is associated with untoward cosmetic effects (e.g., hirsutism, coarsening of facial features, and gingival hypertrophy), and effects on bone metabolism, so it is often avoided in young patients who are likely to require the drug for many years. Carbamazepine can cause leukopenia, aplas-

tic anemia, or hepatotoxicity and would therefore be contraindicated in patients with predispositions to these problems. A major concern with lamotrigine is the occurrence of skin rash during the initiation of therapy. This can be extremely severe and lead to Stevens-Johnson syndrome if unrecognized and if the medication is not discontinued immediately. This risk can be reduced by slow introduction and titration. Lamotrigine must be started slowly when used as add-on therapy with valproic acid, since valproic acid can inhibit its metabolism, thereby substantially prolonging its half-life.

Valproic acid is an effective alternative for some patients with partial seizures, especially when the seizures secondarily generalize. Gastrointestinal side effects are fewer when using the valproate semisodium formulation (Depakote). Valproic acid also rarely causes reversible bone marrow suppression and hepatotoxicity, and laboratory testing is required to monitor toxicity. This drug should generally be avoided in patients with preexisting bone marrow or liver disease. Irreversible, fatal hepatic failure appearing as an idiosyncratic rather than dose-related side effect is a relatively rare complication; its risk is highest in children <2 years old, especially those taking other antiepileptic drugs or with inborn errors of metabolism.

Topiramate, tiagabine, levetiracetam, zonisamide, gabapentin, and oxcarbazepine are additional drugs currently used for the treatment of partial seizures with or without secondary generalization. Until recently, phenobarbital and other barbiturate compounds were commonly used as first-line therapy for many forms of epilepsy. However, the barbiturates frequently cause sedation in adults, hyperactivity in children, and other more subtle cognitive changes; thus, their use should be limited to situations in which no other suitable treatment alternatives exist.

Antiepileptic Drug Selection for Generalized Seizures Valproic acid is currently considered the best initial choice for the treatment of primarily generalized, tonic-clonic seizures. Lamotrigine, followed by carbamazepine and phenytoin, are suitable alternatives. Valproic acid is also particularly effective in absence, myoclonic, and atonic seizures and is therefore the drug of choice in patients with generalized epilepsy syndromes having mixed seizure types. Importantly, both carbamazepine and phenytoin can worsen certain types of generalized seizures, including absence, myoclonic, tonic, and atonic seizures. Ethosuximide is a particularly effective drug for the treatment of uncomplicated absence seizures, but it is not useful for tonic-clonic or partial

seizures. Ethosuximide rarely causes bone marrow suppression, so that periodic monitoring of blood cell counts is required. Although approved for use in partial seizure disorders, lamotrigine appears to be effective in epilepsy syndromes with mixed, generalized seizure types such as JME and Lennox-Gastaut syndrome. Topiramate, zonisamide, and felbamate may have similar broad efficacy. Clinical trials are underway to establish the usefulness of levetiracetam in generalized seizure syndromes.

INITIATION AND MONITORING OF THERAPY

Because the response to any antiepileptic drug is unpredictable, patients should be carefully educated about the approach to therapy. The goal is to prevent seizures and minimize the side effects of therapy; determination of the optimal dose is often a matter of trial and error. This process may take months or longer if the baseline seizure frequency is low. Most anticonvulsant drugs need to be introduced relatively slowly to minimize side effects, and patients should expect that minor side effects such as mild sedation, slight changes in cognition, or imbalance will typically resolve within a few days. Starting doses are usually the lowest value listed under the dosage column in Table 14-9. Subsequent increases should be made only after achieving a steady state with the previous dose (i.e., after an interval of five or more half-lives).

Monitoring of serum antiepileptic drug levels can be very useful for establishing the initial dosing schedule. However, the published therapeutic ranges of serum drug concentrations are only an approximate guide for determining the proper dose for a given patient. The key determinants are the clinical measures of seizure frequency and presence of side effects, not the laboratory values. Conventional assays of serum drug levels measure the total drug (i.e., both free and protein-bound). However, it is the concentration of free drug that reflects extracellular levels in the brain and correlates best with efficacy. Thus, patients with decreased levels of serum proteins (e.g., decreased serum albumin due to impaired liver or renal function) may have an increased ratio of free to bound drug, yet the concentration of free drug may be adequate for seizure control. These patients may have a "subtherapeutic" drug level, but the dose should be changed only if seizures remain uncontrolled, not just to achieve a "therapeutic" level. It is also useful to monitor free drug levels in such patients. In practice, other than during the initiation or modification of therapy, monitoring of antiepileptic drug levels is most useful for documenting compliance.

If seizures continue despite gradual increases to the maximum tolerated dose and documented compliance, then it becomes necessary to switch to another antiepileptic drug. This is usually done by maintaining the patient on the first drug while a second drug is added. The dose of the second drug should be adjusted to decrease seizure frequency without causing toxicity. Once this is achieved, the first drug can be gradually withdrawn (usually over weeks unless there is significant toxicity). The dose of the second drug is then further optimized based on seizure response and side effects. Monotherapy should be the goal whenever possible.

WHEN TO DISCONTINUE THERAPY

Overall, about 70% of children and 60% of adults who have their seizures completely controlled with antiepileptic drugs can eventually discontinue therapy. The following patient profile yields the greatest chance of remaining seizure-free after drug withdrawal: (1) complete medical control of seizures for 1 to 5 years; (2) single seizure type, either partial or generalized; (3) normal neurologic examination, including intelligence; and (4) normal EEG. The appropriate seizure-free interval is unknown and undoubtedly varies for different forms of epilepsy. However, it seems reasonable to attempt withdrawal of therapy after 2 years in a patient who meets all of the above criteria, is motivated to discontinue the medication, and clearly understands the potential risks and benefits. In most cases it is preferable to reduce the dose of the drug gradually over 2 to 3 months. Most recurrences occur in the first 3 months after discontinuing therapy, and patients should be advised to avoid potentially dangerous situations such as driving or swimming during this period.

TREATMENT FOR REFRACTORY EPILEPSY

Approximately one-third of patients with epilepsy do not respond to treatment with a single antiepileptic drug, and it becomes necessary to try a combination of drugs to control seizures. Patients who have focal epilepsy related to an underlying structural lesion or those with multiple seizure types and developmental delay are particularly likely to require multiple drugs. There are currently no clear guidelines for rational polypharmacy, although in theory a combination of drugs with different mechanisms of action may be most useful. In most cases the initial combination therapy combines first-line drugs, i.e., carbamazepine, phenytoin, valproic acid, and lamotrigine. If these drugs are unsuccessful, then the addition of a newer drug such as topiramate or levetiracetam is indicated. Patients with myoclonic seizures resistant to valproic acid may benefit from the addition of clonazepam, and those with absence seizures may respond to a combination of valproic acid and ethosuximide. The same principles concerning the monitoring of therapeutic response, toxicity, and serum levels for monotherapy apply to polypharmacy, and potential drug interactions need to be recognized. If there is no improvement, a third drug can be added while the first two are maintained. If there is a response, the less effective or less well-tolerated of the first two drugs should be gradually withdrawn.

Surgical Treatment For Refractory Epilepsy

Approximately 20% of patients with epilepsy are resistant to medical therapy despite efforts to find an effective combination of antiepileptic drugs. For some, surgery can be extremely effective in substantially reducing seizure frequency and even providing complete seizure control. Understanding the potential value of surgery is especially important when, at the time of diagnosis, a patient has an epilepsy syndrome that is considered likely to be drug-resistant. Rather than submitting the patient to years of unsuccessful medical therapy and the psychosocial trauma and increased mortality associated with ongoing seizures, the patient should have an efficient but relatively brief attempt at medical therapy and then be referred for surgical evaluation.

The most common surgical procedure for patients with temporal lobe epilepsy involves resection of the anteromedial temporal lobe (temporal lobectomy) or a more limited removal of the underlying hippocampus and amygdala (amygdalohippocampectomy). Focal seizures arising from extratemporal regions may be abolished by a focal neocortical resection with precise removal of an identified lesion (lesionectomy). When the cortical region cannot be removed, multiple subpial transection, which disrupts intracortical connections, is sometimes used to prevent seizure spread. Hemispherectomy or multilobar resection is useful for some patients with severe seizures due to hemispheric abnormalities such as hemimegaloencephaly or other dysplastic abnormalities, and corpus callosotomy has been shown to be effective for disabling tonic or atonic seizures, usually when they are part of a mixed-seizure syndrome (e.g., Lennox-Gastaut syndrome).

Presurgical evaluation is designed to identify the functional and structural basis of the patient's seizure disorder. Inpatient video-EEG monitoring is used to define the anatomical location of the seizure focus and to correlate the abnormal electrophysiologic activity with behavioral manifestations of the seizure. Routine scalp or scalp-sphenoidal recordings are usually sufficient for localization, and advances in neuroimaging have made the use of invasive electrophysiologic monitoring such as implanted depth electrodes or subdural electrodes less common. A high-resolution MRI scan is routinely used to identify structural lesions. Functional imaging studies such as SPECT and PET are adjunctive tests that may help verify the localization of an apparent epileptogenic region. Once the presumed location of the seizure onset is identified, additional studies, including neuropsychological testing and the intracarotid amobarbital test (Wada test) may be used to assess language and memory localization and to determine the possible functional consequences of surgical removal of the epileptogenic region. In some cases, the exact extent of the resection to be undertaken is determined by performing cortical mapping at the time of the surgical procedure, allowing for a tailored resection. This involves electrocorticographic recordings made with electrodes on the surface of the brain to identify the extent of epileptiform disturbances. If the region to be resected is within or near brain regions suspected of having sensorimotor or language function, electrical cortical stimulation mapping is performed in the awake patient to determine the function of cortical regions in question in order to avoid resection of so-called eloquent cortex, and thereby minimize postsurgical deficits.

Advances in presurgical evaluation and microsurgical techniques have led to a steady increase in the success of epilepsy surgery. Clinically significant complications of surgery are <5%, and the use of functional mapping procedures has markedly reduced the neurologic sequelae due to removal or sectioning of brain tissue. For example, about 70% of patients treated with temporal lobectomy will become seizure-free, and another 15 to 25% will have at least a 90% reduction in seizure frequency. Marked improvement is also usually seen in patients treated with hemispherectomy for catastrophic seizure disorders due to large hemispheric abnormalities. Postoperatively, patients generally need to remain on antiepileptic drug therapy, but the marked reduction of seizures following surgery can have a very beneficial effect on quality of life.

Vagus Nerve Stimulation (VNS)

VNS is a new treatment option for patients with medically refractory epilepsy who are not candidates for resective brain surgery. The procedure involves placement of a bipolar electrode on the midcervical portion of the left vagus nerve. The electrode is connected to a small, subcutaneous generator located in the infraclavicular region, and the generator is programmed to deliver intermittent electrical pulses to the vagus nerve. Unlike medications, there may be a delay between the initiation of VNS and the appearance of antiseizure effects. The precise mechanism of action of VNS is unknown, although experimental studies have shown that stimulation of vagal nuclei leads to widespread activation of cortical and subcortical pathways and an associated increased seizure threshold. In practice, the efficacy of VNS appears to be no greater than recently introduced anticonvulsant medications. Adverse effects of the surgery are rare, and stimulation-induced side effects, including transient hoarseness, cough, and dyspnea, are usually mild and well tolerated.

STATUS EPILEPTICUS

Status epilepticus refers to continuous seizures or repetitive, discrete seizures with impaired consciousness in the interictal period. The duration of seizure activity sufficient to meet the definition of status epilepticus has traditionally been specified as 15 to 30 min. However, a more practical definition is to consider status epilepticus as a situation in which the duration of seizures prompts the acute use of anticonvulsant therapy, typically when seizures last beyond 5 min.

Status epilepticus is an emergency and must be treated immediately, since cardiorespiratory dysfunction, hyperthermia, and metabolic derangements can develop as a consequence of prolonged seizures, and these can lead to irreversible neuronal injury. Furthermore, CNS injury can occur even when the patient is paralyzed with neuromuscular blockade but continues to have electrographic seizures. The most common causes of status epilepticus are anticonvulsant withdrawal or noncompliance, metabolic disturbances, drug toxicity, CNS infection, CNS tumors, refractory epilepsy, and head trauma.

Generalized status epilepticus is obvious when the patient is having overt convulsions. However, after 30 to 45 min of uninterrupted seizures, the signs may become increasingly subtle. Patients may have mild clonic movements of only the fingers, or fine, rapid movements of the eyes. There may be paroxysmal episodes of tachycardia, hypertension, and pupillary dilation. In such cases, the EEG may be the only method of establishing the diagnosis. Thus, if the patient stops having overt seizures, yet remains comatose, an EEG should be performed to rule out ongoing status epilepticus.

The first step in the management of a patient in status epilepticus is to attend to any acute cardiorespiratory problems or hyperthermia, perform a brief medical and neurologic examination, establish venous access, and send samples for laboratory studies to identify metabolic abnormalities. Anticonvulsant therapy should then begin without delay; a treatment approach is shown in **Fig. 14–4**.

BEYOND SEIZURES: OTHER MANAGEMENT ISSUES

Interictal Behavior

The adverse effects of epilepsy often go beyond the occurrence of clinical seizures, and the extent of these effects depends largely upon the etiology of the seizure disorder, the degree to which the seizures are controlled, and the presence of side effects from antiepileptic therapy. Many patients with epilepsy are completely normal between seizures and able to live highly successful and productive lives. In contrast, patients with seizures secondary to developmental abnormalities or acquired brain injury may have impaired cognitive function and other neurologic deficits. Frequent interictal EEG abnormalities have been shown to be associated with subtle dysfunction of memory and attention. Patients with

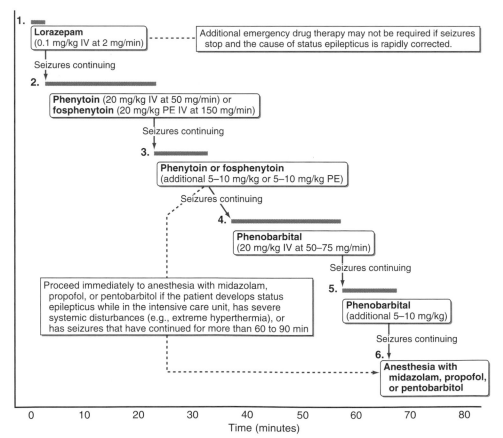

FIGURE 14-4

Pharmacologic treatment of generalized tonic-clonic status epilepticus in adults. IV, intravenous; PE, phenytoin equivalents. The horizontal bars indicate the approximate duration of drug infusions.

many seizures, especially those emanating from the temporal lobe, often note an impairment of short-term memory that may progress over time.

Patients with epilepsy are at risk of developing a variety of psychiatric problems including depression, anxiety, and psychosis. This risk varies considerably depending on many factors, including the etiology, frequency, and severity of seizures and the patient's age and previous history. Depression occurs in ~20% of patients, and the incidence of suicide is higher in epileptic patients than in the general population. Depression should be treated through counseling or medication. The selective serotonin reuptake inhibitors typically have no effect on seizures, while the tricyclic antidepressants may lower the seizure threshold. Anxiety can appear as a manifestation of a seizure, and anxious or psychotic behavior can sometimes be observed as part of a postictal delirium. Postictal psychosis is a rare phenomenon that typically occurs after a period of increased seizure frequency. There is usually a brief lucid interval lasting up to a week, followed by days to weeks of agitated, psychotic behavior. The psychosis will usually resolve spontaneously but may require treatment with antipsychotic or anxiolytic medications.

There is ongoing controversy as to whether some patients with epilepsy (especially temporal lobe epilepsy) have a stereotypical "interictal personality." The predominant view is that the unusual or abnormal personality traits observed in such patients are, in most cases, not due to epilepsy but result from an underlying structural brain lesion, the effects of antiepileptic drugs, or psychosocial factors related to suffering from a chronic disease.

Mortality of Epilepsy

Patients with epilepsy have a risk of death that is roughly two to three times greater than expected in a matched population without epilepsy. Most of the increased mortality is due to the underlying etiology of epilepsy, e.g., tumors or strokes in older adults. However, a significant number of patients die from accidents, status epilepticus, and a syndrome known as *sudden unexpected death in epileptic patients* (SUDEP), which usually affects young people with convulsive seizures and tends to occur at night. The cause of SUDEP is unknown; it may result from brainstem-mediated effects of seizures on cardiac rhythms or pulmonary function.

Psychosocial Issues

There continues to be a cultural stigma about epilepsy, although it is slowly declining in societies with effective health education programs. Many patients with epilepsy harbor fears, such as the fear of becoming mentally retarded or dying during a seizure. These issues need to be carefully addressed by educating the patient about epilepsy and by ensuring that family members, teachers, fellow employees, and other associates are equally well informed. The Epilepsy Foundation of America (1-800-EFA-1000) is a patient advocacy organization and a useful source of educational material.

Employment and Driving

Many patients with epilepsy face difficulty in obtaining or maintaining employment, even when their seizures are well controlled. Federal and state legislation is designed to prevent employers from discriminating against patients with epilepsy, and patients should be encouraged to understand and claim their legal rights. Patients in these circumstances also benefit greatly from the assistance of health providers who act as strong patient advocates.

Loss of driving privileges is one of the most disruptive social consequences of epilepsy. Physicians should be very clear about local regulations concerning driving and epilepsy, since the laws vary considerably among states and countries. In all cases, it is the physician's responsibility to warn patients of the danger imposed on themselves and others while driving if their seizures are uncontrolled (unless the seizures are not associated with impairment of consciousness or motor control). In general, most states allow patients to drive after a seizure-free interval (on or off medications) between 3 months and 2 years.

SPECIAL ISSUES RELATED TO WOMEN AND EPILEPSY

Catamenial Epilepsy

Some women experience a marked increase in seizure frequency around the time of menses. This is thought to reflect either the effects of estrogen and progesterone on neuronal excitability or changes in antiepileptic drug levels due to altered protein binding. Acetazolamide (250 to 500 mg/d) may be effective as adjunctive therapy in some cases when started 7 to 10 days prior to the onset of menses and continued until bleeding stops. Some patients may benefit from increases in antiepileptic drug dosages during this time or from control of the menstrual cycle through the use of oral contraceptives. Natural progestins may be of benefit to a subset of women.

Pregnancy

Most women with epilepsy who become pregnant will have an uncomplicated gestation and deliver a normal baby. However, epilepsy poses some important risks to a pregnancy. Seizure frequency during pregnancy will remain unchanged in ~50% of women, increase in 30%, and decrease in 20%. Changes in seizure frequency are attributed to endocrine effects on the CNS, variations in antiepileptic drug pharmacokinetics (such as acceleration of hepatic drug metabolism or effects on plasma protein binding), and changes in medication compliance. It is useful to see patients at frequent intervals during pregnancy and monitor serum antiepileptic drug levels. Measurement of the unbound drug concentrations may be useful if there is an increase in seizure frequency or worsening of side effects of antiepileptic drugs.

The overall incidence of fetal abnormalities in children born to mothers with epilepsy is 5 to 6%, compared to 2 to 3% in healthy women. Part of the higher incidence is due to teratogenic effects of antiepileptic drugs, and the risk increases with the number of medications used (e.g., 10% risk of malformations with three drugs). A syndrome comprising facial dysmorphism, cleft lip, cleft palate, cardiac defects, digital hypoplasia, and nail dysplasia was originally ascribed to phenytoin therapy, but it is now known to occur with other first-line antiepileptic drugs (i.e., valproic acid and carbamazepine) as well. Also, valproic acid and carbamazepine are associated with a 1 to 2% incidence of neural tube defects compared with a baseline of 0.5 to 1%. Little is currently known about the safety of newer drugs.

Since the potential harm of uncontrolled seizures on the mother and fetus is considered greater than the teratogenic effects of antiepileptic drugs, it is currently recommended that pregnant women be maintained on effective drug therapy. When possible, it seems prudent to have the patient on monotherapy at the lowest effective dose, especially during the first trimester. Patients should also take folate (1 to 4 mg/d), since the antifolate effects of anticonvulsants are thought to play a role in the development of neural tube defects, although the benefits of this treatment remain unproved in this setting.

Enzyme-inducing drugs such as phenytoin, phenobarbital, and primidone cause a transient and reversible deficiency of vitamin K–dependent clotting factors in ~50% of newborn infants. Although neonatal hemorrhage is uncommon, the mother should be treated with oral vitamin K (20 mg daily) in the last 2 weeks of pregnancy, and the infant should receive vitamin K (1 mg) at birth.

Contraception

Special care should be taken when prescribing antiepileptic medications for women who are taking oral contraceptive agents. Drugs such as carbamazepine, phenytoin, phenobarbital, and topiramate can significantly antagonize the effects of oral contraceptives via enzyme induction and other mechanisms. Patients should be advised to consider alternative forms of contraception, or their contraceptive medications should be modified to offset the effects of the antiepileptic medications.

Breast Feeding

Antiepileptic medications are excreted into breast milk to a variable degree. The ratio of drug concentration in breast milk relative to serum is ~80% for ethosuximide, 40 to 60% for phenobarbital, 40% for carbamazepine, 15% for phenytoin, and 5% for valproic acid. Given the overall benefits of breast feeding and the lack of evidence for long-term harm to the infant by being exposed to antiepileptic drugs, mothers with epilepsy can be encouraged to breast feed. This should be reconsidered, however, if there is any evidence of drug effects on the infant, such as lethargy or poor feeding.

ACKNOWLEDGMENT

The editors acknowledge the contributions of Michael J. Aminoff to this chapter in earlier editions of *Harrison's*.

FURTHER READINGS

BLECK TP: Refractory status epilepticus. Curr Opin Crit Care 11:117, 2005

CHANG B, LOWENSTEIN DH: Mechanisms of disease: Epilepsy. N Engl J Med 349:1257, 2003

HIROSE S et al: Genetics of idiopathic epilepsies. Epilepsia 46(Suppl 1):38, 2005

☑ LOWENSTEIN DH: Treatment options for status epilepticus. Curr Opin Pharmacol 5:334, 2005

A concise review of pharmacologic therapies for status epilepticus, including the use of midazolam and propofol in refractory cases.

OGUNI M, OSAWA M: Epilepsy and pregnancy. Epilepsia 45(Suppl 8):37, 2004

☑ PERUCCA E: An introduction to antiepileptic drugs. Epilepsia 46(Suppl 4):31, 2005

An excellent overview of the pharmacology and primary indications of all currently available antiepileptic medications.

TELLEZ-ZENTENO JF et al: Long-term seizure outcomes following epilepsy surgery: A systematic review and meta-analysis. Brain 128:1188, 2005

TOMSON T, BATTINO D: Teratogenicity of antiepileptic drugs: State of the art. Curr Opin Neurol 18:135, 2005

WIEBE S et al: A randomized, controlled trial of surgery for temporal-lobe epilepsy. N Engl J Med 345:311, 2001

WYLLIE E (ed): *The Treatment of Epilepsy: Principles and Practice,* 3d ed. Baltimore, Lippincott Williams & Wilkins, 2001

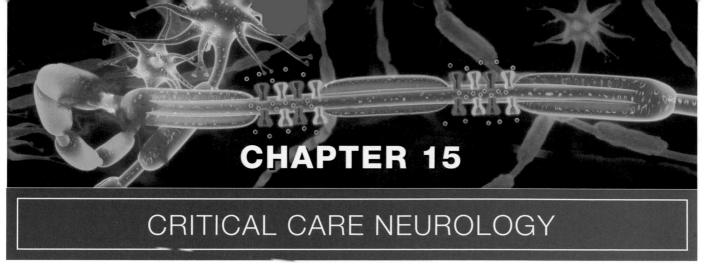

CHAPTER 15

CRITICAL CARE NEUROLOGY

J. Claude Hemphill

Life-threatening neurologic illness may be caused by a primary disorder affecting any region of the neuroaxis or may occur as a consequence of a systemic disorder such as hepatic failure, multisystem organ failure, or cardiac arrest (**Table 15-1**). Neurologic critical care focuses on preservation of neurologic tissue and prevention of secondary brain injury caused by ischemia, edema, and elevated intracranial pressure (ICP).

PATHOPHYSIOLOGY

Brain Edema

Swelling, or edema, of brain tissue occurs with many types of brain injury. The two principal types of edema are vasogenic and cytotoxic. *Vasogenic edema* refers to the influx of fluid and solutes into the brain through an incompetent blood-brain barrier (BBB). In the normal cerebral vasculature, endothelial tight junctions associated with astrocytes create an impermeable barrier (the BBB), through which access into the brain interstitium is dependent upon specific transport mechanisms (Chap. 1). The BBB may be compromised in ischemia, trauma,

infection, and metabolic derangements. Typically, vasogenic edema develops rapidly following injury. *Cytotoxic edema* refers to cellular swelling and occurs in a variety of settings including brain ischemia and trauma. Early astrocytic swelling is a hallmark of ischemia. Brain edema that is clinically significant usually represents a combination of vasogenic and cellular components. Edema can lead to increased ICP as well as tissue shifts and brain displacement from focal processes. These tissue shifts can cause injury by mechanical distraction and compression in addition to the ischemia of impaired perfusion consequent to the elevated ICP.

Ischemic Cascade and Cellular Injury

When delivery of substrates, principally oxygen and glucose, is inadequate to sustain cellular function, a series of interrelated biochemical reactions known as the *ischemic cascade* is initiated. The release of excitatory amino acids, especially glutamate, leads to influx of calcium and sodium ions, which disrupt cellular homeostasis. An increased intracellular calcium concentration may activate proteases and lipases, which then lead to lipid peroxidation and free radical–mediated cell membrane injury. Cytoxic edema ensues, and ultimately necrotic cell death and tissue infarction occur. This pathway to irreversible cell death is common to ischemic stroke, global cerebral ischemia, and traumatic brain injury. *Penumbra* refers to ischemic brain tissue that has not yet undergone irreversible infarction, implying that the region is potentially salvageable if ischemia can be reversed. Factors that may exacerbate ischemic brain injury include systemic hypotension and hypoxia, which further reduce substrate delivery to vulnerable brain tissue, and fever, seizures, and hyperglycemia, which can increase cellular metabolism outstripping compensatory processes. Clinically, these events are known as *secondary brain insults* because they lead to exacerbation of the primary brain injury. Prevention, identification, and treatment of secondary brain insults are fundamental goals of management.

TABLE 15-1

NEUROLOGIC DISORDERS IN CRITICAL ILLNESS

LOCALIZATION ALONG NEUROAXIS	SYNDROME
Central Nervous System	
Brain: Cerebral hemispheres	Global encephalopathy
	Sepsis
	Organ failure — hepatic, renal
	Medication related
	Sedatives/hypnotics/analgesics
	H$_2$ blockers, antihypertensives
	Drug overdose
	Electrolyte disturbance — hyponatremia; hypoglycemia
	Hypotension/hypoperfusion
	Hypoxia
	Meningitis
	Subarachnoid hemorrhage
	Wernicke's disease
	Seizure — postictal or nonconvulsive status
	Hypertensive encephalopathy
	Hypothyroidism — myxedema
	Focal deficits
	Ischemic stroke
	Tumor
	Abscess, subdural empyema
	Subdural/epidural hematoma
Brainstem	Mass effect and compression
	Ischemic stroke, intraparenchymal hemorrhage
	Hypoxia
Spinal cord	Mass effect and compression
	Disc herniation
	Epidural hematoma
	Ischemia — hypotension/embolic
	Subdural empyema
	Trauma, central cord syndrome
Peripheral Nervous System	
Peripheral nerve	
Axonal	Critical illness polyneuropathy
	Possible neuromuscular blocking agent complication
	Metabolic disturbances, uremia — hyperglycemia
	Medication effects — chemotherapeutic, antiretroviral
Demyelinating	Guillian-Barré syndrome
	Chronic inflammatory demyelinating polyneuropathy
Neuromuscular junction	Prolonged effect of neuromuscular blockade
	Medication effects — aminoglycosides
	Myasthenia-gravis, Lambert-Eaton syndrome
Muscle	Septic myopathy
	Cachectic myopathy — with or without disuse atrophy
	Electrolyte disturbances — hypokalemia/hyperkalemia; hypophosphatemia
	Acute quadriplegic myopathy

An alternative pathway of cellular injury is *apoptosis*. This process implies programmed cell death, which may occur in the setting of ischemic stroke, global cerebral ischemia, traumatic brain injury, and possibly intracerebral hemorrhage. Apoptotic cell death can be distinguished histologically from the necrotic cell death of ischemia and is mediated through a different set of biochemical pathways. At present, interventions for prevention and treatment of apoptotic cell death remain less well defined than those for ischemia. Excitotoxicity and mechanisms of cell death are discussed in more detail in Chap. 1.

Cerebral Perfusion and Autoregulation

Brain tissue requires constant perfusion in order to ensure adequate delivery of substrate. The hemodynamic response of the brain has the capacity to preserve perfusion across a wide range of systemic blood pressures. Cerebral perfusion pressure (CPP), defined as the mean systemic arterial pressure (MAP) minus the ICP, provides the driving force for circulation across the capillary beds of the brain. *Autoregulation* refers to the physiologic response whereby cerebral blood flow (CBF) remains relatively constant over a wide range of blood pressures as a consequence of alterations of cerebrovascular resistance (**Fig. 15-1**). If systemic blood pressure drops, cerebral perfusion is preserved through vasodilatation of arterioles in the brain; likewise, arteriolar vasoconstriction occurs at high systemic pressures to prevent hyperperfusion. At the extreme limits of MAP or CPP (high or low), flow becomes directly related to perfusion pressure. These autoregulatory changes occur in the microcirculation and are mediated by vessels below the resolution of those seen on angiography. CBF is also strongly influenced by pH and P_{CO_2}. CBF increases with hypercapnia and acidosis and decreases with hypocapnia and alkalosis. This forms the basis for the use of hyperventilation to lower ICP, and this effect on ICP is mediated through a decrease in intracranial blood volume. Cerebral autoregulation is critical to the normal homeostatic functioning of the brain, and this process may be disordered focally and unpredictably in disease states such as traumatic brain injury and severe focal cerebral ischemia.

Cerebrospinal Fluid and Intracranial Pressure

The cranial contents consist essentially of brain, cerebrospinal fluid (CSF), and blood. CSF is produced principally in the choroid plexus of each lateral ventricle, exits the brain via the foramina of Luschka and Magendi, and flows over the cortex to be absorbed into the venous system along the superior sagittal sinus. Approximately 150 mL of CSF are contained within the ventricles and surrounding the brain and spinal cord; the cerebral blood volume is also ~150 mL. The bony skull offers excellent protection for the brain but allows little tolerance for additional volume. Significant increases in volume eventually result in increased ICP. Obstruction of CSF outflow, edema of cerebral tissue, or increases in volume from tumor or hematoma may increase ICP. Elevated ICP diminishes cerebral perfusion and can lead to tissue ischemia. Ischemia in turn may lead to vasodilatation via autoregulatory mechanisms designed to restore cerebral perfusion. However, vasodilatation also increases cerebral blood volume, which in turn then increases ICP, lowers CPP, and provokes further ischemia (**Fig. 15-2**). This vicious cycle is commonly seen in traumatic brain injury, massive intracerebral hemorrhage, and large hemispheric infarcts with significant tissue shift.

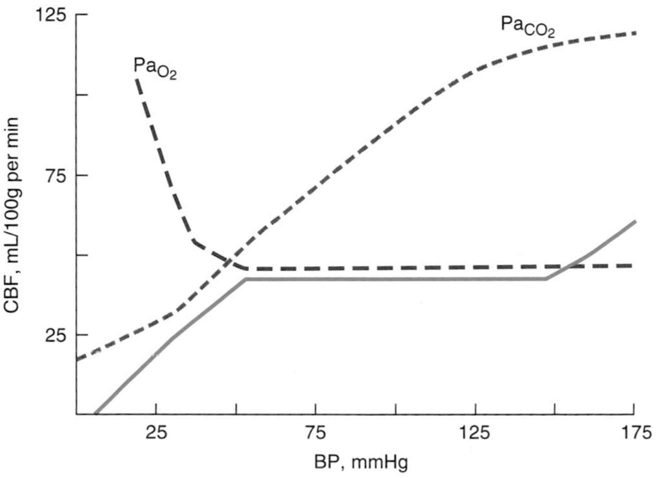

FIGURE 15-1

Autoregulation of cerebral blood flow (solid line). Cerebral perfusion is constant over a wide range of systemic blood pressure. Perfusion is increased in the setting of hypoxia or hypercarbia. BP, blood pressure; CBF, cerebral blood flow. *(Reprinted with permission from Anesthesiology 43:447, 1975. Copyright 1975, Lippincott Company.)*

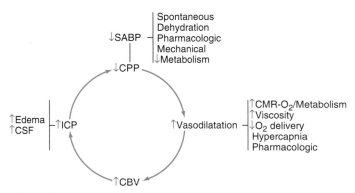

FIGURE 15-2

Ischemia and vasodilatation. Reduced cerebral perfusion pressure (CPP) leads to increased ischemia, vasodilatation, increased intracranial pressure (ICP), and further reductions in CPP, a cycle leading to further neurologic injury. CBV, cerebral blood volume; CMR, cerebral metabolic rate; CSF, cerebrospinal fluid; SABP, systolic arterial blood pressure. *(From MJ Rosner et al: J Neurosurg 83:949, 1995; with permission.)*

APPROACH TO THE PATIENT WITH SEVERE CNS DYSFUNCTION

Critically ill patients with severe central nervous system dysfunction require rapid evaluation and intervention in order to limit primary and secondary brain injury. Initial neurologic evaluation should be performed concurrent with stabilization of basic respiratory, cardiac, and hemodynamic parameters. Significant barriers may exist to neurologic assessment in the critical care unit. Endotracheal intubation and the use of sedative or paralytic agents to facilitate critical care procedures can make clinical assessment challenging.

An impaired level of consciousness is frequent in critically ill patients. The essential first task in assessment is to determine whether the cause of dysfunction is related to a diffuse, usually metabolic, process or whether a focal, usually structural, process is implicated. Examples of diffuse processes include metabolic encephalopathies related to organ failure, drug overdose, or hypoxia-ischemia. Focal processes include ischemic and hemorrhagic stroke and traumatic brain injury, especially with intracranial hematomas. Since these two categories of disorders have fundamentally different causes, treatments, and prognoses, the initial focus is on making this distinction rapidly and accurately. The approach to the confused or comatose patient is discussed in Chap. 8; etiologies are listed in Table 8-1.

Minor focal deficits may be present on the neurologic examination in patients with metabolic encephalopathies. However, the finding of prominent focal signs such as pupillary asymmetry, hemiparesis, gaze palsy, or paraplegia should alert the examiner to the possibility of a structural lesion. All patients with a decreased level of consciousness associated with focal findings should undergo an urgent neuroimaging procedure, as should all patients with coma of unknown etiology. Computed tomographic (CT) scanning is usually the most appropriate initial study because it can be performed quickly in critically ill patients and demonstrates hemorrhage, hydrocephalus, and intracranial tissue shifts well. Magnetic resonance imaging (MRI) may provide more specific information in some situations, such as acute ischemic stroke (diffusion-weighted imaging, DWI) and cerebral venous sinus thrombosis (magnetic resonance venography, MRV). Any suggestion of trauma from the history or examination should alert the examiner to the possibility of cervical spine injury and prompt an imaging evaluation using plain x-rays, MRI, or CT.

Other diagnostic studies are best utilized in specific circumstances, usually when neuroimaging studies fail to reveal a structural lesion and the etiology of the altered mental state remains uncertain. Electroencephalography (EEG) can be important in the evaluation of critically ill patients with severe brain dysfunction. The EEG of metabolic encephalopathy typically reveals generalized slowing. One of the most important uses of EEG is to help exclude inapparent seizures, especially nonconvulsive status epilepticus. Untreated continuous or frequently recurrent seizures may cause neuronal injury, making the diagnosis and treatment of seizure crucial in this patient group. Lumbar puncture (LP) may be necessary to exclude infectious processes, and an elevated opening pressure may be an important clue to cerebral venous sinus thrombosis. In patients with coma or profound encephalopathy, it is preferable to perform a neuroimaging study prior to LP. If bacterial meningitis is suspected, an LP may be performed first or antibiotics may be empirically administered before the diagnostic studies are completed. Standard laboratory evaluation of critically ill patients should include assessment of serum electrolytes (especially sodium and calcium), glucose, renal and hepatic function, complete blood counts, and coagulation. Serum or urine toxicology screens should be performed in patients with encephalopathy of unknown cause. EEG, LP, and other specific laboratory tests are most useful when the mechanism of the altered level of consciousness is uncertain; they are not routinely performed in clear-cut cases of stroke or traumatic brain injury.

Monitoring of ICP can be an important tool in selected patients. Indications for ICP monitoring, as well as specific types of monitors, vary. In general, patients who should be considered for ICP monitoring are those with primary neurologic disorders, such as stroke or traumatic brain injury, who are at significant risk for secondary brain injury due to elevated ICP and decreased CPP. Such patients include those with severe traumatic brain injury resulting in coma [Glasgow Coma Scale (GCS) score of ≤8 (Table 16-1)]; those with large tissue shifts from supratentorial ischemic or hemorrhagic stroke resulting in decreased consciousness; and those with (or at risk for) hydrocephalus from subarachnoid hemorrhage, intraventricular hemorrhage, or posterior fossa stroke. An additional disorder in which ICP monitoring can add important information is fulminant hepatic failure, in which elevated ICP may be treated with barbiturates or, eventually, liver transplantation. In general, ventriculostomy is preferable to ICP monitoring devices that are placed in brain parenchyma, because ventriculostomy allows CSF drainage as a method of treating elevated ICP. However, parenchymal ICP monitoring is most appropriate for patients with diffuse edema and small ventricles (which may make ventriculostomy placement more difficult) or any degree of coagulopathy (in which ventriculostomy carries a higher risk of hemorrhagic complications).

Treatment of Elevated ICP

Elevated ICP may occur in a wide range of disorders including head trauma, intracerebral hemorrhage, subarachnoid hemorrhage with hydrocephalus, and fulminant hepatic failure. Because CSF and blood volume can be redistributed initially, by the time elevated ICP occurs intracranial compliance is severely impaired. At this point, small changes in the volume of CSF, intravascular blood, edema, or a mass lesion may result in significant changes in ICP. Elevated ICP then diminishes cerebral perfusion. This is a fundamental mechanism of secondary ischemic brain injury and constitutes an emergency that requires immediate attention. Specific thresholds of ICP vary, but in general, ICP should be maintained at <20 mmHg and CPP should be maintained at ≥ 70 mmHg.

A number of different interventions may lower ICP, and ideally the selection of treatment will be based on the underlying mechanism responsible for the elevated ICP (**Table 15-2**). For example, in hydrocephalus from subarachnoid hemorrhage, the principal cause of elevated ICP is impairment of CSF drainage. In this setting, ventricular drainage of CSF is likely to be sufficient and most appropriate. In head trauma and stroke, cytotoxic edema may be most responsible, and the use of osmotic diuretics such as mannitol becomes an appropriate early step. As described above, elevated ICP may cause tissue ischemia, and, if cerebral autoregulation is intact, the resulting vasodilatation can lead to a cycle of worsening ischemia. Paradoxically, administration of vasopressor agents to increase mean arterial pressure may actually lower ICP by improving perfusion, thereby allowing autoregulatory vasoconstriction as ischemia is

TABLE 15-2

STEPWISE APPROACH TO TREATMENT OF ELEVATED INTRACRANIAL PRESSURE[a]

Insert ICP monitor — ventriculostomy versus parenchymal device

General goals: maintain ICP < 20 mmHg and CPP > 70 mmHg

For ICP $> 20–25$ mmHg for >5 min:

1. Drain CSF via ventriculostomy (if in place)
2. Elevate head of the bed
3. Osmotherapy — mannitol 25–100 g q4h as needed (maintain serum osmolality <320 mosmol)
4. Glucocorticoids — dexamethasone 4 mg q6h for vasogenic edema from tumor, abscess (avoid glucocorticoids in head trauma, ischemic and hemorrhagic stroke)
5. Sedation (e.g., morphine, propofol, or midazolam); add neuromuscular paralysis if necessary (patient will require endotracheal intubation and mechanical ventilation at this point, if not before)
6. Hyperventilation — to Pa_{CO_2} 30–35 mmHg
7. Pressor therapy — phenylephrine, dopamine, or norepinephrine to maintain adequate MAP to ensure CPP > 70 mmHg (maintain euvolemia to minimize deleterious systemic effects of pressors)
8. Consider second-tier therapies for refractory elevated ICP
   a. High-dose barbiturate therapy ("pentobarb coma")
   b. Aggressive hyperventilation to $Pa_{CO_2} < 30$ mmHg
   c. Hypothermia
   d. Hemicraniectomy

[a]Throughout ICP treatment algorithm, consider repeat head CT to identify mass lesions amenable to surgical evacuation.
Note: CPP, cerebral perfusion pressure; MAP, mean arterial pressure; Pa_{CO_2}, arterial partial pressure of carbon dioxide.

relieved and ultimately decreasing intracranial blood volume.

Early signs of elevated ICP include drowsiness and a diminished level of consciousness. Neuroimaging studies may reveal evidence of edema and mass effect. Hypotonic intravenous fluids should be avoided, and elevation of the head of the bed is recommended. Patients must be carefully observed for risk of aspiration and compromise of the airway as the level of alertness declines. Coma and unilateral pupillary changes are late signs and require immediate intervention. Emergent treatment of elevated ICP is most quickly achieved by intubation and hyperventilation, which causes vasoconstriction and reduces cerebral blood volume. Because of the concern of provoking or worsening cerebral ischemia, hyperventilation is best used for short periods of time until a more definitive treatment can be instituted. Furthermore, the effects of continued hyperventilation on ICP are short-lived, often only for several hours because of the buffering capacity of the cerebral interstitium, and rebound elevated ICP may accompany abrupt discontinuation of hyperventilation. As the level of consciousness declines to coma, the ability to follow the neurologic status of the patient by examination deteriorates and measurement of ICP must be considered. If a ventriculostomy device is in place, direct drainage of CSF to reduce ICP is possible. Finally, high-dose barbiturates or hypothermia are sometimes used for refractory elevated ICP, although these have significant side effects and have not been shown to improve outcome.

Secondary Brain Insults

Patients with primary brain injuries, whether trauma or stroke, are at significant risk for ongoing secondary ischemic brain injury. Because secondary brain injury can be a major determinant of a poor outcome, strategies for minimizing secondary brain insults are an integral part of the critical care of all patients. While elevated ICP may lead to secondary ischemia, most secondary brain injury is mediated through other clinical events that exacerbate the ischemic cascade already initiated by the primary brain injury. Episodes of secondary brain insults are usually not associated with apparent neurologic worsening. Rather, they lead to cumulative injury, which manifests as higher mortality or worsened long-term functional outcome. Thus, clinical strategies involve close monitoring of vital signs and early intervention to prevent secondary ischemia. Avoiding hypotension and hypoxia is critical, as significant hypotensive events (systolic blood pressure < 90 mmHg) as short as 10 min in duration have been shown to adversely influence outcome after traumatic brain injury. Even in patients with stroke or head trauma who do not require ICP monitoring, close attention to adequate cerebral perfusion is warranted. Hypoxia (percutaneous oxygen saturation < 90%), alone or in combination with hypotension, also leads to secondary brain injury. Likewise, fever and hyperglycemia both worsen experimental ischemia and have been associated with worsened clinical outcome after stroke and head trauma. Aggressive control of fever with a goal of normothermia is warranted and can usually be achieved with antipyretic medications and cooling blankets. The use of intravenous insulin infusion is encouraged for control of hyper-

glycemia as this allows better regulation of serum glucose levels than subcutaneous insulin. A reasonable goal is to maintain the serum glucose level at <160 mg/dL, although some experts believe that even tighter control is appropriate. New cerebral monitoring tools that allow continuous evaluation of brain tissue oxygen tension, CBF, and metabolism (via microdialysis) may further improve the management of secondary brain injury.

CRITICAL CARE DISORDERS OF THE CENTRAL NERVOUS SYSTEM ASSOCIATED WITH SYSTEMIC DISEASE

HYPOXIC-ISCHEMIC ENCEPHALOPATHY

This occurs from lack of delivery of oxygen to the brain because of hypotension or respiratory failure. The most common causes are myocardial infarction, cardiac arrest, shock, asphyxiation, paralysis of respiration, and carbon monoxide or cyanide poisoning. In some circumstances, hypoxia may predominate. Carbon monoxide and cyanide poisoning are termed *histotoxic hypoxia* since they cause a direct impairment of the respiratory chain.

Clinical Manifestations

Mild degrees of pure hypoxia, such as occur at high altitudes, cause impaired judgment, inattentiveness, motor incoordination, and, at times, euphoria. However, with hypoxia-ischemia, such as occurs with circulatory arrest, consciousness is lost within seconds. If circulation is restored within 3 to 5 min, full recovery may occur, but if hypoxia-ischemia lasts beyond 3 to 5 min, some degree of permanent cerebral damage is the rule. Except in extreme cases, it may be difficult to judge the precise degree of hypoxia-ischemia, and some patients make a relatively full recovery after even 8 to 10 min of global cerebral ischemia. The distinction between pure hypoxia and hypoxia-ischemia is important, since a Pa_{O_2} as low as 20 mmHg (2.7 kPa) can be well tolerated if it develops gradually and normal blood pressure is maintained, but short durations of very low or absent cerebral circulation may result in permanent impairment.

Clinical examination at different time points after a hypoxic-ischemic insult (especially cardiac arrest) is useful in assessing prognosis for long-term neurologic outcome. The prognosis is better for patients with intact brainstem function, as indicated by normal pupillary light responses and intact oculocephalic (doll's-eyes), oculovestibular (caloric),

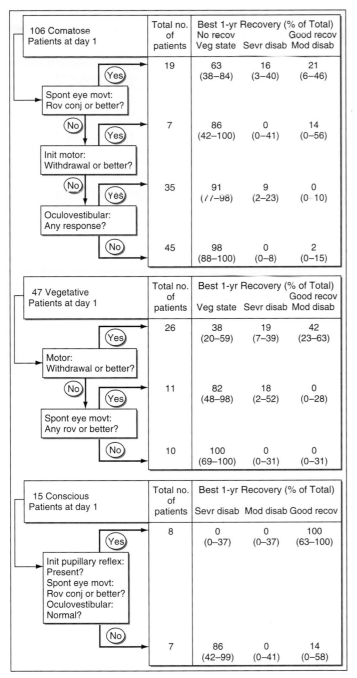

106 Comatose Patients at day 1	Total no. of patients	Best 1-yr Recovery (% of Total) No recov		
		Veg state	Sevr disab	Mod disab Good recov
Spont eye movt: Rov conj or better? — Yes	19	63 (38–84)	16 (3–40)	21 (6–46)
Init motor: Withdrawal or better? — No → Yes	7	86 (42–100)	0 (0–41)	14 (0–56)
Oculovestibular: Any response? — No → Yes	35	91 (77–98)	9 (2–23)	0 (0–10)
No	45	98 (88–100)	0 (0–8)	2 (0–15)

47 Vegetative Patients at day 1	Total no. of patients	Best 1-yr Recovery (% of Total)		
		Veg state	Sevr disab	Good recov Mod disab
Motor: Withdrawal or better? — Yes	26	38 (20–59)	19 (7–39)	42 (23–63)
Spont eye movt: Any rov or better? — No → Yes	11	82 (48–98)	18 (2–52)	0 (0–28)
No	10	100 (69–100)	0 (0–31)	0 (0–31)

15 Conscious Patients at day 1	Total no. of patients	Best 1-yr Recovery (% of Total)		
		Sevr disab	Mod disab	Good recov
Init pupillary reflex: Present? Spont eye movt: Rov conj or better? Oculovestibular: Normal? — Yes	8	0 (0–37)	0 (0–37)	100 (63–100)
No	7	86 (42–99)	0 (0–41)	14 (0–58)

FIGURE 15-3

Clinical examination at day 1 provides useful prognostic information in hypoxic-ischemic encephalopathy. Numbers in parentheses represent 95% confidence intervals. Recov, recovery; veg, vegetative; sev, severe; mod, moderate; spont eye movt, spontaneous eye movement; rov conj, roving conjugate. *(From DE Levy et al: JAMA 253:1420, 1985; with permission.)*

light reflex or absence of a motor response to pain on day 3 following the injury. Electrophysiologically, the finding of bilateral absence of the early cortical somatosensory evoked response (SSEPs) in the first week also conveys a poor prognosis. Whether administration of mild hypothermia after cardiac arrest (see "Treatment") will alter the usefulness of these clinical and electrophysiologic predictors is unknown. Long-term consequences of hypoxic-ischemic encephalopathy include persistent coma or vegetative state (Chap. 8), dementia, visual agnosia, parkinsonism, choreoathetosis, cerebellar ataxia, myoclonus, seizures, and an amnestic state, which may be a consequence of selective damage to the hippocampus.

Pathologic Findings

Principal histologic findings are extensive multifocal or diffuse laminar cortical necrosis, with almost invariable involvement of the hippocampus. Laminar necrosis may be visible by MRI (**Fig. 15-4**). The hippocampal CA1 neurons are vulnerable to even brief episodes of hypoxia-ischemia, perhaps explaining why selective persistent memory deficits may occur after brief cardiac arrest. Scattered small areas of infarction or neuronal loss may be present in the basal ganglia, hypothalamus, or brainstem. In some cases, extensive bilateral thalamic scarring may affect pathways that mediate arousal, and this pathology may be responsible for the persistent vegetative state. A specific form of hypoxic-ischemic encephalopathy, so-called watershed infarcts,

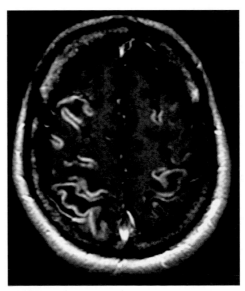

FIGURE 15-4

Laminar cortical necrosis in hypoxic-ischemic encephalopathy. T1-weighted postcontrast magnetic resonance image shows cortical enhancement in a watershed distribution consistent with laminar necrosis.

and corneal reflexes (**Fig. 15-3**). Absence of these reflexes and the presence of persistently dilated pupils that do not react to light are grave prognostic signs. A uniformly dismal prognosis from hypoxic-ischemic coma is conveyed by the clinical findings of absence of pupillary occurs at the distal territories between the major cerebral arteries and can cause cognitive deficits, including visual agnosia, and weakness that is greater in proximal than in distal muscle groups.

Diagnosis

Diagnosis is based upon the history of a hypoxic-ischemic event such as cardiac arrest. Blood pressure < 70 mmHg systolic or Pa_{O_2} < 40 mmHg is usually necessary, although both absolute levels as well as duration of exposure are important determinants of cellular injury. Occasionally the clinical and radiographic features of a hypoxic-ischemic syndrome are seen without documented profound hypotension or hypoxia. Carbon monoxide intoxication can be confirmed by measurement of carboxyhemoglobin and is suggested by a cherry red color of the skin, although the latter is an inconsistent clinical finding.

TREATMENT FOR HYPOXIC-ISCHEMIC ENCEPHALOPATHY

Treatment should be directed at restoration of normal cardiorespiratory function. This includes securing a clear airway, ensuring adequate oxygenation and ventilation, and restoring cerebral perfusion, whether by cardiopulmonary resuscitation, fluid, pressors, or cardiac pacing. Hypothermia may target the neuronal cell injury cascade and has substantial neuroprotective properties in experimental models of brain injury. In two recently reported clinical trials, mild hypothermia (33°C) improved functional outcome in patients who remained comatose after resuscitation from a cardiac arrest. Treatment was initiated within minutes of cardiac resuscitation and continued for 12 h in one study and 24 h in the other. Potential complications of hypothermia treatment include coagulopathy and an increased risk of infection. Based upon these studies, the International Liaison Committee on Resuscitation issued the following advisory statement in 2003: Unconscious adult patients with spontaneous circulation after out-of-hospital cardiac arrest should be cooled to 32 to 34°C for 12 to 24 h when the initial rhythm was ventricular fibrillation.

Severe carbon monoxide intoxication may be treated with hyperbaric oxygen. Anticonvulsants may be needed to control seizures, although these are not usually given prophylactically. Posthypoxic

---

myoclonus may respond to oral administration of clonazepam at doses of 1.5 to 10 mg daily or valproate at doses of 300 mg to 1200 mg daily in divided doses. Myoclonic status epilepticus after a severe hypoxic-ischemic insult portends a universally poor prognosis, even if seizures are controlled.

DELAYED POSTANOXIC ENCEPHALOPATHY

Delayed postanoxic encephalopathy is an uncommon phenomenon in which patients appear to make an initial recovery from hypoxic-ischemic insult but then develop a relapse characterized by apathy, confusion, and agitation. Progressive neurologic deficits may include shuffling gait, diffuse rigidity and spasticity, persistent parkinsonism or myoclonus, and, on occasion, coma and death after 1 to 2 weeks. Widespread cerebral demyelination may be present.

Carbon monoxide and cyanide intoxication can also cause a delayed encephalopathy. Little clinical impairment is evident when the patient first regains consciousness, but a parkinsonian syndrome characterized by akinesia and rigidity without tremor may develop. Symptoms can worsen over months, accompanied by increasing evidence of damage in the basal ganglia as seen on both CT and MRI.

METABOLIC ENCEPHALOPATHIES

Altered mental states, variously described as confusion, delirium, disorientation, and encephalopathy, are present in many patients with severe illness in an intensive care unit (ICU). Older patients are particularly vulnerable to delirium, a confusional state characterized by disordered perception, frequent hallucinations, delusions, and sleep disturbance. This is often attributed to medication effects, sleep deprivation, pain, and anxiety. The term *ICU psychosis* has been used to describe a mental state with profound agitation occurring in this setting. The presence of family members in the ICU may help to calm and orient agitated patients, and in severe cases, low doses of neuroleptics (e.g., haloperidol 0.5 to 1 mg) can be useful. Ultimately, the psychosis resolves with improvement in the underlying illness and a return to familiar surroundings.

In the ICU setting, several metabolic causes of an altered level of consciousness predominate. Hypercarbic encephalopathy can present with headache, confusion, stupor, or coma. Hypoventilation syndrome occurs most frequently in patients with a history of chronic CO_2 retention who are receiving oxygen therapy for emphysema or chronic pulmonary disease. The elevated Pa_{CO_2}

leading to CO_2 narcosis may have a direct anesthetic effect, and cerebral vasodilatation from increased Pa_{CO_2} can lead to increased ICP. Hepatic encephalopathy is suggested by asterixis and can occur in chronic liver failure or acute fulminant hepatic failure. Both hyperglycemia and hypoglycemia can cause encephalopathy, as can hypernatremia and hyponatremia. Confusion, impairment of eye movements, and gait ataxia are the hallmarks of acute Wernicke's disease (see below).

SEPTIC ENCEPHALOPATHY

Pathogenesis

In patients with sepsis, the systemic response to infectious agents leads to the release of circulating inflammatory mediators that appear to contribute to encephalopathy. Critical illness, in association with the systemic inflammatory response syndrome (SIRS), can lead to multisystem organ failure. This syndrome can occur in the setting of apparent sepsis, severe burns, or trauma, even without clear identification of an infectious agent. Many patients with critical illness, sepsis, or SIRS develop encephalopathy without obvious explanation. This condition is broadly termed *septic encephalopathy*. While the specific mediators leading to neurologic dysfunction remain uncertain, it is clear that the encephalopathy is not simply the result of metabolic derangements of multiorgan failure. The cytokines tumor necrosis factor α, interleukin (IL) 1, IL-2, and IL-6 are thought to play a role in this syndrome.

Diagnosis

Septic encephalopathy presents clinically as a diffuse dysfunction of the brain without prominent focal findings. Confusion, disorientation, agitation, and fluctuations in level of alertness are typical. In more profound cases, especially with hemodynamic compromise, the decrease in level of alertness can be more prominent, at times resulting in coma. Hyperreflexia and frontal release signs such as a grasp or snout reflex (Chap. 7) can be seen. Abnormal movements such as myoclonus, tremor, or asterixis can occur. Septic encephalopathy is quite common, occurring in the majority of patients with sepsis and multisystem organ failure. Diagnosis is often difficult because of the multiple potential causes of neurologic dysfunction in critically ill patients, and requires exclusion of structural, metabolic, toxic, and infectious (e.g., meningitis or encephalitis) causes. Although the mortality of patients with septic encephalopathy severe enough to produce coma approaches 50%, this reflects the severity of the underlying critical illness and is not a direct result of the septic encephalopathy. Neurologically, successful treatment of the underlying critical illness almost always

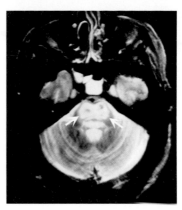

FIGURE 15-5
Central pontine myelinolysis. Axial T2-weighted magnetic resonance scan through the pons reveals a symmetric area of abnormal high signal intensity within the basis pontis (*arrows*).

results in complete resolution of the encephalopathy, without significant residua.

CENTRAL PONTINE MYELINOLYSIS

This disorder typically presents in a devastating fashion as quadriplegia and pseudobulbar palsy. Predisposing factors include severe underlying medical illness or nutritional deficiency; most cases are associated with rapid correction of hyponatremia or with hyperosmolar states. The pathology consists of demyelination without inflammation in the base of the pons, with relative sparing of axons and nerve cells. MRI is useful in establishing the diagnosis (**Fig. 15-5**) and may also identify partial forms that present as confusion, dysarthria, and/or disturbances of conjugate gaze without quadriplegia. Therapeutic guidelines for the restoration of severe hyponatremia should aim for gradual correction, i.e., by ≤10 mmol/L (10 meq/L) within 24 h and 20 mmol/L (20 meq/L) within 48 h.

WERNICKE'S DISEASE

Wernicke's disease is a common and preventable disorder due to a deficiency of thiamine. In the United States, alcoholics account for most cases, but patients with malnutrition due to hyperemesis, starvation, renal dialysis, cancer, or AIDS are also at risk. The characteristic clinical triad is that of ophthalmoplegia, ataxia, and global confusion. However, only one-third of patients with acute Wernicke's disease present with the classic clinical triad. Most patients are profoundly disoriented, indifferent, and inattentive, although rarely they have an agitated delirium related to ethanol withdrawal. If the disease is not treated, stupor, coma, and death may ensue. Ocular motor abnormalities include horizontal nystagmus on lateral gaze, lateral rectus palsy (usually bilateral), conjugate gaze palsies, and rarely ptosis. Gait ataxia probably results from a combination of polyneuropathy, cerebellar involvement, and vestibular paresis. The pupils are usually spared, but they may become miotic with advanced disease.

Wernicke's disease is usually associated with other manifestations of nutritional disease, such as polyneuropathy. Rarely, amblyopia or myelopathy occurs. Tachycardia and postural hypotension may be related to impaired function of the autonomic nervous system or to the co-existence of cardiovascular beriberi. Patients who recover show improvement in ocular palsies within hours after the administration of thiamine, but horizontal nystagmus may persist. Ataxia improves more slowly than the ocular motor abnormalities. Approximately half recover incompletely and are left with a slow, shuffling, wide-based gait and an inability to tandem walk. Apathy, drowsiness, and confusion improve more gradually. As these symptoms recede, an amnestic state with impairment in recent memory and learning may become more apparent (*Korsakoff's psychosis*). Korsakoff's psychosis is frequently persistent; the residual mental state is characterized by gaps in memory, confabulation, and disordered temporal sequencing.

Pathology

Lesions in the periventricular regions of the diencephalon and brainstem as well as the superior vermis of the cerebellum consist of symmetric discoloration of structures surrounding the third ventricle, aqueduct, and fourth ventricle, with petechial hemorrhages in occasional acute cases and atrophy of the mamillary bodies in most chronic cases. There is frequently endothelial proliferation, demyelination, and some neuronal loss. These changes may be detected by MRI scanning (**Fig. 15–6**).

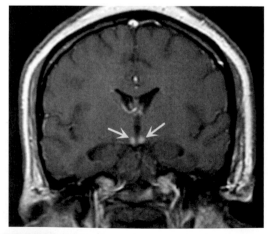

FIGURE 15-6

Wernicke's disease. Coronal T1-weighted postcontrast magnetic resonance image reveals abnormal enhancement of the mammillary bodies (*arrows*), typical of acute Wernicke's encephalopathy.

The amnestic defect is related to lesions in the dorsal medial nuclei of the thalamus.

Pathogenesis

Thiamine is a cofactor of several enzymes, including transketolase, pyruvate dehydrogenase, and α-ketoglutarate dehydrogenase. Thiamine deficiency produces a diffuse decrease in cerebral glucose utilization and results in mitochondrial damage. Glutamate accumulates owing to impairment of α-ketoglutarate dehydrogenase activity and, in combination with the energy deficiency, may result in excitotoxic cell damage.

TREATMENT FOR WERNICKE'S DISEASE

Wernicke's disease is a medical emergency and requires immediate administration of thiamine, in a dose of 100 mg either intravenously or intramuscularly. The dose should be given daily until the patient resumes a normal diet and should be begun prior to treatment with intravenous glucose solutions. Glucose infusions may precipitate Wernicke's disease in a previously unaffected patient or cause a rapid worsening of an early form of the disease. For this reason, thiamine should be administered to all alcoholic patients requiring parenteral glucose.

CRITICAL CARE DISORDERS OF THE PERIPHERAL NERVOUS SYSTEM ASSOCIATED WITH SYSTEMIC DISEASE

Critical illness with disorders of the peripheral nervous system (PNS) arises in two contexts: (1) primary neurologic diseases that require critical care interventions such as intubation and mechanical ventilation, and (2) secondary PNS manifestations of systemic critical illness, often involving multisystem organ failure. The former include acute polyneuropathies such as Guillain-Barré syndrome (Chap. 35), neuromuscular junction disorders including myasthenia gravis (Chap. 36) and botulism, and primary muscle disorders such as polymyositis (Chap. 39). The latter result either from the systemic disease itself or as a consequence of interventions.

General principles of respiratory evaluation in patients with PNS involvement, regardless of cause, include assessment of pulmonary mechanics, such as maximal inspiratory force (MIF) and vital capacity (VC), and evaluation of strength of bulbar muscles. Regardless of the cause of weakness, endotracheal intubation should be considered when the MIF falls to < -25 cmH$_2$O or the VC is <1 L. Also, patients with severe palatal weakness may require endotracheal intubation in order to prevent acute upper airway obstruction or recurrent aspiration. Arterial blood gases and percutaneous oxygen saturation are used to follow patients with potential respiratory compromise from PNS dysfunction. However, intubation and mechanical ventilation should be undertaken based on clinical assessment rather than waiting until oxygen saturation drops or CO$_2$ retention develops from hypoventilation.

NEUROPATHY

While encephalopathy may be the most obvious neurologic dysfunction in critically ill patients, dysfunction of the PNS is also quite common. It is typically present in patients with prolonged critical illnesses lasting several weeks and involving sepsis; clinical suspicion is aroused when there is failure to wean from mechanical ventilation despite improvement of the underlying sepsis and critical illness. *Critical illness polyneuropathy* refers to the most common PNS complication related to critical illness; it is seen in the setting of prolonged critical illness, sepsis, and multisystem organ failure. Neurologic findings include diffuse weakness, decreased reflexes, and distal sensory loss. Electrophysiologic studies demonstrate a diffuse, symmetric, distal axonal sensorimotor neuropathy, and pathologic studies have confirmed axonal degeneration. The precise mechanism of critical illness polyneuropathy remains unclear, but circulating factors such as cytokines, which are associated with sepsis and SIRS, are thought to play a role. It has been reported that up to 70% of patients with the sepsis syndrome have some degree of neuropathy, although far fewer have a clinical syndrome profound enough to cause severe respiratory muscle weakness requiring prolonged mechanical ventilation or resulting in failure to wean. Recent studies suggest that aggressive glycemic control with insulin infusions decreases the risk of critical illness polyneuropathy. Treatment is supportive, with specific intervention directed at treating the underlying illness. While spontaneous recovery is usually seen, the time course may extend over weeks to months and necessitate long-term ventilatory support and care even after the underlying critical illness has resolved.

DISORDERS OF NEUROMUSCULAR TRANSMISSION

A defect in neuromuscular transmission may be a source of weakness in critically ill patients. Myasthenia gravis may be a consideration; however, persistent weakness secondary to impaired neuromuscular junction transmission is almost always due to administration of drugs. A number of medications impair neuromuscular transmission; these include antibiotics, especially aminoglycosides, and beta-blocking agents. In the ICU, the nondepolarizing neuromuscular blocking agents (nd-NMBAs), also known as muscle relaxants, are most commonly responsible. Included in this group of drugs are such agents as pancuronium, vecuronium, rocuronium, and atracurium. They are often used to facilitate mechanical ventilation or other critical care procedures, but with prolonged use persistent neuromuscular blockade may result in weakness even after discontinuation of these agents hours or days earlier. Risk factors for this prolonged action of neuromuscular blocking agents include female sex, metabolic acidosis, and renal failure.

Prolonged neuromuscular blockade does not appear to produce permanent damage to the PNS. Once the offending medications are discontinued, full strength is restored, although this may take days. In general, the lowest dose of neuromuscular blocking agent should be used to achieve the desired result, and, when these agents are used in the ICU, a peripheral nerve stimulator should be used to monitor neuromuscular junction function.

MYOPATHY

Critically ill patients, especially those with sepsis, frequently develop muscle wasting, often in the face of seemingly adequate nutritional support. The assumption has been that this represents a catabolic myopathy brought about as a result of multiple factors, including elevated cortisol and catecholamine release and other circulating factors induced by the SIRS. In this syndrome, known as *cachectic myopathy,* serum creatine kinase levels and electromyography (EMG) are normal. Muscle biopsy shows type II fiber atrophy. Panfascicular muscle fiber necrosis may also occur in the setting of profound sepsis. This so-called *septic myopathy* is characterized clinically by weakness progressing to a profound level over just a few days. There may be associated elevations in serum creatine kinase and urine myoglobin. Both EMG and muscle biopsy may be normal initially but eventually show abnormal spontaneous activity and panfascicular necrosis with an accompanying inflammatory reaction.

Acute quadriplegic myopathy describes a clinical syndrome of severe weakness seen in the setting of glucocorticoid and nd-NMBA use. The most frequent scenario in which this is encountered is the asthmatic patient who requires high-dose glucocorticoids and nd-NMBA to facilitate mechanical ventilation. This muscle disorder is not due to prolonged action of nd–NMBAs at the neuromuscular junction but, rather, is an actual myopathy with muscle damage; it has occasionally been described with high–dose glucocorticoid use alone. Clinically this syndrome is most often recognized when a patient fails to wean from mechanical ventilation despite resolution of the primary pulmonary process. Pathologically, there may be vacuolar changes in both type I and type II muscle fibers with evidence of regeneration. Acute quadriplegic myopathy has a good prognosis. If patients survive their underlying critical illness, the myopathy invariably improves and patients usually return to normal. However, because this syndrome is a result of true muscle damage, not just prolonged blockade at the neuromuscular junction, this process may take weeks or months, and tracheostomy with prolonged ventilatory support may be necessary. At present, it is unclear how to prevent this myopathic complication, except by avoiding use of nd–NMBAs, a strategy not always possible. Monitoring with a peripheral nerve stimulator can help to avoid the overuse of these agents. However, this is more likely to prevent the complication of prolonged neuromuscular junction blockade than it is to prevent this myopathy.

FURTHER READINGS

Holzer M et al: Hypothermia for neuroprotection after cardiac arrest: Systematic review and individual patient data meta-analysis. Crit Care Med 33:414, 2005

The Hypothermia After Cardiac Arrest Study Group: Mild therapeutic hypothermia to improve the neurologic outcome after cardiac arrest. N Engl J Med 346:549, 2002

Latronico N et al: Neuromuscular sequelae of critical illness. Curr Opin Crit Care 11:381, 2005

Review of an important and commonly overlooked neurologic complication of critical illness that is associated with significant morbidity and mortality.

Liou AK et al: To die or not to die for neurons in ischemia, traumatic brain injury and epilepsy: A review on the stress-activated signaling pathways and apoptotic pathways. Prog Neurobiol 69:103, 2003

Nolan JP et al: Therapeutic hypothermia after cardiac arrest: An advisory statement by the Advanced Life Support Task Force of the International Liaison Committee on Resuscitation. Circulation 108:118, 2003

Van den Berghe G et al: Insulin therapy protects the central and peripheral nervous system of intensive care patients. Neurology 64:1348, 2005

Tight glycemic control in critically ill patients decreases frequency of encephalopathy and neuropathy and improves outcome.

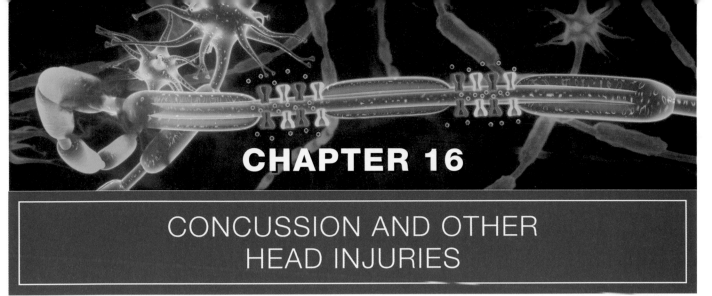

CHAPTER 16

CONCUSSION AND OTHER HEAD INJURIES

Allan H. Ropper

Almost 10 million head injuries occur annually in the United States, about 20% of which are serious enough to cause brain damage. Among men under 35 years, accidents, usually motor vehicle collisions, are the chief cause of death, and >70% of these involve head injury. Furthermore, minor head injuries are so common that almost all physicians will be called upon to provide immediate care or to see patients who are suffering from various sequelae.

Medical personnel caring for head injury patients should be aware that

(1) spinal injury often accompanies head injury, and care must be taken to prevent compression of the spinal cord due to instability of the spinal column;

(2) intoxication is an important accompaniment of traumatic brain injury and, when appropriate, testing should be carried out for drugs and alcohol; and

(3) systemic injuries, including rupture of abdominal organs, may produce vascular collapse or respiratory compromise requiring immediate attention.

TYPES OF HEAD INJURIES

CONCUSSION

This refers to an immediate but transient loss of consciousness that is associated with a short period of amnesia. Patients may appear dazed or report feeling "star struck." It typically occurs after a blunt forward impact that creates a sudden deceleration of the cranium and a movement of the brain within the skull. Severe concussion may precipitate a brief convulsion or autonomic signs such as facial pallor, bradycardia, faintness with mild hypotension, or sluggish pupillary reaction, but most patients are soon neurologically normal. The mechanism of loss of consciousness in concussion is believed to be a transient electrophysiologic dysfunction of the reticular activating system in the upper midbrain caused by rotation of the cerebral hemispheres on the relatively fixed brainstem (Chap. 8).

Gross and light-microscopic changes in the brain are usually absent following concussion, but biochemical and ultrastructural changes, such as mitochondrial ATP depletion and local disruption of the blood-brain barrier, suggest that transient abnormalities occur. Computed tomography (CT) and magnetic resonance imaging (MRI) scans are usually normal; however, ~3% of patients will be found to have an intracranial hemorrhage of some type.

The amnesia of concussion typically occurs in individuals who have experienced at least a few moments of unresponsiveness, but on rare occasions no loss of consciousness is reported. The memory loss spans the time of, and moments before, mild impact injuries but may encompass previous weeks (rarely months) in cases of more severe trauma. In most cases, the extent of retrograde amnesia correlates with the severity of injury. Any anterograde amnesia is usually brief and disappears rapidly in alert patients. Memory is regained in an orderly way from the most distant to recent memories, with islands of amnesia occasionally remaining in severe cases. The mechanism of peritraumatic amnesia is not known. Hysterical posttraumatic amnesia is not uncommon and should be suspected when inexplicable abnormalities of behavior occur, such as recounting events that cannot be recalled on later testing, a bizarre affect, forgetting one's own name, or a persistent anterograde deficit that is excessive in comparison with the degree of injury. For further discussion of amnesia, see Chap. 7.

A single, uncomplicated head injury only infrequently produces permanent neurobehavioral changes in patients who are free of preexisting psychiatric problems and substance abuse. These minor problems in memory and concentration may have an anatomical correlate in small shearing or other microscopic lesions (see below).

CONTUSION, BRAIN HEMORRHAGE, AND AXONAL SHEARING LESIONS

A surface bruise of the brain, or *contusion,* consists of varying degrees of petechial hemorrhage, edema, and tissue destruction. Contusions and deeper hemorrhages result from mechanical forces that displace the hemispheres forcefully relative to the skull by deceleration of the brain against the inner skull, either under a point of impact (coup lesion) or, as the brain swings back, in the antipolar area (contrecoup lesion). Trauma sufficient to cause prolonged unconsciousness usually produces some degree of contusion. Blunt impact, as from an automobile dashboard or from falling forward while drunk, typically causes contusions on the orbital surfaces of the frontal lobes and the anterior and basal portions of the temporal lobes. With lateral forces the contusions are situated on the lateral convexity of the hemispheres. In both instances there may be contrecoup contusions on the opposite side of the impact. The clinical signs are determined by the location and size of the contusion; a hemiparesis or gaze preference is fairly typical. Large bilateral contusions produce coma with extensor posturing. Contusions limited to the frontal lobes cause an abulic-taciturn state, and those in the temporal lobe may cause an aggressive, combative, or delirious syndrome, described below.

Contusions are visible on CT and MRI scans, appearing early as inhomogeneous hyperdensities on CT and as hyperintensities on MRI; the signal changes reflect small scattered areas of cortical and subcortical blood and localized brain edema (**Fig. 16-1**); there is also some degree of subarachnoid bleeding, which may be detected by scans or lumbar puncture.

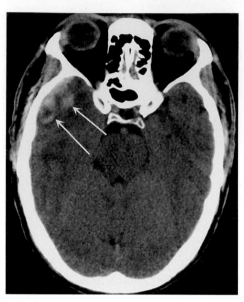

FIGURE 16-1

Traumatic cerebral contusion. Noncontrast CT scan demonstrating a hyperdense hemorrhagic region in the anterior temporal lobe.

Subacutely, contusions acquire a surrounding contrast enhancement that may be mistaken for tumor or abscess. Glial and macrophage reactions may result in scarred, hemosiderin-stained depressions on the surface (*plaques jaunes*) that are the main source of posttraumatic epilepsy.

Torsion or shearing forces in the brain can cause basal ganglial and other deep hematomas independent of surface damage. Large single hemorrhages after minor trauma may be associated with a bleeding diathesis or cerebrovascular amyloidosis in the elderly. For unexplained reasons, deep cerebral hemorrhages may not develop until several days after severe injury. Sudden neurologic deterioration in a comatose patient or a sudden rise in intracranial pressure (ICP) should therefore prompt investigation with a CT scan.

Another type of deep white matter lesion consists of widespread acute disruption, or shearing, of axons at the time of impact. Most characteristic are small areas of tissue disruption in the corpus callosum and dorsolateral pons. The presence of widespread axonal damage of both hemispheres, a state called *diffuse axonal injury,* explains persistent coma and the vegetative state, but small ischemic-hemorrhagic lesions in the midbrain and thalamus are as often the cause. Only severe shearing lesions that contain blood are visualized by CT, usually in the corpus callosum and centrum semiovale (**Fig. 16-2**); however, within days of the injury, MRI scan demonstrates such lesions throughout the white matter with the use of special imaging sequences.

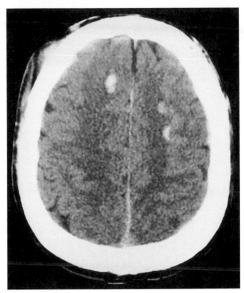

FIGURE 16-2
Multiple small areas of hemorrhage and tissue disruption in the white matter of the frontal lobes on noncontrast CT scan. These appear to reflect an extreme type of the diffuse axonal shearing lesions that occur with closed head injury.

SKULL FRACTURES

A blow to the skull causes a fracture if the elastic tolerance of the bone is exceeded. Intracranial lesions accompany two-thirds of skull fractures, and the presence of a skull fracture increases manyfold the chances of an underlying subdural or epidural hematoma. Consequently, fractures are primarily markers of the site and severity of injury. They provide pathways for entry of bacteria (meningitis) or air (pneumocephalus) to the cerebrospinal fluid (CSF) and for leakage of CSF out through the dura.

Linear fractures, which are most often associated with subdural or epidural hematomas, account for 80% of all skull fractures. They are usually oriented from the point of impact toward the base of the skull. Basilar skull fractures are often extensions of adjacent fractures over the convexity of the skull but may occur independently owing to stresses on the floor of the middle cranial fossa or occiput. They are located parallel to the petrous bone or along the sphenoid bone toward the sella turcica and ethmoidal groove. Although most are uncomplicated, basilar skull fractures can cause CSF leakage, pneumocephalus, and cavernous-carotid fistulas. Hemotympanum (blood behind the tympanic membrane), delayed ecchymosis over the mastoid process (Battle's sign), or periorbital ecchymosis ("racoon sign") all signify fracture of the base of the skull. Because routine x-ray examination may fail to disclose basilar fractures, they should be suspected if these clinical signs are present.

CSF may leak through the cribriform plate or the adjacent sinus and manifest as a watery discharge from the nose (CSF rhinorrhea). Persistent rhinorrhea and recurrent meningitis are indications for surgical repair of torn dura underlying the fracture. The precise site of the leak is often difficult to determine, but useful diagnostic tests include the instillation of water-soluble contrast into the CSF followed by CT with the patient in various positions, and injection of radionuclide compounds or fluorescein into the CSF with an assessment of uptake of these compounds by absorptive nasal pledgets. The site of an intermittent leak is rarely delineated, and most resolve spontaneously. Sellar fractures, even ones associated with serious neuroendocrine dysfunction, are sometimes radiologically occult. Fractures of the dorsum sella may cause sixth or seventh nerve palsies or optic nerve damage. An air-fluid level in the sphenoid sinus suggests a fracture of the sellar floor.

Petrous bone fractures, especially those oriented along the long axis of the bone, may be associated with facial palsy, disruption of ear ossicles, and CSF otorrhea. Transverse petrous fractures are less common; they almost always damage the cochlea or labyrinths and often the facial nerve. External bleeding from the ear is usually from local abrasion of the external canal but can also result from petrous fracture.

Fractures of the frontal bone are often depressed, involving the frontal and paranasal sinuses and the orbits; permanent anosmia results if the olfactory filaments in the cribriform plate are disrupted. Depressed skull fractures are typically compound, but they are often neurologically asymptomatic because the impact energy is dissipated in breaking the bone; however, some are associated with brain contusions and focal neurologic signs caused by damage to the underlying cortical area. Prompt debridement and exploration of compound fractures are required in order to avoid infection.

CRANIAL NERVE INJURIES

The cranial nerves likely to be injured with head trauma include the olfactory, optic, oculomotor, and trochlear nerves; the first and second branches of the trigeminal nerve; and the facial and auditory nerves. Anosmia and an apparent loss of taste (actually a loss of perception of aromatic flavors, with elementary tastes retained) occur in ~10% of persons with serious head injuries, particularly after falls on the back of the head. This sequela results from displacement of the brain and shearing of the olfactory nerve filaments and may occur in the absence of a fracture. Recovery is the rule, leaving residual hyposmia, but if bilateral anosmia persists for several months, the prognosis is poor. Partial optic nerve injuries from closed trauma result in blurring of vision, central or paracentral scotomas, or sector defects. Direct orbital injury may cause short-lived blurred vision for close objects and pupillary paralysis because of reversible iridoplegia. Diplopia limited to downward gaze and corrected when the head is tilted away from the affected eye indicates trochlear nerve damage. It occurs as an isolated problem after minor injury and can develop after a delay of several days. Direct facial nerve injury by a basal fracture is present immediately in 3% of severe injuries; it may also be delayed 5 to 7 days. Fractures through the petrous bone, particularly the less common transverse type, are liable to produce this injury. Delayed facial palsy, the mechanism of which is unknown, has a good prognosis. Injury to the eighth cranial nerve from a fracture of the petrous bone causes loss of hearing, vertigo, and nystagmus immediately after injury. Deafness from nerve injury must be distinguished from that due to rupture of the eardrum, blood in the middle ear, or disruption of the ossicles from fracture through the middle ear. A high-tone hearing loss occurs with direct cochlear concussion.

SEIZURES

Convulsions are surprisingly uncommon immediately after a head injury, but a brief period of tonic extensor posturing or a few clonic movements of the limbs just after the moment of impact may occur. However, the superficial cortical scars that evolve from contusions are highly epileptogenic and may later manifest as seizures, even after many years (Chap. 14). The severity of injury determines the risk of future seizures. It has been estimated that 17% of individuals with brain contusion, subdural hematoma, or prolonged loss of consciousness will develop a seizure disorder and that this risk extends for an indefinite period of time, whereas the risk is only 2% after mild injury. The majority of convulsions in the latter group occur within 5 years of injury.

SUBDURAL AND EPIDURAL HEMATOMAS

Hemorrhages beneath the dura (subdural) or between the dura and skull (epidural) may be associated with contusions and other injuries, making it difficult to determine their relative contribution to the clinical state. However, subdural and epidural hematomas as often occur as the sole manifestation of injury, and each has characteristic clinical and radiologic features. Because the mass effect and the rise in ICP caused by these hemorrhages may be life threatening, it is imperative that hemorrhages be identified immediately by CT or MRI scan and evacuated when appropriate.

Acute Subdural Hematoma

These lesions become symptomatic minutes or hours after injury. Up to one-third of patients have a lucid interval before coma supervenes, but most are drowsy or comatose from the moment of injury. Direct cranial trauma is not required for acute subdural hemorrhage to occur; acceleration forces alone, as from whiplash, are adequate, especially in the elderly and those taking anticoagulant medications. A unilateral headache and slightly enlarged pupil on the same side are frequently but not invariably found. Stupor or coma, a hemiparesis, and unilateral pupillary enlargement are the signs of larger hematomas. In an acutely deteriorating patient with diminished alertness and with pupillary enlargement, burr (drainage) holes or an emergency craniotomy are appropriate. Small subdural hematomas may be asymptomatic and usually do not require evacuation. A subacute syndrome due to subdural hematoma occurs days to weeks after injury with drowsiness, headache, confusion, or mild hemiparesis; it is seen in alcoholics and in the elderly. Subdural hematomas appear as crescentic collections over the convexity of the hemisphere and are located over the frontotemporal region, less often in the inferior middle fossa or over the occipital poles (**Fig. 16–3**).

Interhemispheric, posterior fossa, or bilateral convexity hematomas are less common and are difficult to diagnose clinically, although drowsiness and the signs

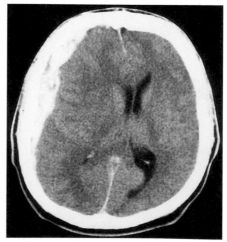

FIGURE 16-3
Acute subdural hematoma in a noncontrast CT scan. The hyperdense clot has an irregular border with the brain and causes more horizontal displacement (mass effect) than might be expected from its thickness. The disproportionate mass effect is the result of the large rostral-caudal extent of these hematomas. Compare to Fig. 16-4.

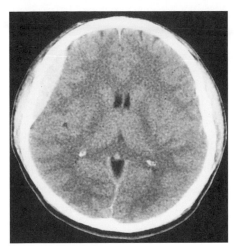

FIGURE 16-4

Acute epidural hematoma. The tightly attached dura is stripped from the inner table of the skull, producing a characteristic lenticular-shaped hemorrhage on CT scan. Epidural hematomas are usually caused by disruption of the middle meningeal artery following fracture of the temporal bone.

expected for each region can be detected (Chap. 7). Larger hematomas are primarily venous in origin, though additional arterial bleeding sites are often found; a few large hematomas, when explored surgically, have an exclusively arterial cause.

Epidural Hematoma (Fig. 16-4)

These evolve more rapidly than subdural hematomas and are therefore more treacherous. They occur in up to 10% of severe head injury cases and are less often associated with underlying cortical damage than are subdural hematomas. Most patients are unconscious when first seen. A "lucid interval" of several minutes to hours before coma supervenes is most characteristic of epidural hemorrhage, but it is still uncommon, and epidural hemorrhage by no means is the only cause of this temporal sequence of events.

Chronic Subdural Hematoma

A history of trauma may or may not be elicited; 20 to 30% of patients recall no head injury, particularly the elderly and those with bleeding diatheses. The causative injury may be trivial and is often forgotten because it was remote. Headache (common but not invariable), slowed thinking, change in personality, a seizure, or a mild hemiparesis emerges weeks or months afterwards. The headache may fluctuate in severity, sometimes with position changes. Many chronic subdural hematomas are

bilateral and produce perplexing clinical syndromes. The initial clinical impression is of a stroke, brain tumor, drug intoxication, depression, or a dementing illness because drowsiness, inattentiveness, and incoherence of thought are more prominent than focal signs such as hemiparesis. Patients with undetected small bilateral subdural hematomas seem to have a low tolerance for surgery, anesthesia, and drugs that depress the nervous system, remaining drowsy or confused for long periods postoperatively. Occasionally a chronic hematoma causes brief episodes of hemiparesis or aphasia that are indistinguishable from transient ischemic attacks.

Skull x-rays are usually normal except for a shift of the calcified pineal body to one side or an occasional unexpected fracture. In long-standing cases the irregular calcification of membranes that surround the collection may be appreciated. CT performed soon after injury (without contrast infusion) shows a low-density mass over the convexity of the hemisphere (**Fig. 16-5**), but between 2 to 6 weeks after the initial bleeding the hemorrhage appears isodense compared to adjacent brain. Bilateral chronic hematomas may fail to be detected because of the absence of lateral tissue shifts; this circumstance is suggested by a "hypernormal" CT scan with fullness of the cortical sulci and small ventricles in an older patient. CT with contrast demonstrates the vascular fibrous capsule surrounding the hemorrhage. MRI reliably identifies either a subacute or chronic hema-

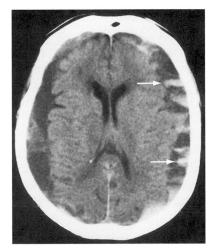

FIGURE 16-5

CT scan of chronic bilateral subdural hematomas of different ages. The collections began as acute hematomas and have become hypodense in comparison to the adjacent brain after a period during which they were isodense and difficult to appreciate. Some areas of resolving blood are contained on the more recently formed collection on the left (*arrows*).

toma. Chronic subdural hematomas can expand gradually and clinically resemble tumors of the brain.

Clinical observation and serial imaging are reasonable in patients with few symptoms and small chronic subdural collections. Treatment with glucocorticoids alone is sufficient in some larger hematomas, but surgical evacuation is more often successful. The fibrous membranes that grow from the dura and encapsulate the region require surgical resection to prevent recurrent fluid accumulation. Small hematomas are largely resorbed, leaving only the organizing membranes.

CLINICAL SYNDROMES AND TREATMENT OF HEAD INJURY

MINOR INJURY

The patient who is fully alert and attentive after head injury but who has one or more symptoms of headache, faintness, nausea, a single episode of emesis, difficulty with concentration, or slight blurring of vision has a good prognosis with little risk of subsequent deterioration. Such patients have usually sustained a concussion and are expected to have a brief amnestic period. Children and young adults are particularly prone to drowsiness, vomiting, and irritability, which is sometimes delayed for several hours after apparently minor injuries. Occasionally, vasovagal syncope follows several minutes to an hour after the injury and may cause undue concern. Constant generalized or frontal headache is common in the days following trauma; it may be migrainous (throbbing and hemicranial) in nature. After several hours of observation, patients with this category of injury may be accompanied home and observed by a family member or friend. Most patients with this syndrome do not have a skull fracture on x-ray or hemorrhage on CT. The decision to perform these tests therefore depends largely on clinical signs suggesting that the impact was severe (e.g., prolonged concussion, periorbital or mastoid hematoma, repeated vomiting, apparent fracture), on the seriousness of other bodily injuries, and on the degree of surveillance that can be anticipated at home. Persistent severe headache and repeated vomiting in the context of normal alertness and no focal neurologic signs are usually benign, but radiologic studies should be obtained and observation in the hospital is justified.

INJURY OF INTERMEDIATE SEVERITY

Patients who are not comatose but who have persistent confusion, behavioral changes, subnormal alertness, extreme dizziness, or focal neurologic signs such as hemiparesis should be admitted to the hospital and soon thereafter have a CT scan. Usually a contusion or hematoma is found. The clinical syndromes most common in this group, in addition to postconcussive drowsiness, headache, dizziness, and vomiting, include (1) delirium with a disinclination to be examined or moved, expletive speech, and resistance if disturbed (anterior temporal lobe contusions); (2) a quiet, disinterested, slowed mental state (abulia) with dull facial appearance and irascibility (inferior frontal and frontopolar contusions); (3) a focal deficit such as aphasia or mild hemiparesis (due to subdural hematoma or convexity contusion, or, less often but frequently missed, carotid artery dissection); (4) confusion with inattention, poor performance on simple mental tasks, and fluctuating or slightly erroneous orientation (associated with several types of injuries, including the first two described above as well as medial frontal contusions and interhemispheric subdural hematoma); (5) repetitive vomiting, nystagmus, drowsiness, and unsteadiness (usually from labyrinthine concussion, but occasionally due to a posterior fossa subdural hematoma or vertebral artery dissection); and (6) diabetes insipidus (damage to the median eminence or pituitary stalk). *It should be emphasized that intermediate-grade injuries are often complicated by drug or alcohol intoxication.*

Clinical observation is necessary to detect increasing drowsiness, change in respiratory pattern, or pupillary enlargement and to ensure restriction of free water (unless there is diabetes insipidus). Most patients in this category improve over several days. During the first week, the state of alertness, memory, and other cognitive functions often fluctuates, and irascibility or agitation is common. Behavioral changes are worse at night, as with many other encephalopathies, and may be treated with small doses of antipsychotic medications. Subtle abnormalities of attention, intellect, spontaneity, and memory tend to return to normal weeks or months after the injury, sometimes surprisingly abruptly; persistent problems in cognition are discussed below.

SEVERE INJURY

Patients who are comatose from the onset require immediate neurologic attention and resuscitation. After intubation, with care taken to avoid deforming the cervical spine, the depth of coma, pupillary size and reactivity, limb movements, and Babinski responses are assessed. As soon as vital functions permit and cervical spine x-rays and a CT scan have been obtained, the patient should be transported to a critical care unit where ICP can be monitored, and where the systemic complications that follow severe brain injury can be treated. The finding of an epidural or subdural hematoma or large intracerebral hemorrhage is an indication for prompt surgery and intracranial decompression in otherwise salvageable patients. Management of raised ICP is discussed in Chap. 15.

TABLE 16-1

GLASGOW COMA SCALE FOR HEAD INJURY

Eye opening (E)	
Spontaneous	4
To loud voice	3
To pain	2
Nil	1
Best motor response (M)	
Obeys	6
Localizes	5
Withdraws (flexion)	4
Abnormal flexion posturing	3
Extension posturing	2
Nil	1
Verbal response (V)	
Oriented	5
Confused, disoriented	4
Inappropriate words	3
Incomprehensible sounds	2
Nil	1

PROGNOSIS

In severe head injury, eye opening, the best motor response of the limbs, and verbal output have been found to be roughly predictive of outcome; these are summarized using the "Glasgow Coma Scale" (**Table 16-1**). Over 85% of patients with aggregate scores of 3 or 4 die within 24 h. However, a number of patients with slightly higher scores and a poor initial prognosis, including a few without pupillary light responses, survive, suggesting that an initially aggressive approach is justified in most patients. Patients <20 years, particularly children, may make remarkable recoveries after having grave early neurologic signs. In one large study of severe head injury, 55% of children had a good outcome at 1 year, compared with 21% of adults. Older age, increased ICP, hypoxia and hypotension, and CT scan evidence of compression of the cisterns surrounding the brainstem and shift of midline structures are all poor prognostic signs. Delayed evacuation of large intracerebral hemorrhages is associated with a poor prognosis. Carrier status for the apolipoprotein E-4 allele is also associated with poor recovery following traumatic brain injury.

POSTCONCUSSION SYNDROME

A structural basis has been sought for the posttraumatic nervous instability termed the *postconcussion syndrome,* which consists of fatigue, dizziness, headache, and diffi-culty in concentration after mild or moderate injury. Most instances are difficult to distinguish from asthenia and depression. Based largely on experimental models, some investigators believe that subtle axonal shearing lesions or yet undefined biochemical alterations account for the cognitive symptoms even when the findings are normal on brain imaging, evoked potentials, and electroencephalogram. In moderate and severe trauma, neuropsychological changes such as difficulty with attention, memory, and other cognitive deficits are undoubtedly present, sometimes severe, but many deficits identified in formal testing are not important for daily functioning. Test scores tend to improve rapidly during the first 6 months after injury, then more slowly for years.

Treatment of the various symptoms of the postconcussive syndrome first requires a symptomatic approach to identify and treat depression and loss of energy, sleeplessness, anxiety, persistent headache, and dizziness. Often, reassurance and treatment directed at anxious depression and sleep problems are all that are required. Care is taken to avoid prolonged use of drugs that produce dependence. Vestibular exercises (Chap. 12) and small doses of vestibular suppressants such as phenergan are helpful when dizziness is the main problem. Patients who after minor or moderate injury report difficulty with memory or with complex cognitive tasks at work may also be reassured that these problems usually improve over 6 to 12 months. It is helpful in this group to obtain focused, serial, and quantified neuropsychological testing in order to adjust the work environment to the patient's current abilities and to document improvement. Whether cognitive exercises are useful is uncertain, but patients certainly report them to be helpful. Previously energetic individuals are usually found to have the best recoveries. In patients with persistent symptoms, the possibility of malingering exists. Physicians should be aware that symptoms tend to persist when litigation regarding the injury is prolonged.

In the absence of adequate data, a common sense approach has been taken to deciding when an athlete who has suffered a concussion should resume athletic activities. Generally, it is advisable to avoid contact sports for several days at least, and for weeks after a second concussion or if there are protracted neurologic symptoms (**Table 16-2**). These guidelines are designed to avoid an extremely rare complication of recurrent head injury, termed the *second impact syndrome,* in which devastating cerebral swelling follows a minor head injury superimposed upon a recent concussion. There is some evidence that repeated concussions in football and soccer players are associated with mild but cumulative cognitive deficits.

TABLE 16-2

GUIDELINES FOR MANAGEMENT OF CONCUSSION IN SPORTS

SEVERITY OF CONCUSSION

Grade 1: Transient confusion, no loss of consciousness (LOC), all symptoms resolve within 15 min.

Grade 2: Transient confusion, no LOC, but concussive symptoms or mental status abnormalities persist longer than 15 min.

Grade 3: Any LOC, either brief (seconds) or prolonged (minutes).

ON-SITE EVALUATION

1. Mental status testing
   a. Orientation — time, place, person, circumstances of injury
   b. Concentration — digits backward, months of year in reverse order
   c. Memory — names of teams, details of contest, recent events, recall of three words and objects at 0 and 5 min

2. Finger-nose-finger with eyes open and closed
3. Pupillary symmetry and reaction
4. Romberg and tandem gait
5. Provocative testing — 40-yard sprint, 5 push ups, 5 sit ups, 5 knee bends (development of dizziness, headaches, or other symptoms is abnormal)

MANAGEMENT GUIDELINES

Grade 1: Remove from contest. Examine immediately and at 5 min intervals. May return to contest if exam clears within 15 min. A second grade 1 concussion eliminates player for 1 week, with return contingent upon normal neurologic assessment at rest and with exercise.

Grade 2: Remove from contest, cannot return for at least 1 week. Examine at frequent intervals on sideline. Formal neurologic exam the next day. If headache or other symptoms persist for 1 week or longer, CT or MRI scan is indicated. After 1 full asymptomatic week, repeat neurologic assessment at rest and with exercise before cleared to resume play. A second grade 2 concussion eliminates player for at least 2 weeks following complete resolution of symptoms.

Grade 3: Transport by ambulance to emergency department if still unconscious or worrisome signs are present; cervical spine stabilization may be indicated. Neurologic exam and, when indicated, CT or MRI scan will guide subsequent management. Hospital admission indicated when signs of pathology are present or if mental status remains abnormal. If findings are normal at the time of the initial medical evaluation, the athlete may be sent home, but daily exams as an outpatient are indicated. A brief (LOC for seconds) grade 3 concussion eliminates player for 1 week, and a prolonged (LOC for minutes) grade 3 concussion for 2 weeks, following complete resolution of symptoms. A second grade 3 concussion should eliminate player from sports for at least 1 month following resolution. Any abnormality on CT or MRI scans should result in termination of the season for the athlete, and return to play at any future time should be discouraged.

Note: CT, computed tomography; MRI, magnetic resonance imaging.
Source: Modified from Quality Standards Subcommittee of the American Academy of Neurology: *The American Academy of Neurology Practice Handbook.* The American Academy of Neurology, St. Paul, MN, 1997.

FURTHER READINGS

BAZARIAN JJ et al: Mild traumatic brain injury in the United States, 1998–2000. Brain Inj 19:85, 2005

BROSHEK DK et al: Sex differences in outcome following sports-related concussion. J Neurosurg 102:856, 2005

LOVELL MR et al: Recovery from concussion in high school athletes. J Neurosurg 98:296, 2003

McCRORY P et al: Summary and agreement statement of the 2nd International Conference on Concussion in Sport, Prague, 2004. Clin J Sport Med 5:48, 2005

MIHALIK JP et al: Posttraumatic migraine characteristics in athletes following sports-related concussion. J Neurosurg 102:850, 2005

ROPPER AH (ed): *Neurological and Neurosurgical Intensive Care,* 4th ed. Philadelphia, Lippincott Williams & Wilkins, 2004

SAVOLA O, HILBLOM M: Early predictors of post-concussion symptoms in patients with mild head injury. Eur J Neurol 10:175, 2003

☑ POVLISHOCK JT, KATZ, DI: Update of neuropathology and neurological recovery after traumatic brain injury. J Head Trauma Rehabil 20:76, 2005

Discusses the spectrum of focal and diffuse pathologies seen in closed head injury and the impact that specific injury patterns have on long-term recovery.

☑ THE BRAIN TRAUMA FOUNDATION: *http://www.braintrauma.org/*

Excellent resource for physicians, patients, and families. Website provides updated protocols for management of traumatic brain injury.

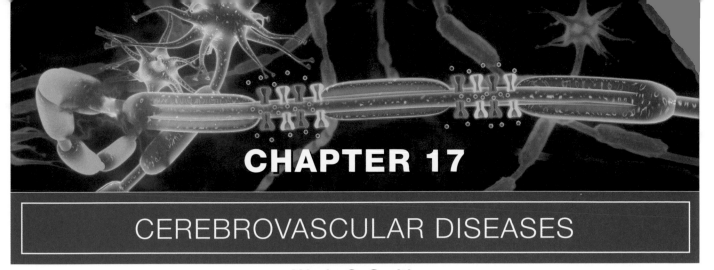

CHAPTER 17

CEREBROVASCULAR DISEASES

Wade S. Smith
S. Claiborne Johnston
J. Donald Easton

Cerebrovascular diseases include some of the most common and devastating disorders: ischemic stroke, hemorrhagic stroke, and cerebrovascular anomalies such as intracranial aneurysms and arteriovenous malformations (AVMs). They cause ~200,000 deaths each year in the United States and are a major cause of disability. The incidence of cerebrovascular diseases increases with age, and the number of strokes is projected to increase as the elderly population grows, with a doubling in stroke deaths in the United States by 2030. Most cerebrovascular diseases are manifest by the abrupt onset of a focal neurologic deficit, as if the patient was "struck by the hand of God." A stroke, or cerebrovascular accident, is defined by this abrupt onset of a neurologic deficit that is attributable to a focal vascular cause. Thus, the definition of stroke is clinical, and laboratory studies including brain imaging are used to support the diagnosis. The clinical manifestations of stroke are highly variable because of the complex anatomy of the brain and its vasculature. *Cerebral ischemia* is caused by a reduction in blood flow that lasts longer than several seconds. Neurologic symptoms are manifest within seconds because neurons lack glycogen, so energy failure is rapid. When blood flow is quickly restored, brain tissue can recover fully and the patient's symptoms are only transient: this is called a *transient ischemic attack* (TIA). Typically the neurologic signs and symptoms of a TIA last for 5 to 15 min but, by definition, must last <24 h. If the cessation of flow lasts for more than a few minutes, *infarction* or death of brain tissue results. Stroke has occurred if the neurologic signs and symptoms last for >24 h. A generalized reduction in cerebral blood flow due to systemic hypotension (e.g., cardiac arrhythmia, myocardial infarction, or hemorrhagic shock) usually produces syncope (Chap. 9). If low cerebral blood flow persists for a longer duration, then infarction in the border zones between the major cerebral artery distributions may develop. In more severe instances, *global hypoxia-ischemia* causes widespread brain injury; the constellation of cognitive sequelae that ensue is called *hypoxic-ischemic encephalopathy* (Chap. 15). *Focal ischemia* or infarction, on the other hand, is usually caused by thrombosis of the cerebral vessels themselves or by emboli from a proximal arterial source or the heart. *Cerebral hemorrhage* produces neurologic symptoms by producing a mass effect on neural structures or from the toxic effects of blood itself.

APPROACH TO THE PATIENT WITH CEREBROVASCULAR DISEASE

Patients with acute stroke often do not seek medical assistance on their own, both because they are rarely in pain, as well as because they may lose the appreciation that something is wrong (*anosagnosia*). It is often a family member or a bystander who calls for help. The rapid evaluation of patients is

233

essential for use of time-sensitive treatments such as thrombolysis. Patients at risk for stroke should be counseled to call emergency medical services immediately if they experience the sudden onset of any of the following: loss of sensory and/or motor function on one side of the body (nearly 85% of ischemic stroke patients have hemiparesis); change in vision, gait, or ability to speak or understand; or if they experience a sudden, severe headache.

There are several common causes of sudden-onset neurologic symptoms that may mimic stroke. An adequate history from an observer that no convulsive activity occurred at the onset reasonably excludes seizure. Tumors may present with acute neurologic symptoms due to hemorrhage, seizure, or hydrocephalus. Surprisingly, migraine can mimic cerebral ischemia, even in patients without a significant migraine history. When it develops without head pain (*acephalgic migraine*), the diagnosis may remain elusive. Patients without any prior history of complicated migraine may develop acephalgic migraine even after age 65. A sensory disturbance is often prominent, and the sensory deficit, as well as any motor deficits, tends to migrate slowly across a limb over minutes. The diagnosis of migraine becomes more secure as the cortical disturbance begins to cross vascular boundaries or if typical visual symptoms are present, such as scintillating scotomata (Chap. 5). At times it may be difficult to make the diagnosis until multiple episodes have occurred leaving behind no residual stroke or magnetic resonance imaging (MRI) changes consistent with stroke. Classically, metabolic encephalopathies produce fluctuating mental status without focal neurologic findings. However, in the setting of prior stroke or brain injury, a patient with fever or sepsis may manifest hemiparesis, which clears rapidly when the infection is remedied. The metabolic process serves to "unmask" a prior deficit.

Once the diagnosis of stroke is made, a brain imaging study is necessary to determine if the cause of stroke is ischemia or hemorrhage (**Fig. 17-1**). Computed tomography (CT) imaging of the brain is the standard imaging modality to detect the presence or absence of intracranial hemorrhage (see "Imaging Studies," below). If the stroke is ischemic, administration of tissue plasminogen activator (tPA) or endovascular mechanical embolectomy may be beneficial in restoring cerebral perfusion (see "Treatment," below). Medical

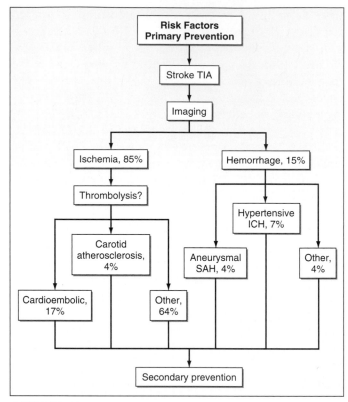

FIGURE 17-1
Schematic approach to acute stroke. Numbers are percentage of all strokes. Abbreviations: TIA, transient ischemic attack; SAH, subarachnoid hemorrhage; ICH, intracerebral hemorrhage.

management to reduce the risk of complications becomes the next priority, followed by plans for secondary prevention. For ischemic stroke, several strategies can reduce the risk of subsequent stroke in all patients, while other strategies are effective for patients with specific causes of stroke such as cardiac embolus and carotid atherosclerosis. For hemorrhagic stroke, aneurysmal subarachnoid hemorrhage (SAH) is the most important treatable condition followed by hypertensive intracranial hemorrhage.

ISCHEMIC STROKE

PATHOPHYSIOLOGY OF ISCHEMIC STROKE

Acute occlusion of an intracranial vessel causes reduction in blood flow to the brain region it supplies. The magnitude of flow reduction is a function of collateral blood flow and this depends on individual vascular anatomy and the site of occlusion. A fall in cerebral blood flow to zero causes death of brain tissue within 4 to 10 min; values <16 to 18 mL/100 g tissue per min cause infarction within an hour; and values <20 mL/100 g tissue per min cause ischemia without infarction unless prolonged for several hours or days. If blood flow is restored prior to a significant amount of cell death, the patient may experience only transient symptoms, i.e., a TIA. Tissue surrounding the core region of infarction is ischemic but reversibly dysfunctional and is referred to as the *ischemic penumbra*. The penumbra may be imaged by using perfusion-diffusion imaging with MRI (see below and Fig. 17-12). The ischemic penumbra will eventually infarct if no change in flow occurs, and hence saving the ischemic penumbra is the goal of revascularization therapies.

Focal cerebral infarction occurs via two distinct pathways: (1) a necrotic pathway in which cellular cytoskeletal breakdown is rapid, due principally to energy failure of the cell, and (2) an apoptotic pathway in which cells become programmed to die. Ischemia-related breakdown of mitochondrial ATP production leads to dysregulation of ion transport, neuronal depolarization, intracellular calcium shifts, and passive water influx, ultimately leading to osmotic lysis and necrotic cell death. In the penumbra region, lesser degrees of ischemia trigger complex excitotoxic and inflammatory cascades involving free radical production, tissue acidosis, and blood-brain barrier disruption. These cascades also appear to initiate apoptotic pathways. Whereas the time frame for necrotic cell death at the core of the infarct is on the order of minutes to hours, irreversible injury in the penumbra occurs over hours to days. The ischemic penumbra is thus an attractive target for therapeutic interventions, although at present, there are no clinically proven strategies that alter these ischemic cascades despite extensive clinical study. It is clear, however, that fever dramatically worsens ischemia, as does hyperglycemia [glucose >11.1 to 16.7 mmol/L (200 to 300 mg/dL)], so it is reasonable to suppress fever and prevent hyperglycemia as much as possible. Hypothermia and other neuroprotective strategies are subjects of continuing clinical research.

TABLE 17-1

CLINICAL MANAGEMENT OF ACUTE STROKE

New onset of neurologic deficit: Stroke or TIA?	Differential diagnosis of new focal deficit 　Stroke or TIA 　Seizure with postictal Todd's paresis 　Tumor 　Migraine 　Metabolic encephalopathy 　Fever/infection and old stroke 　Hyperglycemia 　Hypercalcemia 　Hepatic encephalopathy
Initial assessment and management	ABCs, serum glucose Noncontrast head CT 　Hemorrhage 　　Medical and surgical management 　Tumor or other CNS process 　　Treat as indicated 　Normal or hypodense area consistent with acute ischemic stroke 　　Consider thrombolysis, aspirin 　　Maintain blood pressure and hydrate 　　Admit patient to appropriate level of care depending on concomitant medical problems and airway
Subsequent hospital management	Establish cause of stroke and risk factors Plan for secondary prophylaxis (drugs, risk factor modifications) Obtain physical, occupational, and speech therapy consultation and social work as appropriate Provide nutrition Plan for discharge, including prescriptions for risk factor reduction, including when to institute antihypertensive treatment, and antithrombotic medication prophylaxis

Note: ABCs, airway management, breathing, cardiac status; CNS, central nervous system; CT, computed tomography; TIA, transient ischemic attack.

℞

TREATMENT FOR ISCHEMIC STROKE

Acute Ischemic Stroke

After the clinical diagnosis of stroke is made, an orderly process of evaluation and treatment should follow (**Table 17-1**). The first goal is to prevent or reverse brain injury. After initial stabilization, an emergency noncontrast head CT scan should be performed to differentiate ischemic from hemorrhagic stroke; there are no reliable clinical findings that conclusively separate ischemia from hemorrhage, although a more depressed level of consciousness and higher initial blood pressure favor hemorrhage, and a deficit that remits suggests ischemia. Treatments designed to reverse or lessen the amount of tissue infarction fall within six categories: (1) medical support, (2) thrombolysis, (3) endovascular embolectomy, (4) antiplatelet agents, (5) anticoagulation, and (6) neuroprotection.

MEDICAL SUPPORT

When cerebral infarction occurs, the immediate goal is to optimize cerebral perfusion in the surrounding ischemic penumbra. Attention is also directed toward preventing the common complications of bedridden patients—infections (pneumonia, urinary tract, and skin) and deep venous thrombosis (DVT) with pulmonary embolism. Many physicians use pneumatic compression stockings to prevent DVT; subcutaneous heparin appears to be safe as well.

Because collateral blood flow within the ischemic brain is blood pressure dependent, there is controversy about whether blood pressure should be lowered acutely. Blood pressure should be lowered if there is malignant hypertension or concomitant myocardial ischemia or if blood pressure is >185/110 mmHg and thrombolytic therapy is anticipated. When faced with the competing demands of myocardium and brain, lowering the heart rate with a β_1-adrenergic blocker (such as esmolol or labetolol) can be a first step to decrease cardiac work and maintain blood pressure. Fever is detrimental and should be treated with antipyretics. Serum glucose should be monitored and kept at <6.1 mmol/L (110 mg/dL).

Between 5 and 10% of patients develop enough cerebral edema to cause obtundation or brain herniation. Edema peaks on the second or third day but can cause mass effect for ~10 days. The larger the infarct, the greater the likelihood that clinically significant edema will develop. Special vigilance is warranted for patients with cerebellar infarction. Even small amounts of cerebellar edema can acutely increase intracranial pressure (ICP) in the posterior fossa or directly compress the brainstem. The resulting brainstem compression can result in coma and respiratory arrest and require emergency surgical decompression. Water restriction and intravenous mannitol may be used to raise the serum osmolarity, but hypovolemia should be avoided as this may contribute to hypotension and worsening infarction. Trials are under way to test the clinical benefits of craniotomy and temporary removal of part of the skull (hemicraniectomy) for large hemispheric infarcts with marked cerebral edema.

THROMBOLYSIS

The National Institute of Neurological Disorders and Stroke (NINDS) recombinant tPA (rtPA) Stroke Study showed a clear benefit for intravenous rtPA in selected patients with acute stroke. The NINDS study used intravenous rtPA (0.9 mg/kg to a 90-mg max; 10% as a bolus, then the remainder over 60 min) vs. placebo in patients with ischemic stroke within 3 h of onset. Half of the patients were treated within 90 min. Symptomatic intracerebral hemorrhage occurred in 6.4% of patients on rtPA and 0.6% on placebo. There was a nonsignificant 4% reduction in mortality in patients on rtPA (21% on placebo and 17% on rtPA); there was a significant 12% absolute increase in the number of patients with only minimal disability (32% on placebo and 44% on rtPA.) Thus, despite an increased incidence of symptomatic intracerebral hemorrhage, treatment with intravenous rtPA within 3 h of the onset of ischemic stroke improved clinical outcome.

Results of other trials of rtPA have been negative, perhaps because of the dose of rtPA and timing of its delivery. The European Cooperative Acute Stroke Study (ECASS) I used a higher dose of rtPA (1.2 mg/kg), and ECASS-II tested the NINDS dose of rtPA (0.9 mg/kg; maximum dose, 90 mg) but allowed patients to receive drug up to the sixth hour. No significant benefit was found, but improvement was found in post hoc analyses. The ATLANTIS study (Alteplase Thrombolysis for Acute Noninterventional Therapy in Ischemic Stroke) tested the NINDS dosing of rtPA between 3 and 5 h and found no benefit. Three major trials using streptokinase reported increased mortality for patients receiving streptokinase. Early administration of the fibrinolytic agent ancrod appears to improve outcomes for patients with acute ischemic stroke; although the drug has not been approved for clinical use, its efficacy provides further evidence that thrombolytics should have a role in treatment of acute ischemic stroke.

Because of the marked differences in trial design, including drug and dose used, time to thrombolysis, and severity of stroke, the precise efficacy of intravenous thrombolytics for acute ischemic stroke remains unclear. The risk of intracranial hemorrhage appears to rise with larger strokes, longer times from onset of symptoms, and higher doses of rtPA administered. The established dose of 0.9 mg/kg administered intravenously within 3 h of stroke onset appears safe. Many hospitals have developed expert stroke teams to facilitate this treatment. The drug is now approved in the United States, Canada, and Europe for acute

TABLE 17-2

ADMINISTRATION OF INTRAVENOUS RECOMBINANT TISSUE PLASMINOGEN ACTIVATOR (rtPA) FOR ACUTE ISCHEMIC STROKE[a]

INDICATIONS	CONTRAINDICATIONS
Clinical diagnosis of stroke	Sustained BP > 185/110 despite treatment
Onset of symptoms to time of drug administration ≤3 h	Platelets <100,000; HCT < 25%; glucose < 50 or > 400 mg/dL
CT scan showing no hemorrhage or edema of >1/3 of the MCA territory	Use of heparin within 48 h and prolonged PTT, or elevated INR
	Rapidly improving symptoms
	Prior stroke or head injury within 3 months; prior intracranial hemorrhage
Age ≥18 years	Major surgery in preceding 14 days
Consent by patient or surrogate	Minor stroke symptoms
	Gastrointestinal bleeding in preceding 21 days
	Recent myocardial infarction
	Coma or stupor

Administration of rtPA
Intravenous access with two peripheral IV lines (avoid arterial or central line placement)
Review eligibility for rtPA
Administer 0.9 mg/kg intravenously (maximum 90 mg) IV as 10% of total dose by bolus, followed by remainder of total dose over 1 h
Frequent cuff blood pressure monitoring
No other antithrombotic treatment for 24 h
For decline in neurologic status or uncontrolled blood pressure, stop infusion, give cryoprecipitate, and reimage brain emergently
Avoid urethral catheterization for ≥2 h

[a]See Activase (tissue plasminogen activator) package insert for complete list of contraindications and dosing.
Note: BP, blood pressure; CT, computed tomography; HCT, hematocrit; INR, international normalized ratio; MCA, middle cerebral artery; PTT, partial thromboplastin time.

stroke when given within 3 h from the time the stroke symptoms began, and efforts should be made to give it as early in this 3-h window as possible. The time of stroke onset is defined as the time the patient's symptoms began or the time the patient was last seen as normal. A patient who awakens with stroke has the onset defined as when they went to bed. **Table 17-2** summarizes eligibility criteria and instructions for administration of rtPA.

There is growing interest in using thrombolytics via an intraarterial route to increase the concentration of drug at the clot and minimize systemic bleeding complications. The Prolyse in Acute Cerebral Thromboembolism (PROACT) II trial found benefit for intraarterial pro-urokinase for acute middle cerebral artery (MCA) occlusions up to the sixth hour following onset of stroke. Intraarterial treatment of basilar artery occlusions may also be beneficial for selected patients. Intraarterial administration of a thrombolytic agent for acute ischemic stroke is not approved by the U.S. Food and Drug Administration (FDA); however, many stroke centers offer this treatment based on these data.

ENDOVASCULAR EMBOLECTOMY

Endovascular mechanical embolectomy has recently shown promise as an alternative treatment of acute stroke in patients who have contraindications to thombolytics. The MERCI (Mechanical Embolus Removal in Cerebral Ischemia) trial investigated the ability of a novel endovascular corkscrew embolectomy device to restore patency of occluded intracranial vessels within 8 h of ischemic stroke symptoms. Recanalization of the target vessel occurred in 46% of treated patients, and favorable outcome at 90 days correlated well with successful recanalization. Based upon these data, the FDA recently approved this device for the revascularization of occluded vessels in acute ischemic stroke.

ANTIPLATELET AGENTS

Aspirin is the only antiplatelet agent that has been prospectively studied for the treatment of acute ischemic stroke. The recent large trials, the International Stroke Trial (IST) and the Chinese Acute Stroke Trial (CAST), found that the use of aspirin within 48 h of stroke onset reduced both stroke recurrence risk and mortality minimally. Among 19,435 patients in IST, those allocated to aspirin, 300 mg/d, had slightly fewer deaths within 14 days (9.0 vs. 9.4%), significantly fewer recurrent ischemic strokes (2.8 vs. 3.9%), no excess of hemorrhagic strokes (0.9 vs. 0.8%), and a trend towards a reduction in death or dependence at 6 months (61.2 vs. 63.5%). In CAST, 21,106 patients with ischemic stroke received 160 mg/d of aspirin or a placebo for up to 4 weeks. There were very small reductions in the aspirin group in early mortality (3.3 vs. 3.9%), recurrent ischemic strokes (1.6 vs. 2.1%), and dependency at discharge or death (30.5 vs. 31.6%). These trials demonstrate that the use of aspirin in the treatment of acute ischemic stroke is safe and produces a small net benefit. For every 1000 acute strokes treated with aspirin, about 9 deaths or nonfatal stroke recurrences will be prevented in the first few weeks and ~13 fewer patients will be dead or dependent at 6 months.

Agents that act at the glycoprotein IIb/IIIa receptor are undergoing clinical trials in acute stroke treatment. Early results show that intravenous abciximab can be used safely within 6 h of stroke onset and suggest that it may be effective.

ANTICOAGULATION

The role of anticoagulation in atherothrombotic cerebral ischemia is uncertain. Several trials have investigated antiplatelet versus anticoagulant medications given within 12 to 24 h of the initial event. The U.S. Trial of Organon 10172 in Acute Stroke Treatment (TOAST), an investigational low-molecular-weight heparin, failed to show any benefit over aspirin. Use of subcutaneous unfractionated heparin versus aspirin was tested in IST. Heparin given subcutaneously afforded no additional benefit over aspirin and increased bleeding rates. Several trials of low-molecular-weight heparins have also shown no consistent benefit in acute ischemic stroke. Therefore, trials do not support the use of heparin or other anticoagulants for patients with atherothrombotic stroke.

In spite of the absence of evidence, heparin is still used frequently to treat stroke and TIA, primarily based on beliefs about its impact on pathophysiology. Theoretically, heparin may prevent propagation of clot within a thrombosed vessel or may prevent more emboli from occurring. Heparin is widely used for crescendo TIAs (TIAs that increase in frequency), despite the absence of data from controlled studies regarding this indication. In ~20% of patients with acute stroke, deficits will progress over several hours to 1 to 2 days. Some physicians heparinize all patients with recent mild ischemic stroke in order to prevent some of this worsening, but this practice is discouraged. The bleeding complication rate for 7 days of heparin is about 10%, with a serious bleed rate of ~2%. Clearly the value of this approach must be clarified. Heparinization is generally accomplished by beginning an infusion without bolus and is monitored to maintain the activated partial thromboplastin time (PTT) at approximately twice normal.

NEUROPROTECTION

Neuroprotection is the concept of providing a treatment that prolongs the brain's tolerance to ischemia. Hypothermia is a powerful neuroprotective treatment in patients with cardiac arrest, but it has not been adequately studied in patients with stroke. Drugs that block the excitatory amino acid pathways have been shown to protect neurons and glia in animals, but despite multiple clinical trials, they have not yet been proven to be beneficial in humans. Even so, interest in neuroprotection continues because of the potential for agents to have limited risk, even when administered in the prehospital setting or in conjunction with thrombolytic agents.

Stroke Centers and Rehabilitation

Patient care in comprehensive stroke units followed by rehabilitation services improves neurologic outcomes and reduces mortality. Use of clinical pathways and staff dedicated to the stroke patient can improve care. Stroke teams that provide emergency 24-h evaluation of acute stroke patients for acute medical management and consideration of thrombolysis or endovascular treatments are important.

Proper rehabilitation of the stroke patient includes early physical, occupational, and speech therapy. It is directed toward educating the patient and family about the patient's neurologic deficit, preventing the complications of immobility (e.g., pneumonia, DVT and pulmonary embolism, pressure sores of the skin, and muscle contractures), and providing encouragement and instruction in overcoming the deficit. The goal of rehabilitation is to return the patient to home and to maximize recovery by providing a safe, progressive regimen suited to the individual patient. Additionally, the use of restraint therapy has been shown to improve hemiparesis following stroke, even years following the stroke, suggesting that physical therapy can recruit unused neural pathways. This finding suggests that the human nervous system is more adaptable than originally thought and has stimulated active research into physical and pharmacologic strategies that can enhance long-term neural recovery.

ETIOLOGY OF ISCHEMIC STROKE
(Table 17–3, Fig. 17–2)

Although the initial management of acute ischemic stroke often does not depend on the etiology, establishing

TABLE 17-3

CAUSES OF ISCHEMIC STROKE

COMMON CAUSES	UNCOMMON CAUSES
Thrombosis	Hypercoagulable disorders
Lacunar stroke (small vessel)	Protein C deficiency
Large vessel thrombosis	Protein S deficiency
Dehydration	Antithrombin III deficiency
Embolic occlusion	Antiphospholipid syndrome
Artery-to-artery	Factor V Leiden mutation[a]
Carotid bifurcation	Prothrombin G20210
Aortic arch	mutation[a]
Arterial dissection	Systemic malignancy
Cardioembolic	Sickle cell anemia
Atrial fibrillation	β-Thalassemia
Mural thrombus	Polycythemia vera
Myocardial infarction	Systemic lupus erythematosus
Dilated cardiomyopathy	Homocysteinemia
Valvular lesions	Thrombotic thrombocytopenic
Mitral stenosis	purpura
Mechanical valve	Disseminated intravascular
Bacterial endocarditis	coagulation
Paradoxical embolus	Dysproteinemias
Atrial septal defect	Nephrotic syndrome
Patent foramen ovale	Inflammatory bowel disease
Atrial septal aneurysm	Oral contraceptives
Spontaneous echo contrast	Venous sinus thrombosis[b]
	Fibromuscular dysplasia
	Vasculitis
	Systemic vasculitis (PAN,
	Wegner's, Takayasu's, giant
	cell arteritis)
	Primary CNS vasculitis
	Meningitis (syphilis, tubercu-
	losis, fungal, bacterial,
	zoster)
	Cardiogenic
	Mitral valve calcification
	Atrial myxoma
	Intracardiac tumor
	Marantic endocarditis
	Libman-Sacks endocarditis
	Subarachnoid hemorrhage
	vasospasm
	Drugs: cocaine, amphetamine
	Moyamoya disease
	Eclampsia

[a]Chiefly cause venous sinus thrombosis.
[b]May be associated with any hypercoagulable disorder.
Note: CNS, central nervous system; PAN, polyarteritis nodosa.

a cause is essential in reducing the risk of recurrence. The clinical presentation and examination findings often establish the cause of stroke or narrow the possibilities to a few. Judicious use of laboratory testing and imaging studies completes the initial evaluation. Nevertheless, nearly 30% of strokes remain unexplained despite extensive evaluation.

Clinical examination should be focused on the peripheral and cervical vascular system (carotid auscultation for bruits, blood pressure, and pressure comparison between arms), the heart (dysrhythmia, murmurs), extremities (peripheral emboli), and retina [effects of hypertension and cholesterol emboli (Hollenhorst plaques)]. A complete neurologic examination is performed to localize the site of stroke. An imaging study of the brain is nearly always performed and is required for patients being considered for thrombolysis. A chest x-ray, electrocardiogram (ECG), urinalysis, complete blood count, erythrocyte sedimentation rate, serum electrolytes, blood urea nitrogen, creatinine, blood sugar, serologic test for syphilis, serum lipid profile, prothrombin time, and PTT are often useful and should be considered in all patients. An ECG may demonstrate conduction abnormalities and arrhythmias or reveal evidence of recent myocardial infarction (MI).

Cardioembolic Stroke

Cardioembolism is responsible for ~20% of all ischemic strokes. Stroke caused by heart disease is primarily due to embolism of thrombotic material forming on the atrial or ventricular wall or the left heart valves. These thrombi then detach and embolize into the arterial circulation. The thrombus may fragment or lyse quickly, producing only TIA. Alternatively, the arterial occlusion may last longer, producing stroke. Embolic strokes tend to be sudden in onset, with maximum neurologic deficit at once. With reperfusion following more prolonged ischemia, petechial hemorrhage can occur within the ischemic territory. This is usually of no clinical significance and should be distinguished from frank intracranial hemorrhage into a region of ischemic stroke where the mass effect from the hemorrhage can cause a decline in neurologic function.

Emboli from the heart most often lodge in the MCA, the posterior cerebral artery (PCA), or one of their branches; infrequently, the anterior cerebral artery (ACA) territory is involved. Emboli large enough to occlude the stem of the MCA (3 to 4 mm) lead to large infarcts that involve both deep gray and white matter and some portions of the cortical surface and its underlying white matter. A smaller embolus may occlude a small cortical or penetrating arterial branch. The location and size of an infarct within a vascular territory depend on the extent of the collateral circulation.

The most significant causes of cardioembolic stroke in most of the world are nonrheumatic (often called nonvalvular) atrial fibrillation, MI, prosthetic valves, rheumatic heart disease, and ischemic cardiomyopathy (**Table 17–3**). A few pertinent aspects are highlighted here.

Nonrheumatic atrial fibrillation is the most common cause of cerebral embolism overall. The presumed

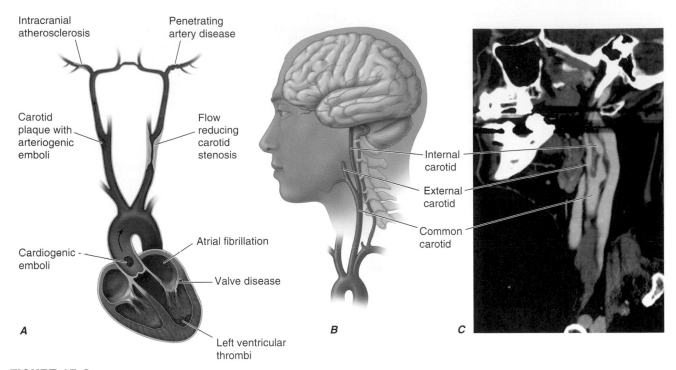

FIGURE 17-2

Pathophysiology of ischemic stroke. **A.** Diagram illustrating the three major mechanisms that underlie ischemic stroke: (1) occlusion of an intracranial vessel by an embolus that arises at a distant site (e.g., cardiogenic sources such as atrial fibrillation or artery-to-artery emboli from carotid atherosclerotic plaque), often affecting the large intracranial vessels; (2) *in situ* thrombosis of an intracranial vessel, typically affecting the small penetrating arteries that arise from the major intracranial arteries; (3) hypoperfusion caused by flow-limiting stenosis of a major extracranial (e.g., internal carotid) or intracranial vessel, often producing "watershed" ischemia. **B.** and **C.** Diagram and reformatted CT angiogram of the common, internal and external carotid arteries. High-grade stenosis of the internal carotid artery, which may be associated with either cerebral emboli or flow-limiting ischemia, was identified in this patient.

stroke mechanism is thrombus formation in the fibrillating atrium or atrial appendage, with subsequent embolization. Patients with atrial fibrillation have an average annual risk of stroke of ~5%. The risk varies according to the presence of certain risk factors, including older age, hypertension, poor left ventricular function, prior cardioembolism, or diabetes. Patients younger than 60 with none of these risk factors have an annual risk for stroke of ~0.5%, while those with most of the factors have a rate of ~15% per year. Left atrial enlargement and congestive heart failure are additional risk factors for formation of atrial thrombi. Rheumatic heart disease usually causes ischemic stroke when there is prominent mitral stenosis or atrial fibrillation. Guidelines for the use of warfarin and aspirin for secondary prevention are based on risk factors (**Table 17-4**).

Recent MI may be a source of emboli, especially when transmural and involving the anteroapical ventricular wall, and prophylactic anticoagulation following MI has been shown to reduce stroke risk. Mitral valve prolapse is not usually a source of emboli unless the prolapse is severe.

Paradoxical embolization occurs when venous thrombi migrate to the arterial circulation, usually via a patent foramen ovale or atrial septal defect. Bubble-contrast echocardiography (intravenous injection of agitated saline coupled with either transthoracic or

TABLE 17-4

CONSENSUS RECOMMENDATION FOR ANTITHROMBOTIC PROPHYLAXIS IN ATRIAL FIBRILLATION		
AGE	**RISK FACTORS[a]**	**RECOMMENDATION**
Age ≤65	≥1	Warfarin INR 2–3
	0	Aspirin
Age 65–75	≥1	Warfarin INR 2–3
	0	Warfarin INR 2–3 or aspirin
Age >75		Warfarin INR 2–3

[a]Risk factors include previous transient ischemic attack or stroke, systemic embolism, hypertension, heart failure, diabetes, clinical coronary artery disease, mitral stenosis or prosthetic mechanical heart valves.
Source: Modified from DE Singer et al: Chest 126 (3Suppl):429, 2004; with permission.

transesophageal echocardiography) can demonstrate a cardiac right-to-left shunt, revealing the conduit for paradoxical embolization. Alternatively, a right-to-left shunt is implied if immediately following intravenous injection of agitated saline, high-intensity transients are observed during transcranial Doppler insonation of the MCA. Both techniques are highly sensitive for detection of right-to-left shunts. Besides venous clot, fat and tumor emboli, bacterial endocarditis, intravenous air, and amniotic fluid emboli associated with delivery may occasionally be responsible for paradoxical embolization. The importance of right-to-left shunt as a cause of stroke is debated, particularly because such shunts occur in ~15% of the general population. Some studies have suggested that the risk is only elevated in the presence of a coexisting atrial septal aneurysm. The presence of a venous source of embolus, most commonly a deep venous thrombus, may provide confirmation of the importance of a right-to-left shunt in a particular case.

Bacterial endocarditis can cause valvular vegetations that can give rise to multiple septic emboli. The appearance of multifocal symptoms and signs in a patient with stroke makes bacterial endocarditis more likely. Infarcts of microscopic size occur, and large septic infarcts may evolve into brain abscesses or cause hemorrhage into the infarct, which generally precludes use of anticoagulation or thrombolytics. Mycotic aneurysms caused by septic emboli give rise to SAH or intracerebral hemorrhage.

Artery-to-Artery Embolic Stroke

Thrombus formation on atherosclerotic plaques may embolize to intracranial arteries producing an artery-to-artery embolic stroke. Alternatively, a diseased vessel may acutely thrombose; the resulting blockage causes stroke by producing ischemia within the region of brain it supplied. Unlike the myocardial vessels, artery-to-artery embolism, rather than thrombosis, appears to be the dominant vascular mechanism causing ischemia. Any diseased vessel may be a source, including the aortic arch, common carotid, internal carotid, vertebral, and basilar arteries. Carotid bifurcation atherosclerosis is the most common source of artery-to-artery embolus, and specific treatments have proven efficacy in reducing risk.

Carotid Atherosclerosis Atherosclerosis within the carotid artery occurs most frequently within the common carotid bifurcation and proximal internal carotid artery. Additionally, the carotid siphon (portion within the cavernous sinus) is also vulnerable to atherosclerosis. Male gender, older age, smoking, hyperten-

TABLE 17-5

RISK FACTORS FOR STROKE

RISK FACTOR	RELATIVE RISK	RELATIVE RISK REDUCTION WITH TREATMENT	NUMBER NEEDED TO TREAT[a]	
			PRIMARY PREVENTION	SECONDARY PREVENTION
Hypertension	2–5	38%	100–300	50–100
Atrial fibrillation	1.8–2.9	68% warfarin 21% aspirin	20–83	13
Diabetes	1.8–6	No proven effect		
Smoking	1.8	50% at 1 year, baseline risk at 5 years post cessation		
Hyperlipidemia	1.8–2.6	10–29%		—
Asymptomatic carotid stenosis	2.0	46–53%	85	N/A
Symptomatic carotid stenosis (70–99%)		65% at 2 years	N/A	12
Symptomatic carotid stenosis (50–69%)		29% at 5 years	N/A	77

[a]Number needed to treat to prevent one stroke annually. Prevention of other cardiovascular outcomes is not considered here.
Note: N/A, not applicable.

sion, diabetes, and hypercholesterolemia are risk factors for carotid disease, as they are for stroke in general (**Table 17-5**). Carotid atherosclerosis produces an estimated 5% of ischemic stroke, and the risk of stroke rises the higher the degree of carotid narrowing.

Carotid disease can be classified by whether the stenosis is symptomatic or asymptomatic and by the degree of stenosis (percent narrowing of the narrowest segment compared to a more distal internal carotid segment). Symptomatic carotid disease implies that the patient has experienced a stroke or TIA within the vascular distribution of the artery, and it is associated with a greater risk of subsequent stroke than asymptomatic stenosis, in which the patient is symptom free and the stenosis is detected through screening. Greater degrees of arterial narrowing are generally associated with a greater risk of stroke.

TREATMENT FOR CAROTID STENOSIS

Surgical Therapy

Surgery for atherosclerotic occlusive disease is largely limited to *carotid endarterectomy* for plaques located at the origin of the internal carotid artery in the neck.

Symptomatic carotid stenosis was studied in the North American Symptomatic Carotid Endarterectomy Trial (NASCET) and the European Carotid Surgery Trial (ECST). Both showed a substantial benefit for surgery in patients with a stenosis of >70%. In NASCET, the average cumulative ipsilateral stroke risk at 2 years was 26% for patients treated medically and 9% for those receiving the same medical treatment plus a carotid endarterectomy. This 17% *absolute* reduction in the surgical group is a 65% *relative* risk reduction favoring surgery (Table 17-5). NASCET also showed a significant benefit for patients with 50 to 70% stenosis, although less robust. ECST found harm for patients with stenosis in the 0 to 30% range treated surgically.

A patient's risk of stroke and possible benefit from surgery are related to the presence of retinal versus hemispheric symptoms, degree of arterial stenosis, extent of associated medical conditions (of note, NASCET and ECST excluded "high risk" patients with significant cardiac, pulmonary, or renal disease), institutional surgical morbidity and mortality, timing of surgery relative to symptoms, and other factors. A recent meta-analysis of the NASCET and ECST trials demonstrated that endarterectomy is most beneficial when performed within 2 weeks of symptom onset. In addition, benefit is more pronounced in patients over 75 years of age, and men appear to benefit more than women.

In summary, a patient with multiple atherosclerosis risk factors, recent symptomatic hemispheric ischemia, high-grade stenosis in the appropriate internal carotid artery, and an institutional perioperative morbidity and mortality rate of ≤6% generally should undergo carotid endarterectomy. If the perioperative stroke rate is >6% for any particular surgeon, however, the benefits of carotid endarterectomy are questionable.

The indications for surgical treatment of *asymptomatic carotid disease* have been clarified by the results of the Asymptomatic Carotid Atherosclerosis Study (ACAS) and the Asymptomatic Carotid Surgery Trial (ACST). ACAS randomized asymptomatic patients with ≥60% stenosis to medical treatment with aspirin or the same medical treatment plus carotid endarterectomy. The surgical group had a risk over 5 years for ipsilateral stroke (and any perioperative stroke or death) of 5.1%, compared to a risk in the medical group of 11%. While this demonstrates a 53% *relative* risk reduction, the *absolute* risk reduction is only 5.9% over 5 years, or 1.2% annually (Table 17-5). Nearly half of

the strokes in the surgery group were caused by preoperative angiograms. The recently published ACST randomized 3120 asymptomatic patients with >60% carotid stenosis to endarterectomy or medical therapy. The 5-year risk of stroke in the surgical group (including perioperative stroke or death) was 6.4%, compared to 11.8% in the medically treated group (46% relative risk reduction and 5.4% absolute risk reduction).

In both ACAS and ACST, the perioperative complication rate was higher in women, perhaps negating any benefit in the reduction of stroke risk within 5 years. It is possible that with longer follow-up, a clear benefit in women will emerge. At present, carotid endarterectomy in asymptomatic women remains particularly controversial.

In summary, the natural history of asymptomatic stenosis is an ~2% per year stroke rate, while symptomatic patients experience a 13% per year risk of stroke. Whether to recommend carotid revascularization for an asymptomatic patient is somewhat controversial and depends on many factors, including patient preference, degree of stenosis, age, gender, and comorbidities. Medical therapy for reduction of atherosclerosis risk factors, including cholesterol-lowering agents and antiplatelet medications, is generally recommended for patients with asymptomatic carotid stenosis. As with atrial fibrillation, it is imperative to counsel the patient about TIAs so their therapy can be revised if they become symptomatic.

Endovascular Therapy

Balloon angioplasty coupled with stenting is being used with increasing frequency to open stenotic carotid arteries and maintain their patency. These techniques can treat carotid stenosis not only at the bifurcation but also near the skull base and in the intracranial segments. The SAPPHIRE trial (Stenting and Angioplasty with Protection in Patients at High Risk for Endarterectomy) randomized high-risk patients (defined as patients with clinically significant coronary or pulmonary disease, contralateral carotid occlusion, restenosis after endarterectomy, contralateral laryngeal nerve palsy, prior radical neck surgery or radiation, or age >80) with symptomatic carotid stenosis >50% or asymptomatic stenosis >80% to either stenting combined with a distal emboli-protection device or endarterectomy. The risk of death, stroke, or myocardial infarction within 30 days and ipsilateral stroke or death within 1 year was 12.2%

in the stenting group and 20.1% in the endarterectomy group ($p = .05$), suggesting that stenting is at the very least comparable to endarterectomy as a treatment option for this patient group. Much of the benefit seen in the stenting group was due to a reduction in peri-procedure myocardial infarction. Multicenter trials are currently underway comparing stenting with endarterectomy in lower risk patients, the population previously studied in the NASCET, ECST, ACAS, and ACST trials (see above).

Bypass Surgery

Extracranial to intracranial (EC-IC) bypass surgery has been proven ineffective for atherosclerotic stenoses that are inaccessible to conventional carotid endarterectomy. However, using more functional techniques [positron emission tomography (PET) imaging] to select patients who may benefit from EC-IC bypass is currently being studied.

Other Causes of Artery-to-artery Embolic Stroke *Intracranial atherosclerosis* produces stroke either by an embolic mechanism or by in situ thrombosis of a diseased vessel. It is more common in patients of Asian and African-American descent. The WASID (Warfarin-Aspirin Symptomatic Intracranial Disease) trial randomized patients with symptomatic stenosis (50–99%) of a major intracranial vessel to medical therapy with either high-dose aspirin (1300 mg/d) or warfarin (target INR, 2.0 to 3.0), with a combined primary end point of ischemic stroke, brain hemorrhage, or death from vascular cause other than stroke. The trial was terminated early because of an increased risk of adverse events related to warfarin anticoagulation. With a mean follow-up of 1.8 years, the primary end point was seen in 22.1% in the aspirin group and 21.8% of the warfarin group. Death from any cause was seen in 4.3% of the aspirin group and 9.7% of the warfarin group; 3.2% of patients on aspirin experienced major hemorrhage, compared to 8.3% of patients taking warfarin.

Given the worrisome natural history of symptomatic intracranial atherosclerosis (in the aspirin arm of the WASID trial, 15% of patients experienced a stroke within the first year, despite current standard aggressive medical therapy), many neurointerventional centers are using intracranial angioplasty coupled with intracranial stenting for symptomatic lesions. This intervention has not been compared with medical therapy for stroke prevention in this patient population, but such clinical trials will likely be conducted in the near future.

Dissection of the internal carotid or vertebral arteries or even vessels beyond the circle of Willis is a common source of embolic stroke in young (age <60 years) patients. The dissection is usually painful and precedes the stroke by several hours or days. Extracranial dissections rarely cause hemorrhage because of the tough adventitia of these vessels. Intracranial dissections, on the other hand, may produce SAH because the adventitia of intracranial vessels is thin and pseudoaneurysms may form, requiring treatment to prevent rerupture. The cause of dissection is usually unknown and recurrence is rare. Ehlers-Danlos type IV, Marfan's disease, cystic medial necrosis, and fibromuscular dysplasia are associated with dissections. Trauma (usually a motor vehicle accident or a sports injury) can cause carotid and vertebral artery dissections. Spinal manipulative therapy is independently associated with vertebral artery dissection and stroke. Most dissections heal spontaneously, and stroke or TIA is uncommon beyond 2 weeks. Although there are no trials comparing anticoagulation to antiplatelet agents, many physicians treat with anticoagulants for 3 to 6 months then convert to antiplatelet therapy after demonstration of vascular recanalization.

Small-Vessel Stroke

The term *lacunar infarction* refers to infarction following atherothrombotic or lipohyalinotic occlusion of a small artery (30 to 300 μm) in the brain. The term *small-vessel stroke* denotes occlusion of such a small penetrating artery and is now the preferred term. Small-vessel strokes account for ~20% of all strokes.

Pathophysiology The MCA stem, the arteries comprising the circle of Willis (A1 segment, anterior and posterior communicating arteries, and P1 segment), and the basilar and vertebral arteries all give rise to 30- to 300-μm branches that penetrate the deep gray and white matter of the cerebrum or brainstem (**Fig. 17-3**). Each of these small branches can occlude either by atherothrombotic disease at its origin or by the development of lipohyalinotic thickening. Thrombosis of these vessels causes small infarcts that are referred to as *lacunes* (Latin for "lake" of fluid noted at autopsy). They range in size from 3 mm to 2 cm. Hypertension and age are the principal risk factors.

Clinical Manifestations The most common *lacunar syndromes* are the following: (1) Pure motor hemiparesis from an infarct in the posterior limb of the internal capsule or basis pontis; the face, arm, and leg are almost always involved; (2) pure sensory stroke from an infarct in the ventral posterolateral thalamus; (3) ataxic hemiparesis from an infarct in the base of the pons; (4) dysarthria and a clumsy hand or arm due to

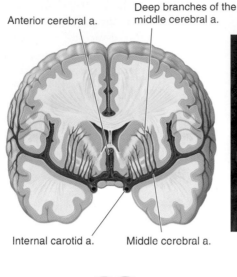

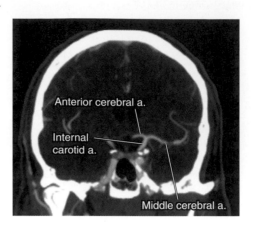

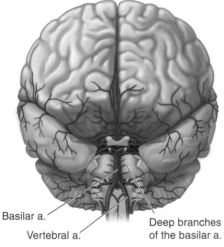

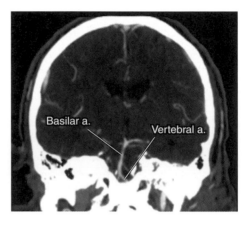

FIGURE 17-3

Diagrams and reformatted CT angiograms in the coronal section illustrating the deep penetrating arteries involved in small-vessel strokes. In the anterior circulation, small penetrating arteries called lenticulostriates arise from the proximal portion of the anterior and middle cerebral arteries and supply deep subcortical structures (*upper panels*). In the posterior circulation, similar arteries arise directly from the vertebral and basilar arteries to supply the brainstem (*lower panels*). Occlusion of a single penetrating artery gives rise to a discrete area of infarct (pathologically termed a "lacune" or lake). Note that these vessels are too small to be visualized on CT angiography.

infarction in the base of the pons or in the genu of the internal capsule; and (5) pure motor hemiparesis with "motor (Broca's) aphasia" due to thrombotic occlusion of a lenticulostriate branch supplying the genu and anterior limb of the internal capsule and adjacent white matter of the corona radiata.

Transient symptoms (small vessel TIAs) may herald a small-vessel infarct; they may occur several times a day and last only a few minutes. Recovery from a small-vessel stroke often begins within hours or days, and over weeks or months may be nearly complete; in some cases, however, there is severe permanent disability. Often, institution of combined antithrombotic treatments does not prevent eventual stroke in "stuttering lacunes."

A large-vessel source (either thrombosis or embolism) may manifest initially as a lacunar syndrome with small-vessel infarction. Therefore, the search for embolic sources (carotid and heart) should not be completely abandoned in the evaluation of these patients. Secondary prevention of lacunar stroke involves risk factor modification, specifically reduction in blood pressure (see "Primary and Secondary Prevention," below).

LESS COMMON CAUSES OF STROKE
(Table 17–3)

Hypercoagulable disorders primarily cause increased risk of venous thrombosis and therefore may cause venous sinus thrombosis. Protein S deficiency and homocysteinemia may cause arterial thromboses as well. Systemic lupus erythematosus with Libman-Sacks endocarditis can be a cause of embolic stroke. These conditions overlap with the antiphospholipid syndrome, which probably requires long-term anticoagulation to prevent further stroke.

Venous sinus thrombosis of the lateral or sagittal sinus or of small cortical veins (cortical vein thrombosis) occurs as a complication of oral contraceptive use, pregnancy and the postpartum period, inflammatory bowel disease, and intracranial infections (meningitis). It is also seen with increased incidence in patients with laboratory-confirmed thrombophilia (Table 17-3) including polycythemia, sickle cell anemia, proteins C and S deficiency, factor V Leiden mutation (resistance to activated protein C), antithrombin III deficiency, homocysteinemia, and the prothrombin G20210 mutation. Women who take oral contraceptives and have the prothrombin G20210 mutation may be at particularly high risk for sinus thrombosis. Patients present with headache, focal neurologic signs (especially paraparesis), and seizures. Often, CT imaging is normal unless an intracranial venous hemorrhage has occurred, but the venous sinus occlusion is readily visualized using magnetic resonance (MR) venography or conventional x-ray angiography. With greater degrees of sinus thrombosis, the patient may develop signs of increased ICP and coma. Intravenous heparin, regardless of the presence of intracranial hemorrhage, has been shown to reduce morbidity and mortality, and the long-term outcome is generally good. Heparin prevents further thrombosis and reduces venous hypertension and ischemia. If an underlying hypercoagulable state is not found, many physicians treat with warfarin sodium for 3 to 6 months then convert to aspirin, depending on the degree of resolution of the venous sinus thrombus. Anticoagulation is often continued indefinitely if thrombophilia is diagnosed.

Fibromuscular dysplasia affects the cervical arteries and occurs mainly in women. The carotid or vertebral arteries show multiple rings of segmental narrowing alternating with dilatation. Occlusion is usually incomplete. The process is often asymptomatic but occasionally is associated with an audible bruit, TIAs, or stroke. The cause and natural history of fibromuscular dysplasia are unknown. TIA or stroke generally occurs only when the artery is severely narrowed or dissects. Anticoagulation or antiplatelet therapy may be helpful.

Temporal (giant cell) arteritis is a relatively common affliction of elderly persons in which the external carotid system, particularly the temporal arteries, becomes the site of a subacute granulomatous inflammation with giant cells. Occlusion of posterior ciliary arteries derived from the ophthalmic artery results in blindness in one or both eyes and can be prevented with glucocorticoids. It

rarely causes stroke as the internal carotid artery is usually not inflamed. Idiopathic giant cell arteritis involving the great vessels arising from the aortic arch (*Takayasu's arteritis*) may cause carotid or vertebral thrombosis; it is rare in the western hemisphere.

Necrotizing (or granulomatous) arteritis, occurring alone or in association with generalized polyarteritis nodosa or Wegener's granulomatosis, involves the distal small branches (<2 mm diameter) of the main intracranial arteries and produces small ischemic infarcts in the brain, optic nerve, and spinal cord. The cerebrospinal fluid often shows pleocytosis, and the protein level is elevated. *Primary central nervous system vasculitis* is rare; small or medium-sized vessels are usually affected. Brain biopsy or high-resolution conventional x-ray angiography is usually required to make the diagnosis (**Fig. 17-4**). Patients with any form of vasculitis may present with insidious progression of combined white and gray matter infarctions, prominent headache, and cognitive decline. Aggressive immunosuppression with glucocorticoids, and often cyclophosphamide, is usually necessary to prevent progression. Depending upon the duration of the disease, many patients can make an excellent recovery.

Drugs, in particular amphetamines and perhaps cocaine, may cause stroke on the basis of acute hypertension and drug-induced vasculitis. Abstinence appears to be the best treatment, as no data exist on use of any treatment. Phenylpropanolamine has been linked with intracranial hemorrhage as has cocaine, perhaps related

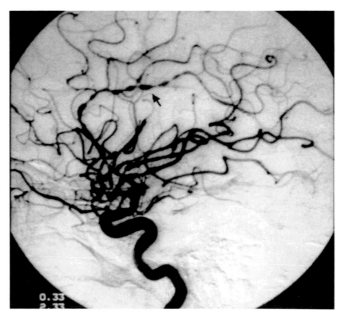

FIGURE 17-4
Cerebral angiogram from a 32-year-old male with central nervous system vasculitis. Dramatic beading (*arrow*) typical of vasculitis is seen.

to a drug-induced vasculitis. Arteritis can also occur as a consequence of bacterial, tuberculous, and syphilitic meningitis.

Moyamoya disease is a poorly understood occlusive disease involving large intracranial arteries, especially the distal internal carotid artery and the stem of the middle and anterior cerebral arteries. Vascular inflammation is absent. The lenticulostriate arteries develop a rich collateral circulation around the occlusive lesion, which gives the impression of a "puff of smoke" (*moyamoya* in Japanese) on conventional x-ray angiography. Other collaterals include transdural anastomoses between the cortical surface branches of the meningeal and scalp arteries. The disease occurs mainly in Asian children or young adults, but the appearance may be identical in adults who have atherosclerosis. The etiology of the childhood form is unknown. Because of the occurrence of intracranial hemorrhage from rupture of the transdural and pial anastomotic channels, anticoagulation is risky. Breakdown of dilated lenticulostriate arteries may produce parenchymal hemorrhage, and progressive occlusion of large surface arteries can occur, producing large-artery distribution strokes. Bypass of extracranial carotid arteries to the dura or MCAs may prevent stroke and hemorrhage.

Reversible posterior leukoencephalopathy can occur in head injury, migraine, sympathomimetic drug use, eclampsia, and the postpartum period. The etiology is unclear but likely involves widespread cerebral segmental vasoconstriction. Patients complain of headache and manifest fluctuating neurologic symptoms and signs, especially visual symptoms. Sometimes cerebral infarction ensues. Conventional x-ray angiography is the only means of establishing the diagnosis, but because angiography itself can cause spasm of vessels, even the existence of this vascular entity is debated.

Binswanger's disease (chronic progressive subcortical encephalopathy) is a rare condition in which infarction of the subcortical white matter occurs subacutely. CT or MRI scans detect periventricular white matter infarcts and gliosis. There is lipohyalinosis in the small arteries of the deep white matter, as in hypertension. There are usually associated lacunar infarcts. Binswanger's disease may represent a type of border zone ischemic infarction in the deep white matter between the penetrating arteries of the circle of Willis and of the cortex. The pathophysiologic basis of the disease is unclear, but it typically occurs in older patients with severe long-standing hypertension.

CADASIL (cerebral autosomal dominant arteriopathy with subcortical infarcts and leukoencephalopathy) is an inherited disorder that presents as small-vessel strokes, progressive dementia, and extensive symmetric white matter changes visualized by MRI. Approximately 40% of patients have migraine with aura, often manifest as transient motor or sensory deficits. Onset is usually in the fourth or fifth decade of life. This autosomal dominant condition is caused by one of several mutations in *Notch-3*, a member of a highly conserved gene family characterized by epidermal growth factor repeats in its extracellular domain. CADASIL is the only monogenic ischemic stroke syndrome so far described. Genetic testing is available.

TRANSIENT ISCHEMIC ATTACKS

TIAs are episodes of stroke symptoms that last only briefly; the current definition of duration is <24 h, but the average duration of a TIA is ~12 min. The causes of TIA are similar to all causes of stroke, but because TIAs may herald stroke they are an important risk factor that should be considered separately. TIAs may arise from emboli to the brain or from in situ thrombosis of an intracranial vessel. With a TIA, the occluded blood vessel reopens and neurologic function is restored. However, infarcts of the brain do occur in 15 to 40% of TIAs even though neurologic signs and symptoms are absent.

In addition to the stroke syndromes discussed below, one specific TIA symptom should receive special notice. *Amaurosis fugax*, or transient monocular blindness, occurs from emboli to the central retinal artery of one eye. This may indicate carotid stenosis as the cause or local ophthalmic artery disease.

The risk of stroke after a TIA is ~10 to 15% in the first 3 months, with most events occurring in the first 2 days. Therefore, urgent evaluation and treatment are justified. Since etiologies for stroke and TIA are identical, evaluation for TIA should parallel that of stroke (Tables 17-1 and 17-3). The improvement characteristic of TIA is a contraindication to thrombolysis. Acute antiplatelet therapy has not been tested specifically after TIA but is likely to be effective and is recommended. No large-scale trial has evaluated acute anticoagulation after TIA, a setting in which the risk of hemorrhage may be lower.

RISK FACTORS FOR ISCHEMIC STROKE

Identification and control of modifiable risk factors is the best strategy to reduce the burden of stroke, as the total number of strokes could be reduced substantially by these means (Table 17-5).

PRIMARY AND SECONDARY PREVENTION
General Principles

A number of medical and surgical interventions, as well as life-style modifications, are available for preventing stroke. Some of these can be widely applied because of their low cost and minimal risk; others are expensive and carry substantial risk but may be valuable for selected high-risk patients.

Evaluation of a patient's *clinical risk profile* can help determine which preventive treatments to offer. In addition to known risk factors for ischemic stroke (above), certain clinical characteristics also contribute to an increased risk of stroke (Table 17-5). NASCET found that even in patients with the same degree of carotid artery stenosis, specifically 70 to 99%, nine prospectively selected risk factors predicted the risk of vascular outcomes in the medically treated patients. The overall risk of stroke was much greater in a high-risk group (those with more than six risk factors) than in a low-risk group (those with fewer than six risk factors). Fully 39% of patients in the high-risk group treated medically experienced an ipsilateral stroke within 2 years. The rate for the low-risk group was less than half that but was still 17%.

Atherosclerosis Risk Factors

Older age, family history of thrombotic stroke, diabetes mellitus, hypertension, tobacco smoking, abnormal blood cholesterol [particularly low high–density lipoprotein (HDL) and/or high low-density lipoprotein (LDL)], and other factors are either proven or probable risk factors for ischemic stroke, largely by their link to atherosclerosis. Risk of second stroke is strongly influenced by prior stroke or TIA, depending on cause. Many cardiac conditions predispose to stroke, including atrial fibrillation and recent MI. Oral contraceptives may increase stroke risk, and certain inherited and acquired hypercoagulable states predispose to stroke. Hypertension is the most significant of the risk factors; in general, all hypertension should be treated. The presence of known cerebrovascular disease is not a contraindication to treatment aimed at achieving normotension. Also, the value of treating systolic hypertension in older patients has been clearly established. Lowering blood pressure to levels below those traditionally defining hypertension appears to reduce the risk of stroke even further. Data are particularly strong in support of thiazide diuretics, angiotensin-converting enzyme inhibitors, and angiotensin receptor blockers.

Several trials have confirmed that statin drugs reduce the risk of stroke even in patients without elevated LDL or low HDL. Although studies specifically targeting primary and secondary prevention of stroke are still underway, results for patients with cardiovascular risk factors or dyslipidemia have been compelling, with a 20 to 30% relative risk reduction for stroke. Therefore, a statin should be considered in all patients with prior ischemic stroke. Tobacco smoking should be discouraged in all

patients. Whether or not tight control of blood sugar in patients with diabetes lowers stroke risk is uncertain.

Antiplatelet Agents

Platelet antiaggregation agents can prevent atherothrombotic events, including TIA and stroke, by inhibiting the formation of intraarterial platelet aggregates. These can form on diseased arteries, induce thrombus formation, and occlude the artery or embolize into the distal circulation. Aspirin, clopidogrel, and the combination of aspirin plus extended-release dipyridamole are the antiplatelet agents most commonly used for this purpose. Ticlopidine has been largely abandoned because of its adverse effects.

Aspirin is the most widely studied antiplatelet agent. Aspirin acetylates platelet cyclooxygenase, which irreversibly inhibits the formation in platelets of thromboxane A_2, a platelet aggregating and vasoconstricting prostaglandin. This effect is permanent and lasts for the usual 8-day life of the platelet. Paradoxically, aspirin also inhibits the formation in endothelial cells of prostacyclin, an antiaggregating and vasodilating prostaglandin. This effect is transient. As soon as aspirin is cleared from the blood, the nucleated endothelial cells again produce prostacyclin. Aspirin in low doses given once daily inhibits the production of thromboxane A_2 in platelets without substantially inhibiting prostacyclin formation. The FDA recommends 50 to 325 mg of aspirin daily for stroke prevention.

Ticlopidine and clopidogrel block the ADP receptor on platelets and thus prevent the cascade resulting in activation of the glycoprotein IIb/IIIa receptor that leads to fibrinogen binding to the platelet and consequent platelet aggregation. Ticlopidine is more effective than aspirin; however, it has the disadvantage of causing diarrhea, skin rash, a low incidence of neutropenia, and thrombotic thrombocytopenic purpura. Clopidogrel is not associated with these important side effects. However, the CAPRIE (Clopidogrel versus Aspirin in Patients at Risk of Ischemic Events) trial, which led to FDA approval, found that it was only marginally more effective than aspirin in reducing risk of stroke. The MATCH (Management of Atherothrombosis with Clopidogrel in High-Risk Patients) study was a large multicenter, randomized double-blind trial that compared clopidogrel in combination with aspirin to clopidogrel alone in the secondary prevention of TIA or stroke. In contrast to studies that have revealed a cardiovascular benefit to such dual antiplatelet therapy, the MATCH trial found no difference in TIA or stroke prevention with this combination but did show a small but significant increase in major bleeding complications (3% vs. 1%). In the MATCH study, almost half of all patients were enrolled more than 1 month after symptom onset;

as the risk of stroke is highest immediately following either TIA or stroke, it is possible that clopidogrel combined with aspirin may be beneficial in this acute period. Ongoing studies are currently addressing this question.

Dipyridamole is an antiplatelet agent that inhibits the uptake of adenosine by a variety of cells, including those of the vascular endothelium. The accumulated adenosine is an inhibitor of aggregation. At least in part through its effects on platelet and vessel wall phosphodiesterases, dipyridamole also potentiates the antiaggregatory effects of prostacyclin and nitric oxide produced by the endothelium and acts by inhibiting platelet phosphodiesterase, which is responsible for the breakdown of cyclic AMP. The resulting elevation in cyclic AMP inhibits aggregation of platelets. Dipyridamole has a controversial history in stroke prevention. The European Stroke Prevention Study-2 showed efficacy of both 50 mg daily of aspirin and extended-release dipyridamole in preventing stroke, and a significantly better risk reduction when the two agents were combined. A combination capsule of extended-release dipyridamole and aspirin is approved for prevention of stroke.

Many large clinical trials have demonstrated clearly that most antiplatelet agents reduce the risk of all important vascular atherothrombotic events (i.e., ischemic stroke, MI, and death due to all vascular causes) in patients at risk for these events. The overall *relative* reduction in risk of nonfatal stroke is about 25 to 30% and of all vascular events is about 25%. The *absolute* reduction varies considerably depending on the particular patient's risk. Individuals at very low risk for stroke seem to experience the same relative reduction, but their risk may be so low that the "benefit" is meaningless. On the other hand, individuals with a 10 to 15% risk of vascular events per year experience a reduction to about 7.5 to 11%.

Aspirin is inexpensive, can be given in low doses, and could be recommended for all adults to prevent both stroke and MI. However, it causes epigastric discomfort, gastric ulceration, and gastrointestinal hemorrhage, which may be asymptomatic or life-threatening. Consequently, not every 40- or 50-year-old should be advised to take aspirin regularly because the risk of atherothrombotic stroke is extremely low and is outweighed by the risk of adverse side effects. Conversely, every patient who has experienced an atherothrombotic stroke or TIA and has no contraindication should be taking an antiplatelet agent regularly because the average annual risk of another stroke is 8 to 10%; another few percent will experience a MI or vascular death. Clearly, the likelihood of benefit far outweighs the risks of treatment.

The choice of antiplatelet agent and dose must balance the risk of stroke, the expected benefit, and the risk and cost of treatment. However, there are no definitive data, and opinions vary. Many authorities believe low-dose (30 to 75 mg daily) and high-dose (650 to 1300 mg daily) aspirin are about equally effective. Some advocate very low doses to avoid adverse effects, and still others advocate very high doses to be sure the benefit is maximal. Most physicians in North America recommend 81 to 325 mg daily, while most Europeans recommend 50 to 100 mg. Similarly, the choice of aspirin, clopidogrel, or dipyridamole plus aspirin must balance the fact that the latter are more effective than aspirin but the cost is higher.

Anticoagulation Therapy and Noncardiogenic Stroke

There are few data to support the use of long-term warfarin for preventing atherothrombotic stroke, for either intracranial or extracranial cerebrovascular disease. The Warfarin-Aspirin Recurrent Stroke Study (WARSS) found no benefit of warfarin sodium (INR 2 to 3) over aspirin, 325 mg, for secondary prevention of stroke but did find a slightly higher bleeding rate in the warfarin group. The WASID study (see above) demonstrated no benefit of warfarin (INR 2 to 3) over aspirin in patients with symptomatic intracranial atherosclerosis, and also found higher bleeding complications.

Anticoagulation Therapy and Embolic Stroke

Several trials have shown that anticoagulation (INR range 2 to 3) in patients with chronic nonvalvular (nonrheumatic) atrial fibrillation prevents cerebral embolism and is safe. For primary prevention and for patients who have experienced stroke or TIA, anticoagulation with warfarin reduces the risk by about 67%, which clearly outweighs the 1% risk per year of a major bleeding complication.

The decision to use anticoagulation for primary prevention is based primarily on risk factors (Table 17-4). The presence of any risk factor tips the balance in favor of anticoagulation.

Because of the high annual stroke risk in untreated rheumatic heart disease, primary prophylaxis against stroke has not been studied in a double-blind fashion. These patients generally receive long-term anticoagulation.

Anticoagulation also reduces the risk of embolism in acute MI. Most clinicians recommend a 3-month course of anticoagulation when there is anterior Q-wave infarction, substantial left ventricular dysfunction, congestive heart failure, mural thrombosis, or atrial fibrillation. Warfarin is recommended long-term if atrial fibrillation persists. Warfarin is currently being studied in patients with congestive heart failure.

Stroke secondary to thromboembolism is one of the most serious complications of prosthetic heart valve implantation. Indications for the intensity of anticoagulation and/or antiplatelet therapy are based upon the type of prosthetic valve and its location. The Seventh American College of Chest Physicians Conference on Antithrombotic Therapy for Valvular Heart Disease published the following guidelines in 2004: (1) for St. Jude Medical bileaflet valves in the aortic position, long-term warfarin with a target INR of 2.5 (range 2.0 to 3.0); (2) for tilting disk valves and bileaflet mechanical valves in the mitral position, long-term warfarin with a target INR of 3.0 (range 2.5 to 3.5); (3) for caged ball or caged disk valves, long-term warfarin with target INR of 3.0 (range 2.5 to 3.5) in combination with aspirin (75 to 100 mg/d); (4), for bioprosthetic valves, warfarin anticoagulation with target INR 2.5 for 3 months, followed by long-term aspirin alone (75 to 100 mg/d), assuming there is no history of atrial fibrillation.

If the embolic source cannot be eliminated, anticoagulation should in most cases be continued indefinitely. Many neurologists recommend combining antiplatelet agents with anticoagulants for patients who "fail" one form of therapy (i.e., have another stroke or TIA). This empirical approach subjects the patient to an increased bleeding risk.

Other Causes of Stroke

■■■ **Carotid Disease** Surgical or endovascular repair of carotid atherosclerosis is preferred over medical therapy for symptomatic carotid artery disease (see section above). Anticoagulation has not been directly compared with antiplatelet therapy for carotid disease.

■■■ **Dural Sinus Thrombosis** Limited evidence exists to support short-term usage of anticoagulants, regardless of the presence of intracranial hemorrhage for venous infarction following sinus thrombosis.

STROKE SYNDROMES

A careful history and neurologic examination can often localize the region of brain dysfunction; if this region corresponds to a particular arterial distribution, the possible causes responsible for the syndrome can be narrowed. This is of particular importance when the patient presents with a TIA and a normal examination. For example, if a patient develops language loss and a right homonymous hemianopia, a search for causes of left middle cerebral emboli should be performed. A finding of an isolated stenosis of the right internal carotid artery in that patient, for example, suggests an asymptomatic carotid stenosis, and the search for other causes of stroke should continue. The following sections describe the clinical findings of cerebral ischemia associated with cerebral vascular territories depicted in Figs. 17-5

through 17-13. Stroke syndromes are divided into: (1) large-vessel stroke within the anterior circulation, (2) large-vessel stroke within the posterior circulation, and (3) small-vessel disease of either vascular bed.

Stroke within the Anterior Circulation

The internal carotid artery and its branches comprise the anterior circulation of the brain. These vessels can be occluded by intrinsic disease of the vessel (e.g., atherosclerosis or dissection) or by embolic occlusion from a proximal source as discussed above. Occlusion of each major intracranial vessel has distinct clinical manifestations.

■■■ **Middle Cerebral Artery** Occlusion of the proximal MCA or one of its major branches is most often due to an embolus (artery-to-artery, cardiac, or of unknown source) rather than intracranial atherothrombosis. Atherosclerosis of the proximal MCA may cause distal emboli to the middle cerebral territory or, less commonly, may produce low-flow TIAs. Collateral formation via leptomeningeal vessels often prevents MCA stenosis from becoming symptomatic.

The cortical branches of the MCA supply the lateral surface of the hemisphere except for (1) the frontal pole and a strip along the superomedial border of the frontal and parietal lobes supplied by the ACA, and (2) the lower temporal and occipital pole convolutions supplied by the PCA (**Figs. 17-5**, 17-7, and 17-8).

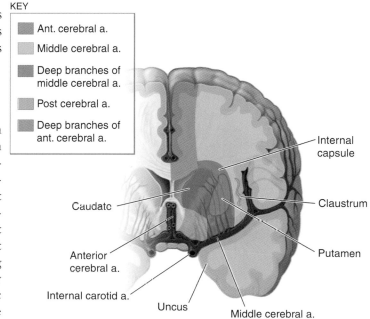

KEY

- ■ Ant. cerebral a.
- ■ Middle cerebral a.
- ■ Deep branches of middle cerebral a.
- ■ Post cerebral a.
- ■ Deep branches of ant. cerebral a.

Internal capsule

Claustrum

Putamen

Caudate

Anterior cerebral a.

Internal carotid a.

Uncus

Middle cerebral a.

FIGURE 17-5

Diagram of a cerebral hemisphere in coronal section showing the deep and superficial territories of the major cerebral vessels.

The proximal MCA (M1 segment) gives rise to penetrating branches (termed *lenticulostriate arteries*) that supply the putamen, outer globus pallidus, posterior limb of the internal capsule, the adjacent corona radiata, and most of the caudate nucleus. In the sylvian fissure, the MCA in most patients divides into *superior* and *inferior* divisions (M2 branches). Branches of the inferior division supply the inferior parietal and temporal cortex, and those from the superior division supply the frontal and superior parietal cortex (**Fig. 17–6**).

If the entire MCA is occluded at its origin (blocking both its penetrating and cortical branches) and the distal collaterals are limited, the clinical findings are contralateral hemiplegia, hemianesthesia, homonymous hemianopia, and a day or two of gaze preference to the ipsi-

lateral side. Dysarthria is common because of facial weakness. When the dominant hemisphere is involved, global aphasia is present also, and when the nondominant hemisphere is affected, anosognosia, constructional apraxia, and neglect are found (Chap. 7).

Complete MCA syndromes occur most often when an embolus occludes the stem of the artery. Cortical collateral blood flow and differing arterial configurations are probably responsible for the development of many partial syndromes. Partial syndromes may also be due to emboli that enter the proximal MCA without complete occlusion, occlude distal MCA branches, or fragment and move distally.

Partial syndromes due to embolic occlusion of a single branch include hand, or arm and hand, weakness

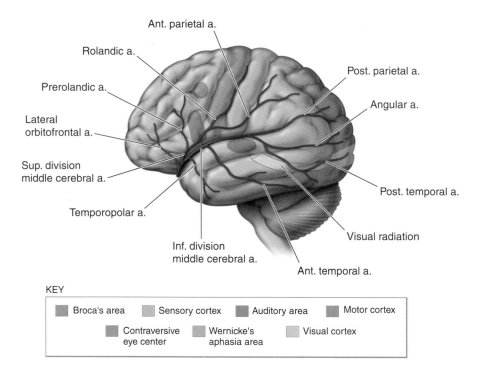

FIGURE 17-6

Diagram of a cerebral hemisphere, lateral aspect, showing the branches and distribution of the middle cerebral artery and the principal regions of cerebral localization. Note the bifurcation of the middle cerebral artery into a superior and inferior division.

Signs and symptoms: *Structures involved*

Paralysis of the contralateral face, arm, and leg; sensory impairment over the same area (pinprick, cotton touch, vibration, position, two-point discrimination, stereognosis, tactile localization, barognosis, cutaneographia): *Somatic motor area for face and arm and the fibers descending from the leg area to enter the corona radiata and corresponding somatic sensory system*

Motor aphasia: *Motor speech area of the dominant hemisphere*

Central aphasia, word deafness, anomia, jargon speech, sensory agraphia, acalculia, alexia, finger agnosia, right-left confusion (the last four comprise the Gerstmann syndrome): *Central, suprasylvian speech area and parietooccipital cortex of the dominant hemisphere*

Conduction aphasia: *Central speech area (parietal operculum)*

Apractognosia of the nondominant hemisphere, anosognosia, hemiasomatognosia, unilateral neglect, agnosia for the left half of external space, dressing "apraxia," constructional "apraxia," distortion of visual coordinates, inaccurate localization in the half field, impaired ability to judge distance, upside-down reading, visual illusions (e.g., it may appear that another person walks through a table): *Nondominant parietal lobe (area corresponding to speech area in dominant hemisphere); loss of topographic memory is usually due to a nondominant lesion, occasionally to a dominant one*

Homonymous hemianopia (often homonymous inferior quadrantanopia): *Optic radiation deep to second temporal convolution*

Paralysis of conjugate gaze to the opposite side: *Frontal contraversive field or projecting fibers* alone (brachial syndrome) or facial weakness with non-fluent (Broca) aphasia (Chap. 7), with or without arm weakness (frontal opercular syndrome). A combination of sensory disturbance, motor weakness, and nonfluent aphasia suggests that an embolus has occluded the proximal superior division and infarcted large portions of the frontal and parietal cortices (Fig. 17-6). If a fluent (Wernicke's) aphasia occurs without weakness, the inferior division of the MCA supplying the posterior part (temporal cortex) of the dominant hemisphere is probably involved. Jargon speech and an inability to comprehend written and spoken language are prominent features, often accompanied by a contralateral, homonymous superior quadrantanopia. Hemineglect or spatial agnosia without weakness indicates that the inferior division of the MCA in the nondominant hemisphere is involved.

Occlusion of a lenticulostriate vessel produces small-vessel (lacunar) stroke within the internal capsule. This produces pure motor stroke or sensory-motor stroke contralateral to the lesion. Ischemia within the genu of the internal capsule causes primarily facial weakness followed by arm then leg weakness as the ischemia moves posterior within the capsule. Alternatively, the contralat-eral hand may become ataxic and dysarthria will be prominent (clumsy hand, dysarthria lacunar syndrome). Lacunar infarction affecting the globus pallidus and putamen often has few clinical signs, but parkinsonism and hemiballismus have been reported.

Anterior Cerebral Artery The ACA is divided into two segments: the precommunal (A1) circle of Willis, or stem, which connects the internal carotid artery to the anterior communicating artery, and the postcommunal (A2) segment distal to the anterior communicating artery (Figs. 17-3 and 17-8). The A1 segment gives rise to several deep penetrating branches that supply the anterior limb of the internal capsule, the anterior perforate substance, amygdala, anterior hypothalamus, and the inferior part of the head of the caudate nucleus (Fig. 17-5).

Occlusion of the proximal ACA is usually well tolerated because of collateral flow through the anterior communicating artery and collaterals through the MCA and PCA. Occlusion of a single A2 segment results in the contralateral symptoms noted in **Fig. 17-7**. If both A2 segments arise from a single anterior cerebral stem

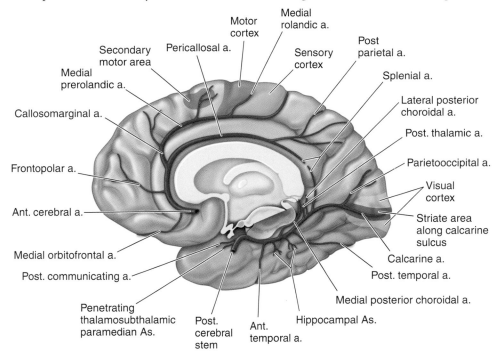

FIGURE 17-7

Diagram of a cerebral hemisphere, medial aspect, showing the branches and distribution of the anterior cerebral artery and the principal regions of cerebral localization.

Signs and symptoms: *Structures involved*

Paralysis of opposite foot and leg: *Motor leg area*

A lesser degree of paresis of opposite arm: *Arm area of cortex or fibers descending to corona radiata*

Cortical sensory loss over toes, foot, and leg: *Sensory area for foot and leg*

Urinary incontinence: *Sensorimotor area in paracentral lobule*

Contralateral grasp reflex, sucking reflex, gegenhalten (paratonic rigidity): *Medial surface of the posterior frontal lobe (?) supplemental motor area*

Abulia (akinetic mutism), slowness, delay, intermittent interruption, lack of spontaneity, whispering, reflex distraction to sights and sounds: *Uncertain localization-probably cingulate gyrus and medial inferior portion of frontal, parietal, and temporal lobes*

Impairment of gait and stance (gait apraxia): *Frontal cortex near leg motor area*

Dyspraxia of left limbs, tactile aphasia in left limbs: *Corpus callosum* (contralateral A1 segment atresia), the occlusion may affect both hemispheres. Profound abulia (a delay in verbal and motor response) and bilateral pyramidal signs with paraparesis and urinary incontinence result.

Anterior Choroidal Artery This artery arises from the internal carotid artery and supplies the posterior limb of the internal capsule and the white matter posterolateral to it, through which pass some of the geniculocalcarine fibers (**Figs.** 17-5 and **17-8**). The complete syndrome of anterior choroidal artery occlusion consists of contralateral hemiplegia, hemianesthesia (hypesthesia), and homonymous hemianopia. However, because this territory is also supplied by penetrating vessels of the proximal MCA and the posterior communicating and posterior choroidal arteries, minimal deficits may occur, and patients frequently recover substantially. Anterior choroidal strokes are usually the result of in situ thrombosis of the vessel, and the vessel is particularly vulnerable to iatrogenic occlusion during surgical clipping of aneurysms arising from the internal carotid artery.

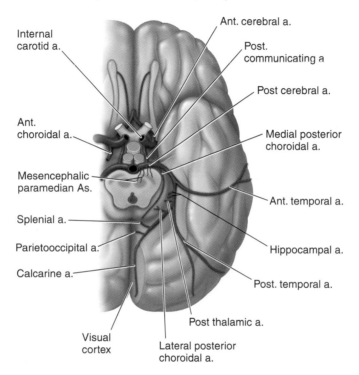

FIGURE 17-8

Inferior aspect of the brain with the branches and distribution of the posterior cerebral artery and the principal anatomic structures shown.

Signs and symptoms: *Structures involved*

Peripheral territory (see also Fig. 17-11). Homonymous hemianopia (often upper quadrantic): *Calcarine cortex or optic radiation nearby.* Bilateral homonymous hemianopia, cortical blindness, awareness or denial of blindness; tactile naming, achromatopia (color blindness), failure to see to-and-fro movements, inability to perceive objects not centrally located, apraxia of ocular movements, inability to count or enumerate objects, tendency to run into things that the patient sees and tries to avoid: *Bilateral occipital lobe with possibly the parietal lobe involved.* Verbal dyslexia without agraphia, color anomia: *Dominant calcarine lesion and posterior part of corpus callosum.* Memory defect: *Hippocampal lesion bilaterally or on the dominant side only.* Topographic disorientation and prosopagnosia: *Usually with lesions of nondominant, calcarine, and lingual gyrus.* Simultagnosia, hemivisual neglect: *Dominant visual cortex, contralateral hemisphere.* Unformed visual hallucinations, peduncular hallucinosis, metamorphopsia, teleopsia, illu-

sory visual spread, palinopsia, distortion of outlines, central photophobia: *Calcarine cortex.* Complex hallucinations: *Usually nondominant hemisphere.*

Central territory. Thalamic syndrome: sensory loss (all modalities), spontaneous pain and dysesthesias, choreoathetosis, intention tremor, spasms of hand, mild hemiparesis: *Posteroventral nucleus of thalamus; involvement of the adjacent subthalamus body or its afferent tracts.* Thalamoperforate syndrome: crossed cerebellar ataxia with ipsilateral third nerve palsy (Claude's syndrome): *Dentatothalamic tract and issuing third nerve.* Weber's syndrome: third nerve palsy and contralateral hemiplegia: *Third nerve and cerebral peduncle.* Contralateral hemiplegia: *Cerebral peduncle.* Paralysis or paresis of vertical eye movement, skew deviation, sluggish pupillary responses to light, slight miosis and ptosis (retraction nystagmus and "tucking" of the eyelids may be associated): *Supranuclear fibers to third nerve, interstitial nucleus of Cajal, nucleus of Darkschewitsch, and posterior commissure.* Contralateral rhythmic, ataxic action tremor; rhythmic postural or "holding" tremor (rubral tremor): *Dentatothalamic tract(?).*

Internal Carotid Artery The clinical picture of internal carotid occlusion varies depending on whether the cause of ischemia is propagated thrombus, embolism, or low flow. The cortex supplied by the MCA territory is affected most often. With a competent circle of Willis, occlusion may go unnoticed. If the thrombus propagates up the internal carotid artery into the MCA or embolizes it, symptoms are identical to proximal MCA occlusion (see above). Sometimes there is massive infarction of the entire deep white matter and cortical surface. When the origins of both the ACA and MCA are occluded at the top of the carotid artery, abulia or stupor occurs with hemiplegia, hemianesthesia, and aphasia or anosognosia. When the PCA arises from the internal carotid artery (a configuration called a *fetal posterior cerebral artery*), it may also become occluded and give rise to symptoms referable to its peripheral territory (Figs. 17-7 and 17-8).

In addition to supplying the ipsilateral brain, the internal carotid artery perfuses the optic nerve and retina via the ophthalmic artery. In about 25% of symptomatic internal carotid disease, recurrent transient monocular blindness (amaurosis fugax) warns of the lesion. Patients typically describe a horizontal shade that sweeps down or up across the field of vision. They may also complain that their vision was blurred in that eye or that the upper or lower half of vision disappeared. In most cases, these symptoms last only a few minutes. Rarely, ischemia or infarction of the ophthalmic artery or central retinal arteries occurs at the time of cerebral TIA or infarction.

A high-pitched prolonged carotid bruit fading into diastole is often associated with tightly stenotic lesions. As the stenosis grows tighter and flow distal to the stenosis becomes reduced, the bruit becomes fainter and may disappear when occlusion is imminent.

Common Carotid Artery All symptoms and signs of internal carotid occlusion may also be present with occlusion of the common carotid artery. Bilateral common carotid artery occlusions at their origin may occur in Takayasu's arteritis.

Stroke within the Posterior Circulation

The posterior circulation is composed of the paired vertebral arteries, the basilar artery, and the paired posterior cerebral arteries. The vertebral arteries join to form the basilar artery at the pontomedullary junction. The basilar artery divides into two posterior cerebral arteries in the interpeduncular fossa (Fig. 17-3). These major arteries give rise to long and short circumferential branches and to smaller deep penetrating branches that supply the cerebellum, medulla, pons, midbrain, subthalamus, thala-mus, hippocampus, and medial temporal and occipital lobes. Occlusion of each vessel produces its own distinctive syndrome.

Posterior Cerebral Artery In 75% of cases, both PCAs arise from the bifurcation of the basilar artery; in 20%, one has its origin from the ipsilateral internal carotid artery via the posterior communicating artery; in 5%, both originate from the respective ipsilateral internal carotid arteries (Fig. 17-3). The precommunal, or P1, segment of the true posterior cerebral artery is atretic in such cases.

PCA syndromes usually result from atheroma formation or emboli that lodge at the top of the basilar artery; posterior circulation disease may also be caused by dissection of either vertebral artery and fibromuscular dysplasia.

Two clinical syndromes are commonly observed with occlusion of the PCA: (1) *P1 syndrome*: midbrain, subthalamic, and thalamic signs, which are due to disease of the proximal P1 segment of the PCA or its penetrating branches (thalamogeniculate, Percheron, and posterior choroidal arteries); and (2) *P2 syndrome*: cortical temporal and occipital lobe signs, due to occlusion of the P2 segment distal to the junction of the PCA with the posterior communicating artery.

P1 Syndromes Infarction usually occurs in the ipsilateral subthalamus and medial thalamus and in the ipsilateral cerebral peduncle and midbrain (Figs. 17-8, 17-13). A third nerve palsy with contralateral ataxia (Claude's syndrome) or with contralateral hemiplegia (Weber's syndrome) may result. The ataxia indicates involvement of the red nucleus or dentatorubrothalamic tract; the hemiplegia is localized to the cerebral peduncle. If the subthalamic nucleus is involved, contralateral hemiballismus may occur. Occlusion of the artery of Percheron produces paresis of upward gaze and drowsiness, and often abulia. Extensive infarction in the midbrain and subthalamus occurring with bilateral proximal PCA occlusion presents as coma, unreactive pupils, bilateral pyramidal signs, and decerebrate rigidity.

Occlusion of the penetrating branches of thalamic and thalamogeniculate arteries produces less extensive thalamic and thalamocapsular lacunar syndromes. The *thalamic Déjerine-Roussy syndrome* consists of contralateral hemisensory loss followed later by an agonizing, searing or burning pain in the affected areas. It is persistent and responds poorly to analgesics. Anticonvulsants (carbamazepine or gabapentin) or tricyclic antidepressants may be beneficial.

P2 Syndromes (See Also Fig. 17-8) Occlusion of the distal PCA causes infarction of the medial temporal and occipital lobes. Contralateral homonymous hemianopia with macula sparing is the usual manifestation. Occasionally, only the upper quadrant of visual field is involved. If the visual association areas are spared and only the calcarine cortex is involved, the patient may be aware of visual defects. Medial temporal lobe and hippocampal involvement may cause an acute disturbance in memory, particularly if it occurs in the dominant hemisphere. The defect usually clears because memory has bilateral representation. If the dominant hemisphere is affected and the infarct extends to involve the splenium of the corpus callosum, the patient may demonstrate alexia without agraphia. Visual agnosia for faces, objects, mathematical symbols, and colors and anomia with paraphasic errors (amnestic aphasia) may also occur in this setting, even without callosal involvement. Occlusion of the posterior cerebral artery can produce *peduncular hallucinosis* (visual hallucinations of brightly colored scenes and objects).

Bilateral infarction in the distal PCAs produces cortical blindness (blindness with preserved pupillary light reaction). The patient is often unaware of the blindness or may even deny it (*Anton's syndrome*). Tiny islands of vision may persist, and the patient may report that vision fluctuates as images are captured in the preserved portions. Rarely, only peripheral vision is lost and central vision is spared, resulting in "gun-barrel" vision. Bilateral visual association area lesions may result in *Balint's syndrome,* a disorder of the orderly visual scanning of the environment (Chap. 7), usually resulting from infarctions secondary to low flow in the "watershed" between the distal posterior and middle cerebral artery territories, as occurs after cardiac arrest. Patients may experience persistence of a visual image for several minutes despite gazing at another scene (*palinopia*). Embolic occlusion of the top of the basilar artery can produce any or all of the central or peripheral territory symptoms. The hallmark is the sudden onset of bilateral signs, including ptosis, pupillary asymmetry or lack of reaction to light, and somnolence.

▇▇▇ Vertebral and Posterior Inferior Cerebellar Arteries The vertebral artery, which arises from the innominate artery on the right and the subclavian artery on the left, consists of four segments. The first (V1) extends from its origin to its entrance into the sixth or fifth transverse vertebral foramen. The second segment (V2) traverses the vertebral foramina from C6 to C2. The third (V3) passes through the transverse foramen and circles around the arch of the atlas to pierce the dura at the foramen magnum. The fourth (V4) segment courses upward to join the other vertebral artery to form the basilar artery; only the fourth segment gives rise to branches that supply the brainstem and cerebellum. The posterior inferior cerebellar artery (PICA) in its proximal segment supplies the lateral medulla and, in its distal branches, the inferior surface of the cerebellum.

Atherothrombotic lesions have a predilection for V1 and V4 segments of the vertebral artery. The first segment may become diseased at the origin of the vessel and may produce posterior circulation emboli; collateral flow from the contralateral vertebral artery or the ascending cervical, thyrocervical, or occipital arteries is usually sufficient to prevent low-flow TIAs or stroke. When one vertebral artery is atretic and an atherothrombotic lesion threatens the origin of the other, the collateral circulation, which may also include retrograde flow down the basilar artery, is often insufficient (Figs. 17-3 and 17-8). In this setting, low-flow TIAs may occur, consisting of syncope, vertigo, and alternating hemiplegia; this state also sets the stage for thrombosis. Disease of the distal fourth segment of the vertebral artery can promote thrombus formation manifest as embolism or with propagation as basilar artery thrombosis. Stenosis proximal to the origin of the posterior inferior cerebellar artery can threaten the lateral medulla and posterior inferior surface of the cerebellum.

If the subclavian artery is occluded proximal to the origin of the vertebral artery, there is a reversal in the direction of blood flow in the ipsilateral vertebral artery. Exercise of the ipsilateral arm may increase demand on vertebral flow, producing posterior circulation TIAs, or "subclavian steal."

Although atheromatous disease rarely narrows the second and third segments of the vertebral artery, this region is subject to dissection, fibromuscular dysplasia, and, rarely, encroachment by osteophytic spurs within the vertebral foramina.

Embolic occlusion or thrombosis of a V4 segment causes ischemia of the lateral medulla. The constellation of vertigo, numbness of the ipsilateral face and contralateral limbs, diplopia, hoarseness, dysarthria, dysphagia, and ipsilateral Horner's syndrome is called the lateral medullary (or Wallenberg's) syndrome (**Fig. 17-9**). Most cases result from ipsilateral vertebral artery occlusion; in the remainder, PICA occlusion is responsible. Occlusion of the medullary penetrating branches of the vertebral artery or PICA results in partial syndromes. *Hemiparesis is not a feature of vertebral artery occlusion.*

Rarely, a *medial medullary syndrome* occurs with infarction of the pyramid and contralateral hemiparesis of the arm and leg, sparing the face. If the medial lemniscus and emerging hypoglossal nerve fibers are involved, contralateral loss of joint position sense and ipsilateral tongue weakness occur.

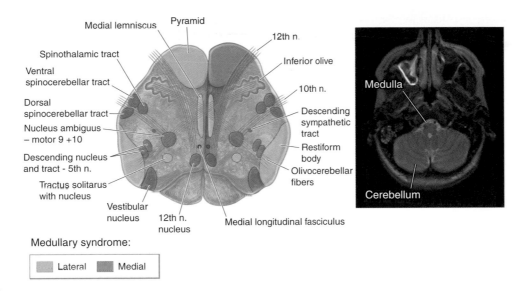

FIGURE 17-9

Axial section at the level of the medulla, depicted schematically on the left, with a corresponding MR image on the right. Note that in Fig. 17-9 through 17-13, all drawings are oriented with the dorsal surface at the bottom, matching the orientation of the brainstem that is commonly seen in all modern neuroimaging studies. Approximate regions involved in medial and lateral medullary stroke syndromes are shown.

Signs and symptoms: *Structures involved*

1. Medial medullary syndrome (occlusion of vertebral artery or of branch of vertebral or lower basilar artery)

   On side of lesion

      Paralysis with atrophy of half the tongue: *Ipsilateral twelfth nerve*

   On side opposite lesion

      Paralysis of arm and leg, sparing face; impaired tactile and proprioceptive sense over half the body: *Contralateral pyramidal tract and medial lemniscus*

2. Lateral medullary syndrome (occlusion of any of five vessels may be responsible-vertebral, posterior inferior cerebellar, superior, middle, or inferior lateral medullary arteries)

   On side of lesion

      Pain, numbness, impaired sensation over half the face: *Descending tract and nucleus fifth nerve*

      Ataxia of limbs, falling to side of lesion: *Uncertain-restiform body, cerebellar hemisphere, cerebellar fibers, spinocerebellar tract(?)*

Nystagmus, diplopia, oscillopsia, vertigo, nausea, vomiting: *Vestibular nucleus*

Horner's syndrome (miosis, ptosis, decreased sweating): *Descending sympathetic tract*

Dysphagia, hoarseness, paralysis of palate, paralysis of vocal cord, diminished gag reflex: *Issuing fibers ninth and tenth nerves*

Loss of taste: *Nucleus and tractus solitarius*

Numbness of ipsilateral arm, trunk, or leg: *Cuneate and gracile nuclei*

On side opposite lesion

   Impaired pain and thermal sense over half the body, sometimes face: *Spinothalamic tract*

3. Total unilateral medullary syndrome (occlusion of vertebral artery): Combination of medial and lateral syndromes

4. Lateral pontomedullary syndrome (occlusion of vertebral artery): Combination of lateral medullary and lateral inferior pontine syndrome

5. Basilar artery syndrome (the syndrome of the lone vertebral artery is equivalent): A combination of the various brainstem syndromes plus those arising in the posterior cerebral artery distribution.

   Bilateral long tract signs (sensory and motor; cerebellar and peripheral cranial nerve abnormalities): *Bilateral long tract; cerebellar and peripheral cranial nerves*

   Paralysis or weakness of all extremities, plus all bulbar musculature: *Corticobulbar and corticospinal tracts bilaterally*

Cerebellar infarction with edema can lead to *sudden respiratory arrest* due to raised ICP in the posterior fossa. Drowsiness, Babinski signs, dysarthria, and bifacial weakness may be absent, or present only briefly, before respiratory arrest ensues. Gait unsteadiness, headache, dizziness, nausea, and vomiting may be the only early symptoms and signs and should arouse suspicion of this impending complication, which may require neurosur-

gical decompression, often with an excellent outcome. Separating these symptoms from those of viral labrynthitis can be a challenge, but headache, neck stiffness, and unilateral dysmetria favor stroke.

BASILAR ARTERY Branches of the basilar artery supply the base of the pons and superior cerebellum and fall into three groups: (1) paramedian, 7 to

10 in number, which supply a wedge of pons on either side of the midline; (2) short circumferential, 5 to 7 in number, which supply the lateral two-thirds of the pons and middle and superior cerebellar peduncles; and (3) bilateral long circumferential (superior cerebellar and anterior inferior cerebellar arteries), which course around the pons to supply the cerebellar hemispheres.

Atheromatous lesions can occur anywhere along the basilar trunk but are most frequent in the proximal basilar and distal vertebral segments. Typically, lesions occlude either the proximal basilar and one or both vertebral arteries. The clinical picture varies depending on the availability of retrograde collateral flow from the posterior communicating arteries. Rarely, dissection of a

vertebral artery may involve the basilar artery and, depending on the location of true and false lumen, may produce multiple penetrating artery strokes.

Although atherothrombosis occasionally occludes the distal portion of the basilar artery, emboli from the heart or proximal vertebral or basilar segments are more commonly responsible for "top of the basilar" syndromes.

Because the brainstem contains many structures in close apposition, a diversity of clinical syndromes may emerge with ischemia, reflecting involvement of the corticospinal and corticobulbar tracts, ascending sensory tracts, and cranial nerve nuclei (**Figs. 17-10**, **17-11**, **17-12**, and **17-13**).

The symptoms of transient ischemia or infarction in the territory of the basilar artery often do not indicate

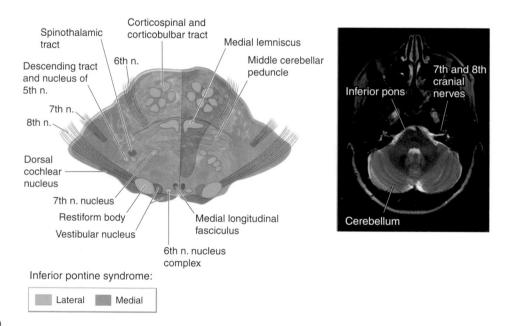

Inferior pontine syndrome:
Lateral   Medial

FIGURE 17-10

Axial section at the level of the inferior pons, depicted schematically on the left, with a corresponding MR image on the right. Approximate regions involved in medial and lateral inferior pontine stroke syndromes are shown.

Signs and symptoms: *structures involved*

1. Medial inferior pontine syndrome (occlusion of paramedian branch of basilar artery)
   On side of lesion
   Paralysis of conjugate gaze to side of lesion (preservation of convergence): *Center for conjugate lateral gaze*
   Nystagmus: *Vestibular nucleus*
   Ataxia of limbs and gait: *Middle cerebellar peduncle (?)*
   Diplopia on lateral gaze: *Abducens nerve*
   On side opposite lesion
   Paralysis of face, arm, and leg: *Corticobulbar and corticospinal tract in lower pons*

   Impaired tactile and proprioceptive sense over half of the body: *Medial lemniscus*
2. Lateral inferior pontine syndrome (occlusion of anterior inferior cerebellar artery)
   On side of lesion
   Horizontal and vertical nystagmus, vertigo, nausea, vomiting, oscillopia: *Vestibular nerve or nucleus*
   Facial paralysis: *Seventh nerve*
   Paralysis of conjugate gaze to side of lesion: *Center for conjugate lateral gaze*
   Deafness, tinnitus: *Auditory nerve or cochlear nucleus*
   Ataxia: *Middle cerebellar peduncle and cerebellar hemisphere*
   Impaired sensation over face: *Descending tract and nucleus fifth nerve*
   On side opposite lesion
   Impaired pain and thermal sense over half the body (may include face): *Spinothalamic tract*

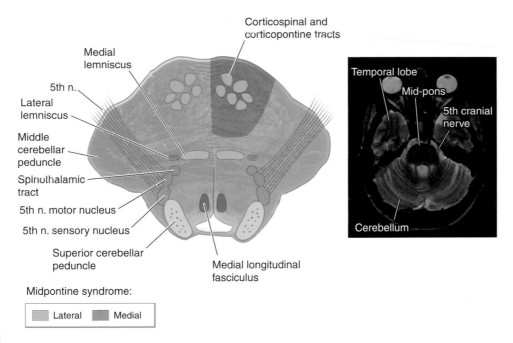

FIGURE 17-11

Axial section at the level of the medial pons, depicted schematically on the left, with a corresponding MR image on the right. Approximate regions involved in medial and lateral midpontine stroke syndromes are shown.

Signs and symptoms: *Structures involved*

1. Medial midpontine syndrome (paramedian branch of mid-basilar artery)
   On side of lesion
      Ataxia of limbs and gait (more prominent in bilateral involvement): *Pontine nuclei*
   On side opposite lesion
      Paralysis of face, arm, and leg: *Corticobulbar and corticospinal tract*

   Variable impaired touch and proprioception when lesion extends posteriorly: *Medial lemniscus*
2. Lateral midpontine syndrome (short circumferential artery)
   On side of lesion
      Ataxia of limbs: *Middle cerebellar peduncle*
      Paralysis of muscles of mastication: *Motor fibers or nucleus of fifth nerve*
      Impaired sensation over side of face: *Sensory fibers or nucleus of fifth nerve*
   On side opposite lesion
      Impaired pain and thermal sense on limbs and trunk: *Spinothalamic tract*

whether the basilar artery itself or one of its branches is diseased, yet this distinction has important implications for therapy. *The picture of complete basilar occlusion, however, is easy to recognize as a constellation of bilateral long tract signs (sensory and motor) with signs of cranial nerve and cerebellar dysfunction.* A "locked-in" state of preserved consciousness with quadriplegia and cranial nerve signs suggests complete pontine and lower midbrain infarction. The therapeutic goal is to identify *impending* basilar occlusion before devastating infarction occurs. A series of TIAs and a slowly progressive, fluctuating stroke are extremely significant as they often herald an atherothrombotic occlusion of the distal vertebral or proximal basilar artery.

TIAs in the proximal basilar distribution may produce vertigo (often described by patients as "swimming," "swaying," "moving," "unsteadiness," or "light-headedness"). Other symptoms that warn of basilar thrombosis include diplopia, dysarthria, facial or circumoral numbness, and hemisensory symptoms. In general, symptoms of basilar branch TIAs affect one side of the brainstem, whereas symptoms of basilar artery TIAs usually affect both sides, though a "herald" hemiparesis has been emphasized as an initial symptom of basilar occlusion. Most often TIAs, whether due to impending occlusion of the basilar artery or a basilar branch, are short-lived (5 to 30 min) and repetitive, occurring several times a day. The pattern suggests intermittent reduction of flow. Many neurologists treat with heparin to prevent clot propagation.

Atherothrombotic occlusion of the basilar artery with infarction usually causes *bilateral* brainstem signs. A gaze paresis or internuclear ophthalmoplegia associated with ipsilateral hemiparesis may be the only manifestation of bilateral brainstem ischemia. More often, unequivocal signs of bilateral pontine disease are present. Complete basilar thrombosis carries a high mortality.

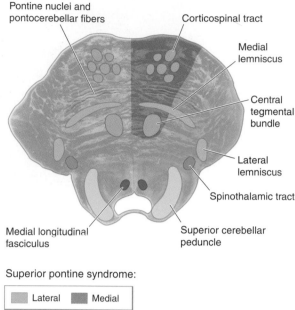
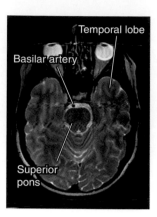

FIGURE 17-12

Axial section at the level of the superior pons, depicted schematically on the left, with a corresponding MR image on the right. Approximate regions involved in medial and lateral superior pontine stroke syndromes are shown.

Signs and symptoms: *Structures involved*

1. Medial superior pontine syndrome (paramedian branches of upper basilar artery)
   On side of lesion
       Cerebellar ataxia (probably): *Superior and/or middle cerebellar peduncle*
       Internuclear ophthalmoplegia: *Medial longitudinal fasciculus*
       Myoclonic syndrome, palate, pharynx, vocal cords, respiratory apparatus, face, oculomotor apparatus, etc.: *Localization uncertain-central tegmental bundle(?), dentate projection(?), inferior olivary nucleus(?)*
   On side opposite lesion
       Paralysis of face, arm, and leg: *Corticobulbar and corticospinal tract*
       Rarely touch, vibration, and position are affected: *Medial lemniscus*

2. Lateral superior pontine syndrome (syndrome of superior cerebellar artery)
   On side of lesion
       Ataxia of limbs and gait, falling to side of lesion: *Middle and superior cerebellar peduncles, superior surface of cerebellum, dentate nucleus*
       Dizziness, nausea, vomiting; horizontal nystagmus: *Vestibular nucleus*
       Paresis of conjugate gaze (ipsilateral): *Pontine contralateral gaze*
       Skew deviation: *Uncertain*
       Miosis, ptosis, decreased sweating over face (Horner's syndrome): *Descending sympathetic fibers*
       Tremor: *Dentate nucleus(?), superior cerebellar peduncle(?)*
   On side opposite lesion
       Impaired pain and thermal sense on face, limbs, and trunk: *Spinothalamic tract*
       Impaired touch, vibration, and position sense, more in leg than arm (there is a tendency to incongruity of pain and touch deficits): *Medial lemniscus (lateral portion)*

Occlusion of a branch of the basilar artery usually causes *unilateral* symptoms and signs involving motor, sensory, and cranial nerves. As long as symptoms remain unilateral, concern over pending basilar occlusion should be reduced.

Occlusion of the superior cerebellar artery results in severe ipsilateral cerebellar ataxia, nausea and vomiting, dysarthria, and contralateral loss of pain and temperature sensation over the extremities, body, and face (spino- and trigeminothalamic tract). Partial deafness, ataxic tremor of the ipsilateral upper extremity, Horner's syndrome, and palatal myoclonus may occur rarely. Partial syndromes occur frequently (Fig. 17-12). With large strokes,

swelling and mass effects may compress the midbrain or produce hydrocephalus; these symptoms may evolve rapidly. Neurosurgical intervention may be lifesaving in such cases.

Occlusion of the anterior inferior cerebellar artery produces variable degrees of infarction because the size of this artery and the territory it supplies vary inversely with those of the PICA. The principal symptoms include: (1) ipsilateral deafness, facial weakness, vertigo, nausea and vomiting, nystagmus, tinnitus, cerebellar ataxia, Horner's syndrome, and paresis of conjugate lateral gaze; and (2) contralateral loss of pain and temperature

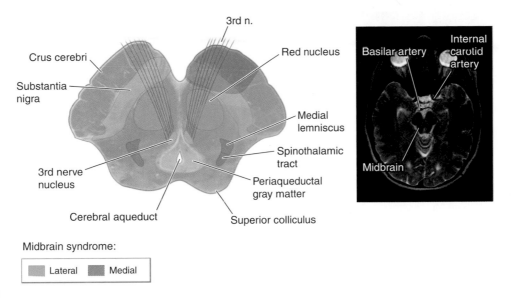

FIGURE 17-13
Axial section at the level of the midbrain, depicted schematically on the left, with a corresponding MR image on the right. Approximate regions involved in medial and lateral midbrain stroke syndromes are shown.
Signs and symptoms: *Structures involved*

1. Medial midbrain syndrome (paramedian branches of upper basilar and proximal posterior cerebral arteries)
   On side of lesion
   　Eye "down and out" secondary to unopposed action of fourth and sixth cranial nerves, with dilated and unresponsive pupil: *Third nerve fibers*
   On side opposite lesion
   　Paralysis of face, arm, and leg: *Corticobulbar and corticospinal tract descending in crus cerebri*

2. Lateral midbrain syndrome (syndrome of small penetrating arteries arising from posterior cerebral artery)
   On side of lesion
   　Eye "down and out" secondary to unopposed action of fourth and sixth cranial nerves, with dilated and unresponsive pupil: *Third nerve fibers and/or third nerve nucleus*
   On side opposite lesion
   　Hemiataxia, hyperkinesias, tremor: *Red nucleus, dentatorubrothalamic pathway*

sensation. An occlusion close to the origin of the artery may cause corticospinal tract signs (Fig. 17-10).

Occlusion of one of the short circumferential branches of the basilar artery affects the lateral two-thirds of the pons and middle or superior cerebellar peduncle, whereas occlusion of one of the paramedian branches affects a wedge-shaped area on either side of the medial pons (Figs. 17-10 through 17-12).

IMAGING STUDIES (See also Chap. 3)

Computed Tomographic Scans

CT radiographic images identify or exclude hemorrhage as the cause of stroke, and they identify extra-parenchymal hemorrhages, neoplasms, abscesses, and other conditions masquerading as stroke. Scans obtained in the first several hours after an infarction generally show no abnormality, and the infarct may not be seen reliably for 24 to 48 h. CT may fail to show small ischemic strokes in the posterior fossa because of bone artifact; small infarcts on the cortical surface may also be missed.

Contrast-enhanced CT scans add specificity by showing contrast enhancement of subacute infarcts and allow visualization of venous structures. Coupled with newer generation scanners, CT angiography (CTA) can be performed with administration of intravenous iodinated contrast allowing visualization of the cervical and intracranial arteries. Carotid disease and intracranial vascular occlusions are readily identified with this method (**Fig. 17-14**). After an intravenous bolus of contrast, deficits in brain perfusion produced by vascular occlusion can also be demonstrated (Fig. 17-14C). CT imaging is also sensitive for detecting subarachnoid hemorrhage, and CTA can readily identify intracranial aneurysms (see below). Because of its speed and wide availability, noncontrast head CT is the imaging modality of choice in patients with acute stroke (Fig. 17-1), and CTA and CT perfusion imaging may also be useful and convenient adjuncts.

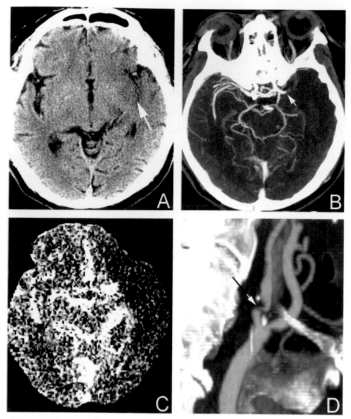

FIGURE 17-14

A. Computed tomography (CT) scan of the brain of a patient with a left middle cerebral artery (MCA) stroke of 3 h duration. As an earliest indicator of infarction, the "insular ribbon sign" is caused by edema (darker signal) within the left insular cortex and basal ganglia (*arrow*). *B*. Embolic occlusion of the MCA imaged with CT angiography during the acute stroke (*arrow*). *C*. Cerebral blood flow measured with CT perfusion; blood flow is reduced over a wider region of brain than appeared edematous in *A*. *D*. CT angiogram of a carotid artery showing high-grade stenosis (*arrow*) from atheroma in another patient.

Magnetic Resonance Imaging (MRI)

MRI reliably documents the extent and location of infarction in all areas of the brain, including the posterior fossa and cortical surface. It also identifies intracranial hemorrhage and other abnormalities but is less sensitive than CT for detecting acute blood. MRI scanners with magnets of higher field strength produce more reliable and precise images. Diffusion-weighted imaging is more sensitive for early brain infarction than standard MR sequences (**Fig. 17-15**), as is FLAIR (fluid–attenuated inversion recovery) imaging (Chap. 3). Using intravenous administration of gadolinium contrast, MR perfusion studies can be performed. Brain regions showing poor perfusion but no abnormality on diffusion are considered equivalent to the ischemic penumbra (see

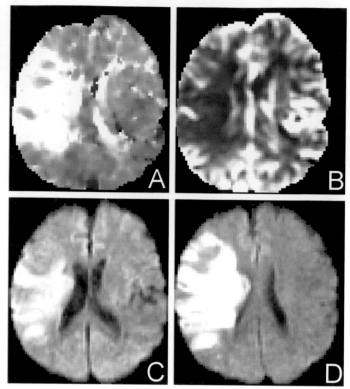

FIGURE 17-15

Magnetic resonance imaging of acute stroke. *A*. Perfusion defect within this right hemisphere (bright signal) imaged after administration of an intravenous bolus of gadolinium contrast. *B*. Cerebral blood flow measured at the same time as in *A*; darker signal reflects decreased blood flow. *C*. Diffusion-weighted image obtained 5 h after onset of a right middle cerebral artery stroke; bright signal indicates regions of restricted diffusion that will progress to infarction. The discrepancy between the region of poor perfusion shown in *A* and *B* and the diffusion deficit, is called *diffusion-perfusion mismatch* and is a measure of the ischemic penumbra. Without specific therapy the region of infarction expands to match the perfusion deficit, as shown in the diffusion weighted image in *D* obtained 5 days later. (*Courtesy of Gregory Albers and Vincent Thijs, MD, Stanford University.*)

"Pathophysiology of Ischemic Stroke," above), and patients showing large regions of mismatch may be better candidates for acute revascularization. MR angiography is highly sensitive for stenosis of extracranial internal carotid arteries and of large intracranial vessels. With higher degrees of stenosis, MR angiography tends to overestimate the degree of stenosis when compared to conventional x-ray angiography. MRI with fat saturation is an imaging sequence used to visualize extra- or intracranial arterial dissection. This sensitive technique images clotted blood within the dissected vessel wall.

MRI is less sensitive for acute blood products than CT and is more expensive and time consuming and less readily available. Claustrophobia also limits its application. Most acute stroke protocols use CT because of these limitations. However, MRI may be useful outside the acute period by more clearly defining the extent and possible source of a stroke.

Cerebral Angiography

Conventional x-ray cerebral angiography is the "gold standard" for identifying and quantifying atherosclerotic stenoses of the cerebral arteries and for identifying and characterizing other pathologies, including aneurysms, vasospasm, intraluminal thrombi, fibromuscular dysplasia, arteriovenous fistula, vasculitis, and collateral channels of blood flow. Endovascular techniques, which are evolving rapidly, can be used to deploy stents within delicate intracranial vessels, to perform balloon angioplasty of stenotic lesions, to treat intracranial aneurysms by embolization, and to open occluded vessels in acute stroke with mechanical embolectomy devices. Recent studies have also documented that intraarterial delivery of thrombolytic agents to patients with acute MCA stroke can effectively recanalize vessels and improve clinical outcomes. Although its use is investigational in many centers, cerebral angiography coupled with endovascular techniques for cerebral revascularization may become routine in the near future. Conventional angiography carries risks of arterial damage, groin hemorrhage, embolic stroke, and renal failure from contrast nephropathy, so it should be reserved for situations where less invasive means are inadequate.

Ultrasound Techniques

Stenosis at the origin of the internal carotid artery can be identified and quantified reliably by ultrasonography that combines a B-mode ultrasound image with a Doppler ultrasound assessment of flow velocity ("duplex" ultrasound). Transcranial Doppler (TCD) assessment of middle, anterior, and posterior cerebral artery flow and of vertebrobasilar flow is also useful. This latter technique can detect stenotic lesions in the large intracranial arteries because such lesions increase systolic flow velocity. In many cases, MR angiography combined with carotid and transcranial ultrasound studies eliminates the need for conventional x-ray angiography in evaluating vascular stenosis. Alternatively, CT angiography of the entire head and neck can be performed during the initial imaging of acute stroke. Because this images the entire arterial system relevant to stroke, with the exception of the heart, much of the clinician's stroke workup can be completed with one imaging study.

Perfusion Techniques

Both xenon techniques (principally xenon–CT) and PET can quantify cerebral blood flow. These tools are generally used for research (Chap. 3) but can be useful for determining the significance of arterial stenosis and planning for revascularization surgery. Single photon emission tomography (SPECT), CT perfusion, and MR perfusion techniques report relative cerebral blood flow. Since CT imaging is used as the initial imaging modality for acute stroke, many centers now combine both CT angiography and CT perfusion imaging together with the noncontrast CT scan. CT perfusion imaging increases the sensitivity and improves accuracy in imaging ischemic brain. Alternatively, MR perfusion can be combined with MR diffusion imaging to identify the ischemic penumbra as the mismatch between these two imaging sequences (Fig. 17-15). The ability to image the ischemic penumbra allows more judicious selection of patients who may or may not benefit from acute interventions such as thrombolysis or investigational neuroprotective strategies.

INTRACRANIAL HEMORRHAGE

Hemorrhages are classified by their location and the underlying vascular pathology. Bleeding into subdural and epidural spaces is principally produced by trauma (Chap. 16). Intraparenchymal, intraventricular, and subarachnoid hemorrhage will be considered here.

DIAGNOSIS

Intracranial hemorrhage is often discovered on noncontrast CT imaging of the brain during the acute evaluation of stroke. Since CT is more sensitive than routine MRI for acute blood, CT imaging is the preferred method for acute stroke evaluation (Table 17-1). The location of the hemorrhage narrows the differential diagnosis to a few entities. **Table 17-6** lists the causes and anatomical spaces involved in hemorrhages.

EMERGENCY MANAGEMENT

Close attention should be paid to airway management since a reduction in the level of consciousness is common. The initial blood pressure should be maintained until the results of the CT scan are reviewed. Patients with acute SAH should have blood pressure lowered to a normal range with nonvasodilating agents such as nicardipine, labetalol, or esmolol. Patients with cerebellar hemorrhages or with depressed mental status and radiographic evidence of hydrocephalus should undergo urgent neurosurgical evaluation. Based on the clinical examination and CT findings, further imaging

TABLE 17-6

CAUSES OF INTRACRANIAL HEMORRHAGE

CAUSE	LOCATION	COMMENTS
Head trauma	Intraparenchymal: frontal lobes, anterior temporal lobes; subarachnoid	Coup and contracoup injury during brain deceleration
Hypertensive hemorrhage	Putamen, globus pallidus, thalamus, cerebellar hemisphere, pons	Chronic hypertension produces hemorrhage from small (~100 μm) vessels in these regions
Transformation of prior ischemic infarction	Basal ganglion, subcortical regions, lobar	Occurs in 1–6% of ischemic strokes with predilection for large hemispheric infarctions
Metastatic brain tumor	Lobar	Lung, choriocarcinoma, melanoma, renal cell carcinoma, thyroid, atrial myxoma
Coagulopathy	Any	Uncommon cause; often associated with prior stroke or underlying vascular anomaly
Drug	Lobar, subarachnoid	Cocaine, amphetamine, phenylpropranolamine
Arteriovenous malformation	Lobar, intraventricular, subarachnoid	Risk is ~2–4% per year for bleeding
Aneurysm	Subarachnoid, intraparenchymal, rarely subdural	Mycotic and nonmycotic forms of aneurysms
Amyloid angiopathy	Lobar	Degenerative disease of intracranial vessels; linkage to Alzheimer's disease, rare in patients <60
Cavernous angioma	Intraparenchymal	Multiple cavernous angiomas linked to chromosome 7q
Dural arteriovenous fistula	Lobar, rarely subarachnoid	Produces bleeding by venous hypertension
Capillary telangiectasias	Usually brainstem	Rare cause of hemorrhage

studies may be necessary, including MRI or conventional x-ray angiography. Stuporous or comatose patients generally are treated presumptively for elevated ICP, with tracheal intubation and hyperventilation, mannitol administration, and elevation of the head of the bed while surgical consultation is obtained (Chap. 15).

SUBARACHNOID HEMORRHAGE

Excluding head trauma, the most common cause of SAH is rupture of a saccular aneurysm. Other causes include bleeding from a vascular anomaly and extension into the subarachnoid space from a primary intracerebral hemorrhage. Some idiopathic SAHs are localized to the perimesencephalic cisterns and are benign; they probably have a venous or capillary source, and angiography is unrevealing.

Saccular ("Berry") Aneurysm

Autopsy and angiography studies have found that about 2% of adults harbor intracranial aneurysms, for a prevalence of 4 million persons in the United States; the aneurysm will rupture, producing SAH, in 25,000 to 30,000 cases per year. For patients who arrive alive at hospital, the mortality rate over the next month is about 45%. Of those who survive, more than half are left with major neurologic deficits as a result of the initial hemorrhage, cerebral vasospasm with infarction, or hydrocephalus. If the patient survives but the aneurysm is not obliterated, the rate of rebleeding is about 20% in the first 2 weeks and about 3% per year afterwards. Given these alarming figures, the major therapeutic emphasis is on preventing the predictable early complications of the SAH.

Unruptured, asymptomatic aneurysms are much less dangerous than a recently ruptured aneurysm. The annual risk of rupture for aneurysms <10 mm in size is ~0.1%, and for aneurysms ≥10 mm in size is ~0.5 to 1%; the surgical morbidity far exceeds these percentages. As more data become available, a true risk-benefit analysis for treating these aneurysms will result.

Giant aneurysms, those >2.5 cm in diameter, occur at the same sites (see below) as small aneurysms and account for 5% of cases. The three most common locations are the terminal internal carotid artery, MCA bifurcation, and top of the basilar artery. Their risk of rupture is about 6% in the first year after identification and may remain high indefinitely. They often cause symptoms by compressing the adjacent brain or cranial nerves.

Mycotic aneurysms are usually located distal to the first bifurcation of major arteries of the circle of Willis. Most result from infected emboli due to bacterial endocarditis causing septic degeneration of arteries and subsequent dilatation and rupture. Whether these lesions should be sought and repaired prior to rupture, or left to heal spontaneously, is controversial.

Pathophysiology Saccular aneurysms occur at the bifurcations of the large to medium-sized intracranial arteries; rupture is into the subarachnoid space in the basal cisterns and often into the parenchyma of the adjacent brain. Approximately 85% of aneurysms occur in the anterior circulation, mostly on the circle of Willis. About 20% of patients have multiple aneurysms, many at mirror sites bilaterally. As an aneurysm develops, it typically forms a neck with a dome. The length of the neck and the size of the dome vary greatly and are factors that are important in planning neurosurgical obliteration or endovascular embolization. The arterial internal elastic lamina disappears at the base of the neck. The media thins, and connective tissue replaces smooth-muscle cells. At the site of rupture (most often the dome) the wall thins, and the tear that allows bleeding is often no more than 0.5 mm long. Aneurysm size and site are important in predicting risk of rupture. Those >7 mm in diameter and those at the top of the basilar artery and at the origin of the posterior communicating artery are at greater risk of rupture.

Clinical Manifestations Most unruptured intracranial aneurysms are completely asymptomatic. Symptoms are usually due to rupture and resultant SAH. At the moment of aneurysmal rupture with major SAH, the ICP suddenly rises. This may account for the sudden transient loss of consciousness that occurs in nearly half of patients. Sudden loss of consciousness may be preceded by a brief moment of excruciating headache, but most patients first complain of headache upon regaining consciousness. In 10% of cases, aneurysmal bleeding is severe enough to cause loss of consciousness for several days. In about 45% of cases, severe headache associated with exertion is the presenting complaint. The patient often calls the headache "the worst headache of my life." Occasionally these ruptures may present as headache of only moderate intensity or as a change in the patient's usual headache pattern. The headache is usually generalized, often with neck stiffness, and vomiting is common.

Although sudden headache in the absence of focal neurologic symptoms is the hallmark of aneurysmal rupture, focal neurologic deficits may occur. Anterior communicating artery or MCA bifurcation aneurysms may rupture into the adjacent brain or subdural space and form a hematoma large enough to produce mass effect. The common deficits that result include hemiparesis, aphasia, and abulia.

Occasionally, prodromal symptoms suggest the location of a progressively enlarging unruptured aneurysm. A third cranial nerve palsy, particularly when associated with pupillary dilatation, loss of ipsilateral (but retained contralateral) light reflex, and focal pain above or behind the eye, may occur with an expanding aneurysm at the junction of the posterior communicating artery and the internal carotid artery. A sixth nerve palsy may indicate an aneurysm in the cavernous sinus, and visual field defects can occur with an expanding supraclinoid carotid or anterior cerebral artery aneurysm. Occipital and posterior cervical pain may signal a posterior inferior cerebellar artery or anterior inferior cerebellar artery aneurysm. Pain in or behind the eye and in the low temple can occur with an expanding MCA aneurysm. Thunderclap headache is a variant of migraine that simulates a SAH. Before concluding that a patient with sudden, severe headache has thunderclap migraine, a definitive workup for aneurysm or other intracranial pathology is required.

Aneurysms can undergo small ruptures and leaks of blood into the subarachnoid space, so-called sentinel bleeds. Sudden unexplained headache at any location should raise suspicion of SAH and be investigated, because a major hemorrhage may be imminent.

Delayed Neurologic Deficits There are four major causes of delayed neurologic deficits: rerupture, hydrocephalus, vasospasm, and hyponatremia.

1. *Rerupture.* The incidence of rerupture of an untreated aneurysm in the first month following SAH is ~30%, with the peak in the first 7 days. Rerupture is associated with a 60% mortality and poor outcome. Early treatment eliminates this risk.

2. *Hydrocephalus.* Acute hydrocephalus can cause stupor and coma. More often, subacute hydrocephalus develops over a few days or weeks and causes progressive drowsiness or slowed mentation (abulia) with incontinence. Hydrocephalus is differentiated from cerebral vasospasm with a CT scan, TCD ultrasound, or conventional x-ray angiography. Hydrocephalus may clear spontaneously or require temporary ventricular drainage. Chronic hydrocephalus may develop weeks to months after SAH and manifest as gait difficulty, incontinence, or impaired mentation. Subtle signs may be a lack of initiative in conversation or a failure to recover independence.

3. *Vasospasm.* Narrowing of the arteries at the base of the brain following SAH causes symptomatic ischemia

and infarction in ~30% of patients and is the major cause of delayed morbidity and death. Signs of ischemia appear 4 to 14 days after the hemorrhage, most often at 7 days. The severity and distribution of vasospasm determine whether infarction will occur.

Delayed vasospasm is believed to result from direct effects of clotted blood and its breakdown products on the artery. In general, the more blood that surrounds the arteries, the greater the chance of symptomatic vasospasm. Spasm of major arteries produces symptoms referable to the appropriate vascular territory (see "Stroke Syndromes," above). All of these focal symptoms may present abruptly, fluctuate, or develop over a few days. In most cases, focal spasm is preceded by a decline in mental status.

Vasospasm can be detected reliably with conventional x-ray angiography, but this invasive procedure is expensive and carries risk of stroke and other complications. TCD ultrasound is based on the principle that the velocity of blood flow within an artery will rise as the lumen diameter is narrowed. By directing the probe along the MCA and proximal ACA, carotid terminus, vertebral, and basilar arteries on a daily or every-other-day basis, vasospasm can be reliably detected and treatments initiated to prevent cerebral ischemia (see below). CT angiography is another method that can reliably detect vasospasm.

Severe cerebral edema in patients with infarction from vasospasm may increase the ICP enough to reduce cerebral perfusion pressure. Treatment is with mannitol and hyperventilation (Chap. 15).

4. *Hyponatremia.* Hyponatremia may be profound and develop quickly in the first 2 weeks following SAH. It usually results from inappropriate secretion of vasopressin and secretion of atrial and brain natriuretic factors, which produce a natriuresis. This "cerebral salt-wasting syndrome" clears over the course of 1 to 2 weeks and, in the setting of SAH, should not be treated with free-water restriction as this may increase the risk of stroke (see below).

Laboratory Evaluation and Imaging (Fig. 17-16)
The hallmark of aneurysmal rupture is blood in the cerebrospinal fluid (CSF). More than 95% of cases have enough blood to be visualized on a high-quality noncontrast CT scan obtained within 72 h. If the scan fails to establish the diagnosis of SAH and no mass lesion or obstructive hydrocephalus is found, a lumbar puncture should be performed to establish the presence of subarachnoid blood. Lysis of the red blood cells and subsequent conversion of hemoglobin to bilirubin stains the spinal fluid yellow within 6 to 12 h of SAH. This xanthochromic spinal fluid peaks in intensity at 48 h and lasts for 1 to 4 weeks, depending on the amount of subarachnoid blood.

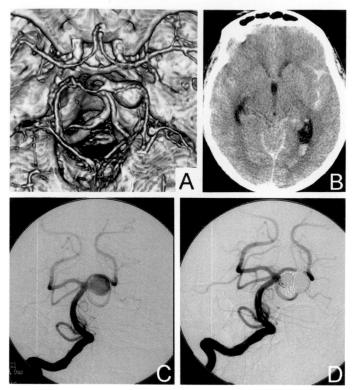

FIGURE 17-16
Subarachnoid hemorrhage. *A.* Computed tomography (CT) angiography revealing an aneurysm of the left superior cerebellar artery. *B.* Noncontrast CT scan at the level of the third ventricle revealing subarachnoid blood in the left sylvian fissure (bright) and within the left lateral ventricle. *C.* Conventional anteroposterior x-ray angiogram of the right vertebral and basilar artery showing the large aneurysm. *D.* Conventional angiogram following coil embolization of the aneurysm, whereby the aneurysm body is filled with platinum delivered through a microcatheter navigated from the femoral artery into the aneurysm neck.

The extent and location of subarachnoid blood on noncontrast CT scan help locate the underlying aneurysm, identify the cause of any neurologic deficit, and predict delayed vasospasm. A high incidence of symptomatic vasospasm in the MCA and ACA has been found when early CT scans show subarachnoid clots >5 × 3 mm in the basal cisterns or layers of blood >1 mm thick in the cerebral fissures. CT scans less reliably predict vasospasm in the vertebral, basilar, or posterior cerebral arteries.

Lumbar puncture prior to an imaging procedure is indicated only if a CT scan is not available at the time of the suspected SAH. Once the diagnosis of hemorrhage from a ruptured saccular aneurysm is suspected, four-vessel conventional x-ray angiography (both carotids and both vertebrals) is generally performed to localize and define the anatomical details of the aneurysm and to determine if other unruptured aneurysms exist (Fig. 17-16).

CT angiography is an alternative method for locating the aneurysm and may be sufficient to plan definitive therapy. At some centers, the ruptured aneurysm can be treated using endovascular techniques at the time of the initial angiogram (see below).

The ECG frequently shows ST-segment and T-wave changes similar to those associated with cardiac ischemia. Prolonged QRS complex, increased QT interval, and prominent "peaked" or deeply inverted symmetric T waves are usually secondary to the intracranial hemorrhage. There is evidence that structural myocardial lesions produced by circulating catecholamines may occur after SAH, causing reversible cardiomyopathy sufficient to cause shock or congestive heart failure. Serious ventricular dysrhythmias are unusual.

Close monitoring (daily or twice daily) of electrolytes is important because hyponatremia can occur precipitously during the first 2 weeks following SAH (see above).

TREATMENT FOR ANEURYSM

Early aneurysm repair prevents rerupture and allows the safe application of techniques to improve blood flow (e.g., induced hypertension and hypervolemia) should symptomatic vasospasm develop. An aneurysm can be "clipped" by a neurosurgeon or "coiled" by a neurointerventional radiologist. Surgical repair involves placing a metal clip across the aneurysm neck, thereby immediately eliminating the risk of rebleeding. This approach requires craniotomy and brain retraction, which is associated with neurologic morbidity. The newer endovascular technique involves placing platinum coils within the aneurysm via a catheter that is passed from the femoral artery. The aneurysm is packed tightly to enhance thrombosis and over time is walled-off from the circulation (Fig. 17-16). The only prospective randomized trial of surgery versus endovascular treatment for ruptured aneurysm, the International Study of Aneurysm Treatment (ISAT), was terminated early when 24% of patients treated with endovascular therapy were dead or dependent at 1 year compared to 31% treated with surgery, a 23% relative reduction. However, some aneurysms have a morphology that is not amenable to coiling, and only a few endovascular centers are available world-wide. Thus, surgery remains an important treatment option.

The medical management of SAH centers on protecting the airway, managing blood pressure before and after aneurysm treatment, preventing rebleeding prior to treatment, managing vasospasm, treating hydrocephalus, treating hyponatremia, and preventing pulmonary embolus.

Intracranial hypertension following aneurysmal rupture occurs secondary to subarachnoid blood, parenchymal hematoma, acute hydrocephalus, or loss of vascular autoregulation. Patients who are stuporous should undergo emergent ventriculostomy to prevent cerebral ischemia from high ICP. Medical therapies designed to combat raised ICP (e.g., mild hyperventilation, mannitol, and sedation) can also be used as needed (Chap. 15). High ICP refractory to treatment is a poor prognostic sign.

Prior to definitive treatment of the ruptured aneurysm, care is required to maintain adequate cerebral perfusion pressure while avoiding excessive elevation of arterial pressure. Occasionally an intracranial hematoma causing neurologic deterioration requires removal.

Because rebleeding is common, all patients who are not candidates for early aneurysm repair are put on bed rest in a quiet room and are given stool softeners to prevent straining. If headache or neck pain is severe, mild sedation and analgesia are prescribed. Extreme sedation is avoided because it can obscure changes in neurologic status. Adequate hydration is necessary to avoid a decrease in blood volume predisposing to brain ischemia.

Seizures are uncommon at the onset of aneurysmal rupture. The quivering, jerking, and extensor posturing that often accompany loss of consciousness are probably related to the sharp rise in ICP or, perhaps, acute generalized vasospasm. However, phenytoin is often given as prophylactic therapy since a seizure may promote rebleeding.

Glucocorticoids may help reduce the head and neck ache caused by the irritative effect of the subarachnoid blood. There is no good evidence that they reduce cerebral edema, are neuroprotective, or reduce vascular injury, and their routine use therefore is not recommended.

Antifibrinolytic agents are not routinely prescribed but may be considered in patients in whom aneurysm treatment cannot proceed immediately. They are associated with a reduced incidence of aneurysmal rerupture but are also associated with an increased incidence of delayed cerebral infarction and DVT.

Vasospasm remains the leading cause of morbidity and mortality following aneurysmal SAH and treatment of the aneurysm. Treatment with the calcium channel antagonist nimodipine (60 mg orally every 4 h) improves outcome, perhaps by preventing ischemic injury rather than reducing the risk of vasospasm. Nimodipine can cause significant hypotension in some patients, which may worsen cerebral ischemia in patients with vasospasm. Symptomatic cerebral vasospasm can also be treated by increasing the cerebral perfusion pressure by raising mean arterial pressure through plasma volume expansion and the judicious use of vasopressor agents, usually phenylephrine or dopamine. Raised perfusion pressure has been associated with clinical improvement in many patients, but high arterial pressure may promote rebleeding in unprotected aneurysms. Treatment with induced hypertension and hypervolemia generally requires monitoring of arterial and central venous pressures. Volume expansion helps prevent hypotension, augments cardiac output, and reduces blood viscosity by reducing the hematocrit. This method is called "triple-H" (hypertension, hemodilution, and hypervolemic) therapy.

If symptomatic vasospasm persists despite optimal medical therapy, intraarterial vasodilators and percutaneous transluminal angioplasty are considered. Vaodilatation following angioplasty appears to be permanent, allowing triple-H therapy to be tapered sooner. The pharmacologic vasodilators (verapamil and nicardipine) do not last more than 8 to 24 h, and therefore multiple treatments may be required until the subarachnoid blood is reabsorbed.

Acute hydrocephalus can cause stupor or coma. It may clear spontaneously or require temporary ventricular drainage. When chronic hydrocephalus develops, ventricular shunting is the treatment of choice.

Free-water restriction is contraindicated in patients with SAH at risk for vasospasm because hypovolemia and hypotension may occur and precipitate cerebral ischemia. Many patients continue to experience a decline in serum sodium despite receiving parenteral fluids containing normal saline. Frequently, supplemental oral salt coupled with normal saline will mitigate hyponatremia, but often patients also require hypertonic saline. Care must be taken not to correct serum sodium too quickly in patients with marked hyponatremia of several days' duration, as central pontine myelinolysis (Chap. 15) may occur.

All patients should have pneumatic compression stockings applied to prevent pulmonary embolism. Systemic heparin is contraindicated in patients with ruptured and untreated aneurysms; it is a relative contraindication following craniotomy, and it may delay thrombosis of a coiled aneurysm.

INTRAPARENCHYMAL HEMORRHAGE

Intraparenchymal hemorrhage is the most common type of intracranial hemorrhage. It accounts for about 10% of all strokes and is associated with a 50% case fatality rate. Incidence rates are particularly high in Asians and African Americans. Hypertension, trauma, and cerebral amyloid angiopathy cause the majority of these hemorrhages. Advanced age and heavy alcohol consumption increase the risk, and cocaine use is one of the most important causes in the young.

Hypertensive Intraparenchymal Hemorrhage

Pathophysiology Hypertensive intraparenchymal hemorrhage (hypertensive hemorrhage or hypertensive intracerebral hemorrhage) usually results from spontaneous rupture of a small penetrating artery deep in the brain. The most common sites are the basal ganglia (especially the putamen), thalamus, deep cerebellum, and pons. When hemorrhages occur in other brain areas or in nonhypertensive patients, greater consideration should be given to hemorrhagic disorders, neoplasms, vascular malformations, and other causes. The small arteries in these areas seem most prone to hypertension-induced vascular injury. The hemorrhage may be small or a large clot may form and compress adjacent tissue, causing herniation and death. Blood may dissect into the ventricular space, which substantially increases morbidity and may cause hydrocephalus.

Most hypertensive intraparenchymal hemorrhages develop over 30 to 90 min, whereas those associated with anticoagulant therapy may evolve for as long as 24 to 48 h. Within 48 h macrophages begin to phagocytize the hemorrhage at its outer surface. After 1 to 6 months, the hemorrhage is generally resolved to a slitlike orange cavity lined with glial scar and hemosiderin-laden macrophages.

Clinical Manifestations Although not particularly associated with exertion, intracerebral hemorrhages almost always occur while the patient is awake and sometimes when stressed. The hemorrhage generally presents as the abrupt onset of focal neurologic deficit. Seizures are uncommon. The focal deficit typically worsens steadily over 30 to 90 min and is associated with a

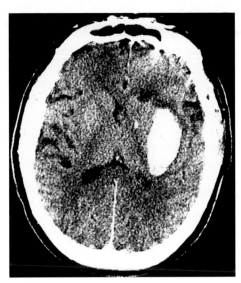

FIGURE 17-17
Transaxial noncontrast computed tomography scan through the region of the basal ganglia reveals a hematoma involving the left putamen in a patient with rapidly progressive onset of right hemiparesis. This is a typical hypertensive hemorrhage.

diminishing level of consciousness and signs of increased ICP, such as headache and vomiting.

The putamen is the most common site for hypertensive hemorrhage, and the adjacent internal capsule is invariably damaged (**Fig. 17-17**). Contralateral hemiparesis is therefore the sentinel sign. When mild, the face sags on one side over 5 to 30 min, speech becomes slurred, the arm and leg gradually weaken, and the eyes deviate away from the side of the hemiparesis. The paralysis may worsen until the affected limbs become flaccid or extend rigidly. When hemorrhages are large, drowsiness gives way to stupor as signs of upper brainstem compression appear. Coma ensues, accompanied by deep, irregular, or intermittent respiration, a dilated and fixed ipsilateral pupil, and decerebrate rigidity. In milder cases, edema in adjacent brain tissue may cause progressive deterioration over 12 to 72 h.

Thalamic hemorrhages also produce a contralateral hemiplegia or hemiparesis from pressure on, or dissection into, the adjacent internal capsule. A prominent sensory deficit involving all modalities is usually present. Aphasia, often with preserved verbal repetition, may occur after hemorrhage into the dominant thalamus, and apractagnosia or mutism occurs in some cases of nondominant hemorrhage. There may also be a homonymous visual field defect. Thalamic hemorrhages cause several typical ocular disturbances by virtue of extension inferiorly into the upper midbrain. These include deviation of the eyes downward and inward so that they appear to be looking at the nose, unequal pupils with absence of light reaction, skew deviation with the eye opposite the hemorrhage displaced downward and medially, ipsilateral Horner's syndrome, absence of convergence, paralysis of vertical gaze, and retraction nystagmus. Patients may later develop a chronic, contralateral pain syndrome (Déjerine-Roussy syndrome).

In pontine hemorrhages, deep coma with quadriplegia usually occurs over a few minutes. There is often prominent decerebrate rigidity and "pin-point" (1 mm) pupils that react to light. There is impairment of reflex horizontal eye movements evoked by head turning (doll's-head or oculocephalic maneuver) or by irrigation of the ears with ice water (Chap. 8). Hyperpnea, severe hypertension, and hyperhidrosis are common. Death often occurs within a few hours, but small hemorrhages are compatible with survival.

Cerebellar hemorrhages usually develop over several hours and are characterized by occipital headache, repeated vomiting, and ataxia of gait. In mild cases there may be no other neurologic signs other than gait ataxia. Dizziness or vertigo may be prominent. There is often paresis of conjugate lateral gaze toward the side of the hemorrhage, forced deviation of the eyes to the opposite side, or an ipsilateral sixth nerve palsy. Less frequent ocular signs include blepharospasm, involuntary closure of one eye, ocular bobbing, and skew deviation. Dysarthria and dysphagia may occur. As the hours pass, the patient often becomes stuporous and then comatose from brainstem compression or obstructive hydrocephalus; immediate surgical evacuation before brainstem compression occurs may be lifesaving. Hydrocephalus from fourth ventricle compression can be relieved by external ventricular drainage, but definitive hematoma evacuation is essential for survival. If the deep cerebellar nuclei are spared, full recovery is common.

Lobar Hemorrhage

Symptoms and signs appear over several minutes. Most lobar hemorrhages are small and cause a restricted clinical syndrome that simulates an embolus to an artery supplying one lobe. For example, the major neurologic deficit with an occipital hemorrhage is hemianopia; with a left temporal hemorrhage, aphasia and delirium; with a parietal hemorrhage, hemisensory loss; and with frontal hemorrhage, arm weakness. Large hemorrhages may be associated with stupor or coma if they compress the thalamus or midbrain. Most patients with lobar hemorrhages have focal headaches, and more than half vomit or are drowsy. Stiff neck and seizures are uncommon.

Other Causes of Intracerebral Hemorrhage

Cerebral amyloid angiopathy is a disease of the elderly in which arteriolar degeneration occurs and amyloid is deposited in the walls of the cerebral arteries. Amyloid angiopathy causes both single and recurrent lobar hemorrhages and is probably the most common cause of lobar hemorrhage in the elderly. It accounts for some intracranial hemorrhages associated with intravenous thrombolysis given for MI. This disorder can be suspected in patients who present with multiple hemorrhages (and infarcts) over several months or years, or in patients with "micro-bleeds" seen on brain MRI sequences sensitive for hemosiderin, but it is definitively diagnosed by demonstration of Congo red staining of amyloid in cerebral vessels. The ε2 and ε4 allelic variations of the apolipoprotein E gene are associated with increased risk of recurrent lobar hemorrhage and may therefore be a marker of amyloid angiopathy and a potential future therapeutic target. Currently, there is no specific therapy, though antiplatelet and anticoagulating agents are typically avoided

Cocaine is a frequent cause of stroke in young (age <45) patients. Intracerebral hemorrhage, ischemic stroke, and SAH are all associated with cocaine use. Angiographic findings vary from completely normal arteries to large-vessel occlusion or stenosis, vasospasm, or changes consistent with vasculitis. The mechanism of cocaine-related stroke is not known, but cocaine enhances sympathetic activity causing acute, sometimes severe, hypertension, and this may lead to hemorrhage. Slightly more than half of cocaine-related intracranial hemorrhages are intracerebral, and the rest are subarachnoid. In cases of SAH, a saccular aneurysm is usually identified. Presumably, acute hypertension causes aneurysmal rupture.

Head injury often causes intracranial bleeding. The common sites are intracerebral (especially temporal and inferior frontal lobes) and into the subarachnoid, subdural, and epidural spaces. Trauma must be considered in any patient with an unexplained acute neurologic deficit (hemiparesis, stupor, or confusion), particularly if the deficit occurred in the context of a fall (Chap. 16).

Intracranial hemorrhages associated with *anticoagulant therapy* can occur at any location; they are often lobar or subdural. Anticoagulant-related intracerebral hemorrhages may evolve slowly, over 24 to 48 h. Coagulopathy should be reversed with fresh-frozen plasma or factor replacement (recombinant factor VIIa) and vitamin K to limit the volume of hemorrhage. When intracerebral hemorrhage is associated with thrombocytopenia (platelet count < 50,000/μL), transfusion of fresh platelets is indicated. Intracerebral hemorrhage associated with *hematologic disorders* (leukemia, aplastic anemia, thrombocytopenic purpura) can occur at any site and may present as multiple intracerebral hemorrhages. Skin and mucous membrane bleeding is usually evident and offers a diagnostic clue.

Hemorrhage into a *brain tumor* may be the first manifestation of neoplasm. Choriocarcinoma, malignant melanoma, renal cell carcinoma, and bronchogenic carcinoma are among the most common metastatic tumors associated with intracerebral hemorrhage. Glioblastoma multiforme in adults and medulloblastoma in children may also have areas of intracerebral hemorrhage.

Hypertensive encephalopathy is a complication of malignant hypertension. In this acute syndrome, severe hypertension is associated with headache, nausea, vomiting, convulsions, confusion, stupor, and coma. Focal or lateralizing neurologic signs, either transitory or permanent, may occur but are infrequent and therefore suggest some other vascular disease (hemorrhage, embolism, or atherosclerotic thrombosis). There are retinal hemorrhages, exudates, papilledema (hypertensive retinopathy), and evidence of renal and cardiac disease. In most cases ICP and CSF protein levels are elevated. The hypertension may be essential or due to chronic renal disease, acute glomerulonephritis, acute toxemia of pregnancy, pheochromocytoma, or other causes. Lowering the blood pressure reverses the process, but stroke can occur, especially if blood pressure is lowered too rapidly. Neuropathologic examination reveals multifocal to diffuse cerebral edema and hemorrhages of various sizes from petechial to massive. Microscopically, there are necrosis of arterioles, minute cerebral infarcts, and hemorrhages. The term *hypertensive encephalopathy* should be reserved for this syndrome and not for chronic recurrent headaches, dizziness, recurrent TIAs, or small strokes that often occur in association with high blood pressure.

Primary intraventricular hemorrhage is rare. It usually begins within the substance of the brain and dissects into the ventricular system without leaving signs of intraparenchymal hemorrhage. Alternatively, bleeding can arise from periependymal veins. Vasculitis, usually polyarteritis nodosa or lupus erythematosus, can produce hemorrhage into any region of the central nervous system; most hemorrhages are associated with hypertension, but the arteritis itself may cause bleeding by disrupting the vessel wall. *Sepsis* can cause small petechial hemorrhages throughout the cerebral white matter. *Moyamoya disease,* mainly an occlusive arterial disease that causes ischemic symptoms, may on occasion produce intraparenchymal hemorrhage, particularly in the young. Hemorrhages into the spinal cord are usually the result of an AVM or metastatic tumor. *Epidural spinal hemorrhage* produces a rapidly evolving syndrome of spinal cord or nerve root compression (Chap. 24). Spinal hemorrhages usually present with sudden back pain and some manifestation of myelopathy.

Laboratory and Imaging Evaluation

The CT scan reliably detects acute focal hemorrhages in the supratentorial space. Small pontine hemorrhages may not be identified because of motion and bone-induced artifact that obscure structures in the posterior fossa. After the first 2 weeks, x-ray attenuation values of clotted blood diminish until they become isodense with surrounding brain. Mass effect and edema may remain. In some cases, a surrounding rim of contrast enhancement appears after 2 to 4 weeks and may persist for months. MRI, though more sensitive for delineating posterior fossa lesions, is generally not necessary in most instances. Images of flowing blood on MRI scan may identify AVMs as the cause of the hemorrhage. MRI, CT angiography, and conventional x-ray angiography are used when the cause of intracranial hemorrhage is uncertain, particularly if the patient is young or not hypertensive and the hematoma is not in one of the four usual sites for hypertensive hemorrhage. For example, hemorrhage into the temporal lobe suggests rupture of a MCA saccular aneurysm.

Since patients typically have focal neurologic signs and obtundation, and often show signs of increased ICP, a lumbar puncture should be avoided as it may induce cerebral herniation.

TREATMENT FOR INTRACEREBRAL HEMORRHAGE

Acute Management

Nearly 50% of patients with a hypertensive intracerebral hemorrhage die, but others may have a good to complete recovery if they survive the initial hemorrhage. The volume and location of the hematoma determine the prognosis. In general, supratentorial hematomas with volumes <30 mL have a good prognosis; 30 to 60 mL, an intermediate prognosis; and >60 mL, a poor prognosis during initial hospitalization. Extension into the ventricular system worsens the prognosis. Except in patients who are on therapeutic anticoagulation or who have a bleeding disorder, at present little can be done about the hemorrhage itself. Hematomas may expand for several hours following the initial hemorrhage, so treating severe hypertension seems reasonable to prevent hematoma progression. Preliminary data suggest that treatment with recombinant factor VIIa, even in patients without coagulopathy, may decrease risk of hematoma expansion and improve clinical outcome; a multicenter randomized trial is currently underway to investigate this hypothesis.

Evacuation of supratentorial hematomas does not appear to improve outcome. The International Surgical Trial in Intracerebral Haemorrhage (STICH) randomized 1033 patients with supratentorial intracerebral hemorrhage to either early surgical evacuation or initial medical management. No benefit was found in the early surgery arm, though analysis was complicated by the fact that 26% of patients in the initial medical management group ultimately had surgery for neurologic deterioration. Overall, these data do not support routine surgical evacuation of supratentorial hemorrhages. Surgical techniques, however, continue to evolve, and minimally invasive endoscopic hematoma evacuation may prove beneficial in future trials.

For cerebellar hemorrhages, a neurosurgeon should be consulted immediately to assist with the evaluation; most cerebellar hematomas >3 cm in diameter will require surgical evacuation. If the patient is alert without focal brainstem signs and if the hematoma is <1 cm in diameter, surgical removal is usually unnecessary. Patients with hematomas between 1 and 3 cm require careful observation for signs of impaired consciousness and precipitous respiratory failure.

Tissue surrounding hematomas is displaced and compressed but not necessarily infarcted. Hence, in survivors, major improvement commonly occurs as the hematoma is reabsorbed and the adjacent tissue regains its function. Careful management of the patient during the acute phase of the hemorrhage can lead to considerable recovery.

Surprisingly, despite large intraparenchymal hemorrhages, ICP is often not elevated. However, if the hematoma causes marked midline shift of structures with consequent obtundation, coma, or hydrocephalus, osmotic agents coupled with induced hyperventilation can be instituted to lower ICP (Chap. 15). These maneuvers will provide enough time to place a ventriculostomy or ICP monitor. Once ICP is recorded, further hyperventilation and osmotic therapy can be tailored to the individual patient. For example, if ICP is found to be high, CSF can be drained from the ventricular space and osmotic therapy continued; persistent or progressive elevation in ICP may prompt surgical evacuation of the clot or withdrawal of support. Alternately, if ICP is normal or only mildly elevated, induced hyperventilation can be reversed and osmotic therapy tapered. Since hyperventilation may actually produce ischemia by cerebral vasoconstriction, induced hyperventilation should be limited to acute resuscitation of the patient with presumptive high ICP and eliminated once other treatments (osmotic therapy or surgical treatments) have been instituted. Glucocorticoids are not helpful for the edema from intracerebral hematoma.

Prevention

Hypertension is the leading cause of primary intracerebral hemorrhage. Prevention is aimed at reducing hypertension, excessive alcohol use, and use of illicit drugs such as cocaine and amphetamines.

VASCULAR ANOMALIES

Vascular anomalies can be divided into congenital vascular malformations and acquired vascular lesions.

CONGENITAL VASCULAR MALFORMATIONS

True *arteriovenous malformations,* venous anomalies, and capillary telangiectasias are lesions that usually remain clinically silent through life. Although most AVMs are congenital, cases of acquired lesions have been reported.

True AVMs are congenital shunts between the arterial and venous systems that may present as headache, seizures, and intracranial hemorrhage. AVMs consist of a tangle of abnormal vessels across the cortical surface or deep within the brain substance. AVMs vary in size from a small blemish a few millimeters in diameter to a large mass of tortuous channels composing an arteriovenous shunt of sufficient magnitude to raise cardiac output. The blood vessels forming the tangle interposed between arteries and veins are usually abnormally thin and do not have a normal structure. AVMs occur in all parts of the cerebral hemispheres, brainstem, and spinal cord, but the largest ones are most frequently in the posterior half of the hemispheres, commonly forming a wedge-shaped lesion extending from the cortex to the ventricle.

Although the lesion is present from birth, bleeding or other symptoms are most common between the ages of 10 and 30, occasionally as late as the fifties. AVMs are more frequent in men, and rare familial cases have been described.

Headache (without bleeding) may be hemicranial and throbbing, like migraine, or diffuse. Focal seizures, with or without generalization, occur in about 30% of cases. Half of AVMs become evident as intracerebral hemorrhages. In most, the hemorrhage is mainly intraparenchymal with extension into the subarachnoid space in some cases. Blood is usually not deposited in the basal cisterns, and symptomatic cerebral vasospasm is rare. The risk of rerupture is about 18% per year and is particularly high in the first few weeks. Hemorrhages may be massive, leading to death, or may be as small as 1 cm in diameter, leading to minor focal symptoms or no deficit. The AVM may be large enough to steal blood away from adjacent normal brain tissue or to increase venous pressure significantly to produce venous ischemia locally and in remote areas of the brain. This is seen most often with large AVMs in the territory of the MCA.

Large AVMs of the anterior circulation may be associated with a systolic and diastolic bruit (sometimes self-audible) over the eye, forehead, or neck and a bounding carotid pulse. Headache at the onset of AVM rupture is not generally as explosive as with aneurysmal rupture. MRI is better than CT for diagnosis, although contrast CT scanning sometimes detects calcification of the AVM. Once identified, conventional x-ray angiography is the "gold standard" for evaluating the precise anatomy of the AVM.

Surgical treatment of symptomatic AVMs, often with preoperative embolization to reduce operative bleeding, is usually indicated for accessible lesions. Stereotaxic radiation, an alternative to surgery, can produce a slow sclerosis of arterial channels over 2 to 3 years.

Patients with asymptomatic AVMs have about a 2% per year risk for hemorrhage. Several angiographic features of the AVM can be used to help predict future bleeding risk. Paradoxically, smaller lesions seem to have a higher hemorrhage rate. The mortality rate with each bleed is about 15%. Given this natural history, surgical treatment is probably indicated for most AVMs that can be treated with reasonable surgical risk.

Venous anomalies are the result of development of anomalous cerebral, cerebellar, or brainstem drainage. These structures, unlike AVMs, are functional venous channels. They are of little clinical significance and should be ignored if found incidentally on brain imaging studies. Surgical resection of these anomalies may result in venous infarction and hemorrhage. Venous anomalies may be associated with cavernous malformations (see below), which do carry some bleeding risk. If resection of a cavernous malformation is attempted, the venous anomaly should not be disturbed.

Capillary telangiectasias are true capillary malformations that often form extensive vascular networks through an otherwise normal brain structure. The pons and deep cerebral white matter are typical locations, and these capillary malformations can be seen in patients with hereditary hemorrhagic telangiectasia (Osler-Rendu-Weber) syndrome. If bleeding does occur, it rarely produces mass effect or significant symptoms. No treatment options exist.

ACQUIRED VASCULAR LESIONS

Cavernous angiomas are tufts of capillary sinusoids that form within the deep hemispheric white matter and brainstem with no normal intervening neural structures. The pathogenesis is unclear. Familial cavernous angiomas have been mapped to several different chromosomal loci; the gene responsible for the 7q-linked form encodes a protein that interacts with a member of the RAS family of GTPases. Cavernous angiomas are typically <1 cm in diameter and are often associated with a venous anomaly. Bleeding is usually of small volume, causing slight mass effect only. The bleeding risk for single cavernous malformations is 0.7 to 1.5% per year and may be higher for patients with prior clinical hemorrhage or multiple malformations. Seizures may occur if the malformation is located near the cerebral cortex. Surgical resection eliminates bleeding risk and may reduce seizure risk, but it is reserved for those malformations that form near the brain surface. Radiation treatment has not been shown to be of benefit.

Dural arteriovenous fistulas are acquired connections usually from a dural artery to a dural sinus. Patients may complain of a pulse-synchronous cephalic bruit ("pulsatile tinnitus") and headache. Depending on the magnitude of the shunt, venous pressures may rise high enough to cause cortical ischemia or venous hypertension and hemorrhage. Surgical and endovascular techniques are usually curative. These fistulas may form because of trauma, but most are idiopathic. There is an association between fistulas and dural sinus thrombosis. Fistulas have been observed to appear months to years following venous sinus thrombosis, suggesting that angiogenesis factors elaborated from the thrombotic process may cause these anomalous connections to form. Alternatively, dural arteriovenous fistulas can produce venous sinus occlusion over time, perhaps from the high pressure and high flow through a venous structure.

FURTHER READINGS

ADAMS HP et al: Guidelines for the early management of patients with ischemic stroke: A scientific statement from the Stroke Council of the American Stroke Association. Stroke 34:1056, 2003

☑ ALBERS GW et al: Antithrombotic and thrombolytic therapy for ischemic stroke. Chest 126(3 Suppl):483S, 2004

Excellent evidence-based guidelines derived from an exhaustive review of the literature.

CHIMOWITZ MI et al: Comparison of warfarin and aspirin for symptomatic intracranial arterial stenosis. N Engl J Med 352:1305, 2005

CHOI JH, MOHR JP: Brain arteriovenous malformations in adults. Lancet Neurol 4:299, 2005

DIENER HC et al: Aspirin and clopidogrel compared with clopidogrel alone after recent ischaemic stroke or transient ischaemic attack in high-risk patients (MATCH): Randomised, double-blind, placebo-controlled trial. Lancet 364:331, 2004

HALLIDAY A et al: Prevention of disabling and fatal strokes by successful carotid endarterectomy in patients without recent neurological symptoms: Randomised controlled trial. Lancet 363:1491, 2004

JOHNSTON SC et al: Recommendations for the endovascular treatment of intracranial aneurysms: A statement for healthcare professionals from the Committee on Cerebrovascular Imaging of the American Heart Association Council on Cardiovascular Radiology. Stroke 33:2536, 2002

KLEINDORFER D et al: Incidence and short-term prognosis of transient ischemic attack in a population-based study. Stroke 36:720, 2005

MAS JL et al: Recurrent cerebrovascular events associated with patent foramen ovale, atrial septal aneurysm, or both. N Engl J Med 345:1740, 2001

MENDELOW AD et al: Early surgery versus initial conservative treatment in patients with spontaneous supratentorial intracerebral haematomas in the International Surgical Trial in Intracerebral Haemorrhage (STICH): A randomised trial. Lancet 365:387, 2005

MOHR JP et al: A comparison of warfarin and aspirin for the prevention of recurrent ischemic stroke. N Engl J Med. 345:1444, 2001

MOLYNEUX A: International Subarachnoid Aneurysm Trial (ISAT) of neurosurgical clipping versus endovascular coiling in 2143 patients with ruptured intracranial aneurysms: A randomised trial. Lancet 360:1267, 2002

NGUYEN-HUYNH MN, JOHNSTON SC: Transient ischemic attack: A neurologic emergency. Curr Neurol Neurosci Rep 5:13, 2005

☑ ROTHWELL PM et al: Endarterectomy for symptomatic carotid stenosis in relation to clinical subgroups and timing of surgery. Lancet 363:915, 2004

This metaanalysis reveals the influence of age, sex, and timing of surgery on outcome of endarterectomy for symptomatic carotid stenosis.

SALEM DN et al: Antithrombotic therapy in valvular heart disease—native and prosthetic. Chest 126: 457S, 2004

SAVITZ SI, CAPLAN LR: Vertebrobasilar disease. N Engl J Med 352:2618, 2005

SINGER DE et al: Antithrombotic therapy in atrial fibrillation. Chest 126(3 Suppl):429, 2004

SMITH WS et al: Safety and efficacy of mechanical embolectomy in acute ischemic stroke: Results of the MERCI trial. Stroke 36:1432, 2005

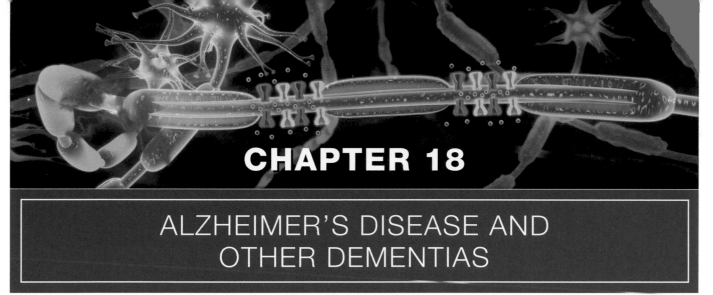

CHAPTER 18

ALZHEIMER'S DISEASE AND OTHER DEMENTIAS

Thomas D. Bird
Bruce L. Miller

Dementia, a syndrome of many causes, affects >4 million Americans and results in a total health care cost of >$100 billion annually. It is defined as an acquired deterioration in cognitive abilities that impairs the successful performance of activities of daily living. Memory is the most common cognitive ability lost with dementia; 10% of persons over age 70 and 20 to 40% of individuals over age 85 have clinically identifiable memory loss. In addition to memory, other mental faculties are also affected in dementia, such as language, visuospatial ability, calculation, judgment, and problem solving. Neuropsychiatric and social deficits develop in many dementia syndromes resulting in depression, withdrawal, hallucinations, delusions, agitation, insomnia, and disinhibition. The common forms of dementia are progressive, but some dementing illnesses are static or fluctuate dramatically from day to day.

MEMORY AND ITS FUNCTIONAL ANATOMY

Memory is a complex function of the brain that uses several storage buffers of differing capacity and duration. It can be divided into three major types: working, episodic, and long-term, or remote, memory. Working memory lasts for <30 s and has a limited storage capacity. Normal individuals can hold seven (plus or minus two) bits of information in working memory where these bits can be manipulated and either discarded or retained as a more permanent memory store. Working memory is highly vulnerable to distraction, requiring attention and vigilance for its maintenance. It is tested by asking the patient to recall digits backwards. The reticular activating system and prefrontal and parietal lobe networks are activated during working memory tasks.

Episodic memory lasts for minutes to many months or even years and binds information about "what," "where," and "when." Normal individuals lay down multiple episodic memories throughout the day, which allow them to move through life connected to previous experiences. On entering this memory buffer, information undergoes a process of consolidation. Significant events are more likely to be consolidated as a more permanent trace. Episodic memory is commonly tested by asking a patient to recall three words after 3 to 5 min. Other simple ways to test episodic memory include determining whether patients can remember what they had for breakfast, how they got to the office, or who examined them earlier in the day. The hippocampal complex is critical for episodic memory, and physiologic changes in synapses in this brain region accompany new episodic memories. Eventually episodic memories become independent of the hippocampal complex and move to neocortex. Anatomically, episodic memory requires the dorsomedial nucleus of the thalamus (damaged in thiamine deficiency) and the medial temporal lobes including the hippocampus and adjacent cortex. Unilateral temporal lobe lesions produce mild to moderate amnesia, while bilateral lesions produce a severe anterograde learning disorder, i.e., an inability to form new episodic memories with retained ability to recall old ones.

Remote, or long-term, memory stores information lasting weeks to a lifetime and contains most of our personal experiences and knowledge. Some information appears to be stored accurately for an indefinite time, whereas other items fade or become distorted. More permanent stores of words, dates, historic facts, or names require the left anterior temporal cortex. The specific localization of other types of long-term memories is unknown, although the neocortex appears to be particularly important. Animal experiments have shown that long-term memory requires new protein synthesis, and the stabilization process probably involves physical changes at neuronal synapses. *Long-term potentiation* (LTP) refers to a long-lasting enhancement of synaptic transmission resulting from repetitive stimulation of excitatory synapses. LTP occurs in the hippocampus, is mediated by N-methyl-D-aspartate (NMDA) receptors, and may serve as the molecular basis for long-term memory storage.

Memory function includes *registration* (encoding or acquisition), *retention* (storage or consolidation), *stabilization* (consolidation), and *retrieval* (decoding or recall). Registration and retrieval are conscious processes. The process of encoding is dependent upon the frontal lobes and hippocampal complex, while the process of retrieval requires the frontal lobes. The hippocampal complex is vulnerable to metabolic insults such as seizures, hypoglycemia, hypoxia, and neurodegenerative processes, which explains why episodic memory deficits are the most common cognitive deficits that follow these varied disorders.

Several additional terms for memory types are sometimes used. *Amnesia* is a term used to describe an impairment in memory function. *Semantic memory* contains unchanging facts, principles, associations, and rules (e.g., the number of days in a week). Injury to the anterior temporal neocortex will lead to loss of semantic memory. *Declarative (explicit) memory* refers to facts about the world and past personal events that must be consciously retrieved to be remembered. Episodic memory is the prototypical declarative, or explicit, memory. *Procedural (implicit) memory* is involved in learning and retaining a skill or procedure such as riding a bicycle, getting dressed, or driving a car. Abilities stored in procedural memory become automatic and do not require conscious implementation. Procedural memory involves areas outside the hippocampus including the basal ganglia, cerebellum, and sensory cortex.

Finally, the term *executive function* refers to mental activity involved in planning, initiating, and regulating behavior. It is considered the central organizing function of the brain that results in systematic, goal-directed activity and is highly dependent upon working memory. Executive functions are active in situations where reflex or automatic behavior is not adequate. Executive functions are presumed to involve the frontal lobes (Chap. 7). Deficits in executive function occur frequently in patients with dementia.

THE CAUSES OF DEMENTIA

The many causes of dementia are listed in **Table 18-1**. The frequency of each condition depends on the age group under study, the access of the group to medical care, the country of origin, and perhaps racial or ethnic background. Alzheimer's disease (AD) is the most common cause of dementia in western countries, representing more than half of demented patients. Vascular disease is the second most common cause of dementia in the United States, representing 10 to 20%. In populations with limited access to medical care, where vascular risk factors are undertreated, the prevalence of vascular dementia can be much higher. Dementia associated with Parkinson's disease is the next most common category, and in many instances these patients suffer from dementia with Lewy bodies (DLB). Chronic intoxications including those resulting from alcohol and prescription drugs are an important, often treatable cause of dementia. Other disorders listed in the table are uncommon but important because many are reversible.

In a study of 1000 persons attending a memory disorders clinic, 19% had a potentially reversible cause of the cognitive impairment and 23% had a potentially reversible concomitant condition. The three most common potentially reversible diagnoses were depression, hydrocephalus, and alcohol dependence.

The single strongest risk factor for dementia is increasing age. The prevalence of disabling memory loss increases with each decade over age 50 and is associated most often with the microscopic changes of AD at autopsy. Slow accumulation of mutations in neuronal mitochondria is also hypothesized to contribute to the increasing prevalence of dementia with age. Nonetheless, some centenarians have intact memory function and no evidence of clinically significant dementia.

Subtle cumulative decline in episodic memory is a natural part of aging. A mild cognitive problem that has begun to interfere with daily activities is no longer part of normal aging and is referred to as *mild cognitive impairment* (MCI). A sizeable proportion of persons with MCI will progress to frank dementia, usually caused by AD. The conversion rate from MCI to AD is ~12% per year. It remains unclear why some individuals show progression and others do not. Factors that predict progression from MCI to AD include a memory deficit >1.5 standard deviations from the norm, family history of dementia, the presence of an apolipoprotein ε4 (Apo ε4) allele, and small hippocampal volumes. A major current area of contention involves whether the use of medications in MCI such as those used to treat AD can decrease the rate of conversion from MCI to dementia.

TABLE 18-1

DIFFERENTIAL DIAGNOSIS OF DEMENTIA

MOST COMMON CAUSES OF DEMENTIA

Alzheimer's disease
Vascular dementia
  Multi-infarct
  Diffuse white matter disease (Binswanger's)

Alcoholism[a]
Parkinson's disease
Drug/medication intoxication[a]

LESS COMMON CAUSES OF DEMENTIA

Vitamin deficiencies
  Thiamine (B$_1$); Wernicke's encephalopathy[a]
  B$_{12}$ (pernicious anemia)[a]
  Nicotinic acid (pellagra)[a]
Endocrine and other organ failure
  Hypothyroidism[a]
  Adrenal insufficiency and Cushing's
    syndrome[a]
  Hypo- and hyperparathyroidism[a]
  Renal failure[a]
  Liver failure[a]
  Pulmonary failure[a]
Chronic infections
  HIV
  Neurosyphilis[a]
  Papovavirus (progressive multifocal
    leukoencephalopathy)
  Prion (Creutzfeldt-Jakob and Gerstmann-
    Sträussler-Scheinker diseases)
  Tuberculosis, fungal, and protozoal[a]
  Whipple's disease[a]
Head trauma and diffuse brain damage
  Dementia pugilistica
  Chronic subdural hematoma[a]
  Postanoxia
  Postencephalitis
  Normal-pressure hydrocephalus[a]
Neoplastic
  Primary brain tumor[a]
  Metastatic brain tumor[a]
  Paraneoplastic limbic encephalitis

Toxic disorders
  Drug, medication, and narcotic
    poisoning[a]
  Heavy metal intoxication[a]
  Dialysis dementia (aluminum)
  Organic toxins
Psychiatric
  Depression (pseudodementia)[a]
  Schizophrenia[a]
  Conversion reaction[a]
Degenerative disorders
  Huntington's disease
  Pick's disease
  Dementia with Lewy bodies
  Progressive supranuclear palsy
    (Steel-Richardson syndrome)
  Multisystem degeneration (Shy-
    Drager syndrome)
  Hereditary ataxias (some forms)
  Motor neuron disease [amyotrophic
    lateral sclerosis (ALS); some forms]
  Frontotemporal dementia
  Cortical basal degeneration
  Multiple sclerosis
  Adult Down's syndrome with
    Alzheimer's
  ALS-Parkinson's-Dementia complex
    of Guam
Miscellaneous
  Sarcoidosis[a]
  Vasculitis[a]
  CADASIL etc
  Acute intermittent porphyria[a]
  Recurrent nonconvulsive seizures[a]
Additional conditions in children or
  adolescents
    Hallervorden-Spatz disease
    Subacute sclerosing panencephalitis
    Metabolic disorders (e.g., Wilson's
      and Leigh's diseases, leukodystro-
      phies, lipid storage diseases, mito-
      chondrial mutations)

[a]Potentially reversible dementia.

The major degenerative dementias include AD, frontotemporal dementia (FTD) and related disorders, DLB, and prion disorders including Creutzfeldt-Jakob disease (CJD). These disorders are all associated with the abnormal aggregation of a specific protein: Aβ_{42} in AD, tau in FTD, α-synuclein in DLB, and PrP in CJD.

APPROACH TO THE PATIENT WITH DEMENTIA

(**Tables** 18-1 and **18-2**) Three major issues should be kept in the forefront: (1) What is the most accurate diagnosis? (2) Is there a treatable or reversible

TABLE 18-2

EVALUATION OF THE PATIENT WITH DEMENTIA

ROUTINE EVALUATION	OPTIONAL FOCUSED TESTS	OCCASIONALLY HELPFUL TESTS
History	Psychometric testing	EEG
Physical examination	Chest x-ray	Parathyroid function
Laboratory tests	Lumbar puncture	Adrenal function
Thyroid function (TSH)	Liver function	Urine heavy metals
Vitamin B$_{12}$	Renal function	RBC sedimentation rate
Complete blood count	Urine toxin screen	Angiogram
Electrolytes	HIV	Brain biopsy
CT/MRI	Apolipoprotein E	SPECT
	RPR or VDRL	PET

DIAGNOSTIC CATEGORIES

REVERSIBLE CAUSES	IRREVERSIBLE/DEGENERATIVE DEMENTIAS	PSYCHIATRIC DISORDERS
Examples	Examples	Depression
Hypothyroidism	Alzheimer's	Schizophrenia
Thiamine deficiency	Frontotemporal dementia	Conversion reaction
Vitamin B$_{12}$ deficiency	Huntington's	
Normal-pressure	Dementia with Lewy bodies	
hydrocephalus	Vascular	
Subdural hematoma	Leukoencephalopathies	
Chronic infection	Parkinson's	
Brain tumor		
Drug intoxication		

ASSOCIATED TREATABLE CONDITIONS

Depression	Agitation
Seizures	Caregiver "burnout"
Insomnia	Drug side effects

Note: PET, positron emission tomography; RPR, rapid plasma reagin (test); SPECT, single photon emission CT; VDRL, Venereal Disease Research Laboratory (test for syphilis).

component to the dementia? (3) Can the physician help to alleviate the burden on caregivers? The major degenerative dementias can usually be distinguished by the initial symptoms; neuropsychological, neuropsychiatric, and neurologic findings; and neuroimaging features (**Table 18-3**).

History

The history should focus on the onset, duration, and tempo of progression of the dementia. In order to make the diagnosis of dementia, as opposed to MCI, activities of daily living must be impaired as a result of the deficit; therefore, interview of a collateral source, usually a family member or close acquaintance, is important.

An acute or subacute onset of confusion may represent delirium and should trigger the search for intoxication, infection, or metabolic derangement. An elderly person with slowly progressive memory

loss over several years is likely to suffer from AD. Nearly 75% of AD patients begin with memory symptoms, but other early symptoms include difficulty with managing money, driving, shopping, following instructions, finding words, or navigating. A change in personality, disinhibition, gain of weight, or food obsession suggests FTD, not AD. FTD is also suggested by the finding of apathy, loss of executive function, progressive abnormalities in speech, or by a relative sparing of memory or spatial abilities. The diagnosis of DLB is suggested by the early presence of visual hallucinations, parkinsonism, delirium, rapid-eye-movement (REM) sleep disorder (the merging of dream states into wakefulness), or *Capgras syndrome,* the delusion that a familiar person has been replaced by an impostor.

A history of sudden stroke with an irregular stepwise progression suggests vascular dementia. In patients suffering from cerebrovascular disease it can

TABLE 18-3

CLINICAL EXMAINATION PEARLS: INITIAL CLINICAL DIFFERENTIATION OF THE MAJOR DEMENTIAS

DISEASE	INITIAL SYMPTOM	MENTAL STATUS	NEUROPSYCHIATRY	NEUROLOGY	IMAGING ON MRI
AD	Memory loss	Episodic memory loss	Initially can be normal	Initially exam can be normal	Entorhinal and hippocampal atrophy
Vascular	Often sudden; variable initial symptoms; apathy, falls, focal weakness	Frontal/executive cognitive slowing; can spare memory	Can include apathy, delusions, anxiety	Usually motor slowing, spasticity; can be normal	Cortical and/or subcortical infarctions, confluent white matter disease
FTD	Apathy; reduced judgment/insight/ speech/language; hyperorality, excessive compulsions. All of which are dependent on which form of FTD presen	Frontal/executive, language; spares drawing	Apathy, disinhibition, hyperorality, euphoria, depression	Vertical gaze palsy, axial rigidity, dystonia, alien hand (due to PSP/CBD overlap)	Frontal and/or temporal atrophy; spares posterior parietal lobe
DLB	Visual hallucinations, REM-sleep disorder, delirium, Capgras syndrome, parkinsonism, fluctuations during the day	Drawing and frontal/executive; spares memory; delirium prone	Formed visual hallucinations, depression, sleep disorder, delusions	Parkinsonism	Posterior parietal; hippocampi larger than in AD
Prion	Dementia, mood changes, anxiety, movement disorder	Variable, frontal/executive, focal cortical, memory	Depression, anxiety	Myoclonus, rigidity, parkinsonism, occasional cerebellar presentations	Cortical ribboning and basal ganglia hyperintensities on diffusion/ flare MRI

Note: AD, Alzheimer's disease; FTD, frontotemporal dementia; PSP, progressive supranuclear palsy; CBD, cortical basal degeneration; DLB, dementia with Lewy bodies; MRI, magnetic resonance imaging.

be difficult to determine whether the dementia is due to AD, vascular dementia, or a mixture of the two. Rapid progression of the dementia in association with motor rigidity and myoclonus suggests a prion disease. Seizures may indicate strokes or neoplasm. Gait disturbance is commonly seen with vascular dementia, Parkinson's disease, or normal-pressure hydrocephalus. Multiple sex partners or intravenous drug use should trigger a search for a central nervous system (CNS) infection, especially in persons with HIV. A history of recurrent head trauma could indicate chronic subdural hematoma, dementia pugilistica, or normal-pressure hydrocephalus. Alcoholism may suggest malnutrition and thiamine deficiency. A remote history of gastric surgery may result in loss of intrinsic factor and vitamin B_{12} deficiency. Certain occupations such as working in a battery or

chemical factory might indicate heavy metal intoxication. A careful review of medications, especially of sedatives and tranquilizers, may raise the issue of chronic drug intoxication or side effects. A family history of dementia is found in Huntington's disease, familial AD, or familial FTD. Depressive signs such as insomnia or weight loss are often seen with pseudo-dementia due to depression, which can also be caused by the recent death of a loved one.

Physical and Neurologic Examination

A thorough examination is essential to document the dementia, look for other signs of nervous system involvement, and search for clues of a systemic disease that might be responsible for the cognitive disorder. AD does not affect motor systems until late in the course. In contrast, some FTD patients develop features of amyotrophic lateral sclerosis (ALS). In DLB, initial symptoms may be the new onset of a parkinsonian syndrome (resting tremor, cogwheel rigidity, bradykinesia, and festinating gait) with the dementia following later, or vice-versa. Corticobasal degeneration (CBD) is associated with dystonia and alien hand (unilateral involuntary movements of the upper limb resembling purposeful actions) and with asymmetric motor deficits or myoclonus. A presentation with unexplained falls, axial rigidity, and gaze deficits suggests progressive supranuclear palsy (PSP). CJD is suggested by diffuse rigidity, an akinetic state, and myoclonus.

Hemiparesis or other focal neurologic deficits may occur in vascular dementia or other focal insults such as neoplasm. Dementia with an associated myelopathy and peripheral neuropathy suggests vitamin B_{12} deficiency. A peripheral neuropathy could also indicate an underlying vitamin deficiency or heavy metal intoxication. Dry cool skin, hair loss, and bradycardia suggest hypothyroidism. Confusion associated with repetitive stereotyped movements may indicate ongoing seizure activity. Hearing impairment or visual loss may produce confusion and disorientation misinterpreted as dementia. Such sensory deficits are common in the elderly and should be screened for in patients with cognitive complaints.

COGNITIVE AND NEUROPSYCHIATRIC EXAMINATION

Brief screening tools such as the mini-mental status examination (MMSE) help to confirm the presence of cognitive impairment and to follow the progression of dementia (Table 18-4). The MMSE is an easily administered 30-point test of cognitive function and contains tests of orientation, working and episodic memory, language comprehension, naming, and copying. In most patients with MCI and some with clinically apparent AD, the MMSE may be normal and a more rigorous set of neuropsychological tests will be required. In addition, the MMSE is weighted heavily toward memory and orientation tasks; dementias such as FTD, in which these areas are often spared until late in the course, may present with profound deficits and a nearly normal MMSE.

Additionally, when the etiology for the dementia syndrome remains in doubt, a specially tailored neuropsychological evaluation should be performed that includes tasks of working and episodic memory, frontal executive tasks, language, visuospatial function, and perception. In AD the deficits involve episodic memory, category generation ("name as many

TABLE 18-4

THE MINI-MENTAL STATUS EXAMINATION

	POINTS
Orientation	
Name: season/date/day/month/year	5 (1 for each name)
Name: hospital/floor/town/state/country	5 (1 for each name)
Registration	
Identify three objects by name and ask patient to repeat	3 (1 for each object)
Attention and calculation	
Serial 7s; subtract from 100 (e.g., 93–86–79–72–65)	5 (1 for each subtraction)
Recall	
Recall the three objects presented earlier	3 (1 for each object)
Language	
Name pencil and watch	2 (1 for each object)
Repeat "No ifs, ands, or buts"	1
Follow a 3-step command (e.g., "Take this paper, fold it in half, and place it on the table")	3 (1 for each command)
Write "close your eyes" and ask patient to obey written command	1
Ask patient to write a sentence	1
Ask patient to copy a design (e.g., intersecting pentagons)	1
Total	30

animals as you can in one minute"), and visuoconstructive ability. Deficits in verbal or visual episodic memory are often the first neuropsychological abnormalities seen with AD, and tasks that require the patient to recall a long list of words or pictures after a predetermined delay will demonstrate deficits in most AD patients. In FTD the earliest deficits often involve frontal executive function or language (speech or naming). DLB patients have more severe deficits in visuospatial function but do better on episodic memory tasks than do patients with AD. Patients with vascular dementia often demonstrate a mixture of frontal executive and visuospatial deficits. In delirium, deficits tend to occur in the areas of attention, working memory, and frontal tasks.

A functional assessment should also be performed. The physician should determine the day-to-day impact of the disorder on the patient's memory, community affairs, hobbies, judgment, dressing, and eating using a collateral source of information. Knowledge of the patient's day-to-day function will help to organize a therapeutic approach with the family.

Other neuropsychiatric assessments are important for diagnosis, prognosis, and treatment. In the early stages of AD mild depressive features, social withdrawal, and denial of illness are the most prominent psychiatric changes. However, patients often maintain their social skills into the middle stages of the illness when delusions, agitation, and sleep disturbance become more common. In FTD dramatic personality change, apathy, overeating, repetitive compulsions, disinhibition, euphoria, and loss of empathy are common. DLB shows formed visual hallucinations that may not be bothersome, delusions related to personal identity, and day-to-day fluctuation. Vascular dementia can present with psychiatric symptoms such as depression, delusions, disinhibition, or apathy.

Laboratory Tests

The choice of laboratory tests in the evaluation of dementia is not straightforward. A reversible or treatable cause must not be missed, yet no single etiology is common; thus a screen must employ multiple tests, each of which has a low yield. Cost/benefit ratios are difficult to assess, and many laboratory screening algorithms for dementia discourage multiple tests. Nevertheless, even a test with only a 1 to 2% positive rate is probably worth undertaking if the alternative is missing a treatable cause of dementia. The algorithm in Table 18-2 lists most screening tests for de-

mentia. For all patients, the routine measurement of thyroid function tests, a vitamin B_{12} level, a complete blood count, electrolytes, VDRL, and a neuroimaging study [computed tomography (CT) or magnetic resonance imaging (MRI)] is recommended.

Neuroimaging studies will identify primary and secondary neoplasms, locate areas of infarction, reveal subdural hematomas, and suggest normal-pressure hydrocephalus or diffuse white matter disease. MRI can provide more information than CT, but either is an appropriate screening tool according to consensus guidelines. Imaging studies also lend support to the diagnosis of AD, especially if there is hippocampal atrophy in addition to diffuse cortical atrophy. Focal frontal and/or anterior temporal atrophy suggest FTD. There is no specific pattern yet determined for DLB, although these patients tend to have less hippocampal atrophy than is seen in AD. Diffusion-weighted MRI will detect abnormalities in the cortical-ribbon and basal ganglia in the vast majority of patients with CJD. Large white matter abnormalities correlate with a vascular etiology for dementia. The role of functional imaging in the diagnosis of dementia is still under study. Single photon emission computed tomography (SPECT) and positron emission tomography (PET) scanning reveal temporal-parietal hypoperfusion or hypometabolism in AD, and frontotemporal hypoperfusion or hypometabolism in FTD, but most of these changes reflect atrophy. Recently, amyloid imaging has shown promise for the diagnosis of AD (**Fig. 18–1**).

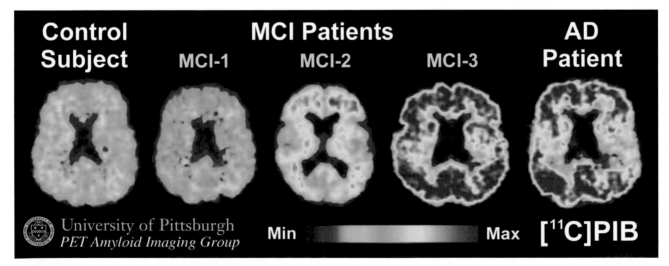

FIGURE 18-1

PET images obtained with the amyloid-imaging agent, Pittsburgh Compound-B ([^{11}C]PIB) in a normal control (far left); three different patients with mild cognitive impairment (MCI; center images); and a mild AD patient (far right). Some MCI patients have control-like levels of amyloid, some have AD-like levels of amyloid, and some have intermediate levels.

Similarly, MRI perfusion and brain activation studies using functional MRI are under study as diagnostic tools.

Lumbar puncture need not be done routinely in the evaluation of dementia but is indicated if CNS infection is a serious consideration. Cerebrospinal fluid (CSF) levels of tau protein are increased and $A\beta_{42}$ amyloid decreased in some AD patients; however, the sensitivity and specificity of these measures are not sufficiently high to warrant routine measurement. CSF levels of protein 14-3-3 are not specific for CJD, and with the advent of new MRI techniques are becoming less useful in this diagnosis. Formal psychometric testing is not necessary in every patient but helps to document the severity of dementia, suggest psychogenic causes, and provide a semiquantitative method for following the disease course. An electroencephalogram (EEG) is rarely helpful except to suggest CJD (repetitive bursts of diffuse high-voltage sharp waves) or an underlying nonconvulsive seizure disorder (epileptiform discharges). Brain biopsy (including meninges) is not advised except to diagnose vasculitis, potentially treatable neoplasms, unusual infections, or systemic disorders such as sarcoid or in young persons where the diagnosis is uncertain. Angiography should be considered when cerebral vasculitis is a possible cause of the dementia.

SPECIFIC DEMENTIAS

ALZHEIMER'S DISEASE

AD is the most common cause of dementia in western countries. Approximately 10% of all persons over the age of 70 have significant memory loss, and in more than half the cause is AD. AD can occur, however, in any decade of adulthood. The annual cost of caring for a single AD patient in an advanced stage of the disease is estimated at $50,000. The disease also exacts a heavy emotional toll on family members and caregivers. AD most often presents with subtle onset of memory loss followed by a slowly progressive dementia that has a course of several years. Pathologically there is diffuse atrophy of the cerebral cortex with secondary enlargement of the ventricular system. Microscopically there are neuritic plaques containing $A\beta$ amyloid, silver-staining neurofibrillary tangles (NFTs) in neuronal cytoplasm, and accumulation of $A\beta$ amyloid in arterial walls of cerebral blood vessels. The identification of four different susceptibility genes has provided a foundation for rapid progress in understanding the biologic basis of AD.

Clinical Manifestations

The cognitive changes with AD tend to follow a characteristic pattern, beginning with memory impairment and spreading to language and visuospatial deficits. However, ~20% of AD patients present with nonmemory complaints such as word-finding, organizational, or navigational difficulty. In the early stages of the disease, the memory loss may go unrecognized or may be ascribed to benign forgetfulness. Once the memory loss begins to mildly affect day-to-day activities or falls to <1.5 standard deviations from normal on standardized memory tasks, the disease is defined as MCI. Slowly the cognitive problems begin to interfere with daily activities, such as keeping track of finances, following instructions on the job, driving, shopping, and housekeeping, making dementia the diagnosis, rather than merely MCI. Some patients are unaware of these difficulties (anosognosia), while others have considerable insight. Change of environment may be bewildering, and the patient may become lost on walks or while driving an automobile. Driving safety evaluation is an important but often frustrating step for the patient. In the middle stages of AD, the patient is unable to work, is easily lost and confused, and requires daily supervision. Social graces, routine behavior, and superficial conversation may be surprisingly retained. Language becomes impaired: first naming, then comprehension, and finally fluency. In some patients, aphasia is an early and prominent feature. Word-finding difficulties and circumlocution may be a problem even when formal testing demonstrates intact naming and fluency. Apraxia emerges and patients have trouble carrying out sequential motor tasks. Visuospatial deficits begin to interfere with dressing, eating, solving simple puzzles, and copying geometric figures. Patients may be unable to perform simple calculations or tell time.

In the late stages of the disease, some persons remain ambulatory but wander aimlessly. Loss of judgment, reason, and cognitive abilities occurs. Delusions are common, usually simple in quality, involving delusions of theft, infidelity, or misidentification. Approximately 10% of AD patients develop the Capgras syndrome, believing that a caregiver has been replaced by an impostor. In contrast to DLB where the Capgras syndrome is an early feature, in AD this syndrome emerges later in the course of the illness. Loss of inhibitions and aggression may alternate with passivity and withdrawal. Sleep-wake patterns are prone to disruption, and nighttime wandering becomes disturbing to the household. Some patients develop a shuffling gait, with generalized muscle rigidity associated with slowness and awkwardness of movement. Patients often look parkinsonian (Chap. 19) but rarely have tremor. In end-stage AD, patients become rigid, mute, incontinent, and bedridden. Help may be needed with the simplest tasks, such as eating, dressing, and toilet function. Hyperactive tendon reflexes may be noted. Myoclonic jerks (sudden brief contractions of various muscles or the whole body) may occur spontaneously or in response to physical or auditory stimulation. Myoclonus raises the possibility of a prion disease (Chap. 32), but the course of AD is much more prolonged. Generalized seizures may also occur. Often, death results from malnutrition, secondary infections, pulmonary emboli, or heart disease. The typical duration of AD is 8 to 10 years, but the course can range from 1 to 25 years. For unknown reasons, some AD patients show a steady downhill decline in function, while others have prolonged plateaus without major deterioration.

Diagnosis

Early in the disease course, other etiologies of dementia should be excluded (see above). Neuroimaging studies (CT and MRI) do not show a single specific pattern with AD and may be normal early in the course of the disease. As AD progresses, diffuse cortical atrophy becomes apparent, and MRI scans show atrophy of the hippocampus (**Fig. 18-2**A, B). Functional imaging studies in AD reveal hypoperfusion or hypometabolism in the posterior temporal-parietal cortex (Fig. 18-2C, D). Amyloid imaging may hold promise for more specific imaging diagnosis. The EEG is normal or shows nonspecific slowing. Routine spinal fluid examination is also normal. The use of blood Apo ε genotyping is discussed under "Genetic Considerations," below.

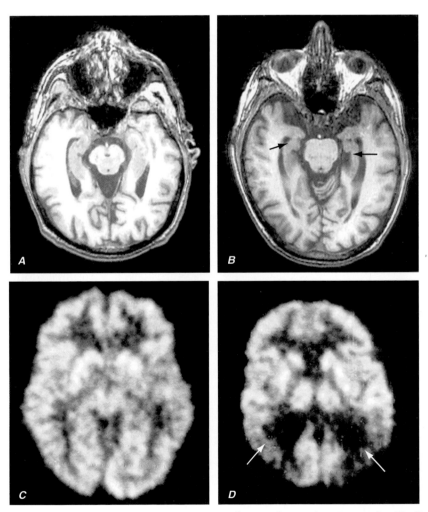

FIGURE 18-2

Alzheimer's disease. Axial T1-weighted MR images through the midbrain of a normal 86-year-old athletic individual (A) and a 77-year-old male (B) with Alzheimer's disease. Note that both individuals have prominent sulci and slight dilatation of the lateral ventricles. However, there is a reduction in the volume of the hippocampus of the patient with Alzheimer's disease (arrows) compared with that of the normal-for-age hippocampus of the older individual. Fluorodeoxyglucose positron emission tomographic scans of a normal control (C) and a patient with Alzheimer's disease (D). Note that the patient with Alzheimer's disease has decreased activity in the parietal lobes bilaterally (arrows), a typical finding in this condition. (Images courtesy of TF Budinger, University of California.)

Slowly progressive decline in memory and orientation, normal results on laboratory tests, and an MRI or CT scan showing only diffuse or posteriorly predominant cortical and hippocampal atrophy are highly suggestive of AD. A clinical diagnosis of AD, reached after careful evaluation, is confirmed at autopsy ~90% of the time, with misdiagnosed cases usually representing one of the other dementing disorders (Table 18-3).

Epidemiology

The most important risk factors for AD are old age and a positive family history. The frequency of AD increases with each decade of adult life, reaching 20 to 40% of the population over the age of 85. A positive family history of dementia suggests a genetic cause of AD. Female gender may also be a risk factor independent of the greater longevity of women. Some AD patients have a past history of head trauma with concussion, but this appears to be a relatively minor risk factor. AD is more common in groups with lower educational attainment, but education influences test-taking ability, and it is clear that AD can affect persons of all intellectual levels. One study found that the capacity to express complex written language in early adulthood correlated with a decreased risk for AD. Numerous environmental factors, including aluminum, mercury, and viruses, have been proposed as causes of AD, but none has been demonstrated to play a significant role. Several studies suggest that the use of nonsteroidal anti-inflammatory agents is associated with a decreased risk of AD, but this has not been confirmed in large prospective studies. Recent work has shown an increased risk of dementia, including AD, in patients with traditional vascular risk factors and elevated markers of inflammation. These studies may provide a link between hypertension, elevated cholesterol and homocysteine levels, diabetes, smoking, and AD, leading to novel primary prevention studies.

Pathology

The most severe pathology is usually found in the hippocampus, temporal cortex, and the acetylcholine-containing nucleus basalis of Meynert (lateral septum). The most important microscopic findings are neuritic "senile" plaques and NFTs. These lesions accumulate in small numbers during normal aging of the brain but occur in excess in AD. Neuritic plaques contain a central core that includes $A\beta$ amyloid, proteoglycans, Apo $\varepsilon4$, α_1 antichymotrypsin, and other proteins. $A\beta$ amyloid is a protein of 39 to 42 amino acids that is derived proteolytically from a larger transmembrane protein, amyloid precursor protein (APP), which has neurotrophic and neuroprotective activity. The normal function of $A\beta$ amyloid is unknown. Soluble amyloid fibrils may represent the initial pathologic event in AD leading to formation of neuritic plaques. The plaque core is surrounded by the debris of degenerating neurons, microglia, and macrophages. The accumulation of $A\beta$ amyloid in cerebral arterioles, termed *amyloid angiopathy,* may lead to cerebral lobar hemorrhages. NFTs are silver-staining, twisted neurofilaments in neuronal cytoplasm that represent abnormally phosphorylated tau protein and appear as paired helical filaments by electron microscopy. Tau is a microtubule-associated protein that may function to assemble and stabilize the microtubules that convey cell organelles, glycoproteins, and other important materials through the neuron. A hyperphosphorylated state of tau impairs its capacity to bind to microtubules. AD is also associated with decreased levels of several proteins and neurotransmitters in the cerebral cortex, especially acetylcholine, its synthetic enzyme choline acetyltransferase, and nicotinic cholinergic receptors. Reduction of acetylcholine may result from degeneration of cholinergic neurons in the nucleus basalis of Meynert that project to many areas of the cortex. There is also reduction in norepinephrine levels in brainstem nuclei such as the locus coeruleus.

GENETIC CONSIDERATIONS Several genes have been found to play important roles in the pathogenesis of at least some cases of AD. The first to be identified was the *APP* gene on chromosome 21. Point mutations in *APP* produce early-onset, autosomal dominant AD. APP is a membrane-spanning protein that is subsequently processed into smaller units, including $A\beta$ amyloid that is deposited in neuritic plaques. $A\beta$ peptide results from cleavage of APP by β- and γ-secretases (**Fig. 18-3**). Only very rare families with AD producing *APP* mutations have been identified. However, adults with trisomy 21 (Down's syndrome) who survive beyond age 40 consistently develop a progressive dementia superimposed upon their baseline mental retardation and accompanied by typical neuropathologic changes of AD. Presumably the extra dose of the *APP* gene on chromosome 21 is the initiating cause of AD in adult Down's syndrome and results in an excess of cerebral amyloid.

Investigation of large families with multigenerational familial AD led to the discovery of two additional AD genes, termed the *presenilins.* Presenilin-1 (*PS-1*) is on chromosome 14 and encodes a protein

Step 1: Cleavage by either α- or β-secretase

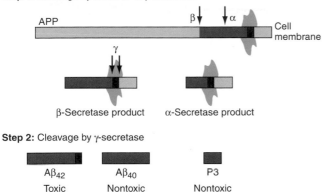

Step 2: Cleavage by γ-secretase

FIGURE 18-3

Amyloid precursor protein (APP) is catabolized by α-, β-, and γ-secretases. A key initial step is the digestion by either β-secretase (BASE) or α-secretase [ADAM10 or ADAM17 (TACE)], producing smaller nontoxic products. Cleavage of the β-secretase product by γ-secretase (step 2) results in either the toxic Aβ42 or the nontoxic Aβ40 peptide; cleavage of the α-secretase product by γ-secretase produces the nontoxic P3 peptide. Excess production of Aβ42 is a key initiator of cellular damage in Alzheimer's disease. Current AD research is focused on developing therapies designed to reduce accumulation of Aβ42 by antagonizing β- or γ-secretases; promoting α-secretase; or clearing Aβ42 that has already formed by use of specific antibodies.

called S182. Mutations in this gene cause an early-onset AD (onset before age 60 and often before age 50) transmitted in an autosomal dominant, highly penetrant fashion. More than 50 different mutations have been found in the *PS-1* gene in families from a wide range of ethnic backgrounds. Presenilin-2 (*PS-2*) is on chromosome 1 and encodes a protein called STM2. Both S182 and STM2 are cytoplasmic neuronal proteins that are widely expressed throughout the nervous system. Patients with mutations in these genes also have elevated plasma levels of Aβ42 amyloid, suggesting a possible link between the presenilins and APP. There is evidence that *PS-1* is involved in the cleavage of APP at the γ-secretase site, and mutations in either gene (*PS-1* or *PS-2*) may disturb this function. Mutations in *PS-1* have thus far proved to be the most common cause of early-onset familial AD, representing 40 to 70% of this relatively rare syndrome. Mutations in the *presenilins* are rarely involved in the more common sporadic cases of late-onset AD occurring in the general population. DNA testing for these uncommon mutations is now possible on a research basis, and mutation analysis of *PS-1* is commercially available. Such testing is likely to be positive only in early-onset

familial cases of AD. Any testing of asymptomatic at-risk individuals should be done only in the context of formal genetic counseling.

A discovery of great importance has implicated the *Apo ε* gene on chromosome 19 in the pathogenesis of late-onset familial and sporadic forms of AD. *Apo ε* is involved in cholesterol transport and has three alleles, designated 2, 3, and 4. The Apo ε4 allele has a strong association with AD in the general population, including sporadic and late-onset familial cases. Approximately 40 to 65% of AD patients, compared to 24 to 30% of the nondemented Caucasian population, has at least one ε4 allele. Many AD patients have no ε4 allele, however, and individuals with ε4 may never develop AD. Nevertheless, it is clear that the Apo ε4 allele, especially in the homozygous 4/4 state, is an important risk factor for AD. It appears to act as a dose-dependent modifier of age of onset, with the earliest onset associated with the ε4/4 homozygous state. Apo ε may be involved with the clearance of amyloid; clearance is least efficient with Apo ε4. Apo ε is present in the neuritic amyloid plaques of AD, and it may be involved in NFT formation, because it binds to tau. Finally, there is suggestive evidence that the ε2 allele may be "protective."

Apo ε testing is not indicated as a predictive test for AD in normal persons. In demented persons who meet clinical criteria for AD, the finding of an ε4 allele increases the reliability of diagnosis; however, its absence does not eliminate the diagnosis of AD.

TREATMENT FOR AD

AD cannot be cured, and no highly effective drug exists. The focus is on judicious use of cholinesterase inhibitor drugs; symptomatic management of behavioral problems; and building rapport with the patient, family members, and other caregivers.

Tacrine (tetrahydroaminoacridine), donepezil, rivastigmine, and galantamine are cholinesterase inhibitors approved by the U.S. Food and Drug Administration (FDA) for treatment of AD. Their pharmacologic action is presumed to be an increase in cerebral levels of acetylcholine. Controlled studies indicate that cholinesterase inhibitors improve caregiver ratings of patients' functioning and decrease the rate of decline in cognitive test scores over periods of up to 3 years. The average patient on an anticholinesterase compound maintains his or her MMSE score at 1 year, whereas a placebo-treated patient declines two to three points over the same time period. Nevertheless, these compounds are only modestly efficacious. In later stages of AD, they may be quite helpful in managing behavioral problems. Tacrine may cause hepatotoxicity, thus it is rarely used. Donepezil avoids liver toxicity and can be administered once daily (5 to 10 mg), offering an advantage over the other cholinesterase inhibitors. There are no large trials comparing the efficacy of these four drugs.

Memantine, an NMDA receptor antagonist, is a novel drug recently approved by the FDA for use in patients with moderate to severe AD. It has been shown to be effective also as an add-on agent in patients already on cholinesterase inhibitors. Most clinicians currently reserve this medication, which has modest benefit, for patients with moderate to severe disease who have continued to progress despite an adequate trial of a cholinesterase inhibitor.

In patients with moderately advanced AD, a prospective trial of the antioxidants selegiline (Chap. 19), α-tocopherol (vitamin E), or both slowed institutionalization and progression to death. Because vitamin E is inexpensive, the doses used in this study of 1000 IU twice daily were offered to many patients with AD. However, the beneficial effects of vitamin E are likely to be small, and recent data questioning the cardiovascular safety of vitamin E have diminished its use.

A controlled trial of an extract of *Ginkgo biloba* found modest improvement in cognitive function in subjects with AD and vascular dementia. This study requires confirmation before *Ginkgo biloba* is considered an effective treatment for dementia because there was a high subject dropout rate and no improvement on a clinician's judgment scale

Exercise has been shown to modestly decrease the rate of decline in AD. Combined with its proven cardiovascular benefits, it has emerged as a mainstay of recommendations by cognitive specialists for AD and other dementia patients.

There has been considerable enthusiasm for a strategy involving vaccination against the Aβ protein. This approach was highly effective in mouse models of AD; amyloid deposits were effectively cleared, and cognitive decline was arrested. The mechanism appears to involve generation of antibodies against Aβ, which cross the blood-brain barrier and eliminate neuritic plaques. Unfortunately, in human trials this approach led to life-threatening meningoencephalitis in some vaccinated individuals, although post-mortem pathology showed decreased burden of amyloid in these patients. Modifications of the vaccine approach are under development.

Several retrospective studies have suggested that nonsteroidal anti-inflammatory agents and statins (HMG-CoA reductase inhibitors) may protect against dementia. Controlled prospective studies using these compounds as well as modification of other classic vascular risk factors are underway.

Mild to moderate depression, common in the early stages of AD, may respond to antidepressant or cholinesterase inhibitors. Selective serotonin reuptake inhibitors (SSRIs) are commonly used due to their low anticholinergic side effects. Generalized seizures should be treated with an appropriate anticonvulsant, such as phenytoin or carbamazepine. For management of behavioral disturbances and suggestions for caregivers, see "General Symptomatic Treatment of the Patient with Dementia," below.

VASCULAR DEMENTIA

Dementia associated with vascular disease appears to be a more common cause of dementia in Asia than in Europe and North America. Individuals who have had several discreet large-vessel strokes may develop chronic cognitive deficits, commonly called *multi-infarct dementia*. The strokes usually involve several different brain regions. The occurrence of dementia appears to depend partly on the total volume of damaged cortex, but it is also more common in individuals with left-hemisphere lesions, independent of any language disturbance. Patients typically report a history of discrete episodes of sudden neurologic deterioration. The recurrent strokes result in a stepwise progression of disease. Neuroimaging studies show multiple areas of infarction. Thus, the history and neuroimaging findings differentiate this condition from AD. However, both AD and multiple infarctions are common and sometimes occur together. With normal aging, there is also an accumulation of amyloid in cerebral blood vessels, leading to a condition called *cerebral amyloid angiopathy of aging* (not associated with dementia), which predisposes older persons to hemorrhagic lobar stroke.

Some individuals with dementia are discovered on MRI to have bilateral subcortical white matter abnormalities, termed *diffuse white matter disease* (or leukoaraiosis), often occurring in association with lacunar infarctions (**Fig. 18-4**). The dementia may be insidious in onset and progress slowly, features that distinguish it from multi-infarct dementia, although other patients can show a stepwise deterioration more typical of multi-infarct dementia. Early symptoms are mild confusion, apathy, changes in personality, depression, psychosis, and memory

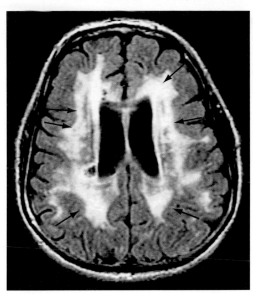

FIGURE 18-4

Diffuse white matter disease. Axial T2-weighted MR image through the lateral ventricles reveals multiple areas of abnormal high signal intensity involving the periventricular white matter as well as the corona radiata. While seen in some individuals with normal cognition, this appearance is more pronounced in patients with dementia of a vascular etiology

or executive deficits. Marked difficulties in judgment and orientation and dependence on others for daily activities develop later. Euphoria, elation, depression, or aggressive behaviors are common. Both pyramidal and cerebellar signs may be present in the same patient. A gait disorder appears in at least half of affected patients. With advanced disease, urinary incontinence and dysarthria with or without other pseudobulbar features (e.g., dysphagia, emotional lability) are frequent. This disorder is a microangiopathy due to occlusive disease of small penetrating cerebral arteries and arterioles. The patients usually, but not always, have a history of hypertension, but any disease causing stenosis of small cerebral vessels may be the critical underlying factor. The term *Binswanger's disease* should be used with caution, because it does not really identify a single entity.

A dominantly inherited form of diffuse white matter disease is known as *cerebral autosomal dominant arteriopathy with subcortical infarcts and leukoencephalopathy* (CADASIL). Clinically there is a progressive dementia developing in the fifth to seventh decades in multiple family members who may also have a history of migraine and recurrent stroke without hypertension. Skin biopsy may show characteristic dense bodies in the media of arterioles. The disease is caused by mutations in the notch 3 gene, and there is a commercially available genetic test. The frequency of this disorder is unknown, and there are no

known treatments. Mitochondrial disorders can also present with strokelike episodes and can selectively injure basal ganglia or cortex. Many such patients show other findings suggestive of a neurologic or systemic disorder such as ophthalmoplegia, retinal degeneration, deafness, myopathy, neuropathy, or diabetes. Diagnosis is difficult, but serum, and especially CSF, levels of lactate and pyruvate may be abnormal, and biopsy of affected tissue is often diagnostic.

Treatment of vascular dementia must be focused on the underlying causes, such as hypertension, atherosclerosis, and diabetes as well as prevention of further vascular events using antiplatelet drugs. Anticholinesterase compounds appear to be useful, as in AD (see above).

FRONTOTEMPORAL DEMENTIA AND RELATED DISORDERS

Frontotemporal Dementia

FTD often begins between 50 and 70 years of age, and in this younger age group its prevalence may approach that of AD. Men and women are equally affected. Unlike AD, behavioral symptoms often predominate in the early stages of FTD. FTD can be sporadic or familial. The clinical heterogeneity is remarkable; patients demonstrate combinations of disinhibition, dementia, apraxia, parkinsonism, and motor neuron disease. In many families with an autosomal dominant pattern of inheritance, mutations in the tau gene on chromosome 17 have been found; in others, the dementia has been linked to 17 but does not involve tau. In still other families, chromosomes 3 and 9 have been linked to FTD.

Early symptoms are divided between cognitive, behavioral, and sometimes motor abnormalities, reflecting degeneration of the anterior frontal and temporal regions, basal ganglia, and motor neurons. Cognitive presentations typically spare memory and involve planning, judgment, or language. Poor business decisions, difficulty organizing work plans, and speech and language deficits emerge. Insight into the disorder is often severely impaired. Common behavioral deficits associated with FTD include apathy, disinhibition, weight gain, food fetishes, compulsions, and euphoria.

Findings at the bedside are dictated by the anatomical localization of the disorder. Asymmetric left frontal cases present with nonfluent aphasias, while left anterior temporal degeneration is characterized by loss of words and concepts related to language (semantic dementia). Nonfluent patients quickly progress to mutism, while those with semantic dementia develop features of visual agnosia, losing the ability to recognize faces, objects, and words (Chap. 7). Copying, calculating, and navigation often remain normal into later in the illness.

These left hemisphere presentations of FTD have been called *primary progressive aphasia*. In contrast, right frontal or temporal cases show profound alterations in social conduct with loss of empathy, disinhibition, and antisocial behaviors predominating. Memory and visuospatial skills are relatively spared in most FTD patients. There is a striking overlap between FTD and PSP, CBD, and motor neuron disease; ophthalmoplegia, dystonia, swallowing symptoms, and fasciculations are common at presentation of FTD or emerge during the course of the illness.

The anatomical hallmark of FTD is a marked atrophy of the temporal and/or frontal lobes, which can be visualized by neuroimaging studies (**Figs. 18-5 and 18-6**). The atrophy is sometimes remarkably asymmetric. A variety of pathologies have been associated with the clinical syndrome. The most consistent microscopic findings include gliosis and neuronal loss, and many cases show swollen or ballooned neurons containing cytoplasmic inclusions that in the majority of cases stain for tau. These aggregates sometimes resemble those found in PSP and CBD; tau is accepted as playing a major role in the pathogenesis of all three conditions. Nearly 80% of FTD patients show involvement of the basal ganglia at autopsy, and 15% go on to develop motor neuron disease, indicating the multisystem nature of this illness. Depletion of seratonergic and glutamatergic neurons is present in many patients. In contrast to AD, the cholinergic system is relatively spared in FTD.

Pick's disease was historically described as a progressive degenerative disorder of the anterior frontal and temporal neocortex accompanied by intracellular inclusions (*Pick's bodies*) that stain positive with silver (argy-

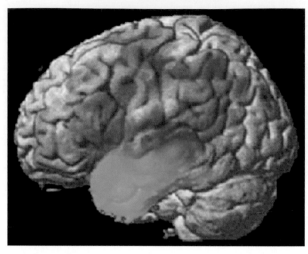

FIGURE 18-6

Voxel-based morphometry (VBM) analysis showing differing patterns of brain atrophy in the frontal variant of frontotemporal dementia (red), temporal variant of frontotemporal dementia (green), and Alzheimer's disease (blue). This technique allows comparison of MRI gray matter volumes between groups of subjects. (*Image courtesy of Marilu Gorno-Tempini, University of California at San Francisco.*)

rophilic) and tau. Many of the τ-positive inclusions in FTD cases, however, are not labeled with silver stains. Although the nomenclature for these patients has remained controversial, the term *FTD* is increasingly used for all patients with frontotemporal degenerations, whereas Pick's disease is used to classify pathologically the subset of FTD cases that show Pick's bodies at autopsy.

The burden on caregivers of FTD patients is extremely high. Treatment is symptomatic, and there are

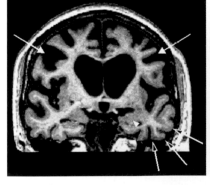 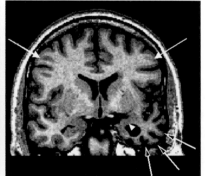

FIGURE 18-5

Frontotemporal dementia (FTD). Coronal MRI sections from one patient with frontally predominant FTD (*left*) and another with temporally predominant FTD (*right*). Prominent atrophy affecting the frontal gyri (*white arrows*) is present in frontally predominant FTD, particularly affecting the right frontal region; note also the thinning of the corpus callosum superior to the lateral ventricles. This patient presented with dysinhibition and antisocial behavior. In the temporally predominant patient, severe atrophy in the left temporal lobe (*open arrows*) and amygdala (*white arrowheads*) is present; this patient presented with progressive aphasia. (*Images courtesy of H Rosen and G Schauer, University of California at San Francisco.*)

currently no therapies known to slow progression or improve cognitive symptoms. Many of the behaviors that accompany FTD such as depression, hyperorality, compulsions, and irritability can be ameliorated with serotonin-modifying antidepressants. The co-association with motor disorders necessitates the careful use antipsychotics, which can exacerbate this problem.

Progressive Supranuclear Palsy

PSP is a degenerative disease that usually begins with falls and a vertical supranuclear gaze paresis and progresses to symmetric rigidity and dementia. A stiff, unstable posture with hyperextension of the neck and slow gait with frequent falls is characteristic. Early in the disease, patients have difficulty with downgaze and lose vertical opticokinetic nystagmus on downward movement of a target. Although patients have very limited voluntary eye movements, oculocephalic reflexes (doll's head maneuver) are retained; thus, the eye movement disorder is supranuclear. Frequent unexplained and sometimes spectacular falls are common secondary to a combination of axial rigidity, inability to look down, and bad judgment. The dementia is similar to FTD with apathy, frontal/executive dysfunction, poor judgment, slowed thought processes, impaired verbal fluency, and difficulty with sequential actions and with shifting from one task to another. These cognitive deficits are usually evident at the time of presentation and often precede the motor syndrome.

PSP is often confused with Parkinson's disease. Dementia does occur in ~20% of Parkinson's disease patients, often secondary to DLB. Furthermore, the behavioral syndromes seen with DLB differ from those of PSP (see below). The occurrence of dementia in Parkinson's disease is more likely with increasing age, increasing severity of extrapyramidal signs, a long duration of disease, and the presence of depression. Cortical atrophy is usually present on brain imaging studies. Neuropathologically, there may be Alzheimer changes in the cortex (amyloid plaques and NFTs), neuronal Lewy body inclusions in both the substantia nigra and the cortex, or no specific microscopic changes other than gliosis and neuronal loss. PSP and Parkinson's disease are discussed in detail in Chap. 19.

Cortical Basal Degeneration

CBD is a slowly progressive dementing illness that typically presents with a unilateral onset with rigidity, dystonia, and apraxia of one arm and hand, sometimes called the "alien hand." Eventually the condition becomes bilateral and includes dysarthria, slow gait, action tremor, and dementia. CBD is discussed in detail in Chap. 19.

DEMENTIA WITH LEWY BODIES

This syndrome is characterized by visual hallucinations, parkinsonism, fluctuating alertness, and falls. Dementia can precede or follow the appearance of parkinsonism. DLB may present in a patient with longstanding Parkinson's disease without cognitive impairment who slowly develops dementia associated with visual hallucinations, parkinsonism, and fluctuating alertness. In other patients the dementia and neuropsychiatric syndrome precede the parkinsonism. Of note, some patients with parkinsonism and dementia who do not have characteristics of DLB are diagnosed with PD-dementia (PDD). This is a more common etiology of dementia than DLB in patients whose memory complaints follow the onset of PD by many years.

DLB patients are highly susceptible to metabolic perturbations, and in some the first manifestation of illness is a delirium, often precipitated by an infection or other systemic disturbance. A delirium induced by L-dopa, prescribed for parkinsonian symptoms attributed to Parkinson's disease, may be the initial clue that the correct diagnosis is DLB. Even without an underlying precipitant, fluctuations can be marked in DLB patients, with the occurrence of episodic confusion admixed with lucid intervals. However, despite the fluctuating pattern, the clinical features persist over a long period of time, unlike delirium, which resolves following correction of the underlying precipitant. Cognitively, DLB patients tend to have relatively better memory, but more severe visuospatial deficits, than individuals with AD.

The key neuropathologic feature is the presence of Lewy bodies throughout the cortex, amygdala, cingulated cortex, and substantia nigra. Lewy bodies are intraneuronal cytoplasmic inclusions that stain with periodic acid–Schiff (PAS) and ubiquitin. Lewy bodies are traditionally found in the substantia nigra of patients with idiopathic Parkinson's disease. A profound cholinergic deficit is present in many patients with DLB and may be a factor responsible for the fluctuations and visual hallucinations present in these patients. In patients without other pathologic features, the condition is referred to as *diffuse Lewy body disease*. In patients whose brains also contain excessive amounts of amyloid plaques and NFTs, the condition is called the *Lewy body variant of AD*. The quantity of Lewy bodies required to establish the diagnosis is not agreed on, but a definite diagnosis requires pathologic confirmation. At autopsy, 10 to 30% of demented patients show cortical Lewy bodies.

Due to the overlap with AD and the cholinergic deficit in DLB, anticholinesterase compounds may be helpful. Exercise programs are also helpful to maximize the motor function of these patients. Antidepressants are often necessary to treat depressive syndromes that accompany DLB. Atypical antipsychotics in low doses are sometimes needed to alleviate psychosis, although even low doses can increase extrapyramidal syndromes, which rarely may be life-threatening. As noted above, patients with DLB are extremely sensitive to dopaminergic medications, which must be carefully titrated; tolerability may be improved by concomitant use of cholinesterase inhibitors.

OTHER CAUSES OF DEMENTIA

Huntington's disease (HD) (Chap. 19) is an autosomal dominant, degenerative brain disorder. A DNA repeat expansion (CAG repeat) of the gene encoding huntingtin on chromosome 4 forms the basis of a diagnostic blood test for the disease gene. The clinical hallmarks of the disease are chorea, behavioral disturbance, and a frontal/executive disorder. Onset is usually in the fourth or fifth decade, but there is a wide range in age of onset, from childhood to >70 years. Memory is frequently not impaired until late in the disease, but attention, judgment, awareness, and executive functions may be seriously deficient at an early stage. Depression, apathy, social withdrawal, irritability, and intermittent disinhibition are common. Delusions and obsessive-compulsive behavior may occur. The disease duration is typically about 15 years but is quite variable. There is no specific treatment,

but the adventitious movements and behavioral changes may partially respond to phenothiazines, haloperidol, or benzodiazepines. Asymptomatic adult children at risk for HD should receive careful genetic counseling prior to DNA testing, because a positive result may have serious emotional and social consequences.

Normal-pressure hydrocephalus (NPH) is a relatively uncommon syndrome consisting of an abnormal gait (ataxic or apractic), dementia (usually mild to moderate), and urinary incontinence. Historically, many individuals who have been treated as having NPH have suffered from other dementias, particularly AD, PSP, vascular dementia, and DLB. Neuroimaging findings in NPH are those of a communicating hydrocephalus with a patent aqueduct of Sylvius (**Fig. 18-7**). In many cases periventricular edema is present. Lumbar puncture findings include an opening pressure in the high-normal range and normal CSF protein, glucose, and cell count. NPH is presumed to be caused by obstruction to normal flow of CSF over the cerebral convexity and delayed absorption into the venous system. The indolent nature of the process results in enlarged lateral ventricles but relatively little increase in CSF pressure. There is presumably stretching and distortion of white matter tracts in the corona radiata, but the exact physiologic cause of the clinical syndrome is unclear. Some patients have a history of conditions producing scarring of the basilar meninges (blocking upward flow of CSF) such as previ-

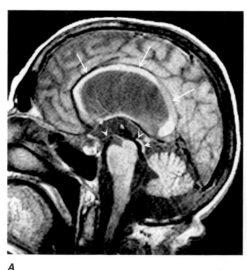

A

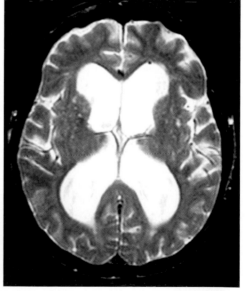

B

FIGURE 18-7

Normal pressure hydrocephalus. *A.* Sagittal T1-weighted MR image demonstrates dilatation of the lateral ventricle and stretching of the corpus callosum (*arrows*), depression of the floor of the third ventricle (*single arrowhead*), and enlargement of the aqueduct (*double arrowheads*). Note the diffuse dilatation of the lateral, third, and fourth ventricles with a patent aqueduct, typical of communicating hydrocephalus. *B.* Axial T2-weighted MR images demonstrate dilatation of the lateral ventricles without generalized cortical atrophy. This patient underwent successful ventriculoperitoneal shunting.

ous meningitis, subarachnoid hemorrhage, or head trauma. Others with longstanding but asymptomatic congenital hydrocephalus may have an adult-onset deterioration in gait or memory that is confused with NPH; in these patients, the aqueduct of Sylvius is small, in contrast to patients with NPH. Unlike in AD, the NPH patient has an early and prominent gait disturbance and no evidence of cortical or hippocampal atrophy on neuroimaging studies. A number of attempts have been made to use various special studies to improve the diagnosis of NPH and predict the success of ventricular shunting. These include radionuclide cisternography (showing a delay in CSF absorption over the convexity) and various attempts to monitor and alter CSF flow dynamics. None has proved to be specific or consistently useful. There is sometimes a transient improvement in gait or cognition following lumbar puncture (or serial punctures) with removal of ≥ 30 mL of CSF, but this finding is not a reliable predictor of post-shunt improvement. Approximately 30 to 50% of patients identified by careful diagnosis as having NPH will show improvement with a ventricular shunting procedure. Gait may improve more than memory. Transient, short-lasting improvement is common. Patients should be carefully selected for this operation, because subdural hematoma and infection are known complications.

Prion diseases such as CJD are rapidly progressive disorders associated with dementia, focal cortical signs, rigidity, and myoclonus. The rapidity of progression seen with CJD is uncommon in AD so that distinction between the two disorders is usually straightforward. CBD and DLB progress more rapidly than AD and are associated with prominent disorders of movement and so are more likely to be mistaken for CJD. Abnormal periodic EEG discharges and cortical and basal ganglia abnormalities on diffusion-weighted MRI are unique diagnostic features of CJD. CSF protein 14-3-3 is not specific for CJD and is often not helpful in the diagnostic workup of these patients. Prion diseases are discussed in detail in (Chap. 32).

Dementia can accompany *chronic alcoholism* (Chap. 42). This may be a result of associated malnutrition, especially of B vitamins and particularly thiamine. However, other as yet poorly defined aspects of chronic alcohol ingestion may also produce cerebral damage. A rare syndrome of dementia and seizures with degeneration of the corpus callosum has been reported primarily in male Italian drinkers of red wine (Marchiafava-Bignami disease).

Thiamine (vitamin B_1) deficiency causes Wernicke's encephalopathy. The clinical presentation is a malnourished individual (frequently but not necessarily alcoholic) with confusion, ataxia, and diplopia from ophthalmoplegia. Thiamine deficiency damages the thalamus, mammillary bodies, midline cerebellum, periaqueductal gray matter of the midbrain, and peripheral nerves. Damage to the dorsomedial thalamic regions correlates most closely with memory loss. Prompt administration of parenteral thiamine may reverse the disease if given in the first few days of symptom onset. However, prolonged untreated thiamine deficiency can result in an irreversible dementia/amnestic syndrome known as *Korsakoff's syndrome.* Here, the patient is unable to recall new information despite normal immediate memory, attention span, and level of consciousness. Memory for new events is seriously impaired, whereas memory of knowledge prior to the illness is relatively intact. Patients are easily confused, disoriented, and incapable of recalling new information for more than a brief interval. Superficially, they may be conversant, entertaining, able to perform simple tasks, and follow immediate commands. Confabulation is common, although not always present, and may result in obviously erroneous statements and elaborations. There is no specific treatment because the previous thiamine deficiency has produced irreversible damage to the medial thalamic nuclei and mammillary bodies. Mammillary body atrophy may be visible on high-resolution MRI.

Vitamin B_{12} deficiency, as can occur in pernicious anemia, causes a macrocytic anemia and may also damage the nervous system (Chap 24). Neurologically it most commonly produces a spinal cord syndrome (myelopathy) affecting the posterior columns (loss of position and vibratory sense) and corticospinal tracts (hyperactive tendon reflexes with Babinski responses); it may also damage peripheral nerves, resulting in sensory loss with depressed tendon reflexes. Damage to cerebral myelinated fibers may also cause dementia. The mechanism of neurologic damage is unclear but may be related to a deficiency of S-adenosylmethionine (required for methylation of myelin phospholipids) due to reduced methionine synthase activity or accumulation of methylmalonate, homocysteine, and propionate, providing abnormal substrates for fatty acid synthesis in myelin. The neurologic signs of vitamin B_{12} deficiency are usually associated with macrocytic anemia, but on occasion may occur in its absence. Treatment with parenteral vitamin B_{12} stops progression of the disease if instituted promptly, but reversal of advanced nervous system damage may not occur.

Other vitamin deficiency syndromes include deficiency of nicotinic acid (pellagra), which is associated with sun-exposed skin rash, glossitis, and angular stomatitis. Severe dietary deficiency of nicotinic acid along with other B vitamins such as pyridoxine may result in spastic paraparesis, peripheral neuropathy, fatigue, irritability, and dementia. This syndrome has been seen in prisoner-of-war and concentration camps. Low serum folate levels appear to be a rough index of malnutrition, but isolated folate deficiency has not been proved to be a specific cause of dementia.

Infections of the CNS usually cause delirium and other acute neurologic syndromes. However, some chronic CNS infections, particularly those associated with chronic meningitis (Chap. 30), may produce a dementing illness. The possibility of chronic infectious meningitis should be suspected in patients presenting with a dementia or behavioral syndrome who also have headache, meningismus, cranial neuropathy, and/or radiculopathy. Between 20 and 30% of patients in the advanced stages of infection with HIV become demented (Chap. 31). Cardinal features include psychomotor retardation, apathy, and impaired memory. This may result from secondary opportunistic infections but can also be caused by direct infection of CNS neurons with HIV. Neurosyphilis was a common cause of dementia in the preantibiotic era; it is now uncommon. Characteristic CSF changes consist of pleocytosis, increased protein, and a positive Venereal Disease Research Laboratory (VDRL) test.

Primary and metastatic neoplasms of the CNS (Chap. 25) usually produce focal neurologic findings and seizures rather than dementia. However, if tumor growth begins in the frontal or temporal lobes, the initial manifestations may be memory loss or behavioral changes. A paraneoplastic syndrome of dementia associated with occult carcinoma (often small cell lung cancer) is termed *limbic encephalitis* (Chap. 27). In this syndrome, confusion, agitation, seizures, poor memory, movement disorders, and dementia occur in association with sensory neuropathy.

A nonconvulsive seizure disorder may underlie a syndrome of confusion, clouding of consciousness, and garbled speech. Psychiatric disease is often suspected, but an EEG demonstrates the seizure discharges. The cognitive disturbance often responds to anticonvulsant therapy.

Systemic diseases: It is important to recognize systemic diseases that indirectly affect the brain and produce chronic confusion or dementia. Such conditions include hypothyroidism; vasculitis; and hepatic, renal, or pulmonary disease. Hepatic encephalopathy may begin with irritability and confusion and slowly progress to agitation, lethargy, and coma.

Isolated vasculitis of the CNS (CNS granulomatous vasculitis) occasionally causes a chronic encephalopathy with confusion, disorientation, and clouding of consciousness. Headache is common, and strokes and cranial neuropathies may occur. Brain imaging studies may be normal or nonspecifically abnormal. CSF studies reveal a mild pleocytosis or elevation in the protein level. Cerebral angiography often shows multifocal stenosis and narrowing of vessels. A few patients have only small-vessel disease that is not revealed on angiography. The angiographic appearance is nonspecific and may be mimicked by atherosclerosis, infec-

tion, or other causes of vascular disease. Brain or meningeal biopsy demonstrates abnormal arteries with endothelial cell proliferation and infiltrates of mononuclear cells. Some patients respond to glucocorticoids or chemotherapy.

Chronic metal exposure may produce a dementing syndrome. The key to diagnosis is to elicit a history of exposure at work, home, or even as a consequence of a medical procedure such as dialysis. Chronic lead poisoning may present as fatigue, depression, and confusion and may be associated with episodic abdominal pain and peripheral neuropathy. Inadequately fired glazed pottery has been reported as a cause. Gray lead lines appear in the gums. There is usually an anemia with basophilic stippling of red cells. The clinical presentation can resemble that of acute intermittent porphyria, including elevated levels of urine porphyrins as a result of the inhibition of δ-aminolevulinic acid dehydrase. The treatment is chelation therapy with agents such as ethylene-diamine tetraacetic acid (EDTA). Chronic mercury poisoning produces dementia, peripheral neuropathy, ataxia, and tremulousness that may progress to choreoathetosis. Chronic arsenic intoxication can produce confusion and memory loss associated with nausea, weight loss, peripheral neuropathy, pigmentation and scaling of the skin, and transverse white lines of the fingernails (Mees' lines). Treatment is chelation therapy with dimercaprol (BAL). Aluminum poisoning has been best documented with the dialysis dementia syndrome, in which water used during renal dialysis was contaminated with excessive amounts of aluminum. A progressive encephalopathy ensued, associated with confusion, aphasia, memory loss, agitation, and, later, lethargy and stupor. Speech arrest and myoclonic jerks were common and associated with severe and generalized EEG changes. The condition has been eliminated by the use of deionized water for dialysis.

Recurrent head trauma in professional boxers may lead to dementia, sometimes called the "punch drunk" syndrome or *dementia pugilistica*. The symptoms can be progressive, beginning late in a boxer's career or even long after retirement. The severity of the syndrome correlates with the length of the boxing career and number of bouts. Early on, a personality change associated with social instability and sometimes paranoia and delusions occurs. Later, memory loss progresses to full dementia, often associated with parkinsonian signs and ataxia or intention tremor. At autopsy, the cerebral cortex may show changes similar to those in AD, although NFTs are usually more prominent than amyloid plaques (which are usually diffuse rather than neuritic). There may also be loss of neurons in the substantia nigra.

Transient global amnesia (TGA) is characterized by the sudden onset of a severe episodic memory deficit, usually occurring in persons over age 50. Often, the memory loss occurs in the setting of an emotional stimulus or physical exertion. During the attack the individual is alert and communicative, general cognition seems intact, and there are no other neurologic signs or symptoms. The patient may seem confused and repeatedly ask about present events. The ability to form new memories returns after a period of hours, and the individual returns to normal with no recall for the period of the attack. Frequently no cause is determined, but cerebrovascular disease, epilepsy (7% in one study), migraine, or cardiac arrhythmia have all been implicated. Recent MRI diffusion imaging of the hippocampus has suggested an ischemic etiology. Approximately one-quarter of patients with TGA have recurrent attacks.

The ALS/parkinsonian/dementia complex of Guam is a rare degenerative disease that has occurred in the Chamorro natives on the island of Guam. Any combination of parkinsonian features, dementia, and motor neuron disease may occur. The most characteristic pathologic features are the presence of NFTs in degenerating neurons of the cortex and substantia nigra and loss of motor neurons in the spinal cord. Epidemiologic evidence supports a possible environmental cause, such as exposure to a neurotoxin with a long latency period. The ALS syndrome is decreasing in frequency on Guam, but a dementing illness with rigidity continues to be seen.

Rarely adult-onset leukodystrophies, neuronal storage diseases, and other genetic disorders can cause dementia late in life. Adult metachromatic leukodystrophy (arylsulfatase A deficiency) can present as a dementia associated with large frontal white matter lesions and usually peripheral neuropathy. Adult presentations of adrenaleukodystrophy have been reported, and in these cases involvement of the spinal cord and posterior white matter is common. This is diagnosed with measurement of very long-chain fatty acids (Chap. 24). The neuronal lipofuscinoses (NCLs) are a genetically heterogeneous group of disorders associated with myoclonus, seizures, and progressive dementia. Diagnosis is made by finding curvilinear inclusions within white blood cells or neuronal tissue.

Psychogenic amnesia for personally important memories is common, although whether this results from deliberate avoidance of unpleasant memories or from unconscious repression is currently unknown. The event-specific amnesia is more likely to occur after violent crimes such as homicide of a close relative or friend or sexual abuse. It may also develop in association with drug or alcohol intoxication and sometimes with schizophrenia. More prolonged psychogenic amnesia occurs in fugue states that also commonly follow severe emotional stress. The patient with a fugue state suffers from a sudden loss of personal identity and may be found wandering far from home. In contrast to organic amnesia, fugue states are associated with amnesia for personal identity and events closely associated with the personal past. At the same time, memory for other recent events and the ability to learn and use new information are preserved. The episodes usually last hours or days and occasionally weeks or months while the patient takes on a new identity. On recovery, there is a residual amnesia for the period of the fugue. Very rarely, selective loss of autobiographical information represents a focal injury in the brain areas involved with these functions.

Psychiatric diseases may mimic dementia. Severely depressed individuals may appear demented, a phenomenon called *pseudodementia*. Memory and language are usually intact when carefully tested in depressed persons, and a significant memory disturbance usually suggests an underlying dementia, even if the patient is depressed. The patient with pseudodementia may feel confused and unable to accomplish routine tasks. Vegetative symptoms are common, such as insomnia, lack of energy, poor appetite, and concern with bowel function. The onset is often abrupt, and the psychosocial milieu may suggest prominent reasons for depression. Such patients respond to treatment of the depression. Schizophrenia is usually not difficult to distinguish from dementia, but occasionally the distinction can be problematic. Schizophrenia usually has a much earlier age of onset (second and third decades) than most dementing illnesses and is associated with intact memory. The delusions and hallucinations of schizophrenia are usually more complex and bizarre than those of dementia. Some chronic schizophrenics develop an unexplained progressive dementia late in life that is not related to AD. Conversely, FTD, HD, vascular dementia, DLB, AD, or leukoencephalopathy can begin with schizophrenia-like features, leading to the misdiagnosis of a psychiatric condition. The later age of onset, presence of significant deficits on cognitive testing, and neuroimaging findings point toward a degenerative condition. Memory loss may also be part of a conversion reaction. In this situation, patients commonly complain bitterly of memory loss, but careful cognitive testing either does not confirm the deficits or demonstrates inconsistent or unusual patterns of cognitive problems. The patient's behavior and "wrong" answers to questions often indicate that he or she understands the question and knows the correct answer.

Medications: Clouding of cognition by chronic drug or medication use, often prescribed by physicians, is an important cause of dementia. Sedatives, tranquilizers, and analgesics, including those with anticholinergic properties, used to treat insomnia, pain, anxiety, or agitation may cause confusion, memory loss, and lethargy, especially in the elderly. Discontinuation of the offending medication often improves mentation.

GENERAL SYMPTOMATIC TREATMENT OF THE PATIENT WITH DEMENTIA

The major goals of management are to treat any correctable causes of the dementia and to provide comfort and support to the patient and caregivers. Removal of sedating or cognition-impairing drugs and medications is often beneficial. If the patient is depressed rather than demented, the depression should be vigorously treated. Patients with degenerative diseases may also be depressed, and that portion of their condition may respond to antidepressant therapy. Antidepressants that are low in cognitive side effects, such as SSRIs (Chap. 41), are advisable when treatment is necessary. Anticonvulsants are used to control seizures.

Agitation, hallucinations, delusions, and confusion are difficult to treat. These behavioral problems represent major causes for nursing home placement and institutionalization. Before treating these behaviors with medications, a thorough search for potentially modifiable environmental or metabolic factors should be sought. Hunger, lack of exercise, toothache, constipation, urinary tract infection, or drug toxicity all represent easily correctable factors that can be treated without psychoactive drugs. Cholinesterase inhibitors themselves may be useful for many neuropsychiatric and behavioral symptoms. Medications that may calm agitation and insomnia without worsening dementia include low-dose haloperidol (0.5 to 2 mg), trazodone, buspirone, or propranolol. The new atypical antipsychotics including risperidone, olanzapine, and quetiapine are increasingly used for patients with difficult behaviors. When patients do not respond it is usually a mistake to advance to higher doses or to use anticholinergics or sedatives (such as barbiturates or benzodiazepines). The few controlled studies comparing drugs with behavioral intervention in the treatment of agitation suggest that both approaches are effective. However, careful, daily, nondrug behavior management is often not available, rendering medication necessary.

A proactive strategy has been shown to reduce the occurrence of delirium in hospitalized patients. This includes frequent orientation, cognitive activities, sleep-enhancement measures, vision and hearing aids, and correction of dehydration.

Nondrug behavior therapy has an important place in the management of dementia. The primary goal is to make the demented patient's life comfortable, uncomplicated, and safe. Memory aids such as notebooks, lists, and posted daily reminders are frequently helpful. It is also useful to stress familiar routines, short-term tasks, walks, and simple physical exercises. For many demented patients, the memory for facts is worse than that for routine activities, and they still may be able to take part in remembered physical activities such as walking, bowling, dancing, and golf. Demented patients usually object to losing control over familiar tasks such as driving, cooking, and handling finances. Attempts to help or take over may be greeted with complaints, depression, or anger. Hostile responses on the part of the caretaker are useless and sometimes harmful. Explanation, reassurance, distraction, and calm statements are more productive responses in this setting. Eventually, tasks such as finances and driving must be assumed by others, and the patient will conform and adjust. Safety is an important issue that includes not only driving but the environment of the kitchen, bathroom, and sleeping area. These areas need to be monitored, supervised, and made as safe as possible. A move to a retirement home, assisted-living center, or nursing home can initially increase confusion and agitation. Repeated reassurance, reorientation, and careful introduction to the new personnel will help to smooth the process. Provision of activities that are known to be enjoyable to the patient can be of considerable benefit. Attention should also be paid to frustration and depression in family members and caregivers. Caregiver guilt and burn-out are common, often resulting in nursing home placement of the patient. Family members often feel overwhelmed and helpless and may vent their frustrations on the patient, each other, and health care providers. Caregivers should be encouraged to take advantage of day-care facilities and respite breaks. Education and counseling about dementia are important. Local and national support groups, such as the Alzheimer's Disease and Related Disorders Association, can be of considerable help.

FURTHER READINGS

BOEVE BF et al: Current management of sleep disturbances in dementia. Curr Neurol Neurosci Rep 2:169, 2002

☑ GILMAN S et al: Clinical effects of Aβ immunization (AN1792) in patients with AD in an interrupted trial. Neurology 64:1553, 2005

Results of first amyloid immunization trial halted secondary to immune-related side effects.

☑ PETERSON RC et al: Vitamin E and donepezil for the treatment of mild cognitive impairment. N Engl J Med 352:2379, 2005

Key paper showing very modest benefit of cholinesterase inhibitors for mild cognitive impairment.

REISBERG B et al: Memantine in moderate to severe Alzheimer's disease. N Engl J Med 348:1333, 2003

ROSEN HJ et al: Utility of clinical criteria in differentiating fron-totemporal lobar degeneration (FTLD) from AD. Neurology 58:1608, 2002

☑ TARIOT PN et al: Memantine treatment in patients with moderate to severe Alzheimer disease already receiving donepezil: A randomized controlled trial. JAMA 291:317, 2004

Establishes a role for memantine as add-on therapy to cholinesterase inhibitor.

WINBECK K et al: DWI in transient global amnesia and TIA: Proposal for an ischemic origin of TIA. J Neurol Neurosurg Psychiatry 76:438, 2005

VERMEER SE et al: Silent brain infarcts and the risk of dementia and cognitive decline. N Engl J Med 348:1215, 2003

YAFFE K et al: The metabolic syndrome, inflammation, and risk of cognitive decline. JAMA 292:2237, 2004

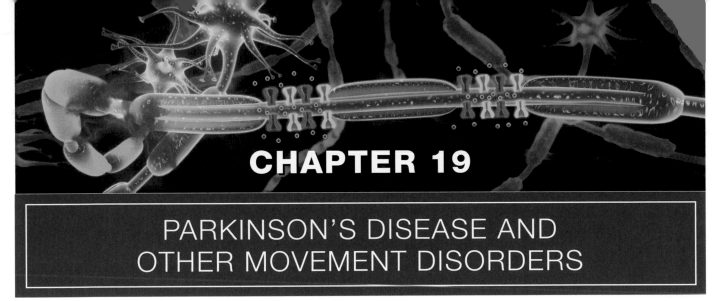

CHAPTER 19

PARKINSON'S DISEASE AND OTHER MOVEMENT DISORDERS

Mahlon R. DeLong

Jorge L. Juncos

PARKINSON'S DISEASE

Parkinson's disease (PD) is the most common example of a family of neurodegenerative disorders characterized by a neuronal accumulation of the presynaptic protein α-synuclein and by variable degrees of *parkinsonism*, defined as a paucity and slowness of movement (*bradykinesia*), tremor at rest, rigidity, shuffling gait, and flexed posture. Nearly all forms of parkinsonism result from a reduction of dopaminergic transmission within the basal ganglia. Sporadic and idiopathic PD account for ~75% of all cases of parkinsonism; the remaining 25% result from genetically defined etiologies and other causes including other neurodegenerative disorders, cerebrovascular disease, and drugs.

EPIDEMIOLOGY

PD afflicts >1 million individuals in the United States (~1% of those >55 years). Its peak age of onset is in the 60s (range is 35 to 85 years), and the course of the illness ranges between 10 and 25 years. Familial clusters of autosomal dominant and recessive forms of PD comprise ~5% of cases (**Table 19–1**). These are characterized by an earlier age of onset (typically before age 50 years) and a longer

TABLE 19-1

FAMILIAL PARKINSON'S DISEASE		
LOCUS	**GENE**	**INHERITANCE**
PARK1	*α-Synuclein*	AD
PARK2	*Parkin*	AR
PARK4	*α-Synuclein* triplication	AD
PARK5	UCHL1	AD
PARK6	PINK1	AR
PARK7	DJ-1	AR
PARK3, 8, 9	Unknown	AD and AR mutations
LRRK2	LRRK2	AD and sporadic
GBA	Glucocerebrosidase	Susceptibility gene

Note: AD, autosomal dominant; AR, autosomal recessive.

course than the more typical "sporadic" PD. Although most patients with PD appear to have no strong genetic determinant, epidemiologic evidence points to a complex interaction between genetic vulnerability and environmental factors. Risk factors include a positive family history, male gender, head injury, exposure to pesticides, consumption of well water, and rural living. Factors linked to a reduced incidence of PD include coffee drinking, smoking, use of nonsteroidal anti-inflammatory drugs, and estrogen replacement in postmenopausal women.

CLINICAL FEATURES

A diagnosis of PD can be made with some confidence in patients who present with at least two of the three cardinal signs—rest tremor, rigidity, and bradykinesia. Tremor is particularly important, as it is present in 85% of patients with true PD; a diagnosis of PD is particularly difficult when tremor is absent. A unilateral and gradual onset of symptoms further supports the diagnosis. Masked facies, decreased eye blinking, stooped posture, and decreased arm swing complete the early picture. The onset may also be heralded by vague feelings of weakness and fatigue, incoordination, aching, and discomfort.

MOTOR FEATURES

The most disabling feature of PD is bradykinesia, which interferes with all aspects of daily living such as walking, rising from a chair, turning in bed, and dressing. Fine motor control is also impaired as evidenced by decreased manual dexterity and handwriting (*micrographia*). Soft speech (*hypophonia*) and sialorrhea are other troubling manifestations of (bulbar) bradykinesia. Rest tremor, at a frequency of 4 to 6 Hz, typically appears unilaterally, first distally, involving the digits and wrist where it may have a "pill-rolling" character. Tremor usually spreads proximally, ipsilaterally, and occasionally to the leg before crossing to the other side after a year or more. It may appear later in the lips, tongue, and jaw but spares the head. Rigidity is felt as a uniform resistance to passive movement about a joint throughout the full range of motion, giving rise to a characteristic "plastic" quality. Brief, regular interruptions of resistance during passive movement, corresponding to subclinical tremor, may give rise to a "cogwheeling" sensation. Dystonia involving the distal arm or leg may occur early in the disease, unrelated to treatment, especially in younger patients. It can also be provoked by antiparkinsonian drug therapy.

Gait disturbance with shuffling short steps and a tendency to turn en bloc is a prominent feature of PD. Festinating gait, a classic parkinsonian sign, results from the combination of flexed posture and loss of postural reflexes, which cause the patient to accelerate in an effort to "catch up" with the body's center of gravity. Freezing of gait, a feature of more advanced PD, occurs commonly at the onset of locomotion (start hesitation), when attempting to change direction or turn around, and upon entering a narrow space such as a doorway.

Abnormalities of balance and posture tend to increase in prominence as the disease progresses. Flexion of the head, stooping and tilting of the upper trunk, and a tendency to hold the arm in a flexed posture while walking are common, as are changes in the posture of the fingers and hands. Postural instability is one of the most disabling features of advanced PD, contributing to falls and injuries and leading to major morbidity and mortality. It can be tested in the office with the "pull-test" (**Fig. 19-1**). Significant postural instability and falls in the first years of the illness, however, strongly suggest a diagnosis other than PD.

NON-MOTOR FEATURES

Non-motor aspects of PD include depression and anxiety, cognitive impairment, sleep disturbances, sensory abnormalities and pain, loss of smell (*anosmia*), and disturbances of autonomic function. Together they may contribute as much to the burden of the disease as the more obvious motor abnormalities. Some of these

---

Testing for Postural Instability

I. Practice session

Explanation must be given that the patient will be pulled forcefully backward to test balance and that the patient must prevent himself or herself from falling, if necessary, by taking a step backward after he or she is pulled. At least one good practice session is carried out before the final test.

II. Patient stance

Patient must be upright and cannot lean forward in any way unless axial flexion prevents upright posture. Patient must not be pulled while off balance from a previous pull. Stance should be with feet comfortably apart.

III. Pull

Patient is pulled briskly and forcefully.

IV. Examiner's response

Examiner is ready to catch the patient but allows enough space to move backward with the patient for at least three steps of recovery. The test is to be performed in a space long enough to differentiate between persistent but recovering retropulsion and no recovery.

FIGURE 19-1

Advanced Examination Pearls: Testing for Postural Instability.
Source: RP Munhox et al. Neurology 62(1):125, 2004, with permission.

(e.g., anosmia, depression, and sleep disorders) may be present long before the onset of motor signs. The physiologic basis of the non-motor signs and symptoms are explained in part by widespread involvement of brainstem, olfactory, thalamic, and cortical structures.

Sensory symptoms most often manifest as a distressing sensation of inner restlessness presumed to be a form of akathisia. Aching pain and discomfort in the extremities can be a prominent presenting symptom or develop when antiparkinson medications are wearing off. Other patients develop a subjective shortness of breath in the absence of any underlying cardiorespiratory pathology.

Sleep disorders are common in PD. Daytime drowsiness and frequent napping are typical signs of sleep disruption. Factors that disrupt sleep include nighttime reemergence of bradykinesia and rigidity, with difficulty turning in bed, as well as tremor and involuntary movements (e.g., myoclonic jerks or periodic leg movements). Restless legs and rapid eye movement–behavioral disorder (RBD) are present in considerable numbers of patients, often preceding the onset of PD. Vivid dreams and hallucinations related to dopaminomimetic therapy may also contribute to sleep disruption. Finally, sleep apnea and other sleep disturbances can occur.

Autonomic dysfunction can produce diverse manifestations, including orthostatic hypotension, constipation, urinary urgency and frequency, excessive sweating, and seborrhea. Orthostatic hypotension is present in many patients resulting from sympathetic denervation of the heart or as a side effect of dopaminomimetic therapy. This rarely leads to syncope unless the patient has developed true autonomic failure or has an unrelated cardiac problem. Drenching sweats may occur in advanced PD, often related to wearing off of medication.

NEUROPSYCHIATRIC SYMPTOMS

Changes in mood, cognition, and behavior are common accompaniments of the later stages of PD and may be the direct result of PD or its comorbid pathologies [e.g., Alzheimer's disease (AD), cortical dementia with Lewy bodies (DLB)], or occur as a side effect of its pharmacotherapy

Depression affects approximately half of patients with PD and can occur at any phase of the illness. It is often difficult to diagnose due to the overlap between the somatic and vegetative symptoms of PD and depression. As a consequence, depression often goes unrecognized and untreated. There is compelling evidence that depression in PD is an intrinsic part of the illness and not simply a reaction to disability. Recognizing even mild depression is particularly important since it can account for otherwise unexplained worsening parkinsonian motor

symptoms, new somatic symptoms, and sleep disruption. Depression can also be induced or aggravated iatrogenically by antiparkinsonian and psychotropic agents used to treat other symptoms. Finally, other causes for depressive symptoms and refractory depression should always be considered, including hypothyroidism, hypogonadism, and vitamin B_{12} deficiency.

Anxiety disorders in PD can appear in isolation or as an accompaniment of depression or progressive cognitive impairment. They can also be due to an akathisia equivalent mediated by "dopamine hunger" due to undertreatment of motor symptoms. The development of drug-induced motor fluctuations can compound the problem by precipitating fluxes in anxiety during the off periods that mimic panic attacks.

Cognitive abnormalities affect many patients with PD. Most are mild to moderate in severity. Difficulties with complex tasks, long-term planning, and memorizing or retrieving new information are common. Although some of these symptoms represent *bradyphrenia* (the cognitive equivalent of bradykinesia), it is now clear that the dysfunction also includes working memory, attention, mental flexibility, visuospatial function, word fluency, and executive functions. Iatrogenic contributors include the indiscriminate use of amantadine or psychotropic, anticholinergic, and dopaminomimetic medications. Depression and intercurrent medical illnesses, such as urinary tract or other infections, are reversible causes of cognitive symptoms in PD.

Whether these nondementing abnormalities form a continuum with the dementias that affect a subset of patients in later stages of the disease is unknown. The incidence of dementia in PD may be as high as six times that in age-matched controls. The presence of significant cognitive impairment may limit therapeutic options and contribute more to overall disability than the motor symptoms in PD. Predictors of dementia include late age of onset, akinetic rigid phenotype, presence of severe depression, persistent hallucinations, and advanced stages of disease.

Psychotic symptoms affect 6 to 40% of patients with PD, depending on the age and prevalence of dementia in the population surveyed. Early symptoms include formed visual hallucinations (usually people and animals) with retained insight. Although depression and dementia are the most important risk factors for psychotic symptoms in PD, the symptoms are often triggered by drug therapy and are dose-dependent. Dopaminomimetics, anticholinergics, amantadine, and selegiline are the chief offenders. Delusions are more disturbing than hallucinations because they place an even heavier burden on the family and caregivers. The prodrome to these psychotic symptoms includes subtle erratic behaviors with temperamental and sometimes unreasonable outbursts.

DIFFERENTIAL DIAGNOSIS

The differential diagnosis of parkinsonian syndromes requires a careful history and physical examination (**Table 19-2**). Neuroimaging with magnetic resonance imaging (MRI) is useful to rule out disorders such as normal pressure hydrocephalus, vascular disease, or mass lesions. Positron emission tomography (PET) is helpful in confirming suspected atypical forms such as corticobasal degeneration. Essential tremor (ET) is sometimes confused with rest tremor in PD, but the absence of other signs of parkinsonism and the bilaterality, higher frequency (8 to 10 Hz), and postural dependency of ET plus significant relief with even a small amount of alcohol help differentiate this from the rest tremor of PD. In individuals under 40 it is important to rule out Wilson's disease. In younger individuals Huntington's disease (HD) sometimes presents with prominent parkinsonian features. Although parkinsonian features are often present in AD, they are greatly outweighed by the cognitive and behavioral disturbances. In DLB, the parkinsonian features are compounded by the early appearance of hallucinations and disturbances in arousal and behavior. Parkinsonism may also develop following exposure to certain neurotoxins such as carbon monoxide or manganese.

The differentiation of sporadic PD from atypical parkinsonism (see below) is the most difficult task, since early in their course these atypical forms often meet diagnostic criteria for PD. Accordingly, it is important not to settle on a definite diagnosis at the first visit. The development of early imbalance and falls suggests progressive supranuclear palsy (PSP); early urinary incontinence, orthostatic hypotension, and dysarthria suggest multiple system atrophy (MSA). The early appearance of drug-induced hallucinations strongly favors the diagnosis of DLB. As a rule the different forms of atypical parkinsonism can be reliably differentiated from sporadic PD within the first 3 to 4 years.

PATHOLOGY

Gross pathologic examination of the brain in PD reveals mild frontal atrophy with loss of the normal dark melanin pigment of the midbrain. Microscopically there is degeneration of the dopaminergic cells with the presence of Lewy bodies (LBs) in the remaining neurons and processes of the substantia nigra pars compacta (SNpc), other brainstem nuclei, and regions such as the medial temporal, limbic, and frontal cortices. LBs have a high concentration of α-synuclein and are the pathologic hallmark of the disorder. Mutations in the α-synuclein gene can cause familial PD by promoting the formation of α-synuclein-positive filaments that aggregate into LBs and Lewy neurites.

The biochemical consequence of dopaminergic cell loss in the SNpc is gradual denervation of the striatum, the main target projection for the SNpc neurons. Other target regions of these neurons include the intralaminar and parafascicular nuclei of the thalamus, the globus pallidus, and the subthalamic nucleus (STN). Dopamine denervation of the striatum leads to many of the motor symptoms of PD. Symptoms develop when striatal dopamine depletion reaches 50 to 70% of normal. Pharmacologic restoration of dopamine transmission is the basis for symptomatic drug treatment of PD.

Although >90% of cases of idiopathic of PD appear to be sporadic, increasing evidence indicates that genetic factors play an important role in many forms PD. Much of this evidence comes from studies of the concordance rates for PD among monozygotic and dizygotic twins.

TABLE 19-2

ADVANCED EXAMINATION PEARLS: HISTORY AND EXAMINATION FEATURES THAT WOULD QUESTION THE DIAGNOSIS OF IDIOPATHIC PARKINSON'S DISEASE	
SYMPTOMS/SIGNS	ALTERNATIVE DIAGNOSIS TO CONSIDER
History	
Falls as the first symptom	PSP
Exposure to neuroleptics	Drug-Induced Parkinsonism
Onset prior to age 40	If PD, think genetic causes
Associated unexplained liver disease	Wilson's Disease
Early hallucinations	Lewy Body Dementia
Sudden onset of Parkinsonism symptoms	Vascular Parkinsonism
Physical Exam	
Dementia as first symptom	Lewy Body Dementia
Prominent orthostasis	MSA-p
Early dysarthria	MSA-c
Lack of tremor	Various Parkinson's-plus Syndromes
High frequency (8-10 Hz) symmetric tremor	Essential Tremor

These studies suggest that heredity plays an important role in cases with age of onset <50 years and a less important role in older patients. The identification of mutations in these families are proving invaluable in refining the correlation between genotypes and phenotypes, in generating animal models to study pathogenesis, and in identifying target pathways for possible therapeutic intervention (Table 19-1).

TREATMENT FOR PD

General Considerations

The goals of therapy in PD are to maintain function and quality of life and to avoid drug-induced complications. Bradykinesia, tremor, rigidity, and abnormal posture respond well to symptomatic therapy early in the course of the illness. In contrast, cognitive symptoms, hypophonia, autonomic dysfunction, and balance difficulties respond poorly. Primary motor disability in PD is often aggravated by secondary disability resulting from physical deconditioning following a sedentary lifestyle. Prevention of secondary disability requires a consistent program of physical activity, thus regular activity is strongly encouraged. Remaining mentally active is probably equally important.

A current priority is to move beyond symptom control to neuroprotective therapies. Unfortunately, no such therapy is yet available, although selegiline (deprenyl) may, in addition to a mild symptomatic effect, have a neuroprotective function. High doses of coenzyme Q_{10} and intrastriatal infusion of neurotrophic factors show promise in early clinical trials. Animal studies have shown that exercise can promote neuroprotection against neurotoxins.

Initiation of Therapy

From a practical standpoint, dopaminomimetic therapy should be initiated as soon as the patient's symptoms begin to interfere with quality of life. The ideal agent for initiation of symptomatic therapy depends on the age and cognitive status of the patient and, to a lesser extent, the patient's clinical type and finances. The choices consist of either a levodopa preparation or a dopamine agonist. Controlled studies support the view that, in early PD, dopamine agonist monotherapy is well tolerated and significantly reduces the risk of later treatment-related complications such as motor fluctuations and dyskinesias. *Motor fluctuations* are the exaggerated ebb and flow of parkinsonian signs experienced by many patients between doses of antiparkinsonian medications. *Dyskinesias* refer to choreiform and dystonic movements that can occur as a peak dose effect or at the beginning or end of the dose (diphasic dyskinesias). More than 50% of patients with PD treated over 5 years with levodopa will develop these complications.

Successful dopamine agonist monotherapy requires a higher dose of the agonist than is typically needed when the agonist is used to supplement levodopa (**Table 19–3**). In both cases titration has to be slow and cautious to avoid unnecessary side effects. Patients benefit greatly from education and support during this titration. Most patients will require the addition of levodopa or another agent within 1 to 3 years of initiating dopamine agonist monotherapy. Preclinical studies suggest that the advantages of dopamine agonist monotherapy can be maintained with agonist-dominant therapy. In this case dopamine agonists continue to provide the bulk of dopaminomimetic therapy, with levodopa playing a supplementary role.

Although dopamine agonist monotherapy is considered the initial treatment of choice for most patients with PD, the long-term benefits noted above must be balanced against a higher incidence of non-motor side effects, especially in older individuals over the age of 70, and a slightly higher level of motor disability than with levodopa. These recommendations may need to be modified in patients with psychotic symptoms or severe daytime sleep disturbances. Older patients and those with akinetic rigid phenotypes of PD have a lower risk of motor complications and dyskinesias compared to the average PD patient and may be satisfactorily treated with levodopa.

Pharmacotherapy of Motor Symptoms

The above advances in the initiation of therapy notwithstanding, levodopa remains the most effective treatment for PD. It significantly improves motor symptoms and increases quality of life and independence. The aim of all dopaminomimetic strategies is to restore dopamine transmission in the striatum. This is accomplished by stimulating postsynaptic receptors (directly with dopamine agonists), increasing dopamine precursor availability (levodopa), blocking the metabolism of levodopa in the periphery and in the brain, and blocking the catabolism of dopamine at the presynaptic terminal (**Fig. 19–2**)

TABLE 19-3

GUIDE TO THE USE OF LEVODOPA FORMULATIONS AND DOPAMINE AGONISTS IN PARKINSON'S DISEASE

		LD DOSE EQUIVALENCY, mg	AVAILABLE STRENGTHS, mg	INITIAL DOSE	OTHER CONSIDERATIONS
CARBIDOPA/LEVODOPA (TYPICAL INITIAL STRENGTH)					
Carbidopa/levodopa IR 25/100	→	100 (anchor dose)	10/100 25/100 25/250	25/100; 0.5 tab tid	Target dose = 3–6 25/100 tabs/d
Carbidopa/levodopa CR 50/200	→	150	25/100 50/200	50/200; one tab bid to tid	Increased bioavailability with food; splitting the tablet negates the CR property
Carbidopa/levodopa/ entacapone 25/100/200	→	120	12.5/50/200, 25/100/200, 37.5/150/200,	25/100/200; one tab bid to tid	Do not split tablets
Carbidopa/levodopa/ phenylalanine (orally disintegrating tablets)	→	100	10/100/3.4, 25/100/3.4, 25/250/8		25/100/3.4 tab tid (same dosing as carbidopa/ levodopa IR) Do not take concomitantly with non-selective MAO inhibitors

				APPROXIMATE TARGET DOSES		
	DA EQUIVALENT TO LD ANCHOR DOSE ABOVE, mg[a]	AVAILABLE STRENGTHS, mg	INITIAL DOSE, mg	AS MONOTHERAPY, mg/d	AS ADJUNCTS TO LD, mg/d	OTHER CONSIDERATIONS
DOPAMINE AGONISTS						
Non-ergot alkaloids						
Ropinirole	5	0.25, 0.5, 1, 2, 3, 4, 5	0.25 tid	12–24	6–16	Hepatic metabolism; potential drug-drug interactions Occasionally associated with "sleep attacks"
Pramipexole	1	0.125, 0.25, 1, 1.5	0.125 tid	1.5–4.5	0.375–3.0	Renal metabolism; dose adjustments needed in renal insufficiency Occasionally associated with "sleep attacks"
Ergot alkaloids						
Pergolide	1	0.05, 0.25, 1.0	0.05 tid	1.5–6	0.3–3	Reports of valvular heart disease; many experts now use exclusively non-ergots; fewer reports of sleep attacks compared to non-ergots
Bromocriptine	2	2.5, 5.0	1.25 bid to tid	7.5–15	3.75–7.5	Rare reports of pulmonary and retroperitoneal fibrosis Relative incidence of sleep attacks not well studied

[a]Equivalency doses are approximations based on clinical experience and may not correlate with the relative in vitro binding properties of these compounds.

Note: LD, levodopa (with carbidopa); IR, immediate release; CR, controlled release; DA, dopamine agonist. Carbidopa/levodopa/entacapone, Stalevo.

Treatment Approach to Newly Diagnosed Idiopathic PD

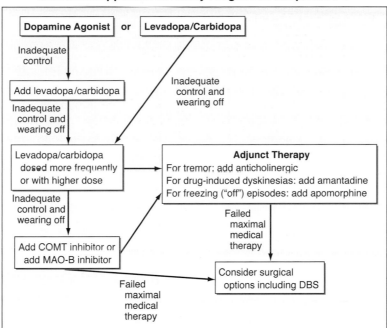

FIGURE 19-2

Treatment approach to newly diagnosed idiopathic Parkinson's disease.

DOPAMINE AGONISTS

Dopamine agonists readily cross the blood–brain barrier and act directly on postsynaptic dopamine receptors (primarily D_2 type). Compared to levodopa, they are longer acting and thus provide a more uniform stimulation of dopamine receptors. They are effective as monotherapeutic agents and as adjuncts to carbidopa/levodopa therapy. They can also be used in combination with anticholinergics and amantadine. Table 19-3 provides a guide to the doses and uses of these agents.

Available agents include two ergot alkaloids, pergolide and bromocriptine, and two non–ergot alkaloids, pramipexole and ropinirole. Apomorphine is now available for subcutaneous injection as rescue therapy to help control motor fluctuations ("off spells") in patients with moderate to advanced disease. These agents are particularly effective in treating bradykinesia and gait disturbances, but they are less effective in treating tremor. Side effects include nausea, postural hypotension, psychiatric symptoms, daytime sedation, and occasional sleep attacks. These can be managed using the above strategies and, in severe cases, through the introduction of peripheral dopamine blockers such as domperidone (not available in the United States) or short courses of trimethobenzamide or dronabinol until the symptoms subside. Patients need to be warned against the potential for sleep attacks, which can occur without warning and have resulted in traffic accidents. This phenomenon has been most often associated with agonists and less so with carbidopa/levodopa. Pergolide has recently been shown to be associated with restrictive valvular heart disease in a significant percentage of patients. This likely represents a class effect of the ergot alkaloids. Patients receiving ergot-derived dopamine agonists should either be switched to non-ergot alkaloids or undergo screening and surveillance echocardiography. When used as adjuncts to levodopa therapy these agents can aggravate dyskinesias if the doses of carbidopa/levodopa are not adjusted accordingly, and they are more expensive than carbidopa/levodopa, which is now available in generic form.

CARBIDOPA/LEVODOPA FORMULATIONS

Carbidopa/levodopa is available in regular, immediate release (IR) formulations (Sinemet, Atamet and others; 10/100 mg, 25/100 mg, and 25/250 mg), controlled release (CR) formulations (Sinemet CR 25/100 mg, 50/200 mg), and more recently as Stalevo (Table 19-3). The latter combines IR carbidopa/levodopa with 200 mg of entacapone (see below). In most individuals, at least 75 mg/d of carbidopa is necessary to block peripheral levodopa decarboxylation into dopamine and thus symptoms of nausea and orthostasis often associated with the initiation of levodopa. Initial target doses of these medications are summarized in the table. Individualized and gradual escalation of these doses is recommended. Initiation of dosing at mealtimes will reduce the incidence and severity of nausea. As patients develop tolerance to nausea and other side effects, these medications can be administered on an empty stomach, which generally leads to a more brisk and predictable absorption.

LEVODOPA AUGMENTATION

Selegiline is a selective and irreversible monoamine oxidase (MAO) B inhibitor with a weak symptomatic effect when used as monotherapy or as an adjunct to carbidopa/levodopa. Typically, selegiline is used as initial therapy or is added to alleviate tremor or levodopa-associated wearing-off. The usual dose is 5 mg with breakfast and lunch. At this dose there is no need for dietary restrictions, as is the case with non-selective and MAO-A inhibitors. A significant side effect of selegiline is insomnia. Older individuals, and those with significant cardiac abnormalities, may benefit from doses as low as 2.5 mg/d. The potential role of selegiline (or desmethylselegiline) as neuroprotective therapy remains controversial.

The catechol O-methyltransferase (COMT) inhibitors entacapone and tolcapone offer yet another strategy to augment the effects of levodopa by blocking the enzymatic degradation of levodopa and dopamine. Entacapone is preferred to tolcapone because of the low but potentially serious incidence of hepatic and hematologic side effects of the latter. When used in conjunction with carbidopa/levodopa, these agents increase the area under the curve of plasma levodopa by >30%. They alleviate wearing-off symptoms and increase by 1 to 2 h the time a patient remains "on" (i.e., well medicated) during the day. The more common side effects are gastrointestinal and hyperdopaminergic, including increased dyskinesias that may require reductions in the dose of carbidopa/levodopa. The dose of entacapone is 200 mg coadministered with each dose of carbidopa/levodopa. The dose of tolcapone is 50 to 200 mg tid.

Anticholinergics and amantadine are appropriate adjuncts to dopaminomimetic therapy. Anticholinergics are particularly useful for controlling rest tremor and dystonia, and amantadine can reduce drug-induced dyskinesias by up to 70%. The mechanisms of action of amantadine are unknown, although there is evidence it has both anticholinergic and dopaminomimetic properties. Recently amantadine has been shown to have weak glutamate antagonist properties, a mechanism thought responsible for reducing drug-induced dyskinesias. The side-effects of amantadine are nausea, headaches, edema, erythema, and livedo reticularis. In older patients, it may aggravate confusion and psychosis. Doses need to be adjusted in patients with renal failure.

Therapy of Non-Motor Symptoms

Patients with frequent nighttime awakenings due to nocturnal akinesia or tremor can be treated with supplemental doses of carbidopa/levodopa at night. A bedtime dose of dopamine agonists helps restless leg symptoms and urinary urgency. Treatment of other bladder symptoms will improve sleep for many elderly patients. Depression typically responds to antidepressants [e.g., tricyclics, selective serotonin reuptake inhibitors (SSRIs)]. The combination of SSRIs and selegiline carries an exceedingly low risk of a hyperserotonergic syndrome (delirium with myoclonus and hyperpyrexia). Electroconvulsive therapy (ECT) is highly effective in drug-refractory cases or in patients intolerant of oral antidepressants. There are several reports indicating that ECT, in addition, has short-term benefit for parkinsonian motor symptoms. Botulinum injections to the salivary glands may help patients with excessive drooling; the side effect of dry mouth may occur.

In patients with psychotic symptoms or confusion, anticholinergics and amantadine should be eliminated first. In severe cases not responding to the above approach, some dopaminomimetics may have to be reduced or eliminated. Further drug simplification and dose reductions should proceed in the following order: selegiline, nocturnal doses of dopamine agonists, Sinemet CR, daytime doses of dopamine agonists, and finally, daytime doses of carbidopa/levodopa. If the patient improves after only a modest reduction of antiparkinsonian therapy, the overall impact on the parkinsonian motor symptoms will be negligible. If in the process parkinsonian symptoms worsen, most specialists initiate treatment with an atypical antipsychotic with a low incidence of extrapyramidal side effects rather than continuing to lower dopaminomimetic therapy. Quetiapine is recommended first because, although not as well studied in PD as clozapine, it has proved to be effective in open-label studies and lacks the small risk of agranulocytosis associated with clozapine. Typical doses of quetiapine are 12.5 to 100 mg/d, and for clozapine 12.5 to 100 mg/d. Both are dosed at night to promote sleep and minimize daytime sedation and orthostasis. Other atypical antipsychotics, such as risperidone and olanzapine, are not well tolerated by most patients with PD because they are associated with dose-dependent parkinsonism. Early evidence suggests that the use of acetylcholinesterase inhibitors may be well tolerated and capable of treating hallucinations and delusions in patients with PD and dementia.

Given the complexity of the above polypharmacy, the management of non-motor symptoms is best carried out in an interdisciplinary setting, coordinated by a neurologist who specializes in PD together with a psychiatrist and the patient's primary care physician.

Neuroprotective Therapy

Reducing the progression of PD through neuroprotective or restorative therapy is a major focus of research. Epidemiologic studies suggest that the chronic use of nonsteroidal anti-inflammatory agents or the use of estrogen replacement in postmenopausal women may delay or prevent the onset of PD through yet unclear mechanisms. From a pharmacologic standpoint, current strategies involve interrupting the cascade of biochemical events that leads to death of dopaminergic cells. The first such clinical trial in PD was the large multicenter DATATOP study in which selegiline monotherapy delayed the need for levodopa therapy by 9 to 12 months in newly diagnosed patients. Most evidence indicates that this delay was due to a mild symptomatic effect of selegiline. Long-term follow-up of the DATATOP cohort revealed that patients who remained on selegiline for 7 years experienced slower motor decline compared to those who were changed to placebo after 5 years. The 7-year patient group was more likely to develop dyskinesias but less likely to develop freezing gait. Finally, the metabolite of selegiline, desmethylselegiline, has been shown in laboratory studies to have powerful neuroprotective effects,

possibly through interactions of glyceraldehyde-3-phosphate dehydrogenase (GAPDH) and other cellular protective (antiapoptotic) factors. Clinical trials to test this agent are under way.

In a recent trial, coenzyme Q_{10}, an antioxidant and a cofactor of complex I of the mitochondrial oxidative chain, appeared to delay progression of early disability in PD. Other potentially neuroprotective agents under investigation are acetyl-levo-carnitine and creatine monohydrate. A large controlled study of the antiglutamatergic agent riluzole (Chap. 21) was prematurely discontinued after a futility analysis revealed little effect on progression of symptoms.

Surgical Treatments

Over the past decade there has been a renaissance in the surgical treatment of PD and other movement disorders. Although both pallidotomy and thalmotomy were performed widely in the 1950s, the introduction of levodopa in the 1960s led to the virtual abandonment of surgery. The resurgence in the use of surgery has been motivated by the fact that after ≥5 years of treatment, many patients develop significant drug-induced motor fluctuations and dyskinesias. Second, advances in understanding of the functional organization of the basal ganglia and the pathophysiologic basis of parkinsonism have provided a clearer rationale for the effectiveness of these procedures and guidance for targeting specific structures. The demonstration, in animal models of PD, that ablation of the STN (subthalamotomy) resulted in a dramatic reduction in all of the cardinal features of parkinsonism was a critical finding.

The selection of suitable patients for surgery is most important, since in general patients with atypical Parkinson's do not have a favorable response. The major indications for surgery are (1) a diagnosis of idiopathic PD, (2) a clear response to levodopa, (3) significant intractable symptoms of PD, and/or (4) drug-induced dyskinesias and wearing-off. Contraindications to surgery include atypical forms of PD, cognitive impairment, major psychiatric illness, substantial medical comorbidities, and advanced age (a relative factor). Signs and symptoms not responding to levodopa, such as postural instability and falling, hypophonia, micrographia, drooling, and autonomic dysfunction, are unlikely to benefit from surgery. As a rule of thumb, the benefits from surgery are unlikely to exceed the benefits of antiparkinson medication. In general, the decision for surgery should be made by a movement disorder neurologist who is part of a team including a neurosurgeon trained in functional neurosurgery, a psychiatrist, a neuropsychologist, and trained technicians.

ABLATION VERSUS DEEP BRAIN STIMULATION (DBS)

The use of ablation (e.g., pallidotomy or thalamotomy) has decreased greatly since the introduction of DBS and is generally reserved for individuals who for medical or economic reasons cannot have DBS. Major advantages of DBS are that it is somewhat less invasive and more reversible than ablation, and in addition may be adjusted to best effect following implantation. Although the choice between the STN and the internal segment of the globus pallidus for DBS has shifted toward the STN, the data to support this are lacking. Several clinical trials are now under way to compare these two targets. The available evidence suggests that both are effective for all the cardinal features of PD as well as for dyskinesias and motor fluctuations. Unilateral stimulation is appropriate for patients with asymmetric disease, although bilateral surgery is generally necessary for patients with more advanced disease and for those with significant bilateral manifestations. Reductions in drug dosages appear to be easier with STN than globus pallidus procedures.

The mechanism of action of DBS remains controversial. Since clinically it appears that ablation and stimulation of a given target have a similar effect, it has been assumed that stimulation caused a functional blockade. It is likely, however, that multiple factors are involved. The basis for improvement may be the replacement of abnormal neural activity by a more tolerable pattern of activity. Following ablation or DBS, the remaining motor systems in the brainstem, thalamus, and cortex are able to compensate more effectively for the abnormal activity associated with the parkinsonian state. Whatever the mechanism, it is clear that these approaches can offer impressive results in properly selected patients.

NEUROTRANSPLANTATION AND OTHER SURGICAL APPROACHES

Despite highly encouraging open-label pilot studies of fetal cell transplantation, this approach has suffered considerable disappointment with the recent publication of the results from two large, well-controlled clinical trials. The first, using sham surgery, showed only modest benefit in patients under 60 and no benefit in those over 60. An unexpected complication in a number of patients was the development of symptomatic dyskinesias, occurring off medication. The second study has shown similar findings with regard to benefit and the development of dyskinesias. A puzzling feature of these studies is the apparent successful grafting observed by PET and autopsy. Because of these disappointing results, the considerable obstacles to obtaining sufficient fetal tissue, and opposition to the use of fetal tissue on ethical grounds, this approach is now viewed as purely investigational. It is hoped that these issues can be addressed with the development of other strategies to enhance dopaminergic cell function (e.g., carotid body cells; stem cells; encapsulated and genetically engineered cells capable of producing levodopa, dopamine, and/or trophic factors). The favorable response from direct infusion of glial cell–derived neurotrophic factor (GDNF) to the putamen in a small number of patients with PD has raised hopes that this approach, or the use of gene-transfer of trophic factors such as GDNF, will succeed. Preliminary studies in primate models of PD have been encouraging in this regard.

DEMENTIA IN PARKINSON'S DISEASE

As noted above, the incidence of dementia in PD may be as high as six times that in the general non-PD population. Approximately a quarter of patients will develop dementia of the Alzheimer type simply due to the overlap of these two common age-related disorders. Pathologically, the incidence of AD-type findings in postmortem tissue from patients dying with PD is as high as 40%. Conversely, 25% of AD patients have at least mild clinical parkinsonian features such as rigidity and bradykinesia, and ≥60% have coexistent α-synuclein pathology in the cortex. Patients with PD-dementia (PDD) typically have the akinetic/rigid form of the disorder where tremor is less prominent than in idiopathic PD. The course of PDD is more rapid and the management is more difficult than in PD due to the high incidence of cognitive side effects from antiparkinsonian therapy, particularly anticholinergics and amantadine. Central dopaminomimetic toxicity can present in many ways, ranging from sleep disruption with daytime sleepiness, personality changes, depression and mental dullness, episodic confusion, hallucinations, and disruptive behaviors. There is increasing evidence suggesting that cholinesterase inhibitors may be beneficial for patients with PDD.

DLB is an increasingly recognized form of dementia with prominent parkinsonian features. The dementia may precede or follow closely the parkinsonian syndrome. In patients presenting with parkinsonian features, the dementia is often heralded by levodopa-induced sedation, myoclonus, and hallucinations. Early on, the phenotype can be indistinguishable from PD. Features that help differentiate this entity from PD include the presence of an action rather than a rest tremor, a rapidly fading response to levodopa, and rapidly fluctuating, spontaneous, and drug-induced problems with arousal. Another feature of DLB is the higher incidence of neuropsychiatric symptoms than in idiopathic PD. These symptoms include apathy, personality changes, depression, fixed delusions, and hallucinations. Finally, patients with DLB exhibit a heightened sensitivity to drug-induced parkinsonism (DIP) when exposed to any dopamine blocker. The progression of symptoms in DLB is intermediate between the PD and PD/AD overlap. DLB is discussed in detail in Chap. 18.

OTHER PARKINSONIAN DISORDERS

PARKINSONIAN DISORDERS ASSOCIATED WITH ABNORMAL METABOLISM OF α-SYNUCLEIN (α-SYNUCLEINOPATHIES)

Multiple System Atrophy

MSA represents a sporadic group of disorders characterized by varying degrees of parkinsonism and cerebellar, corticospinal, and autonomic dysfunction. The average age of onset is 50 years (earlier than in PD), and the median survival 6 to 9 years. The clinical presentation is highly varied and may begin with any of the above clinical signs. The unifying pathologic hallmark is the presence of α-synuclein-positive inclusions located in various brain regions.

Clinical Phenotypes With disease progression, 90% percent of patients exhibit parkinsonian signs, 80% signs of autonomic failure, and a similarly high percentage exhibit upper motor neuron signs. Tremor is common but, unlike in PD, this and other parkinsonian signs are more likely to present symmetrically. Parkinsonian symptoms are typically poorly responsive to dopaminergic therapy, although some patients may respond favorably for years. Drug-induced dyskinesias typically involve the face and neck rather than the trunk and limbs, as is the case in PD. Corticospinal signs consist of spasticity, involving the legs more than the arms, and pseudobulbar palsy. This aspect of the illness may mimic primary lateral sclerosis with lower motor neurons being occasionally involved. A few patients develop myoclonus.

Signs of autonomic failure include orthostatic hypotension, leg swelling not due to drug therapy, changes in sweating patterns, and autonomic storms with diaphoresis and flushing. Orthostatic hypotension can present with dizziness, faintness, or syncope. Once patients are successfully treated for syncope, they often develop fatigue and lassitude. This is due in part to chronic tissue hypoperfusion caused by marginal blood pressures while sitting or standing. More aggressive management of the blood pressure is warranted but not always successful. Urinary symptoms include urgency, retention, and incontinence. In men impotence is one of the earliest and most prominent signs. The autonomic dysfunction can precede or follow the development of other neurologic signs by several years. Dementia may not be as frequent as in PD.

The clinical phenotype of MSA can fall into one of two broad categories, termed *MSA-p* (prominent parkinsonism at onset) and *MSA-c* (prominent cerebellar involvement at onset). Disorders that now have been reclassified as part of this new naming scheme include striatonigral degeneration (SND), olivopontocerebellar atrophy (OPCA), and progressive autonomic failure without or with parkinsonism (Shy-Drager syndrome) Patients presenting with a relatively pure form of akinetic rigid parkinsonism and a limited response to levodopa are designated as having MSA-p. The diagnosis is difficult. Individuals with other signs such as ataxia, upper motor neuron and corticobulbar involvement, myoclonus, oculomotor abnormalities, peripheral neuropathy, and deafness fit into the category of MSA-c. This phenotype is notably heterogeneous, with sporadic and hereditary forms. The sporadic forms are more likely to form part of the spectrum referred to in this section, with the hereditary forms usually representing one of the spinocerebellar ataxias (Chap. 20). Although the above categories remain clinically useful, it should be noted that as disease progresses, there tends to be more clinical and pathologic overlap than separation between these entities.

The spectrum of disease in MSA is determined by the location and density of the LB pathology. For instance, in PD the LBs are confined to neurons in the brainstem, and in DLB to the brainstem, cortex, and hippocampus. In MSA these deposits take the form of glial α-synuclein-positive intracytoplasmic inclusions in the substantia nigra, putamen, inferior olives, pontine nuclei, pigmented nuclei of the brainstem, the intermediolateral nucleus of the spinal cord, and the cerebellum. In addition in MSA there are myelin degeneration and oligodendroglia containing argyrophilic glial cytoplasmic inclusions that are immunoreactive for ubiquitin and α-synuclein. Similar inclusions can be found in neuronal cell bodies and processes.

Several diagnostic tests help differentiate MSA from PD and other parkinsonian syndromes. In MSA-c, brain MRI reveals prominent atrophy of the cerebellum, pons, and olivary eminence of the medulla. In MSA-p, prominent volume loss and T2-weighted image hyperintensity in the putamen, globus pallidus, and white matter may be present. Commercially available genetic tests are available for many of the spinocerebellar ataxias (Chap. 20) that present with features that overlap those of MSA-c.

TREATMENT

Early in the course of the illness parkinsonian features may respond to dopaminomimetic agents. These have to be used with caution due to their tendency to provoke orthostatic hypotension. Treatment of orthostatic hypotension and other autonomic symptoms is discussed in Chap. 22.

PARKINSONIAN DISORDERS ASSOCIATED WITH ABNORMALITIES OF TAU METABOLISM (TAUOPATHIES)

As in the synucleopathies, the discovery that a group of familial and sporadic disorders with pathology involving the microtubule-associated protein tau has helped classify a group of disorders characterized by atypical parkinsonism and dementia. In the less common familial forms, mutations in the *tau* gene have been linked to rare forms of parkinsonism and to frontotemporal dementia, another tauopathy discussed in Chap. 18. This discussion will focus on two entities that typically present with movement disorders. The first, PSP, has not been linked to mutations in the *tau* gene but is associated with overrepresentation of the H1 *tau* gene haplotype. These and other findings support the view that abnormal processing of tau may be directly linked to the pathogenesis of sporadic and familial tauopathies.

Progressive Supranuclear Palsy

This is a sporadic neurodegenerative disorder of unknown etiology associated with tau pathology. It presents in the sixth to seventh decades and progresses faster than PD, with death in 5 to 10 years. Risk factors include head trauma, vascular disease, dietary exposure to benzyl-tetrahydroisoquinolines (TIQ, reticuline), and beta-carbolines (reports from the West Indies).

PSP is characterized by akinetic rigid parkinsonism, dizziness, unsteadiness, slowness, falls, and pseudobulbar dysarthria. Tremor is distinctly uncommon. Supranuclear eye movement abnormalities affecting downgaze occur first, followed by variable limitations of upward and horizontal eye movement. Because the vestibular ocular reflex ("doll's eyes" maneuver) and the Bell's reflex (elevation and abduction of eyes on attempted lid closure) are intact, these abnormalities are termed *supranuclear*. Neurologic examination often reveals prominent stare and furrowed brow, axial (especially nuchal) and proximal distal limb rigidity and dystonia, as well as upper motor neuron and occasional cerebellar signs. Virtually all patients develop frontal-type cognitive dysfunction (Chap. 18), and a significant number may develop dementia with distinct subcortical features (e.g., abulia, mental inflexibility, and defects in memory retrieval). Brain MRI reveals midbrain atrophy (superior colliculus), and PET studies show symmetric frontal and striatal hypometabolism. Although some response may occur to levodopa and other antiparkinson medications, especially early in the course, treatment is generally not highly effective. The diagnosis is made on clinical grounds.

Pathologically, PSP is characterized by deposition of neurofibrillary tangles histochemically positive for tau (mostly 4-repeat tau) and negative for amyloid or α-synuclein. The deposits are associated with varying degrees of degeneration in the brainstem, basal ganglia, and cerebellum. There is loss of dopamine and dopamine receptors due to intrinsic striatal damage. This is thought to account for the poor response to therapy.

Corticobasal Degeneration (CBD)

CBD, another sporadic tauopathy, is less common and has a broader range of clinical presentations than PSP. As with most atypical forms of parkinsonism, it begins insidiously in the sixth to seventh decades with varying degrees of asymmetric progressive apraxia, rigidity, dystonia, bradykinesia, and myoclonic jerks with or without cortical sensory loss. The "alien limb" phenomenon, consisting of involuntary purposeful movements of a hand or limb, is a characteristic sign present in many cases. The disorder progresses to become bilateral over 2 to 5 years, leading to total incapacity with, ultimately, paraplegia in flexion. A significant number of cases present with frontotemporal dementia or progressive aphasia, followed by asymmetric cortical sensory signs, including abnormalities of graphesthesia and astereognosis (Chap. 18). Brain MRI reveals focal cortical loss in the contralateral superior frontal and parietal lobes with corresponding hypometabolic changes on PET scan, as well as hyperintense signal abnormalities in white matter and sometimes atrophy of the corpus callosum. Treatment is largely ineffective.

Grossly, CBD is a focal cortical degenerative process with asymmetric pathology and volume loss in the parietal and frontal regions. Most of the damage is in the dorsal peri-Rolandic, superior frontal, and superior parietal cortices, whereas cases with aphasia show abnormalities in the peri-Sylvian regions. Histologically, gliosis and swollen (ballooned) achromatic neurons and neuronal loss are present in these cortical regions as well as in the nigra, caudate, putamen, and thalamus. Recent clinicopathologic evidence indicates the syndrome can occur in the absence of basal ganglia or nigral degeneration.

SECONDARY PARKINSONISM

Drug-Induced Parkinsonism

DIP closely resembles PD except for the tremor, which is generally (but not always) less prominent. It is commonly due to neuroleptics, some atypical antipsychotics, lithium carbonate, or antiemetic agents (especially metochlopramide). Less common causes include valproic acid and, more recently, fluoxetine. DIP can be induced as well by the chronic administration of antihypertensive agents such as reserpine and alpha-methyldopa. Exposure to manganese, carbon monoxide or disulfides, cyanide, and methanol can also lead to a parkinsonian state. The severity of the parkinsonian symptoms usually correlates with the dose or exposure to a medication or toxin. If due to medication, the symptoms tend to disappear within days to weeks after stopping the offending agent but may be permanent. Patients with permanent symptoms may have been in the process of developing parkinsonism. DIP may respond to anticholinergic agents, amantadine, and levodopa.

Vascular Parkinsonism

The concept of vascular or atherosclerotic parkinsonism remains a topic of controversy. Generally, patients with vascular parkinsonism exhibit an akinetic-rigid syndrome with short mincing steps without tremor. Most have neurologic signs distinguishable from those associated with PD, including upper motor neuron signs, pseudobulbar palsy, or dementia. A poor response to levodopa therapy is characteristic. Imaging studies are heterogeneous and may reveal basal ganglia lacunes or multiple infarcts. The hypertensive and diabetic microangiopathy and diffuse white matter disease (Chap. 17) typically present with patchy, confluent or diffuse white matter in the centrum semiovale. Other causes of microangiopathy can also rarely be a cause. The premortem diagnosis of

these disorders is difficult to make with certainty, given the absence of disease markers.

TREMOR

Tremor is defined as an "approximately rhythmic and roughly sinusoidal movement of variable amplitude and frequency" (Elble and Koller). Not all tremors are abnormal; most are involuntary with occasional voluntary tremors occurring in malingerers. Individuals with conversion disorders may show partial control over their tremor symptom. Physiologic tremor is a normal high-frequency, low-amplitude tremor notable only during hyperadrenergic states. Parkinsonian rest tremor is discussed above. Cerebellar kinetic tremor is discussed in Chap. 20. Kinetic tremors can be postural, action, or both. Postural tremor is most prominent when the arms are held in front of the chest. Action or intention tremor is most notable when reaching to a target. Most tremor disorders have a predominant tremor type and a variable representation of other tremor types.

ESSENTIAL TREMOR

ET is perhaps the most common movement disorder, affecting 5 to 10 million adults and a few children in the United States. It is characterized by a 6- to 12-Hz postural and kinetic tremor affecting the arms in almost all cases (Table 19–4). In order of decreasing frequency, other body parts that can also be involved include the head (titubation), legs, the larynx (voice tremor), and the trunk. Diagnosis is made on clinical grounds. An autosomal dominant inheritance pattern is likely; thus a positive family history is very helpful, as is a history of partial response to alcohol consumption. Drugs that can aggravate any tremor include valproic acid, lithium, β-adrenergic agonists, methylxanthines, thyroxin, glucocorticoids, tricyclic antidepressants, and serotonin reuptake blockers. Withdrawal from drugs associated with tolerance, or medical conditions such as thyrotoxicosis and other enhanced adrenergic states, can amplify physiologic tremor, mimic pathologic tremors, or aggravate ET.

Compared to PD, symptoms of ET are generally bilateral from onset and the course slower. A small subset of patients has comorbid PD. ET can nonetheless be associated with significant disability, depending on amplitude of the tremor and the body region involved. Anxiety disorders are comorbid in a significant number of cases, and, as in all movement disorders, symptoms and signs worsen during emotional and physiologic stress. There is no consensus with respect to any pathology associated with ET, and diagnostic imaging of the brain is normal.

TABLE 19-4

ADVANCED EXAMINATION PEARLS: DIFFERENTIATING ESSENTIAL TREMOR FROM PARKINSONIAN TREMOR		
	ESSENTIAL TREMOR	**PARKINSONIAN TREMOR**
Speed	5–10 Hz	4–6 Hz
Symmetry	Bilateral	Usually asymmetric
Most common component	Postural	Rest
Other Parkinsonian symptoms	Absent	Present
Helped with alcohol	Usually	Rarely
Family history	Present Often	Usually absent

TREATMENT FOR ET

There is no cure for ET, but symptoms can be managed adequately with pharmacologic interventions in ~50% of cases and with surgical interventions in 80% of patients. Primidone and propranolol are the first-line treatments for ET; both have shown efficacy in double-blind, placebo-controlled studies. Primidone (50 to 750 mg/d) is often highly effective. The starting dose should be 25 mg (one-half of a 50-mg tab) at bedtime, with slowly increasing doses to minimize sedation. Propranolol (40 to 320 mg/d) is better tolerated but no more effective and is contraindicated in patients with asthma, bradycardia, and some cardiac conduction defects. Additional medications with potential efficacy (with or without the primary agents) include benzodiazepines, gabapentin, topiramate, and botulinum toxin injections to affected muscle groups. Approximately 80% of patients resistant or intolerant to pharmacotherapy respond to thalamotomy or to deep brain stimulation of the ventral intermediate nucleus of the thalamus.

HYPERKINETIC DISORDERS

Hyperkinetic movement disorders encompass a wide variety of involuntary movements, which may occur in isolation or in combination. Hyperkinesias have a wide spectrum of severity ranging from subtle restlessness to the violent movements of hemiballismus and the highly complex and emotionally laden vocal tics and coprolalia in Tourette syndrome.

HEMIBALLISMUS/HEMICHOREA

Hemiballismus, a dramatic disorder, is typically acute in onset and ranges from mild chorea to the wild flinging movements of ballism. Hemiballismus may be viewed as a large-amplitude, violent form of chorea affecting the proximal more than the distal limbs. The most common cause is a lesion of the subthalamic nucleus, most often a hypertensive lacunar stroke. Other cerebral lesions associated with hemiballismus and hemichorea include cortical, thalamic, and basal ganglia infarcts or lesions and demyelinating disease. Medical management of hemiballismus consists of supportive care to avoid injuries, exhaustion, and dehydration. The condition is difficult to treat pharmacologically but the drugs most consistently beneficial are tetrabenazine (not available in the United States), haloperidol, propranolol, phenytoin, clonazepam, and baclofen. Although hemiballismus was once thought to carry a poor prognosis, with proper treatment there is a high likelihood of survival and improvement over weeks to months. In intractable cases, pallidotomy or thalamotomy can be highly effective.

CHOREA/HUNTINGTON'S DISEASE

The term *chorea* ("dance") refers to arrhythmic involuntary, irregular movements that are typically sudden and brief and that seem to flow from one part of the body to another. There are a number of etiologies of chorea including those classified as metabolic, vascular, and genetic in origin. Huntington's disease (HD), the prototypic hereditary disorder associated with chorea, is a fatal autosomal dominant disorder characterized by progressive motor, emotional, and cognitive dysfunction. Onset is typically between the ages of 35 and 45 years (range 3 to 70). HD occurs worldwide, with a prevalence of 10 cases per 100,000. It is caused by mutations in the

Huntington's gene on the short arm of chromosome 4, specifically an expanding and unstable polyglutamine repeat (CAG) in its coding sequence. The gene encodes the highly conserved cytoplasmic protein huntingtin, which is present in all neurons.

Clinical Features

A clinical diagnosis of HD can be made readily in cases with a positive family history and an insidious onset of chorea with variable degrees of dementia and emotional symptoms. When chorea is combined with slower writhing movements or dystonic posturing, the term *choreoathetosis* is often used. Examples of other involuntary movements that may be confused with chorea include myoclonus and tics. Myoclonic jerks are lightning fast but lack the rhythmic flow of activity seen in chorea. While patients with myoclonic jerks commonly lose motor control and drop objects, this rarely happens with chorea or tics. Unlike chorea and myoclonus, motor tics can be readily suppressed voluntarily.

The clinical course of HD can last 15 to 20 years. In the early stages the chorea is focal and segmental (i.e., increased blinking, grimacing) but progresses to involve multiple body parts. The chorea typically peaks within 10 years and is gradually replaced by bradykinesia, rigidity, and dystonia. In 6 to 10% of cases HD may present with a parkinsonian syndrome rather than with chorea (Westphalt variant). The latter cases typically have an early onset (e.g., <20 years). The behavioral and cognitive disturbances characteristic of HD most often account for the brunt of the patient's disability and most of the hardship to the family. Approximately one-third develop dysthymia or an affective disorder; one-third an intermittent explosive disorder; and the remaining third substance-abuse problems, sexual dysfunction, antisocial personality traits, or schizophreniform symptoms. Depression with suicidal tendencies is not uncommon. Even the minority who may not manifest behavioral problems ultimately succumb to dementia.

The diagnosis of HD is confirmed with genetic testing, which is also helpful in the differential diagnosis of chorea of unknown etiology and in cases of atypical dementia or psychosis. Genetic testing is also used for genetic counseling in adults but is usually not necessary in symptomatic individuals if there is genetic or pathologic confirmation of HD in other family members. Other conditions important in the differential diagnosis of HD include so-called senile chorea occurring in older individuals, benign hereditary chorea in younger individuals, and neuroacanthocytosis, a progressive autosomal recessive degeneration of the basal ganglia associated with acanthocytosis of red cells in the peripheral smear and normal plasma lipoproteins. Ancillary diagnostic measures include MRI to determine if there is caudate atrophy. Other diagnostic measures may be helpful in atypical cases without a clear family history and in cases where the genetic testing results are indeterminate. These tests include PET, which typically reveals decreased striatal metabolic activity before atrophy is apparent, and neuropsychologic testing.

Pathology and Pathophysiology

The neuropathology of HD consists of widespread cerebral atrophy with prominent involvement of the striatum and cerebral cortex. Neuronal loss and gliosis are maximal in the caudate initially, with lesser involvement of the cortex and other subcortical structures. Although the mechanism of cell death in HD remains unclear, there is now experimental evidence to support the hypothesis that abnormal glutamatergic transmission with excitotoxicity of striatal cells bearing glutamate receptors plays a role.

TREATMENT FOR HD

Treatment should involve a multidisciplinary team that can provide social, medical, neuropsychiatric, and genetic guidance to patients and families throughout the course of the illness. Although dopamine blockers are moderately effective for chorea, they may aggravate bradykinesia and dystonia. Atypical antipsychotics such as clozapine, risperidone, and olanzapine are better tolerated but may not be as effective. The indications for treating chorea include interference with activities of daily living and social embarrassment.

Depression responds to conventional antidepressant therapy. The therapy needs to be monitored carefully since it can produce mania or precipitate suicide, a particularly serious problem in HD. Anxiety responds to benzodiazepines as well as to effective treatment of depression. Long-acting benzodiazepines are favored over short-acting ones because of the lesser potential for abuse and paradoxical excitation.

Psychosis can be treated with atypical neuroleptics clozapine (50 to 600 mg/d), quetiapine (100 to 600 mg/d), and risperidone (2 to 8 mg/d). These medications control dyskinesias as well as traditional neuroleptics but have fewer extrapyramidal side effects. When these drugs cannot be tolerated, smaller doses combined with tetrabenazine can be tried. There is currently no adequate treatment for the motor and cognitive decline of HD.

DYSTONIA

Clinical Features

Dystonia is a syndrome consisting of involuntary muscular contractions that result in twisting and repetitive movements and/or abnormal postures. Dystonia comprises a large and heterogeneous group of disorders. Although dystonia is one of the more common movement disorders, it is also one of the most frequently under- and misdiagnosed due to its highly variable presentations. The prevalence is not certain because of underreporting but probably exceeds 300,000 cases in the United States, a prevalence equal to that of multiple sclerosis.

Co-contraction of agonist and antagonist muscles is a fundamental feature of dystonia, distinguishing it from chorea, tics, and other dyskinesias. Also, unlike other hyperkinetic movement disorders, dystonia is characteristically present during attempted voluntary movement (so-called action dystonia). It is also associated with "overflow," the abnormal spread of activation to muscles other than those required for the intended movement. As with most movement disorders, dystonia is exacerbated by stress and fatigue. A unique feature of dystonia is that it can often be attenuated by sensory (tactile or proprioceptive) input (so-called sensory tricks). For instance, in patients with torticollis, placing a finger on the chin or the hand on the neck may reduce the twisting movements or abnormal postures. Another common feature of primary dystonia is the presence of dystonic tremor, which may appear in a form resembling essential tremor or as a succession of rapid dystonic movements.

The dystonias can be classified according to: (1) age of onset (childhood vs. adult), (2) region of the body involved, and (3) etiology. Using an etiologic scheme, similar to that used for PD, the dystonias may be divided into primary, secondary, dystonia-plus syndromes, and hereditary degenerative disorders.

PRIMARY DYSTONIA

Primary dystonia includes syndromes in which dystonia is the only clinical manifestation of the disease (other than tremor), and no pathologic changes are evident. Primary dystonia is often inherited and a number of genes have been identified. The major childhood disorder in this group is idiopathic torsion dystonia (ITD), or Oppenheim's dystonia. Sporadic adult-onset focal dystonias are the most common forms of primary dystonia.

Oppenheim's Dystonia

ITD is an autosomal dominant hereditary disorder affecting primarily Ashkenazi Jewish families (up to 90% of all cases of dystonia) but also present in non-Jewish families. The gene is located on chromosome 9q34 and results in a loss of glutamic acid in the protein Torsin A. The penetrance is about 30%. Families with ITD may exhibit either generalized or focal dystonia. The age of onset is typically in childhood for generalized and later for focal dystonia. The first signs of dystonia generally occur in the foot during walking or in the arms during voluntary movement. Dystonia later occurs at rest, leading to postural abnormalities. It usually spreads to the arm on the same side before spreading to the other side of the body. The age of onset is typically later in cases in which the symptoms begin in the arm or neck. In late-onset ITD the dystonia tends to remain focal, in contrast to early-onset forms that usually become generalized.

Focal Dystonias

The most common forms of dystonia are the focal dystonias, which present primarily in adults. These may affect (1) the eyelids, causing them to close involuntarily (*blepharospasm*); (2) the neck and shoulders (*cervical dystonia*), causing the neck to twist to the side (*torticollis*), forward (*anterocollis*), or backward (*retrocollis*); (3) the lower face and jaw or a syndrome causing the jaw to move incessantly (*oromandibular dystonia*); and (4) the larynx (*spasmodic dysphonia*), causing the voice to have a strained and discontinuous quality due to involuntary closing of the vocal cords with phonation. The combination of lower facial and jaw dystonia (*Meige's syndrome*) is not uncommon. Another type of task-specific focal dystonia affects the hand and forearm in specific activities such as handwriting (writer's cramp), typing, or playing a musical instrument (musician's cramp). Dystonia can, in fact, occur in almost any situation involving repetitive activities of the hand or other body parts. The focal dystonias are still often misdiagnosed as psychiatric or orthopedic problems.

The role of hereditary and environmental factors in adult-onset focal dystonia is not well understood. There is now mounting evidence that in some cases dystonia can develop from peripheral factors such as trauma to peripheral nerves. In addition to peripheral injury, discrete cerebral lesions, typically involving the basal ganglia but also the thalamus, cortex, or brainstem, can cause unilateral dystonia. The most frequent cause is a cerebral infarction but trauma, tumor, and other lesions may be accountable. In the case of infarction, the onset of dystonia is typically delayed by weeks to months as the associated hemiparesis clears.

SECONDARY DYSTONIAS

Secondary dystonias are largely due to drugs and other environmental factors. The drug-induced phenomena include levodopa-induced dystonia as well as acute and tardive dystonia associated with dopamine receptor blockers (see "Drug-Induced Movement Disorders," below). External factors producing dystonia include cerebral palsy (athetoid form), cerebral trauma, peripheral nerve injury, cerebral hypoxia, some infectious and postinfectious states, and toxic exposure to manganese, cyanide, and 3-nitro proprionic acid.

Dystonia-Plus Syndromes

Two types of dystonia-plus syndromes deserve mention—dopamine-responsive dystonia (DRD) and myoclonic dystonia. DRD is a dominantly inherited disorder associated with mutations in the gene for cyclohydrolase I (*GTPCH*), the rate-limiting enzyme in the synthesis of the tyrosine hydroxylase cofactor tetrahydrobiopterin. Tyrosine hydroxylase is the rate-limiting enzyme for dopamine synthesis. DRD typically presents in childhood beginning in the legs and spreading to the arms. Marked diurnal fluctuations are common. In the typical case a child aged between 4 and 8 develops a stiff-legged gait that worsens as the day progresses but improves dramatically on awakening from sleep. Some patients exhibit parkinsonism and signs of spasticity. In late-onset cases the presentation may consist of parkinsonism instead of dystonia. Patients have an excellent response to levodopa and a non-progressive course. DRD may be misdiagnosed as "athetoid" cerebral palsy, "spastic" paraplegia, or parkinsonism. Although rare, DRD is so responsive to levodopa that many feel that a trial of levodopa is warranted in all cases of dystonia.

The hereditary syndrome of myoclonic dystonia (also called hereditary dystonia with lightning jerks) is not always easily distinguished from primary dystonia or heredity essential myoclonus. It is distinguished not only by its character but also by its responsiveness to alcohol.

The hereditary degenerative diseases that may manifest dystonia typically present with more prominent parkinsonian features and include Wilson's disease, HD, PD, corticobasal degeneration (CBD), progressive supranuclear palsy (PSP), the Lubag form of dystonia-parkinsonism (DYT3), Leigh's disease, and other mitochondrial encephalopathies.

Pathophysiology

There is now considerable evidence for a loss of inhibition at multiple levels in the central nervous system (CNS), including the cortex, brainstem, and spinal cord, in patients with both generalized and focal dystonia. Dystonia appears to result primarily from dysfunction within the basal ganglia. As in PD, both ablation and DBS of the internal segment of the globus pallidus are effective in ameliorating the abnormal motor signs. Experimental studies in humans and animals have demonstrated a degradation of sensorimotor representation in the cortex, suggesting a disturbance of neuroplasticity.

TREATMENT FOR DYSTONIA

Treatment for dystonia is for the most part symptomatic except in the rare instances such as Wilson's disease or DRD, where known mechanisms are present and specific therapies are available. The available treatments include physical and emotional support, physical therapy and neurorehabilitation, drugs, and surgery including bilateral DBS. The importance of education and supportive care must be recognized. Sensory retraining in humans with focal dystonias has resulted in a substantial recovery of function in some patients. Patients with generalized dystonia benefit from a team approach in a specialized center.

Pharmacotherapy

Anticholinergic drugs are the most effective forms of treatment for generalized primary dystonia. Trihexyphenidyl is most commonly used. Doses ≥ 120 mg/d in children may be necessary, with a usual range of 20 to 50 mg/d. Adults can rarely tolerate these high doses. The limiting factors include constipation, dry mouth, blurred vision, and urinary retention as well as impaired short-term memory, confusion, and hallucinations. Benzodiazepines, including clonazepam or diazepam, are also effective for dystonia, alone or in combination with anticholinergics. Dosages are raised slowly until benefits are obtained or side effects, including sedation, ataxia, and confusion, prevent further escalation. Baclofen, a drug similar to the naturally occurring neurotransmitter γ-aminobutyric acid (GABA), is also effective for treating both focal and generalized dystonia. Relatively high doses are required (60 to 100 mg); however, side effects are often limiting. A baclofen pump for intrathecal infusion may be helpful for such cases. Dystonia involving the legs and trunk is most responsive to this form of therapy. Unfortunately, sustained benefits are not the rule and complications are not infrequent. Dopaminergic drugs are occasionally beneficial in both generalized and focal dystonias, but the most dramatic effects are seen in individuals with DRD, who experience a dramatic and sustained improvement with even a small dose of levodopa.

Paradoxically, a fair percentage of patients with generalized dystonia (and craniocervical dystonia) respond to dopaminergic antagonists, such as haloperidol or pimozide. Sometimes the combination of tetrabenazine, pimozide, and trihexyphenidyl is effective.

Botulinum Toxin

Although the focal dystonias are generally poorly responsive to drugs, they often respond dramatically to botulinum toxin injected into the affected muscle groups. Botulinum toxin can also be used in generalized dystonia for the occasional treatment of focal problems. Botulinum toxin acts by blocking the release of acetylcholine at the neuromuscular junction, resulting in dose-dependent weakness. Repeated injections are required every 2 to 5 months. Botulinum toxin serotypes A and B are now available, providing an alternative should resistance develop to either serotype.

Surgical Approaches

Prior to the introduction of botulinum toxin, peripheral denervation procedures, such as dorsal or anterior cervical rhizotomy and selective peripheral denervation, were commonly performed, primarily for the treatment of cervical dystonia. These are now performed far less frequently, generally in patients with cervical dystonia who fail botulinum toxin injections. Stereotactic surgery is used primarily for severe generalized dystonia unresponsive to other treatments. In recent years following the success in PD, pallidotomy and bilateral DBS of the pallidum are being used with promising results. The best candidates for surgery appear to be individuals with primary (DYT1) dystonia. Patients with secondary forms of dystonia are less likely to benefit. Bilateral surgery is usually necessary to obtain control of axial dystonia.

TOURETTE SYNDROME

The most common disorder characterized by tics is Tourette syndrome (TS), a neurodevelopmental disorder with neurologic and behavioral manifestations. The true prevalence of TS disorders is unknown but has been estimated at 0.05%. In addition to tics, approximately half of patients develop comorbidities, specifically obsessive-compulsive disorder (OCD) and attention-deficit hyperactivity disorder (ADHD).

Clinical Features

A *tic* is a brief, rapid, repetitive, and seemingly purposeless stereotyped action that may involve one or more muscle groups. Tics are divided into motor or vocal types, depending on the affected muscle group, and into simple and complex, depending on the number of muscle groups involved and the associated behaviors. They can range from the barely detectable and easily rationalized "nervous habits" such as blinking, twitching of the nose, and jerking of the neck, to the complex, emotionally laden, and sometimes offensive utterances of a minority of patients (*coprolalia*). Tics can be associated with brief focal sensory experiences termed *sensory tics* that commonly affect the face, head, and neck areas. Some tics may be difficult to distinguish from other fast "jerky" movements, such as chorea and myoclonus, but are unique in that they can be voluntarily inhibited for a brief period of time.

Developmentally, attentional problems develop before school and tics present during the first years of school. OCD symptoms develop later, just before or during adolescence. Tics and ADHD symptoms tend to stabilize with aging. The OCD symptoms have a more variable course.

The inheritance pattern of TS best fits the model of a major gene or genes with low penetrance, modifier genes, and a phenotype influenced by environmental factors. The risk of a family with one affected child of having another is 25%. No specific gene has been linked to TS, however. In PET studies using selective dopamine D_2-receptor ligands, alleles of this gene have been shown to modify symptom severity.

TREATMENT FOR TS

Tic symptoms have been ascribed to an overactivity of dopaminergic circuits. Accordingly dopamine blockers have consistently improved symptoms. Tics are not the most disabling feature of the illness, and treatment is generally indicated only when tics interfere with quality of life. The typical antipsychotics, fluphenazine, haloperidol, and pimozide, thought to be very effective at treating tics, have been associated with extrapyramidal symptoms and school phobias. More recently, selected atypical antipsychotics have been shown to control tic symptoms and to have a lower incidence of these complications compared to typical antipsychotics. Drugs in this category include risperidone (0.5 to 4 mg/d), olanzapine (5 to 30 mg/d), and ziprasidone (80 to 200 mg/d). Other treatments for tics include clonidine (0.1 to 0.4 mg/d or the equivalent as transdermal patch), guanifencine (0.5 to 2 mg/d), and clonazepam (0.5 to 4.0 mg/d). Botulinum toxin injections can be effective in controlling focal tics involving small muscle groups. In general, symptoms of anxiety and OCD should be treated first since their control may preclude the need to treat the tics (Chap. 41).

MYOCLONUS

Myoclonus is a rapid, brief, irregular movement that is usually multifocal. Mycoclonus can occur spontaneously or at rest, in response to sensory stimuli, or with voluntary movements. It is a symptom that occurs in a wide variety of metabolic and neurologic disorders. Posthypoxic intention myoclonus (Lance-Adams) is a special myoclonus that occurs as a sequel to cerebral anoxia. Myoclonus can result from encephalitis and prion diseases or more commonly from diverse metabolic etiologies including chronic renal failure, hepatic failure, electrolyte disturbances, or encephalopathies due to respiratory failure. Myoclonus is also a feature of certain types of epilepsy (Chap. 14). Palatal and segmental myoclonus are uncommon and caused by structural disease of the brainstem or spinal cord at the level of the abnormal movement.

DRUG-INDUCED HYPERKINETIC DISORDERS

This important group of iatrogenic and mostly reversible movement disorders is primarily associated with drugs that directly or indirectly affect central dopaminergic transmission. CNS stimulants, levodopa, dopamine agonists, and dopamine receptor blockers are the most common offending agents. The mechanism of acute and subacute movement disorders appears to result from idiosyncratic extensions of the intended action of the compound. By contrast, the mechanism of delayed or tardive dyskinesia (TD) syndromes remains more obscure.

DRUG-INDUCED MOVEMENT DISORDERS

Acute

Reactions in this category include acute dystonia in response to dopamine antagonists, which appears most frequently in a generalized form in children and in a focal form (e.g., blepharospasm, torticollis, or oromandibular dystonia) in adults. These movements can be readily treated with the parenteral administration of anticholinergics (benztropine, diphenhydramine, or antiemetics includ-

ing metoclopramide) or benzodiazepines (lorazepam or diazepam). Other acute movement disorders include dyskinesias, stereotypic behaviors, and tics after exposure to CNS stimulants such as methylphenidate, dextroamphetamine, and pemoline.

Subacute

Probably the most common of these reactions is neuroleptic-induced akathisia, a state of motor restlessness with a feeling of restlessness and a need to move, which tends to alleviate the symptoms temporarily. Therapy consists of removing the offending agent(s). When this is not possible, symptoms can be ameliorated with benzodiazepines, anticholinergics, beta blockers, and, in some cases, dopamine agonists.

Tardive

Tardive movement disorders such as TD are primarily due to chronic exposure to central dopamine blockers. The movements are most often choreatic, affecting first the mouth, lips, and tongue and later the trunk and limbs. In a fully developed case there can be head nodding, pelvic rocking, and fine movements of the fingers and toes. The diaphragm is affected rarely, producing respiratory distress. Other tardive syndromes include tardive dystonia, which generally presents with more axial than appendicular involvement; tardive akathisia; tardive tics; and even tardive tremor.

Approximately one-third of patients with TD remit within 3 months of stopping neuroleptic therapy, and in most patients the movements will gradually remit within 5 years. Patients at risk of permanent TD include the elderly, the edentulous, and those with underlying organic cerebral dysfunction. Patients with affective illnesses appear more likely to develop TD than patients with schizophrenia. Since treatment of TD is most often unsatisfactory and frustrating for both patient and physician, it is critical that typical antipsychotics be used judiciously and that, once started, their continued need be reassessed periodically. Abrupt drug cessation may result in "withdrawal dyskinesias," which presage the development of frank TD.

TREATMENT FOR DRUG-INDUCED DISORDERS

Atypical antipsychotics (clozapine, risperidone, olanzepine, quetiapine, ziprasidone, and aripiprazole) significantly lower the risk of TD compared to typical antipsychotics. Accordingly, if withdrawal of the offending antipsychotic is not possible, replacing traditional with atypical antipsychotics should be tried. Furthermore, it appears that atypical antipsychotics can successfully block the dyskinesias themselves. Elimination of stimulants and anticholinergics will also alleviate dyskinesias. In refractory cases, choreatic TD can be treated with the catecholamine depletors reserpine and tetrabenazine. Reserpine should be started at 0.125 mg/d and escalated slowly as needed up to 6 mg/d. Tetrabenazine should be started at 12.5 mg/d and gradually increased as necessary up to 200 mg/d. The elderly are less likely to tolerate the dose-dependent sedation and orthostatic hypotension associated with these drugs. Approximately 15% of patients on catecholamine depletors develop depression with chronic use of reserpine. Another strategy employs GABAergic medications such as baclofen (40 to 80 mg/d), clonazepam (1 to 8 mg/d), or valproic acid (750 to 3,000 mg/d). The latter strategy is particularly helpful in patients with tardive dystonia, which may also benefit from anticholinergic therapy and botulinum toxin injections.

Neuroleptic Malignant Syndrome (NMS)

This serious complication of neuroleptic medications occurs in 1 to 2% of treated individuals; the mortality rate may be as high as 20%. Muscle rigidity with myonecrosis; an altered mental status resembling catatonia; and autonomic dysfunction with hyperthermia, tachycardia, and a labile blood pressure constitute the principal manifestations. Symptoms typically evolve subacutely over several days and usually occur in the first few weeks following initial exposure to the drug, but can develop anytime. NMS can also be precipitated by the abrupt withdrawal of antiparkinson medications.

TREATMENT

Treatment begins with immediate cessation of the offending antipsychotic drug as well as lithium and anticholinergic agents, which appear to increase the risk of NMS. Careful monitoring of body temperature, hydration, electrolytes (especially K^+), and blood pressure are essential. Specific pharmacologic agents include dopamine agonists or levodopa, amantadine, and benzodiazepines as well as dantrolene. Supportive measures include antipyretics, cooling blankets, fluids, and measures to maintain blood pressure.

FURTHER READINGS

AHLSKOG JE: Slowing Parkinson's disease progression: Recent dopamine agonist trials. Neurology 60:381, 2003

DAWSON TM, DAWSON VL: Molecular pathways of neurodegeneration in Parkinson's disease. Science 302:819, 2003

☑ ERIKSEN JL et al: Molecular pathogenesis of Parkinson's disease. Arch Neurol 62:353, 2005

A nice review of current genetics and pathogenesis of PD.

PAHWA R, LYONS K: ESSENTIAL TREMOR: Differential diagnosis and current therapy. Am J Med 115:134, 2003

SIDEROWF A, STERN M: Update on Parkinson's disease. Ann Intern Med 138:651, 2003

☑ VAN CAMP G et al: Treatment of Parkinson's disease with pergolide and relation to restrictive valvular heart disease. Lancet 363: 1179, 2004

Established risk of valvular abnormalities with ergot-derived dopamine agonists

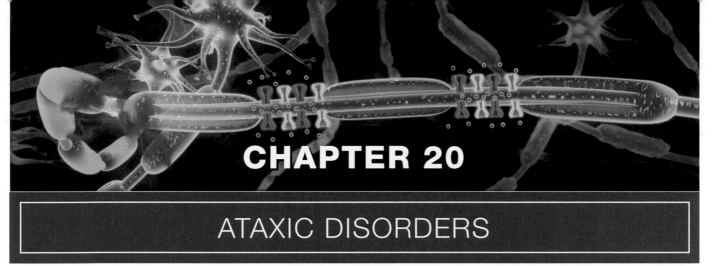

CHAPTER 20

ATAXIC DISORDERS

Roger N. Rosenberg

Symptoms and signs of ataxia consist of gait impairment, unclear ("scanning") speech, visual blurring due to nystagmus, hand incoordination, and tremor with movement. These result from the involvement of the cerebellum and its afferent and efferent pathways, including the spinocerebellar pathways, and the fronto-pontocerebellar pathway originating in the rostral frontal lobe. In the patient who presents with ataxia, the rate and pattern of the development of cerebellar symptoms help to narrow the diagnostic possibilities (**Table 20-1**). A gradual and progressive increase in symptoms with bilateral and symmetric involvement suggests a biochemical, metabolic, immune, or toxic etiology. Conversely, focal, unilateral symptoms with headache and impaired level of consciousness accompanied by ipsilateral cranial nerve palsies and contralateral weakness imply a space-occupying cerebellar lesion (**Table 20-2**).

SYMMETRIC ATAXIA

Progressive and symmetric ataxia can be classified with respect to onset as acute (over hours or days), subacute (weeks or months), or chronic (months to years). Acute and reversible ataxias include those caused by intoxication with alcohol, phenytoin, lithium, barbiturates, and other drugs. Intoxication caused by toluene exposure, gasoline sniffing, glue sniffing, spray painting, or exposure to methyl mercury or bismuth are additional causes of acute or subacute ataxia, as is treatment with cytotoxic chemotherapeutic drugs such as fluorouracil and paclitaxel. Patients with a postinfectious syndrome (especially after varicella) may develop gait ataxia and mild dysarthria, both of which are reversible (Chap. 28). Rare infectious causes of acquired ataxia include poliovirus, coxsackievirus, echovirus, Epstein-Barr virus, toxoplasmosis, *Legionella,* and Lyme disease.

The subacute development of ataxia of gait over weeks to months (degeneration of the cerebellar vermis) may be due to the combined effects of alcoholism and malnutrition, particularly with deficiencies of vitamins B_1 and B_{12}. Hyponatremia has also been associated with ataxia. Paraneoplastic cerebellar ataxia is associated with a number of different tumors (and autoantibodies) such as breast and ovarian cancers (anti-Yo), small-cell lung cancer (anti-PQ type voltage-gated calcium channel), and Hodgkin's disease (anti-Tr) (Chap. 27). Another paraneoplastic syndrome associated with myoclonus and opsoclonus occurs with breast (anti-Ri) and lung cancers and neuroblastoma. For all of these paraneoplastic ataxias, the neurologic syndrome may be the presenting symptom of the cancer. Another immune-mediated progressive ataxia is associated with anti-gliadin (and anti-endomysium) antibodies and the HLA DQB1*0201 haplotype; in some affected patients, biopsy of the small intestine reveals villous atrophy consistent with gluten-sensitive enteropathy. Finally, subacute progressive ataxia may be caused by a prion disorder, especially when an infectious etiology, such as transmission from contaminated human growth hormone, is responsible (Chap. 32).

Chronic symmetric gait ataxia suggests an inherited ataxia (discussed below), a metabolic disorder, or a chronic infection. Hypothyroidism must always be considered as a readily treatable and reversible form of gait ataxia. Infectious diseases that can present with ataxia are meningovascular syphilis and tabes dorsalis due to degeneration of the posterior columns and spinocerebellar pathways in the spinal cord.

TABLE 20-1

ACQUIRED CEREBELLAR ATAXIAS

ETIOLOGY	TESTS TO CONSIDER
Acute onset (hours to days)	
Cerebellar infarction	MRI of brain
Cerebellar hemorrhage or subdural hematoma	CT or MRI of brain
Migraine (mainly children)	
Medication effects (especially anticonvulsants, lithium, barbiturates)	
Postinfectious cerebellitis, especially following varicella	
Viral infections (including HIV, PML, rubella, SSPE)	JC virus PCR in CSF for PML
Miller-Fisher syndrome	anti-GQ1b Ab
Subacute (days to weeks)	
Cerebellar tumor	CT w/contrast or MRI
Cerebellar abscess	CT w/contrast or MRI
Multiple sclerosis	MRI brain
Encephalomyelitis	MRI brain
Hydrocephalus	CT of Brain
Toxins (solvents such as toluene, glue sniffing)	
Bacterial infections (Whipple's, Lyme, *Mycoplasma, Legionella*)	LP and culture or PCR, small bowel bx for Whipple's
Mycobacterial infections	LP and culture
Vitamin deficiencies (vitamin E especially, also B_{12} and B_1)	Vitamin levels
Chronic (months to years)	
Alcoholic cerebellar degeneration	
Paraneoplastic (including anti-Yo, anti-Ri, anti-Gad especially)	LP for Ab titers
Hypothyroidism	TSH
Prion disease including CJD, GSS	Brain biopsy
Wilson's disease	Ceruloplasmin, 24-h urinary copper, liver biopsy, ophthalmologic examination
Heavy metal poisoning (especially thallium, mercury, lead)	Serum levels
Ataxia associated with anti-gliadin antibodies	Anti-gliadin Abs

Abbreviations: Ab, antibody; CJD, Creutzfeldt-Jakob disease; CSF, cerebrospinal fluid; CT, computed tomography; GSS, Gerstmann-Sträussler-Scheinker (disease); LP, lumbar puncture; MRI, magnetic resonance imaging; PCR, polymerase chain reaction; PML, progressive multifocal leukoencephalopathy; SSPE, subacute sclerosing panencephalitis; TSH, thyroid-stimulating hormone.

FOCAL ATAXIA

Acute focal ataxia commonly results from cerebrovascular disease, usually ischemic infarction, or cerebellar hemorrhage. These lesions typically produce cerebellar symptoms ipsilateral to the injured cerebellum and may be associated with an impaired level of consciousness due to brainstem compression and increased intracranial pressure; ipsilateral pontine signs, including sixth and seventh nerve palsies, may be present. Focal and worsening signs of acute ataxia should also prompt consideration of a posterior fossa subdural hematoma, bacterial abscess, or primary or metastatic cerebellar tumor. Computed tomography (CT) or magnetic resonance imaging (MRI) studies will reveal clinically significant processes of this type. Many of these lesions represent true neurologic emergencies, as sudden herniation, either rostrally through the tentorium or caudal herniation of cerebellar tonsils through the foramen magnum, can occur and is usually devastating. Acute surgical decompression may be required (Chap. 15). Lymphoma or progressive multifocal leukoencephalopathy (PML) in a patient with AIDS may present with an acute or subacute focal

TABLE 20-2

GENOTYPE CLASSIFICATION OF THE SPINOCEREBELLAR ATAXIAS

NAME	LOCUS	PHENOTYPE
SCA 1 (autosomal dominant type 1)	6p22-p23 with CAG repeats (exonic) Ataxin-1	Ataxia with ophthalmoparesis, pyramidal and extrapyramidal findings
SCA2 (autosomal dominant type 2)	12q23-q24.1 with CAG repeats (exonic)	Ataxia with slow saccades and minimal pyramidal and extrapyramidal findings
Machado-Joseph disease/SCA3 (autosomal dominant type 3)	Ataxin-2 14q24.3-q32 with CAG repeats (exonic) MJD-ataxin-3	Ataxia with opthalmoparesis and variable pyramidal, extrapyramidal, and amyotrophic signs
SCA4 (autosomal dominant type 4)	16q24-ter	Ataxia with normal eye movements, sensory axonal neuropathy, and pyramidal signs
SCA5 (autosomal dominant type 5)	Centromeric region of chromosome II	Ataxia and dysarthria
SCA6 (autosomal dominant type 6)	19p13.2 with CAG repeats in α_{1A}-voltage—dependent calcium channel gene (exonic)	Ataxia and dysarthria, nystagmus, mild proprioceptive sensory loss
SCA7 (autosomal dominant type 7)	3p14.1-p21.1 with CAG repeats (exonic) Ataxin-7	Ophthalmoparesis, visual loss, ataxia, dysarthria, extensor plantar response, pigmentary retinal degeneration
SCA8 (autosomal dominant type 8)	13q21 with CTG repeats; noncoding	Gait ataxia, dysarthria, nystagmus, leg spasticity, and reduced vibratory sensation
SCA10 (autosomal dominant type 10)	22q; ATTCT repeat; noncoding	Gait ataxia, dysarthria, nystagmus; partial complex and generalized motor seizures; polyneuropathy
SCA11 (autosomal dominant type 11)	15q14-q21.3 by linkage	Slowly progressive gait and extremity ataxia, dysarthria, vertical nystagmus, hyperreflexia
SCA12 (autosomal dominant type 12)	5q31-q33 by linkage; CAG repeat; protein phosphatase 2A	Tremor, decreased movement, increased reflexes, dystonia, ataxia, dysautonomia, dementia, dysarthria
SCA13 (autosomal dominant type 13)	19q13.3-q14.4	Mutation unknown
SCA14 (autosomal dominant type 14)	19q-13.4	Mutation unknown
SCA15 (autosomal dominant type 15)	Mutation unknown in 1 family; other known loci were excluded	Gait and extremity ataxia, dysarthria
SCA16 (autosomal dominant type 16)	8q22.1-24.1	Mutation unknown; pure cerebellar ataxia and head tremor, gait ataxia, and dysarthria; horizontal gaze-evoked nystagmus
SCA17 (autosomal dominant type 17)	6q27; CAG expansion in the TATA-binding protein (TBP) gene	Gait ataxia, dementia, parkinsonism, dystonia, chorea, seizures; MRI shows cerebral and cerebellar atrophy
SCA18 (autosomal dominant type 18)	7q22-q32	Ataxia, motor/sensory neuropathy
SCA19 (autosomal dominant type 19)	1p21-q21	Ataxia, tremor, cognitive impairment, myoclonus
SCA20 (autosomal dominant type 20)	Chromosome 11	Dysarthria as initial sign; dentate nucleus calcifications seen as low signal on MRI
SCA21 (autosomal dominant type 21)	7p21.3-p15.1	Ataxia, extrapyramidal features of akinesia, rigidity, tremor, cognitive defect
SCA23 (autosomal dominant type 23)	20p13-p12.3	Slowly progressive isolated SCA with gait and speech problems prominent
Dentatorubropallidoluysian atrophy (autosomal dominant)	12p12-ter with CAG repeats (exonic) Atrophin	Ataxia, choreoathetosis, dystonia, seizures, myoclonus, dementia
Friedreich's ataxia (autosomal recessive)	9q13-q21.1 with intronic GAA repeats Frataxin	Ataxia, areflexia, extensor plantar responses, position sense deficits, cardiomyopathy, diabetes mellitus, scoliosis, foot deformities; defective iron transport from mitochondria

(Continued)

TABLE 20-2 *(Continued)*

NAME	LOCUS	PHENOTYPE
Friedreich's ataxia (autosomal recessive)	8q13.1-q13.3; (α-TTP deficiency)	Same as phenotype that maps to 9q but associated with vitamin E deficiency
Autosomal recessive spastic ataxia of Charlevoix-Saguenay (ARSACS)	Chromosome 13; SACS gene; loss of Sacsin peptide activity	Childhood onset of ataxia, spasticity, dysarthria, distal muscle wasting, foot deformity, retinal striations, mitral valve prolapse
Kearns-Sayre syndrome (sporadic)	mtDNA deletion and duplication mutations	Ptosis, ophthalmoplegia, pigmentary retinal degeneration, cardiomyopathy, diabetes mellitus, deafness, heart block, increased CSF protein, ataxia
Myoclonic epilepsy and ragged red fiber syndrome (MERRF) (maternal inheritance)	Mutation in mtDNA of the tRNA^{lys} at 8344; also mutation at 8356	Myoclonic epilepsy, ragged red fiber myopathy, ataxia
Mitochondrial encephalopathy, lactic acidosis, and stroke syndrome (MELAS) (maternal inheritance)	tRNA^{leu} mutation at 3243; also at 3271 and 3252	Headache, stroke, lactic acidosis, ataxia
Leigh's disease; subacute necrotizing encephalopathy (maternal inheritance or autosomal recessive)	mtDNA complex V defect (ATPase gene at 8993) or mitochondrial protein synthesis defect (both maternally inherited); or complex IV defect (autosomal recessive)	Obtundation, hypotonia, cranial nerve defects, respiratory failure, hyperintense signals on T2-weighted MRI in basal ganglia, cerebellum, or brainstem; ataxia
Episodic ataxia, type 1 (EA-1) (autosomal dominant)	12p; potassium channel gene, *KCNA1*	Episodic ataxia for minutes; provoked by startle or exercise; with facial and hand myokymia; cerebellar signs are not progressive; responds to phenytoin
Episodic ataxia, type 2 (EA-2) (autosomal dominant)	19p-13(*CACNA1A*) (allelic with SCA6) (α_{1A}-voltage—dependent calcium channel subunit)	Episodic ataxia for days; provoked by stress, fatigue; with down-gaze nystagmus; cerebellar atrophy results; progressive cerebellar signs; responds to acetazolamide
Ataxia telangiectasia (autosomal recessive)	11q22-23; *ATM* gene for regulation of cell cycle; mitogenic signal transduction and meiotic recombination	Telangiectasia, ataxia, dysarthria, pulmonary infections, neoplasms of lymphatic system; IgA and IgG deficiencies; diabetes mellitus, breast cancer
Infantile-onset spinocerebellar ataxia of Nikali et al. (autosomal recessive)	10q23.3-q24.1	Infantile ataxia, sensory neuropathy; athetosis, hearing deficit, ophthalmoplegia, optic atrophy; primary hypogonadism in females
Hypocoeruloplasminemia with ataxia and dysarthria (autosomal recessive)	Coeruloplasmin gene; 3q23-q25 (trp 858 ter)	Gait ataxia and dysarthria; hyperreflexia; cerebellar atrophy by MRI; iron deposition in cerebellum, basal ganglia, thalamus, and liver; onset in the 4th decade
Spinocerebellar ataxia with neuropathy (SCAN1) (autosomal recessive)	Tryosyl-DNA phosphodiesterase-1 (TDP-1) 14q31-q32	Onset in 2d decade; gait ataxia, dysarthria, seizures, cerebellar vermis atrophy on MRI, dysmetria

Abbreviations: MRI, magnetic resonance imaging; CSF, cerebrospinal fluid.

cerebellar syndrome. Chronic etiologies of progressive ataxia include multiple sclerosis (Chap. 28) and congenital lesions such as a Chiari malformation (Chap. 24) or a congenital cyst of the posterior fossa (Dandy–Walker syndrome).

THE INHERITED ATAXIAS

These may show autosomal dominant, autosomal recessive, or maternal (mitochondrial) modes of inheritance. A genomic classification has now largely superseded previous ones based on clinical expression alone.

Although the clinical manifestations and neuropathologic findings of cerebellar disease dominate the clinical picture, there may also be characteristic changes in the basal ganglia, brainstem, spinal cord, optic nerves, retina, and peripheral nerves. In large families with dominantly inherited ataxias, many gradations are observed from purely cerebellar manifestations to mixed cerebellar and brainstem disorders, cerebellar and basal ganglia syndromes, and spinal cord or peripheral nerve disease. Rarely, dementia is present as well. The clinical picture may be homogeneous within a family with dominantly inherited ataxia, but sometimes most affected family members show one characteristic syndrome, while one or several members have an entirely different phenotype.

AUTOSOMAL DOMINANT ATAXIAS

The autosomal spinocerebellar ataxias (SCAs) include SCA types 1 through 23, dentatorubropallidoluysian atrophy (DRPLA), and episodic ataxia (EA) types 1 and 2. SCA1, SCA2, SCA3 [Machado-Joseph disease (MJD)], SCA6, SCA7, and SCA17 are caused by CAG triplet repeat expansions in different genes. The clinical phenotypes of these SCAs overlap. The genotype has become the "gold standard" for diagnosis and classification. CAG encodes glutamine, and these expanded CAG triplet repeat expansions result in expanded polyglutamine proteins, termed *ataxins,* that produce a toxic gain of function with autosomal dominant inheritance.

SCA1

███ **Symptoms and Signs** SCA1 (previously referred to as *olivopontocerebellar atrophy*) is characterized by the development in early or middle adult life of progressive cerebellar ataxia of the trunk and limbs, impairment of equilibrium and gait, slowness of voluntary movements, scanning speech, nystagmoid eye movements, and oscillatory tremor of the head and trunk. Dysarthria, dysphagia, and oculomotor and facial palsies may also occur. Extrapyramidal symptoms include rigidity, an immobile face, and parkinsonian tremor. The reflexes are usually normal, but knee and ankle jerks may be lost, and extensor plantar responses may occur. Dementia may be noted but is usually mild. Impairment of sphincter function is common, with urinary and sometimes fecal incontinence. Cerebellar and brainstem atrophy are evident on MRI (**Fig. 20-1**).

Marked shrinkage of the ventral half of the pons, disappearance of the olivary eminence on the ventral surface of the medulla, and atrophy of the cerebellum are the pathologic hallmarks of this condition. Variable loss of Purkinje cells, reduced numbers of cells in the molecular and granular layer, demyelination of the middle

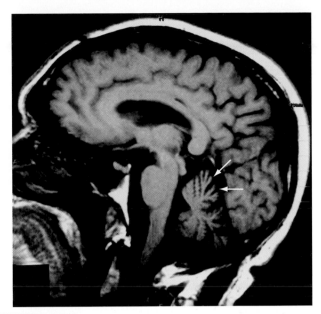

FIGURE 20-1

Sagittal MRI of the brain of a 60-year-old man with gait ataxia and dysarthria due to SCA1, illustrating cerebellar atrophy (*arrows*).

cerebellar peduncle and the cerebellar hemispheres, and severe loss of cells in the pontine nuclei and olives are found on histologic examination. Degenerative changes in the striatum, especially the putamen, and loss of the pigmented cells of the substantia nigra may be found in cases with extrapyramidal features. More widespread degeneration in the central nervous system (CNS), including involvement of the posterior columns and the spinocerebellar fibers, is often present.

SCA1 encodes a gene product, called ataxin-1, which is a novel protein of unknown function. The mutant allele has 40 CAG repeats located within the coding region, whereas alleles from unaffected individuals have ≤36 repeats.

SCA2

███ **Symptoms and Signs** Another clinical phenotype, SCA2, has been described in Cubans. These patients probably are descendants of a common ancestor, and the population may be the largest homogeneous group of patients with ataxia yet described. The age of onset ranges from 2 to 65 years, and there is considerable clinical variability within families. Although neuropathologic and clinical findings are compatible with a diagnosis of SCA1, including slow saccadic eye movements, ataxia, dysarthria, parkinsonian rigidity, optic disk pallor, mild spasticity, and retinal degeneration, SCA2 is a unique form of cerebellar degenerative disease.

The gene in SCA2 families also contains the CAG repeat expansions coding for a polyglutamine-containing protein, ataxin-2. Normal alleles contain 15 to 32 repeats; mutant alleles have 35 to 77 repeats.

Machado-Joseph Disease/SCA3

MJD was first described among the Portuguese and their descendants in New England and California. Subsequently, MJD has been found in families from Portugal, Australia, Brazil, Canada, China, England, France, India, Israel, Italy, Japan, Spain, Taiwan, and the United States. In most populations, it is the most common autosomal dominant ataxia.

■■■ **Symptoms and Signs** MJD has been classified into three clinical types. In type I MJD (amyotrophic lateral sclerosis–parkinsonism–dystonia type), neurologic deficits appear in the first two decades and involve weakness and spasticity of extremities, especially the legs, often with dystonia of the face, neck, trunk, and extremities. Patellar and ankle clonus are common, as are extensor plantar responses. The gait is slow and stiff, with a slightly broadened base and lurching from side to side; this gait results from spasticity, not true ataxia. There is no truncal titubation. Pharyngeal weakness and spasticity cause difficulty with speech and swallowing. Of note is the prominence of horizontal and vertical nystagmus, loss of fast saccadic eye movements, hypermetric and hypometric saccades, and impairment of upward vertical gaze. Facial fasciculations, facial myokymia, lingual fasciculations without atrophy, ophthalmoparesis, and ocular prominence are common early manifestations.

In type II MJD (ataxic type), true cerebellar deficits of dysarthria and gait and extremity ataxia begin in the second to fourth decades along with corticospinal and extrapyramidal deficits of spasticity, rigidity, and dystonia. Type II is the most common form of MJD. Ophthalmoparesis, upward vertical gaze deficits, and facial and lingual fasciculations are also present. Type II MJD can be distinguished from the clinically similar disorders SCA1 and SCA2.

Type III MJD (ataxic-amyotrophic type) presents in the fifth to the seventh decades with a pancerebellar disorder that includes dysarthria and gait and extremity ataxia. Distal sensory loss involving pain, touch, vibration, and position senses and distal atrophy are prominent, indicating the presence of peripheral neuropathy. The deep tendon reflexes are depressed to absent, and there are no corticospinal or extrapyramidal findings.

The mean age of onset of symptoms in MJD is 25 years. Neurologic deficits invariably progress and lead to death from debilitation within 15 years of onset, especially in patients with types I and II disease. Usually, patients retain full intellectual function.

The major pathologic findings are variable loss of neurons and glial replacement in the corpus striatum and severe loss of neurons in the pars compacta of the substantia nigra. A moderate loss of neurons occurs in the dentate nucleus of the cerebellum and in the red nucleus. Purkinje cell loss and granule cell loss occur in the cerebellar cortex. Cell loss also occurs in the dentate nucleus and in the cranial nerve motor nuclei. Sparing of the inferior olives distinguishes MJD from other dominantly inherited ataxias.

The gene for MJD maps to 14q24.3-q32. Unstable CAG repeat expansions are present in the MJD gene coding for a polyglutamine-containing protein named ataxin-3, or MJD-ataxin. An earlier age of onset is associated with longer repeats.

SCA6

Genomic screening for CAG repeats in other families with autosomal dominant ataxia and vibratory and proprioceptive sensory loss have yielded another locus. Of interest is that different mutations in the same gene for the α_{1A} voltage-dependent calcium channel subunit (CACNLIA4; also referred to as the *CACNA1A* gene) at 19p13 result in different clinical disorders. CAG repeat expansions (21 to 27 in patients; 4 to 16 triplets in normal individuals) result in late-onset progressive ataxia with cerebellar degeneration. Missense mutations in this gene result in familial hemiplegic migraine. Nonsense mutations resulting in termination of protein synthesis of the gene product yield hereditary paroxysmal cerebellar ataxia or EA. Some patients with familial hemiplegic migraine develop progressive ataxia and also have cerebellar atrophy.

Dentatorubropallidoluysian Atrophy

DRPLA has a variable presentation that may include progressive ataxia, choreoathetosis, dystonia, seizures, myoclonus, and dementia. DRPLA is due to unstable CAG triplet repeats in the open reading frame of a gene named *atrophin* located on chromosome 12p12-ter. Larger expansions are found in patients with earlier onset. The number of repeats is 49 in patients with DRPLA and ≤ 26 in normal individuals. Anticipation occurs in successive generations, with earlier onset of disease in association with an increasing CAG repeat number in children who inherit the disease from their father.

AUTOSOMAL RECESSIVE ATAXIAS

Friedreich's Ataxia

This is the most common form of inherited ataxia, comprising one-half of all hereditary ataxias. It can occur in a classic form or in association with a genetically determined vitamin E deficiency syndrome; the two forms are clinically indistinguishable.

Symptoms and Signs Friedreich's ataxia presents before 25 years of age with progressive staggering gait, frequent falling, and titubation. The lower extremities are more severely involved than the upper ones. Dysarthria occasionally is the presenting symptom; rarely, progressive scoliosis, foot deformity, nystagmus, or cardiopathy is the initial sign.

The neurologic examination reveals nystagmus, loss of fast saccadic eye movements, truncal titubation, dysarthria, dysmetria, and ataxia of trunk and limb movements. Extensor plantar responses (with normal tone in trunk and extremities), absence of deep tendon reflexes, and weakness (greater distally than proximally) are usually found. Loss of vibratory and proprioceptive sensation occurs. The median age of death is 35 years. Women have a significantly better prognosis than men.

Cardiac involvement occurs in 90% of patients. Cardiomegaly, symmetric hypertrophy, murmurs, and conduction defects are reported. Moderate mental retardation or psychiatric syndromes are present in a small percentage of patients. A high incidence of diabetes mellitus (20%) is found and is associated with insulin resistance and pancreatic β-cell dysfunction. Musculoskeletal deformities are common and include pes cavus, pes equinovarus, and scoliosis. MRI of the spinal cord shows atrophy (**Fig. 20-2**).

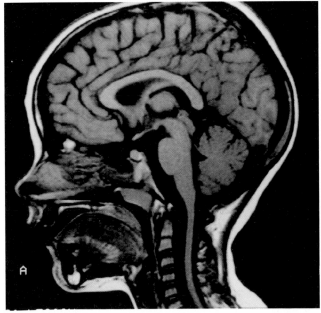

FIGURE 20-2
Sagittal MRI of the brain and spinal cord of a patient with Friedreich's ataxia, demonstrating spinal cord atrophy.

The primary sites of pathology are the spinal cord, dorsal root ganglion cells, and the peripheral nerves. Slight atrophy of the cerebellum and cerebral gyri may occur. Sclerosis and degeneration occur predominantly in the spinocerebellar tracts, lateral corticospinal tracts, and posterior columns. Degeneration of the glossopharyngeal, vagus, hypoglossal, and deep cerebellar nuclei is described. The cerebral cortex is histologically normal except for loss of Betz cells in the precentral gyri. The peripheral nerves are extensively involved, with a loss of large myelinated fibers. Cardiac pathology consists of myocytic hypertrophy and fibrosis, focal vascular fibromuscular dysplasia with subintimal or medial deposition of periodic acid–Schiff (PAS)–positive material, myocytopathy with unusual pleomorphic nuclei, and focal degeneration of nerves and cardiac ganglia.

The classic form of Friedreich's ataxia has been mapped to 9q13-q21.1, and the mutant gene, *frataxin,* contains expanded GAA triplet repeats in the first intron. There is homozygosity for expanded GAA repeats in >95% of patients. Normal persons have 7 to 22 GAA repeats, and patients have 200 to 900 GAA repeats. A more varied clinical syndrome has been described in compound heterozygotes who have one copy of the GAA expansion and the other copy a point mutation in the *frataxin* gene. When the point mutation is located in the region of the gene that encodes the amino-terminal half of frataxin, the phenotype is milder, often consisting of a spastic gait, retained or exaggerated reflexes, no dysarthria, and mild or absent ataxia.

Patients with Friedreich's ataxia have undetectable or extremely low levels of *frataxin* mRNA, as compared with carriers and unrelated individuals; thus, disease appears to be caused by a loss of expression of the frataxin protein. Frataxin is a mitochondrial protein involved in iron homeostasis. Mitochondrial iron accumulation due to loss of the iron transporter coded by the mutant *frataxin* gene results in oxidized intramitochondrial iron. Excess oxidized iron results in turn in the oxidation of cellular components and irreversible cell injury.

Ataxia Telangiectasia

Symptoms and Signs Patients with ataxia telangiectasia (AT) present in the first decade of life with progressive telangiectatic lesions associated with deficits in cerebellar function and nystagmus. The neurologic manifestations correspond to those in Friedreich's disease, which should be included in the differential diagnosis. Truncal and limb ataxia, dysarthria, extensor plantar responses, myoclonic jerks, areflexia, and distal sensory deficits may develop. There is a high incidence of recurrent pulmonary infections and neoplasms of the lymphatic and reticuloendothelial system in patients with AT. Thymic hypoplasia with cellular and humoral (IgA and IgG2) immunodeficiencies, premature aging, and endocrine disorders such as type 1 diabetes mellitus are described. There is an increased incidence of lymphomas, Hodgkin's disease, acute leukemias of the T cell type, and breast cancer.

The most striking neuropathologic changes include loss of Purkinje, granule, and basket cells in the cerebellar cortex as well as of neurons in the deep cerebellar nuclei. The inferior olives of the medulla may also have neuronal loss. There is a loss of anterior horn neurons in the spinal cord and of dorsal root ganglion cells associated with posterior column spinal cord demyelination. A poorly developed or absent thymus gland is the most consistent defect of the lymphoid system.

The gene for AT (the *ATM* gene) encodes a protein that is similar to several yeast and mammalian phosphatidylinositol-3'-kinases involved in mitogenic signal transduction, meiotic recombination, and cell cycle control. Defective DNA repair in AT fibroblasts exposed to ultraviolet light has been demonstrated. The discovery of *ATM* will make possible the identification of heterozygotes who are at risk for cancer (e.g., breast cancer) and permit early diagnosis.

Mitochondrial Ataxias

Spinocerebellar syndromes have been identified with mutations in mitochondrial DNA (mtDNA). Thirty pathogenic mtDNA point mutations and 60 different types of mtDNA deletions are known, several of which cause or are associated with ataxia (Chap. 39).

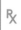

TREATMENT FOR ATAXIA

The most important goal in management of patients with ataxia is to identify treatable disease entities. Mass lesions must be recognized promptly and treated appropriately. Paraneoplastic disorders can often be identified by the clinical patterns of disease that they produce, measurement of specific autoantibodies, and uncovering the primary cancer; these disorders are often refractory to therapy, but some patients improve following removal of the tumor or immunotherapy (Chap. 27). Ataxia with anti-gliadin antibodies and gluten-sensitive enteropathy may improve with a gluten-free diet. Malabsorption syndromes leading to vitamin E deficiency may lead to ataxia. The vitamin E deficiency form of Friedreich's ataxia must be consid-

ered, and serum vitamin E levels measured. Vitamin E therapy is indicated for these rare patients. Vitamin B_1 and B_{12} levels in serum should be measured, and the vitamins administered to patients having deficient levels. Hypothyroidism is easily treated. The cerebrospinal fluid should be tested for a syphilitic infection in patients with progressive ataxia and other features of tabes dorsalis. Similarly, antibody titers for Lyme disease and *Legionella* should be measured, and appropriate antibiotic therapy should be instituted in antibody-positive patients. Aminoacidopathies, leukodystrophies, urea-cycle abnormalities, and mitochondrial encephalomyopathies may produce ataxia, and some dietary or metabolic therapies are available for these disorders. The deleterious effects of diphenylhydantoin and alcohol on the cerebellum are well known, and these exposures should be avoided in patients with ataxia of any cause.

There is no proven therapy for any of the autosomal dominant ataxias. There is preliminary evidence that idebenone, a free-radical scavenger, can improve myocardial hypertrophy in patients with classic Friedreich ataxia; there is no current evidence, however, that it improves neurologic function. Iron chelators and antioxidant drugs are potentially harmful in Friedreich's patients as they may increase heart muscle injury. Acetazolamide can reduce the duration of symptoms of episodic ataxia. At present, identification of an at-risk person's genotype, together with appropriate family and genetic counseling, can reduce the incidence of these cerebellar syndromes in future generations.

FURTHER READINGS

HADJIVASSILIOU M et al: Gluten ataxia in perspective: Epidemiology, genetic susceptibility and clinical characteristics. Brain 136:685, 2003

LYNCH DR et al: Friedreich ataxia: Effects of genetic understanding on clinical evaluation and therapy. Arch Neurol 59:743, 2002

☑ ROSENBERG RN, PAULSON HL: The inherited ataxias, in *The Molecular and Genetic Basis of Neurologic and Psychiatric Disease*, 3rd ed, RN Rosenberg et al (eds). Philadelphia, Elsevier Science, and Boston, Butterworth-Heinemann, 2003

A complete list and description of all of the known inherited ataxias.

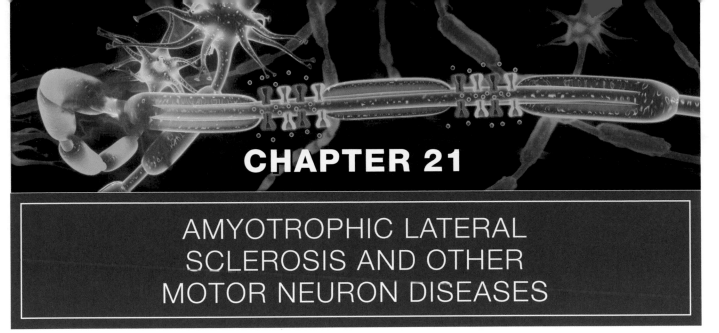

CHAPTER 21

AMYOTROPHIC LATERAL SCLEROSIS AND OTHER MOTOR NEURON DISEASES

Robert H. Brown, Jr.

AMYOTROPHIC LATERAL SCLEROSIS

Amyotrophic lateral sclerosis (ALS) is the most common progressive motor neuron disease. It is a prime example of a neurodegenerative disease and is arguably the most devastating of the neurodegenerative disorders.

Pathology

The pathologic hallmark of motor neuron disorders is death of lower motor neurons (consisting of anterior horn cells in the spinal cord and their brainstem homologues innervating bulbar muscles) and upper, or corticospinal, motor neurons (originating in layer five of the motor cortex and descending via the pyramidal tract to synapse with lower motor neurons, either directly or indirectly via interneurons) (**Fig. 21-1**). Although at its onset ALS may involve selective loss of function of only upper or lower motor neurons, it ultimately causes progressive loss of both types. Indeed, in the absence of clear involvement of both upper and lower motor neurons, the diagnosis of ALS is questionable.

Other motor neuron diseases involve only particular subsets of motor neurons (**Table 21-1**). Thus, in bulbar palsy and spinal muscular atrophy (SMA; also called progressive muscular atrophy), the lower motor neurons of brainstem and spinal cord, respectively, are most severely involved. By contrast, pseudobulbar palsy and primary lateral sclerosis (PLS) affect only upper motor neurons innervating the brainstem and spinal cord.

In each of these diseases, the affected motor neurons undergo shrinkage, often with accumulation of the pigmented lipid (lipofuscin) that normally develops in these cells with advancing age. In ALS, the motor neuron cytoskeleton is typically affected early in the illness. Focal enlargements are frequent in proximal motor axons; ultrastructurally, these "spheroids" are composed of accumulations of neurofilaments. Also seen is proliferation of astroglia and microglia, the inevitable accompaniment of all degenerative processes in the central nervous system (CNS).

The death of the peripheral motor neurons in the brainstem and spinal cord leads to denervation and consequent atrophy of the corresponding muscle fibers. In the early phases of the illness denervated muscle can be reinnervated by sprouting of nearby distal motor nerve terminals, although reinnervation in this disease is considerably less extensive than in most other disorders affecting motor neurons (e.g., poliomyelitis, peripheral neuropathy). As denervation progresses, muscle atrophy is readily recognized in muscle biopsies and on clinical examination. This is the basis for the term *amyotrophy*. The loss of cortical motor neurons results in thinning of the corticospinal tracts that travel via the internal capsule

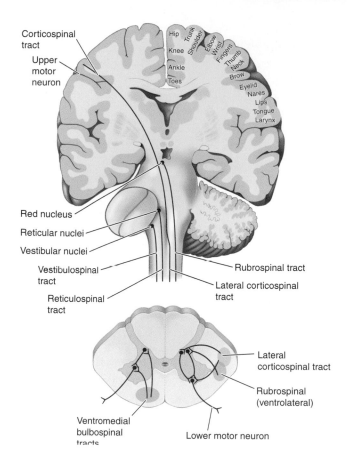

FIGURE 21-1

The corticospinal and bulbospinal upper motor neuron pathways. Upper motor neurons have their cell bodies in layer V of the primary motor cortex (the precentral gyrus, or Brodmann's area 4) and in the premotor and supplemental motor cortex (area 6). The upper motor neurons in the primary motor cortex are somatotopically organized as illustrated on the right side of the figure.

Axons of the upper motor neurons descend through the subcortical white matter and the posterior limb of the internal capsule. Axons of the *pyramidal* or *corticospinal system* descend through the brainstem in the cerebral peduncle of the midbrain, the basis pontis, and the medullary pyramids. At the cervicomedullary junction, most pyramidal axons decussate into the contralateral corticospinal tract of the lateral spinal cord, but 10 to 30% remain ipsilateral in the anterior spinal cord. Pyramidal neurons make direct monosynaptic connections with lower motor neurons. They innervate most densely the lower motor neurons of hand muscles and are involved in the execution of learned, fine movements. Corticobulbar neurons are similar to corticospinal neurons but innervate brainstem motor nuclei.

Bulbospinal upper motor neurons influence strength and tone but are not part of the pyramidal system. The descending *ventromedial bulbospinal pathways* originate in the tectum of the midbrain (tectospinal pathway), the vestibular nuclei (vestibulospinal pathway), and the reticular formation (reticulospinal pathway). These pathways influence axial and proximal muscles and are involved in the maintenance of posture and integrated movements of the limbs and trunk. The descending *ventrolateral bulbospinal pathways,* which originate predominantly in the red nucleus (rubrospinal pathway), facilitate distal limb muscles. The bulbospinal system is sometimes referred to as the *extrapyramidal upper motor neuron system*. In all figures, nerve cell bodies and axon terminals are shown, respectively, as closed circles and forks.

TABLE 21-1

SPORADIC MOTOR NEURON DISEASES
CHRONIC
Upper and lower motor neurons
Amyotrophic lateral sclerosis
Predominantly upper motor neurons
Primary lateral sclerosis
Predominantly lower motor neurons
Multifocal motor neuropathy with conduction block
Motor neuropathy with paraproteinemia or cancer
Motor-predominant peripheral neuropathies
Other
Associated with other degenerative disorders
Secondary motor neuron disorders
ACUTE
Poliomyelitis
Herpes zoster
Coxsackie virus
West Nile Virus

(**Fig. 21-2**) and brainstem to the lateral and anterior white matter columns of the spinal cord. The loss of fibers in the lateral columns and resulting fibrillary gliosis impart a particular firmness (*lateral sclerosis*). A remarkable feature of the disease is the selectivity of neuronal cell death. By light microscopy, the entire sensory apparatus, the regulatory mechanisms for the control and coordination of movement, and the components of the brain that are needed for cognitive processes remain intact. However, immunostaining indicates that neurons bearing ubiquitin, a marker for degeneration, are also detected in nonmotor systems. Moreover, studies of glucose metabolism also indicate that there is neuronal dysfunction outside of the motor system in this disorder. Within the motor system, there is some selectivity of involvement. Thus, motor neurons required for ocular motility remain unaffected, as do the parasympa-

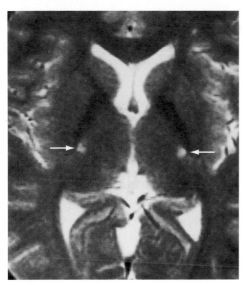

FIGURE 21-2

Amyotrophic lateral sclerosis. Axial T2-weighted MRI scan through the lateral ventricles of the brain reveals abnormal high signal intensity within the corticospinal tracts (*arrows*). This MRI feature represents an increase in water content in myelin tracts undergoing Wallerian degeneration secondary to cortical motor neuronal loss. This finding is commonly present in ALS but can also be seen in AIDS-related encephalopathy, infarction, or other disease processes that produce corticospinal neuronal loss in a symmetric fashion.

thetic neurons in the sacral spinal cord that innervate the sphincters of the bowel and bladder.

Clinical Manifestations

The manifestations of ALS are somewhat variable depending on whether corticospinal neurons or lower motor neurons in the brainstem and spinal cord are more prominently involved. With lower motor neuron dysfunction and early denervation, typically the first evidence of the disease is insidiously developing asymmetric weakness, usually first evident distally in one of the limbs. A detailed history often discloses recent development of cramping with volitional movements, typically in the early hours of the morning (e.g., while stretching in bed). Weakness caused by denervation is associated with progressive wasting and atrophy of muscles and, particularly early in the illness, spontaneous twitching of motor units, or fasciculations. In the hands, a preponderance of extensor over flexor weakness is common. When the initial denervation involves bulbar rather than limb muscles, the problem at onset is difficulty with chewing, swallowing, and movements of the face and tongue. Early involvement of the muscles of respiration may lead to death before the disease is far advanced elsewhere. With prominent corticospinal involvement, there is hyperactivity of the muscle-stretch reflexes (tendon jerks) and, often, spastic resistance to passive movements of the affected limbs. Patients with significant reflex hyperactivity complain of muscle stiffness often out of proportion to weakness. Degeneration of the cortico-bulbar projections innervating the brainstem results in dysarthria and exaggeration of the motor expressions of emotion. The latter leads to involuntary excess in weeping or laughing (so-called pseudobulbar affect).

Virtually any muscle group may be the first to show signs of disease, but, as time passes, more and more muscles become involved until ultimately the disorder takes on a symmetric distribution in all regions. It is characteristic of ALS that, regardless of whether the initial disease involves upper or lower motor neurons, both will eventually be implicated. Even in the late stages of the illness, sensory, bowel and bladder, and usually cognitive functions are preserved. Even when there is severe brainstem disease, ocular motility is spared until the very late stages of the illness. Although dementia is not traditionally considered as a component of ALS, signs of frontotemporal dementia (Chap. 18) are present in some individuals with familial or sporadic ALS.

A committee of the World Federation of Neurology has established diagnostic guidelines for ALS. Essential for the diagnosis is simultaneous upper and lower motor neuron involvement with progressive weakness, and the exclusion of all alternative diagnoses. The disorder is ranked as "definite" ALS when three or four of the following are involved: bulbar, cervical, thoracic, and lumbosacral motor neurons. When two sites are involved, the diagnosis is "probable," and when only one site is implicated, the diagnosis is "possible." An exception is made for those who have progressive upper and lower motor neuron signs at only one site and a mutation in the gene encoding superoxide dismutase (SOD1; below).

Epidemiology

The illness is relentlessly progressive, leading to death from respiratory paralysis; the median survival is from 3 to 5 years. There are very rare reports of stabilization or even regression of ALS. In most societies there is an incidence of 1 to 3 per 100,000 and a prevalence of 3 to 5 per 100,000. Several endemic foci of higher prevalence exist in the western Pacific (e.g., in specific regions of Guam or Papua New Guinea). In the United States and Europe, males are somewhat more frequently affected than females. While ALS is overwhelmingly a sporadic disorder, some 5 to 10% of cases are inherited as an autosomal dominant trait.

Familial ALS

Several forms of selective motor neuron disease are inheritable. The most common is familial ALS (FALS). Apart from its inheritance as an autosomal dominant trait, it is clinically indistinguishable from sporadic ALS. Genetic studies have identified mutations in the gene encoding the cytosolic, copper- and zinc-binding enzyme SOD1 as the cause of one form of FALS. However, this accounts for only 20% of inherited cases of ALS. Rare mutations in other genes are also clearly implicated in ALS-like diseases. Another familial, adult-onset disorder that may mimic aspects of ALS is Kennedy's syndrome caused by mutations in the androgen receptor.

Differential Diagnosis

Because ALS is currently untreatable, it is imperative that potentially remediable causes of motor neuron dysfunction be excluded. This is particularly true in cases that are atypical by virtue of (1) restriction to either upper or lower motor neurons, (2) involvement of neurons other than motor neurons, and (3) evidence of motor neuronal conduction block on electrophysiologic testing. Electromyographic and nerve conduction studies (EMG/NCS) are essential for the diagnosis of ALS and other motor neuron diseases.

Compression of the cervical spinal cord or cervicomedullary junction from tumors in the cervical region or at the foramen magnum or from cervical spondylosis with osteophytes projecting into the vertebral canal can produce weakness, wasting, and fasciculations in the upper limbs and spasticity in the legs, closely resembling ALS. The absence of cranial nerve involvement may be helpful in differentiation, although some foramen magnum lesions may compress the twelfth cranial (hypoglossal) nerve, with resulting paralysis of the tongue. Absence of pain or of sensory changes, normal bowel and bladder function, normal imaging studies of the spine, and normal cerebrospinal fluid (CSF) all favor ALS. Where doubt exists, magnetic resonance imaging (MRI) scans should be performed to visualize the cervical spinal cord.

Another important entity in the differential diagnosis of ALS is *multifocal motor neuropathy with conduction block* (MMCB), discussed below. A diffuse, lower motor axonal neuropathy mimicking ALS sometimes evolves in association with hematopoietic disorders such as lymphoma. In this clinical setting, the presence of an M-component in serum should prompt consideration of a bone marrow biopsy. Lyme disease may also cause an axonal, lower motor neuropathy.

Other treatable disorders that occasionally mimic ALS are chronic lead poisoning, hyperparathyroidism, and thyrotoxicosis. These disorders may be suggested by the patient's social or occupational history or by unusual clinical features. When the family history is positive, disorders involving the genes encoding cytosolic SOD1, hexosaminidase A, or α-glucosidase deficiency must be excluded. These are readily identified by appropriate laboratory tests. Benign fasciculations are occasionally a source of concern because on inspection they resemble the fascicular twitchings that accompany motor neuron degeneration. The absence of weakness, atrophy, or denervation phenomena on electrophysiologic examination usually excludes ALS or other serious neurologic disease. Patients who have recovered from poliomyelitis may experience a delayed deterioration of motor neurons that presents clinically with progressive weakness, atrophy, and fasciculations. Its cause is unknown, but it is thought to reflect sublethal prior injury to motor neurons by poliovirus.

TREATMENT FOR ALS

No treatment arrests the underlying pathologic process in ALS. The drug riluzole (100 mg/d) was approved for ALS because it produces a modest lengthening of survival. In one trial, the survival rate at 18 months with riluzole was similar to placebo at 15 months. The mechanism of this effect is not known with certainty; riluzole may reduce excitotoxicity by diminishing glutamate release. Riluzole is generally well tolerated; nausea, dizziness, weight loss, and elevated liver enzymes occur occasionally. Several agents have failed in clinical trials in human ALS including brain-derived neurotrophic factor, glial-derived neurotrophic factor, the anti-glutamate compound topiramate, and creatine. The latter was somewhat surprising as creatine was proven to be beneficial in transgenic ALS mice, perhaps by augmenting intracellular ATP stores. Insulin-like growth factor 1 (IGF-1) produced inconsistent results in ALS patients and is undergoing further clinical trials. COX-2 inhibitors and minocycline are also currently undergoing clinical trials because of success in a mouse model of ALS.

In the absence of a primary therapy for ALS, a variety of rehabilitative aids may substantially assist ALS patients. Foot-drop splints facilitate ambulation by obviating the need for excessive hip flexion and by preventing tripping on a floppy foot. Finger extension splints can potentiate grip. Respiratory support may be life-sustaining. For patients electing against long-term ventilation by tracheostomy, positive-pressure ventilation by mouth or nose provides transient (several weeks) relief from hypercarbia and hypoxia. Also extremely beneficial for some patients is a respiratory device (Inexsufflator or Cough Assist Device) that produces an artificial cough. This is highly effective in clearing airways and preventing aspiration pneumonia. When bulbar disease prevents normal chewing and swallowing, gastrostomy is uniformly helpful, restoring normal nutrition and hydration. Fortunately, an increasing variety of speech synthesizers are now available to augment speech when there is advanced bulbar palsy. These facilitate oral communication and may be effective for telephone use. Peudobulbar affect in ALS patients was shown to be palliated by a combination of quinidine (30 mg) and dextromethorphan (30 mg) twice daily.

SELECTED LOWER MOTOR NEURON DISORDERS

In these motor neuron diseases, the peripheral motor neurons are affected without evidence of involvement of the corticospinal motor systems.

X-LINKED SPINOBULBAR MUSCULAR ATROPHY (KENNEDY'S DISEASE)

This is an X-linked lower motor neuron disorder in which progressive weakness and wasting of limb and bulbar muscles begins in males in mid-adult life and is conjoined with androgen insensitivity manifested by gynecomastia and reduced fertility. In addition to gynecomastia, which may be subtle, two findings distinguishing this disorder from ALS are the absence of signs of pyramidal tract disease (spasticity) and the presence of a subtle sensory neuropathy in some patients. The underlying molecular defect is an expanded trinucleotide repeat (-CAG-) in the first exon of the androgen receptor gene on the X chromosome. DNA testing is available. An inverse correlation appears to exist between the number of –CAG– repeats and the age of onset of the disease.

ADULT TAY-SACH'S DISEASE

Several reports have described adult-onset, predominantly lower motor neuropathies arising from deficiency of the enzyme hexosaminidase A (Hx A). These tend to be distinguishable from ALS because they are very slowly progressive; dysarthria and radiographically evident

cerebellar atrophy may be prominent. In rare cases, spasticity may also be present, although it is generally absent.

SPINAL MUSCULAR ATROPHY

The SMAs are a family of selective lower motor neuron diseases of early onset. Despite some phenotypic variability (largely in age of onset), the defect in the majority of families with SMA maps to a locus on chromosome 5 encoding a putative motor neuron survival protein (SMN, for survival motor neuron) that is important in the formation and trafficking of RNA complexes across the nuclear membrane. Neuropathologically these disorders are characterized by extensive loss of large motor neurons; muscle biopsy reveals evidence of denervation atrophy. Several clinical forms exist.

Infantile SMA (SMA I, Werdnig-Hoffmann Disease) has the earliest onset and most rapidly fatal course. In some instances it is apparent even before birth, as indicated by decreased fetal movements late in the third trimester. Though alert, afflicted infants are weak and floppy (hypotonic) and lack muscle stretch reflexes. Death generally ensues within the first year of life. *Chronic childhood SMA* (SMA II) begins later in childhood and evolves with a more slowly progressive course. *Juvenile SMA* (SMA III, Kugelberg-Welander disease) manifests during late childhood and runs a slow, indolent course. Unlike most denervating diseases, in this chronic disorder weakness is greatest in the proximal muscles; indeed, the pattern of clinical weakness can suggest a primary myopathy such as limb-girdle dystrophy. Electrophysiologic and muscle biopsy evidence of denervation distinguish SMA III from the myopathic syndromes.

MULTIFOCAL MOTOR NEUROPATHY WITH CONDUCTION BLOCK

In this disorder lower motor neuron function is regionally and chronically disrupted by remarkably focal blocks in conduction. Many cases have elevated serum titers of monoclonal and polyclonal antibodies to ganglioside GM1; it is hypothesized that the antibodies produce selective, focal, paranodal demyelination of motor neurons. MMCB is not typically associated with corticospinal signs. In contrast with ALS, MMCB may respond dramatically to therapy such as intravenous immunoglobulin or chemotherapy; it is thus imperative that MMCB be excluded when considering a diagnosis of ALS. EMG/NCS can usually make this distinction.

OTHER FORMS OF LOWER MOTOR NEURON DISEASE

In individual families, other syndromes characterized by selective lower motor neuron dysfunction in an SMA-like pattern have been described. There are rare X-linked and autosomal dominant forms of apparent SMA. There is an ALS variant of juvenile onset, the Fazio-Londe syndrome, that involves mainly the musculature innervated by the brainstem.

SELECTED DISORDERS OF THE UPPER MOTOR NEURON

PRIMARY LATERAL SCLEROSIS

This exceedingly rare disorder arises sporadically in adults in mid- to late life. Clinically PLS is characterized by progressive spastic weakness of the limbs, preceded or followed by spastic dysarthria and dysphagia, indicating combined involvement of the corticospinal and corticobulbar tracts. Fasciculations, amyotrophy, and sensory changes are absent; neither electromyography nor muscle biopsy shows denervation. On neuropathologic examination there is selective loss of the large pyramidal cells in the precentral gyrus and degeneration of the corticospinal and corticobulbar projections. The peripheral motor neurons and other neuronal systems are spared. The course of PLS is variable; while long-term survival is documented, the course may be as aggressive as in ALS, with ~3-year survival from onset to death. Early in its course, PLS raises the question of multiple sclerosis or other demyelinating diseases such as adrenoleukodystrophy as diagnostic considerations. A myelopathy suggestive of PLS is infrequently seen with infection with the retrovirus human T cell lymphotropic virus (HTLV-I). The clinical course and laboratory testing will distinguish these possibilities.

FAMILIAL SPASTIC PARAPLEGIA

FSP usually arises in the third or fourth decade and is characterized by progressive spastic weakness beginning in the distal lower extremities. FSP patients typically have a long survival, presumably because respiratory function is spared. Late in the illness there may be urinary urgency and incontinence and sometimes fecal incontinence; sexual function tends to be preserved. In pure forms of FSP, ataxia, posterior column sensory loss, and amyotrophy are absent or minimal; however, in some patients, minor sensory changes (impaired vibration and position sense) may be observed in late stages. Some family members may have spasticity without clinical symptoms. It is now apparent that defects at numerous loci underlie both dominantly

and recessively inherited forms of FSP; most adult-onset cases have autosomal dominant inheritance and are due to mutations in the protein spastin.

CLINICAL PEARLS

EMG/NCS essential for the diagnosis of ALS and other motor neuron diseases

Cervical spine disease can mimic motor neuron disease; consider MRI

Fasciculations without weakness or atrophy are common and usually benign

If a family history of a similar disorder is present, consider familial ALS or familial spastic paraplegia (FSP)

WEB SITES

Several web sites provide valuable information on ALS including those offered by the Muscular Dystrophy Association (www.mdausa.org), the Amyotrophic Lateral Sclerosis Association (www.alsa.org), and the World Federation of Neurology and the Neuromuscular Unit At Washington University in St. Louis(www.neuro.wustl.edu/neuromuscular).

FURTHER READINGS

☑ BROOKS BR et al: Treatment of pseudobulbar affect in ALS with dextromethorphan/quinidine: A randomized trial. Neurology 63:1364, 2004

Effectiveness of a compound for pseudobulbar affect in ALS patients is demonstrated.

CLEVELAND DW, ROTHSTEIN JD: From Charcot to Lou Gehrig: Deciphering selective motor neuron death in ALS. Nat Rev Neurosci 2:806, 2001

HADANO S et al: A gene encoding a putative GTPase regulator is mutated in familial amyotrophic lateral sclerosis. Nat Genet 29:166, 2001

LAMBRECHTS D et al: VEGF is a modifier of amyotrophic lateral sclerosis in mice and humans and protects motoneurons against ischemic death. Nat Genet 34(4):384, 2003

PULS I et al: Mutant dynactin in motor neuron disease. Nat Genet 33:455, 2003

YANG Y et al: The gene encoding alsin, a protein with three guanine-nucleotide exchange factor domains, is mutated in a form of recessive amyotrophic lateral sclerosis. Nat Genet 29:160, 2001

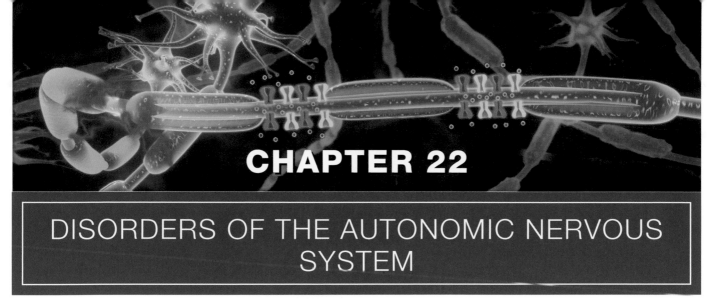

CHAPTER 22

DISORDERS OF THE AUTONOMIC NERVOUS SYSTEM

Phillip A. Low
John W. Engstrom

The autonomic nervous system (ANS) innervates the entire neuraxis and permeates all organ systems. It regulates blood pressure (BP), heart rate, sleep, and bladder and bowel function. It operates in the background, so that its full importance becomes recognized only when ANS function is compromised, resulting in dysautonomia.

ANATOMICAL ORGANIZATION

The activity of the autonomic nervous system is regulated by central neurons responsive to diverse afferent inputs. After central integration of afferent information, autonomic outflow is adjusted to permit the functioning of the major organ systems in accordance with the needs of the organism as a whole. Connections between the cerebral cortex and the autonomic centers in the brainstem coordinate autonomic outflow with higher mental functions.

The preganglionic neurons of the parasympathetic nervous system leave the central nervous system (CNS) in the third, seventh, ninth, and tenth cranial nerves as well as the second and third sacral nerves, while the preganglionic neurons of the sympathetic nervous system exit the spinal cord between the first thoracic and the second lumbar segments (**Fig. 22-1**). The postganglionic neurons, located in ganglia outside the CNS, give rise to the postganglionic autonomic nerves that innervate organs and tissues throughout the body. Responses to sympathetic and parasympathetic stimulation are frequently antagonistic (**Table 22-1**), reflecting highly coordinated interactions within the CNS; the resultant changes in parasympathetic and sympathetic activity provide more precise control of autonomic responses than could be achieved by the modulation of a single system.

Acetylcholine (ACh) is the preganglionic neurotransmitter for both divisions of the ANS as well as the postganglionic neurotransmitter of the parasympathetic neurons. Norepinephrine (NE) is the neurotransmitter of the postganglionic sympathetic neurons, except for cholinergic neurons innervating the eccrine sweat glands.

CLINICAL EVALUATION

CLASSIFICATION

Disorders of the ANS may result from pathology of either the CNS or the peripheral nervous system (PNS) (**Table 22-2**). Signs and symptoms may result from interruption of the afferent limb, CNS processing centers, or efferent limb of reflex arcs controlling autonomic responses. For example, a lesion of the medulla produced by a posterior fossa tumor can impair BP responses to postural changes and result in orthostatic hypotension (OH). OH can also be caused by lesions of the spinal cord or peripheral vasomotor nerve fibers (e.g., diabetic autonomic neuropathy). The site of reflex interruption is usually established by the clinical context in which the dysautonomia arises, combined with judicious use of ANS testing and neuroimaging

Parasympathetic   **Sympathetic**

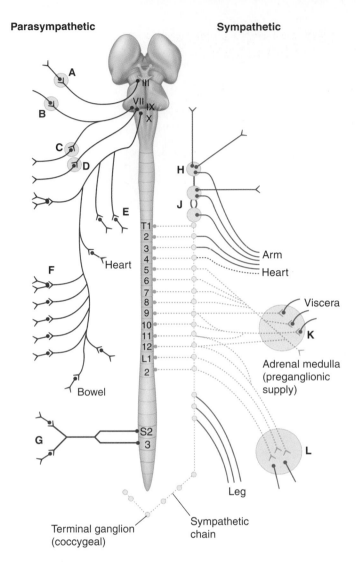

TABLE 22-1

FUNCTIONAL CONSEQUENCES OF NORMAL ANS ACTIVATION

	SYMPATHETIC	PARASYMPATHETIC
Heart rate	Increased	Decreased
Blood pressure	Increased	Mildly decreased
Bladder	Increased sphincter tone	Voiding (decreased tone)
Bowel motility	Decreased motility	Increased
Lung	Bronchodilation	Bronchoconstriction
Sweat glands	Sweating	—
Pupils	Dilation	Constriction
Adrenal glands	Catecholamine release	—
Sexual function	Ejaculation, orgasm	Erection
Lacrimal glands	—	Tearing
Parotid glands	—	Salivation

Some syndromes do not fit easily into any classification scheme.

SYMPTOMS OF AUTONOMIC DYSFUNCTION

Clinical manifestations result from a loss of function (e.g., impaired baroreflexes leading to OH), overactivity (e.g., hyperhidrosis, hypertension, tachycardia), or loss of regulation (e.g., autonomic dysreflexia) of autonomic circuits. The disorder may be widespread or regional in distribution. An autonomic history focuses on systemic functions (BP, heart rate, sleep, thermoregulation) and individual organ systems (pupils, bowel, bladder, sexual function). More formal assessment is possible using a standardized instrument such as the autonomic symptom profile. It is also important to recognize the modulating effects of age and gender. For instance, OH commonly results in lightheadedness in the young, whereas cognitive slowing is much more important in the elderly. Specific symptoms of orthostatic intolerance are quite diverse (**Table 22–3**). Autonomic symptoms may vary dramatically, reflecting the dynamic nature of autonomic control over homeostatic function. For example, OH might be manifest only in the early morning, following a meal, or with exercise, depending upon the regional vascular bed affected by dysautonomia.

Early symptoms may be overlooked. Impotence, although not specific for autonomic failure, often heralds autonomic failure in men and may precede other symptoms by years. A decrease in the frequency of spontaneous early morning erections may occur months before loss of nocturnal penile tumescence and development of total impotence. Bladder dysfunction may

Parasympathetic system
from cranial nerves III, VII, IX, X and from sacral nerves 2 and 3

A Ciliary ganglion
B Sphenopalatine (pterygopalatine) ganglion
C Submandibular ganglion
D Otic ganglion
E Vagal ganglion cells in the heart wall
F Vagal ganglion cells in bowel wall
G Pelvic ganglia

Sympathetic system
from T1-L2
Preganglionic fibers ··········
Postganglionic fibers ———

H Superior cervical ganglion
J Middle cervical ganglion and inferior cervical (stellate) ganglion including T1 ganglion
K Coeliac and other abdominal ganglia
L Lower abdominal sympathetic ganglia

FIGURE 22-1
Schematic representation of the autonomic nervous system. (*Redrawn from M Moskowitz: Clin Endocrinol Metab 6(3):745, 1977, with permission from Elsevier.*)

studies. Important elements of the clinical context include the presence or absence of CNS signs (pathophysiology and prognosis differ), association with sensory or motor polyneuropathy, family history, and pathologic findings.

TABLE 22-2

CLASSIFICATION OF CLINICAL AUTONOMIC DISORDERS

I. Autonomic disorders with brain involvement
  A. Associated with multisystem degeneration
    1. Multisystem degeneration: autonomic failure clinically prominent
      a. Multiple system atrophy (MSA)
      b. Parkinson's disease with autonomic failure
      c. Diffuse Lewy body disease (some cases)
    2. Multisystem degeneration: autonomic failure clinically not usually prominent
      a. Parkinson's disease
      b. Other extrapyramidal disorders (inherited spinocerebellar atrophies, progressive supranuclear palsy, corticobasal degeneration, Machado-Joseph disease)
  B. Unassociated with multisystem degeneration
    1. Disorders mainly due to cerebral cortex involvement
      a. Frontal cortex lesions causing urinary/bowel incontinence
      b. Partial complex seizures
    2. Disorders of the limbic and paralimbic circuits
      a. Shapiro's syndrome (agenesis of corpus callosum, hyperhidrosis, hypothermia)
      b. Autonomic seizures
    3. Disorders of the hypothalamus
      a. Wernicke-Korsakoff syndrome
      b. Diencephalic syndrome
      c. Neuroleptic malignant syndrome
      d. Serotonin syndrome
      e. Fatal familial insomnia
      f. Antidiuretic hormone (ADH) syndromes (diabetes insipidus, inappropriate ADH)
      g. Disturbances of temperature regulation (hyperthermia, hypothermia)
      h. Disturbances of sexual function
      i. Disturbances of appetite
      j. Disturbances of BP/HR and gastric function
      k. Horner's syndrome
    4. Disorders of the brainstem and cerebellum
      a. Posterior fossa tumors
      b. Syringobulbia and Arnold-Chiari malformation
      c. Disorders of BP control (hypertension, hypotension)
      d. Cardiac arrhythmias
      e. Central sleep apnea
      f. Baroreflex failure
      g. Horner's syndrome
II. Autonomic disorders with spinal cord involvement
  A. Traumatic tetraplegia
  B. Syringomyelia
  C. Subacute combined degeneration
  D. Multiple sclerosis
  E. Amyotrophic lateral sclerosis
  F. Tetanus
  G. Stiff-man syndrome
  H. Spinal cord tumors
III. Autonomic neuropathies
  A. Acute/subacute autonomic neuropathies
    1 Subacute autoimmune autonomic neuropathy (panautonomic neuropathy, pandysautonomia)
      a. Subacute paraneoplastic autonomic neuropathy
      b. Guillain-Barré syndrome
      c. Botulism
      d. Porphyria

(Continued)

TABLE 22-2 *(Continued)*

CLASSIFICATION OF CLINICAL AUTONOMIC DISORDERS

      e. Drug-induced autonomic neuropathies
      f. Toxic autonomic neuropathies

  B. Chronic peripheral autonomic neuropathies
    1. Distal small fiber neuropathy
    2. Combined sympathetic and parasympathetic failure
      a. Amyloid
      b. Diabetic autonomic neuropathy
      c. Autoimmune autonomic neuropathy (paraneoplastic and idiopathic)
      d. Sensory neuronopathy with autonomic failure
      e. Familial dysautonomia (Riley-Day syndrome)

Note: BP, blood pressure; HR, heart rate.

appear early in men and women, particularly in those with CNS involvement. Brain and spinal cord disease above the level of the lumbar spine results first in nocturia, urinary frequency, and small bladder volumes, and eventually incontinence (upper motor neuron or spastic bladder). Disease of PNS autonomic nerve fibers to and from the bladder results in large bladder volumes, urinary frequency, and overflow incontinence (lower motor neuron bladder or flaccid bladder). Measurement of bladder volume (postvoid residual) is a useful bedside test for distinguishing between upper and lower motor neuron bladder dysfunction in the early stages of dysautonomia. Gastrointestinal autonomic dysfunction typically presents as severe constipation. Diarrhea occurs occasionally (as in diabetes mellitus) due to rapid transit of contents or uncoordinated small-bowel motor activity, or on an osmotic basis from bacterial overgrowth associated with small-bowel stasis. Impaired glandular secretory function may cause difficulty with food intake due to decreased salivation or with eye irritation due to decreased lacrimation. Occasionally, temperature elevation and vasodilation can result from anhidrosis because sweating is normally important for heat dissipation.

OH (also called "postural hypotension") is often the most disabling feature of autonomic dysfunction. The prevalence of OH is relatively high, especially when OH associated with aging and diabetes is included (**Table 22-4**). OH can cause a variety of symptoms including dimming or loss of vision, lightheadedness, diaphoresis, diminished hearing, pallor, and weakness. Syncope results when the drop in BP impairs cerebral perfusion. Other manifestations of impaired baroreflexes are supine hypertension, a heart rate that is fixed regardless of posture, postprandial hypotension, and an excessively high nocturnal BP. Many patients with OH have a preceding diagnosis of hypertension, reflecting the great importance of baroreflexes in maintaining postural and supine normotension. A recent study from France found that patients with neurogenic OH had difficulty tolerating a severe summer heat wave. The most common causes of OH are not neurologic in origin; these must be distinguished from the neurogenic causes (**Table 22-5**).

TABLE 22-3

SYMPTOMS OF ORTHOSTATIC INTOLERANCE

Lightheadedness (dizziness)	88%
Weakness or tiredness	72%
Cognitive difficulty (thinking/concentrating)	47%
Blurred vision	47%
Tremulousness	38%
Vertigo	37%
Pallor	31%
Anxiety	29%
Palpitations	26%
Clammy feeling	19%
Nausea	18%

Source: From Low et al.

TABLE 22-4

PREVALENCE OF ORTHOSTATIC HYPOTENSION IN DIFFERENT DISORDERS

DISORDER	PREVALENCE
Aging	14–20%
Diabetic neuropathy	10%
Other autonomic neuropathies	10–50 per 100,000
Multiple system atrophy	5–15 per 100,000
Pure autonomic failure	10–30 per 100,000

TABLE 22-5

NONNEUROGENIC CAUSES OF ORTHOSTATIC HYPOTENSION

Cardiac pump failure
  Myocardial infarction
  Myocarditis
  Constrictive pericarditis
  Aortic stenosis
  Tachyarrhythmias
  Bradyarrhythmias
  Salt-losing nephropathy
  Adrenal insufficiency
  Diabetes insipidus
  Venous obstruction
Reduced intravascular volume
  Straining of heavy lifting,
    urination, defecation
  Dehydration
  Diarrhea, emesis
  Hemorrhage
  Burns
Metabolic
  Adrenocortical insufficiency
  Hypoaldosteronism
  Pheochromocytoma
  Severe potassium depletion

Venous pooling
  Alcohol
  Postprandial dilation of splanchnic vessel beds
  Vigorous exercise with dilation of skeletal vessel beds
  Heat: hot environment, hot showers and baths, fever
  Prolonged recumbancy or standing
  Sepsis
Medications
  Antihypertensives
  Diuretics
  Vasodilators: nitrates, hydralazine
  Alpha- and beta-blocking agents
  CNS sedatives: barbiturates, opiates
  Tricylic antidepressants
  Phenothiazines

APPROACH TO THE PATIENT WITH OH

The first step in the evaluation of symptomatic OH is the exclusion of treatable causes. The history should include a review of medications that may cause OH (e.g., diuretics, antihypertensives, antidepressants, phenothiazines, ethanol, narcotics, insulin, barbiturates, and calcium channel blocking agents). However, the precipitation of OH by medications may also be the first sign of an underlying autonomic disorder. The history may reveal an underlying cause for symptoms (e.g., diabetes, Parkinsonism) or specific underlying mechanisms (e.g., cardiac pump failure, reduced intravascular volume). The relationship of symptoms to meals (splanchnic pooling), standing on awakening in the morning (intravascular volume depletion), ambient warming (vasodilatation), or exercise (muscle arteriolar vasodilatation) should be sought.

Physical examination includes measurement of supine and standing pulse and BP. OH is defined as a sustained drop in systolic (≥ 20 mmHg) or diastolic (≥ 10 mmHg) BP within 3 min of standing up. In nonneurogenic causes of OH (such as hypovolemia), the BP drop is accompanied by a compensatory increase in heart rate of >15 beats/min.

An important clinical clue that the patient has neurogenic OH is the aggravation or precipitation of OH by autonomic stressors (such as a meal, hot bath, and exercise). Neurologic evaluation should include a mental status examination (to exclude neurodegenerative disorders), cranial nerve examination (impaired downgaze is found with progressive supranuclear palsy), abnormal pupils (Horner's or Adie's pupils), motor examination (Parkinson's disease and parkinsonian syndromes), and sensory examination (polyneuropathies). In patients without a clear initial diagnosis, follow-up neurologic examinations and repeat laboratory evaluations over 1 to 2 years may reveal an evolution of findings that enables a specific diagnosis to be made.

Disorders of autonomic function should be considered in patients with symptoms of altered sweating (hyperhidrosis or hypohidrosis), gastroparesis (bloating, nausea, vomiting of old food), constipation, impotence, or bladder dysfunction (urinary frequency, hesitancy, or incontinence).

Autonomic Testing

Autonomic function tests (**Table 22-6**) are helpful when the history and physical examination findings

TABLE 22-6

NEURAL PATHWAYS UNDERLYING SOME STANDARDIZED AUTONOMIC TESTS

TEST EVALUATED	PROCEDURE	AUTONOMIC FUNCTION
HRBD	6 deep breaths/min	Cardiovagal function
Valsalva ratio	Expiratory pressure, 40 mmHg for 10–15 s	Cardiovagal function
QSART	Axon-reflex test 4 limb sites	Postganglionic sudomotor function
BP$_{BB}$ to VM	BP$_{BB}$ response to VM	Adrenergic function: baroreflex adrenergic control of vagal and vasomotor function
HUT	BP$_{BB}$ and heart rate response to HUT	Adrenergic and cardiovagal responses to HUT

Note: HRDB, heart rate response to deep breathing; BP$_{BB}$, beat-to-beat blood pressure; QSART, quantitative sudomotor axon-reflex test; VM, Valsalva maneuver; HUT, head-up tilt.

are inconclusive, when detection of subclinical involvement is important to evaluate the extent and severity of abnormalities, or to follow the course of an autonomic disorder or its response to therapy.

HEART RATE VARIATION WITH DEEP BREATHING

This is a test of parasympathetic influence, via the vagus nerve, on cardiovascular function. Results are influenced by the subject's posture, rate and depth of respiration [6 breaths per minute and a forced vital capacity (FVC) > 1.5 L are optimal], age, medications, and hypocapnea. Interpretation of results requires comparison of test data with results from normal individuals collected under the same test conditions. For example, the lower limit of normal heart rate variation with deep breathing in persons <20 years is >15 to 20 beats/min, but for persons over age 60 it is 5 to 8 beats/min. As a consequence, heart rate variation with deep breathing (respiratory sinus arrhythmia) is abolished by the administration of atropine but is unaffected by sympathetic blockade (e.g., propranolol).

VALSALVA RESPONSE

This response (Table 22-6) assesses integrity of the baroreflex control of heart rate (parasympathetic) and BP (adrenergic). The response is obtained with the subject supine. A constant expiratory pressure of 40 mmHg is maintained for 15 s while measuring changes in heart rate and beat-to-beat BP. There are

four phases of BP and heart rate response to the Valsalva maneuver. Phases I and III are mechanical and related to changes in intrathoracic and intraabdominal pressure. In early phase II, reduced venous return results in a fall in stroke volume and BP, counteracted by a combination of reflex tachycardia and increased total peripheral resistance. Increased total peripheral resistance arrests the BP drop ~5 to 8 s after the onset of the maneuver. Late phase II begins with a progressive rise in BP to or above baseline. Venous return and cardiac output return to normal in phase IV. Persistent peripheral arteriolar vasoconstriction and increased cardiac adrenergic tone results in a temporary BP overshoot and phase IV bradycardia (mediated by the baroreceptor reflex).

Autonomic function during the Valsalva maneuver can be measured using beat-to-beat blood pressure or heart rate changes. The Valsalva ratio is defined as the maximum phase II tachycardia divided by the minimum phase IV bradycardia. The ratio reflects cardiovagal function.

SUDOMOTOR FUNCTION

Sweating is induced by release of ACh from sympathetic postganglionic fibers. The quantitative sudomotor axon reflex test (QSART) is a measure of regional autonomic function mediated by ACh-induced sweating. A reduced or absent response indicates a lesion of the postganglionic sudomotor axon. For example, sweating may be reduced in the legs as a result of peripheral neuropathy (e.g., in diabetes) before other signs of autonomic dysfunction emerge. The thermoregulatory sweat test (TST) is a qualitative measure of regional sweat production in response to an elevation of body temperature. An indicator powder placed on the anterior body surface changes color with sweat production during temperature elevation. The pattern of color changes is a measure of regional sweat secretion. Combining TST and QSART results will determine the site of the lesion. A postganglionic lesion is present if both QSART and TST show absent sweating. In a preganglionic lesion, QSART is intact but TST shows anhidrosis. Measurement of galvanic skin responses in the limbs after an induced electrical potential is a qualitative test for detecting the presence or absence of sweating.

ORTHOSTATIC BP RECORDINGS

Beat-to-beat BP measurements determined in supine, 70° tilt, and tilt-back positions are useful to quantitate orthostatic failure of BP control. It is important to allow a 20-min period of supine rest before assessing changes in BP during tilting. The BP change combined with heart rate monitoring can be useful for the evaluation of patients with suspected OH or unexplained syncope or to detect vagally mediated syncope.

PHARMACOLOGIC TESTS

Pharmacologic assessments can help localize an autonomic defect to the CNS or the PNS. A useful method to evaluate the systemic adrenergic response is the measurement of plasma NE, first with the patient supine and then after standing for at least 5 min. Supine values are reduced in postganglionic disorders (such as autonomic neuropathy or pure autonomic failure) and may fail to increase in preganglionic or postganglionic disorders (e.g., multiple system atrophy).

Administration of tyramine (releases NE from postganglionic terminals) and phenylephrine (denervation supersensitivity—directly acting α_1-agonist) is often used to evaluate postganglionic adrenergic function. In a postganglionic lesion, the response to tyramine is reduced and there is an excessive response to subthreshold doses of phenylephrine. Other strategies include ganglionic blockade with trimethaphan (greater fall in resulting BP with a preganglionic lesion) or administration of arginine vasopressin (to evaluate afferent central pathways).

MULTIPLE SYSTEM ATROPHY

Multiple system atrophy (MSA) is an uncommon entity that comprises autonomic failure (OH and/or a neurogenic bladder are required for diagnosis) combined with either striatonigral degeneration (Shy-Drager syndrome) or sporadic olivopontocerebellar atrophy (Chap. 19). The parkinsonism is usually unassociated with rest tremor and is not responsive to levodopa. Levodopa-induced dyskinesia is also uncommon. Autonomic function tests can usually differentiate MSA from Parkinson's disease in that the severity and distribution of autonomic failure is more severe and generalized in MSA. Cardiac postganglionic adrenergic innervation, measured as labeled metaiodobenzylguanidine (MIBG) uptake on single photon emission computed tomography or fluorodopamine on positron emission tomography (PET), is markedly impaired in the dysautonomia of Parkinson's disease but is normal in MSA.

MSA generally progresses relentlessly to death 7 to 10 years after onset. Neuropathologic changes include primary neuronal degeneration with loss of neurons and gliosis in many CNS regions, including the brainstem, the cerebellum, the striatum, and the intermediolateral cell column of the thoracolumbar spinal cord.

Autonomic dysfunction is also a common feature in dementia with Lewy bodies; the severity is usually less than that found in MSA or Parkinson's disease.

SPINAL CORD

Spinal cord lesions from any cause may result in focal autonomic deficits or autonomic hyperreflexia. Spinal cord transection or hemisection may be attended by autonomic hyperreflexia affecting bowel, bladder, sexual, temperature-regulation, or cardiovascular functions. Dangerous increases or decreases in body temperature may result from inability to experience the sensory accompaniments of heat or cold exposure below the level of the injury. Quadriparetic patients exhibit both supine hypertension and OH after upward tilting. Markedly increased autonomic discharge can be elicited by bladder pressure or stimulation of the skin or muscles; suprapubic palpation of the bladder, a distended bladder, catheter insertion, catheter obstruction, or urinary infection are common and correctable precipitants. This phenomenon, termed *autonomic dysreflexia,* affects 85% of patients with a traumatic spinal cord lesion above the C6 level. In patients with supine hypertension, BP can be lowered by tilting the head upward. Vasodilator drugs may be used to treat acute elevations in BP. Clonidine is used prophylactically to reduce the hypertension resulting from bladder stimulation. Sudden, dramatic increases in BP can lead to intracranial hemorrhage and death.

PERIPHERAL NERVE AND NEUROMUSCULAR JUNCTION DISORDERS

Peripheral neuropathies (Chap. 33; Table 22-2) are the most common cause of chronic autonomic insufficiency. Neuropathies that affect small myelinated and unmyelinated fibers of the sympathetic and parasympathetic nerves occur in diabetes mellitus, amyloidosis, chronic alcoholism, porphyria, and Guillain-Barré syndrome. Neuromuscular junction disorders include botulism and Lambert-Eaton syndrome.

Diabetes Mellitus

Autonomic neuropathy typically begins ~10 years after the onset of diabetes and slowly progresses. The earliest autonomic abnormalities, typically asymptomatic, consist of vagal disturbances, which can be detected as reduced heart rate variation with deep breathing, and loss of distal sudomotor function, detected by QSART. Loss of small myelinated and unmyelinated nerve fibers in the splanchnic distribution, carotid sinus, and vagus nerves is characteristic. In advanced disease, widespread enteric neuropathy can cause profound disturbances in gut motility (gastroparesis), nausea and vomiting, malnutrition, achlorhydria, and bowel incontinence. Other symptoms can include impotence, urinary incontinence, pupillary abnormalities, and OH. Typical symptoms and signs of hypoglycemia may fail to appear because damage to the sympathetic innervation of the adrenal gland can result in a lack of epinephrine release. Insulin increases flow through arteriovenous shunts and may also aggravate OH. Autonomic dysfunction may lengthen the QT interval, increasing the risk of sudden death due to cardiac arrhythmia. Hyperglycemia appears to be a direct risk factor for autonomic involvement in diabetes. Biochemical and pharmacologic studies in diabetic neuropathy are compatible with autonomic failure localized to the PNS.

Amyloidosis

Autonomic neuropathy occurs in both sporadic and familial forms of amyloidosis. The AL (immunoglobulin light chain) type is associated with primary amyloidosis or amyloidosis secondary to multiple myeloma. The ATTR type, with transthyretin as the primary protein component, is responsible for the most common form of inherited amyloidosis. Although patients usually present

with a distal painful neuropathy accompanied by sensory loss, autonomic insufficiency can precede the development of the polyneuropathy or occur in isolation. Diagnosis can be made by a combination of serum protein electrophoresis studies on blood and urine, tissue biopsy (abdominal fat pad, rectal, or nerve) to search for amyloid deposits, and genetic testing for transthyretin in familial cases. Treatment of the ATTR type with liver transplantation may be helpful for familial cases; use of melphalan and stem cell transplantation for primary amylodiosis yields mixed results. Death is usually due to cardiac or renal impairment. Postmortem studies reveal amyloid deposition in many organs, including two sites that contribute to autonomic failure: intraneural blood vessels and autonomic ganglia. Pathologic examination reveals a loss of unmyelinated and myelinated nerve fibers.

Alcoholic Neuropathy

Abnormalities in parasympathetic vagal and efferent sympathetic function are usually mild in individuals with alcoholic neuropathy. Pathologic changes can be demonstrated in the parasympathetic (vagus) and sympathetic fibers and in ganglia. OH is usually due to brainstem involvement. Impotence is a major problem, but concurrent gonadal hormone abnormalities may obscure the parasympathetic component. Clinical symptoms of autonomic failure generally appear when the polyneuropathy is severe and there is usually coexisting Wernicke's encephalopathy. Autonomic involvement may contribute to the high mortality rates associated with alcoholism.

Porphyria

Although each of the porphyrias can cause autonomic dysfunction, the condition is most extensively documented in the acute intermittent type. Autonomic symptoms include tachycardia, sweating, urinary retention, hypertension, and, less commonly, hypotension. Other prominent symptoms include anxiety, abdominal pain, nausea, and vomiting. Abnormal autonomic function can occur both during acute attacks and during remissions. Elevated catecholamine levels during acute attacks correlate with the degree of tachycardia and hypertension.

Guillain-Barré Syndrome

BP fluctuations and arrhythmias can be severe (Chap. 35). It is estimated that 2 to 10% of patients seriously ill with Guillain-Barré syndrome suffer fatal cardiovascular collapse. Gastrointestinal autonomic involvement is common. Abnormal sweating, sphincter disturbance, and pupillary dysfunction also occur. Demyelination has been described in the vagus and glossopharyngeal nerves, the sympathetic chain, and the white rami communicantes. The presence of autonomic involvement is not clearly related to the severity of motor or sensory involvement.

Autoimmune Autonomic Neuropathy

The development of serologic testing for the ganglionic ACh receptor (A_3 AChR) autoantibody, which is a putative effector of autoimmune dysautonomia, now allows definition of the entity of autoimmune autonomic neuropathy (AAN). This disorder presents as the subacute development of autonomic failure with OH, enteric neuropathy (gastroparesis, ileus, constipation/diarrhea), and cholinergic failure; the latter consists of loss of sweating, sicca complex, and a tonic pupil. In general, the antibody titer correlates with the severity of autonomic failure. Symptoms of cholinergic failure are also predictive of a high antibody titer. Onset of the neuropathy follows a viral infection in approximately half of cases. Some patients appear to respond to immunotherapy. The spectrum of AAN is broader than originally thought, and some antibody-positive cases have an insidious onset and slow progression with a pure autonomic failure (see below) phenotype.

AAN can have a paraneoplastic basis. The clinical features of the autonomic neuropathy may be indistinguishable from the nonparaneoplastic form, or a coexisting paraneoplastic syndrome, such as cerebellar involvement or dementia, may be present. The neoplasm may be truly occult, possibly suppressed by the autoantibody.

Botulism

Botulinum toxin binds presynaptically to cholinergic nerve terminals and, after uptake into the cytosol, blocks ACh release. Manifestations consist of motor paralysis and autonomic disturbances that include blurred vision, dry mouth, nausea, unreactive or sluggishly reactive pupils, constipation, and urinary retention.

PURE AUTONOMIC FAILURE (PAF)

This sporadic syndrome consists of postural hypotension, impotence, bladder dysfunction, and defective sweating. The disorder begins in the middle decades and occurs in women more often than men. The symptoms can be disabling, but the disease does not shorten life span. The clinical and pharmacologic characteristics suggest primary involvement of postganglionic sympathetic neurons. There is a severe reduction in the density of neurons within sympathetic ganglia that results in low supine plasma NE levels and noradrenergic supersensitivity. Recent studies have questioned the specificity of

PAF as a distinct clinical entity. Some cases are ganglionic antibody–positive and thus represent a type of AAN. Between 10 and 15% of cases evolve into MSA.

POSTURAL ORTHOSTATIC TACHYCARDIA SYNDROME (POTS)

This syndrome is characterized by symptomatic orthostatic intolerance (not OH) and by either an increase in heart rate to >120 beats/min or an increase of 30 beats/min with standing that subsides on sitting or lying down. Women are affected approximately five times more often than men, and most develop the syndrome between the ages of 15 and 50 years. Approximately half of affected patients report an antecedent viral infection. Syncopal symptoms (lightheadedness, weakness, blurred vision) combined with those of autonomic overactivity (palpitations, tremulousness, nausea) are common. Recurrent unexplained episodes of dysautonomia and fatigue also occur. The pathogenesis is unclear in most cases; hypovolemia, venous pooling, impaired brainstem regulation, or α-receptor supersensitivity may play a role. In one affected individual, a mutation in the NE transporter, which resulted in impaired NE clearance from synapses, was responsible. Some cases are due to an underlying limited autonomic neuropathy. Although ~80% of patients improve, only one-quarter eventually resume their usual daily activities (including exercise and sports). Expansion of fluid volume and postural training (see "Treatment") are initial approaches to treatment. When these approaches are inadequate, midodrine, fludrocortisone, phenobarbital, beta blockers, or clonidine have been used with some success.

INHERITED DISORDERS

There are five known hereditary sensory and autonomic neuropathies (HSAN I–V). The most important ones are HSAN I and HSAN III (Riley-Day syndrome; familial dysautonomia). HSAN I is dominantly inherited and often presents as a distal small-fiber neuropathy (burning feet syndrome). The responsible gene, on chromosome 9q, is designated SPTLC1. SPTLC is an important enzyme in the regulation of ceramide. Cells from HSAN I patients affected by mutation of SPTLCI produce higher-than-normal levels of glucosyl ceramide, perhaps triggering apoptosis.

HSAN III, an autosomal recessive disorder of infants and children that occurs among Ashkenazi Jews, is much less prevalent than HSAN I. Decreased tearing, hyperhidrosis, reduced sensitivity to pain, areflexia, absent fungiform papillae on the tongue, and labile BP may be present. Episodic abdominal crises and fever are common. Pathologic examination of nerves reveals a loss of small myelinated and unmyelinated nerve fibers. The defective gene, named *IKBKAP*, is also located on the long arm of chromosome 9. Pathogenic mutations may prevent normal transcription of important molecules in neural development.

PRIMARY HYPERHIDROSIS

This syndrome presents with excess sweating of the palms of the hands and soles of the feet and affects 0.6 to 1.0% of the population. The etiology is unclear, but there may be a genetic component. While not dangerous, the condition can be socially embarrassing (e.g., shaking hands) or disabling (e.g., inability to write without soiling the paper). Onset of symptoms is usually in adolescence; the condition tends to improve with age. Topical antiperspirants are occasionally helpful. More useful are potent anticholinergic drugs such as glycopyrrolate, 1 to 2 mg tid. T2 ganglionectomy or sympathectomy is successful in >90% of patients with palmar hyperhidrosis. The advent of endoscopic transaxillary T2 sympathectomy has lowered the complication rate of the procedure. The most common postoperative complication is compensatory hyperhidrosis, which improves spontaneously over months; other potential complications include recurrent hyperhidrosis (16%), Horner's syndrome (<2%), gustatory sweating, wound infection, hemothorax, and intercostal neuralgia. Local injection of botulinum toxin has also been used to block cholinergic, postganglionic sympathetic fibers to sweat glands in patients with palmar hyperhidrosis. This approach is limited by the need for repetitive injections (the effect usually lasts 4 months before waning), pain with injection, the high cost of botulinum toxin, and the possibility of temporary intrinsic hand muscle weakness.

MISCELLANEOUS

Other conditions associated with autonomic failure include infections, poisoning (organophosphates), malignancy, and aging. Disorders of the hypothalamus can affect autonomic function and produce abnormalities in temperature control, satiety, sexual function, and circadian rhythms.

REFLEX SYMPATHETIC DYSTROPHY AND CAUSALGIA

The failure to identify a primary role of the ANS in the pathogenesis of these disorders has resulted in a change of nomenclature. Complex regional pain syndrome (CRPS) types I and II are now used in place of reflex sympathetic dystrophy (RSD) and causalgia, respectively.

CRPS type I is a regional pain syndrome that usually develops after tissue trauma. Examples of associated trauma include myocardial infarction, minor shoulder or limb injury, and stroke. *Allodynia* (the perception of a nonpainful stimulus as painful), *hyperpathia* (an exaggerated pain response to a painful stimulus), and spontaneous pain occur. The symptoms are unrelated to the severity of the initial trauma and are not confined to the distribution of a single peripheral nerve. CRPS type II is a regional pain syndrome that develops after injury to a peripheral nerve, usually a major nerve trunk. Spontaneous pain initially develops within the territory of the affected nerve but eventually may spread outside the nerve distribution.

Pain is the primary clinical feature of CRPS. Vasomotor dysfunction, sudomotor abnormalities, or focal edema may occur alone or in combination but must be present for diagnosis. Limb pain syndromes that do not meet these criteria are best classified as "limb pain—not otherwise specified." In CRPS, localized sweating (increased resting sweat output) and changes in blood flow may produce temperature differences between affected and unaffected limbs.

CRPS type I (RSD) has classically been divided into three clinical phases but is now considered to be more variable. Phase I consists of pain and swelling in the distal extremity occurring within weeks to 3 months after the precipitating event. The pain is diffuse, spontaneous, and either burning, throbbing, or aching in quality. The involved extremity is warm and edematous, and the joints are tender. Increased sweating and hair growth develop. In phase II (3 to 6 months after onset), thin, shiny, cool skin appears. After an additional 3 to 6 months (phase III), atrophy of the skin and subcutaneous tissue plus flexion contractures complete the clinical picture.

The natural history of typical CRPS may be more benign than reflected in the literature. A variety of surgical and medical treatments have been developed, with conflicting reports of efficacy. Clinical trials suggest that early mobilization with physical therapy or a brief course of glucocorticoids may be helpful for CRPS type I. Other medical treatments that have been used include the use of adrenergic blockers, nonsteroidal anti-inflammatory drugs (NSAIDs), calcium channel blockers, phenytoin, opioids, and calcitonin. Stellate ganglion blockade is a commonly used invasive therapeutic technique that often provides temporary pain relief, but the efficacy of repetitive blocks is uncertain.

TREATMENT FOR ORTHOSTATIC HYPOTENSION

Management of autonomic failure is aimed at specific treatment of the cause and alleviation of symptoms. Of particular importance is the removal of drugs or amelioration of underlying conditions that cause or aggravate the autonomic symptom. For instance, OH can be caused or aggravated by angiotensin-converting enzyme inhibitors, calcium channel blocking agents, tricyclic antidepressants, levodopa, alcohol, or insulin.

Patient Education

OH can be asymptomatic or symptomatic. Neurogenic OH requires treatment, but only a minority of patients require pharmacologic treatment. All patients should be taught the mechanisms of postural normotension (volume status, resistance and capacitance bed, autoregulation) and the nature of orthostatic stressors (time of day and the influence of meals, heat, standing, and exercise). Patients should learn to recognize orthostatic symptoms early in their evolution (especially subtle cognitive symptoms, weakness, and fatigue) and to modify activities that provoke episodes. Other helpful measures may include keeping a BP log, dietary education (salt/fluids), monitoring urine volume and sodium excretion, or recognizing medications and situations to avoid. Learning physical countermaneuvers that reduce standing OH, practicing postural and resistance training, and learning to manage worsening OH in specific situations and at specific times are helpful measures.

Symptomatic Treatment

Nonpharmacologic approaches are summarized in **Table 22-7**. Adequate intake of salt and fluids to produce a voiding volume between 1.5 to 2.5 L of urine (containing >170 meq of Na+) each 24 h is essential. Sleeping with the head of the bed elevated will minimize the effects of supine nocturnal hypertension. Prolonged recumbency should be avoided when possible. Patients are advised to sit

TABLE 22-7

INITIAL TREATMENT OF ORTHOSTATIC HYPOTENSION (OH)
Patient education: mechanisms and stressors of OH
High-salt diet (10–20 g/d)
High-fluid intake (2 L/D)
Elevate head of bed 10 cm (4 in.)
Maintain postural stimuli
Learn physical countermaneuvers
Correct anemia

with legs dangling over the edge of the bed for several minutes before attempting to stand in the morning; other postural stresses should be similarly approached in a gradual manner. Physical countermaneuvers that can reduce OH include leg-crossing, with maintained contraction of leg muscles for 30 s. Such maneuvers compress leg veins and increase systemic resistance. Compressive garments such as compression stockings and abdominal binders may be helpful; some patients find these uncomfortable. Anemia should be corrected, if necessary, with erythropoietin, administered subcutaneously at doses of 25 to 75 U/kg three times per week. The hematocrit increases after 2 to 6 weeks. A weekly maintenance dose is usually necessary. The increased intravascular volume that accompanies the rise in hematocrit can exacerbate supine hypertension.

If these measures are not sufficient, drug treatment might be necessary. Midodrine is effective but can aggravate supine hypertension at higher doses. The drug is a directly acting α_1-agonist that does not cross the blood-brain barrier. It has a duration of action of 2 to 4 h. The usual dose is 5 to 10 mg orally tid, but some patients respond best to a decremental dose (e.g., 15 mg on awakening, 10 mg at noon, and 5 mg in the afternoon). Midodrine should not be taken after 6 P.M. Side effects include pruritus, uncomfortable piloerection, and supine hypertension. Pyridostigmine appears to improve OH without aggravating supine hypertension by enhancing ganglionic transmission (maximal when orthostatic, minimal supine). Fludrocortisone will reduce OH, but it aggravates supine hypertension. At doses between 0.1 mg/d and 0.3 mg bid orally, it enhances renal sodium conservation and increases the sensitivity of arterioles to NE. Susceptible patients may develop fluid overload, congestive heart failure, supine hypertension, or hypokalemia. Potassium supplements are often necessary with chronic administration of fludrocortisone. Sustained elevations of supine BP >180/110 mmHg should be avoided.

Postprandial OH may respond to several measures. Frequent, small, low-carbohydrate meals may diminish splanchnic shunting of blood after meals and reduce postprandial OH. Prostaglandin inhibitors (ibuprofen or indomethacin) taken with meals or midodrine (10 mg with the meal) can be helpful. The somatostatin analogue octreotide can be useful in the treatment of postprandial syncope by inhibiting the release of gastrointestinal peptides that have vasodilator and hypotensive effects. The subcutaneous dose ranges from 25 μg bid to 100 to 200 μg tid.

The patient should be taught to self-treat transient worsening of OH. Drinking two 250-mL (8-oz) glasses of water can raise standing BP 20 to 30 mmHg for about 2 h, beginning ~20 min after the fluid load. The patient can increase intake of salt and fluids (bouillon treatment), increase use of physical countermaneuvers, temporarily resort to a full-body stocking (compression pressure 30 to 40 mmHg), or increase the dose of midodrine. Supine hypertension (>180/110 mmHg) can be self-treated by avoiding the supine position and reducing fludrocortisone. A daily glass of wine, if requested by the patient, can be taken shortly before bedtime. If these simple measures are not adequate, drugs to be considered include oral hydralazine (25 mg qhs), oral procardia (10 mg qhs), or a nitroglycerin patch.

ACKNOWLEDGMENTS

In the previous edition, Lewis Landsberg and James B. Young contributed the section on the anatomical organization of the autonomic nervous system.

FURTHER READINGS

Burns TM et al: Adynamic ileus in severe Guillain-Barré syndrome. Muscle Nerve 24:963, 2001

Gordon VM et al: Hemodynamic and symptomatic effects of acute interventions on tilt in patients with postural tachycardia syndrome. Clin Auton Res 10:29, 2000

☑ Klein CM et al: The spectrum of autoimmune autonomic neuropathies. Ann Neurol 53:752, 2003

Clinical and serologic features in a case series.

☑ Low PA et al: Autonomic dysfunction in peripheral nerve disease. Muscle Nerve 27:646, 2003

Review of acute and chronic autoimmune neuropathies; approach to the patient.

Pathak A et al: Heat related morbidity in patients with orthostatic hypotension and primary autonomic failure. Mov Disord 66:21, 2005.

Shannon JR et al: Orthostatic intolerance and tachycardia associated with norepinephrine-transporter deficiency. N Engl J Med 342:541, 2000

Singer W et al: Acetylcholinesterase inhibition—a novel approach in the treatment of neurogenic orthostatic hypotension. J Neurol Neurosurg Psychiatry 74:1294, 2003

☑ Thaisetthawatkul P et al: Autonomic dysfunction in dementia with Lewy bodies. Neurology 62(10):1804, 2004

Description of orthostatic hypotension and sweating abnormalities in dementia with Lewy bodies.

Vernino S et al: Autoantibodies to ganglionic acetylcholine receptors in autoimmune autonomic neuropathies. N Engl J Med 343:847, 2000

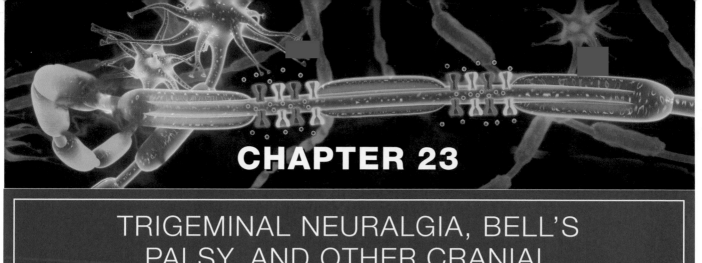

CHAPTER 23

TRIGEMINAL NEURALGIA, BELL'S PALSY, AND OTHER CRANIAL NERVE DISORDERS

M. Flint Beal
Stephen L. Hauser

Symptoms and signs of cranial nerve pathology are common in internal medicine. They often develop in the context of a widespread neurologic disturbance, and in such situations cranial nerve involvement may represent the initial manifestation of the illness. In other disorders, involvement is largely restricted to one or several cranial nerves; these distinctive disorders are reviewed in this chapter. Disorders of ocular movement are discussed in Chap. 11; disorders of hearing in Chap. 12; and vertigo and disorders of vestibular function in Chap. 9.

FACIAL PAIN OR NUMBNESS

ANATOMICAL CONSIDERATIONS

The trigeminal (fifth cranial) nerve supplies sensation to the skin of the face and anterior half of the head (**Fig. 23-1**). Its motor part innervates the masseter and pterygoid masticatory muscles.

TRIGEMINAL NEURALGIA (TIC DOULOUREUX)

Clinical Manifestations

Trigeminal neuralgia is characterized by excruciating paroxysms of pain in the lips, gums, cheek, or chin and, very rarely, in the distribution of the ophthalmic division of the fifth nerve. The pain seldom lasts more than a few seconds or a minute or two but may be so intense that the patient winces, hence the term *tic*. The paroxysms, experienced as single jabs or clusters, tend to recur frequently, both day and night, for several weeks at a time. They may occur spontaneously or with movements of affected areas evoked by speaking, chewing, or smiling. Another characteristic feature is the presence of trigger zones, typically on the face, lips, or tongue, that provoke attacks; patients may report that tactile stimuli—e.g., washing the face, brushing the teeth, or exposure to a draft of air—generate excruciating pain. *An essential feature of trigeminal neuralgia is that objective signs of sensory loss cannot be demonstrated on examination.*

Trigeminal neuralgia is relatively common, with an estimated annual incidence of 4.5 per 100,000 individuals. Middle-aged and elderly persons are affected primarily, and ~60% of cases occur in women. Onset is typically sudden, and bouts tend to persist for weeks or months before remitting spontaneously. Remissions may be longlasting, but in most patients the disorder ultimately recurs.

Pathophysiology

Symptoms result from ectopic generation of action potentials in pain-sensitive afferent fibers of the fifth cranial nerve root just before it enters the lateral surface of the pons. Compression or other pathology in the nerve

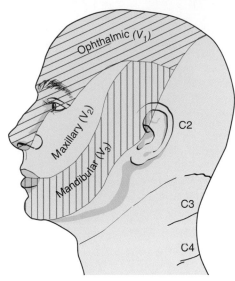

FIGURE 23-1

The three major sensory divisions of the trigeminal nerve consist of the ophthalmic, maxillary, and mandibular nerves.

leads to demyelination of large myelinated fibers that do not themselves carry pain sensation but become hyperexcitable and electrically coupled with smaller unmyelinated or poorly myelinated pain fibers in close proximity; this may explain why tactile stimuli, conveyed via the large myelinated fibers, can stimulate paroxysms of pain. Compression of the trigeminal nerve root by a blood vessel, most often the superior cerebellar artery or on occasion a tortuous vein, is the source of trigeminal neuralgia in a substantial proportion of patients. In cases of vascular compression, age-related brain sagging and increased vascular thickness and tortuosity may explain the prevalence of trigeminal neuralgia in later life.

Differential Diagnosis

Trigeminal neuralgia must be distinguished from other causes of face and head pain (Chap. 5) and from pain arising from diseases of the jaw, teeth, or sinuses. Pain from migraine or cluster headache tends to be deep seated and steady, unlike the superficial stabbing quality of trigeminal neuralgia; rarely, cluster headache is associated with trigeminal neuralgia, a syndrome known as *cluster-tic.* In temporal arteritis, superficial facial pain is present but is not typically shock-like, the patient frequently complains of myalgias and other systemic symptoms, and an elevated erythrocyte sedimentation rate (ESR) is usually present. When trigeminal neuralgia develops in a young adult or is bilateral, multiple sclerosis is a key consideration, and in such cases the cause is a demyelinating plaque at the root entry zone of the fifth nerve in the pons; often,

evidence of facial sensory loss can be found on careful examination. Cases that are secondary to mass lesions—such as aneurysms, neurofibromas, or meningiomas—also usually produce objective signs of sensory loss in the trigeminal nerve distribution (trigeminal neuropathy, see below).

Laboratory Evaluation

An ESR is indicated if temporal arteritis is suspected. In typical cases of trigeminal neuralgia, neuroimaging studies are not necessary.

TREATMENT FOR FACIAL PAIN

Drug therapy with carbamazepine is effective in ~50 to 75% of patients. Carbamazepine should be started as a single daily dose of 100 mg taken with food, and increased gradually (by 100 mg daily every 1 to 2 days) until substantial (>50%) pain relief is achieved. Most patients require a maintenance dose of 200 mg qid. Doses >1200 mg daily provide no additional benefit. Dizziness, imbalance, sedation, and rare cases of agranulocytosis are the most important side effects of carbamazepine. If treatment is effective, it is usually continued for ~1 month and then tapered as tolerated. If carbamazepine is not well tolerated or is ineffective, phenytoin, 300 to 400 mg daily, can be tried. Baclofen may also be administered, either alone or in combination with carbamazepine or phenytoin. The initial dose is 5 to 10 mg tid, gradually increasing as needed to 20 mg qid.

If drug treatment fails, surgical therapy should be offered. The most widely applied procedure creates a heat lesion of the trigeminal (gasserian) ganglion or nerve, a method termed *radiofrequency thermal rhizotomy.* Injection of glycerol in Meckel's cave is a method preferred by some surgeons. Either procedure produces short-term relief in >95% of patients; however, long-term studies indicate that pain recurs in a substantial percentage of treated patients. Complications are infrequent in experienced hands. These procedures result in partial numbness of the face and carry a risk of corneal denervation with secondary keratitis when used for first-division trigeminal neuralgia.

A third treatment, microvascular decompression, requires a suboccipital craniotomy. This procedure has a >70% efficacy rate and a low rate of pain recurrence in responders; in a small number of cases, there is perioperative damage to the eighth or seventh nerve. High-resolution magnetic resonance angiography may be useful preoperatively to visualize the relationships between the fifth cranial nerve root and nearby blood vessels.

TRIGEMINAL NEUROPATHY

A variety of diseases may affect the trigeminal nerve (**Table 23-1**). Most present with sensory loss on the face or with weakness of the jaw muscles. Deviation of the jaw on opening indicates weakness of the pterygoids on the side to which the jaw deviates. Some cases are due to Sjögren's syndrome or a collagen-vascular disease such as systemic lupus erythematosus, scleroderma, or mixed connective tissue disease. Among infectious causes, herpes zoster and leprosy should be considered. Tumors of the middle cranial fossa (meningiomas), of the trigeminal nerve (schwannomas), or of the base of the skull (metastatic tumors) may cause a combination of motor and sensory signs. Lesions in the cavernous sinus can affect the first and second divisions of the trigeminal nerve, and lesions of the superior orbital fissure can affect the first (ophthalmic) division; the accompanying corneal anesthesia increases the risk of ulceration (neurokeratitis).

Loss of sensation over the chin (mental neuropathy) can be the only manifestation of systemic malignancy. Rarely, an idiopathic form of trigeminal neuropathy is observed. It is characterized by numbness and paresthesia, sometimes bilaterally, with loss of sensation in the territory of the trigeminal nerve but without weakness of the jaw. Gradual recovery is the rule. Tonic spasm of the masticatory muscles, known as *trismus*, is symptomatic of tetanus or may occur in patients treated with phenothiazine drugs.

FACIAL WEAKNESS

ANATOMICAL CONSIDERATIONS (Fig. 23-2)

The seventh cranial nerve supplies all the muscles concerned with facial expression. The sensory component is small (the nervus intermedius); it conveys taste sensation from the anterior two-thirds of the tongue and probably cutaneous impulses from the anterior wall of the external auditory canal. The motor nucleus of the seventh nerve lies anterior and lateral to the abducens nucleus. After leaving the pons, the seventh nerve enters the internal auditory meatus with the acoustic nerve. The nerve continues its course in its own bony channel, the facial canal, and exits from the skull via the stylomastoid foramen. It then passes through the parotid gland and subdivides to supply the facial muscles.

A complete interruption of the facial nerve at the stylomastoid foramen paralyzes all muscles of facial expression. The corner of the mouth droops, the creases and skin folds are effaced, the forehead is unfurrowed, and the eyelids will not close. Upon attempted closure of the lids, the eye on the paralyzed side rolls upward (*Bell's phenomenon*). The lower lid sags and falls away from the conjunctiva, permitting tears to spill over the cheek. Food collects between the teeth and lips, and saliva may dribble from the corner of the mouth. The patient complains of a heaviness or numbness in the face, but sensory loss is rarely demonstrable and taste is intact.

If the lesion is in the middle ear portion, taste is lost over the anterior two-thirds of the tongue on the same side. If the nerve to the stapedius is interrupted, there is hyperacusis (sensitivity to loud sounds). Lesions in the internal auditory meatus may affect the adjacent auditory and vestibular nerves, causing deafness, tinnitus, or dizziness. Intrapontine lesions that paralyze the face usually affect the abducens nucleus as well, and often the corticospinal and sensory tracts.

If the peripheral facial paralysis has existed for some time and recovery of motor function is incomplete, a continuous diffuse contraction of facial muscles may appear. The palpebral fissure becomes narrowed, and the nasolabial fold deepens. Attempts to move one group of facial muscles may result in contraction of all (associated movements, or *synkinesis*). Facial spasms, initiated by movements of the face, may develop (*hemifacial spasm*). Anomalous regeneration of seventh nerve fibers may result in other troublesome phenomena. If fibers originally

TABLE 23-1

TRIGEMINAL NERVE DISORDERS	
Nuclear (brainstem) lesions	Peripheral nerve lesions
Multiple sclerosis	Nasopharyngeal
Stroke	carcinoma
Syringobulbia	Trauma
Glioma	Guillain-Barré syndrome
Lymphoma	Sjögren's syndrome
Preganglionic lesions	Collagen-vascular diseases
Acoustic neuroma	Sarcoidosis
Meningioma	Leprosy
Metastasis	Drugs (stilbamidine,
Chronic meningitis	trichloroethylene)
Cavernous carotid	Idiopathic trigeminal
aneurysm	neuropathy
Gasserian ganglion lesions	
Trigeminal neuroma	
Herpes zoster	
Infection (spread from otitis	
media or mastoiditis)	

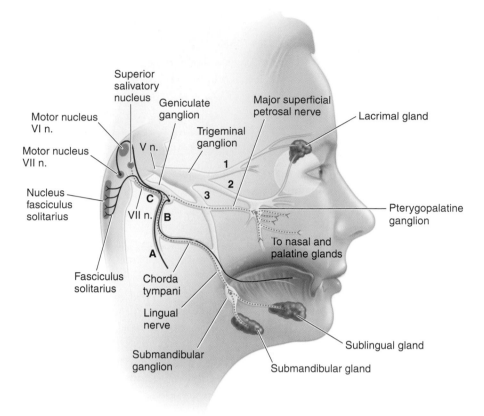

FIGURE 23-2

The facial nerve. A, B, and C denote lesions of the facial nerve at the stylomastoid foramen, distal and proximal to the geniculate ganglion, respectively. Green lines indicate the parasympathetic fibers, red line indicates motor fibers, and purple lines indicate visceral afferent fibers (taste). (*Adapted from Carpenter, 1978.*)

connected with the orbicularis oculi come to innervate the orbicularis oris, closure of the lids may cause a retraction of the mouth, or if fibers originally connected with muscles of the face later innervate the lacrimal gland, anomalous tearing ("crocodile tears") may occur with any activity of the facial muscles, such as eating. Another facial synkinesia is triggered by jaw opening, causing closure of the eyelids on the side of the facial palsy (jaw-winking).

BELL'S PALSY

The most common form of facial paralysis is *Bell's palsy.* The annual incidence of this idiopathic disorder is between 11 and 40 per 100,000 annually, or about 1 in 60 persons in a lifetime.

Clinical Manifestations

The onset of Bell's palsy is fairly abrupt, maximal weakness being attained by 48 h as a general rule. Pain behind the ear may precede the paralysis for a day or two. Taste sensation may be lost unilaterally, and hyperacusis

may be present. In some cases there is mild cerebrospinal fluid lymphocytosis. Magnetic resonance imaging (MRI) may reveal swelling and uniform enhancement of the geniculate ganglion and facial nerve, and, in some cases, entrapment of the swollen nerve in the temporal bone. Approximately 80% of patients recover within a few weeks or months. Electromyography may be of some prognostic value; evidence of denervation after 10 days indicates that there has been axonal degeneration and that there will be a long delay (3 months, as a rule) before regeneration occurs and that it may be incomplete. The presence of incomplete paralysis in the first week is the most favorable prognostic sign.

Pathophysiology

Bell's palsy is associated with the presence of herpes simplex virus type 1 DNA in endoneurial fluid and posterior auricular muscle, suggesting that a reactivation of this virus in the geniculate ganglion may be responsible. However, a causal role for herpes simplex virus in Bell's palsy is unproven.

Differential Diagnosis

There are many other causes of facial palsy that must be considered in the differential diagnosis of Bell's palsy. Tumors that invade the temporal bone (carotid body, cholesteatoma, dermoid) may produce a facial palsy, but the onset is insidious and the course progressive. The *Ramsay Hunt syndrome,* presumably due to herpes zoster of the geniculate ganglion, consists of a severe facial palsy associated with a vesicular eruption in the pharynx, external auditory canal, and other parts of the cranial integument; often the eighth cranial nerve is affected as well. *Acoustic neuromas* frequently involve the facial nerve by local compression. Infarcts, demyelinating lesions of multiple sclerosis, and tumors are the common pontine lesions that interrupt the facial nerve fibers; other signs of brainstem involvement are usually present. Bilateral facial paralysis (facial diplegia) occurs in *Guillain-Barré syndrome* (Chap. 35) and also in a form of sarcoidosis known as *uveoparotid fever (Heerfordt syndrome).* Lyme disease is a frequent cause of facial palsies in endemic areas. The rare *Melkersson-Rosenthal syndrome* consists of a triad of recurrent facial paralysis, recurrent—and eventually permanent—facial (particularly labial) edema, and less constantly, plication of the tongue; its cause is unknown. Leprosy frequently involves the facial nerve, and facial neuropathy may also occur in diabetes mellitus.

All these forms of nuclear or peripheral facial palsy must be distinguished from the supranuclear type. In the latter, the frontalis and orbicularis oculi muscles are involved less than those of the lower part of the face, since the upper facial muscles are innervated by corticobulbar pathways from both motor cortices, whereas the lower facial muscles are innervated only by the opposite hemisphere. In supranuclear lesions there may be a dissociation of emotional and voluntary facial movements, and often some degree of paralysis of the arm and leg or an aphasia (in dominant hemisphere lesions) is conjoined.

Laboratory Evaluation

The diagnosis of Bell's palsy can usually be made clinically in patients with (1) a typical presentation, (2) no risk factors or preexisting symptoms for other causes of facial paralysis, (3) absence of cutaneous lesions of herpes zoster in the external ear canal, and (4) a normal neurologic examination with the exception of the facial nerve. Particular attention to the eighth cranial nerve, which courses near to the facial nerve in the pontomedullary junction and in the temporal bone, and to other cranial nerves is essential. In atypical or uncertain cases, an ESR, testing for diabetes mellitus, a Lyme titer, angiotensin-converting enzyme and chest x-ray for possible sarcoidosis, or MRI scanning may be indicated.

TREATMENT FOR BELL'S PALSY

Symptomatic measures include (1) the use of paper tape to depress the upper eyelid during sleep and prevent corneal drying, and (2) massage of the weakened muscles. A course of glucocorticoids, given as prednisone 60 to 80 mg daily during the first 5 days and then tapered over the next 5 days, appears to shorten the recovery period and modestly improve the functional outcome. In one double-blind study, patients treated within 3 days of onset with both prednisone and acyclovir (400 mg five times daily for 10 days) had a better outcome than patients treated with prednisone alone.

OTHER MOTOR DISORDERS OF THE FACE

Hemifacial spasm consists of painless irregular involuntary contractions on one side of the face. Symptoms may develop as a sequela to Bell's palsy but may also be due to an irritative lesion of the facial nerve (e.g., an acoustic neuroma, an aberrant artery that compresses the nerve, or a basilar artery aneurysm). However, in the most common form of hemifacial spasm, the cause and pathology are unknown. Hemifacial spasm can be treated successfully with carbamazepine or, if this drug fails, with baclofen. Refractory cases due to vascular compression usually respond to surgical decompression of the facial nerve. *Blepharospasm* is an involuntary recurrent spasm of both eyelids that occurs in elderly persons as an isolated phenomenon or with varying degrees of spasm of other facial muscles. Severe, persistent cases of blepharospasm can be treated by local injection of botulinum toxin into the orbicularis oculi; the spasms are relieved for 3 to 4 months, and the injections can be repeated. *Facial myokymia* refers to a fine rippling activity of the facial muscles; it may be caused by multiple sclerosis or follow Guillain-Barré syndrome (Chap. 35).

Facial hemiatrophy occurs mainly in females and is characterized by a disappearance of fat in the dermal and subcutaneous tissues on one side of the face. It usually begins in adolescence or early adult years and is slowly progressive. In its advanced form, the affected side of the face is gaunt, and the skin is thin, wrinkled, and rather brown. The facial hair may turn white and fall out, and the sebaceous glands become atrophic. The muscles and bones are not involved as a rule. Sometimes the atrophy becomes bilateral. The condition is a form of lipodystrophy. Treatment is cosmetic, consisting of transplantation of skin and subcutaneous fat.

OTHER CRANIAL NERVE DISORDERS

GLOSSOPHARYNGEAL NEURALGIA

This form of neuralgia involves the ninth (glossopharyngeal) and sometimes portions of the tenth (vagus) cranial nerves. It resembles trigeminal neuralgia in many respects but is much less common. The pain is intense and paroxysmal; it originates on one side of the throat, approximately in the tonsillar fossa. In some cases the pain is localized in the ear or may radiate from the throat to the ear because of involvement of the tympanic branch of the glossopharyngeal nerve. Spasms of pain may be initiated by swallowing or coughing. There is no demonstrable motor or sensory deficit; the glossopharyngeal nerve supplies taste sensation to the posterior third of the tongue and, together with the vagus nerve, sensation to the posterior pharynx. Cardiac symptoms—bradycardia, hypotension, and fainting—have been reported. Medical therapy is similar to that for trigeminal neuralgia, and carbamazepine is generally the first choice. If drug therapy is unsuccessful, surgical procedures, including microvascular decompression if vascular compression is evident, or rhizotomy of glossopharyngeal and vagal fibers in the jugular bulb is frequently successful.

Very rarely, herpes zoster involves the glossopharyngeal nerve. Glossopharyngeal neuropathy in conjunction with vagus and accessory nerve palsies may also occur with a tumor or aneurysm in the posterior fossa or in the jugular foramen. Hoarseness due to vocal cord paralysis, some difficulty in swallowing, deviation of the soft palate to the intact side, anesthesia of the posterior wall of the pharynx, and weakness of the upper part of the trapezius and sternocleidomastoid muscles make up the jugular foramen syndrome (**Table 23–2**).

DYSPHAGIA AND DYSPHONIA

When the intracranial portion of one vagus (tenth cranial) nerve is interrupted, the soft palate droops ipsilaterally and does not rise in phonation. There is loss of the gag reflex on the affected side, as well as of the "curtain movement" of the lateral wall of the pharynx, whereby the faucial pillars move medially as the palate rises in saying "ah." The voice is hoarse and slightly nasal, and the vocal cord lies immobile midway between abduction and adduction. Loss of sensation at the external auditory meatus and the posterior pinna may also be present.

The pharyngeal branches of both vagal nerves may be affected in diphtheria; the voice has a nasal quality, and regurgitation of liquids through the nose occurs during the act of swallowing.

The vagus nerve may be involved at the meningeal level by neoplastic and infectious processes and within

TABLE 23-2

CRANIAL NERVE SYNDROMES

SITE	CRANIAL NERVES	USUAL CAUSE
Sphenoid fissure (superior orbital)	III, IV, first division V, VI	Invasive tumors of sphenoid bone; aneurysms
Lateral wall of cavernous sinus	III, IV, first division V, VI, often with proptosis	Infection, thrombosis, aneurysm, or fistula of cavernous sinus; invasive tumors from sinuses and sella turcica; benign granuloma responsive to glucocorticoids
Retrosphenoid space	II, III, IV, V, VI	Large tumors of middle cranial fossa
Apex of petrous bone	V, VI	Petrositis; tumors of petrous bone
Internal auditory meatus	VII, VIII	Tumors of petrous bone (dermoids, etc.); infectious processes; acoustic neuroma
Pontocerebellar angle	V, VII, VIII, and sometimes IX	Acoustic neuroma; meningioma
Jugular foramen	IX, X, XI	Tumors and aneurysms
Posterior laterocondylar space	IX, X, XI, XII	Tumors of parotid gland and carotid body and metastatic tumors
Posterior retroparotid space	IX, X, XI, XII and Horner syndrome	Tumors of parotid gland, carotid body, lymph nodes; metastatic tumor; tuberculous adenitis

the medulla by tumors, vascular lesions (e.g., the lateral medullary syndrome), and motor neuron disease. This nerve may be involved by infection with herpes zoster virus. Polymyositis and dermatomyositis, which cause hoarseness and dysphagia by direct involvement of laryngeal and pharyngeal muscles, may be confused with diseases of the vagus nerves. Also, dysphagia is a symptom in some patients with myotonic dystrophy.

The recurrent laryngeal nerves, especially the left, are most often damaged as a result of intrathoracic disease. Aneurysm of the aortic arch, an enlarged left atrium, and tumors of the mediastinum and bronchi are much more frequent causes of an isolated vocal cord palsy than are intracranial disorders. However, a substantial number of cases of recurrent laryngeal palsy remain idiopathic.

When confronted with a case of laryngeal palsy, the physician must attempt to determine the site of the lesion. If it is intramedullary, there are usually other signs, such as ipsilateral cerebellar dysfunction, loss of pain and temperature sensation over the ipsilateral face and contralateral arm and leg, and an ipsilateral Horner syndrome. If the lesion is extramedullary, the glossopharyngeal and spinal accessory nerves are frequently involved (jugular foramen syndrome). If it is extracranial in the posterior laterocondylar or retroparotid space, there may be a combination of ninth, tenth, eleventh, and twelfth cranial nerve palsies and a Horner syndrome (Table 23-2). If there is no sensory loss over the palate and pharynx and no palatal weakness or dysphagia, the lesion is below the origin of the pharyngeal branches, which leave the vagus nerve high in the cervical region; the usual site of disease is then the mediastinum.

NECK WEAKNESS

Isolated involvement of the accessory (eleventh cranial) nerve can occur anywhere along its route, resulting in partial or complete paralysis of the sternocleidomastoid and trapezius muscles. More commonly, involvement occurs in combination with deficits of the ninth and tenth cranial nerves in the jugular foramen or after exit from the skull (Table 23-2). An idiopathic form of accessory neuropathy, akin to Bell's palsy, has been described, and it may be recurrent in some cases. Most but not all patients recover.

TONGUE PARALYSIS

The hypoglossal (twelfth cranial) nerve supplies the ipsilateral muscles of the tongue. The nucleus of the nerve or its fibers of exit may be involved by intramedullary lesions such as tumor, poliomyelitis, or most often motor neuron disease. Lesions of the basal meninges and the occipital bones (platybasia, invagination of occipital condyles, Paget's disease) may compress the nerve in its extramedullary course or in the hypoglossal canal.

Isolated lesions of unknown cause can occur. Atrophy and fasciculation of the tongue develop weeks to months after interruption of the nerve.

MULTIPLE CRANIAL NERVE PALSIES

Several cranial nerves may be affected by the same disease process. In this situation, the main clinical problem is to determine whether the lesion lies within the brainstem or outside it. Lesions that lie on the surface of the brainstem are characterized by involvement of adjacent cranial nerves (often occurring in succession) and late and rather slight involvement of the long sensory and motor pathways and segmental structures lying within the brainstem. The opposite is true of primary lesions within the brainstem. The extramedullary lesion is more likely to cause bone erosion or enlargement of the foramens of exit of cranial nerves. The intramedullary lesion involving cranial nerves often produces a crossed sensory or motor paralysis (cranial nerve signs on one side of the body and tract signs on the opposite side).

Involvement of multiple cranial nerves outside the brainstem is frequently the result of diabetes or trauma, localized infections such as herpes zoster, infectious and noninfectious (especially carcinomatous) causes of meningitis (Chap. 29), granulomatous diseases such as Wegener's granulomatosis, Behçet's disease, enlarging saccular aneurysms, or tumors. Among the tumors, nasopharyngeal cancers, lymphomas, neurofibromas, meningiomas, chordomas, cholesteatomas, carcinomas, and sarcomas have all been observed to involve a succession of lower cranial nerves. Owing to their anatomical relationships, the multiple cranial nerve palsies form a number of distinctive syndromes, listed in Table 23-2. Sarcoidosis is the cause of some cases of multiple cranial neuropathy, and chronic glandular tuberculosis the cause of a few others. Platybasia, basilar invagination of the skull, and the adult Chiari malformation are additional causes. A purely motor disorder without atrophy always raises the question of myasthenia gravis (Chap. 36). As noted above, Guillain-Barré syndrome commonly affects the facial nerves bilaterally. In the Fisher variant of the Guillain-Barré syndrome, oculomotor paresis occurs with ataxia and areflexia in the limbs (Chap. 35). Wernicke encephalopathy can cause a severe ophthalmoplegia combined with other brainstem signs.

The *cavernous sinus syndrome* (**Fig. 23-3**) is a distinctive and frequently life-threatening disorder. It often presents as orbital or facial pain; orbital swelling and chemosis due to occlusion of the ophthalmic veins; fever; oculomotor neuropathy affecting the third, fourth, and sixth cranial nerves; and trigeminal neuropathy affecting the ophthalmic (V_1) and occasionally the maxillary (V_2) divisions of the trigeminal nerve. Cavernous sinus thrombosis, often se-

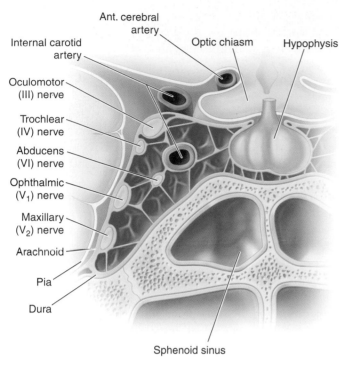

Internal carotid artery
Ant. cerebral artery
Optic chiasm
Hypophysis
Oculomotor (III) nerve
Trochlear (IV) nerve
Abducens (VI) nerve
Ophthalmic (V₁) nerve
Maxillary (V₂) nerve
Arachnoid
Pia
Dura
Sphenoid sinus

FIGURE 23-3
Anatomy of the cavernous sinus in coronal section, illustrating the location of the cranial nerves in relation to the vascular sinus, internal carotid artery (which loops anteriorly to the section), and surrounding structures.

condary to infection from orbital cellulitis (frequently *Staphylococcus aureus*), a cutaneous source on the face, or sinusitis (especially with mucormycosis in diabetic patients), is the most frequent cause; other etiologies include aneurysm of the carotid artery, a carotid-cavernous fistula (orbital bruit may be present), meningioma, nasopharyngeal carcinoma, other tumors, or an idiopathic granulomatous disorder (Tolosa-Hunt syndrome). The two cavernous sinuses directly communicate via intercavernous channels, thus involvement on one side may extend to become bilateral. Early diagnosis is essential, especially when due to infection, and treatment depends upon the underlying etiology. In infectious cases, prompt administration of broad-spectrum antibiotics, drainage of any abscess cavities, and

identification of the offending organism is essential. Anticoagulant therapy may benefit cases of primary thrombosis. Repair or occlusion of the carotid artery may be required for treatment of fistulas or aneurysms. The Tolosa-Hunt syndrome generally responds to glucocorticoids.

An idiopathic form of multiple cranial nerve involvement on one or both sides of the face is occasionally seen. The syndrome consists of a subacute onset of boring facial pain, followed by paralysis of motor cranial nerves. The clinical features overlap those of the Tolosa-Hunt syndrome and appear to be due to idiopathic inflammation of the dura mater, which may be visualized by MRI. The syndrome is frequently responsive to glucocorticoids.

ACKNOWLEDGMENT

The authors acknowledge the contributions of Dr. Joseph B. Martin to this chapter in previous editions.

FURTHER READINGS

CARPENTER MB: *Core Text of Neuroanatomy,* 2d ed. Baltimore, Williams & Wilkins, 1978

GILDEN DH: Clinical practice. Bell's palsy. N Engl J Med 23:1323, 2004

GROGAN PM, GRONSETH GS: Practice parameter: Steroids, acyclovir, and surgery for Bell's palsy (an evidence-based review). Report of the Quality Standards Subcommittee of the American Academy of Neurology. Neurology 56:830, 2001

Evidence-based guidelines for treatment of Bell's palsy.

LOVE S, COAKHAM HB: Trigeminal neuralgia: Pathology and pathogenesis. Brain 124:2347, 2002

PATEL A et al: Microvascular decompression in the management of glossopharyngeal neuralgia: Analysis of 217 cases. Neurosurgery 50:705, 2002

SWEENEY CJ, GILDEN DH: Ramsay Hunt syndrome. J Neurol Neurosurg Psychiatry 71:149, 2001

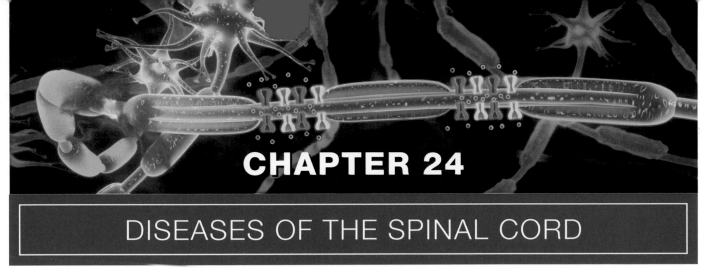

CHAPTER 24

DISEASES OF THE SPINAL CORD

Stephen L. Hauser

Allan H. Ropper

Diseases of the spinal cord are frequently devastating. They can produce quadriplegia, paraplegia, and sensory deficits far beyond the damage they would inflict elsewhere in the nervous system because the spinal cord contains, in a small cross-sectional area, almost the entire motor output and sensory input of the trunk and limbs. Many spinal cord diseases are reversible if recognized and treated at an early stage (**Table 24-1**); thus, they are among the most critical of neurologic emergencies. The efficient use of diagnostic procedures, guided by a knowledge of the anatomy and the clinical features of common spinal cord diseases, is required for a successful outcome.

APPROACH TO THE PATIENT WITH SPINAL CORD DISEASE

Spinal Cord Anatomy Relevant to Clinical Signs

The spinal cord is a thin, tubular extension of the central nervous system contained within the bony spinal canal. It originates at the medulla and continues caudally to the conus medullaris at the lumbar level; its fibrous extension, the filum terminale, terminates at the coccyx. The adult spinal cord is ~46 cm (18 in.) long, oval or round in shape, and enlarged in the cervical and lumbar regions, where neurons that innervate the upper and lower extremities, respectively, are located. The white matter tracts containing ascending sensory and descending motor pathways are located peripherally, whereas nerve cell bodies are clustered in an inner region shaped like a four-leaf clover that surrounds the central canal (anatomically an extension of the fourth ventricle). The membranes that cover the spinal cord—the pia, arachnoid, and dura—are continuous with those of the brainstem and cerebral hemispheres.

The spinal cord has 31 segments, each defined by an exiting ventral motor root and entering dorsal sensory root. During embryologic development, growth of the cord lags behind that of the vertebral column, and in the adult the spinal cord (conus segments) ends at approximately the first lumbar vertebral body. The lower spinal nerves take an increasingly downward course to exit via intervertebral foramina. The first seven pairs of cervical spinal nerves exit above the same-numbered vertebral bodies,

TABLE 24-1

SOME TREATABLE SPINAL CORD DISORDERS

Compressive
  Epidural, intradural, or intramedullary neoplasm
  Epidural abscess
  Epidural hemorrhage
  Cervical spondylosis
  Herniated disc
  Posttraumatic compression by fractured or
    displaced vertebra or hemorrhage
Vascular
  Arteriovenous malformation
  Antiphospholipid syndrome and other hypercoagulable
    states
Inflammatory
  Multiple sclerosis including neuromyelitis optica
  Transverse myelitis
  Sarcoidosis
  Vasculitis
Infectious
  Viral: VZV, HSV-1 and -2, CMV, HIV, HTLV-I, others
  Bacterial and mycobacterial: *Borrelia, Listeria,*
    syphilis, others
  Mycoplasma pneumoniae
  Parasitic: schistosomiasis, toxoplasmosis
Developmental
  Syringomyelia
  Meningomyelocoele
  Tethered cord syndrome
Metabolic
  Vitamin B_{12} deficiency (subacute combined
    degeneration)
  Adrenomyeloneuropathy

Note: VZV, varicella-zoster virus; HSV, herpes simplex virus; CMV cytomegalovirus; HT human T cell lymphotropic virus.

whereas all the subsequent nerves exit below the same-numbered vertebral bodies; this situation is due to the presence of eight cervical spinal cord segments but only seven cervical vertebrae. The relationship between spinal cord segments and the corresponding vertebral bodies is shown in **Table 24-2.** These relationships assume particular importance for localization of lesions that cause spinal cord compression; a T10 spinal cord level, for example, indicates involvement of the cord adjacent to the seventh or eighth thoracic vertebral body. In addition, at every level the main ascending and descending tracts are somatotopically organized with a laminated distribution that reflects the origin or destination of nerve fibers.

LEVEL OF THE LESION (Fig. 24-1)

The presence of a horizontally defined level below which sensory, motor, and/or autonomic function

TABLE 24-2

SPINAL CORD LEVELS RELATIVE TO THE VERTEBRAL BODIES

SPINAL CORD LEVEL	CORRESPONDING VERTEBRAL BODY
Upper cervical	Same as cord level
Lower cervical	1 level higher
Upper thoracic	2 levels higher
Lower thoracic	2 to 3 levels higher
Lumbar	T10-T12
Sacral	T12-L1
Coccygeal	L1

is impaired is a hallmark of spinal cord disease. A sensory level is sought by asking the patient to identify a pinprick or cold stimulus (i.e., a dry tuning fork after immersion in cold water) applied to the low back and sequentially moved up toward the neck on each side. The presence of a sensory level indicates damage to the spinothalamic tract, but the lesion is located one to two segments above the perceived level of a unilateral spinal cord lesion and at the level of the lesion when bilateral. That is the result of the ascent of second-order sensory fibers, which originate in the dorsal horn, proceed to cross anterior to the central canal, and join the opposite spinothalamic tract. Lesions that transect the descending corticospinal and other motor tracts cause paraplegia or quadriplegia, with increased muscle tone, exaggerated deep tendon reflexes, and extensor plantar signs (the upper motor neuron syndrome). Such lesions also typically produce autonomic disturbances consisting of disturbed sweating and bladder, bowel, and sexual dysfunction.

The uppermost level of a spinal cord lesion can also be localized by attention to the *segmental signs* corresponding to disturbed motor or sensory innervation by an individual cord segment. A band of altered sensation (hyperalgesia or hyperpathia) at the upper end of the sensory disturbance, fasciculations or atrophy in muscles innervated by one or several segments, or a diminished or absent deep tendon reflex may be noted. These signs also occur with focal root or peripheral nerve disorders; thus, segmental signs are most useful when they occur with signs of long tract damage. With severe and acute transverse lesions, the limbs initially may be flaccid rather than spastic. This state of "spinal shock" lasts for several days, rarely for weeks, and should not be mistaken for extensive damage to many segments of the cord or for a polyneuropathy.

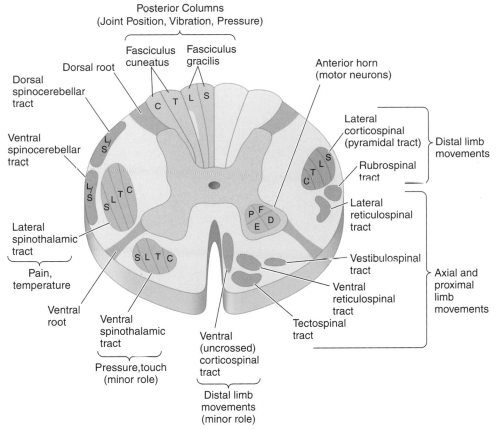

FIGURE 24-1

Transverse section through the spinal cord, composite representation, illustrating the principal ascending (*left*) and descending (*right*) pathways. The lateral and ventral spinothalamic tracts ascend contralateral to the side of the body that is innervated. C, cervical; T, thoracic; L, lumbar; S, sacral; P, proximal; D, distal; F, flexors; E, extensors.

The main features of transverse damage at each level of the spinal cord are summarized below.

Cervical Cord   Extensive lesions near the junction of the cervical cord and medulla are usually fatal owing to involvement of adjacent medullary vasomotor and respiratory centers. Upper cervical cord lesions produce quadriplegia and weakness of the diaphragm. Breathing is possible only by use of accessory muscles of respiration. Lesions at C4-C5 produce quadriplegia; at C5-C6, there is loss of power and reflexes in the biceps; at C7 weakness is found in finger and wrist extensors and triceps; and at C8, finger and wrist flexion are impaired. A Horner's syndrome (miosis, ptosis, and facial hypohidrosis) may accompany a cervical cord lesion at any level.

Thoracic Cord   Lesions here are localized by the sensory level on the trunk and midline back pain if it accompanies the syndrome. The sensory dermatomes of the body are shown in **Fig. 33-1**. useful markers are the nipples (T4) and umbilicus (T10). Leg weakness and disturbances of bladder and bowel function accompany the paralysis. Lesions at T9-T10 paralyze the lower, but not the upper, abdominal muscles, resulting in upward movement of the umbilicus when the abdominal wall contracts (Beevor's sign).

Lumbar Cord   The lumbar and sacral cord segments are small and are situated behind the T12 to L1 vertebrae. Lesions at L2-L4 paralyze flexion and adduction of the thigh, weaken leg extension at the knee, and abolish the patellar reflex. Lesions at L5–S1 paralyze movements of the foot and ankle, flexion at the knee, and extension of the thigh, and abolish the ankle jerk (S1).

Sacral Cord/Conus Medullaris   The conus medullaris is the tapered caudal termination of the spinal cord, comprising the lower sacral and single coccygeal segments. The conus syndrome is distinctive, consisting of bilateral saddle anesthesia (S3–S5), prominent bladder and bowel dysfunction (urinary retention and incontinence with lax anal tone), and impotence. The bulbocavernosus (S2–S4) and anal (S4–S5) reflexes are absent (Chap. 2). Muscle strength is largely preserved. Lesions of the conus must be distinguished from those of the cauda equina, the cluster of nerve roots derived from the lower cord. Cauda equina lesions are characterized by low back or radicular pain, asymmetric leg weakness and sensory loss, variable areflexia in the lower extremities, and relative sparing of bowel and bladder function. Mass lesions in the lower spinal canal often produce a mixed clinical picture in which elements of both cauda equina and conus medullaris syndromes coexist; the typical cause is an ependymoma in that region. Cauda equina syndromes are discussed in Chap. 6.

Special Patterns of Spinal Cord Disease

The location of the major ascending and descending pathways of the spinal cord are shown in Fig. 24-1. Most fiber tracts—including the posterior columns and the spinocerebellar and pyramidal tracts—are situated on the side of the body they innervate. Afferent fibers mediating pain and temperature sensation ascend the spinothalamic tract contralateral to the side they supply. The anatomical relationships of these various fiber tracts produce characteristic clinical syndromes that provide clues to the underlying disease process.

Brown-Sequard Hemicord Syndrome   This consists of ipsilateral weakness (corticospinal tract) and loss of joint position and vibratory sense (posterior column), with contralateral loss of pain and temperature sense (spinothalamic tract) one or two levels below the lesion. Segmental signs, such as radicular pain, muscle atrophy, or loss of a deep tendon reflex, are unilateral. This classic syndrome is rare, and partial forms are more commonly encountered.

Central Cord Syndrome   The central cord syndrome results from damage to the gray matter nerve cells and crossing spinothalamic tracts near the central canal. In the cervical cord, the central cord syndrome produces arm weakness out of proportion to leg weakness and a "dissociated" sensory loss signifying a loss of pain and temperature sense in a cape distribution over the shoulders, lower neck, and upper trunk in contrast to intact light touch, joint position, and vibration sense in these regions. Trauma, syringomyelia, tumors, and anterior spinal artery ischemia are main causes.

Anterior Spinal Artery Syndrome   Infarction of the cord is generally the result of occlusion or diminished flow in this artery. The result is extensive bilateral tissue destruction that spares the posterior columns. All spinal cord functions—motor, sensory, and autonomic—are lost below the level of the lesion, with the striking exception of retained vibration and position sensation.

Lesions of the Foramen Magnum   Partial lesions in this area interrupt decussating pyramidal tract fibers destined for the legs, which cross below those of the arms, resulting in a "crural paresis" of the lower limbs. Compressive lesions near the foramen magnum may produce weakness of the ipsilateral shoulder and arm followed by weakness of the ipsilateral leg, then the contralateral leg, and finally the contralateral arm (an "around the clock" pattern that may begin in any of the four limbs). There is typically suboccipital pain spreading to the neck and shoulders.

Intramedullary and Extramedullary Syndromes   It is useful to differentiate intramedullary processes, arising within the substance of the cord, from extramedullary ones that compress the spinal cord or its vascular supply. The differentiating features are only relative and serve as rough guides to clinical decision-making. With extramedullary lesions, radicular pain is often prominent, and there are early sacral sensory loss (lateral spinothalamic tract) and spastic weakness in the legs (corticospinal tract); this is due to the superficial location of the leg fibers in the corticospinal tract. Intramedullary lesions tend to produce poorly localized burning pain rather than radicular pain and spare sensation in the perineal and sacral areas ("sacral sparing") reflecting the laminated configuration of the spinothalamic tract with these fibers outermost; corticospinal tract signs appear later. Regarding extramedullary lesions, a further distinction is made between extradural and intradural masses, as the former are generally malignant and the latter benign (neurofibroma being the common cause); for this reason, a long duration of symptoms favors an intradural origin.

ACUTE AND SUBACUTE SPINAL CORD DISEASES

The initial symptom is often focal neck or back pain, followed by various combinations of paresthesias, sensory loss, motor weakness, and sphincter disturbance evolving over hours to several days. There may be mild sensory symptoms only or a devastating functional transection of the cord. Partial forms may selectively involve the posterior columns, anterior spinothalamic tracts, or one hemicord. Paresthesias or numbness may begin in the feet and ascend either symmetrically or asymmetrically, earlier in one leg than in the other; these symptoms may initially raise a question of Guillain-Barré syndrome, but involvement of the trunk with a sharply demarcated spinal cord level indicates the myelopathic nature of the process. In severe cases, areflexia indicating spinal shock may be present, but hyperreflexia soon supervenes; persistent areflexic paralysis indicates necrosis over multiple segments of the spinal cord.

APPROACH TO THE PATIENT

DISTINGUISHING COMPRESSIVE FROM NONCOMPRESSIVE MYELOPATHY

The first priority is to identify a treatable mass lesion. The common causes in this category are tumor, epidural abscess or hematoma, herniated disc, or other vertebral pathology. Epidural compression due to malignancy or abscess often causes warning signs of neck or back pain, bladder disturbances, and sensory symptoms that precede the development of paralysis. Spinal subluxation, hemorrhage, and noncompressive etiologies such as infarction are more likely to produce myelopathy without antecedent symptoms. Magnetic resonance imaging (MRI) with contrast of the clinically suspected level of pathology is the initial diagnostic procedure; in some cases it is appropriate to image the entire spine (cervical through sacral regions) to search for additional, clinically silent, lesions. Once compressive lesions have been excluded, noncompressive causes of acute myelopathy that are intrinsic to the cord are considered: primarily vascular, inflammatory, and infectious etiologies.

COMPRESSIVE MYELOPATHIES

Neoplastic Spinal Cord Compression

In adults, most neoplasms are epidural in origin, resulting from metastases to the adjacent spinal bones. The propensity of solid tumors to metastasize to the vertebral column probably reflects the high percentage of bone marrow lo-

cated in the axial skeleton. Almost any malignant tumor can metastasize to the spinal column, with breast, lung, prostate, kidney, lymphoma, and plasma cell dyscrasia being particularly frequent. The thoracic cord is most commonly involved; exceptions are metastases from prostate and ovarian cancer, which occur disproportionately in the sacral and lumbar vertebrae, perhaps resulting from spread through Batson's plexus, a network of veins along the anterior epidural space. Retroperitoneal neoplasms (especially lymphomas or sarcomas) enter the spinal canal through the intervertebral foramina; they produce radicular pain and other signs of root involvement prior to cord compression.

Pain is the initial symptom; it may be either aching and localized or sharp and radiating in quality. The pain typically worsens with movement, coughing, or sneezing and characteristically awakens patients at night. A recent onset of persistent back pain, particularly if in the thoracic spine (which is uncommonly involved by spondylosis), should prompt consideration of vertebral metastasis. Rarely, pain is mild or absent. Pain typically precedes signs of cord compression by weeks or even months. However, once cord compression occurs, it usually advances rapidly. Plain radiographs of the spine and radionuclide bone scans have only a limited role in diagnosis because they do not identify 15 to 20% of metastatic vertebral lesions and fail to detect paravertebral masses that reach the epidural space through the intervertebral foramina. MRI provides excellent anatomical resolution of the site and extent of spinal tumors **(Fig. 24-2)**; MRI has largely replaced computed

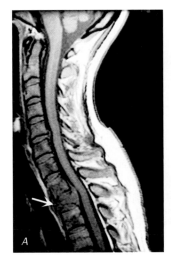
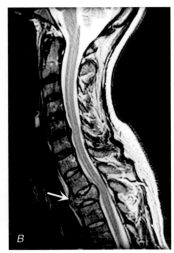

FIGURE 24-2

Epidural spinal cord compression due to breast carcinoma. Sagittal T1-weighted (*A*) and T2-weighted (*B*) MRI scans through the cervicothoracic junction reveal a compression fracture of the second thoracic vertebral body with posterior displacement and compression of the upper thoracic spinal cord. The low-intensity bone marrow signal in *A* signifies replacement by tumor.

tomography (CT) and myelography in the diagnosis of epidural masses. MRI can often distinguish between malignant lesions and other masses—epidural abscess, tuberculoma, or epidural hemorrhage, among others—that present in a similar fashion. Vertebral metastases are usually hypointense relative to a normal bone marrow signal on T1-weighted MRI scans; after the administration of gadolinium, contrast enhancement may "normalize" the appearance of the tumor by increasing its intensity to that of normal bone marrow. Infections of the spinal column (osteomyelitis and related disorders) are distinctive in that, unlike tumor, they may cross the disk space.

It is important to convey to the radiologist an estimate of the urgency of the imaging procedure requested. If signs of spinal cord involvement are present, imaging should be obtained promptly. If there are radicular symptoms but no evidence of myelopathy, it is usually safe, if necessary, to defer imaging for 24 to 48 h. With back or neck pain only, imaging studies may be obtained within a few days. Up to 40% of patients who present with symptomatic disease at one level are found to have asymptomatic epidural disease elsewhere; thus, the length of the spine should be imaged when epidural malignancy is in question.

compression fracture contributes to cord compression. A good response to radiotherapy can be expected in individuals who are ambulatory at presentation; new weakness is prevented, and some recovery of motor function occurs in approximately half of treated patients. Fixed motor deficits—paraplegia or quadriplegia—once established for >12 h, do not usually improve, and beyond 48 h the prognosis for substantial motor recovery is poor.

In contrast to tumors of the epidural space, most intradural mass lesions are slow-growing and benign. Meningiomas and neurofibromas account for most of these lesions, with occasional cases representing chordoma, lipoma, dermoid, or sarcoma. Meningiomas (**Fig. 24-3**) are often located posterior to the thoracic cord or near the foramen magnum, although they can arise from the meninges anywhere along the spinal canal. Neurofibromas are benign tumors of the nerve

TREATMENT FOR SPINAL CORD COMPRESSION

Management includes glucocorticoids to reduce cord edema, local radiotherapy (initiated as early as possible) to the symptomatic lesion, and specific therapy for the underlying tumor type. Glucocorticoids (dexamethasone, 40 mg daily) can be administered before the imaging study if the clinical suspicion is strong and continued at a lower dose (20 mg daily in divided doses) until radiotherapy (a total of 3000 cGy administered in 15 daily fractions) is completed. Radiotherapy appears to be as effective as surgery, even for classically radioresistant metastases. Biopsy of the epidural mass is unnecessary in patients with known preexisting cancer, but the procedure may be indicated if a history of underlying cancer is lacking. Surgery, either decompression or vertebral body resection, should be considered when signs of cord compression worsen despite radiotherapy, when the maximum tolerated dose of radiotherapy has been delivered previously to the site, or when a vertebral

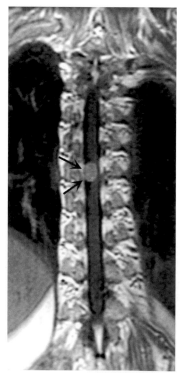

FIGURE 24-3

MRI of a thoracic meningioma. Coronal T1-weighted post-contrast image through the thoracic spinal cord demonstrates intense enhancement of a well-circumscribed extramedullary mass (*arrows*) which displaces the spinal cord to the left, widening the cistern adjacent to the mass.

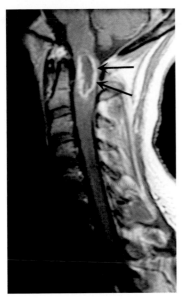

FIGURE 24-4

MRI of an intramedullary astrocytoma. Sagittal T1-weighted post-contrast image through the cervical spine demonstrates expansion of the upper cervical spine by a mass lesion emanating from within the spinal cord at the cervicomedullary junction. Irregular peripheral enhancement occurs within the mass (*arrows*).

sheath that typically arise near the posterior root; when multiple, neurofibromatosis is the likely etiology. Symptoms usually begin with radicular sensory symptoms followed by an asymmetric, progressive spinal cord syndrome. Therapy is by surgical resection.

Primary intramedullary tumors of the spinal cord are uncommon. They typically present as central cord or hemicord syndromes, often in the cervical region; there may be poorly localized burning pain in the extremities and sparing of sacral sensation. In adults, most of these lesions are ependymomas, hemangioblastomas, or low-grade astrocytomas (**Fig. 24-4**). Complete resection of an intramedullary ependymoma is often possible with microsurgical techniques. Debulking of an intramedullary astrocytoma can also be helpful, as these are often slowly growing lesions; the value of adjunctive radiotherapy is uncertain. Secondary (metastatic) intramedullary tumors are seen on most oncology services.

Spinal Epidural Abscess

Spinal epidural abscess presents as a clinical triad of pain, fever, and rapidly progressive weakness. Prompt recognition of this distinctive and treatable process will in most cases prevent permanent sequelae. Aching pain is almost always present, either over the spine or in a radicular pattern. The duration of pain prior to presentation is

generally ≤2 weeks but may on occasion be several months or longer. Fever is usual, accompanied by an elevated white blood cell count and sedimentation rate. As the abscess expands, further spinal cord damage results from venous congestion and thrombosis in the epidural space. Once weakness and other signs of myelopathy appear, progression may be rapid. A more chronic granulomatous form of abscess is also known.

Risk factors include an impaired immune status (diabetes mellitus, renal failure, alcoholism, malignancy), intravenous drug abuse, and infections of the skin or other tissues. Two-thirds of epidural infections result from hematogenous spread from the skin (furunculosis), soft tissue (pharyngeal or dental abscesses), or deep viscera (bacterial endocarditis). One-third result from direct extension of a local infection to the subdural space; examples of local predisposing conditions are vertebral osteomyelitis; decubitus ulcers; or iatrogenic complications of lumbar puncture, epidural anesthesia, or spinal surgery. Most cases are due to *Staphylococcus aureus*; gram-negative bacilli, *Streptococcus,* anaerobes, and fungi can also cause epidural abscesses. Tuberculosis from an adjacent vertebral source remains an important cause in the underdeveloped world. MRI scans (**Fig. 24-5**) localize the abscess and exclude other causes of myelopathy. Lumbar puncture is not required but may be indicated if encephalopathy or other clinical signs raise the question of

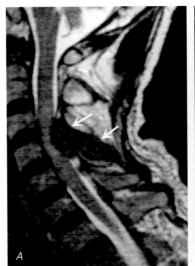
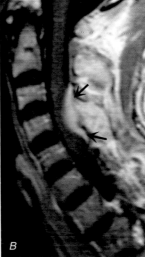

FIGURE 24-5

MRI of a spinal epidural abscess due to tuberculosis. *A.* Sagittal T2-weighted free spin-echo MR sequence. A hypointense mass replaces the posterior elements of C3 and extends epidurally to compress the spinal cord (*arrows*). *B.* Sagittal T1-weighted image after contrast administration reveals a diffuse enhancement of the epidural process (*arrows*) with extension into the epidural space.

associated meningitis, a feature that is found in <25% of cases. In such situations, the level of the puncture should be planned to minimize the risk of inducing meningitis by passage of the needle through infected tissue, or herniation from decompression below an area of obstruction to the flow of cerebrospinal fluid (CSF). A high cervical tap is often the safest approach. CSF abnormalities in subdural abscess consist of pleocytosis with a preponderance of polymorphonuclear cells, an elevated protein level, and a reduced glucose level, but the responsible organism is not cultured unless there is an associated meningitis. Blood cultures are positive in <25% of cases.

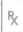

TREATMENT FOR SPINAL EPIDURAL ABSCESS

Treatment is by decompressive laminectomy with debridement combined with long-term antibiotic treatment. Surgical evacuation prevents development of paralysis and may improve or reverse paralysis in evolution, but it is unlikely to improve deficits of more than several days' duration. Antibiotics should be started empirically before surgery and then modified on the basis of culture results; medication is continued for at least 4 weeks. If surgery is contraindicated or if there is a fixed paraplegia or quadriplegia that is unlikely to improve following surgery, long-term administration of systemic and oral antibiotics can be used; in such cases, the choice of antibiotics may be guided by results of blood cultures. However, paralysis may develop or progress during antibiotic therapy; thus, initial surgical management remains the treatment of choice unless the abscess is very limited in size and causes no neurologic signs.

Epidural Hematoma

Hemorrhage into the epidural (or subdural) space causes an acute onset of focal or radicular pain followed by variable signs of a spinal cord or conus medullaris disorder. Therapeutic anticoagulation, trauma, tumor, or blood dyscrasias are predisposing conditions. Rare cases complicate lumbar puncture or epidural anesthesia, sometimes in association with use of low-molecular-weight heparin. MRI and CT confirm the clinical suspicion and can delineate the extent of the bleeding. Extrinsic spinal cord compression from any cause is an urgent condition, and appropriate treatment consists of prompt reversal of any underlying clotting disorder and surgical decompression. Surgery may be followed by

substantial recovery, especially in patients with some preservation of motor function preoperatively. Because of the risk of hemorrhage, lumbar puncture should be avoided whenever possible in patients with thrombocytopenia or other coagulopathies.

Hematomyelia

Hemorrhage into the substance of the spinal cord is a rare result of trauma, intraparenchymal vascular malformation (see below), vasculitis due to polyarteritis nodosa or systemic lupus erythematosus (SLE), bleeding disorders, or a spinal cord neoplasm. Hematomyelia presents as an acute painful transverse myelopathy. With large lesions, extension into the subarachnoid space may occur, resulting in subarachnoid hemorrhage (Chap. 17). Diagnosis is made by MRI. Therapy is supportive, and surgical intervention is generally not useful. An exception is hematomyelia due to an underlying vascular malformation, in which selective spinal angiography may be indicated, followed by surgery to evacuate the clot and remove the underlying vascular lesion.

NONCOMPRESSIVE MYELOPATHIES

Acute transverse myelopathies (ATM) are rapidly progressive spinal cord syndromes with limb weakness, incontinence, and bilateral sensory loss accompanied by a sensory level and not due to cord compression. The time from onset to maximum symptoms is often hours or a few days, but some cases progress more slowly, over several weeks. Five general causes of ATM need to be considered: spinal cord infarction; systemic disorders including SLE and sarcoidosis; infectious (especially viral) causes; demyelinating diseases such as multiple sclerosis or neuromyelitis optica; and idiopathic transverse myelitis. The evaluation begins with a lumbar puncture and a search for systemic disease that may underlie the myelopathy (**Table 24–3**).

Spinal Cord Infarction

The cord is supplied by three arteries that course vertically over its surface: a single anterior spinal artery and paired posterior spinal arteries. At each segment, paired penetrating vessels branch from the anterior spinal artery to supply the anterior two-thirds of the spinal cord; the posterior spinal arteries, which often become less distinct below the midthoracic level, supply the posterior columns. Rostrally, the spinal arteries arise from the vertebral arteries. During embryogenesis, arterial feeders arise at each segmental level, but most involute before birth; generally, between three and eight major feeders remain, arising from the vertebral, subclavian,

TABLE 24-3

EVALUATION OF ACUTE TRANSVERSE MYELOPATHY

1. MRI of spinal cord with and without contrast (exclude compressive causes).
2. CSF studies: Cell count, protein, glucose, IgG index/synthesis rate, oligoclonal bands, VDRL; Gram's stain, acid-fast bacilli, and India ink stains; PCR for VZV, HSV-2, HSV-1, EBV, CMV, HHV-6, enteroviruses, HIV; antibody for HTLV-I, *B. burgdorferi*, *M. pneumoniae,* and *Chlamydia pneumoniae;* viral, bacterial, mycobacterial, and fungal cultures.
3. Blood studies for infection: HIV; RPR; IgG and IgM enterovirus antibody; IgM mumps, measles, rubella, group B arbovirus, *Brucella melitensis, Chlamydia psittaci, Bartonella henselae,* schistosomal antibody; cultures for *B. melitensis.* Also consider nasal/pharyngeal/anal cultures for enteroviruses; stool O&P for *Schistosoma* ova.
4. Immune-mediated disorders: ESR; ANA: ENA; dsDNA; rheumatoid factor; anti-SSA; anti-SSB, complement levels; antiphospholipid and anticardiolipin antibodies; p-ANCA; antimicrosomal and antithyroglobulin antibodies; if Sjögren syndrome suspected, Schirmer test, salivary gland scintography, and salivary/lacrimal gland biopsy.
5. Sarcoidosis: Serum angiotensin-converting enzyme; serum Ca; 24 hour urine Ca; chest x-ray; chest CT; total body gallium scan; lymph node biopsy.
6. Demyelinating disease: Brain MRI scan, evoked potentials.
7. Vascular causes: CT myelogram; spinal angiogram.

Note: VDRL, Venereal Disease Research Laboratory; PCR, polymerase chain reaction; VZV, varicella-zoster virus; HHV, human herpes virus; RPR, rapid plasma reagin (test); O&P, ova and parasites; ESR, erythrocyte sedimentation rate; ANA, antinuclear antibodies; ENA, epithelial neutrophil-activity (protein).

intercostal (from the aorta), iliac, and sacral arteries. In addition to the vertebral arteries, anterior spinal artery feeders arise at C6, at an upper thoracic level, and, most consistently, at T11–L2 (artery of Adamkiewicz).

Spinal cord ischemia can occur at any level; however, the presence of the artery of Adamkiewicz creates a watershed of marginal blood flow in the upper-thoracic segments. With systemic hypotension, cord infarction occurs at the level of greatest ischemic risk, often T3-T4, and also at boundary zones between the anterior and posterior spinal artery territories. The latter may result in an acute—or more commonly progressive—syndrome of weakness and spasticity with little sensory change, superficially resembling amyotrophic lateral sclerosis (ALS).

Acute infarction in the territory of the anterior spinal artery produces paraplegia or quadriplegia, dissociated sensory loss affecting pain and temperature sense but sparing vibration and position sense, and loss of sphincter control. Onset may be sudden and dramatic but more typically is progressive over minutes or a few hours, quite unlike stroke in the cerebral hemispheres. Sharp midline or radiating back pain localized to the area of ischemia is frequent. Partial infarction of one anterior hemicord (hemiplegia or monoplegia and crossed pain and temperature loss) may also occur. Areflexia due to spinal shock is often present initially; with time, hyperreflexia and spasticity appear. Infarction in the territory of the posterior spinal arteries, resulting in loss of posterior column function, also occurs and may be underrecognized as a cause of obscure loss of position and vibration sense.

Spinal cord infarction is associated with aortic atherosclerosis, dissecting aortic aneurysm (chest or back pain with diminished pulses in legs), or hypotension from any cause. Cardiogenic emboli; vasculitis related to collagen vascular disease, particularly SLE and the antiphospholipid antibody syndrome (see below); and surgical interruption of aortic aneurysms are other causative conditions. Occasional cases develop by an unknown mechanism that leads to embolism of nucleus pulposus material into spinal vessels. In a substantial number of cases, no cause can be found, and thromboembolism in arterial feeders is suspected. The MRI may not demonstrate limited infarctions of the cord but is more often abnormal at the affected level.

Therapy is directed at treatment of any predisposing condition. In cord infarction due to presumed thromboembolism, acute anticoagulation is probably not indicated, with the exception of the unusual transient ischemic attack or incomplete infarction with a stuttering or progressive course. The antiphospholipid antibody syndrome is treated with anticoagulation.

Immune-Mediated Diseases

ATM occurs in ~1% of patients with SLE and may appear as the presenting manifestation of SLE. In some patients the ATM may be preceded or followed by optic neuritis (neuromyelitis optica; Chap. 28). Antiphospholipid antibodies are present in nearly two-thirds of patients with SLE-associated ATM. CSF is usually normal or shows a lymphocytic pleocytosis; oligoclonal bands are generally negative. Possible responses to glucocorticoids and/or cyclophosphamide have been reported. Other immune-mediated disorders associated with ATM include Sjögren's syndrome, mixed connective tissue disease, Behçet's syndrome, and vasculitis with perinuclear antineutrophilic cytoplasmic (p-ANCA) antibodies.

Another important consideration is sarcoid myelopathy, in which a large edematous swelling of the spinal cord may mimic tumor; there is almost always enhancement of the lesion and the adjacent surface of the cord. The CSF profile consists of variable lymphocytic pleocytosis, and oligoclonal bands are present in one-third of cases. The diagnosis of sarcoid affecting the spinal cord is particularly difficult when systemic manifestations of sarcoid are meager or absent (50% of cases) or when other neurologic manifestations of the disease—such as cranial neuropathy, hypothalamic involvement, or meningeal enhancement visualized by MRI—are lacking. Whenever neurosarcoid is considered, a careful slit-lamp examination of the eye to search for uveitis, chest x-ray and CT to assess pulmonary involvement and mediastinal lymphadenopathy, serum angiotensin-converting enzyme (positive in only one-quarter of cases), serum calcium, and a gallium scan may be indicated. Initial treatment is with oral glucocorticoids; immunosuppressant drugs are used for resistant cases.

Recurrent episodes of myelitis are usually due to an immune-mediated disease such as SLE or sarcoid, a demyelinating disease, or infection with herpes simplex virus (HSV) type 2 (below).

Infectious and Parainfectious Myelitis

Many viruses have been associated with an acute myelitis that is caused by direct infection of the spinal cord. Herpes zoster is the most common viral cause of acute myelitis; HSV types 1 and 2, Epstein-Barr virus (EBV), cytomegalovirus (CMV), and rabies virus are other well-described etiologies. HSV-2 can produce a distinctive syndrome of recurrent sacral myelitis in association with outbreaks of genital herpes which mimics multiple sclerosis (MS). Poliomyelitis is the prototypic virus that produces acute infection of the spinal cord. In some cases it may be appropriate to begin specific therapy based upon the suspicion that a particular viral agent might be responsible for myelitis, pending laboratory confirmation. Herpes zoster, HSV, and EBV myelitis are treated with acyclovir (10 mg/kg tid for 10 to 14 days); CMV with ganciclovir (5 mg/kg IV bid) plus foscarnet (60 mg/kg IV tid) or with cidofovir (5 mg/kg per week for 2 weeks).

Bacterial and mycobacterial etiologies are less common than viral causes. Almost any pathogenic species may be responsible, including *Listeria monocytogenes, Borrelia burgdorferi* (Lyme disease), and *Treponema pallidum* (syphilis). *Mycoplasma pneumoniae* may be underrecognized as a cause of ATM.

Schistosomiasis is an important cause of parasitic myelitis in endemic areas. The myelitis is intensely inflammatory and granulomatous in nature, caused by a local response to tissue-digesting enzymes from the ova of the parasite. Toxoplasmosis can occasionally cause a focal myelopathy, and this diagnosis should be considered, particularly in patients with AIDS.

Other cases of myelitis, termed *postinfectious myelitis,* or *postvaccinial myelitis,* follow an infection or vaccination. Many infectious agents have been implicated, including influenza, measles, varicella, rubeola, and mumps. As in the related disorder, acute disseminated encephalomyelitis (Chap. 28), postinfectious transverse myelitis often begins as the patient appears to be recovering from the infection, but an infectious agent cannot be isolated from the nervous system or spinal fluid. These features suggest that the myelitis represents an autoimmune disorder triggered by infection and is not due to direct infection of the spinal cord.

Demyelinating Diseases

Multiple sclerosis (Chap. 28) may present as ATM, particularly in individuals of Asian or African ancestry. In Caucasians, MS rarely causes ATM (e.g., transverse myelitis with acute bilateral signs) but is a common cause of acute partial myelopathy. Unlike infectious and parainfectious ATM, MS-associated ATM is usually not associated with fever, rash, or other manifestations of an antecedent infection. Neuromyelitis optica (Devic's disease; Chap. 28) is a demyelinating syndrome related to MS that presents as ATM associated with optic neuritis; the optic neuritis is often bilateral and may precede or follow the myelitis by weeks or months. A neuromyelitis optica syndrome is also associated with SLE (see above) and other immune-mediated diseases, and with the antiphospholipid syndrome.

MRI findings in MS-associated ATM consist of mild swelling and edema of the cord and diffuse or multifocal areas of abnormal signal on T2-weighted sequences, often extending over several cord segments. Contrast enhancement, indicating disruption in the blood-brain barrier associated with inflammation, is present in acute cases. A brain MRI should be obtained to assess the likelihood that the myelitis represents an initial attack of MS. A normal scan indicates that the risk of evolution to MS is low—~10% over 5 years; by contrast, the finding of multiple periventricular T2-bright lesions indicates a risk of >50%. The CSF may be normal, but more often there is a mild pleocytosis, occasionally up to several hundred mononuclear cells per microliter. CSF protein levels are normal or at most mildly elevated; oligoclonal banding is a variable finding but, when present, implicates MS.

There are no adequate trials of therapy for MS-associated ATM. Intravenous methylprednisolone (500 mg qd for 3 days) followed by oral prednisone (1 mg/kg per day for several weeks, then gradual taper) is the initial treatment of choice; a course of plasma exchange may be tried if glucocorticoids are ineffective.

Idiopathic Transverse Myelitis

In approximately one-quarter of cases of ATM, no underlying cause can be identified. Some will later manifest additional symptoms of a systemic immune-mediated disease such as SLE or a demyelinating disorder. In cases associated with inflammation (e.g., contrast enhancement of the lesion by spinal MRI or CSF pleocytosis) but not evidence of infection, glucocorticoids and plasma exchange are the first and second options, as for demyelinating causes (above).

CHRONIC MYELOPATHIES

SPONDYLITIC MYELOPATHY

Spondylitic myelopathy is one of the most common causes of gait difficulty in the elderly. Neck and shoulder pain with stiffness are early symptoms; impingement of bone and soft tissue overgrowth on nerve roots results in radicular arm pain, most often in a C5 or C6 distribution. Compression of the cervical cord produces a slowly progressive spastic paraparesis, at times asymmetric, and often accompanied by paresthesias in the feet and hands. Vibratory sense is diminished in the legs, and occasionally there is a sensory level for vibration on the upper thorax. In some cases coughing or straining produces leg weakness or radiating arm or shoulder pain. Dermatomal sensory loss in the arms, atrophy of intrinsic hand muscles, increased deep tendon reflexes in the legs, and extensor plantar responses are common. Urinary urgency or incontinence occurs in advanced cases. A tendon reflex in the arms is often diminished at some level; the biceps is most often affected (C5-C6). In individual cases, radicular, myelopathic, or combined signs may predominate. The diagnosis should be considered in cases of progressive cervical myelopathy, paresthesias of the feet and hands, or wasting of the hands.

Diagnosis is best made by MRI. Extrinsic cord compression is appreciated on axial views, and T2-weighted sequences may reveal areas of high signal intensity within the cord adjacent to the site of compression. Definitive therapy consists of surgical relief of the compression. Posterior laminectomy or an anterior approach with resection of the protruded disc material may be required. A cervical collar may be very helpful in milder cases. Cervical spondylosis and related degenerative diseases of the spine are discussed in Chap. 6.

VASCULAR MALFORMATIONS

Although uncommon, vascular malformations of the cord are important lesions because they represent a treatable cause of progressive myelopathy. Arteriovenous malformations (AVMs) are most often located posteriorly, within the dura or along the surface of the cord, at or below the midthoracic level. The typical presentation is a middle-aged man with a progressive myelopathy. The myelopathy may worsen slowly or rapidly or may have periods of apparent remission with superimposed worsenings, resembling MS. Acute deterioration due to hemorrhage into the spinal cord or subarachnoid space may also occur. At presentation, most patients have sensory, motor, and bladder disturbances. The motor disorder may predominate and produce a mixture of upper and lower motor neuron signs, simulating amyotrophic lateral sclerosis (ALS). Pain, either dysesthesias or radicular pain, is also common. Other symptoms suggestive of AVM include intermittent claudication (symptoms that appear with exercise and are relieved by rest), or symptoms that change with posture, menses, or fever. A rare AVM syndrome presents as a progressive thoracic myelopathy with paraparesis developing over weeks or several months, associated with abnormally thick, hyalinized vessels (Foix-Alajouanine syndrome).

Spinal bruits are infrequent but should be sought at rest and after exercise. High-resolution MRI with contrast administration detects most AVMs (**Fig. 24-6**). A small number of AVMs not detected by MRI may be

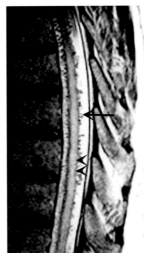 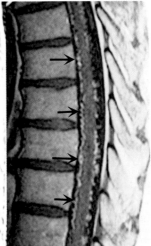

FIGURE 24-6

Arteriovenous malformation. Sagittal MR scans of the thoracic spinal cord: T2 fast spin-echo technique (*left*) and T1 post-contrast image (*right*). On the T2-weighted image (*left*), abnormally high signal intensity is noted in the central aspect of the spinal cord (*arrowheads*). Numerous punctate flow voids indent the dorsal and ventral spinal cord (*arrow*). These represent the abnormally dilated venous plexus supplied by a dural arteriovenous fistula. After contrast administration (*right*), multiple, serpentine, enhancing veins (*arrows*) on the ventral and dorsal aspect of the thoracic spinal cord are visualized, diagnostic of arteriovenous fistula. This patient was a 54-year-old man with a 4-year history of progressive paraparesis.

visualized by CT myelography as enlarged vessels along the surface of the cord. Definitive diagnosis requires selective spinal angiography, which will also define the feeding vessels and the extent of the malformation. Spinal angiography should be considered when the clinical suspicion of an AVM is high, even when myelography is unrevealing. Embolization with occlusion of the major feeding vessels may stabilize a progressive neurologic deficit or produce a gradual recovery.

RETROVIRUS-ASSOCIATED MYELOPATHIES

The myelopathy associated with the human T cell lymphotropic virus type I (HTLV-I), formerly called tropical spastic paraparesis, presents as a slowly progressive spastic paraparesis with variable sensory and bladder disturbance. The myelopathy typically implicates a thoracic level. Approximately half of patients have back or leg pain. The signs may be asymmetric, often lacking a well-defined sensory level; the only sign in the arms is hyperreflexia. The onset is generally insidious, and the tempo of progression is variable, but most patients are nonambulatory within 10 years of onset. This presentation may resemble primary progressive MS or a thoracic AVM. Diagnosis is made by demonstration of HTLV-I–specific antibody in serum by enzyme-linked immunosorbent assay (ELISA), confirmed by radioimmunoprecipitation or Western blot analysis. There is no effective treatment, but symptomatic therapy for spasticity and bladder symptoms may be helpful.

A progressive myelopathy may also occur in AIDS, characterized by vacuolar degeneration of the posterior and lateral tracts resembling subacute combined degeneration (see below).

SYRINGOMYELIA

Syringomyelia is a developmental, slowly enlarging cavitary expansion of the cervical cord that produces progressive myelopathy. Symptoms begin insidiously in adolescence or early adulthood, progress irregularly, and may undergo spontaneous arrest for several years; most patients acquire a cervical-thoracic scoliosis. More than half of all cases are associated with Chiari type 1 malformations in which the cerebellar tonsils protrude through the foramen magnum and into the cervical spinal canal. The pathophysiology of the syrinx is controversial. Some interference with the normal flow of CSF seems likely. Acquired cavitations of the cord are also termed *syrinx cavities*; these may follow trauma, myelitis, chronic arachnoiditis due to tuberculosis and other etiologies, or necrotic spinal cord tumors.

The classic presentation is of a central cord syndrome with dissociated sensory loss and areflexic weakness in the upper limbs. The sensory deficit consists of loss of pain and temperature sensation with sparing of touch and vibration which is "suspended" over the nape of the neck, shoulders, and upper arms in a cape distribution or is in the hands. Most cases begin asymmetrically with unilateral sensory loss in the hands and unappreciated burns. Muscle wasting in the lower neck, shoulders, arms, and hands with asymmetric or absent reflexes reflects extension of the cavity to the anterior horns. As the lesion enlarges, spasticity and weakness of the legs, bladder and bowel dysfunction, and, in some cases, a Horner's syndrome appear. Thoracic kyphoscoliosis is a frequent additional finding. Some patients develop facial numbness and sensory loss from damage to the descending tract of the trigeminal nerve (C2 level or above). With Chiari malformations, cough, headache, and neck, arm, or facial pain are common. Extension of the syrinx into the medulla, syringobulbia, may present as palatal or vocal cord paralysis, dysarthria, horizontal or vertical nystagmus, episodic dizziness, and/or tongue weakness.

MRI scans accurately identify developmental and acquired syrinx cavities and their associated spinal cord enlargement (**Fig. 24–7**). MRI scans of the brain and the entire spinal cord should be obtained to delineate the full

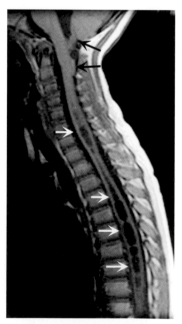

FIGURE 24-7

MRI of a syringomyelia associated with a Chiari malformation. Sagittal T1-weighted image through the cervical and upper thoracic spine demonstrates descent of the cerebellar tonsils and vermis below the level of the foramen magnum (*black arrows*). Within the substance of the cervical and thoracic spinal cord, a CSF collection dilates the central canal (*white arrows*).

longitudinal extent of the syrinx, assess posterior fossa structures, and determine whether hydrocephalus is present. If a Chiari malformation is not found, a contrast-enhanced MRI scan should be obtained to search for abnormal enhancement from an associated spinal cord tumor.

TREATMENT FOR CHRONIC MYELOPATHIES

Treatment is generally unsatisfactory. Syringomyelia associated with tonsillar herniation is treated with posterior fossa decompression, generally consisting of suboccipital craniectomy, upper cervical laminectomy, and placement of a dural graft. If obstruction of fourth ventricular outflow is present, flow may be reestablished by enlargement of the opening. If the syrinx cavity is large, some surgeons recommend direct decompression of the fluid cavity, but the added benefit of this procedure is uncertain, and morbidity may occur. With Chiari malformations, shunting of hydrocephalus should generally precede any attempt to correct the syrinx. Surgery may stabilize the neurologic deficit; some patients have improvement postoperatively. Syringomyelia secondary to trauma or infection is treated with a decompression and drainage procedure in which a small shunt is inserted between the syrinx cavity and the subarachnoid space. Syringomyelia due to an intramedullary spinal cord tumor is managed by resection of the tumor, if feasible; decompression of the cyst cavity may produce temporary relief, but recurrence is common.

MULTIPLE SCLEROSIS

Spinal cord involvement is common in MS. It may develop acutely as an exacerbation in a patient with known MS or appear as the presenting manifestation of the disease (see above). Chronic progressive myelopathy is the most frequent cause of disability in both primary progressive and secondary progressive forms of MS. Involvement is typically asymmetric, producing motor, sensory, and bladder/bowel disturbances. Diagnosis is facilitated by identification of earlier attacks that may not be initially recalled by the patient; by MRI, CSF and evoked response testing; and by exclusion of other conditions. The diagnosis may be particularly difficult to establish in patients with primary progressive MS. Therapy with interferon β or glatiramer acetate is indicated for patients with coexisting relapses of MS. MS is discussed in Chap. 28.

SUBACUTE COMBINED DEGENERATION (VITAMIN B$_{12}$ DEFICIENCY)

This treatable myelopathy presents with parasthesias in the hands and feet, early loss of vibration and position sensation, and a progressive spastic and ataxic weakness. Loss of reflexes due to a superimposed peripheral neuropathy, present in many patients, is an important diagnostic clue. Optic atrophy and irritability and other mental changes may be prominent in advanced cases and on occasion are the presenting symptoms (megaloblastic madness). The myelopathy of subacute combined degeneration tends to be diffuse rather than focal; signs are generally symmetric and reflect predominant involvement of the posterior and lateral tracts, including Romberg's sign. The diagnosis is confirmed by the finding of macrocytic red cells, a low serum B$_{12}$ concentration, elevated levels of homocysteine and methylmalonic acid in uncertain cases, and a positive Schilling test.

TABES DORSALIS

The classic syndromes of tabes dorsalis and meningovascular syphilis of the spinal cord are rare but must be considered in the differential diagnosis of spinal cord disorders. The most common symptoms of tabes are characteristic fleeting and repetitive lancinating pains, which occur primarily in the legs and less commonly in the back, thorax, abdomen, arms, and face. Ataxia of the legs and gait due to loss of position sense occurs in half of patients. Paresthesias, bladder disturbances, and acute abdominal pain with vomiting (visceral crisis) occur in 15 to 30% of patients. The cardinal signs of tabes are loss of reflexes in the legs, impaired position and vibratory sense, Romberg's sign, and bilateral Argyll Robertson pupils, which fail to constrict to light but react with accommodation. In the modern era, diabetic polyradiculopathy simulates tabes.

FAMILIAL SPASTIC PARAPLEGIA (Chap. 21)

Some cases of progressive myelopathy are genetic in origin. More than 20 different loci have been identified, including autosomal dominant, autosomal recessive, and X-linked forms. Most patients present with progressive spasticity and weakness in the legs; the syndrome is usually but not always symmetric. Sensory symptoms and signs are usually absent or mild. Sphincter disturbances may be present. In some families in which the condition is referred to as "complicated" familial spastic paraplegia, additional neurologic signs, e.g., nystagmus, ataxia, or optic atrophy, occur. Onset may be as early as the first year of life or as late as middle adulthood. The causative mutations responsible for several forms of familial spastic paraplegia are now known. The most common of these is a mutation in spastin (chromosome 2p; autosomal dominant). No therapies are currently available.

ADRENOMYELONEUROPATHY

This X-linked disorder, a variant of adrenoleukodystrophy, most commonly presents as a progressive spastic paraparesis beginning in early adulthood; some patients also have a mild peripheral neuropathy. Affected males usually have a history of adrenal insufficiency beginning in childhood. Rare heterozygous females may also present with adult-onset myelopathy. Diagnosis is usually made by demonstration of elevated levels of very long chain fatty acids in plasma and in cultured fibroblasts. The responsible gene, located at Xq17-28, encodes a protein involved in peroxysomal transport. Steroid replacement is indicated if hypoadrenalism is present, and bone marrow transplantation has been attempted for this condition, although without clear evidence of efficacy.

OTHER CHRONIC MYELOPATHIES

Primary lateral sclerosis (Chap. 21) is a degenerative disorder characterized by progressive spasticity with weakness, often accompanied by dysarthria and dysphonia. Sensory function is spared. The disorder resembles ALS, but there is no evidence of a lower motor neuron disturbance. Toxic causes of spastic myelopathy include (1) lathyrism due to ingestion of chick peas containing the excitotoxin β-N-oxalylaminoalanine (BOAA) and seen primarily in the underdeveloped world, and (2) nitrous oxide inhalation producing a myelopathy identical to subacute combined degeneration. SLE, Sjögren's syndrome, and sarcoid, as mentioned above, have all been associated with progressive myelopathy, which may involve the cord even without evidence of overt systemic disease. Cancer-related causes include chronic paraneoplastic myelopathy or radiation injury; metastases to the cord are probably more common than either of these. Finally, as in ATM, in some patients the etiology of a chronic myelopathy may not be determined initially. A cause can often be identified through periodic reassessment.

MEDICAL REHABILITATION OF SPINAL CORD DISORDERS

The prospects for recovery from an acute spinal cord lesion fade after ~6 months. There are currently no effective means to promote repair of injured spinal cord tissue. Promising experimental approaches include the use of factors that influence reinnervation by axons of the corticospinal tract, nerve graft bridges that promote reinnervation across spinal cord lesions, and the local injection of stem cells. The disability associated with irreversible spinal cord damage is determined primarily by the level of the lesion and by whether the disturbance in function is complete or incomplete (**Table 24-4**). Even a complete high cervical cord lesion may be compatible with a productive life. Development of a rehabilitation plan framed by realistic expectations, and attention to the neurologic, medical, and psychological complications that commonly arise, are primary goals of treatment.

Many of the usual symptoms associated with medical illnesses, especially somatic and visceral pain, may be lacking because of the destruction of afferent pain pathways. Unexplained fever, worsening of spasticity, or deterioration in neurologic function should prompt a search for infection, thrombophlebitis, or an intraabdominal pathology; these etiologies are far more likely to be responsible than primary neurologic events such as meningitis, secondary syringomyelia, or chronic arachnoiditis. The loss of normal thermoregulation and inability to maintain normal body temperature can produce recurrent fever (*quadriplegic fever*), although most episodes of fever are due to infection of the urinary tract, lung, skin, or bone.

TABLE 24-4

EXPECTED NEUROLOGIC FUNCTION FOLLOWING COMPLETE CORD LESIONS

LEVEL	SELF-CARE	TRANSFERS	MAXIMUM MOBILITY
High quadriplegia (C1-C4)	Dependent on others; requires respiratory support	Dependent on others	Motorized wheelchair
Low quadriplegia (C5-C8)	Partially independent with adaptive equipment	May be dependent or independent	May use manual wheelchair, drive an automobile with adaptive equipment
Paraplegia (below T1)	Independent	Independent	Ambulates short distances with aids

Source: Adapted from JF Ditunno, CS Formal: Chronic spinal cord injury. N Engl J Med 330:550, 1994; with permission.

Bladder dysfunction generally results from loss of supraspinal innervation of the detrusor muscle of the bladder wall and the sphincter musculature. Detrusor spasticity is treated with anticholinergic drugs (oxybutinin, 2.5 to 5 mg qid) or tricyclic antidepressants with anticholinergic properties (imipramine, 25 to 200 mg/d). Failure of the sphincter muscle to relax during bladder emptying (urinary dyssynergia) may be managed with the α-adrenergic blocking agent terazosin hydrochloride (1 to 2 mg tid or qid), with intermittent catheterization, or, if that is not feasible, by use of a condom catheter in men or a permanent indwelling catheter. Surgical options include the creation of an artificial bladder by isolating a segment of intestine that can be catheterized intermittently (enterocystoplasty) or can drain continuously to an external appliance (urinary conduit). Bladder areflexia due to acute spinal shock or conus lesions is best treated by catheterization.

Bladder paralysis predisposes the patient to urinary tract infection. Bacteriuria due to asymptomatic colonization is extremely common and is generally not treated. Prophylaxis with antiseptics or antibiotics is a controversial practice. Urinary tract infections may present only as foul-smelling urine or a change in voiding pattern; the development of high fever or other systemic signs often indicates pyelonephritis. Bowel regimens and disimpaction are necessary in most patients to ensure at least biweekly evacuation and avoid colonic distention or obstruction.

High cervical cord lesions cause various degrees of mechanical respiratory failure requiring artificial ventilation. In cases of incomplete respiratory failure, chest physical therapy is useful, and a negative-pressure cuirass may alleviate atelectasis, particularly if the major lesion is below C4. With severe respiratory failure, tracheal intubation, followed by tracheotomy, provides tracheal access for ventilation and suctioning. Phrenic nerve pacing may be an option in some patients with lesions at C5 or above.

Patients with acute cord injury are at high risk for venous thrombosis and pulmonary embolism. During the first 2 weeks, use of calf-compression devices and anticoagulation with heparin (5000 U subcutaneously every 12 h) or warfarin (INR, 2 to 3) are recommended. In cases of persistent paralysis, anticoagulation should probably be continued for 3 months.

Prophylaxis against decubitus ulcers should involve frequent changes in position in a chair or bed, the use of special mattresses, and cushioning of areas where pressure sores often develop, such as the sacral prominence and heels. Early treatment of ulcers with careful cleansing, surgical or enzyme debridement of necrotic tissue, and appropriate dressing and drainage may prevent infection of adjacent soft tissue or bone.

Spasticity is aided by stretching exercises to maintain mobility of joints. Drug treatment is effective but may result in reduced function, as some patients depend upon spasticity as an aid to stand, transfer, or walk. Baclofen (15 to 240 mg/d in divided doses) is the most effective drug; it acts by facilitating GABA-mediated inhibition of motor reflex arcs. Diazepam acts by a similar mechanism and is useful for leg spasms that interrupt sleep (2 to 4 mg at bedtime). For nonambulatory patients, the direct muscle inhibitor dantrolene (25 to 100 mg qid) may be used, but it is potentially hepatotoxic. In severe cases, intrathecal baclofen administered via an implanted pump, botulinum toxin injections, or dorsal rhizotomy may be required to control spasticity.

A dramatic paroxysmal autonomic hyperreflexia may occur following lesions above the major splanchnic sympathetic outflow at T6. Headache, flushing, and diaphoresis above the level of the lesion, and hypertension with bradycardia or tachycardia, are the major symptoms. The trigger is typically a noxious stimulus—for example, bladder or bowel distention, a urinary tract infection, or a decubitus ulcer—below the level of the cord lesion. Treatment consists of removal of offending stimuli; ganglionic blocking agents (mecamylamine, 2.5 to 5 mg) or other short-acting antihypertensive drugs are useful in some patients.

Attention to these details allows longevity and a productive life for patients with myelopathy.

FURTHER READINGS

DE SEZE J et al: Acute myelopathies: Clinical, laboratory and outcome profiles in 79 cases. Brain 124:1509, 2001

KALB RG: Getting the spinal cord to think for itself. Arch Neurol 60:805, 2003

☑ KAPLIN AI et al: Diagnosis and management of acute myelopathies. Neurologist 11:2, 2005

  Up-to-date review of etiology and management.

PRASAD D, SCHIFF D: Malignant spinal-cord compression Lancet Oncol 6:15, 2005

TRANSVERSE MYELITIS CONSORTIUM WORKING GROUP: Proposed diagnostic criteria and nosology of acute transverse myelitis. Neurology 59:499, 2002

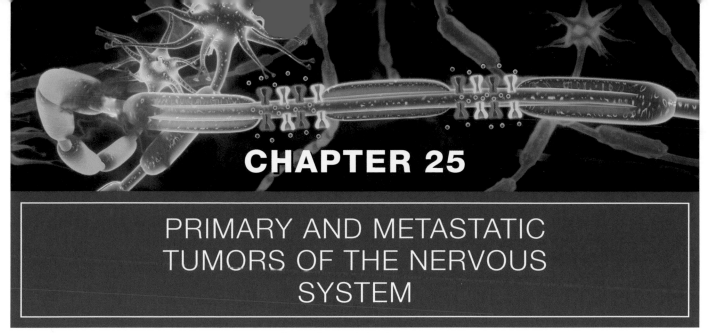

CHAPTER 25

PRIMARY AND METASTATIC TUMORS OF THE NERVOUS SYSTEM

Stephen M. Sagar
Mark A. Israel

Malignant primary tumors of the central nervous system (CNS) occur in ~16,500 individuals and account for an estimated 13,000 deaths in the United States annually, a mortality rate of 6 per 100,000. An approximately equal number of benign tumors of the CNS are diagnosed, with a much lower mortality rate. Glial tumors account for 50 to 60% of primary brain tumors, meningiomas for 25%, schwannomas for 10%, and all other CNS tumors for the remainder.

Brain and vertebral metastases from systemic cancer are more prevalent than primary CNS tumors. About 15% of patients who die of cancer (80,000 individuals each year in the United States) have symptomatic brain metastases; an additional 5% suffer spinal cord involvement. Brain and spinal metastases therefore pose a major problem in the management of systemic cancer.

BRAIN TUMORS

APPROACH TO THE PATIENT WITH A BRAIN TUMOR

CLINICAL FEATURES

Brain tumors usually present with one of three syndromes: (1) subacute progression of a focal neurologic deficit; (2) seizure; or (3) nonfocal neurologic disorder such as headache, dementia, personality change, or gait disorder. The presence of systemic symptoms such as malaise, weight loss, anorexia, or fever suggests a metastatic rather than a primary brain tumor.

Progressive focal neurologic deficits result from compression of neurons and white matter tracts by expanding tumor and surrounding edema. Less commonly, a brain tumor presents with a sudden stroke-like onset of a focal neurologic deficit.

Although this presentation may be caused by hemorrhage into the tumor, often no hemorrhage can be demonstrated and the mechanism is obscure. Tumors frequently associated with hemorrhage include high-grade gliomas and metastatic melanoma and choriocarcinoma.

Seizures may result from disruption of cortical circuits. Tumors that invade or compress the cerebral cortex, even small meningiomas, are more likely to be associated with seizures than subcortical neoplasms. Nonfocal neurologic dysfunction usually reflects increased intracranial pressure (ICP), hydrocephalus, or diffuse tumor spread. Tumors in some areas of the brain may produce behavioral disorders; for example, frontal lobe tumors may present with personality change, dementia, or depression.

Headache may result from focal irritation or displacement of pain-sensitive structures (Chap. 5) or from a generalized increase in ICP. A headache that worsens rather than abates with recumbency is suggestive of a mass lesion. Headaches from increased ICP are usually holocephalic and episodic, occurring more than once a day. They typically develop rapidly over several minutes, persist for 20 to 40 min, and subside quickly. They may awaken the patient from a sound sleep, generally 60 to 90 min after retiring, or may be precipitated by coughing, sneezing, or straining. Vomiting may occur with severe headaches. As elevated ICP becomes sustained, the headache becomes continuous but varying in intensity. Elevated ICP may cause papilledema (Chap. 11), although it is often not present in infants or some older patients.

The Karnofsky performance scale is useful in assessing and following patients with brain tumors. A score ≥70 indicates that the patient is ambulatory and independent in self-care activities; it is often taken as a level of function justifying aggressive therapy.

LABORATORY EXAMINATION

Primary brain tumors typically do not produce serologic abnormalities such as an elevated sedimentation rate or tumor-specific antigens associated with systemic cancers. In contrast, metastases to the nervous system, depending on the type and extent of the primary tumor, may be associated with systemic signs of malignancy. Lumbar puncture may precipitate brain herniation in patients with mass lesions and should be performed only in patients with suspected CNS infection or meningeal metastasis. Findings in the cerebrospinal fluid (CSF) of patients with primary and metastatic nervous system tumors may include raised opening pressure, elevated protein level, and a mild lymphocytic pleocytosis. The CSF rarely contains malignant cells, with the important exceptions of leptomeningeal metastases, primary CNS lymphoma, and primitive neuroectodermal tumors, including medulloblastoma.

NEUROIMAGING

Computed tomography (CT) and magnetic resonance imaging (MRI) can reveal mass effect and contrast enhancement. Mass effect reflects the volume of neoplastic tissue as well as surrounding edema. Brain tumors typically produce a vasogenic pattern of edema, with accumulation of excess water in white matter. Contrast enhancement reflects a breakdown of the blood-brain barrier within the tumor, permitting leakage of contrast agent. Low-grade gliomas typically do not exhibit contrast enhancement. MR spectroscopy is emerging as a tool to distinguish primary brain tumors from other mass lesions and to differentiate glioma from lymphoma.

Positron emission tomography (PET) and single-photon emission computed tomography (SPECT) have ancillary roles in the imaging of brain tumors, primarily in distinguishing tumor recurrence from tissue necrosis that can occur after irradiation (see below). Electroencephalography (EEG) has a role in the evaluation of patients with seizures. Functional imaging with PET, MRI, or magnetoencephalography may be of use in surgical or radiosurgical planning to define the anatomical relationship of the tumor to critical brain regions such as the primary motor or language cortex.

TREATMENT FOR BRAIN TUMORS

SYMPTOMATIC

Glucocorticoids decrease the volume of edema surrounding brain tumors and improve neurologic function; dexamethasone (12 to 20 mg/d in divided doses orally or intravenously) is used because it has relatively little mineralocorticoid activity.

Tumors that involve the cerebral cortex or hippocampus may produce epilepsy. Anticonvulsants are therefore used therapeutically and sometimes prophylactically; phenytoin, carbamazepine, and valproic acid are equally effective, although in practice newer agents, such as levetiracetam, with fewer drug interactions are used increasingly. If the tumor is subcortical in location, prophylactic anticonvulsants are unnecessary.

Gliomas and primary CNS lymphomas are associated with an increased risk for deep vein thrombosis and pulmonary embolism, probably because these tumors secrete procoagulant factors into the systemic circulation. Even though hemorrhage within gliomas is a frequent histopathologic finding, patients appear to be at no increased risk for symptomatic intracranial bleeding following treatment with an anticoagulant. Prophylaxis with low-dose subcutaneous heparin should be considered for patients with brain tumors who have lower limb immobility, which places them at risk for deep venous thrombosis.

PRIMARY BRAIN TUMORS

ETIOLOGY

Exposure to ionizing radiation is the only well-documented environmental risk factor for the development of gliomas. A number of hereditary syndromes are associated with an increased risk of brain tumors (**Table 25-1**). Genes that contribute to the development of brain tumors, as well as other malignancies, fall into two general classes, *tumor-suppressor genes* and *protooncogenes*. Whereas germ-line mutations of tumor-suppressor genes are rare, somatic mutations are almost invariably found in malignant tumors, including brain tumors. Likewise, the activation of protooncogenes occurs frequently in brain tumors. Moreover, cytogenetic analysis often reveals characteristic changes. In astrocytic tumors, DNA is commonly lost on chromosomes 10p, 17p, 13q, and 9. Oligodendrogliomas frequently have deletions of 1p and 19q. In meningiomas portions of 22q, which contains the gene for neurofibromatosis (NF) type 2, are often lost. In approximately one-third of glioblastomas, there is amplification of the *EGFR* gene.

TABLE 25-1

HEREDITARY SYNDROMES ASSOCIATED WITH BRAIN TUMORS

SYNDROME	GENE (LOCUS)	GENE PRODUCT (FUNCTION)	NERVOUS SYSTEM NEOPLASMS
Neurofibromatosis type 1 (von Recklinghausen's Disease)[a]	NF1 (17q)	Neurofibromin (GTPase activating protein)	Neuroma, schwannoma, meningioma, optic glioma
Neurofibromatosis type 2[a]	NF2 (22q)	Merlin (cytoskeletal protein)	Schwannoma, glioma, ependymoma, meningioma
Tuberous sclerosis	TSC1 (9q) TSC2 (16p)	Hamartin (unknown function) Tuberin (GTPase activating protein)	Astrocytoma
von Hippel–Lindau[a]	VHL (3p)	pVHL (modulator of cellular hypoxic response)	Hemangioblastoma of retina, cerebellum and spinal cord; pheochromocytoma
Li-Fraumeni[a]	p53 (17p)	TP53 (cell cycle and transcriptional regulator)	Malignant glioma
Retinoblastoma[a]	RB1 (13q)	RB (cell cycle regulator)	Retinoblastoma, pineoblastoma, malignant glioma
Turcot	APC (5q) (adenomatous polyposis coli)	APC (cell adhesion)	Medulloblastoma, malignant glioma
Gorlin (basal cell nevus syndrome)	PTCH (9q) (patched)	PTH (developmental regulator)	Medulloblastoma
Multiple endocrine neoplasia 1 (Werner syndrome)[a]	MEN1 (11q13)	Menin (cofactor for transcription)	Pituitary adenoma, malignant schwannoma

[a]Genetic testing possible.

The particular constellation of genetic alterations varies among individual gliomas, even those that are histologically indistinguishable. Moreover, gliomas are genetically unstable. Genetic abnormalities tend to accumulate with time, and these changes correspond with an increasingly malignant phenotype. There are at least two genetic routes for the development of malignant glioma. One route involves the progression, generally over years, from a low-grade astrocytoma with deletions of chromosome 17 and inactivation of the *p53* gene to a malignant glioma with additional chromosomal alterations. The second route is characterized by the de novo appearance of a malignant glioma with amplification of the *EGFR* gene and an intact *p53* gene. In both pathways, inactivation of the *PTEN* gene as a result of the loss of chromosome 10 occurs frequently.

ASTROCYTOMAS

Tumors with astrocytic cytologic features are the most common primary intracranial neoplasms (**Fig. 25-1**). The most widely used histologic grading system is the World Health Organization four-tiered grading system. Grade I is reserved for special histologic variants of astrocytoma that have an excellent prognosis after surgical excision. These include *juvenile pilocytic astrocytoma*, *subependymal giant cell astrocytoma* (which occurs in patients with tuberous sclerosis), and *pleiomorphic xanthoastrocytoma*. At the other extreme is grade IV, *glioblastoma multiforme*, a clinically aggressive tumor. *Astrocytoma* (grade II) and *anaplastic astrocytoma* (grade III) are intermediate in their histologic and clinical manifestations. The histologic features associated with higher grade are hypercellularity, nuclear and cytoplasmic atypia, endothelial proliferation, mitotic activity, and necrosis. Endothelial proliferation and necrosis are predictors of aggressive behavior.

A limitation of all grading schemes, especially when applied to a single biopsy, is that astrocytic tumors are histologically variable from region to region, and their histopathology may change with time. It is common for low-grade astrocytomas to progress over time to a higher histopathologic grade and a more aggressive clinical course.

Quantitative measures of mitotic activity also correlate with prognosis. The proliferation index can be determined by immunohistochemical staining with antibodies to the proliferating cell nuclear antigen (PCNA) or with a monoclonal antibody termed *Ki-67*, which recognizes a histone protein expressed in proliferating but not

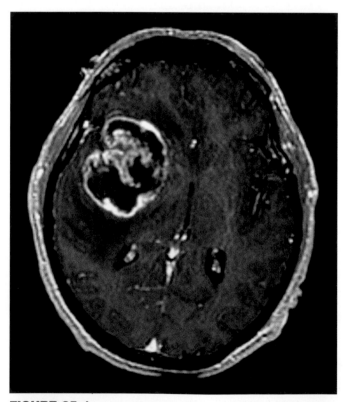
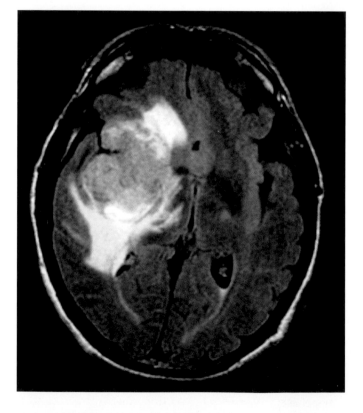

FIGURE 25-1

Malignant astrocytoma. Axial T1-weighted gadolinium-enhanced *(left)* and T2-weighted FLAIR *(right)* MRI sequences demonstrating a right frontal mass with heterogeneous signal and rim-enhancement found on biopsy to represent a glioblastoma multiforme (GBM).

quiescent cells. These measures provide estimates of DNA synthesis and correlate with malignant clinical behavior of the tumor.

The overall prognosis is poor. In a representative Finnish population, the median survival was 93.5 months for patients with grade I or II astrocytomas, 12.4 months for patients with grade III (anaplastic astrocytoma), and 5.1 months for patients with grade IV (glioblastoma) tumors. In the United States, the median survival of patients with high-grade brain tumors is ~12 months. Clinical features that correlate with poor prognosis include age >65 and a poor functional status, as defined by the Karnofsky performance scale.

Low-Grade Astrocytoma

Low-grade astrocytomas are more common in children than adults. Pilocytic astrocytoma, named for its characteristic spindle-shaped cells, is the most common childhood brain tumor. It frequently occurs in the cerebellum. Typically, this tumor is cystic and well demarcated from adjacent brain. Complete surgical excision usually produces long-term, disease-free survival.

The optimal management of grade II astrocytomas is controversial. For patients who are symptomatic from mass effect or poorly controlled epilepsy, surgical excision can relieve symptoms. For patients who are asymptomatic or minimally symptomatic at presentation, a diagnostic biopsy should be performed and, when surgically feasible, the tumor may be resected. The indications for postoperative radiation therapy are uncertain. In many centers, when only a biopsy or partial resection is possible, postoperative external beam radiation therapy is administered, whereas it is not used if a gross total tumor resection can be achieved. Other centers reserve radiation therapy for tumor recurrence or progression, at which time the tumor may display a more malignant phenotype. No role for chemotherapy in the management of low-grade astrocytoma has been defined.

High-Grade Astrocytoma

The large majority of astrocytomas arising in adults are high grade, supratentorial, and do not have a clearly defined margin. Neoplastic cells migrate away from the main tumor mass and infiltrate adjacent brain, often tracking along white matter pathways. Imaging studies do not indicate the full extent of this infiltrating tumor. These tumors are eventually fatal, although prolonged survival occurs in a few patients. Longer survival correlates with younger age, better performance status, and greater extent of surgical resection. Late in their course, gliomas, especially those located in the posterior fossa, can metastasize along CSF pathways to the spine. Metastases outside the CNS are rare.

High-grade astrocytomas are managed with glucocorticoids, surgery, radiation therapy, and chemotherapy. Dexamethasone is generally administered at the time of diagnosis and continued for the duration of radiation therapy. After completion of radiation therapy, dexamethasone is tapered to the lowest tolerated dose.

Because astrocytomas infiltrate adjacent normal brain, total surgical excision is not possible. Surgery is indicated to obtain tissue for pathologic diagnosis and to control mass effect. Moreover, retrospective studies indicate that the extent of tumor resection correlates with survival, at least in younger patients. Therefore, accessible astrocytomas are resected aggressively in patients <65 years old who are in good general medical condition.

Postoperative radiation therapy prolongs survival and improves quality of life, although the duration of benefit is only a few months. Treated with dexamethasone alone following surgery, the mean survival of patients <65 years with glioblastoma is 7 to 9 months. Survival is prolonged to 11 to 13 months with radiation therapy. Focal brain irradiation is less toxic and is as effective as whole-brain radiation for primary glial tumors. Radiation is generally administered to the tumor mass, as defined by contrast enhancement on a CT or MRI scan, plus a 3- to 4-cm margin. A total dose of 5000 to 7000 cGy is administered in 25 to 35 equal fractions, 5 days per week.

The roles of stereotaxic radiosurgery and interstitial brachytherapy in glioma treatment are uncertain. *Stereotaxic radiosurgery* is the administration of a focused high dose of radiation to a precisely defined volume of tissue in a single treatment. Stereotaxic radiosurgery can potentially achieve tumor ablation within the treated volume. A major limitation of stereotaxic radiosurgery is that it can be used for only relatively small tumors, generally <4 cm in maximum diameter. *Interstitial brachytherapy*, the implantation of radioactive material into the tumor mass, is generally reserved for tumor recurrence because of its associated toxicity—in particular, necrosis of adjacent brain tissue.

Chemotherapy is marginally effective and is often used as an adjuvant therapy following surgery and radiation therapy. Nitrosoureas, including carmustine (BCNU) and lomustine (CCNU), and temozolomide are the most effective available agents. Temozolomide is an orally administered alkylating agent, has activity against gliomas, and is generally better tolerated than the nitrosoureas. Experimental approaches include intraarterial infusion of chemotherapy, the implantation of chemotherapy-releasing wafers or injection of chemotherapeutic agents into the tumor resection cavity, and administration of chemotherapy after disruption of the blood-brain barrier.

Gliomatosis cerebri is a rare form of astrocytoma in which there is diffuse infiltration of the brain by malignant astrocytes without a focal enhancing mass. It generally presents as a multifocal CNS syndrome or a more generalized disorder including dementia, personality change, or seizures. Neuroimaging studies are often nonspecific, and biopsy is required to establish the diagnosis. Gliomatosis cerebri is treated with whole-brain radiation therapy or temozolomide; in selected patients, radiation to the entire neuroaxis is employed.

OLIGODENDROGLIOMAS

Oligodendrogliomas, which comprise about 15% of gliomas in adults, have a more benign course and are more responsive to cytotoxic treatment than astrocytomas. Five-year survival is >50%, and 10-year survival is 15 to 43%.

Oligodendrogliomas occur chiefly in supratentorial locations; in adults, ~30% contain areas of calcification (**Fig. 25-2**). Many gliomas contain mixtures of cells with astrocytic and oligodendroglial features. If this mixed histology is prominent, the tumor is termed a *mixed glioma* or an *oligoastrocytoma*. The greater the oligodendroglial component, the more benign the clinical course. As a rule, oligodendrogliomas are less infiltrative than astrocytomas, permitting more complete surgical excision. Histologic features of mitoses, necrosis, and nuclear atypia are associated with a more aggressive clinical course. If these features are prominent, the tumor is termed an *anaplastic oligodendroglioma*.

Surgery, at minimum a stereotaxic biopsy, is necessary to establish a diagnosis. Many oligodendrogliomas are amenable to gross total surgical resection. In addition, oligodendrogliomas may respond dramatically to systemic combination chemotherapy with procarbazine, lomustine, and vincristine (PCV) or to single-agent chemotherapy with temozolomide. Oligodendrogliomas with deletions of chromosome 1p always respond to PCV, but only ~25% of oligodendrogliomas lacking 1p deletion respond to chemotherapy. The simultaneous deletion of 1p and 19q predicts a durable response to chemotherapy (>31 months on average) and survival >10 years. Many centers therefore use 1p deletion as an indication for adjuvant or neo-adjuvant chemotherapy and reserve external beam irradiation for tumor recurrence.

EPENDYMOMAS

In adults ependymomas are typically located in the spinal canal, especially in the lumbosacral region. They typically arise from the filum terminale of the spinal cord and have a myxopapillary histology, with a papillary arrangement of cells and mucin production. In children, ependymomas occur within the ventricles, most often the fourth ventricle, and have a different histology, typically with ependymal rosettes. Ependymomas with histologic signs of malignancy, including cellular atypia, frequent mitotic

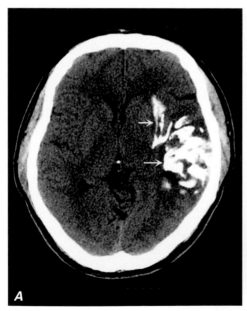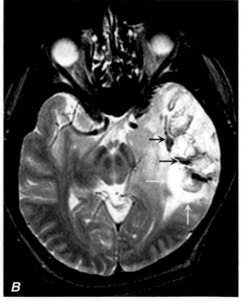

FIGURE 25-2

Oligodendroglioma. **A**. Noncontrast CT scan reveals a calcified mass involving the left temporal lobe (*arrows*) associated with mild mass effect but little edema. **B**. An MR T2-weighted image demonstrates a heterogeneous mass with hypointense signal (*black arrows*) surrounded by a zone of higher signal intensity (*white arrows*), consistent with a calcified temporal lobe mass. The tumor extends into the left medial temporal lobe and compresses the midbrain.

figures, or a high labeling index virtually always recur after surgical resection. Imaging with CT or MRI scans reveals ependymomas as uniformly enhancing masses that are relatively well demarcated from adjacent neural tissue. Ependymomas may metastasize via CSF pathways: brain tumor metastases that spread to the spinal cord by this means are termed *drop metastases*.

Following the gross total excision of an ependymoma, the prognosis is excellent. The 5-year disease-free survival is >80%. However, many ependymomas cannot be totally excised, and postoperative focal external beam radiation or stereotaxic radiosurgery is used. Whether focal radiation is adequate or whether the entire neuraxis needs to be irradiated is not known.

GERMINOMAS

These tumors most commonly present during the second decade of life, generally at sites within or adjacent to the third ventricle, including the pineal region. Germinomas are the most frequent variety of *germ cell tumor*, a tumor type arising in midline structures and including *teratoma*, yolk sac tumor (*endodermal sinus tumor*), *embryonal carcinoma*, and *choriocarcinoma*. Germinomas of the CNS may be benign but are more often aggressive and invasive. Due to their location, patients frequently present with hypothalamic-pituitary dysfunction including diabetes insipidus, visual field deficits, disturbances of memory or mood, or hydrocephalus (Chap. 26). Neuroimaging demonstrates germinomas to be uniformly enhancing masses that may not have well-defined borders. The treatment of choice is complete surgical resection. For unresectable tumors, a stereotaxic biopsy is performed for diagnosis, and focal radiation is the primary therapy. When the extent of disease or very young age precludes radiotherapy as primary treatment, platinum-based chemotherapy may decrease tumor size and facilitate subsequent radiation therapy of residual disease or recurrent tumor. Prognosis depends on the histology and surgical resectability of the tumor. Germinomas are generally radiosensitive and chemosensitive. Five-year survival is >85%.

MEDULLOBLASTOMAS AND PRIMITIVE NEUROECTODERMAL TUMORS (PNET)

These highly cellular malignant tumors are thought to arise from neural precursor cells. Medulloblastomas of the posterior fossa are the most frequent malignant brain tumor of children. *PNET* is a term applied to tumors histologically indistinguishable from medulloblastoma but occurring either in adults or supratentorially in children. In adults, >50% present in the posterior fossa. These tumors frequently disseminate along CSF pathways.

If possible, these tumors should be surgically excised, although outcome is not related to the extent of surgery. In adults, surgical excision of a PNET should be followed by chemotherapy and irradiation of the entire neuraxis, with a boost in radiation dose to the primary tumor. If the tumor is not disseminated at presentation, the prognosis is generally favorable. Aggressive treatment can result in prolonged survival, although half of adult patients relapse within 5 years of treatment.

CNS LYMPHOMA

Primary CNS Lymphoma

These are high-grade B cell malignancies that present within the neuraxis without evidence of systemic lymphoma. They occur most frequently in immunocompromised individuals, specifically organ transplant recipients or patients with AIDS. In immunocompromised patients, CNS lymphomas are invariably associated with Epstein-Barr virus infection of the tumor cells.

In immunocompetent patients, neuroimaging studies most often reveal a uniformly enhancing mass lesion. In immunocompromised patients, primary CNS lymphoma is likely to be multicentric and exhibit ring enhancement or to arise in the meninges (**Fig. 25-3**). Stereotaxic needle biopsy can be used to establish the diagnosis. CSF cytology is often obtained but sensitivity is not high. Leptomeningeal involvement is present in ~15% of patients at presentation and in 50% at some time during the course of the illness. Moreover, the disease extends to the eyes in up to 15% of patients. Therefore, a slit-lamp examination and, if indicated, anterior chamber paracentesis or vitreous biopsy is necessary to define radiation ports.

The prognosis of primary CNS lymphoma is poor compared to histologically similar lymphoma occurring outside the CNS. Many patients experience a dramatic clinical and radiographic response to glucocorticoids; however, relapse almost invariably occurs within weeks. The mainstay of definitive therapy is chemotherapy including high-dose methotrexate. This may be followed in patients <60 years with whole-brain irradiation. Whole-brain irradiation is postponed as long as possible in patients >60 because of the risk of dementia as a manifestation of late-delayed radiation toxicity. Intrathecal chemotherapy with methotrexate can be added if leptomeningeal disease is present. Other agents including rituximab and temozolomide may have a place in initial chemotherapy. Despite aggressive therapy, >90% of patients develop recurrent CNS disease. Historically, the survival of immunocompetent patients with CNS lymphoma has been ~18 months but is now longer with the use of systemic chemotherapy. In organ transplant recipients, reversal of the immunosuppressed state

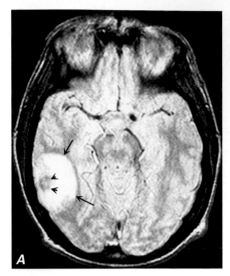
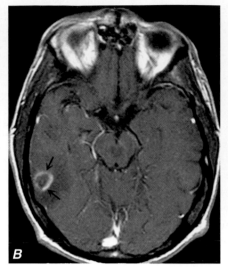
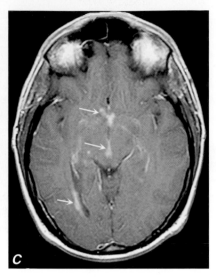

FIGURE 25-3

CNS lymphoma. **A**. Proton density–weighted MR image through the temporal lobe demonstrates a low signal intensity nodule (*small arrows*) surrounded by a ring of high signal intensity edema (*larger arrows*). **B**. T1-weighted contrast-enhanced axial MRI demonstrates ring enhancement surrounded by a nonenhanced rim of edema. In this patient with AIDS, a solitary lesion of this type is consistent with either lymphoma or toxoplasmosis; the presence of multiple lesions favors toxoplasmosis. **C**. In a different patient with lymphomatous meningitis, an axial postcontrast T1-weighted MRI through the midbrain demonstrates multiple areas of abnormal enhancement in periventricular and subependymal regions (*arrows*). Lymphoma tends to spread subependymally at interfaces of CSF and brain parenchyma.

can improve outcome. Survival with AIDS-related primary CNS lymphoma is very poor, generally <3 months; pretreatment performance status, the degree of immunosuppression, and the extent of CNS dissemination at diagnosis all appear to influence outcome.

Secondary CNS Lymphoma

Secondary CNS lymphoma is a manifestation of systemic disease and almost always occurs in adults with progressive B cell lymphoma or B cell leukemia who have tumor involvement of bone, bone marrow, testes, or the cranial sinuses. Leptomeningeal lymphoma is usually detectable with contrast-enhanced CT or gadolinium-enhanced MRI of the brain and spine or by CSF examination. Treatment consists of systemic chemotherapy, intrathecal chemotherapy, and CNS irradiation. It is usually possible to suppress the leptomeningeal disease effectively, although the overall prognosis is determined by the course of the systemic lymphoma.

PITUITARY ADENOMAS   See Chap. 26

MENINGIOMAS

Meningiomas are derived from mesoderm, probably from cells giving rise to the arachnoid granulations. These tumors are usually benign and attached to the dura. They may invade the skull but only infrequently invade the brain. Meningiomas most often occur along the sagittal sinus, over the cerebral convexities, in the cerebellar-pontine angle, and along the dorsum of the spinal cord. They are more frequent in women than men, with a peak incidence in middle age.

Meningiomas may be found incidentally on a CT or MRI scan or may present with a focal seizure, a slowly progressive neurologic deficit, or symptoms of raised ICP. The radiologic image of a dural-based, extraaxial mass with dense, uniform contrast enhancement is essentially diagnostic, although a dural metastasis must also be considered (**Fig. 25-4**). A meningioma may have a "dural tail," a streak of dural enhancement flanking the main tumor mass; however, this finding may also be present with other dural tumors.

Total surgical resection of benign meningiomas is curative. If a total resection cannot be achieved, local external beam radiotherapy or stereotaxic radiosurgery reduces the recurrence rate to <10%. For meningiomas that are not surgically accessible, targeted radiosurgery or heavy particle radiation should be considered. Small asymptomatic meningiomas incidentally discovered in older patients can safely be followed radiologically; these tumors grow at an average rate of ~0.24 cm in diameter per year and only rarely become symptomatic.

Rare meningiomas invade the brain or have histologic evidence of malignancy such as nuclear pleomorphism and cellular atypia. A high mitotic index is also predictive of aggressive behavior. *Hemangiopericytoma*, although not strictly a meningioma, is a meningeal tumor with an

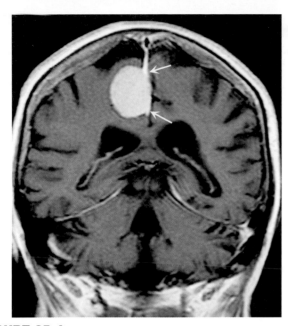

FIGURE 25-4

Meningioma. Coronal postcontrast T1-weighted MR image demonstrates an enhancing extraaxial mass arising from the falx cerebri (*arrows*). There is a "dural tail" of contrast enhancement extending superiorly along the intrahemispheric septum.

especially aggressive behavior. Meningiomas with features of aggressiveness and hemangiopericytomas, even if totally excised by gross inspection, frequently recur and should receive postoperative radiotherapy. Chemotherapy has no proven benefit.

SCHWANNOMAS

These tumors are also called *neuromas*, *neurinomas*, or *neurolemmomas*. They arise from Schwann cells of nerve roots, most frequently in the eighth cranial nerve (*vestibular schwannoma*, formerly termed *acoustic schwannoma*). The fifth cranial nerve is the second most frequent site; however, schwannomas may arise from any cranial or spinal root except the optic and olfactory nerves, which are myelinated by oligodendroglia rather than Schwann cells. NF type 2 (see below) strongly predisposes to vestibular schwannoma. Schwannomas of spinal nerve roots also occur in patients with NF type 2 as well as patients with NF type 1.

Eighth nerve schwannomas typically arise from the vestibular division of the nerve. They are densely and uniformly enhancing neoplasms on MRI (**Fig. 25–5**). Vestibular schwannomas enlarge the internal auditory canal, an imaging feature that helps distinguish them from other cerebellopontine angle masses. Because the vestibular system adapts to slow destruction of the

eighth nerve, vestibular schwannomas characteristically present as progressive unilateral hearing loss rather than with dizziness or other vestibular symptoms. Unexplained unilateral hearing loss merits evaluation with audiometry and either brainstem auditory evoked potentials or an MRI scan (Chap. 12). As a vestibular schwannoma grows, it can compress the cerebellum, pons, or facial nerve. With rare exceptions schwannomas are histologically and clinically benign.

Whenever possible, schwannomas should be surgically excised. When the tumors are small, it is usually possible to preserve hearing in the involved ear. In the case of large tumors, the patient is usually deaf at presentation; nonetheless, surgery is indicated to prevent further compression of posterior fossa structures. Stereotaxic radiosurgery is also effective treatment for schwannoma and has a complication rate equivalent to that of surgery.

OTHER BENIGN BRAIN TUMORS

Epidermoid tumors are cystic tumors with proliferative epidermal cells at the periphery and more mature epidermal cells towards the center of the cyst. The mature cells desquamate into the liquid center of the cyst. Epidermoid tumors are thought to arise from embryonic epidermal rests within the cranium. They occur extraaxially near the midline, in the middle cranial fossa, the suprasellar region, or the cerebellopontine angle. These well-demarcated lesions are amenable to complete surgical excision. Postoperative radiation therapy is unnecessary.

Dermoid cysts are thought to arise from embryonic rests of skin tissue trapped within the CNS during closure of the neural tube. The most frequent locations are in the midline supratentorially or at the cerebellopontine angle. Histologically, they are composed of all elements of the dermis, including epidermis, hair follicles, and sweat glands; they frequently calcify. Treatment is surgical excision.

Craniopharyngiomas are thought to arise from remnants of Rathke's pouch, the mesodermal structure from which the anterior pituitary gland is derived (Chap. 26). Craniopharyngiomas typically present as suprasellar masses. Histologically, craniopharyngiomas resemble epidermoid tumors; they are usually cystic, and in adults 80% are calcified. Because of their location, they may present as growth failure in children, endocrine dysfunction in adults, or visual loss in either age group. Treatment is surgical excision; postoperative external beam radiation or stereotaxic radiosurgery is added if total surgical removal cannot be achieved.

Colloid cysts are benign tumors of unknown cellular origin that occur within the third ventricle and can obstruct CSF flow, leading occasionally to drop attacks or episodes of obtundation. *Rare benign primary brain tu-*

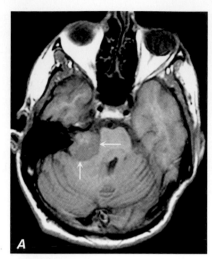
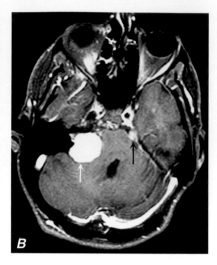

FIGURE 25-5

Vestibular schwannoma. **A**. Axial noncontrast MR scan through the cerebellopontine angle demonstrates an extraaxial mass that extends into a widened internal auditory canal, displacing the pons (*arrows*). **B**. Postcontrast T1-weighted image demonstrates intense enhancement of the vestibular schwannoma (*white arrow*). Abnormal enhancement of the left fifth nerve (*black arrow*) most likely represents another schwannoma in this patient with neurofibromatosis type 2.

mors include neurocytomas, subependymomas, and pleomorphic xanthoastrocytomas. Surgical excision of these neoplasms is the primary treatment and can be curative.

NEUROCUTANEOUS SYNDROMES

This group of genetic disorders, also known as the *phakomatoses*, produces a variety of developmental abnormalities of skin along with an increased risk of nervous system tumors (Table 25-1). These disorders are inherited as autosomal dominant conditions with variable penetrance.

NEUROFIBROMATOSIS TYPE 1 (VON RECKLINGHAUSEN'S DISEASE)

NF1 is characterized by cutaneous *neurofibromas*, pigmented lesions of the skin called *café au lait spots*, freckling in non–sun-exposed areas such as the axilla, hamartomas of the iris termed *Lisch nodules*, and pseudoarthrosis of the tibia. Neurofibromas are benign peripheral nerve tumors composed of proliferating Schwann cells and fibroblasts. They present as multiple, palpable, rubbery, cutaneous tumors. They are generally asymptomatic; however, if they grow in an enclosed space, e.g., the intervertebral foramen, they may produce a compressive radiculopathy or neuropathy. Aqueductal stenosis with hydrocephalus,

scoliosis, short stature, hypertension, epilepsy, and mental retardation may also occur.

Patients with NF1 are at increased risk of developing nervous system neoplasms, including plexiform neurofibromas, optic pathway gliomas, ependymomas, meningiomas, astrocytomas, and pheochromocytomas. Neurofibromas may undergo secondary malignant degeneration and become sarcomatous.

Mutation of the *NF1* gene on chromosome 17 causes von Recklinghausen's disease. The *NF1* gene is a tumor-suppressor gene; it encodes a protein, *neurofibromin*, which modulates signal transduction through the *ras* GTPase pathway.

NEUROFIBROMATOSIS TYPE 2

NF2 is characterized by the development of bilateral vestibular schwannomas in >90% of individuals who inherit the gene. Patients with NF2 also have a predisposition for the development of meningiomas, gliomas, and schwannomas of cranial and spinal nerves. In addition, a characteristic type of cataract, juvenile posterior subcapsular lenticular opacity, occurs in NF2. Multiple café au lait spots and peripheral neurofibromas occur only rarely.

In patients with NF2, vestibular schwannomas usually present with progressive unilateral deafness early in the third decade of life. Bilateral vestibular schwannomas are generally detectable by MRI at that time (**Fig. 25–6**). Surgical management is designed to treat the underlying tumor and preserve hearing as long as possible.

This syndrome is caused by mutation of the *NF2* gene on chromosome 22q; *NF2* encodes a protein called *neurofibromin 2*, *schwannomin*, or *merlin*, with homology to a family of cytoskeletal proteins that includes moesin, ezrin, and radixin.

TUBEROUS SCLEROSIS (BOURNEVILLE'S DISEASE)

Tuberous sclerosis is characterized by cutaneous lesions, seizures, and mental retardation. The cutaneous lesions include adenoma sebaceum (facial angiofibromas), ash leaf–shaped hypopigmented macules (best seen under ultraviolet illumination with a Wood's lamp), shagreen patches (yellowish thickenings of the skin over the lumbosacral region of the back), and depigmented nevi. On neuroimaging studies, the presence of subependymal nodules, which may be calcified, is characteristic. Patients inheriting the tuberous sclerosis gene are at increased risk of developing ependymomas and childhood astrocytomas, of which >90% are *subependymal giant cell astrocytomas*. These are benign neoplasms that may develop in the retina or along the border of the lateral ventricles. They may obstruct the foramen of Monro and produce hydrocephalus, necessitating their removal. Rhabdomyomas of the myocardium and angiomyomas of the kidney, liver, adrenals, and pancreas may also occur.

Treatment is symptomatic. Anticonvulsants for seizures, shunting for hydrocephalus, and behavioral and educational strategies for mental retardation are the mainstays of management.

Mutations at both 9q(*TSC-1*) and 16p(*TSC-2*) are associated with tuberous sclerosis. The mutated genes encode *tuberins*, proteins that modulate the GTPase activity of other cellular proteins.

VON HIPPEL–LINDAU SYNDROME

This syndrome consists of retinal, cerebellar, and spinal hemangioblastomas, which are slowly growing cystic tumors. Hypernephroma, renal cell carcinoma, pheochromocytoma, and benign cysts of the kidneys, pancreas, epididymis, or liver may also occur. Erythropoietin production by hemangioblastomas may result in polycythemia. The von Hippel–Lindau (*VHL*) gene on chromosome 3p is a tumor suppressor that encodes a protein with multiple functions, including mediating signal transduction in response to cellular hypoxia.

TUMORS METASTATIC TO BRAIN

MECHANISMS OF BRAIN METASTASES

The large majority of brain metastases disseminate by hematogenous spread. The anatomical distribution of brain metastases generally parallels regional cerebral blood flow, with a predilection for the gray matter–white matter junction and for the border zone

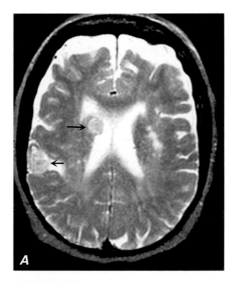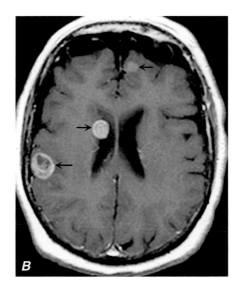

FIGURE 25-6

Brain metastasis. **A**. Axial T2-weighted MRI through the lateral ventricles reveals two isodense masses, one in the subependymal region and one near the cortex (*arrows*). **B**. T1-weighted postcontrast image at the same level as *A* reveals enhancement of the two masses seen on the T2-weighted image as well as a third mass in the left frontal lobe (*arrows*).

between middle cerebral and posterior cerebral artery distributions. The lung is the most common origin of brain metastases; both primary lung cancer (adenocarcinoma and small cell lung cancer) and cancers metastatic to the lung can metastasize to the brain. Breast cancer (especially ductal carcinoma) has a propensity to metastasize to the cerebellum and the posterior pituitary gland. Moreover, breast cancer that metastasizes to bone tends not to metastasize to the brain. Other common origins of brain metastases are gastrointestinal malignancies and melanoma (**Table 25-2**). Certain less common tumors have a special propensity to metastasize to brain, including germ cell tumors and thyroid cancer. By contrast, prostate cancer, ovarian cancer, and Hodgkin's disease rarely metastasize to the brain.

EVALUATION OF METASTASES FROM KNOWN CANCER

On MRI scans brain metastases typically appear as well-demarcated, approximately spherical lesions that are hypointense or isointense relative to brain on T1-weighted images and bright on T2-weighted images. They invariably enhance with gadolinium, reflecting extravasation of gadolinium through tumor vessels that lack a blood-tumor barrier (Fig. 25-6). Small metastases often enhance uniformly. Larger metastases typically produce ring enhancement surrounding a central mass of nonenhancing necrotic tissue that develops as the metastasis outgrows its blood supply. Metastases are surrounded by variable amounts of edema. Blood products may also be seen, reflecting hemorrhage of abnormal tumor vessels.

The radiologic appearance of a brain metastasis is not specific. The differential diagnosis of ring-enhancement lesions includes brain abscess, radiation necrosis, toxoplasmosis, granulomas (tuberculosis, sarcoidosis), demyelinating lesions, primary brain tumors, primary CNS lymphoma, stroke, hemorrhage, and trauma. Contrast-enhanced CT scanning is less sensitive than MRI for the detection of brain metastases. Cytologic examination of the CSF is not indicated, since intraparenchymal brain metastases almost never shed cells into the CSF. Measuring CSF levels of tumor markers such as carcinoembryonic antigen (CEA) is rarely helpful in management.

BRAIN METASTASES WITHOUT A KNOWN PRIMARY TUMOR

In general hospital populations, up to one-third of patients presenting with brain metastases do not have a known underlying cancer. These patients generally present with either a seizure or a progressive neurologic deficit. Neuroimaging studies demonstrate one or multiple ring-enhancement lesions. In individuals who are not immunocompromised and not at risk for brain abscesses, this radiologic pattern is most likely due to brain metastasis.

Diagnostic evaluation begins with a search for the primary tumor. Blood tests should include CEA and liver function tests. Examination of the skin for melanoma and the thyroid gland for masses should be carried out. A CT scan of the chest, abdomen, and pelvis or whole-body PET scan should be obtained. If these are all negative, further imaging studies, including bone scan, other radionuclide scans, mammography, and upper and lower gastrointestinal barium studies, are unlikely to be productive. The search for a primary cancer most often discloses lung cancer, particularly small cell lung cancer, or melanoma. In 30% of patients no primary tumor can be identified, even after extensive evaluation.

TABLE 25-2

FREQUENCY OF NERVOUS SYSTEM METASTASES BY COMMON PRIMARY TUMORS			
SITE OF PRIMARY TUMOR	BRAIN METASTASES, %	LEPTOMENINGEAL METASTASES, %	SPINAL CORD COMPRESSION, %
Lung	40	24	18
Breast	19	41	24
Melanoma	10	12	4
Gastrointestinal tract	7	13	6
Genitourinary tract	7		18
Other	17	10	30

A tissue diagnosis is essential. If a primary tumor is found, it will usually be more accessible to biopsy than a brain lesion. If a single brain lesion is found in a surgically accessible location, if a primary tumor is not found, or if the primary tumor is in a location difficult to biopsy, the brain metastasis should be biopsied or resected.

TREATMENT FOR TUMORS METASTATIC TO BRAIN

Once a systemic cancer metastasizes to the brain it is, with rare exception, incurable. Therapy is therefore palliative, designed to prevent disability and suffering and, if possible, to prolong life. Published outcome studies have focused on survival as the primary end point, leaving questions regarding quality of life unanswered. There is, however, widespread agreement that glucocorticoids, anticonvulsants, and radiation therapy improve the quality of life for many patients. The roles of surgery and chemotherapy are less well established.

General Measures

Glucocorticoids frequently ameliorate symptoms of brain metastases. Improvement is often dramatic, occurs within 24 h, and is sustained with continued administration, although the toxicity of glucocorticoids is cumulative. Therefore, if possible, a more definitive therapy for metastases should be instituted to permit withdrawal of glucocorticoid therapy. One-third of patients with brain metastases have one or more seizures. Anticonvulsants are used empirically for seizure prophylaxis when supratentorial metastases are present.

Specific Measures
RADIATION THERAPY

Radiation is the primary treatment for brain metastases. Since multiple microscopic deposits of tumor cells throughout the brain are likely to be present in addition to metastases visualized by neuroimaging studies, whole-brain irradiation is usually used. Its benefit has been established in controlled studies, but no clear dose response has been shown. Usually, 30 to 37.5 Gy is administered in 10 to 15 fractions; an additional dose ("boost") of focal irradiation to a single or large metastasis may also be administered. Stereotaxic radiosurgery is of benefit in patients with four or fewer metastases demonstrable by MRI.

SURGERY

Up to 40% of patients with brain metastases have only a single tumor mass identified by CT. Accessible single metastases are usually surgically excised as a palliative measure. If the systemic disease is under control, total resection of a single brain lesion has been demonstrated to improve survival and minimize disability. Survival appears to be improved if surgery is followed by whole-brain irradiation.

CHEMOTHERAPY

Brain metastases of certain tumors, including breast cancer, small cell lung cancer, and germ cell tumors, are often responsive to systemic chemotherapy. Although metastases frequently do not respond as well as the primary tumor, dramatic responses to systemic chemotherapy or hormonal therapy may occur in some cases. In patients who are neurologically stable, two to four cycles of systemic chemotherapy may be administered initially to reduce tumor mass and render the residual tumor more amenable to radiation therapy. Even if a complete radiologic remission is achieved from chemotherapy, whole-brain irradiation should then be administered.

EXPERIMENTAL THERAPIES

These include gene therapy, immunotherapy, intraarterial chemotherapy, and chemotherapy administered following osmotic disruption of the blood-brain barrier.

LEPTOMENINGEAL METASTASES

Leptomeningeal metastases are also called *carcinomatous meningitis*, *meningeal carcinomatosis*, and, in the cases of specific tumors, *leukemic meningitis* or *lymphomatous meningitis*. Clinical evidence of leptomeningeal metastases is present in 8% of patients with metastatic solid tumors; at necropsy, the prevalence is as high as 19%. Among solid tumors, adenocarcinomas of the breast, lung, and gastrointestinal tract and melanoma are the most common cause of leptomeningeal metastases (Table 25-2). In one-quarter of patients the systemic cancer is under control; thus effective control of leptomeningeal disease can improve the quality and duration of life.

Cancer usually metastasizes to the meninges via the bloodstream. Alternatively, a superficially located parenchymal brain metastasis may shed cells directly into the subarachnoid space. Some tumors, including squamous cell carcinoma of the skin and some non-Hodgkin's lymphomas, have a propensity to grow along peripheral nerves and may seed the meninges by that route.

CLINICAL FEATURES

Leptomeningeal metastases present with signs and symptoms at multiple levels of the nervous system, most often in a setting of known systemic malignancy. Encephalopathy is frequent, and cranial neuropathy or spinal radiculopathy from nodular nerve root compression is characteristic. Hydrocephalus results from obstruction of CSF outflow. Focal neurologic deficits from coexisting intraparenchymal metastases may occur.

LABORATORY EVALUATION

Leptomeningeal metastases are diagnosed by cytologic demonstration of malignant cells in the CSF, by MRI demonstration of nodular tumor deposits in the meninges or diffuse meningeal enhancement (**Fig. 25-7**), or by meningeal biopsy. CSF findings are usually those of an inflammatory meningitis, consisting of lymphocytic pleocytosis, elevated protein levels, and normal or low CSF glucose. A complete MRI examination of the neuraxis may demonstrate hydrocephalus due to obstruction of CSF pathways and identify nodular meningeal metastases.

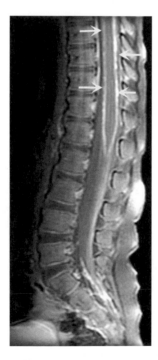

FIGURE 25-7
Carcinomatous meningitis. Sagittal postcontrast MRI through the lower thoracic region demonstrates diffuse pial enhancement along the surface of the spinal cord (*arrows*), typical of CSF spread of neoplasm.

TREATMENT FOR LEPTOMENINGEAL METASTASES

In selected patients, intrathecal chemotherapy or focal external beam radiotherapy to sites of nodular leptomeningeal disease is employed. Although the prognosis of leptomeningeal metastases is poor, ~20% of patients treated aggressively for leptomeningeal metastases can expect a response of >6 months. Intrathecal therapy exposes meningeal tumor implants to high concentrations of chemotherapy with minimal systemic toxicity. Methotrexate can be safely administered intrathecally and is effective against leptomeningeal metastases from a variety of solid tumors and lymphoma; cytarabine and thiotepa are alternative agents. Intrathecal chemotherapy may be administered either by repeated lumbar puncture or through an indwelling Ommaya reservoir, which consists of a catheter in one lateral ventricle attached to a reservoir implanted under the scalp. If there is a question of patency of CSF pathways, a radionuclide flow study through the reservoir may be performed.

Large, nodular deposits of tumor on the meninges or along nerve roots are unlikely to respond to intrathecal chemotherapy, as the barrier to diffusion is too great. Therefore, external beam radiation is employed. Hydrocephalus is treated with a ventriculoperitoneal shunt, although seeding of the peritoneum by tumor is a risk.

MALIGNANT SPINAL CORD COMPRESSION

Spinal cord compression from solid tumor metastases usually results from expansion of a vertebral metastasis into the epidural space. Primary tumors that frequently metastasize to bone include lung, breast, and prostate cancer. Back pain is usually the first symptom and is prominent at presentation in 90% of patients. The pain is typically dull, aching, and may be associated with localized tenderness. If a nerve root is compressed, radicular pain is also present. The thoracic cord is most often affected. Weakness, sensory loss, and autonomic dysfunction (urinary urgency and incontinence, fecal incontinence, and sexual impotence in men) are the hallmarks of spinal cord compression. Once signs of spinal cord compression appear, they tend to progress rapidly. It is thus essential to recognize and treat this serious complication of malignancy promptly in order to prevent irreversible neurologic deficits. Diagnosis and management are discussed in Chap. 24.

METASTASES TO THE PERIPHERAL NERVOUS SYSTEM

Systemic cancer may compress or invade peripheral nerves. Compression of the brachial plexus may occur by direct extension of Pancoast's tumors (cancer of the apex of the lung) or by extension of local lymph node metastases of breast or lung cancer or lymphoma. The lumbosacral plexus may be compressed by the retroperitoneal spread of prostate or ovarian cancer or lymphoma. Skull metastases may compress cranial nerve branches as they pass through the skull, and pituitary metastases may extend into the cavernous sinus. The epineurium generally provides an effective barrier to invasion of the peripheral nerves by solid tumors, but certain tumors characteristically invade and spread along peripheral nerves. Squamous cell carcinoma of the skin may spread along the trigeminal nerve and extend intracranially. Non-Hodgkin's lymphoma may be neurotrophic and cause polyradiculopathy or a syndrome resembling mononeuropathy multiplex. Focal external beam radiation may reduce pain, prevent irreversible loss of peripheral nerve function, and possibly restore function.

In patients with cancer who have brachial or lumbosacral plexopathy, it may be difficult to distinguish tumor invasion from radiation injury. High radiation dose or the presence of myokymia (rippling contractions of muscle) suggests radiation injury, whereas pain suggests tumor. Radiographic imaging studies may be equivocal, and surgical exploration is sometimes required.

COMPLICATIONS OF THERAPY

RADIATION TOXICITY

The nervous system is vulnerable to injury by therapeutic radiation. Histologically, there is demyelination, degeneration of small arterioles, and eventually brain infarction and necrosis.

Acute radiation injury occurs during or immediately after therapy. It is rarely seen with current protocols of external beam radiation but may occur after stereotaxic radiosurgery. Manifestations include headache, sleepiness, and worsening of preexisting neurologic deficits.

Early delayed radiation injury occurs within 4 months of therapy. It is associated with an increased white matter T2 signal on MRI scans. In children, the *somnolence syndrome* is a common form of early delayed radiation injury in which somnolence and ataxia develop after whole-brain irradiation. Irradiation of the cervical spine

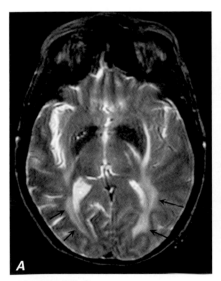 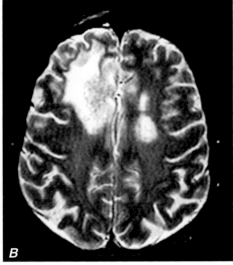 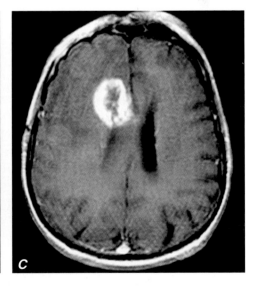

FIGURE 25-8

Radiation injury. *A*. Late-delayed radiation injury 1 year after whole-brain radiation (5500 cGy). T2-weighted MR image at the level of the temporal lobes reveals high signal intensity abnormality in periventricular white matter (*arrows*). *B* and *C*. Focal radiation necrosis 3 years after radiotherapy (7000 cGy) for carcinoma of the nasopharynx. Axial T2-weighted MRI (*B*) demonstrates a mass in the right frontal lobe with surrounding vasogenic edema. Abnormal signal changes are also present on the left. T1-weighted postcontrast MRI (*C*) reveals a heterogeneously enhancing mass in the right cingulate gyrus.

may cause Lhermitte's phenomenon, an electricity-like sensation evoked by neck flexion. Acute and early delayed radiation injury are self-limited and glucocorticoid-responsive disorders that do not appear to increase the risk of late radiation injury.

Late delayed radiation injury produces permanent damage to the nervous system. It occurs >4 months (generally 8 to 24 months) after completion of therapy; onset 15 years after therapy has been described. After whole-brain irradiation, progressive dementia can occur, sometimes accompanied by gait apraxia. White matter signal abnormalities are present on MRI studies (**Fig. 25-8**). Following focal brain irradiation, radiation necrosis occurs within the radiation field producing a contrast-enhancing (frequently ring-enhancing) mass. MRI or CT scans are often unable to distinguish radiation necrosis from recurrent tumor, but PET or SPECT scans may demonstrate that glucose metabolism is increased in tumor tissue but decreased in radiation necrosis. Magnetic resonance spectroscopy may demonstrate a high lactate concentration with relatively low choline concentration in areas of necrosis. Biopsy is frequently required to establish the correct diagnosis. Peripheral nerves, including the brachial and lumbosacral plexuses, may also develop late delayed radiation injury.

If untreated, radiation necrosis of the CNS may act as an expanding mass lesion, although it may resolve spontaneously or after treatment with glucocorticoids. Progressive radiation necrosis is best treated with surgical resection if the patient has a life expectancy of at least 6 months and a Karnofsky performance score >70. There are anecdotal reports that anticoagulation with heparin or warfarin may be beneficial. Radiation injury also accelerates the development of atherosclerosis in large arteries, but an increase in the risk of stroke becomes significant only years after radiation treatment.

Endocrine dysfunction frequently follows exposure of the hypothalamus or pituitary gland to therapeutic radiation. Growth hormone is the pituitary hormone most sensitive to radiation therapy, and thyroid-stimulating hormone is the least sensitive; ACTH, prolactin, and the gonadotropins have an intermediate sensitivity.

Development of a second neoplasm is another risk of therapeutic radiation that generally occurs many years after radiation exposure. Depending on the irradiated field, the risk of gliomas, meningiomas, sarcomas, and thyroid cancer is increased.

COMPLICATIONS OF CHEMOTHERAPY

Chemotherapy regimens used to treat primary brain tumors have generally included a nitrosourea or temozolomide and are well tolerated. Infrequently, nitrosoureas and other drugs used to treat CNS neoplasms cause altered mental states (e.g., confusion, depression), ataxia, and seizures. Chemotherapy for systemic malignancy is a more frequent cause of nervous system toxicity. Cisplatin commonly produces tinnitus and high-frequency bilateral hearing loss, especially in younger patients. At cumulative doses, >450 mg/m^2, cisplatin can produce a symmetric, large-fiber axonal neuropathy that is predominantly sensory; paclitaxel (Taxol) produces a similar picture. Fluorouracil and high-dose cytarabine can cause cerebellar dysfunction that resolves after discontinuation of therapy. Vincristine, which is commonly used to treat lymphoma, may cause an acute ileus and is frequently associated with development of a progressive distal, symmetric sensory-motor neuropathy with foot drop and paresthesias.

FURTHER READINGS

BEHIN A et al: Primary brain tumors in adults. Lancet 361:323, 2003

BYRNE TN: Response of low-grade oligodendroglial tumors to temozolomide. J Neurooncol 70:279, 2004

GLANTZ M et al: Temozolomide as an alternative to irradiation for elderly patients with newly diagnosed malignant gliomas. Cancer 97:2262, 2003

☑ LEBRUN C et al: Long-term outcome of oligodendrogliomas. Neurology 62:1783, 2004

A study detailing survival data for patients with oligodendrogliomas.

☑ OHGAKI H: Genetic pathways to glioblastomas. Neuropathology 25:1, 2005

Review of molecular mechanisms leading to the development of malignant astrocytomas.

ZHU Y, PARADA LF: The molecular and genetic basis of neurological tumors. Nat Rev Cancer 2:616, 2002

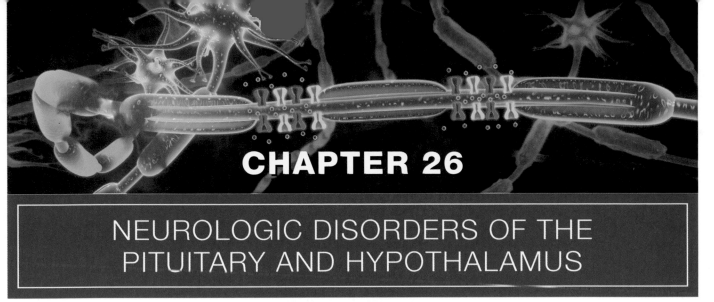

CHAPTER 26

NEUROLOGIC DISORDERS OF THE PITUITARY AND HYPOTHALAMUS

Shlomo Melmed
J. Larry Jameson
Gary L. Robertson

The pituitary is often referred to as the "master gland" because, together with the hypothalamus, it orchestrates the complex regulatory functions of multiple other endocrine glands.

The anterior pituitary gland produces six major hormones: (1) prolactin (PRL), (2) growth hormone (GH), (3) adrenocorticotropin hormone (ACTH), (4) luteinizing hormone (LH), (5) follicle-stimulating hormone (FSH), and (6) thyroid-stimulating hormone (TSH). Pituitary hormones are secreted in a pulsatile manner, reflecting stimulation by an array of specific hypothalamic releasing factors. Each of these pituitary hormones elicits specific responses in peripheral target tissues. The hormonal products of these peripheral glands, in turn, exert feedback control at the level of the hypothalamus and pituitary to modulate pituitary function (**Fig. 26-1**). Pituitary tumors cause characteristic hormone excess syndromes. Hormone deficiency may be inherited or acquired. Fortunately, efficacious treatments exist for the various pituitary hormone excess and deficiency syndromes. Nonetheless, these diagnoses are often elusive, emphasizing the importance of recognizing subtle clinical manifestations and performing the correct laboratory diagnostic tests.

The neurohypophysis, or posterior pituitary gland, is formed by axons that originate in large cell bodies in the supraoptic and paraventricular nuclei of the hypothalamus. It produces two hormones: (1) arginine vasopressin (AVP), also known as antidiuretic hormone; and (2) oxytocin. AVP acts on the renal tubules to reduce water loss by concentrating the urine. Oxytocin stimulates postpartum milk letdown in response to suckling. AVP deficiency causes diabetes insipidus (DI), characterized by the production of large amounts of dilute urine. Excessive or inappropriate AVP production predisposes to hyponatremia if water intake is not reduced in parallel with urine output.

ANATOMY

The pituitary gland weighs ~600 mg and is located within the sella turcica ventral to the diaphragma sella; it comprises anatomically and functionally distinct anterior and posterior lobes. The sella is contiguous to vascular and neurologic structures, including the cavernous sinuses, cranial nerves, and optic chiasm. Thus, expanding intrasellar pathologic processes may have significant central mass effects in addition to their endocrinologic impact.

Hypothalamic neural cells synthesize specific releasing and inhibiting hormones that are secreted directly into the portal vessels of the pituitary stalk. Blood supply of the pituitary gland is derived from the superior and inferior hypophyseal arteries (**Fig. 26-2**). The hypothalamic-pituitary portal plexus provides the major blood source for the anterior pituitary, allowing reliable transmission of hypothalamic peptide pulses without significant

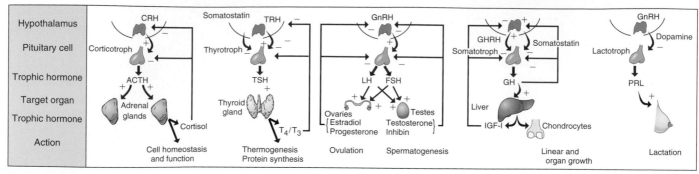

FIGURE 26-1

Diagram of pituitary axes. Hypothalamic hormones regulate anterior pituitary trophic hormones that, in turn, determine target gland secretion. Peripheral hormones feed back to regulate hypothalamic and pituitary hormones. For abbreviations, see text.

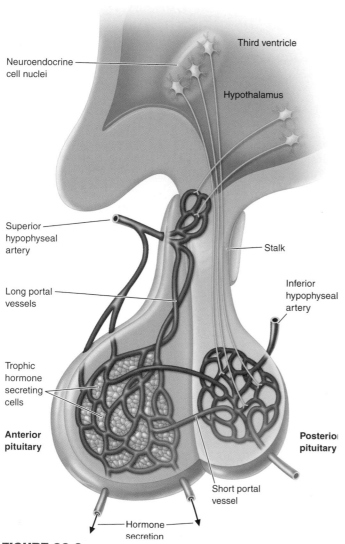

FIGURE 26-2

Diagram of hypothalamic-pituitary vasculature: The hypothalamic nuclei produce hormones that traverse the portal system and impinge on anterior pituitary cells to regulate pituitary hormone secretion. Posterior pituitary hormones are derived from direct neural extensions.

systemic dilution; consequently, pituitary cells are exposed to sharp spikes of releasing factors and in turn release their hormones as discrete pulses (**Fig. 26-3**).

The posterior pituitary is supplied by the inferior hypophyseal arteries. In contrast to the anterior pituitary, the posterior lobe is directly innervated by hypothalamic neurons (supraopticohypophyseal and tuberohypophyseal nerve tracts) via the pituitary stalk. Thus, posterior pituitary production of vasopressin (antidiuretic hormone; ADH) and oxytocin is particularly sensitive to neuronal damage by lesions that affect the pituitary stalk or hypothalamus.

HYPOTHALAMIC AND ANTERIOR PITUITARY INSUFFICIENCY

Hypopituitarism results from impaired production of one or more of the anterior pituitary trophic hormones. Reduced pituitary function can result from inherited disorders; more commonly, it is acquired and reflects the mass effects of tumors or the consequences of inflammation or vascular damage. These processes may also impair synthesis or secretion of hypothalamic hormones, with resultant pituitary failure (**Table 26-1**).

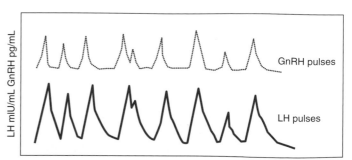

FIGURE 26-3

Hypothalamic gonadotropin-releasing hormone (GnRH) pulses induce secretory pulses of luteinizing hormone (LH).

TABLE 26-1

ETIOLOGY OF HYPOPITUITARISM[a]

Development/structural
  Transcription factor defect
  Pituitary dysplasia/aplasia
  Congenital CNS mass, encephalocele
  Primary empty sella
  Congenital hypothalamic disorders (septo-optic
    dysplasia, Prader-Willi syndrome, Laurence-
    Moon-Biedl syndrome, Kallmann syndrome)
Traumatic
  Surgical resection
  Radiation damage
  Head injuries
Neoplastic
  Pituitary adenoma
  Parasellar mass (meningioma, germinoma,
    ependymoma, glioma)
  Rathke's cyst
  Craniopharyngioma
  Hypothalamic hamartoma, gangliocytoma
  Pituitary metastases (breast, lung, colon carcinoma)
  Lymphoma and leukemia
  Meningioma
Infiltrative/inflammatory
  Hemochromatosis
  Lymphocytic hypophysitis
  Sarcoidosis
  Histiocytosis X
  Granulomatous hypophysitis
Vascular
  Pituitary apoplexy
  Pregnancy-related (infarction with diabetes;
    postpartum necrosis)
  Sickle cell disease
  Arteritis
Infections
  Fungal (histoplasmosis)
  Parasitic (toxoplasmosis)
  Tuberculosis
  Pneumocystis carinii

[a]Trophic hormone failure associated with pituitary compression or destruction usually occurs sequentially GH > FSH > LH > TSH > ACTH. During childhood, growth retardation is often the presenting feature, and in adults hypogonadism is the earliest symptom.

ACQUIRED HYPOPITUITARISM

Hypopituitarism may be caused by accidental or neurosurgical trauma; vascular events such as apoplexy; pituitary or hypothalamic neoplasms such as pituitary adenomas, craniopharyngiomas, or metastatic tumors; inflammatory disease such as lymphocytic hypophysitis; infiltrative disorders such as sarcoidosis, hemochromatosis, and tuberculosis; or irradiation.

Hypothalamic Infiltration Disorders

These disorders—including sarcoidosis, histiocytosis X, amyloidosis, and hemochromatosis—frequently involve both hypothalamic and pituitary neuronal and neurochemical tracts. Consequently, DI occurs in half of patients with these disorders. Growth retardation is seen if attenuated GH secretion occurs before pubertal epiphyseal closure. Hypogonadotropic hypogonadism and hyperprolactinemia are also common.

Inflammatory Lesions

Pituitary damage and subsequent dysfunction can be seen with chronic infections such as tuberculosis, opportunistic fungal infections associated with AIDS, and in tertiary syphilis. Other inflammatory processes, such as granulomas or sarcoidosis, may mimic a pituitary adenoma. These lesions may cause extensive hypothalamic and pituitary damage, leading to trophic hormone deficiencies.

Cranial Irradiation

Cranial irradiation may result in long-term hypothalamic and pituitary dysfunction, especially in children and adolescents, as they are more susceptible to damage following whole-brain or head and neck therapeutic irradiation. The development of hormonal abnormalities correlates strongly with irradiation dosage and the time interval after completion of radiotherapy. Up to two-thirds of patients ultimately develop hormone insufficiency after a median dose of 50 Gy (5000 rad) directed at the skull base. The development of hypopituitarism occurs over 5 to 15 years and usually reflects hypothalamic damage rather than absolute destruction of pituitary cells. Though the pattern of hormone loss is variable, GH deficiency is most common, followed by gonadotropin and ACTH deficiency. When deficiency of one or more hormones is documented, the possibility of diminished reserve of other hormones is likely. Accordingly, anterior pituitary function should be evaluated over the long term in previously irradiated patients, and replacement therapy instituted when appropriate (see below).

Lymphocytic Hypophysitis

This occurs mainly in pregnant or postpartum women; it usually presents with hyperprolactinemia and magnetic resonance imaging (MRI) evidence of a prominent pituitary mass resembling an adenoma, with mildly elevated PRL levels. Pituitary failure caused by diffuse lymphocytic infiltration may be transient or permanent but requires immediate evaluation and treatment. Rarely, isolated pituitary hormone deficiencies have been described, suggesting a selective autoimmune process targeted to specific cell types. Most patients manifest symptoms of progressive mass effects with headache and visual disturbance. The erythrocyte sedimentation rate is often elevated. As the MRI image may be indistinguishable from that of a pituitary adenoma, hypophysitis should be considered in a postpartum woman with a newly diagnosed pituitary mass before embarking on unnecessary surgical intervention. The inflammatory process often resolves after several months of glucocorticoid treatment, and pituitary function may be restored, depending on the extent of damage.

Pituitary Apoplexy

Acute intrapituitary hemorrhagic vascular events can cause substantial damage to the pituitary and surrounding sellar structures. Pituitary apoplexy may occur spontaneously in a preexisting adenoma (usually nonfunctioning); postpartum (Sheehan's syndrome); or in association with diabetes, hypertension, sickle cell anemia, or acute shock. The hyperplastic enlargement of the pituitary during pregnancy increases the risk for hemorrhage and infarction. Apoplexy is an endocrine emergency that may result in severe hypoglycemia, hypotension, central nervous system (CNS) hemorrhage, and death. Acute symptoms may include severe headache with signs of meningeal irritation, bilateral visual changes, ophthalmoplegia, and, in severe cases, cardiovascular collapse and loss of consciousness. Pituitary computed tomography (CT) or MRI may reveal signs of intratumoral or sellar hemorrhage, with deviation of the pituitary stalk and compression of pituitary tissue.

Patients with no evident visual loss or impaired consciousness can be observed and managed conservatively with high-dose glucocorticoids. Those with significant or progressive visual loss or loss of consciousness require urgent surgical decompression. Visual recovery after surgery is inversely correlated with the length of time after the acute event. Therefore, severe ophthalmoplegia or visual deficits are indications for early surgery. Hypopituitarism is very common after apoplexy.

Empty Sella

A partial or apparently totally empty sella is often an incidental MRI finding. These patients usually have normal pituitary function, implying that the surrounding rim of pituitary tissue is fully functional. Hypopituitarism, however, may develop insidiously. Pituitary masses may undergo clinically silent infarction with development of a partial or totally empty sella by cerebrospinal fluid (CSF) filling the dural herniation. Rarely, functional pituitary adenomas may arise within the rim of pituitary tissue, and these are not always visible on MRI.

PRESENTATION AND DIAGNOSIS

The clinical manifestations of hypopituitarism depend on which hormones are lost and the extent of the hormone deficiency. GH deficiency causes growth disorders in children and leads to abnormal body composition in adults. Gonadotropin deficiency causes menstrual disorders and infertility in women and decreased sexual function, infertility, and loss of secondary sexual characteristics in men. TSH and ACTH deficiency usually develop later in the course of pituitary failure. TSH deficiency causes growth retardation in children and features of hypothyroidism in children and in adults. The secondary form of adrenal insufficiency caused by ACTH deficiency leads to hypocortisolism with relative preservation of mineralocorticoid production. PRL deficiency causes failure of lactation. When lesions involve the posterior pituitary, polyuria and polydipsia reflect loss of vasopressin secretion. Epidemiologic studies have documented an increased mortality rate in patients with longstanding pituitary damage, primarily from increased cardiovascular and cerebrovascular disease.

LABORATORY INVESTIGATION

Biochemical diagnosis of pituitary insufficiency is made by demonstrating low levels of trophic hormones in the setting of low target hormone levels. For example, low free thyroxine in the setting of a low or inappropriately normal TSH level suggests secondary hypothyroidism. Similarly, a low testosterone level without elevation of gonadotropins suggests hypogonadotropic hypogonadism. Provocative tests may be required to assess pituitary reserve (**Table 26-2**). GH responses to insulin-induced hypoglycemia, arginine, L-dopa, growth hormone–releasing hormone (GHRH), or growth hormone–releasing peptides (GHRPs) can be used to assess GH reserve. PRL and TSH responses to thyrotropin–releasing hormone (TRH) reflect lactotrope and thyrotrope function. Corticotropin-releasing hormone (CRH) administration induces ACTH release, and administration of synthetic ACTH (cortrosyn) evokes adrenal cortisol release as an indirect indicator of pituitary ACTH reserve. ACTH reserve is most reliably assessed during insulin-induced hypoglycemia. However, this test should be performed cautiously in patients with suspected adrenal insufficiency because of increased risk of hypoglycemia and hypotension. Insulin-induced hypoglycemia is contraindicated in patients with coronary heart disease or seizure disorders.

TABLE 26-2

TESTS OF PITUITARY INSUFFICIENCY

HORMONE	TEST	BLOOD SAMPLES	INTERPRETATION
Growth hormone	Insulin tolerance test: Regular insulin (0.05–0.15 U/kg IV)	−30, 0, 30, 60, 120 min for glucose and GH	Glucose <40 mg/dL; GH should be >3 μg/L
	GHRH test: 1 μg/kg IV	0, 15, 30, 45, 60, 120 min for GH	Normal response is GH >3 μg/L
	L-Arginine test: 30 g IV over 30 min	0, 30, 60, 120 min for GH	Normal response is GH >3 μg/L
	L-dopa test: 500 mg PO	0, 30, 60, 120 min for GH	Normal response is GH >3 μg/L
Prolactin	TRH test: 200–500 μg IV	0, 20, and 60 min for TSH and PRL	Normal prolactin is >2 μg/L and increase >200% of baseline
ACTH	Insulin tolerance test: Regular insulin (0.05–0.15 U/kg IV)	−30, 0, 30, 60, 90 min for glucose and cortisol	Glucose <40 mg/dL; Cortisol should increase by >7 μg/dL or to >20 μg/dL
	CRH test: 1 μg/kg ovine CRH IV at 0800 h	0, 15, 30, 60, 90, 120 min for ACTH and cortisol	Basal ACTH increases 2- to 4-fold and peaks at 20–100 pg/mL; Cortisol levels >20–25 μg/dL
	Metyrapone test: Metyrapone (30 mg/kg) at midnight	Plasma 11-deoxycortisol and cortisol at 8 A.M.; ACTH can also be measured	Plasma cortisol should be <4 μg/dL to assure an adequate response; Normal response is 11-deoxycortisol >7.5 μg/dL or ACTH >75 pg/mL
	Standard ACTH stimulation test: ACTH 1-24 (Cosyntropin), 0.25 mg IM or IV	0, 30, 60 min for cortisol and aldosterone	Normal response is cortisol >21 μg/dL and aldosterone response of >4 ng/dL above baseline
	Low-dose ACTH test: ACTH 1-24 (Cosyntropin), 1 μg IV	0, 30, 60 min for cortisol	Cortisol should be >21 μg/dL
	3-day ACTH stimulation test consists of 0.25 mg ACTH 1-24 given IV over 8 h each day		Cortisol >21 μg/dL
TSH	Basal thyroid function tests: T_4, T_3, TSH	Basal tests	Low free thyroid hormone levels in the setting of TSH levels that are not appropriately increased
	TRH test: 200–500 μg IV	0, 20, 60 min for TSH and PRL	TSH should increase by >5 mU/L unless thyroid hormone levels are increased
LH, FSH	LH, FSH, testosterone, estrogen	Basal tests	Basal LH and FSH should be increased in postmenopausal women; Low testosterone levels in the setting of low LH and FSH
	GnRH test: GnRH (100 μg) IV	0, 30, 60 min for LH and FSH	In most adults, LH should increase by 10 IU/L and FSH by 2 IU/L; Normal responses are variable
Multiple hormones	Combined anterior pituitary test: GHRH (1 μg/kg), CRH (1 μg/kg), GnRH (100 μg), TRH (200 μg) are given IV	−30, 0, 15, 30, 60, 90, 120 min for GH, ACTH, cortisol, LH, FSH, and TSH	Combined or individual releasing hormone responses must be elevated in the context of basal target gland hormone values and may not be diagnostic (see text)

Note: For abbreviations, see text.

BEGIN

TREATMENT FOR HYPOPITUITARISM

Hormone replacement therapy, including glucocorticoids, thyroid hormone, sex steroids, growth hormone, and vasopressin, is usually free of complications. Treatment regimens that mimic physiologic hormone production allow for maintenance of satisfactory clinical homeostasis. Effective dosage schedules are outlined in **Table 26-3**. Patients in need of glucocorticoid replacement require careful dose adjustments during stressful events such as acute illness, dental procedures, trauma, and acute hospitalization.

TABLE 26-3

HORMONE REPLACEMENT THERAPY FOR ADULT HYPOPITUITARISM[a]

TROPHIC HORMONE DEFICIT	HORMONE REPLACEMENT
ACTH	Hydrocortisone (10–20 mg A.M.; 10 mg P.M.) Cortisone acetate (25 mg A.M.; 12.5 mg P.M.) Prednisone (5 mg A.M.; 2.5 mg P.M.)
TSH	L-Thyroxine (0.075–0.15 mg daily)
FSH/LH	Males Testosterone enanthate (200 mg IM every 2 weeks) Testosterone skin patch (5 mg/d) Females Conjugated estrogen (0.65–1.25 mg qd for 25 days) Progesterone (5–10 mg qd) on days 16–25 Estradiol skin patch (0.5 mg, every other day) For fertility: Menopausal gonadotropins, human chorionic gonadotropins
GH	Adults: Somatotropin (0.3–1.0 mg SC qd) Children: Somatotropin [0.02–0.05 (mg/kg per day)]
Vasopressin	Intranasal desmopressin (5–20 μg twice daily) Oral (300–600 μg qd)

[a]All doses shown should be individualized for specific patients and should be reassessed during stress, surgery, or pregnancy.
Note: For abbreviations, see text.

HYPOTHALAMIC, PITUITARY, AND OTHER SELLAR MASSES

PITUITARY TUMORS

Pituitary adenomas are the most common cause of pituitary hormone hypersecretion and hyposecretion syndromes in adults. They account for ~10% of all intracranial neoplasms. At autopsy, up to a quarter of all pituitary glands harbor an unsuspected microadenoma (<10 mm diameter). Similarly, pituitary imaging detects small pituitary lesions in at least 10% of normal individuals.

Pathogenesis

Pituitary adenomas are benign neoplasms that arise from one of the five anterior pituitary cell types. The clinical and biochemical phenotype of pituitary adenomas depend on the cell type from which they are derived. Thus, tumors arising from lactotrope (PRL), somatotrope (GH), corticotrope (ACTH), thyrotrope (TSH), or gonadotrope (LH, FSH) cells hypersecrete their respective hormones (**Table 26-4**). Plurihormonal tumors that express combinations of GH, PRL, TSH, ACTH, and the glycoprotein hormone α subunit may be diagnosed by careful immunocytochemistry or may manifest as clinical syndromes that combine features of these hormonal hypersecretory syndromes. Morphologically, these tumors may arise from a single polysecreting cell type or consist of cells with mixed function within the same tumor.

Hormonally active tumors are characterized by autonomous hormone secretion with diminished responsiveness to the normal physiologic pathways of inhibition. Hormone production does not always correlate with tumor size. Small hormone-secreting adenomas may cause significant clinical perturbations, whereas larger adenomas that produce less hormone may be clinically silent and remain undiagnosed (if no central compressive effects occur). About one-third of all adenomas are clinically nonfunctioning and produce no distinct clinical hypersecretory syndrome. Most of these arise from gonadotrope cells and may secrete small amounts of α- and β-glycoprotein hormone subunits or, very rarely, intact circulating gonadotropins. True pituitary carcinomas with documented extracranial metastases are exceedingly rare.

Genetic Syndromes Associated with Pituitary Tumors

Several familial syndromes are associated with pituitary tumors, and the genetic mechanisms for some of these have been unraveled.

TABLE 26-4

CLASSIFICATION OF PITUITARY ADENOMAS[a]

ADENOMA CELL ORIGIN	HORMONE PRODUCT	CLINICAL SYNDROME
Lactotrope	PRL	Hypogonadism, galactorrhea
Gonadotrope	FSH, LH, subunits	Silent or hypogonadism
Somatotrope	GH	Acromegaly/gigantism
Corticotrope	ACTH	Cushing's disease
Mixed growth hormone and prolactin cell	GH, PRL	Acromegaly, hypogonadism, galactorrhea
Other plurihormonal cell	Any	Mixed
Acidophil stem cell	PRL, GH	Hypogonadism, galactorrhea, acromegaly
Mammosomatotrope	PRL, GH	Hypogonadism, galactorrhea, acromegaly
Thyrotrope	TSH	Thyrotoxicosis
Null cell	None	Pituitary failure
Oncocytoma	None	Pituitary failure

[a]Hormone-secreting tumors are listed in decreasing order of frequency. All tumors may cause local pressure effects, including visual disturbances, cranial nerve palsy, and headache.

Note: For abbreviations, see text.

Source: Adapted from S Melmed, in JL Jameson (ed): *Principles of Molecular Medicine*, Totowa, Humana Press, 1998.

Multiple endocrine neoplasia (MEN) 1 is an autosomal dominant syndrome characterized primarily by a genetic predisposition to parathyroid, pancreatic islet, and pituitary adenomas. MEN1 is caused by inactivating germline mutations in *MENIN*, a constitutively expressed tumor-suppressor gene located on chromosome 11q13. Loss of heterozygosity (LOH), or a somatic mutation of the remaining normal *MENIN* allele, leads to tumorigenesis. About half of affected patients develop prolactinomas; acromegaly and Cushing's syndrome are less commonly encountered.

Carney syndrome is characterized by spotty skin pigmentation, myxomas, and endocrine tumors including testicular, adrenal, and pituitary adenomas. Acromegaly occurs in about 20% of patients. A subset of patients have mutations in the R1α regulatory subunit of protein kinase A (*PRKAR1A*).

McCune-Albright syndrome consists of polyostotic fibrous dysplasia, pigmented skin patches, and a variety of endocrine disorders, including GH-secreting pituitary tumors, adrenal adenomas, and autonomous ovarian function. Hormonal hypersecretion is due to constitutive cyclic AMP production caused by inactivation of the GTPase activity of $G_s\alpha$. The $G_s\alpha$ mutations occur postzygotically, leading to a mosaic pattern of mutant expression.

Familial acromegaly is a rare disorder in which family members may manifest either acromegaly or gigantism.

The disorder is associated with LOH at a chromosome 11q13 locus distinct from that of *MENIN*.

OTHER SELLAR MASSES

Craniopharyngiomas are derived from Rathke's pouch. They arise near the pituitary stalk and commonly extend into the suprasellar cistern. These tumors are often large, cystic, and locally invasive. Many are partially calcified, providing a characteristic appearance on skull x-ray and CT images. More than half of all patients present before age 20, usually with signs of increased intracranial pressure, including headache, vomiting, papilledema, and hydrocephalus. Associated symptoms include visual field abnormalities, personality changes and cognitive deterioration, cranial nerve damage, sleep difficulties, and weight gain. Anterior pituitary dysfunction and DI are common. About half of affected children present with growth retardation.

Treatment usually involves transcranial or transsphenoidal surgical resection followed by postoperative radiation of residual tumor. This approach can result in long-term survival and ultimate cure, but most patients require lifelong pituitary hormone replacement. If the pituitary stalk is uninvolved and can be preserved at the time of surgery, the incidence of subsequent anterior pituitary dysfunction is significantly diminished.

Developmental failure of Rathke's pouch obliteration may lead to *Rathke's cysts,* which are small (<5 mm) cysts entrapped by squamous epithelium; these cysts are found in about 20% of individuals at autopsy. Although Rathke's cleft cysts do not usually grow and are often diagnosed incidentally, about a third present in adulthood with compressive symptoms, DI, and hyperprolactinemia due to stalk compression. Rarely, internal hydrocephalus develops. The diagnosis is suggested preoperatively by visualizing the cyst wall on MRI, which distinguishes these lesions from craniopharyngiomas. Cyst contents range from CSF-like fluid to mucoid material. *Arachnoid cysts* are rare and generate an MRI image isointense with cerebrospinal fluid.

Sella chordomas usually present with bony clival erosion, local invasiveness, and, on occasion, calcification. Normal pituitary tissue may be visible on MRI, distinguishing chordomas from aggressive pituitary adenomas. Mucinous material may be obtained by fine-needle aspiration.

Meningiomas arising in the sellar region may be difficult to distinguish from nonfunctioning pituitary adenomas. Meningiomas typically enhance on MRI and may show evidence of calcification or bony erosion. Meningiomas may cause compressive symptoms.

Histiocytosis X comprises a variety of syndromes associated with foci of eosinophilic granulomas. DI, exophthalmos, and punched-out lytic bone lesions (*Hand-Schüller-Christian disease*) are associated with granulomatous lesions visible on MRI, as well as a characteristic axillary skin rash. Rarely, the pituitary stalk may be involved.

Pituitary metastases occur in ~3% of cancer patients. Blood-borne metastatic deposits are found almost exclusively in the posterior pituitary. Accordingly, diabetes insipidus can be a presenting feature of lung, gastrointestinal, breast, and other pituitary metastases. About half of pituitary metastases originate from breast cancer; about 25% of patients with breast cancer have such deposits. Rarely, pituitary stalk involvement results in anterior pituitary insufficiency. The MRI diagnosis of a metastatic lesion may be difficult to distinguish from an aggressive pituitary adenoma; the diagnosis may require histologic examination of excised tumor tissue. Primary or metastatic lymphomas, leukemias, and plasmacytomas also occur within the sella.

Hypothalamic hamartomas and *gangliocytomas* may arise from astrocytes, oligodendrocytes, and neurons with varying degrees of differentiation. These tumors may overexpress hypothalamic neuropeptides including gonadotropin-releasing hormone (GnRH), GHRH, or CRH. In GnRH-producing tumors, children present with precocious puberty, psychomotor delay, and laughing-associated seizures. Medical treatment of GnRH-producing hamartomas with long-acting GnRH analogues effectively suppresses gonadotropin secretion and controls premature pubertal development. Rarely, hamartomas are also associated with craniofacial abnormalities; imperforate anus; cardiac, renal, and lung disorders; and pituitary failure (*Pallister-Hall syndrome*). Hypothalamic hamartomas are often contiguous with the pituitary, and preoperative MRI diagnosis may not be possible. Histologic evidence of hypothalamic neurons in tissue resected at transsphenoidal surgery may be the first indication of a primary hypothalamic lesion.

Hypothalamic gliomas and *optic gliomas* occur mainly in childhood and usually present with visual loss. Adults have more aggressive tumors; about a third are associated with neurofibromatosis.

Brain germ-cell tumors may arise within the sellar region. These include *dysgerminomas,* which are frequently associated with DI and visual loss. They rarely metastasize. *Germinomas, embryonal carcinomas, teratomas,* and *choriocarcinomas* may arise in the parasellar region and produce hCG. These germ-cell tumors present with precocious puberty, DI, visual field defects, and thirst disorders. Many patients are GH-deficient with short stature.

METABOLIC EFFECTS OF HYPOTHALAMIC LESIONS

Lesions involving the anterior and preoptic hypothalamic regions cause paradoxical vasoconstriction, tachycardia, and hyperthermia. Acute hyperthermia is usually due to a hemorrhagic insult, but poikilothermia may also occur. Central disorders of thermoregulation result from posterior hypothalamic damage. The *periodic hypothermia syndrome* comprises episodic attacks of rectal temperatures <30°C, sweating, vasodilation, vomiting, and bradycardia. Damage to the ventromedial nuclei by craniopharyngiomas, hypothalamic trauma, or inflammatory disorders may be associated with *hyperphagia* and *obesity.* This region appears to contain an energy-satiety center where melanocortin receptors are influenced by leptin, insulin, proopiomelanocortin products, and gastrointestinal peptides. Hypothalamic gliomas in early childhood may be associated with a diencephalic syndrome characterized by progressive severe emaciation and growth failure. Polydipsia and hypodipsia are associated with damage to central osmo-receptors located in preoptic nuclei. Slow-growing hypothalamic lesions can cause increased somnolence and disturbed sleep cycles as well as obesity, hypothermia, and emotional outbursts. Lesions of the central hypothalamus may stimulate sympathetic neurons, leading to elevated serum catecholamine and cortisol levels. These patients are predisposed to cardiac arrhythmias, hypertension, and gastric erosions.

EVALUATION

Local Mass Effects

Clinical manifestations of sellar lesions vary, depending on the anatomical location of the mass and direction of its extension (**Table 26-5**). The dorsal roof of the sella presents the least resistance to soft tissue expansion from within the confines of the sella, consequently, pituitary adenomas frequently extend in a suprasellar direction. Bony invasion may ultimately occur as well.

Headaches are common features of small intrasellar tumors, even with no demonstrable suprasellar extension. Because of the confined nature of the pituitary, small changes in intrasellar pressure stretch the dural plate; however, the severity of the headache correlates poorly with adenoma size or extension.

Suprasellar extension can lead to visual loss by several mechanisms, the most common being compression of the optic chiasm, but direct invasion of the optic nerves or obstruction of CSF flow leading to secondary visual disturbances also occurs. Pituitary stalk compression by a hormonally active or inactive intrasellar mass may compress the portal vessels, disrupting pituitary access to the hypothalamic hormones and dopamine; this results in hyperprolactinemia and concurrent loss of other pituitary hormones. This "stalk section" phenomenon may also be caused by trauma, whiplash injury with posterior clinoid stalk compression, or skull base fractures. Lateral mass invasion may impinge on the cavernous sinus and compress its neural contents, leading to cranial nerve III, IV, and VI palsies as well as effects on the ophthalmic and maxillary branches of the fifth cranial nerve. Patients may present with diplopia, ptosis, ophthalmoplegia, and decreased facial sensation, depending on the extent of neural damage. Extension into the sphenoid sinus indicates that the pituitary mass has eroded through the sellar floor. Aggressive tumors rarely invade the palate roof and cause nasopharyngeal obstruction, infection, and CSF leakage. Both temporal

TABLE 26-5

FEATURES OF SELLAR MASS LESIONS[a]

IMPACTED STRUCTURE	CLINICAL IMPACT
Pituitary	Hypogonadism
	Hypothyroidism
	Growth failure and adult hyposomatotropism
	Hypoadrenalism
Optic chiasm	Loss of red perception
	Bitemporal hemianopia
	Superior or bitemporal field defect
	Scotoma
	Blindness
Hypothalamus	Temperature dysregulation
	Appetite and thirst disorders
	Obesity
	Diabetes insipidus
	Sleep disorders
	Behavioral dysfunction
	Autonomic dysfunction
Cavernous sinus	Opthalmoplegia ± ptosis or diplopia
	Facial numbness
Frontal lobe	Personality disorder
	Anosmia
Brain	Headache
	Hydrocephalus
	Psychosis
	Dementia
	Laughing seizures

[a]As the intrasellar mass expands, it first compresses intrasellar pituitary tissue, then usually invades dorsally through the dura to lift the optic chiasm or laterally to the cavernous sinuses. Bony erosion is rare, as is direct brain compression. Microadenomas may present with headache.

and frontal lobes may be invaded, leading to uncinate seizures, personality disorders, and anosmia. Direct hypothalamic encroachment by an invasive pituitary mass may cause important metabolic sequelae, precocious puberty or hypogonadism, DI, sleep disturbances, dysthermia, and appetite disorders.

MRI

Sagittal and coronal T1-weighted spin-echo MRI imaging, before and after administration of gadolinium, allows precise visualization of the pituitary gland with clear delineation of the hypothalamus, pituitary stalk, pituitary tissue and surrounding suprasellar cisterns, cavernous sinuses, sphenoid sinus, and optic chiasm. Pituitary gland height ranges from 6 mm in children to 8 mm in adults; during pregnancy and puberty, the height may reach 10 to 12 mm. The upper aspect of the adult pituitary is flat or slightly concave, but in adolescent and pregnant individuals this surface may be convex, reflecting physiologic pituitary enlargement. The stalk should be vertical. CT scan is indicated to define the extent of bony erosion or the presence of calcification.

The soft tissue consistency of the pituitary gland is slightly heterogeneous on MRI. Anterior pituitary signal intensity resembles that of brain matter on T1-imaging (**Fig. 26-4**). Adenoma density is usually lower than that of surrounding normal tissue on T1-weighted imaging, and the signal intensity increases with T2-weighted images. The high phospholipid content of the posterior pituitary results in a "pituitary bright spot."

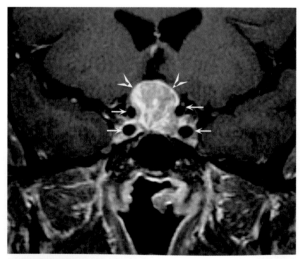

FIGURE 26-4
Pituitary adenoma. Coronal T1-weighted postcontrast MR image shows a homogeneously enhancing mass (*arrowheads*) in the sella turcica and suprasellar region compatible with a pituitary adenoma; the small arrows outline the carotid arteries.

Sellar masses are commonly encountered as incidental findings on MRI, and most of these are pituitary adenomas (incidentalomas). In the absence of hormone hypersecretion, these small lesions can be safely monitored by MRI, which is performed annually and then less often if there is no evidence of growth. Resection should be considered for incidentally discovered macroadenomas, as about one-third become invasive or cause local pressure effects. If hormone hypersecretion is evident, specific therapies are indicated. When larger masses (>1 cm) are encountered, they should also be distinguished from nonadenomatous lesions. Meningiomas are often associated with bony hyperostosis; craniopharyngiomas may be calcified and are usually hypodense, whereas gliomas are hyperdense on T2-weighted images.

Ophthalmologic Evaluation

Because optic tracts may be contiguous to an expanding pituitary mass, reproducible visual field assessment that uses perimetry techniques should be performed on all patients with sellar mass lesions that abut the optic chiasm. Bitemporal hemianopia or superior bitemporal defects are classically observed, reflecting the location of these tracts within the inferior and posterior part of the chiasm. Homonymous cuts are postchiasmal and monocular field cuts are prechiasmal. Loss of red perception is an early sign of optic tract pressure. Early diagnosis reduces the risk of blindness, scotomas, or other visual disturbances.

Laboratory Investigation

The presenting clinical features of functional pituitary adenomas (e.g., acromegaly, prolactinomas, or Cushing's disease) should guide the laboratory studies (**Table 26-6**). However, for a sellar mass with no obvious clinical features of hormone excess, laboratory studies are geared towards determining the nature of the tumor and assessing the possible presence of hypopituitarism. When a pituitary adenoma is suspected based on MRI, initial hormonal evaluation usually includes: (1) basal PRL; (2) insulin-like growth factor (IGF) I; (3) 24-h urinary free cortisol (UFC) and/or overnight oral dexamethasone (1 mg) suppression test; (4) α-subunit, FSH, and LH levels; and (5) thyroid function tests. Additional hormonal evaluation may be indicated based on the results of these tests. Pending more detailed assessment of hypopituitarism, a menstrual history, testosterone level, 8 A.M. cortisol, and thyroid function tests usually identify patients with pituitary hormone deficiencies that require hormone replacement before further testing or surgery.

TABLE 26-6

SCREENING TESTS FOR FUNCTIONAL PITUITARY ADENOMAS

	TEST	COMMENTS
Acromegaly	Serum IGF-I	Interpret IGF-I relative to age- and gender-matched controls
	Oral glucose tolerance test with GH obtained at 0, 30, and 60 min	Normal subjects should suppress growth hormone to <1 μg/L
Prolactinoma	Exclude medications	MRI of the sella should be ordered if prolactin is elevated
Cushing's disease	24-h urinary free cortisol	Ensure urine collection is total and accurate
	Dexamethasone (1 mg) at 11 P.M. and fasting plasma cortisol measured at 8 A.M.	Normal subjects suppress to <5 μg/dL
	ACTH assay	Distinguishes adrenal adenoma (ACTH suppressed) from ectopic ACTH or Cushing's disease (ACTH normal or elevated)

Note: For abbreviations, see text.

Histologic Evaluation

Immunohistochemical staining of pituitary tumor specimens obtained at transsphenoidal surgery confirms clinical and laboratory studies and provides a histologic diagnosis when hormone studies are equivocal and in cases of clinically nonfunctioning tumors. Occasionally, ultrastructural assessment by electron microscopy is required for diagnosis.

TREATMENT FOR SELLAR MASSES

Overview

Successful management of sellar masses requires accurate diagnosis as well as selection of optimal therapeutic modalities. Most pituitary tumors are benign and slow-growing. Clinical features result from local mass effects and hormonal hypo- or hypersecretion syndromes caused directly by the adenoma or as a consequence of treatment. Thus, life-long management and follow-up are necessary for these patients.

MRI technology with gadolinium enhancement for pituitary visualization, new advances in transsphenoidal surgery and in stereotactic radiotherapy (including gamma-knife radiotherapy), and novel therapeutic agents have improved pituitary tumor management. The goals of pituitary tumor treatment include normalization of excess pituitary secretion, amelioration of symptoms and signs of hormonal hypersecretion syndromes, and shrinkage

or ablation of large tumor masses with relief of adjacent structure compression. Residual anterior pituitary function should be preserved and can sometimes be restored by removing tumor mass. Ideally, adenoma recurrence should be prevented.

Transsphenoidal Surgery

Transsphenoidal rather than transfrontal resection is the desired surgical approach for pituitary tumors, except for the rare invasive suprasellar mass surrounding the frontal or middle fossa, the optic nerves, or invading posteriorly behind the clivus. Intraoperative microscopy facilitates visual distinction between adenomatous and normal pituitary tissue, as well as microdissection of small tumors that may not be visible by MRI (**Fig. 26-5**). Transsphenoidal surgery also avoids the cranial invasion and manipulation of brain tissue required by subfrontal surgical approaches. Endoscopic techniques with three-dimensional intraoperative localization have improved visualization and access to tumor tissue. The endoscopic approach is also less traumatic, as the technique is endonasal and does not require a transsphenoidal retractor.

In addition to correction of hormonal hypersecretion, pituitary surgery is indicated for mass lesions that impinge on surrounding structures. Surgical decompression and resection are required for an expanding pituitary mass accompanied by persistent headache, progressive visual field defects, cranial nerve palsies, internal hydrocephalus, and,

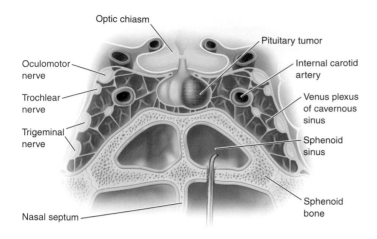

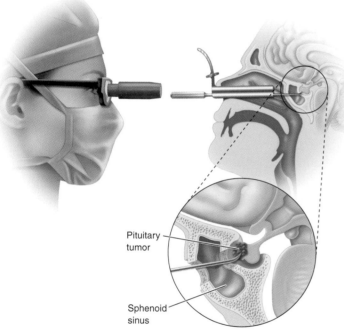

FIGURE 26-5

Transsphenoidal resection of pituitary mass via the endonasal approach. (Adapted from *Fahlbusch R: Endocrinol Metab Clin 21:669, 1992.*)

occasionally, intrapituitary hemorrhage and apoplexy. Transsphenoidal surgery is sometimes used for pituitary tissue biopsy and histologic diagnosis.

Whenever possible, the pituitary mass lesion should be selectively excised; normal tissue should be manipulated or resected only when critical for effective dissection. Nonselective hemihypophysectomy or total hypophysectomy may be indicated if no mass lesion is clearly discernible, multifocal lesions are present, or the remaining nontumorous pituitary tissue is obviously necrotic. This strategy increases the likelihood of hypopituitarism and the need for lifelong hormonal replacement.

Preoperative local compression signs, including visual field defects or compromised pituitary function, may be reversed by surgery, particularly when these deficits are not long-standing. For large and invasive tumors, it is necessary to determine the optimal balance between maximal tumor resection and preservation of anterior pituitary function, especially for preserving growth and reproductive function in younger patients. Similarly, tumor invasion outside of the sella is rarely amenable to surgical cure; the surgeon must judge the risk:benefit ratio of extensive tumor resection.

Tumor size and the degree of invasiveness largely determine the incidence of surgical complications. Operative mortality is about 1%. Transient DI and hypopituitarism occur in up to 20% of patients. Permanent DI, cranial nerve damage, nasal septal perforation, or visual disturbances may be encountered in up to 10% of patients. CSF leaks occur in 4% of patients. Less common complications include carotid artery injury, loss of vision, hypothalamic damage, and meningitis. Permanent side effects are rarely encountered after surgery for microadenomas.

Radiation

Radiation is used either as a primary therapy for pituitary or parasellar masses or, more commonly, as an adjunct to surgery or medical therapy. Focused megavoltage irradiation is achieved by precise MRI localization, using a high-voltage linear accelerator and accurate isocentric rotational arcing. A major determinant of accurate irradiation is to reproduce the patient's head position during multiple visits and to maintain absolute head immobility. A total of <50 Gy (5000 rad) is given as 180-cGy (180 rad) fractions split over about 6 weeks. Stereotactic radiosurgery delivers a large single high-energy dose from a cobalt-60 source (gamma knife), linear accelerator, or cyclotron. Long-term effects of gamma-knife surgery are as yet unknown.

The role of radiation therapy in pituitary tumor management depends on multiple factors including the nature of the tumor, age of the patient, and the availability of surgical and radiation expertise. Because of its relatively slow onset of action, radiation therapy is usually reserved for postsurgical management. As an adjuvant to surgery, radiation is used to treat residual tumor and in an attempt to prevent regrowth. Irradiation offers the only effective means for ablating significant residual tumor tissue derived from nonfunctioning tumors. PRL-, GH-, and ACTH-secreting tumor tissues are also amenable to medical therapy.

In the short term, radiation may cause transient nausea and weakness. Alopecia and loss of taste and smell may be more long-lasting. Failure of pituitary hormone synthesis is common in patients who have undergone head and neck or pituitary-directed irradiation. More than 50% of patients develop failure of GH, ACTH, TSH, and/or gonadotropin secretion within 10 years, usually due to hypothalamic damage. Lifelong follow-up with testing of anterior pituitary hormone reserve is therefore necessary after radiation treatment. Optic nerve damage with impaired vision due to optic neuritis is reported in about 2% of patients who undergo pituitary irradiation. Cranial nerve damage is uncommon now that radiation doses are ≤ 2 Gy (200 rad) at any one treatment session and the maximum dose is <50 Gy (5000 rad). The advent of stereotactic radiotherapy may reduce damage to adjacent structures. The cumulative risk of developing a secondary tumor after conventional radiation is 1.3% after 10 years and 1.9% after 20 years.

Medical Therapy

Medical therapy for pituitary tumors is highly specific and depends on tumor type. For prolactinomas, dopamine agonists are the treatment of choice. For acromegaly and TSH-secreting tumors, somatostatin analogues and, occasionally, dopamine agonists are indicated. ACTH-secreting tumors and nonfunctioning tumors are generally not responsive to medication and require surgery and/or irradiation.

FURTHER READINGS

ATTANUSIO AF et al: Human growth hormone replacement in adult hypopituitary patients. J Clin Endocrinol Metab 87:1600, 2002

☑ COULDWELL WT: Transsphenoidal and transcranial surgery for pituitary adenomas. J Neurooncol 69:237, 2004

Review of current pituitary surgical approaches.

KALTSAS GA et al: Clinical review: Diagnosis and management of pituitary carcinomas. J Clin Endocrinol Metab 90:3089, 2005

MELMED S et al: Consensus guidelines for acromegaly management. J Clin Endocrinol Metab 87:4054, 2002

OLSON LE, ROSENFELD MG: Perspective: Genetic and genomic approaches in elucidating mechanisms of pituitary development. Endocrinology 143:2007, 2002

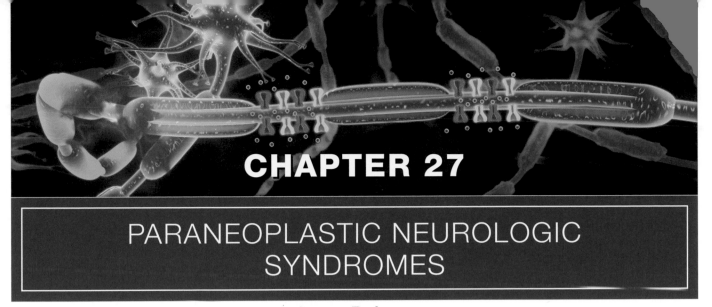

CHAPTER 27

PARANEOPLASTIC NEUROLOGIC SYNDROMES

Josep Dalmau
Myrna R. Rosenfeld

Paraneoplastic neurologic disorders (PNDs) are cancer-related syndromes that can affect any part of the nervous system (**Table 27-1**). They are remote effects of cancer, caused by mechanisms other than metastasis or by any of the complications of cancer such as coagulopathy, stroke, metabolic and nutritional conditions, infections, and side effects of cancer therapy. In 60% of patients the neurologic symptoms precede the cancer diagnosis. Overall, clinically disabling PNDs occur in 0.5 to 1% of all cancer patients, but they occur in 2 to 3% of patients with neuroblastoma or small cell lung cancer (SCLC), and in 30 to 50% of patients with thymoma or sclerotic myeloma.

PATHOGENESIS

Most PNDs are mediated by immune responses triggered by the tumor expression of neuronal proteins (onconeuronal antigens). In PNDs of the central nervous system

(CNS), many antibody-associated immune responses have been identified (**Table 27-2**). These antibodies usually react with the patient's tumor, and their detection in serum or cerebrospinal fluid (CSF) strongly predicts the presence of cancer (**Fig. 27-1**). The target antigens are usually intracellular proteins with roles in neuronal development and function. Some of the antibodies react with epitopes located in critical protein domains, disrupting protein function leading to neuronal apoptosis. In addition to onconeuronal antibodies, most PNDs of the CNS are associated with infiltrates of CD4+ and CD8+ T cells, microglial activation, gliosis, and variable neuronal loss. The infiltrating T cells are often in close contact with neurons undergoing degeneration, suggesting a primary pathogenic role. T cell–mediated cytotoxicity may contribute directly to cell death in these PNDs. Thus both humoral and cellular immune mechanisms participate in the pathogenesis of many PNDs. This complex immunopathogenesis may underlie the resistance of many of these conditions to therapy.

Only three of the antibodies listed in Table 27-2 have been shown to play a direct pathogenic role in PNDs; all produce distinctive disorders of the peripheral nervous system. These are: antibodies to P/Q-type voltage-gated calcium channels (VGCC) in patients with the Lambert-Eaton myasthenic syndrome (LEMS); antibodies to acetylcholine receptors in patients with myasthenia gravis; and antibodies to voltage-gated potassium channels (VGKC) in some patients with peripheral nerve hyperexcitability (neuromyotonia). Common features of these three antibodies are that they target cell-surface molecules and that their passive transfer to animals reproduces the disorders. Plasma exchange or immunomodulation with intravenous immunoglobulin (IVIg) usually produces neurologic improvement. Each of these disorders can occur without cancer, and therefore detection of these antibodies does not predict the presence of cancer.

TABLE 27-1

PARANEOPLASTIC SYNDROMES OF THE NERVOUS SYSTEM

Syndromes of the brain, brainstem, and cerebellum
   Focal encephalitis
      Cortical encephalitis
      Limbic encephalitis
      Brainstem encephalitis
      Cerebellar dysfunction
      Autonomic dysfunction
   Paraneoplastic cerebellar degeneration
   Opsoclonus-myoclonus
Syndromes of the spinal cord
   Subacute necrotizing myelopathy
   Motor neuron dysfunction
   Myelitis
   Stiff-person syndrome
Syndromes of dorsal root ganglia
   Sensory neuronopathy
Multiple levels of involvement
   Encephalomyelitis[a], sensory neuronopathy, autonomic dysfunction
Syndromes of peripheral nerve
   Chronic and subacute sensorimotor peripheral neuropathy
   Vasculitis of nerve and muscle
   Neuropathy associated with malignant monoclonal gammopathies
   Peripheral nerve hyperexcitability
   Autonomic neuropathy
Syndromes of the neuromuscular junction
   Lambert-Eaton myasthenic syndrome
   Myasthenia gravis
Syndromes of the muscle
   Polymyositis/dermatomyositis
   Acute necrotizing myopathy
Syndromes affecting the visual system
   Cancer-associated retinopathy (CAR)
   Melanoma-associated retinopathy (MAR)
   Uveitis (usually in association with encephalomyelitis)

[a]Includes cortical, limbic, or brainstem encephalitis, cerebellar dysfunction, myelitis.

Other PNDs are likely immune-mediated although their antigens are unknown. These include several syndromes of inflammatory neuropathies and myopathies. In addition, many patients with typical PND syndromes are antibody-negative.

For still other PNDs, the cause remains quite obscure. These include, among others, several neuropathies that occur in the terminal stages of cancer and a number of neuropathies associated with plasma cell dyscrasias or lymphoma without evidence of inflammatory infiltrates or deposits of immunoglobulin, cryoglobulin, or amyloid.

APPROACH TO THE PATIENT WITH PNDs

The diagnosis and management of PNDs may be difficult for several reasons. First, it is common for symptoms to appear before the presence of a tumor is known. Second, the neurologic syndrome can evolve in a rapidly progressive fashion, producing a severe and usually irreversible neurologic deficit in a short period of time. There is evidence that prompt tumor control improves the course of PNDs. Therefore, the major concern of the physician is to recognize a disorder promptly as paraneoplastic in order to identify and treat the tumor.

PND of the Central Nervous System and Dorsal Root Ganglia

When symptoms involve brain, spinal cord, or dorsal root ganglia, the suspicion of PND is usually based on a combination of clinical, radiologic, and CSF findings. In these cases, a biopsy of the affected tissue is often difficult to obtain, and although useful to rule out other disorders (e.g., metastasis, infection), neuropathologic findings are not specific for PND. Furthermore, there are no specific radiologic or electrophysiologic tests that are diagnostic of PND. The presence of antineuronal antibodies (Table 27-2) may help in the diagnosis with the following caveats: (1) antibodies are detected in only 40 to 50% of PNDs of the CNS; (2) antibodies may be present in both the serum and CSF, but in some patients only the CSF is positive (especially with antibodies to Tr and Ma proteins); (3) antibodies (usually at low titer) are present in a variable proportion of cancer patients without PND; (4) there is an imperfect correlation between antibody titers and the course of the neurologic disorder; (5) several antibodies may associate with a similar syndrome, with the antibody specificity often correlating with the tumor type (e.g., cerebellar degeneration is associated with anti-Tr antibodies if the tumor is Hodgkin's disease but with anti-Yo antibodies if the tumor is ovarian or breast cancer); and (6) several antibodies may be present in the serum or CSF of the same patient (e.g., anti-Hu and anti-CV$_2$/CRMP5, or less frequently anti-Ri).

Magnetic resonance imaging (MRI) and CSF studies are important to rule out neurologic

TABLE 27-2

PARANEOPLASTIC ANTINEURONAL ANTIBODIES, ASSOCIATED SYNDROMES AND CANCERS

ANTIBODY	SYNDROME	ASSOCIATED CANCERS
Anti-Hu (ANNA-1)	PEM (including cortical, limbic, brainstem encephalitis, cerebellar dysfunction, myelitis), PSN, autonomic dysfunction	SCLC, other neuroendocrine tumors
Anti-Yo (PCA-1)	PCD	Ovary and other gynecologic cancers, breast
Anti-Ri (ANNA-2)	PCD, brainstem encephalitis, opsoclonus-myoclonus	Breast, gynecological, SCLC
Anti-Tr	PCD	Hodgkin's lymphoma
Anti-Zic	PCD, encephalomyelitis	SCLC and other neuroendocrine tumors
Anti-CV$_2$/CRMP5	PEM, PCD, chorea, peripheral neuropathy, uveitis	SCLC, thymoma, other
Anti-Ma proteins[a]	Limbic, hypothalamic, brainstem encephalitis (infrequently PCD)	Germ-cell tumors of testis, lung cancer, other solid tumors
Anti-amphiphysin	Stiff-person syndrome, PEM	Breast, SCLC
Anti-VGCC[b]	LEMS, PCD	SCLC, lymphoma
Anti-AChR[b]	MG	Thymoma
Anti-VGKC[b]	Peripheral nerve hyperexcitability (neuromyotonia)	Thymoma, SCLC, others
Anti-recoverin	Cancer-associated retinopathy (CAR)	SCLC and other
Anti-bipolar cells of the retina	Melanoma-associated retinopathy (MAR)	Melanoma

[a]Patients with antibodies to Ma2 are usually men with testicular cancer. Patients with additional antibodies to other Ma proteins are men or women with a variety of solid tumors.
[b]These antibodies can occur with or without a cancer association.

Note: PEM: paraneoplastic encephalomyelitis; PCD, paraneoplastic cerebellar degeneration; PSN, paraneoplastic sensory neuronopathy; LEMS, Lambert-Eaton myasthenic syndrome; MG, myasthenia gravis; VGCC, voltage-gated calcium channel; AChR, acetylcholine receptor; VGKC, voltage-gated potassium channel; SCLC, small-cell lung cancer.

complications due to the direct spread of cancer, particularly metastatic and leptomeningeal disease. In most PNDs the MRI findings are nonspecific. Paraneoplastic limbic encephalitis is usually associated with characteristic MRI abnormalities in the mesial temporal lobes (see below), but similar findings can occur with other disorders [e.g., systemic lupus erythematosus, human herpesvirus (HHV) 6 encephalitis]. The CSF profile of patients with PND of the CNS or dorsal root ganglia typically consists of mild to moderate pleocytosis (<200 mononuclear cells, predominantly lymphocytes), an increase in the protein concentration, intrathecal synthesis of IgG, and a variable presence of oligoclonal bands.

PND of Nerve and Muscle

If symptoms involve peripheral nerve, neuromuscular junction, or muscle, the diagnosis of a specific PND is usually established on clinical, electrophysiologic, and pathologic grounds. The clinical history, accompanying symptoms (e.g., anorexia, weight loss), and type of syndrome dictate the studies and degree of effort needed to demonstrate a neoplasm. For example, the frequent association of LEMS with SCLC should lead to a chest and abdomen computed tomography or body positron emission tomography (PET) scan and, if negative, periodic tumor screening for at least 3 years after the neurologic diagnosis. In contrast, the weak association of polymyositis with cancer calls into question the need for repeated cancer screenings in this situation. Serum and urine immunofixation studies should be considered in patients with peripheral neuropathy of unknown cause; detection of a monoclonal gammopathy suggests the need for additional studies to uncover a B cell or plasma cell malignancy. In paraneoplastic neuropathies, diagnostically useful antineuronal antibodies are limited to anti-CV$_2$/CRMP5 and anti-Hu.

For any type of PND, if antineuronal antibodies are negative, the diagnosis relies on the demonstration of cancer and the exclusion of other cancer-related or independent neurologic disorders. Body PET scans often uncover tumors undetected by other tests.

SPECIFIC PARANEOPLASTIC NEUROLOGIC SYNDROMES (Table 27-3)

PARANEOPLASTIC ENCEPHALOMYELITIS AND FOCAL ENCEPHALITIS

The term *encephalomyelitis* describes an inflammatory process with multifocal involvement of the nervous system, including brain, brainstem, cerebellum, and spinal cord. It is often associated with dorsal root ganglia and

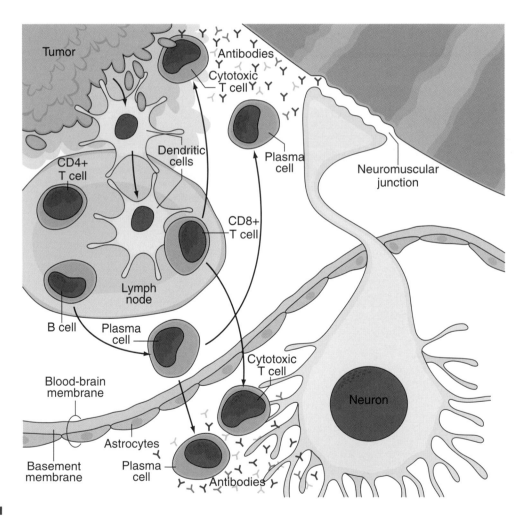

FIGURE 27-1

Proposed mechanism for pathogenesis of paraneoplasic neurologic disorders involves a tumor not in the nervous system expressing a neuronal protein. When tumor cells migrate to lymph nodes, antigen-specific CD4+, CD8+, and B cells are produced against this neuronal protein. These immune cells then can react against this same protein that exists normally in the central or peripheral nervous system, leading to neurologic symptoms. (After Darnell RB, Posner JB: Mechanisms of disease: Paraneoplastic syndromes involving the nervous system. N Engl J Med 349:1543, 2003, with permission.)

autonomic dysfunction. For any given patient, the clinical manifestations are determined by the area or areas predominantly involved, but pathology almost always reveals abnormalities (inflammatory infiltrates, neuronal loss, gliosis) beyond the symptomatic regions. Several clinicopathologic syndromes may occur alone or in combination: (1) *cortical encephalitis,* which may present as "epilepsia partialis continua"; (2) *limbic encephalitis,* characterized by confusion, depression, agitation, anxiety, severe short-term memory deficits, partial complex seizures, and dementia; the MRI usually shows unilateral or bilateral medial temporal lobe abnormalities, best seen with T2 and fluid-attenuated inversion recovery sequences, and occasionally enhancing with gadolinium; (3) *brainstem encephalitis,* resulting in eye movement disorders (nystagmus, opsoclonus, supranuclear or nuclear paresis), cranial nerve paresis, dysarthria, dysphagia, and central autonomic dysfunction; (4) *cerebellar gait and limb ataxia;* (5) *myelitis,* which may cause lower or upper motor neuron symptoms, myoclonus, muscle rigidity, and spasms; and (6) *autonomic dysfunction* as a result of involvement of the neuraxis at multiple levels, including

TABLE 27-3

A GUIDE TO ANTIBODY-ASSOCIATED PARANEOPLASTIC AND NON-PARANEOPLASTIC SYNDROMES[a]

	ANTIBODIES		
	PARANEOPLASTIC		
SYNDROME	FREQUENT	INFREQUENT	NON-PARANEOPLASTIC
Limbic encephalitis	Ma2, Hu, CV$_2$/CRMP5	Tr, VGKC	VGKC
Cerebellar degeneration	Yo, Tr, P/Q VGCC, Hu, *Zic*, Ri, CV$_2$/CRMP5, Mal-2	*mGluR1*	Gliadin GAD
Hypothalamic, brainstem encephalitis	Ma2, Hu	CV$_2$/CRMP5	
Encephalomyelitis	Hu, *Zic*	CV$_2$/CRMP5, Ri, amphiphysin	
Chorea	CV$_2$/CRMP5		
Opsoclonus-myoclonus	Ri	Hu, Ma2, Yo,	
Stiff-person syndrome	Amphiphysin	*Gephyrin*, Ri	GAD
PNH (neuromyotonia)	VGKC		VGKC
Myasthenia gravis	AChR, titin		AChR, MuSK
EMS	P/Q-type VGCC	*MysB*	P/Q-type VGCC
Sensory neuronopathy	Hu		
Axonal sensorimotor neuropathy	Hu, CV$_2$/CRMP5		Monoclonal gammopathy (M protein)[b]
Autonomic neuropathy	Hu	CV$_2$/CRMP5, ganglionic AChR	Ganglionic AChR
Predominant sensory demyelinating neuropathy		MAG, ganglioside antibodies: often present with Waldenström's macroglobulinemia	MAG, ganglioside antibodies, often present with MGUS
Paraneoplastic retinopathy	Recoverin (CAR), **anti-bipolar cell antibodies** (*MAR*)	*Tubby-like protein 1, PNR*	

[a]Antibodies have been validated by more than one laboratory and/or the protein sequence of the target antigen is known.
[b]The M protein usually does not have specific antibody activity.
Note: Italics indicate that commercial testing for these antibodies is not available. PNH, peripheral nerve hyperexcitability; CAR, cancer-associated retinopathy; MAR, melanoma-associated retinopathy;

PNR, photoreceptor-specific nuclear receptor; MGUS, monoclonal gammopathy of uncertain significance; VGKC, voltage-gated potassium channel; GAD, glutamic acid decarboxylase; AChR, acetylcholine receptor; LEMS, Lambert-Eaton myasthenic syndrome; VGCC, voltage-gated calcium channel; MAG, myelin-associated glycoprotein.

hypothalamus, brainstem, and autonomic nerves (see autonomic neuropathy). Cardiac arrhythmias, postural hypotension, or central hypoventilation are frequent causes of death in patients with encephalomyelitis.

Paraneoplastic encephalomyelitis and focal encephalitis are usually associated with SCLC, but many other cancers have also been reported. Patients with SCLC and these syndromes usually have anti-Hu antibodies in serum and CSF. Anti-CV_2/CRMP5 antibodies occur less frequently; some of these patients may develop chorea or uveitis. Antibodies to Ma proteins are associated with limbic and brainstem encephalitis and occasionally with cerebellar symptoms; prominent hypothalamic dysfunction, hypersomnia, and cataplexy can also occur. MRI abnormalities are frequent, including those described with limbic encephalitis and variable involvement of the hypothalamus, basal ganglia, or brainstem. The oncologic associations of these antibodies are shown in Table 27-2.

All types of paraneoplastic encephalitis and encephalomyelitis, except limbic encephalitis, respond poorly to treatment. Stabilization of symptoms or partial neurologic improvement may occasionally occur, particularly if there is a satisfactory response of the tumor to treatment. The roles of plasma exchange, IVIg, and immunosuppression have not been established. Rare patients with limbic encephalitis have shown dramatic improvement after treatment, but it is not known whether remission of the cancer, glucocorticoids, or IVIg was responsible.

PARANEOPLASTIC CEREBELLAR DEGENERATION

This disorder is often preceded by a prodrome that may include dizziness, oscillopsia, blurry or double vision, nausea, and vomiting. A few days or weeks later, dysarthria, gait and limb ataxia, and variable dysphagia can appear. The examination usually shows downbeating nystagmus and, rarely, opsoclonus. Brainstem dysfunction, upgoing toes, or a mild neuropathy may occur, but more often the symptoms and signs are restricted to the cerebellum. Early in the course, MRI studies are usually normal; in some patients a transient enhancement of the cerebellar cortex has been noted. Later, the MRI typically reveals cerebellar atrophy. The disorder results from extensive degeneration of Purkinje cells, with variable involvement of other cerebellar cortical neurons, deep cerebellar nuclei, and spinocerebellar tracts. An immune-mediated pathogenesis is supported by CSF findings and biopsy studies obtained during the early stage of the disorder. The tumors more frequently involved are SCLC, cancer of the breast and ovary, and Hodgkin's lymphoma.

Anti-Yo antibodies in patients with breast and gynecologic cancers and anti-Tr antibodies in patients with Hodgkin's lymphoma are the two paraneoplastic antibodies typically associated with prominent or pure cerebellar degeneration. Antibodies to P/Q-type VGCC occur in some patients with SCLC and cerebellar dysfunction; only some of these patients develop LEMS. A subacute cerebellar ataxia can also be the presenting symptom of paraneoplastic encephalomyelitis; in this syndrome, symptoms of widespread CNS involvement eventually occur. Of note, a variable degree of cerebellar dysfunction can be associated with virtually any type of antibody-related PND of the CNS (Table 27-2). A number of single case reports have described neurologic improvement after tumor removal, plasma exchange, IVIg, cyclophosphamide, or glucocorticoids. However, large series of patients with well-defined antibody-positive paraneoplastic cerebellar degeneration show that these disorders rarely improve with any treatment.

PARANEOPLASTIC OPSOCLONUS-MYOCLONUS SYNDROME

Opsoclonus is a disorder of eye movement characterized by involuntary, chaotic saccades that occur in all directions of gaze; it is frequently associated with myoclonus and ataxia. Opsoclonus-myoclonus may be cancer-related or idiopathic. When the cause is paraneoplastic, the tumors involved are usually cancer of the lung and breast in adults and neuroblastoma in children. The pathologic substrate of opsoclonus-myoclonus is unclear. The majority of SCLC patients do not harbor antineuronal antibodies. A small subset of patients with ataxia, opsoclonus, and other eye movement disorders develop anti-Ri antibodies; in rare instances muscle rigidity, autonomic dysfunction, and dementia also occur. The tumor most frequently involved in anti-Ri-associated syndromes is breast cancer; however, only 50% of patients with anti-Ri antibodies develop opsoclonus.

If the tumor is not successfully treated, the paraneoplastic opsoclonus-myoclonus syndrome in adults often progresses to encephalopathy, coma, and death. In addition to treating the tumor, symptoms may respond to immunotherapy (glucocorticoids and/or IVIg).

At least 50% of children with opsoclonus-myoclonus have an underlying neuroblastoma. Hypotonia, ataxia, behavioral changes, and irritability are frequent accompanying symptoms. Although some patients harbor anti-Hu antibodies, most are antibody-negative. Neurologic symptoms often improve with treatment of the tumor (including chemotherapy) and with glucocorticoids, adrenocorticotropic hormone (ACTH), plasma exchange, and IVIg. The response to treatment varies; patients who do not improve with glucocorticoids may respond to ACTH. Neurologic relapses are frequent, and many patients are left with psychomotor retardation and behavioral and sleep problems.

PARANEOPLASTIC SYNDROMES OF THE SPINAL CORD

The number of reports of paraneoplastic spinal cord syndromes, such as *subacute motor neuronopathy* and *acute necrotizing myelopathy,* has decreased in recent years. This may represent a true decrease in incidence, due to improved and prompt oncologic interventions, or may be because of the identification of nonparaneoplastic etiologies; e.g., subacute necrotizing myelopathy may occur with herpes simplex virus (HSV) infection, usually HSV-2.

Some patients with cancer develop *upper* or *lower motor neuron dysfunction* or both, resembling amyotrophic lateral sclerosis. Because paraneoplastic antibody markers are lacking, it is unclear whether these disorders have a paraneoplastic etiology or simply coincide with the presence of cancer. There are isolated case reports of cancer patients with motor neuron dysfunction who had neurologic improvement after tumor treatment. A more than coincidental association occurs between lymphoma and motor neuron dysfunction. A search for lymphoma should be undertaken in patients with a motor neuron syndrome who are found to have a monoclonal protein in serum or CSF or an increased protein concentration in the CSF.

Paraneoplastic myelitis may present with upper or lower motor neuron symptoms, segmental myoclonus, and rigidity. This syndrome can appear as the presenting manifestation of encephalomyelitis and may be associated with SCLC and serum anti-Hu, anti-CV$_2$/CRMP5, or anti-amphiphysin antibodies.

Paraneoplastic myelopathy can also produce several syndromes characterized by prominent muscle stiffness and rigidity. The spectrum ranges from focal symptoms in one or several extremities (*stiff-limb syndrome* or *stiff-person syndrome*) to a disorder that also affects the brainstem (known as *encephalomyelitis with rigidity*) and likely has a different pathogenesis.

PARANEOPLASTIC STIFF-PERSON SYNDROME

This disorder is characterized by progressive muscle rigidity, stiffness, and painful spasms triggered by auditory, sensory, or emotional stimuli. Rigidity mainly involves the lower trunk and legs, but it can affect the upper extremities and neck. Symptoms improve with sleep and general anesthetics. Electrophysiologic studies demonstrate continuous motor unit activity. Antibodies associated with the stiff-person syndrome target proteins [glutamic acid

decarboxylase (GAD), amphiphysin] involved in the function of inhibitory synapses utilizing γ-aminobutyric acid (GABA) or glycine as neurotransmitters. Paraneoplastic stiff-person syndrome and amphiphysin antibodies are often related to breast cancer. By contrast, antibodies to GAD may occur in some cancer patients but are much more frequently present in the non-paraneoplastic disorder. Optimal treatment of stiff-person syndrome requires therapy of the underlying tumor, glucocorticoids, and symptomatic use of drugs that enhance GABA-ergic transmission (diazepam, baclofen, sodium valproate, vigabatrin). A benefit of IVIg has been demonstrated for the non-paraneoplastic disorder but remains to be established for the paraneoplastic syndrome.

PARANEOPLASTIC SENSORY NEURONOPATHY OR DORSAL ROOT GANGLIONOPATHY

This syndrome is characterized by sensory deficits that may be symmetric or asymmetric, painful dysesthesias, radicular pain, and decreased or absent reflexes. All modalities of sensation and any part of the body including face and trunk can be involved. Specialized sensations such as taste and hearing can also be affected. Electrophysiologic studies show decreased or absent sensory nerve potentials with normal or near-normal motor conduction velocities. Symptoms result from an inflammatory, likely immune-mediated, process that targets the dorsal root ganglia, causing neuronal loss, proliferation of satellite cells, and secondary degeneration of the posterior columns of the spinal cord. The dorsal nerve roots, and less frequently the anterior nerve roots and peripheral nerves, may also be involved.

This disorder often precedes or is associated with encephalomyelitis and autonomic dysfunction and has the same immunologic and oncologic associations, i.e., anti-Hu antibodies and SCLC. As with anti-Hu-associated encephalomyelitis, the therapeutic approach focuses on prompt treatment of the tumor. Glucocorticoids occasionally produce clinical stabilization or improvement. The benefit of IVIg and plasma exchange is not proved.

PARANEOPLASTIC PERIPHERAL NEUROPATHIES

These disorders may develop any time during the course of the neoplastic disease. Neuropathies occurring at late stages of cancer or lymphoma usually cause mild to moderate sensorimotor deficits due to axonal degeneration of unclear etiology. These neuropathies are often masked by concurrent neurotoxicity from chemotherapy and other cancer therapies. In contrast, the neuropathies that develop in the early stages of cancer often show a rapid progression, sometimes with a relapsing and remitting course, and evidence of inflammatory infiltrates and axonal loss or demyelination in biopsy studies. If demyelinating features predominate (Chaps. 33, 35), IVIg or glucocorticoids may improve symptoms. These neuropathies are not usually associated with antineuronal antibodies. Occasionally anti-CV_2/CRMP5 antibodies are present; detection of anti-Hu suggests concurrent dorsal root ganglionitis.

Guillain-Barré syndrome and *brachial plexitis* have occasionally been reported in patients with lymphoma, but there is no clear evidence of a paraneoplastic association.

Malignant monoclonal gammopathies include: (1) multiple myeloma and sclerotic myeloma associated with IgG or IgA monoclonal proteins; and (2) Waldenström's macroglobulinemia, B cell lymphoma, and chronic B cell lymphocytic leukemia associated with IgM monoclonal proteins. These disorders may cause neuropathy by a variety of mechanisms, including compression of roots and plexuses by metastasis to vertebral bodies and pelvis, deposits of amyloid in peripheral nerves, and paraneoplastic mechanisms. The paraneoplastic variety has several distinctive features. Approximately half of patients with sclerotic myeloma develop a sensorimotor neuropathy with predominantly motor deficits, resembling a chronic inflammatory demyelinating neuropathy (Chap. 35); some patients develop elements of the POEMS syndrome (*p*olyneuropathy, *o*rganomegaly, *e*ndocrinopathy, *M* protein, *s*kin changes). Treatment of the plasmacytoma or sclerotic lesions usually improves the neuropathy. In contrast, the sensorimotor or sensory neuropathy associated with multiple myeloma rarely responds to treatment. Between 5 and 10% of patients with Waldenström's macroglobulinemia develop a distal symmetric sensorimotor neuropathy with predominant involvement of large sensory fibers. These patients may have IgM antibodies in their serum against myelin-associated glycoprotein (Chap. 35). In addition to treating the Waldenström's macroglobulinemia, other therapies may improve the neuropathy, including plasma exchange, IVIg, chlorambucil, cyclophosphamide, fludarabine, or rituximab.

Vasculitis of the nerve and muscle causes a painful symmetric or asymmetric distal sensorimotor neuropathy with variable proximal weakness. It predominantly affects elderly men and is associated with an elevated erythrocyte sedimentation rate and increased CSF protein concentration. SCLC and lymphoma are the primary tumors involved. Pathology demonstrates axonal degeneration and T cell infiltrates involving the small vessels of the nerve and muscle. Immunosuppressants (glucocorticoids and cyclophosphamide) often result in neurologic improvement.

Peripheral nerve hyperexcitability (neuromyotonia, or Isaacs' syndrome) is characterized by spontaneous and continuous muscle fiber activity of peripheral nerve origin. Clinical features include cramps, muscle twitching (fasciculations or myokymia), stiffness, delayed muscle relaxation (pseudomyotonia), and spontaneous or evoked carpal or pedal spasms. The involved muscles may be hypertrophic, and some patients develop paresthesias and hyperhydrosis. CNS dysfunction, including mood changes, sleep disorder, or hallucinations, may occur. The electromyogram (EMG) shows fibrillations; fasciculations; and doublet, triplet, or multiplet single unit (myokymic) discharges that have a high intraburst frequency. An immune pathogenesis is suggested by the frequent presence of serum antibodies to VGKC. The disorder often occurs without cancer; if paraneoplastic, benign and malignant thymomas and SCLC are the usual tumors. Some patients with thymoma develop acetylcholine receptor antibodies with or without myasthenia gravis. Diphenylhydantoin, carbamazepine, and plasma exchange improve symptoms.

The *cramps-fasciculation syndrome* resembles neuromyotonia, but the EMG does not show myokymic discharges. It may also occur with thymoma, lung cancer, and antibodies to VGKC.

Paraneoplastic autonomic neuropathy usually develops as a component of other disorders, such as LEMS and encephalomyelitis. It may rarely occur as a pure or predominantly autonomic neuropathy with adrenergic or cholinergic dysfunction at the pre- or postganglionic levels. Patients can develop several life-threatening complications, such as gastrointestinal paresis with pseudoobstruction, cardiac dysrhythmias, and postural hypotension. Other symptoms include dry mouth, erectile dysfunction, anhidrosis, and sphincter dysfunction. The disorder has been reported to occur in association with several tumors, including SCLC, cancer of the pancreas or testis, carcinoid tumors, and lymphoma. Because autonomic symptoms can also be the presenting feature of encephalomyelitis, serum anti-Hu and anti-CV_2/CRMP5 antibodies should also be sought. Serum antibodies to ganglionic acetylcholine receptors have been reported in this syndrome, but they also occur without a cancer association. (See also Table 22-2.)

LAMBERT-EATON MYASTHENIC SYNDROME

LEMS is discussed in Chap. 36.

MYASTHENIA GRAVIS

For discussion of myasthenia gravis, see Chap. 36.

POLYMYOSITIS-DERMATOMYOSITIS

Polymyositis and dermatomyositis are discussed in detail in Chap. 39.

ACUTE NECROTIZING MYOPATHY

Patients with this syndrome develop myalgias and rapid progression of weakness involving the extremities and the pharyngeal and respiratory muscles, often resulting in death. Serum muscle enzymes are elevated, and muscle biopsy shows extensive necrosis with minimal or absent inflammation and sometimes deposits of complement. The disorder occurs as a paraneoplastic manifestation of a variety of cancers including SCLC and cancer of the gastrointestinal tract, breast, kidney, and prostate, among others. Glucocorticoids or treatment of the underlying tumor rarely control the disorder.

PARANEOPLASTIC VISUAL SYNDROMES

This group of disorders involves the retina and, less frequently, the uvea and optic nerves. The term *cancer-associated retinopathy* is used to describe paraneoplastic cone and rod dysfunction characterized by photosensitivity, progressive loss of vision and color perception, central or ring scotomas, night blindness, and attenuation of photopic and scotopic responses in the electroretinogram (ERG). The most commonly associated tumor is SCLC. Melanoma-associated retinopathy affects patients with metastatic cutaneous melanoma. Patients develop the acute onset of night blindness and shimmering, flickering, or pulsating photopsias that often progress to visual loss. The ERG demonstrates reduction in the b-wave amplitude. Paraneoplastic optic neuritis and uveitis are very uncommon and can develop in association with encephalomyelitis. Some patients with paraneoplastic uveitis harbor anti-CV_2/CRMP5 antibodies.

Some paraneoplastic retinopathies are associated with serum antibodies that specifically react with the subset of retinal cells undergoing degeneration, supporting an immune-mediated pathogenesis (Table 27-2). Paraneoplastic retinopathies usually fail to improve with treatment, although rare responses to glucocorticoids, plasma exchange, and IVIg have been reported.

FURTHER READINGS

CHAN JW: Paraneoplastic retinopathies and optic neuropathies. Surv Ophthalmol 48:12, 2003

DROPCHO EJ: Remote neurologic manifestations of cancer. Neurol Clin 20:85, 2002

☑ ———: Update on paraneoplastic syndromes. Curr Opin Neurol 18:331, 2005

An up-to-date reference detailing paraneoplastic neurologic syndromes.

GRAUS F et al. Recommended diagnostic criteria for paraneoplastic neurological syndromes. J Neurol Neurosurg Psychiatry 75:1135, 2004

☑ Rosenfeld MR, Dalmau J: Current therapy of paraneoplastic syndromes. Curr Treat Opt Neurol 5:69, 2003

Outlines approaches to treatment of neurologic paraneoplastic syndromes.

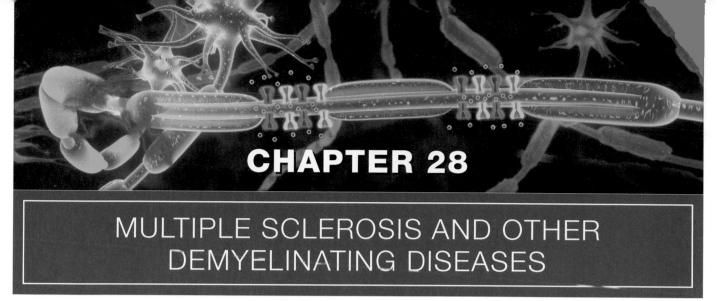

CHAPTER 28

MULTIPLE SCLEROSIS AND OTHER DEMYELINATING DISEASES

Stephen L. Hauser
Douglas S. Goodin

Demyelinating disorders are characterized by inflammation and selective destruction of central nervous system (CNS) myelin. The peripheral nervous system (PNS) is spared, and most patients have no evidence of an associated systemic illness.

MULTIPLE SCLEROSIS

Multiple sclerosis (MS) is characterized by a triad of inflammation, demyelination, and gliosis (scarring); the course can be relapsing-remitting or progressive. Lesions of MS are typically disseminated in time and location. MS affects ~350,000 Americans and 1.1 million individuals worldwide. In western societies, MS is second only to trauma as a cause of neurologic disability in early to middle adulthood. Manifestations of MS vary from a benign illness to a rapidly evolving and incapacitating disease requiring profound life-style adjustments.

PATHOGENESIS

Anatomy

MS lesions (plaques) vary in size from 1 or 2 mm to several centimeters. Acute MS lesions are characterized by perivenular cuffing with inflammatory mononuclear cells, predominantly T cells and macrophages, which also infiltrate the surrounding white matter. At sites of inflammation, the blood-brain barrier (BBB) is disrupted but, unlike vasculitis, the vessel wall is preserved. In more than half of cases, myelin-specific autoantibodies promote demyelination and stimulate macrophages and microglial cells (bone marrow–derived CNS phagocytes) that scavenge the myelin debris. As lesions evolve, astrocytes proliferate (gliosis). Surviving oligodendrocytes or those that differentiate from precursor cells may partially remyelinate the surviving naked axons, producing so-called shadow plaques. Ultrastructural studies of MS lesions suggest that fundamentally different underlying pathologies may exist in different patients. Heterogeneity has been observed in terms of: (1) whether the inflammatory cell infiltrate is associated with deposition of antibody and activation of complement, and (2) whether the target of the immunopathologic process is the myelin sheath itself or the cell body of the oligodendrocyte. Although sparing of axons is typical of MS, partial or total axonal destruction can also occur. Indirect evidence suggests that axonal loss is a major cause of irreversible neurologic disability in MS.

Physiology

Nerve conduction in myelinated axons occurs in a saltatory manner, with the nerve impulse jumping from one node of Ranvier to the next without depolarization of

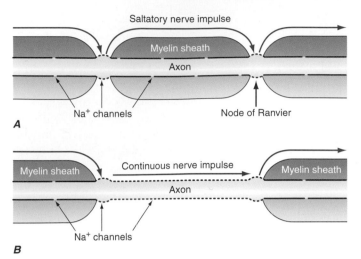

FIGURE 28-1

Nerve conduction in myelinated and demyelinated axons. *A.* Saltatory nerve conduction in myelinated axons occurs with the nerve impulse jumping from one node of Ranvier to the next. Sodium channels are concentrated at the nodes where axonal depolarization occurs. *B.* Following demyelination, the sodium channels are redistributed along the axon, thereby supporting continuous propagation of the nerve action potential in this region.

the axonal membrane underlying the myelin sheath between nodes (**Fig. 28-1**). This produces considerably faster conduction velocities (~70 m/s) than the slow velocities (~1 m/s) produced by continuous propagation in unmyelinated nerves. Conduction block occurs when the nerve impulse is unable to traverse the demyelinated segment. This can happen when the resting axon membrane becomes hyperpolarized due to the exposure of voltage-dependent potassium channels that are normally buried underneath the myelin sheath. A temporary conduction block often follows a demyelinating event before the sodium channels (originally concentrated at the nodes) have had a chance to redistribute themselves along the naked axon (Fig. 28-1). This redistribution ultimately allows the continuous propagation of nerve action potentials through the demyelinated segment but, before this happens, the leakage currents are too large for the nerve impulse to jump the internode distance and conduction fails. On occasion, conduction block is incomplete, affecting, for example, high- but not low–frequency volleys of impulses. Variable conduction block can occur with raised body temperature or metabolic alterations and may explain clinical fluctuations (typical of MS) that vary from hour to hour or in association with fever or exercise. Conduction slowing occurs when the demyelinated segments support only (slow) continuous nerve impulse propagation.

Epidemiology

MS is approximately twice as common in women as in men. The age of onset is typically between 20 and 40 years (slightly later in men than in women). Rarely, it can begin as early as 2 years of age or as late as the eighth decade.

The highest known prevalence for MS (250 per 100,000) occurs in the Orkney islands, located north of Scotland, and similarly high rates are found throughout northern Europe, the northern United States, and Canada. By contrast, the prevalence is low in Japan (2 per 100,000), in other parts of Asia, in equatorial Africa, and in the Middle East. In general, prevalence increases with increasing distance from the equator, although certain exceptions are notable. Thus, the incidence of MS in the Eskimo population of Alaska is rare compared to the incidence in Caucasians living at similar latitudes. Similarly, native South Africans have a markedly lower prevalence compared to South Africans of European descent who live in the same geographic area. However, distinctive migration patterns of certain populations may artifactually suggest a relationship between MS and climate. Thus, when Scandanavians migrated to the United States or when the Scots migrated to New Zealand, they tended to migrate preferentially to places (e.g., the northern United States or southern New Zealand) with similar climates to their native lands. Such considerations point to potential genetic mechanisms (see below) rather than to an influence of temperate climate per se.

Changes in Incidence/prevalence Studies from the United States, Europe, Australia, and the Middle East suggest that the prevalence of MS may be increasing, although improved methods of diagnosis may account for the apparent change. Other reports suggest that individuals who move from an area of high prevalence to one of low prevalence (or vice versa) before the age of 15 years adopt the risk of MS in their new environment, whereas if they move after this age, they retain the risk of their native land. The reliability of these observations is uncertain, although, if correct, they would suggest an environmental factor in the pathogenesis of MS.

Reported Clusters Clusters of MS cases are occasionally reported. Often these apparent epidemics cannot be distinguished easily from chance occurrences, although some reports (e.g., the clustering of MS cases in the Faeroe Islands after British occupation during World War II) are more convincing than others. Such clustering, however, seems to be rare.

The Relationship of MS to Trauma and Stress

The existing evidence does not support any association of trauma with either MS onset or exacerbation. Similarly, a relationship between stress and either onset or exacerbation of MS has not been established, although this area is not easily studied because of difficulties in quantifying stress.

A genetic susceptibility to MS exists, as evidenced by the following observations:

1. The prevalence of MS differs among ethnic groups residing in the same environment.
2. First-, second-, and third-degree relatives of MS patients are at increased risk for the disease. Siblings of affected individuals have a lifetime risk of 2 to 5%, whereas the risk to parents or children of affected individuals is somewhat lower.
3. Twin studies demonstrate concordance rates of 25 to 30% in monozygotic twins compared to only 2 to 5% in dizygotic twins (similar to the risk in nontwin siblings).

The inheritance of MS cannot be explained by a simple genetic model. Susceptibility is probably polygenic, with each gene contributing a relatively small amount to the overall risk. It is also likely that genetic heterogeneity (different susceptibilities among individuals) also exists. The major histocompatibility complex (MHC) on chromosome 6p21 (encoding proteins involved in presenting peptide antigens to T cells) is the most important MS susceptibility region identified to date. MS susceptibility is associated with the class II region of the MHC, specifically with the DR2 (DRB1*1501) allele and its corresponding haplotype. Other genetic regions implicated in MS susceptibility are located on chromosomal regions 19q35 and 17q13.

Immunology

An autoimmune cause for MS is supported by the laboratory model of experimental allergic encephalomyelitis (EAE) and by studies of the immune system in MS patients.

Autoreactive T Lymphocytes Myelin basic protein (MBP) is an important T cell antigen in EAE and probably also in human MS. Activated MBP-reactive T cells are often found in the blood or cerebrospinal fluid (CSF) of MS patients and, occasionally, also in MS lesions. Moreover, DR2 may influence the autoimmune response because it binds with high affinity to a fragment of MBP (spanning amino acids 89 to 96), stimulating T cell responses to this self-protein.

Autoantibodies Autoantibodies, directed against myelin antigens such as myelin oligodendrocyte glycoprotein (MOG), probably act in concert with a pathogenic T cell response to cause the demyelinating lesions in many patients. Recent evidence suggests that the presence of anti-MOG antibodies in the serum of patients with a clinically isolated syndrome (CIS) is highly predictive of the development of MS in the future. Also, evidence of an abnormal humoral immune response is present in the CSF of MS patients. Membrane attack complexes (from complement-mediated antibody damage) can be detected in CSF, and elevated CSF immunoglobulin (synthesized locally) is characteristic of MS. Oligoclonal antibody (derived from expansion of a selected group of plasma cells) is present in most cases. Oligoclonal immunoglobulin is also detected in other chronic inflammatory conditions, including infections, and thus is not specific to MS. The pattern of banding is unique to each individual, and attempts to identify the targets of these antibodies have been unsuccessful.

Triggers Magnetic resonance imaging (MRI) has demonstrated bursts of disease activity 7 to 10 times more frequently than is clinically apparent. This finding indicates that there is a large reservoir of subclinical disease activity in MS, especially during the early stages of the disease. The triggers causing these bursts are unknown, although the fact that patients may experience relapses after nonspecific upper respiratory infections suggests that either molecular mimicry between viruses and myelin antigens or viral superantigens activating pathogenic T cells may play a role in MS pathogenesis.

Microbiology

As noted above, epidemiologic evidence supports the role of an environmental exposure in MS. MS risk also correlates with high socioeconomic status, which may reflect improved sanitation and delayed initial exposures to infectious agents. By analogy, some viral infections (e.g., poliomyelitis and measles viruses) produce neurologic sequelae more frequently when the age of initial infection is delayed. The best studied experimental model of virus-induced demyelinating disease is infection with Theiler virus, a murine coronavirus similar to measles, which produces a chronic oligodendrocyte infection with multifocal perivascular lymphocytic infiltration and demyelination, closely resembling lesions of MS.

High antibody titers against many viruses have been reported in serum and CSF of MS patients, including measles, herpes simplex, varicella, rubella, Epstein-Barr, and influenza C and some parainfluenza strains. Numerous viruses and bacteria (or their genomic sequences) have been recovered from MS tissues and fluids. Most recently human herpes virus type 6 (HHV-6) and *Chlamydia pneumoniae* have been implicated, although a causal role for any infectious agent in MS remains unproven.

CLINICAL MANIFESTATIONS

The onset of MS may be abrupt or insidious. Symptoms may be severe or seem so trivial that a patient may not seek medical attention for months or years. Indeed, at autopsy some individuals who were asymptomatic during life will be found, unexpectedly, to have MS. In other cases an MRI scan obtained for an unrelated reason may show evidence of asymptomatic MS. Symptoms of MS are extremely varied and depend upon the location of lesions within the CNS (**Table 28-1**). Examination generally reveals evidence of neurologic dysfunction, often in asymptomatic locations. For example, a patient may present with symptoms in one leg and signs in both.

Weakness of the limbs may manifest as loss of strength or dexterity, fatigue, or a disturbance of gait. Exercise-induced weakness is a characteristic symptom of MS. The weakness is of the upper motor neuron type and is frequently accompanied by other pyramidal signs such as spasticity, hyperreflexia and Babinski signs. Occasionally, a tendon reflex may be lost (simulating a lower motor neuron lesion) if an MS lesion disrupts the afferent reflex fibers in the spinal cord.

Spasticity is often associated with spontaneous and movement-induced muscle spasms. More than 30% of MS patients have moderate to severe spasticity, especially in the legs. It is often accompanied by painful spasms and can interfere with a patient's ability to ambulate or work or with self-care. Occasionally, spasticity may provide nonvolitional support for the body weight during ambulation. In these cases, treatment of spasticity may actually do more harm than good.

Optic neuritis (ON) generally presents as diminished visual acuity, dimness, or decreased color perception (desaturation) in the central field of vision. These symptoms may be mild or may progress to severe visual loss. Rarely, there is complete loss of light perception. Visual symptoms are generally monocular but may occur bilaterally. Periorbital pain (aggravated by eye movement) often precedes or accompanies the visual loss. An afferent pupillary defect may be found. Funduscopic examination may be normal or reveal optic disc swelling (papillitis). Pallor of the optic disc (optic atrophy) commonly follows ON. Uveitis is rare and should raise the possibility of alternative diagnoses. ON is discussed in Chap. 11.

Visual blurring in MS may result from ON or diplopia. Visual blurring that resolves when either eye is covered is due to diplopia.

Diplopia may result from internuclear ophthalmoplegia (INO) or from palsy of the sixth cranial nerve (rarely the third or fourth). An INO consists of impaired adduction of one eye due to a lesion in the ipsilateral medial longitudinal fasciculus (Chap. 11). Prominent nystagmus is often observed in the abducting eye, along with a small skew deviation. A bilateral INO is particularly suggestive of MS. Other common gaze disturbances in MS include: (1) a horizontal gaze palsy, (2) a "one and a half" syndrome (horizontal gaze palsy plus an INO), and (3) acquired pendular nystagmus.

Sensory symptoms are varied and include both paresthesias (e.g., tingling, prickling sensations, formications, "pins and needles," or painful burning) and hypesthesia (e.g., reduced sensation, numbness or a "dead" feeling). Unpleasant sensations (e.g., feelings that body parts are swollen, wet, raw, or tightly wrapped) are also common. Sensory impairment of the trunk and legs below a

TABLE 28-1

INITIAL SYMPTOMS OF MS			
SYMPTOM	**PERCENT OF CASES**	**SYMPTOM**	**PERCENT OF CASES**
Sensory loss	37	Lhermitte	3
Optic neuritis	36	Pain	3
Weakness	35	Dementia	2
Paresthesias	24	Visual loss	2
Diplopia	15	Facial palsy	1
Ataxia	11	Impotence	1
Vertigo	6	Myokymia	1
Paroxysmal attacks	4	Epilepsy	1
Bladder	4	Falling	1

Source: After WB Matthews et al, *McAlpine's Multiple Sclerosis*, New York, Churchill Livingstone, 1991.

horizontal line on the torso (a sensory level) suggests that the spinal cord is the origin of the sensory disturbance. It is often accompanied by a bandlike sensation of tightness around the torso. Pain is a common symptom of MS, experienced by >50% of patients. Pain can occur anywhere on the body and can change locations over time.

Ataxia usually manifests as cerebellar tremors (Chap. 20). Ataxia may also involve the head and trunk or the voice, producing a characteristic cerebellar dysarthria (scanning speech). The true extent of cerebellar involvement may be difficult to determine in an individual patient, because motor and sensory deficits can affect coordination and weakness may interfere with coordination testing.

Bladder and bowel dysfunction arise from different causes and frequently different types of dysfunction coexist. During normal reflex voiding, relaxation of the bladder sphincter (α-adrenergic innervation) is coordinated with contraction of the detrusor muscle in the bladder wall (muscarinic cholinergic innervation). Stoppage of the urinary stream is accomplished with a coordinated sphincter contraction and detrusor relaxation. Bladder-stretch (during filling) activates this reflex, which is inhibited by supraspinal (voluntary) input. Symptoms of bladder dysfunction are present in >90% of MS patients and, in a third, dysfunction results in weekly or more frequent episodes of incontinence.

Detrusor hyperreflexia, due to impairment of suprasegmental inhibition, causes urinary frequency, urgency, nocturia, and uncontrolled bladder emptying. *Detrusor sphincter dyssynergia,* due to loss of synchronization between detrusor and sphincter muscles, causes difficulty in initiating and/or stopping the urinary stream, thereby producing hesitancy. It can also lead to urinary retention, large postvoid residual volumes, overflow incontinence, and recurrent infection.

Constipation occurs in >30% of patients. Fecal urgency or *bowel incontinence* is less common (15%) but can be socially debilitating.

Cognitive dysfunction can include memory loss, impaired attention, difficulties in problem-solving, slowed information processing, and problems shifting between cognitive tasks. Euphoria (elevated mood) was once thought to be characteristic of MS but is actually uncommon, occurring in <20% of patients. Cognitive dysfunction sufficient to impair activities of daily living also occurs but is rare.

Depression, experienced by 50 to 60% of patients, can be reactive, endogenous, or part of the illness itself and can contribute to fatigue. Suicide in MS patients is 7.5-fold more common than in age-matched controls.

Fatigue is experienced by 90% of patients and is moderate or severe in half. Symptoms include generalized motor weakness, limited ability to concentrate, extreme lassitude, loss of energy, decreased endurance, and an overwhelming sense of exhaustion that requires the patient to rest or fall asleep. Fatigue (either alone or with other symptoms) is the most common reason for work-related disability in MS. Fatigue can be exacerbated by elevated temperatures, by depression, by expending exceptional effort to accomplish basic activities of daily living, or by sleep disturbances (e.g., from frequent nocturnal awakenings to urinate). MS-related fatigue may be maximum during mid-afternoon or continuous throughout the day, and it is often difficult to treat.

Sexual dysfunction is common in MS. Men report impotence, less desire, impaired genital sensation, impaired ejaculation, and inability to achieve/maintain an erection. Women report genital numbness, diminished orgasmic response, decreased libido, unpleasant sensations during intercourse, and diminished vaginal lubrication. Adductor spasticity (in women) can also interfere with intercourse, and urinary incontinence (in either men or women) can be problematic.

Facial weakness due to a lesion in the intraparenchymal pathway of the seventh cranial nerve may resemble idiopathic Bell's palsy. However, unlike Bell's palsy, facial weakness in MS is generally not associated with ipsilateral loss of taste sensation or retroauricular pain (Chap. 23).

Vertigo may appear suddenly and resemble acute labyrinthitis. A brainstem rather than end-organ origin is suggested by the presence of coexisting trigeminal or facial nerve involvement; vertical nystagmus; or nystagmus that has no latency to onset, no direction reversal, and doesn't fatigue. Hearing loss may also occur in MS but is uncommon.

Ancillary Symptoms

Heat sensitivity refers to neurologic symptoms produced by an elevation of the body's core temperature. For example, transient unilateral visual blurring or loss may occur during a hot shower or with physical exercise (*Uhthoff's symptom*). It is common for MS symptoms to worsen transiently, sometimes dramatically, during febrile illnesses (see pseudoexacerbation, below). Such heat-related symptoms probably result from transient conduction block (see above).

Lhermitte's symptom is the electric shock–like sensation (evoked by neck flexion or other movement) that radiates down the back into the legs. Rarely, it radiates into the arms. It is generally self-limited but may persist for years. Lhermitte's symptom can also occur with other disorders of the cervical spine (e.g., cervical spondylosis).

Paroxysmal symptoms are distinguished by their brief duration (30 s to 2 min), high frequency (5 to 40 episodes per day), lack of any alteration of consciousness or change in background electroencephalogram during episodes, and a self-limited course (generally lasting weeks to months). They may be precipitated by hyperventilation or movement. These syndromes include Lhermitte's symptom; tonic contractions of a limb, face, or trunk (tonic seizures); paroxysmal dysarthria/ataxia; paroxysmal sensory disturbances; and several other less well characterized syndromes. Paroxysmal symptoms probably result from spontaneous discharges, arising at the edges of demyelinated plaques, and spreading ephaptically to adjacent white matter tracts.

Trigeminal neuralgia, hemifacial spasm, and glossopharyngeal neuralgia can occur when the demyelinating lesion involves the root entry (or exit) zone of the fifth, seventh, and ninth cranial nerve, respectively. *Trigeminal neuralgia* (tic douloureux) is a very brief lancinating facial pain often triggered by an afferent input from the face or teeth. Most cases of trigeminal neuralgia are not MS-related. However, the occurrence of atypical features (Chap. 23) such as the onset before age 50 years, bilateral symptoms, objective sensory loss, or nonparoxysmal pain should raise concerns that a symptomatic cause such as MS is responsible.

Facial myokymia consists of either persistent rapid flickering contractions of the facial musculature (especially the lower portion of the orbicularis oculus) or a contraction that slowly spreads across the face. It results from lesions of the corticobulbar tracts or brainstem course of the facial nerve.

DISEASE COURSE

Four clinical types of MS have been described (**Fig. 28-2**):

1. *Relapsing/remitting MS* (RRMS) accounts for 85% of MS cases at onset and is characterized by discrete attacks that generally evolve over days to weeks (rarely over hours). Often, but not invariably, there is complete recovery over the ensuing weeks to months (Fig. 28-2*A*). However, when ambulation is severely impaired during an attack, approximately half will fail to improve. Between attacks, patients are neurologically stable.
2. *Secondary progressive MS* (SPMS) always begins as RRMS (Fig. 28-2*B*). At some point, however, the RRMS clinical course changes so that the patient experiences a steady deterioration in function unassociated with acute attacks (which may continue or cease during the progressive phase). SPMS produces a greater amount of fixed neurologic disability than RRMS. Approximately 50% of patients with RRMS will have developed SPMS after 15 years, and longer follow-up points indicate that the great majority of RRMS ultimately evolves into SPMS. Thus, SPMS appears to represent a late-stage of the same underlying illness as RRMS.

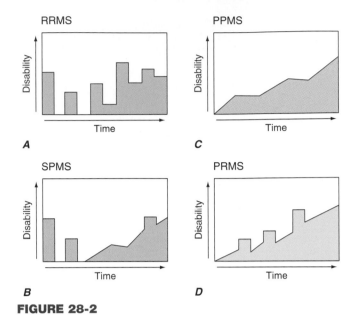

FIGURE 28-2

Clinical course of multiple sclerosis (MS). *A.* Relapsing/remitting MS. *B.* Secondary progressive MS. *C.* Primary progressive MS. *D.* Progressive/relapsing MS.

3. *Primary progressive MS* (PPMS) accounts for ~15% of cases. These patients do not experience attacks but only a steady functional decline from disease onset (Fig. 28-2*C*). Compared to RRMS, the sex distribution is more even, the disease begins later in life (mean age, ~40 years), and disability develops faster. Whether PPMS is an unusual phenotype of the same underlying illness as RRMS or whether these are distinct illnesses is unknown.
4. *Progressive/relapsing MS* (PRMS) overlaps PPMS and SPMS and accounts for ~5% of MS patients. Like patients with PPMS, these patients experience a steady deterioration in their condition from disease onset. However, like SPMS patients, they experience occasional attacks superimposed upon their progressive course (Fig. 28-2*D*). The early stages of PRMS are indistinguishable from those of PPMS (i.e., until the first clinical attack).

DIAGNOSIS

There is no definitive diagnostic test for MS. Diagnostic criteria for clinically definite MS require documentation of two or more episodes of symptoms and two or more signs that reflect pathology in anatomically noncontiguous white matter tracts of the CNS (**Table 28-2**). Symptoms must last for >24 h and occur as distinct episodes that are separated by a month or more. At least one of the two required signs must be present on neurologic examination. The second may be documented by certain abnormal paraclinical tests such as MRI or evoked potentials (EPs). In patients who experience gradual progression of disability for ≥6 months without superimposed relapses,

TABLE 28-2

DIAGNOSTIC CRITERIA FOR MS

1. Examination must reveal *objective* abnormalities of the CNS.
2. Involvement must reflect predominantly disease of white matter long tracts, usually including (a) pyramidal pathways, (b) cerebellar pathways, (c) medial longitudinal fasciculus, (d) optic nerve, and (e) posterior columns.
3. Examination or history must implicate involvement of two or more areas of the CNS.
   a. MRI may be used to document a second lesion when only one site of abnormality has been demonstrable on examination. A confirmatory MRI must have either four lesions involving the white matter or three lesions if one is periventricular in location. Acceptable lesions must be >3 mm in diameter. For patients older than 50 years, two of the following criteria must also be met: (a) lesion size >5 mm, (b) lesions adjacent to the bodies of the lateral ventricles, and (c) lesion(s) present in the posterior fossa.
   b. Evoked response testing may be used to document a second lesion not evident on clinical examination.
4. The clinical pattern must consist of (a) two or more separate episodes of worsening involving different sites of the CNS, each lasting at least 24 h and occurring at least 1 month apart, or (b) gradual or stepwise progression over at least 6 months if accompanied by increased IgG synthesis or two or more oligoclonal bands. MRI may be used to document dissemination in time if a new T2 lesion of a Gd-enhancing lesion is seen 3 or more months after a clinically isolated syndrome.
5. The patient's neurologic condition could not better be attributed to another disease.

Diagnostic Categories

1. *Definite MS:* All five criteria fulfilled.
2. *Probable MS:* All five criteria fulfilled except (a) only one objective abnormality despite two symptomatic episodes or (b) only one symptomatic episode despite two or more objective abnormalities.
3. *At risk for MS:* Criteria 1, 2, 3, and 5 fulfilled: patient has only one symptomatic episode and one objective abnormality.

Note: CNS, central nervous system: MRI, magnetic resonance imaging; Gd, gadolinium.

DIAGNOSTIC TESTS

Magnetic Resonance Imaging

MRI has revolutionized the diagnosis and management of MS (**Fig. 28-3**); characteristic abnormalities are found in >95% of patients. An increase in vascular permeability from a breakdown of the BBB is detected by leakage of intravenous gadolinium (Gd) into the parenchyma. Such leakage occurs early in the development of an MS lesion and serves as a useful marker of inflammation. Gd-enhancement persists for up to 3 months, and the residual MS plaque remains visible indefinitely as a focal area of hyperintensity (a lesion) on spin-echo (T2-weighted) and proton-density images. Lesions are frequently oriented perpendicular to the ventricular surface, corresponding to the pathologic pattern of perivenous demyelination (Dawson's fingers). Lesions are multifocal within the brain, brainstem, and spinal cord. Lesions in the anterior corpus callosum are helpful diagnostically because this site is usually spared in cerebrovascular disease. Different criteria for the use of MRI in the diagnosis of MS have been proposed (Table 28-2).

The total volume of T2-weighted signal abnormality (the "burden of disease") shows a significant (albeit weak) correlation with clinical disability. Approximately one-third of T2-weighted lesions appear as hypointense lesions (black holes) on T1-weighted imaging. Black holes may be a better marker of irreversible demyelination and axonal loss than T2 hyperintensities, although even this measure depends upon the timing of the image acquisition (e.g., most acute Gd-enhancing T2 lesions are T1 dark).

Newer MRI measures such as brain atrophy, magnetization transfer ratio (MTR) imaging and proton magnetic resonance spectroscopic imaging (MRSI) may ultimately serve as surrogate markers of clinical disability. For example, MRSI can quantitate molecules such as N-acetyl aspartate (NAA), which is a marker of axonal integrity, and MTR may be able to distinguish demyelination from edema.

Evoked Potentials

EP testing assesses function in afferent (visual, auditory, and somatosensory) or efferent (motor) CNS pathways. EPs use computer averaging to measure CNS electric potentials evoked by repetitive stimulation of selected peripheral nerves or of the brain. These tests provide the most information when the pathways studied are clinically uninvolved. For example, in a patient with a remitting and relapsing spinal cord syndrome with sensory deficits in the legs, an abnormal somatosensory EP following posterior tibial nerve stimulation provides little new information. By contrast, an abnormal visual EP in this circumstance would permit a diagnosis of clinically definite MS (Table 28-2). Abnormalities on one or more EP modalities occur in 80 to 90% of MS patients. EP abnormalities are not specific to MS, although a marked delay in the latency of a specific EP component (as opposed to a reduced amplitude) is suggestive of demyelination.

documentation of intrathecal IgG and visual EP testing may be used to support the diagnosis.

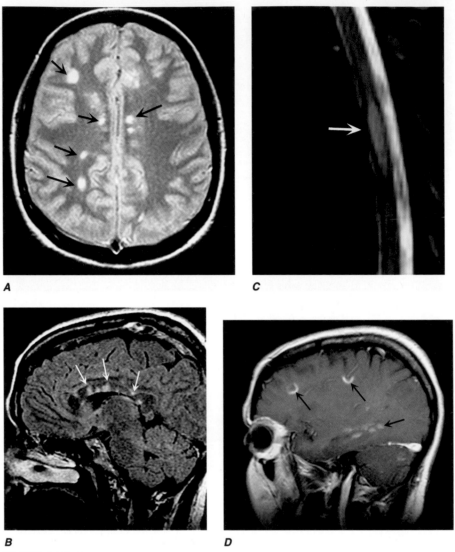

FIGURE 28-3

MRI findings in MS. *A*. Axial first-echo image from T2-weighted sequence demonstrates multiple bright signal abnormalities in white matter, typical for MS. *B*. Sagittal T2-weighted FLAIR (fluid attenuated inversion recovery) image in which the high signal of CSF has been suppressed. CSF appears dark, while areas of brain edema or demyelination appear high in signal as shown here in the corpus callosum (*arrows*). Lesions in the anterior corpus callosum are frequent in MS and rare in vascular disease. *C*. Sagittal T2-weighted fast spin echo image of the thoracic spine demonstrates a fusiform high signal intensity lesion in the mid-thoracic spinal cord. *D*. Sagittal T1-weighted image obtained after the intravenous administration of gadolinium DTPA reveals focal areas of blood-brain barrier disruption, identified as high-signal-intensity regions (*arrows*).

Cerebrospinal Fluid

CSF abnormalities found in MS include a mononuclear cell pleocytosis and an increased level of intrathecally synthesized IgG. The total CSF protein is usually normal or slightly elevated. Various formulas distinguish intrathecally synthesized IgG from IgG that may have entered the CNS passively from the serum. One formula (the CSF IgG index) expresses the ratio of IgG to albumin in the CSF divided by the same ratio in the serum. A more complicated formula, the IgG synthesis rate, makes certain assumptions but uses the same serum and CSF IgG and albumin measurements to calculate the rate of CNS IgG synthesis. The measurement of oligoclonal banding (OCB) in the CSF also assesses intrathecal production of IgG. OCBs are detected by agarose gel electrophoresis. Two or more OCBs are found in 75 to 90% of patients with MS. OCBs may be absent at the onset of MS, and in individual patients the number of bands present may increase with time. It is important that paired serum samples be studied to exclude a peripheral (i.e., non-CNS) origin of any OCBs detected in the CSF.

A mild CSF pleocytosis (>5 cells/μL) is present in ~25% of cases, usually in young patients with RRMS. A pleocytosis of >75 cells/μL, the presence of polymorphonuclear leukocytes, or a protein concentration of >1.0 g/L (>100 mg/dL) in CSF should raise concern that the patient may not have MS.

DIFFERENTIAL DIAGNOSIS

No single clinical sign or test is diagnostic of MS. The diagnosis is readily made in a young adult with relapsing and remitting symptoms involving different areas of CNS white matter. The possibility of an alternative diagnosis should always be considered (**Table 28-3**), particularly when (1) symptoms are localized exclusively to the posterior fossa, craniocervical junction, or spinal cord; (2) the patient is <15 or >60 years of age; (3) the clinical course

TABLE 28-3

DISORDERS THAT CAN MIMIC MS
Acute disseminated encephalomyelitis (ADEM)
Antiphospholipid antibody syndrome
Behçet's disease
Cerebral autosomal dominant arteriopathy, subcortical infarcts, and leukoencephalopathy (CADASIL)
Congenital leukodystrophies (e.g., adrenoleukodystrophy, metachromatic leukodystrophy)
Human immunodeficiency virus (HIV) infection
Ischemic optic neuropathy (arteritic and nonarteritic)
Lyme disease
Mitochondrial encephalopathy with lactic acidosis and stroke (MELAS)
Neoplasms (e.g., lymphoma, glioma, meningioma)
Sarcoid
Sjögren's syndrome
Stroke and ischemic cerebrovascular disease
Syphilis
Systemic lupus erythematosus and related collagen vascular disorders
Tropical spastic paraparesis (HTLV I/II infection)
Vascular malformations (especially spinal dural AV fistulas)
Vasculitis (primary CNS or other)
Vitamin B_{12} deficiency

Note: HTLV, human T cell leukemia/lymphoma virus; AV, arteriovenous; CNS, central nervous system.

is progressive from onset; (4) the patient has never experienced visual, sensory, or bladder symptoms; or (5) laboratory findings (e.g., MRI, CSF, or EPs) are atypical. Similarly, uncommon or rare symptoms in MS (e.g., aphasia, parkinsonism, chorea, isolated dementia, severe muscular atrophy, peripheral neuropathy, episodic loss of consciousness, fever, headache, seizures, or coma) should increase concern about an alternative diagnosis. Diagnosis is also difficult in patients with a rapid or explosive (stroke-like) onset or with mild symptoms and a normal neurologic examination. Rarely, intense inflammation and swelling may produce a mass lesion that mimics a primary or metastatic tumor. The specific tests required to exclude alternative diagnoses will vary with each clinical situation; however, an erythrocyte sedimentation rate, serum B_{12} level, antinuclear antibody (ANA), and Venereal Disease Research Laboratory (VDRL) test should probably be obtained in all patients with suspected MS.

PROGNOSIS

Most patients with MS experience progressive neurologic disability. Fifteen years after onset, only 20% of patients have no functional limitation; half will have progressed to SPMS and will require assistance with ambulation. Twenty-five years after onset, $>80\%$ of MS patients will have reached this level of disability. In 1998, it was estimated that the total annual economic burden of MS in the United States exceeded $6.8 billion.

However, even if the prognosis for disability is grave for the average patient, the prognosis in an individual is difficult to establish. Certain clinical features suggest a more favorable prognosis. Patients with ON or sensory symptoms at onset, patients who recover completely from early attacks, patients <40 years at onset (but not beginning in childhood), women, patients with RRMS, patients with fewer than two relapses in the first year of illness, and patients with minimal impairment after 5 years do better than patients without these clinical features. By contrast, patients with truncal ataxia, action tremor, pyramidal symptoms, or a progressive disease course are more likely to become disabled. A purely progressive disease course carries a graver outlook at all disease stages than does a disease course accompanied by occasional relapses.

Importantly, some MS patients have a benign variant of MS and never develop neurologic disability. The likelihood of having benign MS is thought to be $<20\%$, although it may be underestimated by existing natural history studies. One recent study of patients with benign MS 15 years after onset reported that, although most patients had developed disability by 25 years, those patients with entirely normal neurologic examinations maintained their benign course.

In patients with their first demyelinating event (i.e., a clinically isolated syndrome), the brain MRI provides prognostic information. With three or more typical T2-weighted lesions, the risk of developing MS after 10 years is 70 to 80%. Conversely, with a normal brain MRI, the likelihood of developing MS is <20%. Similarly, two or more Gd-enhancing lesions at baseline is highly predictive of future MS, as is the appearance of either new T2-weighted lesions or new Gd enhancement ≥3 months after the episode. Typical abnormalities on EP testing and CSF examination provide similar prognostic information, although these relationships are not as well characterized.

Mortality as a direct consequence of MS is uncommon, although it has been estimated that the 25-year survival is only 85% of expected. Death can occur during an acute MS attack, although this is distinctly rare. More commonly, death occurs as a complication of MS (e.g., pneumonia in a debilitated individual). Death also results from suicide.

Effect of Pregnancy

Pregnant MS patients experience fewer attacks than expected during gestation (especially in the last trimester) but more attacks than expected in the first 3 months postpartum. When considering the pregnancy year as a whole (i.e., 9 months pregnancy plus 3 months postpartum), the overall disease course is unaffected. Decisions about childbearing should thus be made based upon (1) the mother's physical state, (2) her ability to care for the child, and (3) the availability of social support. Disease-modifying therapy is generally discontinued during pregnancy, although the actual risk from the interferons and glatiramer acetate (see below) appears to be quite low.

TREATMENT FOR MS

Current therapy for MS can be divided into several categories: (1) treatment of acute attacks as they occur (2) treatment with disease-modifying agents that reduce the biological activity of MS, and (3) symptomatic therapy. Treatments that promote remyelination or neural repair do not currently exist but would be highly desirable.

The Kurtzke Expanded Disability Status Score (EDSS) is a measure of neurologic impairment in MS (**Table 28-4**). The EDSS provides a useful snapshot of the disease status of a patient at a given time and a composite picture of the disease course over time. Most patients with EDSS scores <3.5 have RRMS, walk normally, and are not disabled; by contrast, patients with EDSS scores >5.5 have progressive MS (SPMS or PPMS) and are gait-impaired and occupationally disabled.

TABLE 28-4

SCORING SYSTEM FOR MS

Kurtzke Expanded Disability Status Score (EDSS)

0.0 = Normal neurologic exam [all grade 0 in functional status (FS)]	6.0 = Unilateral assistance required to walk about 100 m with or without resting
1.0 = No disability, minimal signs in one FS (i.e., grade 1)	6.5 = Constant bilateral assistance required to walk about 20 m without resting
1.5 = No disability, minimal signs in more than one FS (more than one grade 1)	7.0 = Unable to walk beyond about 5 m even with aid; essentially restricted to wheelchair; wheels self and transfers alone
2.0 = Minimal disability in one FS (one FS grade 2, others 0 or 1)	7.5 = Unable to take more than a few steps; restricted to wheelchair; may need aid to transfer
2.5 = Minimal disability in two FS (two FS grade 2, other 0 or 1)	8.0 = Essentially restricted to bed or chair or perambulated in wheelchair, but out of bed most of day; retains many self-care functions; generally has effective use of arms
3.0 = Moderate disability in one FS (one FS grade 3, others 0 or 1) or mild disability in three or four FS (three/four FS grade 2, others 0 or 1) though fully ambulatory	8.5 = Essentially restricted to bed much of the day; has some effective use of arm(s); retains some self-care functions
3.5 = Fully ambulatory but with moderate disability in one FS (one grade 3) and one or two FS grade 2; or two FS grade 3; or five FS grade 2 (others 0 or 1)	9.0 = Helpless bed patient; can communicate and eat
4.0 = Ambulatory without aid or rest for ≥500 m	9.5 = Totally helpless bed patient; unable to communicate or eat
4.5 = Ambulatory without aid or rest for ≥300 m	10.0 = Death due to MS
5.0 = Ambulatory without aid or rest for ≥200 m	
5.5 = Ambulatory without aid or rest for ≥100 m	

TABLE 28-4 *(Continued)*

SCORING SYSTEM FOR MS

Functional Status (FS) Score

A. Pyramidal functions
    0 = Normal
    1 = Abnormal signs without disability
    2 = Minimal disability
    3 = Mild or moderate paraparesis or hemiparesis, or severe monoparesis
    4 = Marked paraparesis or hemiparesis, moderate quadriparesis, or monoplegia
    5 = Paraplegia, hemiplegia, or marked quadriparesis
    6 = Quadriplegia
B. Cerebellar functions
    0 = Normal
    1 = Abnormal signs without disability
    2 = Mild ataxia
    3 = Moderate truncal or limb ataxia
    4 = Severe ataxia all limbs
    5 = Unable to perform coordinated movements due to ataxia
C. Brainstem functions
    0 = Normal
    1 = Signs only
    2 = Moderate nystagmus or other mild disability
    3 = Severe nystagmus, marked extraocular weakness, or moderate disability of other cranial nerves
    4 = Marked dysarthria or other marked disability
    5 = Inability to swallow or speak
D. Sensory functions
    0 = Normal
    1 = Vibration or figure-writing decrease only, in 1 or 2 limbs
    2 = Mild decrease in touch or pain or position sense, and/or moderate decrease in vibration in 1 or 2 limbs, or vibratory decrease alone in 3 or 4 limbs
    3 = Moderate decrease in touch or pain or position sense, and/or essentially lost vibration in 1 or 2 limbs, or mild decrease in touch or pain, and/or moderate decrease in all proprioceptive tests in 3 or 4 limbs
    4 = Marked decrease in touch or pain or loss of proprioception, alone or combined, in 1 or 2 limbs

or moderate decrease in touch or pain and/or severe proprioceptive decrease in more than 2 limbs
    5 = Loss (essentially) of sensation in 1 or 2 limbs or moderate decrease in touch or pain and/or loss of proprioception for most of the body below the head
    6 = Sensation essentially lost below the head
E. Bowel and bladder functions
    0 = Normal
    1 = Mild urinary hesitancy, urgency, or retention
    2 = Moderate hesitancy, urgency, retention of bowel or bladder, or rare urinary incontinence
    3 = Frequent urinary incontinence
    4 = In need of almost constant catheterization
    5 = Loss of bladder function
    6 = Loss of bowel and bladder function
F. Visual (or optic) functions
    0 = Normal
    1 = Scotoma with visual acuity (corrected) better than 20/30
    2 = Worse eye with scotoma with maximal visual acuity (corrected) of 20/30 to 20/59
    3 = Worse eye with large scotoma, or moderate decrease in fields, but with maximal visual acuity (corrected) of 20/60 to 20/99
    4 = Worse eye with marked decrease of fields and maximal acuity (corrected) of 20/100 to 20/200; grade 3 plus maximal acuity of better eye of 20/60 or less
    5 = Worse eye with maximal visual acuity (corrected) less than 20/200; grade 4 plus maximal acuity of better eye of 20/60 or less
    6 = Grade 5 plus maximal visual acuity of better eye of 20/60 or less
G. Cerebral (or mental) functions
    0 = Normal
    1 = Mood alteration only (does not affect EDSS score)
    2 = Mild decrease in mentation
    3 = Moderate decrease in mentation
    4 = Marked decrease in mentation
    5 = Chronic brain syndrome — severe or incompetent

Source: After JF Kurtzke: Rating neurologic impairment in multiple sclerosis: An expanded disability status scale (EDSS). Neurology 33:1444, 1983.

Acute Attacks or Initial Demyelinating Episodes

When patients experience an acute deterioration, it is important to consider whether this change reflects new disease activity or a "pseudoexacerbation" resulting from an increase in ambient temperature, fever, or an infection. In such instances, glucocorticoid treatment is inappropriate. Glucocorticoids are used to manage either first attacks or acute exacerbations. They provide short-term clinical benefit by reducing the severity and shortening the duration of attacks. Whether treatment provides any long-term benefit on the course of the illness is less clear. As a result, mild attacks are often not treated. Physical and occupational therapy can help with mobility and manual dexterity.

Glucocorticoid treatment is administered as intravenous methylprednisolone, 500 to 1000 mg/d for 3 to 5 days, either without a taper or followed by a course of oral prednisone beginning at a dose of 60 to 80 mg/d and gradually tapered over 2 weeks. Outpatient treatment is usually possible. If intravenous therapy is unavailable or inconvenient, oral glucocorticoids can be substituted.

Side effects of short-term glucocorticoid therapy include fluid retention, potassium loss, weight gain, gastric disturbances, acne, and emotional lability. Concurrent use of a low-salt, potassium-rich diet and avoidance of potassium-wasting diuretics is advisable. Lithium carbonate (300 mg orally bid) may help to manage emotional lability and insomnia associated with glucocorticoid therapy. Patients with a history of peptic ulcer disease may require cimetidine (400 mg bid) or ranitidine (150 mg bid).

Plasma exchange (7 exchanges: 54 mL/kg or 1.1 plasma volumes per exchange, every other day for 14 days) may benefit patients with fulminant attacks of demyelination (not only MS) that are unresponsive to glucocorticoids. However, because the cost is high, and the evidence of efficacy is preliminary, plasma exchange should be considered only in selected cases.

Disease-Modifying Therapies for Relapsing Forms of MS (RRMS SPMS with Exacerbations)

Four such agents are approved in the United States: (1) interferon (IFN)-β1a (Avonex), (2) IFN-β1a (Rebif); (3) IFN-β1b (Betaseron); and (4) glatiramer acetate (Copaxone). Each of these treatments is also used in SPMS patients who still experience attacks, because SPMS can be difficult to distinguish from RRMS and the clinical trials suggest that such patients also derive therapeutic benefit. In phase III clinical trials, recipients of IFN-β1b, IFN-β1a, and glatiramer acetate experienced ~30% fewer clinical exacerbations and fewer new MRI lesions compared to placebo recipients. Mitoxantrone (Novantrone), an immune suppressant, has also been approved in the United States, although, because of its potential toxicity, it is generally reserved for patients with progressive disability who have failed other treatments.

INTERFERON β AND GLATIRAMER ACETATE

IFN-β is a class I interferon originally identified by its antiviral properties. Efficacy in MS, however, probably results from immunomodulatory properties including: (1) downregulating expression of MHC molecules on antigen-presenting cells; (2) inhibiting proinflammatory and increasing regulatory cytokine levels; (3) inhibition of T cell proliferation; and (4) limiting the trafficking of inflammatory cells in the CNS. Glatiramer acetate is a synthetic, random polypeptide composed of four amino acids (L-glutamic acid, L-lysine, L-alanine, and L-tyrosine). Its mechanism of action may include: (1) induction of antigen-specific suppressor T cells; (2) binding to MHC molecules, thereby displacing bound MBP; or (3) altering the balance between proinflammatory and regulatory cytokines.

IFN-β reduces the attack rate (whether measured clinically or by MRI) in MS patients. It also improves disease severity measures such as EDSS progression and MRI-documented disease burden. The efficacy of IFN-β in SPMS patients is less convincing than the efficacy in RRMS patients. IFN-β should be considered in patients with either RRMS or SPMS with superimposed relapses. In patients with SPMS but without relapses, efficacy has not been established. Higher IFN-β doses appear to have slightly greater efficacy but are also more likely to induce neutralizing antibodies, which may reduce the clinical benefit (see below).

Glatiramer acetate also reduces the attack rate (whether measured clinically or by MRI) in RRMS. Glatiramer acetate may also benefit disease severity measures, although this is less well established than for the relapse rate. Therefore, glatiramer acetate should be considered in RRMS patients. However, its usefulness in progressive disease is entirely unknown.

The long-term efficacy of these treatments remains largely unknown. For the interferons, clear-cut beneficial effects in reducing the relapse rate and, more substantially, in reducing CNS inflammation inferred by MRI have not been matched by similar success in treating patients with progressive symptoms (see below). This discordance has led to a reconsideration of the MS disease process as having two separate phases: inflammatory and neurodegenerative. In this model, the former leads to attacks and the latter to progression. It is likely that a gradual loss of axons underlies progressive MS symptoms, and this process could hypothetically result from loss of trophic influences provided by intact myelin. If true, then an MS attack early in the course might lead to a progressive symptom many years later. Because of this possibility, many experts currently believe that very early treatment with a disease-modifying drug is appropriate for most MS patients. It is reasonable to delay initiating treatment in patients with (1) normal neurologic examinations; (2) a single attack or a low attack frequency; and (3) a low burden of disease as assessed by brain MRI. Untreated patients need to be followed closely with periodic brain MRI scans; the need for therapy is reassessed if the scans reveal evidence of ongoing, subclinical disease.

Most treated patients with relapsing forms of MS receive IFN-β as first-line therapy. Regardless of which agent is chosen first, treatment should probably be altered in patents who continue to

have frequent attacks or progressive disability (**Fig. 28-4**). The value of combination therapy is unknown.

IFN-β1a (Avonex), 30 μg, is administered by intramuscular injection once every week. IFN-β1a (Rebif), 44 μg, is administered by subcutaneous injection three times per week. IFN-β1b (Betaseron), 250 μg, is administered by subcutaneous injection every other day. Glatiramer acetate, 20 mg, is administered by subcutaneous injection every day. Common side effects of IFN-β therapy include flulike symptoms (e.g., fevers, chills, and myalgias) and mild abnormalities on routine laboratory evaluation (e.g., elevated liver function tests or lymphopenia). Rarely, more severe hepatotoxicity may occur. Subcutaneous IFN-β also causes reactions at the injection site (e.g., pain, redness, induration, or, rarely, skin

Algorithm for MS Therapy

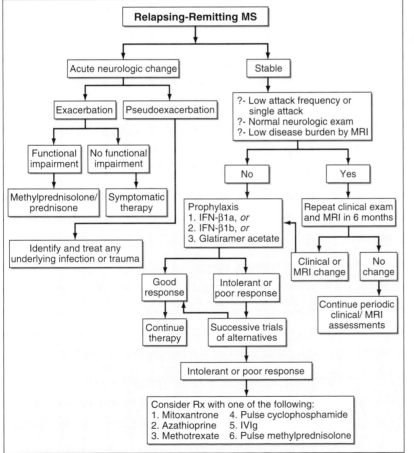

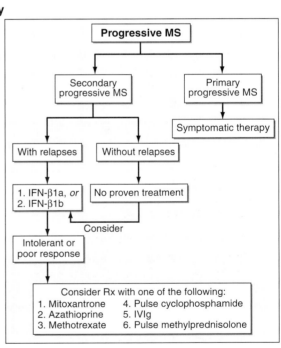

A

B

FIGURE 28-4

Therapeutic decision making for MS.

necrosis). Side effects can usually be managed with concomitant nonsteroidal anti-inflammatory medications and with the use of an auto-injector. Depression, increased spasticity, and cognitive changes have been reported, although these symptoms can also be due to the underlying disease. In any event, side effects to IFN-β therapy usually subside with time.

Approximately 2 to 10% of IFN-β1a (Avonex) recipients, 15 to 25% of IFN-β1a (Rebif) recipients, and 30 to 40% of IFN-β1b (Betaseron) recipients develop neutralizing antibodies to IFN-β, which may disappear over time. Some evidence suggests that neutralizing antibodies reduce efficacy, especially for MRI outcomes. The current clinical data, however, are quite conflicting. Moreover, there are few situations where measurement of antibodies is necessary. Thus, for a patient doing well on therapy, the presence of antibodies should not matter. Conversely, for a patient doing poorly on therapy, alternative treatment should be considered, even if there are no detectable antibodies.

Injection site reactions also occur with glatiramer acetate but are less severe than with IFN-β1b. Approximately 15% of patients experience one or more episodes of flushing, chest tightness, dyspnea, palpitations, and anxiety after injection. This systemic reaction is unpredictable, brief (duration <1 h), and tends not to recur.

MITOXANTRONE HYDROCHLORIDE

Mitoxantrone (Novantrone), an anthracenedione, exerts its antineoplastic action by (1) intercalating into DNA and producing both strand breaks and interstrand cross-links, (2) interfering with RNA synthesis and, (3) inhibiting topoisomerase II (involved in DNA repair). The U.S. Food and Drug Administration (FDA) approved mitoxantrone on the basis of a single (relatively small) phase III clinical trial in Europe, in addition to an even smaller phase II study completed earlier. Mitoxantrone received (from the FDA) the broadest indication of any current treatment for MS. Thus, mitoxantrone is indicated for use in SPMS, in PRMS, and in patients with worsening RRMS (defined as patients whose neurologic status remains significantly abnormal between MS attacks). Despite this broad indication, however, the data supporting its efficacy are weaker than for other approved therapies.

Mitoxantrone can produce cardiac problems (e.g., cardiomyopathy, reduced left ventricular ejection fraction, and irreversible congestive heart failure). As a result, a cumulative dose >140 mg/m^2 is not recommended. At currently approved doses (12 mg/m^2 every 3 months), the maximum duration of therapy can be only 2 to 3 years. Furthermore, >40% of women will experience amenorrhea, which may be permanent. Finally, there is risk of acute leukemia, and this complication has already been reported in several mitoxantrone-treated MS patients.

Given these risks, mitoxantrone should not be used as a first-line agent in either RRMS or relapsing SPMS. It is reasonable to consider mitoxantrone in selected patients with a progressive course who have failed other approved therapies.

NATALIZUMAB

This therapy is a humanized monoclonal antibody that binds to α_4-integrin on lymphocytes, inhibiting the attachment of T cells to endothelial cells and their migration across the BBB. Natalizumab was approved by the FDA in November 2004, based upon 1-year data from ongoing clinical studies suggesting that natalizumab was approximately twice as effective as other disease-modifying therapies in preventing MS attacks. It is administered by infusion every 4 weeks. Hypersensitivity reactions, which may be severe, occur in ~1% of recipients, and ~6% of recipients develop neutralizing antibodies that may reduce the efficacy of this therapy. Unfortunately, natalizumab was temporarily withdrawn from the market in March, 2005, after two MS patients treated with natalizumab and IFN-1a in combination (and a third patient with Crohn's disease treated with natalizumab and other chemotherapeutic drugs) developed the viral infection progressive multifocal leukoencephalopathy.

Disease-Modifying Therapies for SPMS without Relapses

High-dose IFN-β probably has a beneficial effect in patients with SPMS who are still experiencing acute relapses. IFN-β is probably ineffective in patients with SPMS who are not having acute attacks.

Although mitoxantrone has been approved for patients with progressive MS, this is not the population studied in the pivotal trial. Therefore no evidence-based recommendation can be made with regard to its use in this setting.

PPMS

No currently available therapies have shown any promise for treating PPMS at this time. A phase III clinical trial of glatiramer acetate in PPMS was recently stopped because of an apparent lack of efficacy. A trial of mitoxantrone in PPMS is in progress.

Off-Label Treatment Options for RRMS and SPMS

Azathioprine (2 to 3 mg/kg body weight) has been used primarily in SPMS. Meta-analysis of published trials suggests that azathioprine is marginally effective at lowering relapse rates, although a benefit on disability progression has not been demonstrated.

Methotrexate (7.5 to 20 mg/wk) was shown in one study to slow the progression of upper extremity dysfunction in SPMS. Because of the possibility of developing irreversible liver damage, some experts recommend a blind liver biopsy after 2 years of therapy.

Cyclophosphamide (700 mg/m^2, every other month) may be helpful for treatment-refractory patients who are (1) otherwise in good health, (2) ambulatory, and (3) <40 years of age. Because cyclophosphamide can be used for periods in excess of 3 years, it may be preferable to mitoxantrone in these circumstances.

Intravenous immunoglobulin (IVIg), administered in monthly pulses (up to 1 g/kg) for up to 2 years, appears to reduce annual exacerbation rates. However, its use is limited because of its high cost, questions about optimal dose, and uncertainty about its effect on long-term disability outcome.

Methylprednisolone, administered in one study as monthly high-dose intravenous pulses, reduced disability progression (see above).

Other Therapeutic Claims

Many purported treatments for MS have never been subjected to scientific scrutiny. These include dietary therapies (e.g., the Swank diet in addition to others), megadose vitamins, calcium orotate, bee stings, cow colostrum, hyperbaric oxygen, procarin (a combination of histamine and caffeine), chelation, acupuncture, acupressure, various Chinese herbal remedies, and removal of mercury amalgam tooth fillings, among many others. Patients should avoid costly or potentially hazardous unproven treatments. Many such treatments lack biologic plausibility. For example, no reliable case of mercury poisoning resembling typical MS has ever been described.

Although potential roles for human herpes virus 6 and/or chlamydia have been suggested for MS, these reports are unconfirmed, and treatment with antiviral agents or antibiotics is not currently appropriate.

Symptomatic Therapy

Potassium channel blockers (e.g., 4-aminopyridine, 10 to 40 mg/d; and 3,4-di-aminopyridine, 40 to 80 mg/d) may be helpful for *weakness,* especially for heat-sensitive symptoms. At high doses they may cause seizures. These agents are not FDA-approved but can be obtained from compounding pharmacies around the United States.

Ataxia/tremor is often intractable. Clonazepam, 1.5 to 20 mg/d; mysoline, 50 to 250 mg/d; propranalol, 40 to 200 mg/d; or ondansetron, 8 to 16 mg/d may help. Wrist-weights occasionally reduce tremor in the arm or hand. Thalamotomy or deep brain stimulation has been tried with mixed success.

Spasticity and *spasms* may improve with physical therapy, regular exercise, and stretching. Avoidance of triggers (e.g., infections, fecal impactions, bed sores) is extremely important. Effective medications include lioresal (20 to 120 mg/d), diazepam (2 to 40 mg/d), tizanidine (8 to 32 mg/d), dantroline (25 to 400 mg/d), and cyclobenzaprine hydrochloride (10 to 60 mg/d). For severe spasticity, a lioresal pump (delivering medication directly into the CSF) can provide substantial relief.

Pain is treated with anticonvulsants (carbamazepine, 100 to 1000 mg/d; phenytoin, 300 to 600 mg/d; or gabapentin, 300 to 3600 mg/d), antidepressants (amitriptyline, 25 to 150 mg/d; nortryptiline, 25 to 150 mg/d; desipramine, 100 to 300 mg/d; or venlafaxine, 75 to 225 mg/d), or antiarrhythmics (mexiletine, 300 to 900 mg/d). If these approaches fail, patients should be referred to a comprehensive pain management program.

Bladder dysfunction management is best guided by urodynamic testing. Evening fluid restriction or frequent voluntary voiding may help *detrusor hyperreflexia.* If these methods fail, propantheline bromide (10 to 15 mg/d), oxybutinin (5 to 15 mg/d), hycosamine sulfate (0.5 to 0.75 mg/d), or tolteridine tartrate (2 to 4 mg/d) may help. Coadministration of pseudoephedrine (30 to 60 mg) is sometimes beneficial.

Detrusor/sphyncter dyssynergia may respond to phenoxybenzamine (10 to 20 mg/d) or terazosin hydrochloride (1 to 20 mg/d). Loss of reflex bladder wall contraction may respond to bethanecol (30 to 150 mg/d). However, both conditions often require catheterization.

Urinary tract infections should be treated promptly. Patients with large postvoid residual urine volumes are predisposed to infections. Prevention by urine acidification (with cranberry juice or vitamin C) inhibits some bacteria. Prophylactic administration of antibiotics is sometimes necessary but may lead to colonization by resistant organisms. Intermittent catheterization may help to prevent recurrent infections.

Treatment of *constipation* includes high-fiber diets and fluids. Natural or other laxatives may help. *Fecal incontinence* may respond to a reduction in dietary fiber.

Depression should be treated. Useful drugs include the selective serotonin reuptake inhibitors (fluoxitine, 20 to 80 mg/d, or sertraline, 50 to 200 mg/d); the tricyclic antidepressants (amitriptyline, 25 to 150 mg/d, nortryptiline, 25 to 150 mg/d, or desipramine, 100 to 300 mg/d); and the non-tricyclic antidepressants (venlafaxine, 75 to 225 mg/d).

Fatigue may improve with assistive devices, help in the home, or successful management of spasticity. Patients with frequent nocturia may benefit from anticholinergic medication at bedtime. Primary MS fatigue may respond to amantadine (200 mg/d), pemoline (37.5 to 75 mg/d), methylphenidate (5 to 25 mg/d), or modafinil (100 to 400 mg/d).

Cognitive problems may respond to the cholinesterase inhibitor donepezil hydrochloride (10 mg/d).

Paroxysmal symptoms respond dramatically to low-dose anticonvulsants (acetazolamide, 200 to 600 mg/d; carbamazepine, 50 to 400 mg/d; phenytoin, 50 to 300 mg/d; or gabapentin, 600 to 1800 mg/d).

Heat sensitivity may respond to heat-avoidance, air conditioning, or cooling garments.

Sexual dysfunction may be helped by lubricants to aid in genital stimulation and sexual arousal. Management of pain, spasticity, fatigue, and bladder/bowel dysfunction may also help. Sildenafil (50 to 100 mg) taken 1 to 2 h before sex is now the standard treatment for maintaining erections.

Promising Experimental Therapies

Numerous clinical trials are currently underway. These include: (1) combination therapies; (2) higher-dose IFN-β than currently prescribed; (3) monoclonal antibodies against CD52 to induce global lymphocyte depletion, or against CD20 to deplete B cells selectively; (4) use of statins as immunomodulators; (5) estriol to induce a pregnancy-like state; (6) bone marrow transplants; and (7) Schwann cell transplants.

CLINICAL VARIANTS OF MS

Neuromyelitis optica (NMO), or Devic's syndrome, consists of separate attacks of acute ON and myelitis. ON may be unilateral or bilateral and precede or follow an attack of myelitis by days, months, or years. In contrast to MS, patients with NMO do not experience brainstem, cerebellar, and cognitive involvement, and the brain MRI is typically normal. A focal enhancing region of swelling and cavitation, extending over three or more spinal cord segments, is typically seen on MRI. Histopathology of these lesions may reveal areas of necrosis and thickening of blood vessel walls. In the serum of some patients with NMO, autoantibodies have been identified that bind to brain endothelia and recognize the aquaporin-4 water channel localized to astrocyte foot processes at the BBB. NMO, which is uncommon in Caucasians compared with Asians and Africans, is best understood as a syndrome with diverse causes. Some patients have a systemic autoimmune disorder, often systemic lupus erythematosus, Sjögren's syndrome, p-ANCA (perinuclear antineutrophil cytoplasmic antibody) associated vasculitis, or mixed connective tissue disease. In others, onset may be associated with acute infection with varicella-zoster virus or HIV. More frequently, however, NMO is idiopathic and probably represents an MS variant.

Occasional patients present with apparent NMO but have periventricular MRI changes indicating typical MS. Furthermore, in the MS disease model EAE, immunization with peptides of MOG can produce an NMO-like disorder. Disease-modifying therapies for MS have not been rigorously studied in NMO. Acute attacks are usually treated with high-dose glucocorticoids as for MS exacerbations (see above). Because of the possibility that NMO is antibody-mediated, plasma exchange has also been used empirically for acute episodes that fail to respond to glucocorticoids. Immunosuppressants or interferons are sometimes used in the hope that further relapses will be prevented.

Acute MS (Marburg's variant) is a fulminant demyelinating process that progresses to death within 1 to 2 years. Typically, there are no remissions. Diagnosis is established by biopsy or at autopsy, revealing widespread demyelination, axonal loss, edema, and macrophage infiltration. Discrete plaques may also be seen. Recent evidence strongly supports an antibody-mediated process in the demyelinating lesions. Marburg's variant does not seem to follow infection or vaccination, and it is unclear whether this syndrome represents an extreme form of MS or another disease altogether. No controlled trials of therapy exist; high-dose glucocorticoids, plasma exchange, and cyclophosphamide have been tried, with uncertain benefit.

ACUTE DISSEMINATED ENCEPHALOMYELITIS (ADEM)

ADEM has a monophasic course and is frequently associated with antecedent immunization (postvaccinal encephalomyelitis) or infection (postinfectious encephalomyelitis). The hallmark of ADEM is the presence of widely scattered small foci of perivenular inflammation and demyelination. In its most explosive form, acute hemorrhagic leukoencephalitis of Weston Hurst, the lesions are vasculitic and hemorrhagic, and the clinical course is devastating.

Postvaccinal encephalomyelitis may follow the administration of smallpox and certain rabies vaccines. Postinfectious encephalomyelitis is most frequently associated with the viral exanthems of childhood. Infection with measles virus is the most common antecedent (1 in 1000 cases). Worldwide, measles encephalomyelitis is still common, although use of the live measles vaccine has dramatically reduced its incidence in developed countries. An ADEM-like illness rarely follows vaccination with live measles vaccine (1 to 2 in 10^6 immunizations). ADEM is now most frequently associated with varicella (chickenpox) infections (1 in 4000 to 10,000 cases). It may also follow infection with rubella, mumps, influenza, parainfluenza, and infectious mononucleosis viruses and with *Mycoplasma*. Some patients may have a nonspecific upper respiratory infection or no known antecedent illness.

An autoimmune response to MBP can be detected in the CSF from many patients with ADEM. This response has been most clearly established after rabies vaccination and infection with measles virus. With measles infection, the induction of immune responses to a variety of CNS antigens may occur, but only the response to MBP correlates with the development of ADEM. Many cases of postvaccinal encephalomyelitis may result from sensitization with brain material that contaminates the viral vaccines. Attempts to demonstrate direct viral invasion of the CNS have been unsuccessful.

CLINICAL MANIFESTATIONS

In severe cases, onset is abrupt, and progression rapid (hours to days). In postinfectious ADEM, the neurologic syndrome generally begins late in the course of the viral illness as the exanthem is fading. Fever reappears, and headache, meningismus, and lethargy progressing to coma may develop. Seizures are common. Signs of disseminated neurologic disease are consistently present (e.g., hemiparesis or quadriparesis, extensor plantar responses, lost or hyperactive tendon reflexes, sensory loss and brainstem involvement). In ADEM due to chickenpox, cerebellar involvement is often conspicuous. CSF protein is modestly elevated [0.5 to 1.5 g/L (50 to 150 mg/dL)]. Lymphocytic pleocytosis, generally 200 cells/μL, occurs in 80% of patients. Occasional patients have higher counts or a mixed polymorphonuclear-lymphocytic pattern during the initial days of the illness. Transient CSF oligoclonal banding has been reported. MRI may reveal extensive gadolinium enhancement of white matter in brain and spinal cord.

DIAGNOSIS

The diagnosis is easily established when there is a history of recent vaccination or exanthematous illness. In severe cases with predominantly cerebral involvement, acute encephalitis due to infection with herpes simplex or other viruses may be difficult to exclude. The simultaneous onset of disseminated symptoms and signs is common in ADEM and rare in MS. Similarly, meningismus, drowsiness or coma, or seizures suggest ADEM rather than MS. Unlike in MS, in ADEM optic nerve involvement is generally bilateral and transverse myelopathy complete. MRI findings that may support a diagnosis of ADEM include extensive and relatively symmetric white matter abnormalities and Gd enhancement of all abnormal areas, indicating active disease and a monophasic course.

TREATMENT FOR ADEM

Initial treatment is with high-dose glucocorticoids as for exacerbations of MS (see above). Patients who fail to respond may benefit from a course of plasma exchange or intravenous immunoglobulin. The prognosis reflects the severity of the underlying acute illness. Measles encephalomyelitis is associated with a mortality rate of 5 to 20%, and most survivors have permanent neurologic sequelae. Children who recover may have persistent seizures and behavioral and learning disorders.

FURTHER READINGS

GOODIN DS et al: Disease modifying therapies in multiple sclerosis: Report of the Therapeutics and Technology Assessment Subcommittee of the American Academy of Neurology. Neurology 58:169, 2002

■ LENNON VA et al: IgG marker of optic-spinal multiple sclerosis binds to the aquaporin-4 water channel. J Exp Med 202:473, 2005

Antibodies to vascular endothelium may be useful as a serologic test for opticospinal variants of MS and Devic's disease.

MILLER D et al: Clinically isolated syndromes suggestive of multiple sclerosis, Part 1: Natural history, pathogenesis, diagnosis and prognosis. Lancet Neurol 4:281, 2005

———— et al: Clinically isolated syndromes suggestive of multiple sclerosis, Part 2: Non-conventional MRI, recovery processes, and management. Lancet Neurol 4:341, 2005

O'CONNOR KC et al: Antibodies from inflamed central nervous system tissue recognize myelin oligodendrocyte glycoprotein. J Immunol 175:1974, 2005

OKSENBERG J et al: Mapping multiple sclerosis susceptibility to the HLA-DR locus in African Americans. Am J Hum Genet 74:160, 2004

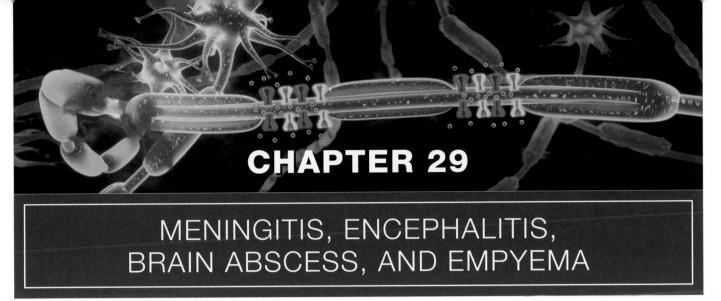

CHAPTER 29

MENINGITIS, ENCEPHALITIS, BRAIN ABSCESS, AND EMPYEMA

Karen L. Roos

Kenneth L. Tyler

Acute infections of the nervous system are among the most important problems in medicine because early recognition, efficient decision-making, and rapid institution of therapy can be lifesaving. These distinct clinical syndromes include acute bacterial meningitis, viral meningitis, encephalitis, focal infections such as brain abscess and subdural empyema, and infectious thrombophlebitis. Each may present with a nonspecific prodrome of fever and headache, which in a previously healthy individual may initially be thought to be benign, until (with the exception of viral meningitis) altered consciousness, focal neurologic signs, or seizures appear. Key goals of early management are to emergently distinguish between these conditions, identify the responsible pathogen, and initiate appropriate antimicrobial therapy.

APPROACH TO THE PATIENT WITH INFECTION OF THE NERVOUS SYSTEM

(**Fig. 29-1**) The first task is to identify whether an infection predominantly involves the subarachnoid space ("meningitis") or whether there is evidence of either generalized or focal involvement of brain tissue in the cerebral hemispheres, cerebellum, or brainstem. When brain tissue is directly injured by a viral infection the disease is referred to as "en-

cephalitis," whereas focal bacterial, fungal, or parasitic infections involving brain tissue are classified as either "cerebritis" or "abscess," depending on the presence or absence of a capsule.

Nuchal rigidity is the pathognomonic sign of meningeal irritation and is present when the neck resists passive flexion. Kernig's and Brudzinski's signs are also classic signs of meningeal irritation. *Kernig's sign* is elicited with the patient in the supine position.

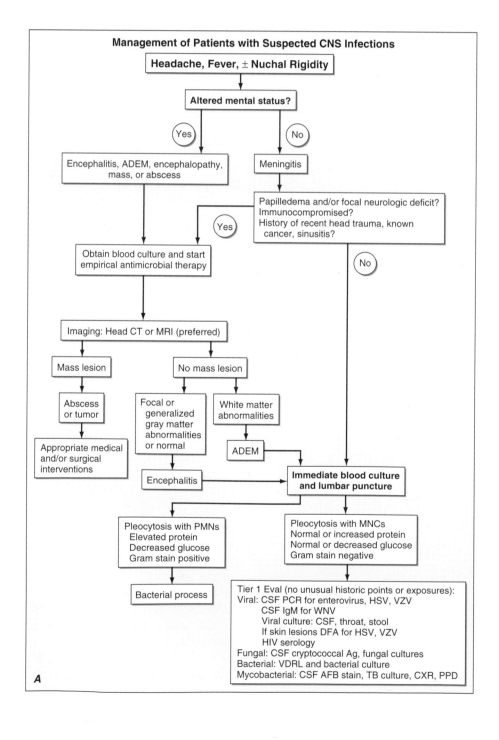

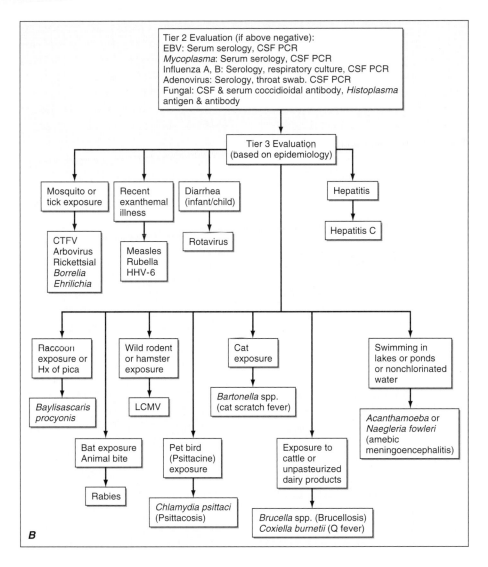

FIGURE 29-1

Algorithm for management of patients with suspected CNS infections. ADEM, acute disseminated encephalomyelitis; CT, computed tomography; MRI, magnetic resonance imaging; PMNs, polymorphonuclear leukocytes; MNCs, mononuclear cells; CSF, cerebrospinal fluid; PCR, polymerase chain reaction; HSV, herpes simplex virus; VZV, varicella-zoster virus; WNV, West Nile Virus; DFA, direct fluorescent antibody; Ag, antigen; VDRL, Venereal Disease Research Laboratory; AFB, acid-fast bacillus; TB, tuberculosis; CXR, chest x-ray; PPD, purified protein derivative; EBV, Epstein-Barr virus; CTFV, Colorado tick fever virus; HHV, human herpesvirus; LCMV, lymphocytic choriomeningitis virus.

The thigh is flexed on the abdomen, with the knee flexed; attempts to passively extend the knee elicit pain when meningeal irritation is present. *Brudzinski's sign* is elicited with the patient in the supine position and is positive when passive flexion of the neck results in spontaneous flexion of the hips and knees. Although commonly tested on physical examinations, the sensitivity and specificity of Kernig's and Brudzinski's signs are uncertain. Both may be absent or reduced in very young or elderly patients, immunocompromised individuals, or patients with a severely depressed mental status. The high prevalence of cervical spine disease in older individuals may result in false-positive tests for nuchal rigidity.

Initial management can be guided by several considerations:

1. Empirical therapy should be initiated promptly whenever bacterial meningitis is a significant diagnostic consideration.

2. All patients who have had recent head trauma, are immunocompromised, have known malignant lesions or central nervous system (CNS) neoplasms, or have focal neurologic findings including papilledema or a depressed level of consciousness should undergo computed tomography (CT) or magnetic resonance imaging (MRI) of the brain prior to lumbar puncture (LP). In these cases empirical antibiotic therapy should not be delayed pending test results but should be administered prior to neuroimaging and LP.

3. A significantly depressed mental status (e.g., somnolence, coma), seizures, or focal neurologic deficits only rarely occur in viral ("aseptic") meningitis; patients with these symptoms should be hospitalized for further evaluation and treated empirically for bacterial and viral meningoencephalitis.

4. Immunocompetent patients with a normal level of consciousness, no prior antimicrobial treatment, and a cerebrospinal fluid (CSF) profile consistent with viral meningitis (lymphocytic pleocytosis and a normal glucose concentration) can often be treated as outpatients, if appropriate contact and monitoring can be ensured. Failure of a patient with suspected viral meningitis to improve within 48 h should prompt a reevaluation including follow-up neurologic and general medical examination and repeat imaging and laboratory studies, often including a second LP.

ACUTE BACTERIAL MENINGITIS

DEFINITION

Bacterial meningitis is an acute purulent infection within the subarachnoid space. It is associated with a CNS inflammatory reaction that may result in decreased consciousness, seizures, raised intracranial pressure (ICP), and stroke. The meninges, the subarachnoid space (SAS), and the brain parenchyma are all frequently involved in the inflammatory reaction (*meningoencephalitis*).

EPIDEMIOLOGY

Bacterial meningitis is the most common form of suppurative CNS infection, with an annual incidence in the United States of >2.5 cases/100,000 population. The epidemiology of bacterial meningitis has changed significantly in recent years, reflecting a dramatic decline in the incidence of meningitis due to *Haemophilus influenzae*, and a smaller decline in that due to *Neisseria meningitidis*, following the introduction and increasingly widespread use of vaccines for both these organisms. Currently, the organisms most commonly responsible for community-acquired bacterial meningitis are *Streptococcus pneumoniae* (~50%), *N. meningitidis* (~25%), group B streptococci (~15%), and *Listeria monocytogenes* (~10%). *H. influenzae* now accounts for <10% of cases of bacterial meningitis in most series.

ETIOLOGY

S. pneumoniae is the most common cause of meningitis in adults >20 years of age, accounting for nearly half the reported cases (1.1 per 100,000 persons per year). There are a number of predisposing conditions that increase the risk of pneumococcal meningitis, the most important of which is pneumococcal pneumonia. Additional risk factors include coexisting acute or chronic pneumococcal sinusitis or otitis media, alcoholism, diabetes, splenectomy, hypogammaglobulinemia, complement deficiency, and head trauma with basilar skull fracture and CSF rhinorrhea. Mortality remains ~20% despite antibiotic therapy.

N. meningitidis accounts for 25% of all cases of bacterial meningitis (0.6 cases per 100,000 persons per year) and for up to 60% of cases in children and young adults between the ages of 2 and 20. The presence of petechial or purpuric skin lesions can provide an important clue to the diagnosis of meningococcal infection. In some patients the disease is fulminant, progressing to death within hours of symptom onset. Infection may be initiated by nasopharyngeal colonization, which can result in either an asymptomatic carrier state or invasive meningococcal disease. The risk of invasive disease following nasopharyngeal colonization depends on both bacterial virulence factors and host immune defense mechanisms, including the host's capacity to produce antimeningococcal antibodies and to lyse meningococci by both the classic and alternative complement pathways. Individuals with deficiencies of any of the complement components, including properdin, are highly susceptible to meningococcal infections.

Enteric gram-negative bacilli are an increasingly common cause of meningitis in individuals with chronic and debilitating diseases such as diabetes, cirrhosis, or alcoholism and in those with chronic urinary tract infections. Gram-negative meningitis can also complicate neurosurgical procedures, particularly craniotomy.

Group B streptococcus, or *S. agalactiae,* was previously responsible for meningitis predominantly in neonates, but it has been reported with increasing frequency in individuals >50 years of age, particularly those with underlying diseases.

L. monocytogenes has become an increasingly important cause of meningitis in neonates (<1 month of age), pregnant women, individuals >60 years, and immunocompromised individuals of all ages. Infection is acquired by ingesting foods contaminated by *Listeria*. Foodborne human listerial infection has been reported from contaminated coleslaw, milk, soft cheeses, and several types of "ready-to-eat" foods including delicatessen meat and uncooked hotdogs.

The frequency of *H. influenzae* type b meningitis in children has declined dramatically since the introduction of the Hib conjugate vaccine, although rare cases of Hib meningitis in vaccinated children have been reported. More frequently, *H. influenzae* causes meningitis in unvaccinated children and adults.

Staphylococcus aureus and coagulase-negative staphylococci are important causes of meningitis that follows invasive neurosurgical procedures, particularly shunting procedures for hydrocephalus, or that occurs as a complication of the use of subcutaneous Ommaya reservoirs for administration of intrathecal chemotherapy.

PATHOPHYSIOLOGY

The most common bacteria that cause meningitis, *S. pneumoniae* and *N. meningitidis,* initially colonize the nasopharynx by attaching to nasopharyngeal epithelial cells. Bacteria are transported across epithelial cells in membrane-bound vacuoles to the intravascular space or invade the intravascular space by creating separations in the apical tight junctions of columnar epithelial cells. Once in the bloodstream, bacteria are able to avoid phagocytosis by neutrophils and classic complement–mediated bactericidal activity because of the presence of a polysaccharide capsule. Bloodborne bacteria can reach the intraventricular choroid plexus, directly infect choroid plexus epithelial cells, and gain access to the CSF. Some bacteria, such as *S. pneumoniae,* can adhere to cerebral capillary endothelial cells and subsequently migrate through or between these cells to reach the CSF. Bacteria are able to multiply rapidly within CSF because of the absence of effective host immune defenses. Normal CSF contains few white blood cells (WBCs) and relatively small amounts of complement proteins and immunoglobulins. The paucity of the latter two prevents effective opsonization of bacteria, an essential prerequisite for bacterial phagocytosis by neutrophils. Phagocytosis of bacteria is further impaired by the fluid nature of CSF, which is less conducive to phagocytosis than a solid tissue substrate.

A critical event in the pathogenesis of bacterial meningitis is the inflammatory reaction induced by the invading bacteria. Many of the neurologic manifestations and complications of bacterial meningitis result from the immune response to the invading pathogen rather than from direct bacteria-induced tissue injury. As a result, neurologic injury can progress even after the CSF has been sterilized by antibiotic therapy.

During the very early stages of meningitis there is an increase in cerebral blood flow, soon followed by a decrease in cerebral blood flow and a loss of cerebrovascular autoregulation. Narrowing of the large arteries at the base of the brain due to encroachment by the purulent exudate in the subarachnoid space and infiltration of the arterial wall by inflammatory cells with intimal thickening (*vasculitis*) also occur and may result in ischemia and infarction, obstruction of branches of the middle cerebral artery by thrombosis, thrombosis of the major cerebral venous sinuses, and thrombophlebitis of the cerebral cortical veins. The combination of interstitial, vasogenic, and cytotoxic edema leads to raised ICP and coma. Cerebral herniation usually results from the effects of cerebral edema, either focal or generalized; hydrocephalus and dural sinus or cortical vein thrombosis may also play a role.

CLINICAL PRESENTATION

Meningitis can present as either an acute fulminant illness that progresses rapidly in a few hours or as a subacute infection that progressively worsens over several days. The classic clinical triad of meningitis is fever, headache, and nuchal rigidity ("stiff neck"). Each of these signs and symptoms occurs in >90% of cases. Alteration in mental status occurs in >75% of patients and can vary from lethargy to coma. Nausea, vomiting, and photophobia are also common complaints.

Seizures occur as part of the initial presentation of bacterial meningitis or during the course of the illness in 20 to 40% of patients. Focal seizures are usually due to focal arterial ischemia or infarction, cortical venous thrombosis with hemorrhage, or focal edema. Generalized seizure activity and status epilepticus may be due to hyponatremia, cerebral anoxia, or, less commonly, the toxic effects of antimicrobial agents such as high-dose penicillin.

Raised ICP is an expected complication of bacterial meningitis and is the major cause of obtundation and coma in this disease. More than 90% of patients will have a CSF opening pressure > 180 mmH$_2$O, and 20% have opening pressures > 400 mmH$_2$O. Signs of increased ICP include a deteriorating or reduced level of consciousness, papilledema, dilated poorly reactive pupils, sixth nerve palsies, decerebrate posturing, and the Cushing reflex (bradycardia, hypertension, and irregular respirations). The most disastrous complication of increased ICP is cerebral herniation. The incidence of herniation in patients with bacterial meningitis has been reported to occur in as few as 1% to as many as 8% of cases.

Specific clinical features may provide clues to the diagnosis of individual organisms and are discussed in more detail in specific chapters devoted to individual pathogens. The most important of these clues is the rash of meningococcemia, which begins as a diffuse erythematous maculopapular rash resembling a viral exanthem, but the skin lesions of meningococcemia rapidly become petechial. Petechiae are found on the trunk and lower extremities, in the mucous membranes and conjunctiva, and occasionally on the palms and soles.

DIAGNOSIS

When bacterial meningitis is suspected, blood cultures should be immediately obtained and empirical antimicrobial therapy initiated without delay. The diagnosis of bacterial meningitis is made by examination of the CSF (**Table 29-1**). The need to obtain neuroimaging studies (CT or MRI) prior to LP requires clinical judgment. In an immunocompetent patient with no known history of recent head trauma, a normal level of consciousness, and no evidence of papilledema or focal neurologic deficits, it is safe to perform LP without prior neuroimaging studies. If LP is delayed in order to obtain neuroimaging studies, empirical antibiotic therapy should be initiated after blood cultures are obtained. Antibiotic therapy initiated a few hours prior to LP will not significantly alter the CSF WBC count or glucose concentration, nor is it likely to prevent visualization of organisms by Gram's stain.

TABLE 29-1

CEREBROSPINAL FLUID (CSF) ABNORMALITIES IN BACTERIAL MENINGITIS	
Opening pressure	>180 mmH$_2$O
White blood cells	10/μL to 10,000/μL; neutrophils predominate
Red blood cells	Absent in nontraumatic tap
Glucose	<2.2 mmol/L (<40 mg/dL)
CSF/serum glucose	<0.4
Protein	>0.45 g/L (>45 mg/dL)
Gram's stain	Positive in >60%
Culture	Positive in >80%
Latex agglutination	May be positive in patients with meningitis due to *S. pneumoniae, N. meningitidis, H. influenzae* type b, *E. coli*, group B streptococci
Limulus lysates	Positive in cases of gram-negative meningitis
PCR for bacterial DNA	Research test

Note: PCR, polymerase chain reaction.

The classic CSF abnormalities in bacterial meningitis (Table 29-1) are (1) polymorphonuclear (PMN) leukocytosis (>100 cells/μL in 90%), (2) decreased glucose concentration [<2.2 mmol/L (<40 mg/dL) and/or CSF/serum glucose ratio of <0.4 in ~60%], (3) increased protein concentration [>0.45 g/L (>45 mg/dL) in 90%], and (4) increased opening pressure (>180 mmH$_2$O in 90%). CSF bacterial cultures are positive in >80% of patients, and CSF Gram's stain demonstrates organisms in >60%.

CSF glucose concentrations <2.2 mmol/L (<40 mg/dL) are abnormal, and a CSF glucose concentration of zero can be seen in bacterial meningitis. Use of the CSF/serum glucose ratio corrects for hyperglycemia that may mask a relative decrease in the CSF glucose concentration. The CSF glucose concentration is low when the CSF/serum glucose ratio is <0.6. A CSF/serum glucose ratio <0.4 is highly suggestive of bacterial meningitis but may also be seen in other conditions, including fungal, tuberculous, and carcinomatous meningitis. It takes from 30 min to several hours for CSF glucose concentration to reach equilibrium with blood glucose concentrations; therefore, administration of 50 mL of 50% glucose (D50) prior to LP, as commonly occurs in emergency room settings, is unlikely to alter CSF glucose concentration significantly unless more than a few hours have elapsed between glucose administration and LP.

The latex agglutination (LA) test for the detection of bacterial antigens of *S. pneumoniae, N. meningitidis, H. influenzae* type b, group B streptococcus, and *Escherichia coli* K1 strains in the CSF is very useful for making a rapid diagnosis of bacterial meningitis, especially in patients who have been pretreated with antibiotics and in whom CSF Gram's stain and culture are negative. The CSF LA test has a *specificity* of 95 to 100% for *S. pneumoniae* and *N. meningitidis,* so a positive test is virtually diagnostic of bacterial meningitis caused by these organisms. However, the *sensitivity* of the CSF LA test is only 70 to 100% for detection of *S. pneumoniae* and 33 to 70% for detection of *N. meningitidis* antigens, so a negative test does not exclude infection by these organisms. The Limulus amebocyte lysate assay is a rapid diagnostic test for the detection of gram-negative endotoxin in CSF, and thus for making a diagnosis of gram-negative bacterial meningitis. The test has a specificity of 85 to 100% and a sensitivity approaching 100%. Thus, a positive Limulus amebocyte lysate assay occurs in virtually all patients with gram-negative bacterial meningitis, but false-positives may occur. CSF polymerase chain reaction (PCR) tests are not as useful in the diagnosis of bacterial meningitis as they are in the diagnosis of viral CNS infections. A CSF PCR test has been developed for detecting DNA from bacteria in CSF, but its sensitivity and specificity need to be better characterized before its role in diagnosis can be defined.

Almost all patients with bacterial meningitis will have neuroimaging studies performed during the course of their illness. MRI is preferred over CT because of its superiority in demonstrating areas of cerebral edema and ischemia. In patients with bacterial meningitis, diffuse meningeal enhancement is often seen after the administration of gadolinium. Meningeal enhancement is not diagnostic of meningitis but occurs in any CNS disease associated with increased blood-brain barrier permeability.

Petechial skin lesions, if present, should be biopsied. The rash of meningococcemia results from the dermal seeding of organisms with vascular endothelial damage, and biopsy may reveal the organism on Gram's stain.

DIFFERENTIAL DIAGNOSIS

Viral meningoencephalitis, and particularly herpes simplex virus (HSV) encephalitis, can mimic the clinical presentation of bacterial meningitis (see "Encephalitis," below). HSV encephalitis typically presents with headache, fever, altered consciousness, focal neurologic deficits (e.g., dysphasia, hemiparesis), and focal or generalized seizures. The findings on CSF studies, neuroimaging, and electroencephalogram (EEG) distinguish HSV encephalitis from bacterial meningitis. The typical CSF profile with viral CNS infections is a lymphocytic pleocytosis with a normal glucose concentration, in contrast to PMN pleocytosis and hypoglycorrhachia characteristic of bacterial meningitis. MRI abnormalities (other than meningeal enhancement) are not seen in uncomplicated bacterial meningitis. By contrast, in HSV encephalitis parenchymal changes, especially in orbitofrontal and medial temporal lobes, are usually found. Some patients with HSV encephalitis have a distinctive periodic pattern on EEG (see below).

Rickettsial disease can resemble bacterial meningitis. Rocky Mountain spotted fever (RMSF) is transmitted by a tick bite and caused by the bacteria *Rickettsia rickettsii*. The disease may present acutely with high fever, prostration, myalgia, headache, and nausea and vomiting. Most patients develop a characteristic rash within 96 h of the onset of symptoms. The rash is initially a diffuse erythematous maculopapular rash that may be difficult to distinguish from that of meningococcemia. It progresses to a petechial rash, then to a purpuric rash, and, if untreated, to skin necrosis or gangrene. The color of the lesions changes from bright red to very dark red, then yellowish-green to black. The rash typically begins in the wrist and ankles, and then spreads distally and proximally within a matter of a few hours and involves the palms and soles. Diagnosis is made by immunofluorescent staining of skin biopsy specimens.

Focal suppurative CNS infections (see below), including subdural and epidural empyema and brain abscess, should also be considered, especially when focal neurologic findings are present. MRI should be performed promptly in all patients with suspected meningitis who have focal features, both to detect the intracranial infection and to search for associated areas of infection in the sinuses or mastoid bones.

A number of noninfectious CNS disorders can mimic bacterial meningitis. Subarachnoid hemorrhage (SAH; Chap. 17) is generally the major consideration. Other possibilities include chemical meningitis due to rupture of tumor contents into the CSF (e.g., from a cystic glioma, craniopharyngioma epidermoid or dermoid cyst); drug-induced hypersensitivity meningitis; carcinomatous or lymphomatous meningitis; meningitis associated with inflammatory disorders such as sarcoid, systemic lupus erythematosus (SLE), and Behçet disease; pituitary apoplexy; and uveomeningitic syndromes (Vogt-Koyanagi-Harada syndrome).

Subacutely evolving meningitis (Chap. 30) may on occasion be considered in the differential diagnosis of acute meningitis. The principal causes include *Mycobacterium tuberculosis, Cryptococcus neoformans, Histoplasma capsulatum, Coccidioides immitis,* and *Treponema pallidum.*

TREATMENT

Empirical Antimicrobial Therapy (Table 29-2)

Bacterial meningitis is a medical emergency. The goal is to begin antibiotic therapy within 60 min of a patient's arrival in the emergency room. Empirical antimicrobial therapy is initiated in patients with suspected bacterial meningitis before the results of CSF Gram's stain and culture are known. *S. pneumoniae* and *N. meningitidis* are the most common etiologic organisms of community-acquired bacterial meningitis. Due to the emergence of penicillin- and cephalosporin-resistant *S. pneumoniae,* empirical therapy of community-acquired bacterial meningitis in children and adults should include a third-generation cephalosporin (e.g., ceftriaxone or cefotaxime) and vancomycin. Ceftriaxone or cefotaxime provide good coverage for susceptible *S. pneumoniae,* group B streptococci, and *H. influenzae* and adequate coverage for *N. meningitidis.* Cefepime is a broad-spectrum fourth-generation cephalosporin with in vitro activity similar to that of cefotaxime or ceftriaxone against *S. pneumoniae* and *N. meningitidis* and greater activity against

TABLE 29-2

ANTIBIOTICS USED IN EMPIRICAL THERAPY OF BACTERIAL MENINGITIS AND FOCAL CNS INFECTIONS[a]

INDICATION	ANTIBIOTIC
Preterm infants to infants <1 month	Ampicillin + cefotaxime
Infants 1–3 mos	Ampicillin + cefotaxime or ceftriaxone
Immunocompetent children > 3 mos and adults <55	Cefotaxime or ceftriaxone + vancomycin
Adults > 55 and adults of any age with alcoholism or other debilitating illnesses	Ampicillin + cefotaxime or ceftriaxone + vancomycin
Hospital-acquired meningitis, posttraumatic or postneurosurgery meningitis, neutropenic patients, or patients with impaired cell-mediated immunity	Ampicillin + ceftazidime + vancomycln

Antimicrobial Agent	TOTAL DAILY DOSE AND DOSING INTERVAL	
	Child (>1 month)	Adult
Ampicillin	200 (mg/kg)/d, q4h	12 g/d, q4h
Cefepime	150 (mg/kg)/d, q8h	6 g/d, q8h
Cefotaxime	200 (mg/kg)/d, q6h	12 g/d, q4h
Ceftriaxone	100 (mg/kg)/d, q12h	4 g/d, q12h
Ceftazidime	150 (mg/kg)/d, q8h	6 g/d, q8h
Gentamicin	7.5 (mg/kg)/d, q8h[b]	7.5 (mg/kg)/d, q8h
Meropenem	120 (mg/kg)/d, q8h	3 g/d, q8h
Metronidazole	30 (mg/kg)/d, q6h	1500–2000 mg/d, q6h
Nafcillin	100–200 (mg/kg)/d, q6h	9–12 g/d, q4h
Penicillin G	400,000 (U/kg)/d, q4h	20–24 million U/d, q4h
Vancomycin	60 (mg/kg)/d, q6h	2 g/d, q12h[b]

[a]All antibiotics are administered intravenously; doses indicated assume normal renal and hepatic function.
[b]Doses should be adjusted based on serum peak and trough levels: gentamicin therapeutic level: peak: 5–8 μg/mL; trough:<2 μg/mL; vancomycin therapeutic level: peak: 25–40 μg/mL; trough: 5–15 μg/mL.

Enterobacter spp. and *Pseudomonas aeruginosa*. In clinical trials, cefepime has been demonstrated to be equivalent to cefotaxime in the treatment of penicillin-sensitive pneumococcal and meningococcal meningitis, but its efficacy in bacterial meningitis caused by penicillin- and cephalosporin-resistant pneumococcal organisms, *Enterobacter* spp., and *P. aeruginosa* has not been established. Ampicillin should be added to the empirical regimen for coverage of *L. monocytogenes* in individuals <3 months of age, those >55, or those with suspected impaired cell-mediated immunity because of chronic illness, organ transplantation, pregnancy, malignancies, or immunosuppressive therapy. In hospital-acquired meningitis, and particularly meningitis following neurosurgical procedures, staphylococci and gram-negative organisms including *P. aeruginosa* are the most common etiologic organisms. In these patients, empirical therapy should include a combination of vancomycin and ceftazidime. Ceftazidime should be substituted for ceftriaxone or cefotaxime in neurosurgical patients and in neutropenic patients, as ceftazidime is the only cephalosporin with adequate activity against CNS infection with *P. aeruginosa*. Meropenem is a carbapenem antibiotic that is highly active in vitro against *L. monocytogenes*, has been demonstrated to be effective in cases of meningitis caused by *P. aeruginosa*, and shows good activity against penicillin-resistant pneumococci. In experimental pneumococcal meningitis, meropenem was comparable to ceftriaxone and inferior to vancomycin in sterilizing CSF cultures. The number of patients with bacterial meningitis enrolled in clinical trials of meropenem has not been sufficient to definitively assess the efficacy of this antibiotic.

Specific Antimicrobial Therapy (Table 29-3)
MENINGOCOCCAL MENINGITIS

Although ceftriaxone and cefotaxime provide adequate empirical coverage for *N. meningitidis,* penicillin G remains the antibiotic of choice for meningococcal meningitis caused by susceptible strains. Isolates of *N. meningitidis* with moderate resistance to penicillin have been identified, but patients infected with these strains have still been successfully treated with penicillin. CSF isolates of *N. meningitidis* should be tested for penicillin and ampicillin susceptibility, and if resistance is found, cefotaxime or ceftriaxone should be substituted for penicillin. A 7-day course of intravenous antibiotic therapy is adequate for uncomplicated meningococcal meningitis. The index case and all close contacts should receive chemoprophylaxis with a 2-day regimen of rifampin (600 mg every 12 h for 2 days in adults and 10 mg/kg every 12 h for 2 days in children >1 year). Rifampin is not recommended in pregnant women. Alternatively, adults can be treated with one dose of ciprofloxacin (750 mg), one dose of azithromycin (500 mg), or one intramuscular dose of ceftriaxone (250 mg). Close contacts are defined as those individuals who have had contact with oropharyngeal secretions either through kissing or by sharing toys, beverages, or cigarettes.

PNEUMOCOCCAL MENINGITIS

Antimicrobial therapy of pneumococcal meningitis is initiated with a cephalosporin (ceftriaxone, cefotaxime, or cefepime) and vancomycin. All CSF isolates of *S. pneumoniae* should be tested for sensitivity to penicillin and the cephalosporins. Once the results of antimicrobial susceptibility tests are known, therapy can be modified accordingly (Table 29-3). For *S. pneumoniae* meningitis, an isolate of *S. pneumoniae* is considered to be susceptible to penicillin with a minimal inhibitory concentration (MIC) < 0.06 μg/mL, to have intermediate resistance when the MIC is 0.1 to 1.0 μg/mL, and to be highly resistant when the MIC > 1.0 μg/mL. Isolates of *S. pneumoniae* that have cephalosporin MICs ≤ 0.5 μg/mL are considered sensitive to the cephalosporins (cefotaxime, ceftriaxone, cefepime). Those with MICs of 1 μg/mL are considered to have intermediate resistance, and those with MICs ≥ 2 μg/mL are considered resistant. For meningitis due to pneumococci with cefotaxime or ceftriaxone MICs ≤ 0.5 μg/mL, treatment with cefotaxime or ceftriaxone is usually adequate. If the MIC > 1 μg/mL, vancomycin is the antibiotic of choice. Rifampin can be added to vancomycin for its synergistic effect but is inadequate as monotherapy because resistance develops rapidly when it is used alone.

Patients with *S. pneumoniae* meningitis should have a repeat LP performed 24 to 36 h after the initiation of antimicrobial therapy to document sterilization of the CSF. Failure to sterilize the CSF after 24 to 36 h of antibiotic therapy should be considered presumptive evidence of antibiotic resistance. Patients with penicillin- and cephalosporin-resistant strains of *S. pneumoniae* who do not respond to intravenous vancomycin alone may benefit from the addition of intraventricular vancomycin. The intraventricular route of administration is preferred over the intrathecal route because adequate concentrations of vancomycin in the cerebral ventricles are not always achieved with intrathecal administration. A 2-week course of intravenous antimicrobial therapy is recommended for pneumococcal meningitis.

L. MONOCYTOGENES MENINGITIS

Meningitis due to this organism is treated with ampicillin for at least 3 weeks (Table 29-3). Gentamicin is

TABLE 29-3

ANTIMICROBIAL THERAPY OF CNS BACTERIAL INFECTIONS BASED ON PATHOGEN[a]

ORGANISM	ANTIBIOTIC
Neisseria meningitides	
Penicillin-sensitive	Penicillin G or Ampicillin
Penicillin-resistant	Ceftriaxone or cefotaxime
Streptococcus pneumoniae	
Penicillin-sensitive	Penicillin G
Penicillin-intermediate	Ceftriaxone or cefotaxime
Penicillin-resistant	(Ceftriaxone or cefotaxime) + vancomycin
Gram-negative bacilli (except *Pseudomonas* spp.)	Ceftriaxone or cefotaxime
Pseudomonas aeruginosa	Ceftazidime
Staphylococci spp.	
Methicillin-sensitive	Nafcillin
Methicillin-resistant	Vancomycin
Listeria monocytogenes	Ampicillin + gentamicin
Haemophilus influenzae	Ceftriaxone or cefotaxime
Streptococcus agalactiae	Penicillin G or ampicillin
Bacteroides fragilis	Metronidazole
Fusobacterium spp.	Metronidazole

[a]Doses are as indicated in Table 29-2.

often added (2 mg/kg loading dose, then 5.1 mg/kg per day given every 8 h and adjusted for serum levels and renal function). The combination of trimethoprim [10 to 20 (mg/kg)/d] and sulfamethoxazole [50 to 100 (mg/kg)/d] given every 6 h may provide an alternative in penicillin-allergic patients.

STAPHYLOCOCCAL MENINGITIS

Meningitis due to susceptible strains of *S. aureus* or coagulase-negative staphylococci is treated with nafcillin (Table 29-3). Vancomycin is the drug of choice for methicillin-resistant staphylococci and for patients allergic to penicillin. In these patients, the CSF should be monitored during therapy. If the CSF is not sterilized after 48 h of intravenous vancomycin therapy, then either intrathecal or intraventricular vancomycin, 20 mg once daily, can be added.

GRAM-NEGATIVE BACILLARY MENINGITIS

The third-generation cephalosporins, cefotaxime, ceftriaxone, and ceftazidime, are equally efficacious for the treatment of gram-negative bacillary meningitis, with the exception of meningitis due to *P. aeruginosa,* which should be treated with ceftazidime (Table 29-3). A 3-week course of intravenous antibiotic therapy is recommended for meningitis due to gram-negative bacilli.

Adjunctive Therapy

The release of bacterial cell-wall components by bactericidal antibiotics leads to the production of the inflammatory cytokines interleukin (IL) 1 and tumor necrosis factor (TNF) in the subarachnoid space. Dexamethasone exerts its beneficial effect by inhibiting the synthesis of IL-1 and TNF at the level of mRNA, decreasing CSF outflow resistance, and stabilizing the blood-brain barrier. The rationale for giving dexamethasone 20 min before antibiotic therapy is that dexamethasone inhibits the production of TNF by macrophages and microglia only if it is administered before these cells are activated by endotoxin. Dexamethasone does not alter TNF production once it has been induced. The results of clinical trials of dexamethasone therapy in children, predominantly with meningitis due to *H. influenzae* and *S. pneumoniae,* have demonstrated its efficacy in decreasing meningeal inflammation and neurologic sequelae such as the incidence of sensorineural hearing loss.

A prospective European trial of adjunctive therapy for acute bacterial meningitis in 301 adults found that dexamethasone reduced the number of unfavorable outcomes (15% vs. 25%, $p = .03$) including death (7% vs. 15%, $p = .04$). The benefits were most striking in patients with pneumococcal meningitis. Dexamethasone (10 mg intravenously) was administered 15 to 20 min before the first dose of an antimicrobial agent, and the same dose was repeated every 6 h for 4 days. These results were confirmed in a second trial of dexamethasone in adults with pneumococcal meningitis. Therapy with dexamethasone should ideally be started 20 min before, or not later than concurrent with, the first dose of antibiotics. It is unlikely to be of significant benefit if started >6 h after antimicrobial therapy has been initiated. Dexamethasone may decrease the penetration of vancomycin into CSF, and it delays the sterilization of CSF in experimental models of *S. pneumoniae* meningitis. As a result, its potential benefit should be carefully weighed when vancomycin is the antibiotic of choice. Alternatively, vancomycin can be administered by the intraventricular route.

Increased Intracranial Pressure

Emergency treatment of increased ICP includes elevation of the patient's head to 30 to 45°, intubation and hyperventilation (Pa_{CO_2} 25 to 30 mmHg), and mannitol. Patients with increased ICP should be managed in an intensive care unit; accurate ICP measurements are best obtained with an ICP monitoring device. Treatment of increased intracranial pressure is discussed in detail in Chap. 15.

PROGNOSIS

Mortality is 3 to 7% for meningitis caused by *H. influenzae, N. meningitidis,* or group B streptococci; 15% for that due to *L. monocytogenes*; and 20% for *S. pneumoniae.* In general, the risk of death from bacterial meningitis increases with (1) decreased level of consciousness on admission, (2) onset of seizures within 24 h of admission, (3) signs of increased ICP, (4) young age (infancy) and age >50, (5) the presence of comorbid conditions including shock and/or the need for mechanical ventilation, and (6) delay in the initiation of treatment. Decreased CSF glucose concentration [<2.2 mmol/L (<40 mg/dL)] and markedly increased CSF protein concentration [>3 g/L (>300 mg/dL)] have been predictive of increased mortality and poorer outcomes in some series. Moderate or severe sequelae occur in ~25% of survivors, although the exact incidence varies with the infecting organism. Common sequelae include decreased intellectual function, memory impairment, seizures, hearing loss and dizziness, and gait disturbances.

ACUTE VIRAL MENINGITIS

CLINICAL MANIFESTATIONS

Viral meningitis presents as fever, headache, and meningeal irritation coupled with an inflammatory CSF profile (see below). Fever may be accompanied by malaise, myalgia, anorexia, nausea and vomiting, abdominal pain, and/or diarrhea. It is not uncommon to see a mild degree of lethargy or drowsiness. The presence of more profound alterations in consciousness, such as stupor, coma, or marked confusion, should prompt consideration of alternative diagnoses. Similarly, seizures or other focal neurologic signs or symptoms suggest involvement of the brain parenchyma and do not occur in uncomplicated viral meningitis. The headache associated with viral meningitis is usually frontal or retroorbital and often associated with photophobia and pain on moving the eyes. Nuchal rigidity is present in most cases but may be mild and present only near the limit of neck anteflexion. Evidence of severe meningeal irritation, such as Kernig's and Brudzinski's signs, is generally absent.

ETIOLOGY

Enteroviruses account for 75 to 90% of aseptic meningitis cases in most series (**Table 29-4**). Viruses belonging to the *Enterovirus* genus are members of the family Picornaviridae and include the coxsackieviruses, echoviruses, polioviruses, and human enteroviruses 68 to 71. Using a variety of diagnostic techniques including CSF PCR tests, culture, and serology, a specific viral cause can be found in 75 to 90% of cases of viral meningitis. CSF cultures are positive in 30 to 70% of patients, the frequency of isolation depending on the specific viral agent. Approximately two-thirds of culture-negative cases of aseptic meningitis have a specific viral etiology identified by CSF PCR testing (see below).

EPIDEMIOLOGY

The exact incidence of viral meningitis in the United States is impossible to determine since most cases go unreported to public health authorities, although a reasonable estimate would be ~75,000 cases per year. In temperate climates, there is a substantial increase in cases during the summer and early fall months, reflecting the seasonal predominance of enterovirus and arthropod-borne encephalitis virus ("arbovirus") infections, with a peak monthly incidence of about 1 reported case per 100,000 population. The dramatic seasonal predilections of some viruses causing meningitis provide a valuable clue to diagnosis (**Table 29-5**).

LABORATORY DIAGNOSIS

CSF Examination

The most important laboratory test in the diagnosis of viral meningitis is examination of the CSF. The typical profile is a lymphocytic pleocytosis (25 to 500 cells/μL), a normal or slightly elevated protein concentration [0.2 to 0.8 g/L (20 to 80 mg/dL)], a normal glucose concentration, and a normal or mildly elevated opening pressure (100 to 350 mmH$_2$O). Organisms are *not* seen on Gram's or acid-fast stained smears or India ink preparations of CSF. Rarely, PMNs may predominate in the first 48 h of illness,

TABLE 29-4

VIRUSES CAUSING ACUTE MENINGITIS AND ACUTE ENCEPHALITIS		
COMMON	**LESS COMMON**	**RARE**
Acute Meningitis		
Enteroviruses	HSV-1	Adenoviruses
Arboviruses	LCMV	CMV
HIV	VZV	EBV
HSV-2		Influenza A, B, parainfluenza, mumps, rubella
Acute Encephalitis		
Arboviruses	CMV	Adenoviruses, CTFV, hepatitis C,
Enteroviruses	EBV	influenza A, LCMV, parainfluenza,
HSV-1	HIV	rabies, rotavirus, rubella
	Mumps	

Note: CMV, cytomegalovirus; CTFV, Colorado tick fever virus; EBV, Epstein-Barr virus; HSV, herpes simplex virus; LCMV, lymphocytic choriomeningitis virus; VZV, varicella-zoster virus.

TABLE 29-5

SEASONAL PREVALENCE OF VIRUSES COMMONLY CAUSING MENINGITIS			
SUMMER/EARLY FALL	**FALL/WINTER**	**WINTER/SPRING**	**NONSEASONAL**
Arboviruses	LCMV	Mumps	HSV
Enteroviruses			HIV

Note: Abbreviations are as in Table 29-4.

especially in patients with infections due to echovirus 9, West Nile virus or Eastern equine encephalitis virus, or mumps. Recent studies suggest that in some patients with West Nile virus infection, PMN pleocytosis can persist for up to a week before shifting to a lymphocytic pleocytosis. Despite these exceptions, the presence of a CSF PMN pleocytosis in a patient with suspected viral meningitis should always prompt consideration of an alternative diagnosis including bacterial meningitis or parameningeal infections. The total CSF cell count in viral meningitis is typically 25 to 500/μL, although cell counts of several thousand per microliter are occasionally seen, especially with infections due to lymphocytic choriomeningitis virus (LCMV) and mumps virus. The CSF glucose concentration is typically normal in viral infections, although it may be decreased in 10 to 30% of cases due to mumps as well as in cases due to LCMV. Rare instances of decreased CSF glucose concentration occur in cases of meningitis due to echoviruses and other enteroviruses, HSV type 2, and varicella-zoster virus (VZV). As a rule, a lymphocytic pleocytosis with a low glucose concentration should suggest fungal, listerial, or tuberculous meningitis or noninfectious disorders (e.g., sarcoid, neoplastic meningitis).

Polymerase Chain Reaction Amplification of Viral Nucleic Acid

Amplification of viral-specific DNA or RNA from CSF using PCR amplification has become the single most important method for diagnosing CNS viral infections. In both enteroviral and HSV infections of the CNS, PCR has become the diagnostic procedure of choice and is substantially more sensitive than viral cultures. HSV PCR is also an important diagnostic test in patients with recurrent episodes of "aseptic" meningitis, many of whom have amplifiable HSV DNA in CSF despite negative viral cultures. CSF PCR is also used routinely to diagnose CNS viral infections caused by cytomegalovirus (CMV), Epstein-Barr virus (EBV), and VZV.

CSF Culture

The overall results of CSF culture for the diagnosis of viral infection are disappointing, presumably because of the generally low concentration of infectious virus present and the need to customize isolation procedures for individual viruses. For viral isolation, 2 mL of CSF should be brought promptly to the microbiology laboratory, where it should be refrigerated and processed as speedily as possible. CSF specimens for viral isolation should never be stored in a −20°C freezer since viruses are often unstable at this temperature, and most freezers have "frostfree" warm-up cycles that are detrimental to viral stability. Storage for >24 h is probably best done in a −70°C freezer.

Other Sources for Viral Isolation

Viruses may also be isolated from sites and body fluids other than CSF, including throat, stool, blood, and urine. Enteroviruses and adenoviruses may be found in feces; arboviruses, some enteroviruses, and LCMV, in blood; mumps and CMV, in urine; and enteroviruses, mumps, and adenoviruses, in throat washings. During enteroviral infections, viral shedding in stool may persist for several weeks. The presence of enterovirus in stool is not diagnostic and may result from residual shedding from a previous enteroviral infection; it also occurs in some asymptomatic individuals during enteroviral epidemics.

Serologic Studies

For some viruses, including many arboviruses such as West Nile virus (WNV), serologic studies remain a crucial diagnostic tool. Serum serologic studies are less useful for viruses such as HSV, VZV, CMV, and EBV for which the prevalence of antibody seropositivity in the general population is high. Diagnosis of acute viral infection can be made by documenting seroconversion between acute-phase and convalescent sera (typically obtained after 2 to 4 weeks) or by demonstrating the presence of virus-specific IgM antibodies. Documentation of intrathecal synthesis of virus-specific antibodies, as shown by an increased IgG index or the presence of IgM antibodies in CSF, is often significantly more useful than serum serology alone and can provide presumptive evidence of CNS infection. Although serum and CSF IgM antibodies generally persist for only a few months after acute infection, there are exceptions to this rule. For example, WNV IgM has been shown to persist in some patients for >1 year following acute infection. Unfortunately, the delay between onset of infection and the generation by the host of a virus-specific antibody response often means that serologic data are useful mainly for the retrospective establishment of a specific diagnosis, rather than in urgent diagnosis or management.

Agarose electrophoresis or isoelectric focusing of CSF γ globulins may reveal the presence of oligoclonal bands. These bands have been found in association with a number of viral infections, including infections with HIV, human T cell lymphotropic virus (HTLV) type I, VZV, mumps, subacute sclerosing panencephalitis (SSPE), and progressive rubella panencephalitis. The associated antibodies are often directed against viral proteins. The finding of oligoclonal bands may be of some diagnostic utility, since typically they are not seen with arbovirus, enterovirus, or HSV infections. Oligoclonal bands are also encountered in certain noninfectious neurologic diseases (e.g., multiple sclerosis) and may be found in nonviral infections (e.g., syphilis, Lyme borreliosis).

Other Laboratory Studies

All patients with suspected viral meningitis should have a complete blood count and differential; liver function tests; and measurement of the erythrocyte sedimentation rate (ESR), blood urea nitrogen (BUN), and plasma levels of electrolytes, glucose, creatinine, creatine kinase, aldolase, amylase, and lipase. Abnormalities in specific test results may suggest particular etiologic diagnoses. MRI, CT, EEG, evoked response studies, electromyography (EMG), and nerve conduction studies are not necessary in most cases. They are best used selectively when atypical presentations or unusual features present diagnostic problems.

DIFFERENTIAL DIAGNOSIS

The most important issue in the differential diagnosis is the exclusion of nonviral causes that can mimic viral meningitis. The major categories of disease that should always be considered and excluded are (1) bacterial meningitis and other infectious meningidities (e.g., *Mycoplasma, Listeria, Brucella, Coxiella,* and *Rickettsia*); (2) parameningeal infections or partially treated bacterial meningitis; (3) nonviral infectious meningitides where cultures may be negative (e.g., fungal, tuberculous, parasitic, or syphilitic disease); (4) neoplastic meningitis; and (5) meningitis secondary to noninfectious inflammatory diseases such as sarcoid, Behçet's disease, and the uveomeningitic syndromes.

SPECIFIC VIRAL ETIOLOGIES

Enteroviruses are the most common cause of viral meningitis (>75% of cases in which a specific etiology can be identified) and should be considered the most likely cause of viral meningitis when a typical case occurs in the summer months, especially in a child (<15 years). However, despite their summer predominance, sporadic cases of enteroviral CNS infection are seen year-round. The physical examination should include a careful search for exanthemata, hand-foot-mouth disease, herpangina, pleurodynia, myopericarditis, and hemorrhagic conjunctivitis, which may be stigmata of enterovirus infections. PCR amplification of enteroviral RNA from CSF has become the diagnostic procedure of choice for these infections.

Arbovirus infections typically occur in the summer months, may have clear circumscribed geographic localization, and occur in both endemic and epidemic form, all factors reflecting the ecology of their transmission through infected insect vectors (Table 29-5). Arboviral meningitis should be considered when clusters of meningitis cases occur in a restricted geographic region during the summer or early fall. WNV infection should be suspected when bird deaths precede clusters of human cases of meningitis or encephalitis in an area known to harbor the virus. A history of tick exposure or travel or residence in the appropriate geographic area should suggest the possibility of Colorado tick fever virus or Powassan virus infection, although nonviral diseases producing meningitis (e.g., Lyme disease) or headache with meningismus (e.g., RMSF) may also present this way.

HSV-2 meningitis occurs in ~25% of women and 11% of men at the time of an initial (primary) episode of genital herpes. Of these patients, 20% go on to have recurrent attacks of meningitis. In some series, HSV-2 has been the most important cause of aseptic meningitis in adults, especially women, and overall it is probably second only to enteroviruses as a cause of viral meningitis. Although HSV-2 can be cultured from CSF during a first episode of meningitis, cultures are invariably negative during recurrent episodes of HSV-2 meningitis. Diagnosis depends on amplification of HSV-2 DNA from CSF by PCR. Almost all cases of recurrent HSV meningitis are due to HSV-2, although rare cases due to HSV-1 have been reported. Most cases of benign recurrent lymphocytic meningitis, including cases previously diagnosed as "Mollaret's meningitis," appear to be due to HSV. Genital lesions may not be present, and most patients give no history of genital herpes. CSF cultures are negative, although HSV DNA can be amplified from CSF by PCR during attacks of meningitis but not during symptom-free intervals.

VZV meningitis should be suspected in the presence of concurrent chickenpox or shingles. However, it is important to recognize that in some series up to 40% of VZV meningitis cases have been reported to occur in the absence of rash. The frequency of VZV as a cause of meningitis is extremely variable, ranging from as low as 3% to as high as 20% in different series. In addition to meningitis, encephalitis (see below), and shingles (see below), VZV can also produce acute cerebellar ataxia. This typically occurs in children and presents with the abrupt onset of limb and truncal ataxia. A similar syndrome occurs less commonly in association with EBV and enteroviral infection. PCR has rapidly become a major tool in the diagnosis of VZV CNS infections. In patients with negative CSF PCR results, the diagnosis of VZV CNS infection can be made by the demonstration of VZV-specific intrathecal antibody synthesis and/or the presence of VZV CSF IgM antibodies, or by positive CSF cultures.

EBV infections may also produce aseptic meningitis, with or without accompanying evidence of the infectious mononucleosis syndrome. The diagnosis may be suggested by the finding of atypical lymphocytes in the CSF or an atypical lymphocytosis in peripheral blood. The demonstration of IgM antibody to viral capsid antigen (VCA), or antibody to the diffuse (D) component of early antigen (EA) in the absence of or preceding detectable antibody to nuclear antigen (EBNA), are indicative of acute EBV infection. EBV is almost never cultured from CSF, but EBV DNA can be amplified from CSF in some patients with EBV-associated CNS infections. HIV-infected patients with primary CNS lymphoma may have a positive CSF PCR for EBV DNA even in the absence of meningoencephalitis.

HIV meningitis should be suspected in any patient with known or identified risk factors for HIV infection. Aseptic meningitis is a common manifestation of primary exposure to HIV and occurs in 5 to 10% of cases. In some patients, seroconversion may be delayed for several months; however, detection of the presence of HIV genome by PCR or p24 protein establishes the diagnosis. HIV can be cultured from CSF in some patients. Cranial nerve palsies, most commonly involving cranial nerves V, VII, or VIII, are more common in HIV meningitis than in other viral infections. For further discussion of HIV infection, see Chap. 31.

Mumps should be considered when meningitis occurs in the late winter or early spring, especially in males (male/female ratio 3:1). With the widespread use of the live attenuated mumps vaccine in the United States since 1967, the incidence of mumps meningitis has fallen by >95%. Rare cases of mumps vaccine–associated meningitis have been reported, but they are not usually seen after vaccination with the attenuated Jeryl-Lynn strain of virus used in the United States. The presence of orchitis, oophoritis, parotitis, pancreatitis, or elevations in serum lipase and amylase are suggestive but can be found with other viruses, and their absence does not exclude the diagnosis. Clinical meningitis occurs in 5% of patients with parotitis, but only 50% of patients with meningitis have associated parotitis. Mumps infection confers lifelong immunity, so a documented history of previous infection excludes this diagnosis. The presence of hypoglycorrhachia, found in 10 to 30% of patients, may be an additional diagnostic clue, once other causes have been excluded (see above). Up to 25% of patients may have a PMN-predominant CSF pleocytosis, and CSF abnormalities may persist for months. Diagnosis is typically made by isolation of virus from CSF and/or demonstration of seroconversion between acute-phase and convalescent sera.

LCMV infection should be considered when aseptic meningitis occurs in the late fall or winter, and in individuals with a history of exposure to house mice (*Mus musculus*), pet or laboratory rodents (e.g., hamsters), or their excreta. Some patients have an associated rash, pulmonary infiltrates, alopecia, parotitis, orchitis, or myopericarditis. Laboratory clues to the diagnosis of LCMV, in addition to the clinical findings noted above, may include the presence of leukopenia, thrombocytopenia, or abnormal liver function tests. Some cases present with a marked CSF pleocytosis (>1000 cells/μL) and hypoglycorrachia (<30%).

TREATMENT FOR VIRAL MENINGITIS

In the usual case of viral meningitis, treatment is symptomatic and hospitalization is not required. Exceptions include patients with deficient humoral immunity, neonates with overwhelming infection, and patients in whom the clinical or CSF profile suggests the possibility of a bacterial or other nonviral cause of infection. Patients with suspected bacterial meningitis should receive appropriate empirical therapy pending culture results (see above). Patients usually prefer to rest undisturbed in a quiet, darkened room. Analgesics can be used to relieve headache, which is often reduced by the initial diagnostic LP. Antipyretics may help to reduce fever, which rarely exceeds 40°C. Hyponatremia may develop as a result of inappropriate vasopressin secretion [syndrome of inappropriate secretion of antidiuretic hormone (SIADH)], so fluid and electrolyte status should be monitored. Repeat LP is indicated only in patients whose fever and symptoms fail to resolve after a few days, in patients with an initial PMN pleocytosis or hypoglycorhachia, or if there is doubt about the initial diagnosis.

Oral or intravenous acyclovir may be of benefit in patients with meningitis caused by HSV-1 or -2 and in cases of severe EBV or VZV infection. Data concerning treatment of HSV, EBV, and VZV meningitis are extremely limited. Seriously ill patients should probably receive intravenous acyclovir (30 mg/kg per day in three divided doses) for 7 days. Oral acyclovir (800 mg, five times daily), famciclovir (500 mg, tid), or valacyclovir (1000 mg, tid) for a week may be tried in less severely ill patients, although data on efficacy are lacking. Patients with HIV meningitis should receive highly active antiretroviral therapy (Chap. 31).

Patients with viral meningitis who are known to have deficient humoral immunity (e.g. X-linked agammaglobulinemia), and who are not already receiving either intramuscular γ-globulin or intravenous immunoglobulin (IVIg), should be treated with these agents. Intraventricular administration of immunoglobulin through an Ommaya reservoir has been tried in some patients with chronic enteroviral meningitis who have not responded to intramuscular or intravenous immunoglobulin.

An experimental drug, pleconaril (Viropharma Inc., VP 63843), has shown efficacy against a variety of enteroviral infections and has good oral bioavailability and excellent CNS penetration. Ongoing clinical trials in patients with enteroviral meningitis suggest that pleconaril decreases the duration of symptoms compared to placebo. Since most cases of enteroviral CNS infection are benign and self-limited, the indications for pleconaril therapy need to be better defined. Antiviral treatment might benefit patients with chronic CNS enteroviral infections in the setting of agammaglobulinemia or those who develop poliomyelitis as a complication of polio vaccine administration.

Vaccination is an effective method of preventing the development of meningitis and other neurologic complications associated with poliovirus, mumps, and measles infection. A live attenuated VZV vaccine (Varivax) is available in the United States. Clinical studies indicate an effectiveness rate of 70 to 90% for this vaccine, but a booster may be required to maintain immunity. An inactivated varicella vaccine is available for transplant recipients.

PROGNOSIS

In adults, the prognosis for full recovery from viral meningitis is excellent. Rare patients complain of persisting headache, mild mental impairment, incoordination, or generalized asthenia for weeks to months. The outcome in infants and neonates (<1 year) is less certain; intellectual impairment, learning disabilities, hearing loss, and other lasting sequelae have been reported in some studies.

VIRAL ENCEPHALITIS

DEFINITION

In contrast to viral meningitis, where the infectious process and associated inflammatory response are limited largely to the meninges, in encephalitis the brain parenchyma is also involved. Many patients with encephalitis also have evidence of associated meningitis (meningoencephalitis) and, in some cases, involvement of the spinal cord or nerve roots (encephalomyelitis, encephalomyeloradiculitis).

CLINICAL MANIFESTATIONS

In addition to the acute febrile illness with evidence of meningeal involvement characteristic of meningitis, the patient with encephalitis commonly has confusion, behaviroral abnormalities, an altered level of consciousness, and evidence of either focal or diffuse neurologic signs and symptoms. Any degree of altered consciousness may occur, ranging from mild lethargy to deep coma. Patients with encephalitis may have hallucinations, agitation, personality change, behavioral disorders, and, at times, a frankly psychotic state. Focal or generalized seizures occur in many patients with severe encephalitis. Virtually every possible type of focal neurologic disturbance has been reported in viral encephalitis; the signs and symptoms reflect the sites of infection and inflammation. The most commonly encountered focal findings are aphasia, ataxia, hemiparesis (with hyperactive tendon reflexes and extensor plantar responses), involuntary movements (e.g., myoclonic jerks, tremor), and cranial nerve deficits (e.g., ocular palsies, facial weakness). Involvement of the hypothalamic-pituitary axis may result in temperature dysregulation, diabetes insipidus, or the development of SIADH. Despite the clear neuropathologic evidence that viruses differ in the regions of the CNS they injure, it is often impossible to distinguish reliably on clinical grounds alone one type of viral encephalitis (e.g., that caused by HSV) from others (see "Differential Diagnosis," below).

ETIOLOGY

In the United States, there are ~20,000 reported cases of encephalitis per year; the actual number is likely to be significantly higher. Hundreds of viruses are capable of causing encephalitis, although only a limited subset is responsible for most cases in which a specific cause is identified (Table 29-4). The same organisms responsible for aseptic meningitis are also responsible for encephalitis, although their relative frequencies differ. The most important viruses causing sporadic cases of encephalitis in immunocompetent adults are HSV-1 (**Fig. 29-2**), VZV and, less commonly, enteroviruses. Epidemics of encephalitis are caused by arboviruses, which belong to several different viral taxonomic groups including *Alphaviruses* (e.g. Eastern equine encephalitis virus, Western equine encephalitis virus), *Flaviviruses* (e.g., WNV, St. Louis encephalitis virus, Powassan virus), and *Bunyaviruses* (e.g., California encephalitis virus serogroup, LaCrosse virus). Historically, the largest number of cases of arbovirus encephalitis in the United States has been due to St. Louis encephalitis virus and the California encephalitis virus serogroup. However, in 2002, WNV produced the largest epidemic of encephalitis ever recorded in the United States, with 4156 cases and 284 deaths. New causes of viral encephalitis are constantly appearing, as evidenced by the recent outbreak of 257 cases of encephalitis with a 40% mortality rate in Malaysia caused by Nipah virus, a new member of the Paramyxovirus family.

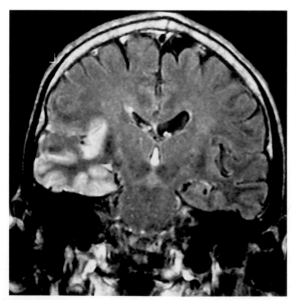

FIGURE 29-2

Coronal FLAIR magnetic resonance image from a patient with herpes simplex encephalitis. Note the area of increased signal in the temporal lobe (left) confined predominantly to the gray matter. This patient had predominantly unilateral disease; bilateral lesions are more common but may be quite asymmetric in their intensity.

LABORATORY DIAGNOSIS

CSF Examination

CSF examination should be performed in all patients with suspected viral encephalitis unless contraindicated by the presence of severely increased ICP. The characteristic CSF profile is indistinguishable from that of viral meningitis and consists of a lymphocytic pleocytosis, a mildly elevated protein concentration, and a normal glucose concentration. A CSF pleocytosis (>5 cells/μL) occurs in >95% of patients with documented viral encephalitis. In rare cases, a pleocytosis may be absent on the initial LP but present on subsequent LP's. Patients who are severely immunocompromised by HIV infection, glucocorticoid or other immunosupressant drugs, chemotherapy, or lymphoreticular malignancies may fail to mount a CSF inflammatory response. CSF cell counts exceed 500/μL in only about 10% of patients with encephalitis. Infections with certain arboviruses (e.g., Eastern equine encephalitis or California encephalitis viruses), mumps, and LCMV may occasionally result in cell counts >1000/μL, but this degree of pleocytosis should suggest the possibility of nonviral infections or other inflammatory processes. Atypical lymphocytes in the CSF may be seen in EBV infection and less commonly with other viruses, including CMV, HSV, and enteroviruses. The presence of substantial numbers of PMNs after the first 48 h should prompt consideration of bacterial infection, leptospirosis, amebic infection, and noninfectious processes such as acute hemorrhagic leukoencephalitis. PMN pleocytosis that can persist for up to a week has also been reported in cases of WNV encephalitis. Large numbers of CSF PMNs may be present in patients with viral encephalitis due to Eastern equine encephalitis virus, echovirus 9, and, more rarely, other enteroviruses. About 20% of patients with encephalitis will have a significant number of red blood cells (>500/μL) in the CSF in a nontraumatic tap. The pathologic correlate of this finding may be a hemorrhagic encephalitis of the type seen with HSV, Colorado tick fever virus, and occasionally California encephalitis virus. A decreased CSF glucose concentration is distinctly unusual in viral encephalitis and should suggest the possibility of bacterial, fungal, tuberculous, parasitic, leptospiral, syphilitic, sarcoid, or neoplastic meningitis. Rare patients with mumps, LCMV, or advanced HSV encephalitis may have low CSF glucose concentrations.

CSF PCR

CSF PCR has become the primary diagnostic test for CNS infections caused by CMV, EBV, VZV and enteroviruses (see "Viral Meningitis," above). The sensitivity and specificity of CSF PCRs vary with the virus being tested. Recent studies with HSV encephalitis indicate that the sensitivity (~98%) and specificity (~94%) of CSF PCR equal or exceed those of brain biopsy. It is important to recognize that CSF HSV PCR results need to be interpreted after considering the likelihood of disease in the patient being tested, the timing of the test in relationship to onset of symptoms, and the prior use of antiviral therapy. A negative HSV CSF PCR test performed in a patient with a high likelihood of HSV encephalitis based on clinical and laboratory tests significantly reduces the likelihood of HSV encephalitis but does not exclude it. There have been several recent reports of initially negative CSF HSV PCR tests that were obtained early (≤72 h) following symptom onset, that became positive when repeated 1 to 3 days later. The frequency of positive CSF HSV PCRs in patients with herpes encephalitis also decreases as a function of the duration of illness, with only ~20% of cases remaining positive after ≥14 days. PCR results are generally not affected by ≤1 week of antiviral therapy. In one study 98% of CSF specimens remained PCR-positive during the first week of initiation of antiviral therapy, but the numbers fell to ~50% by 8 to 14 days and to ~21% by >15 days after initiation of therapy.

The sensitivity and specificity of CSF PCR tests for viruses other than herpes simplex have not been definitively characterized. Enteroviral CSF PCR appears to have a sensitivity and specificity of >95%. The specificity of EBV CSF PCR has not been established, and apparent false-positive results can occur in patients with CNS lymphoma and in patients with inflammatory CSF specimens. In patients with CNS infection due to VZV, CSF antibody and PCR studies should be considered complementary, as several cases with positive serologies and negative PCR studies have been reported. In the case of WNV infection, CSF PCR is considerably less sensitive (~70% sensitivity) than detection of WNV-specific CSF IgM in diagnosis of WNV encephalitis.

CSF Culture

Attempts to culture viruses from the CSF in cases of encephalitis are often disappointing. Cultures are invariably negative in cases of HSV-1 encephalitis.

Serologic Studies and Antigen Detection

The basic approach to the serodiagnosis of viral encephalitis is identical to that discussed earlier for viral meningitis. In patients with HSV encephalitis, both antibodies to HSV-1 glycoproteins and glycoprotein antigens have been detected in the CSF. Optimal detection of both HSV antibodies and antigen typically occurs after the first week of illness, limiting the utility of these tests in acute diagnosis. Nonetheless, CSF HSV antibody

testing may be of value in selected patients whose illness is >1 week in duration and who are CSF PCR-negative for HSV. Demonstration of WNV IgM antibodies is diagnostic of WNV encephalitis, as IgM antibodies do not cross the blood-brain barrier and their presence in CSF is therefore indicative of intrathecal synthesis.

MRI, CT, EEG

Patients with suspected encephalitis almost invariably undergo neuroimaging studies and often EEG. These tests help identify or exclude alternative diagnoses and assist in the differentiation between a focal, as opposed to a diffuse, encephalitic process. Focal findings in a patient with encephalitis should always raise the possibility of HSV encephalitis. Examples of focal findings include: (1) areas of increased signal intensity in the frontotemporal, cingulate, or insular regions of the brain on T2-weighted, fluid-attenuated inversion recovery (FLAIR), or diffusion-weighted MRI images (Fig. 29-2); (2) temporoparietal areas of low absorption, mass effect, and contrast enhancement on CT; or (3) periodic focal temporal lobe spikes on a background of slow or low-amplitude ("flattened") activity on EEG. Approximately 10% of patients with PCR-documented HSV encephalitis will have a normal MRI, although nearly 90% will have abnormalities in the temporal lobe. CT is less sensitive than MRI and is normal in up to 33% of patients. The addition of FLAIR and diffusion-weighted images to the standard MRI sequences enhances sensitivity. EEG abnormalities occur in >90% of PCR-documented cases of HSV encephalitis; they typically involve the temporal lobes but are often nonspecific. Some patients with HSV encephalitis have a distinctive EEG pattern consisting of periodic, stereotyped, sharp-and-slow complexes originating in one or both temporal lobes and repeating at regular intervals of 2 to 3 s. The periodic complexes are typically noted between the second and the fifteenth day of the illness and are present in two-thirds of pathologically proven cases of HSV encephalitis.

Significant MRI abnormalities are found in only ~30% of patients with WNV encephalitis, a frequency significantly less than that of HSV encephalitis. When present, abnormalities often involve deep brain structures including the thalamus, basal ganglia, and brainstem rather than the cortex. Patients with VZV encephalitis may show areas of hemorrhagic infarction reflecting the tendency of this virus to produce a CNS vasculopathy rather than a true encephalitis.

Brain Biopsy

Brain biopsy is now generally reserved for patients in whom CSF PCR studies fail to lead to a specific diagnosis, who have focal abnormalities on MRI, and who continue to show progressive clinical deterioration despite treatment with acyclovir and supportive therapy. The isolation of HSV from brain tissue obtained at biopsy was once considered the "gold standard" for the diagnosis of HSV encephalitis, although with the advent of CSF PCR tests for HSV it is rarely necessary to perform brain biopsy for this purpose. The need for brain biopsy to diagnose other forms of viral encephalitis has also declined greatly with the widespread availability of CSF PCR diagnostic tests for EBV, CMV, VZV, and enteroviruses. When biopsy is performed, the tissue is cultured for virus and examined histopathologically and ultrastructurally. Tissue should be taken from a site that appears to be significantly involved on the basis of clinical and laboratory criteria. Although brain biopsy is not an innocuous procedure, the mortality rate is low (<0.2%) and serious complications occur in only 0.5 to 2.0% of cases. Potential morbidity, in addition to that related to general anesthesia, includes local bleeding and edema, the development of a seizure focus, and wound dehiscence or infection.

DIFFERENTIAL DIAGNOSIS

Some of the most common illnesses masquerading as viral encephalitis, as identified in multicenter clinical trials using brain biopsy as a diagnostic standard, were vascular diseases; abscess and empyema; fungal, parasitic, rickettsial, and tuberculous infections; tumors; Reye's syndrome; toxic encephalopathy; subdural hematoma; and SLE. Acute disseminated encephalomyelitis (ADEM), limbic encephalitis, prion diseases, and Hashimoto's encephalopathy are additional considerations. Of the nonviral infections, particular attention should be paid to *Listeria, Mycoplasma, Leptospira, Cryptococcus,* and *Mucor* infections, as well as to toxoplasmosis and tuberculosis.

Meningoencephalitis caused by ameba can also mimic viral encephalitis. Infection caused by *Naegleria fowleri* usually causes an acute syndrome (primary amebic meningoencephalitis), whereas that caused by *Acanthamoeba* and *Balamuthia* more typically produces subacute or chronic granulomatous amebic meningoencephalitis. *Naegleria* thrive in warm iron-rich pools of water including those found in drains, canals, and both natural and man-made outdoor pools. Infection has typically occurred in immunocompetent children with a history of swimming in potentially infected water. The presentation is of an acute encephalitis, with a CSF neutrophilic pleocytosis and hypoglycorrhachia identical to that seen in bacterial meningitis. Motile trophozoites can be seen in a wet mount of warm fresh CSF. No effective treatment has been identified, and mortality approaches 100%.

There have also been several recent reports of encephalitis caused by the raccoon pinworm *Baylisascaris procyonis.* Clues to the diagnosis include a history of raccoon exposure, and especially of playing in or eating dirt potentially contaminated with raccoon feces. Most patients are children, and many have an associated eosinophilia.

Infection with *Bartonella* species, the agents of cat scratch fever, can also produce a meningoencephalitis. In some recent surveys, *Bartonella* infection has been the most common bacterial infection mimicking viral encephalitis. Infection is transmitted by the bite or scratch of a cat, with an increased risk associated with kittens and feral cats. Patients often develop regional lymphadenopathy; 2 to 4% of infected patients develop encephalopathy, retinitis, or less commonly cranial or peripheral neuropathy. CSF shows a lymphocytic pleocytosis with normal glucose in about one-third of cases, the remainder having no abnormalities or only mild protein elevation. Neuroimaging results are nonspecific, and diagnosis is based on serology. Antibiotic therapy is of uncertain value in immunocompetent hosts, although doxycycline (200 mg daily for 3 months) is often tried in patients with CNS disease.

Once nonviral causes of encephalitis have been excluded, the major diagnostic challenge is to distinguish HSV from other viruses that cause encephalitis. This distinction is particularly important because in virtually every other instance the therapy is supportive, whereas specific and effective antiviral therapy is available for HSV, and its efficacy is enhanced when it is instituted early in the course of infection. HSV encephalitis should be considered when clinical features suggesting involvement of the inferomedial frontotemporal regions of the brain are present, including prominent olfactory or gustatory hallucinations, anosmia, unusual or bizarre behavior or personality alterations, or memory disturbance. HSV encephalitis should always be suspected in patients with focal findings on clinical examination, neuroimaging studies, or EEG. The diagnostic procedure of choice in these patients is CSF PCR analysis for HSV. A positive CSF PCR establishes the diagnosis, and a negative test dramatically reduces the likelihood of HSV encephalitis (see above).

The anatomical distribution of lesions may provide an additional clue to diagnosis. Patients with rapidly progressive encephalitis and prominent brainstem signs, symptoms, or neuroimaging abnormalities may be infected by flaviviruses (WNV, Japanese encephalitis virus), HSV, rabies or *L. monocytogenes.* Significant involvement of deep gray matter structures including the basal ganglia and thalamus should also suggest possible flavivirus infection. These patients may present clinically with prominent movement disorders (tremor, myoclonus) or Parkinson's disease–like features. Patients with WNV infection can also present with acute poliomyelitis-like areflexic paralysis, as can patients infected with enterovirus 71 and less commonly other enteroviruses. Despite an aggressive World Health Organization poliovirus eradication initiative, cases of wild-type poliovirus-induced poliomyelitis continue to be reported in at least seven countries worldwide: Egypt, Somalia, Niger, Nigeria, India, Pakistan, and Afghanistan. Rare cases continue to occur in the United States in nonvaccinated individuals exposed to vaccine strains of virus that have reverted to virulence. A recent outbreak of poliomyelitis on Hispaniola (the Dominican Republic and Haiti) has been attributed to vaccine strain–derived viruses that have reverted to virulence after apparently recombining with other circulating enteroviruses. Acute ascending paralysis resembling Guillain-Barré syndrome but associated with CSF pleocytosis can occur with HIV infection, rabies, and WNV infection.

Epidemiologic factors may provide important clues. Particular attention should be paid to the season of the year (Table 29-5); the age of the patient (**Table 29-6**); the geographic location and travel history (Table 29-6); and possible exposure to animal bites or scratches, rodents, and ticks. Although transmission from the bite of an infected dog remains the most common cause of rabies worldwide, in the United States very few cases of dog rabies occur, and the most common risk factor is exposure to bats—although a clear history of a bite or scratch is often lacking. The classic clinical presentation of encephalitic (furious) rabies is of fever and autonomic hyperactivity with fluctuating mental status. Phobic spasms of the larynx, pharynx, neck muscles, and diaphragm can be triggered by attempts to swallow water (*hydrophobia*) or by inspiration (*aerophobia*). Patients may also present with paralytic (dumb) rabies characterized by acute ascending paralysis. Patients with rabies have a CSF lymphocytic pleocytosis and may show areas of increased T2 signal abnormality in the brainstem, hippocampus, and hypothalamus. Diagnosis can be made by finding rabies virus antigen in brain tissue or in the neural innervation of hair follicles at the nape of the neck. PCR amplification of viral nucleic acid from CSF and saliva or tears may also enable diagnosis. Serology is frequently negative in both serum and CSF in the first week after onset of infection, which limits its acute diagnostic utility. No specific therapy is available, and cases are almost invariably fatal, with isolated survivors having devastating neurologic sequelae.

Morbidity and Mortality Weekly Reports provides regular information about the prevalence of particular viruses causing encephalitis by season and region of the country. State public health authorities provide another valuable resource concerning isolation of particular agents in individual regions. Deaths in crows and other corvid birds in the local area have preceded human infection by WNV during outbreaks in the United States. Details of the occurrence of WNV in mosquitoes, birds, horses, and humans can be found on the Centers for Disease Control and Prevention (CDC) and U.S. Geological Survey (USGS) websites (and *http://westnilemaps.usgs.gov/*).

TREATMENT FOR VIRAL ENCEPHALITIS

Specific antiviral therapy should be initiated when appropriate. Vital functions, including respiration and blood pressure, should be monitored continuously

TABLE 29-6

FEATURES OF SELECTED ARBOVIRUS ENCEPHALITIDES

FEATURE	WNV	WEE	EEE	VEE	SLE	CE
Region	All	West, midwest	Atlantic and Gulf coasts	SW, W	All	East and NC
Age	Adults > 60	Infants, adults > 50	Children, adults > 60	Adults	Adults > 60	Children
Deaths	7%	3–15%	50–75%	1%	2–20%	<1%
Sequelae	?	Common	80%	Rare	20%	Rare
Vector	M	M	M	M	M	M
Animal reservoir	B	B	B	H, sm M	B	sm M

Note: WNV, West Nile virus; WEE, Western equine encephalitis (virus); EEE, Eastern equine encephalitis (virus); VEE, Venezuelan equine encephalitis (virus); SLE, St. Louis encephalitis; CE, California encephalitis (virus); B, bird; H, horse; M, mosquito; NC, north central United States; sm M, small mammal; SW, southwest; W, west.

and supported as required. In the initial stages of encephalitis, many patients will require care in an intensive care unit. Basic management and supportive therapy should include careful monitoring of ICP, fluid restriction and avoidance of hypotonic intravenous solutions, and suppression of fever. Seizures should be treated with standard anticonvulsant regimens, and prophylactic therapy should be considered in view of the high frequency of seizures in severe cases of encephalitis. As with all seriously ill, immobilized patients with altered levels of consciousness, encephalitis patients are at risk for aspiration pneumonia, stasis ulcers and decubiti, contractures, deep venous thrombosis and its complications, and infections of indwelling lines and catheters.

Acyclovir is of benefit in the treatment of HSV and should be started empirically in patients with suspected viral encephalitis while awaiting viral diagnostic studies. Treatment should be discontinued in patients found not to have HSV encephalitis, with the possible exception of patients with severe encephalitis due to VZV or EBV. HSV, VZV, and EBV all encode an enzyme, deoxypyrimidine (thymidine) kinase, that phosphorylates acyclovir to produce acyclovir-5′-monophosphate. Host cell enzymes then phosphorylate this compound to form a triphosphate derivative. It is the triphosphate that acts as an antiviral agent by inhibiting viral DNA polymerase and by causing premature termination of nascent viral DNA chains. The specificity of action depends on the fact that uninfected cells do not phosphorylate significant amounts of acyclovir to acyclovir-5′-monophosphate. A second level of specificity is provided by the fact that the acyclovir triphosphate is a more potent inhibitor of viral DNA polymerase than of the analogous host cell enzymes.

Adults should receive a dose of 10 mg/kg of acyclovir intravenously every 8 h (30 mg/kg per day total dose) for a minimum of 14 days. Although no studies directly addressing this issue are yet available, repeating the CSF PCR after completion of acyclovir therapy should be considered. Patients with a persisting positive CSF PCR for HSV after completing a standard course of acyclovir therapy should be treated for an additional 7 days, followed by a repeat CSF PCR test. Neonatal HSV CNS infection is less responsive to acyclovir therapy than HSV encephalitis in adults; it is recommended that neonates with HSV encephalitis receive 20 mg/kg of acyclovir every 8 h (60 mg/kg per day total dose) for a minimum of 21 days.

Prior to intravenous administration, acyclovir should be diluted to a concentration ≤7 mg/mL. (A 70-kg person would receive a dose of 700 mg, which would be diluted in a volume of 100 mL.) Each dose should be infused slowly over 1 h rather than by rapid or bolus infusion, to minimize the risk of renal dysfunction. Care should be taken to avoid extravasation or intramuscular or subcutaneous administration. The alkaline pH of acyclovir can cause local inflammation and phlebitis (9%). Dose adjustment is required in patients with impaired renal glomerular filtration. Penetration into CSF is excellent, with average drug levels ~50% of serum levels. Complications of therapy include elevations in BUN and creatinine levels (5%), thrombocytopenia (6%), gastrointestinal toxicity (nausea, vomiting, diarrhea) (7%), and neurotoxicity (lethargy or obtundation, disorientation, confusion, agitation, hallucinations, tremors, seizures) (1%). Acyclovir resistance may be mediated by changes in either the viral deoxypyrimidine kinase or DNA polymerase. To date, acyclovir-resistant isolates have not been a significant clinical problem in immunocompetent individuals. However, there have been reports of clinically virulent acyclovir-resistant HSV isolates from sites outside the CNS in immunocompromised individuals, including those with AIDS.

Oral antiviral drugs with efficacy against HSV, VZV, and EBV, including acyclovir, famciclovir, and valacyclovir, have not been evaluated in the treatment of encephalitis either as primary therapy or as supplemental therapy following completion of a course of parenteral acyclovir. An NIAID/NINDS-sponsored phase III trial of supplemental oral valacyclovir therapy (2 g, tid for 3 months) following the initial 14- to 21-day course of therapy with parenteral acyclovir has recently been initiated by the Collaborative Antiviral Study Group (CASG) in patients with HSV encephalitis (CASG 204); it may help clarify the role of extended oral antiviral therapy.

Both ganciclovir and foscarnet have been shown to be effective in the treatment of CMV-related CNS infections. These drugs are often used in combination. Cidofovir (see below) may provide an alternative in patients who fail to respond to ganciclovir and foscarnet, although data concerning its use in CMV CNS infections are extremely limited.

Ganciclovir is a synthetic nucleoside analogue of 2′-deoxyguanosine. The drug is preferentially phosphorylated by virus-induced cellular kinases. Ganciclovir triphosphate acts as a competitive inhibitor of the CMV DNA polymerase, and its incorporation into nascent viral DNA results in premature chain termination. Following intravenous administration, CSF concentrations of ganciclovir are 25 to 70% of coincident plasma levels. The usual dose for treatment of severe neurologic illnesses is 5 mg/kg every 12 h given intravenously at a constant rate over 1 h. Induction therapy is followed by maintenance therapy of 5 mg/kg every day for an indefinite period. Induction therapy should be continued until patients show a decline in CSF pleocytosis and a reduction in CSF CMV DNA copy number on quantitative PCR testing (where available). Doses should be adjusted in patients with renal insufficiency. Treatment is often limited by the development of granulocytopenia and thrombocytopenia (20 to 25%), which may require reduction in or discontinuation of therapy. Gastrointestinal side effects including nausea, vomiting, diarrhea, and abdominal pain occur in ~20% of patients. Some patients treated with ganciclovir for CMV retinitis have developed retinal detachment, but the causal relationship to ganciclovir treatment is unclear.

Foscarnet is a pyrophosphate analogue that inhibits viral DNA polymerases by binding to the pyrophosphate-binding site. Following intravenous infusion, CSF concentrations range from 15 to 100% of coincident plasma levels. The usual dose for serious CMV-related neurologic illness is 60 mg/kg every 8 h administered by constant infusion over 1 h. Induction therapy for 14 to 21 days is followed by maintenance therapy (60 to 120 mg/kg per day). Induction therapy may need to be extended in patients who fail to show a decline in CSF pleocytosis and a reduction in CSF CMV DNA copy number on quantitative PCR tests (where available). Approximately one-third of patients develop renal impairment during treatment, which is reversible following discontinuation of therapy in most, but not all, cases. This is often associated with elevations in serum creatinine and proteinuria and is less frequent in patients who are adequately hydrated. Many patients experience fatigue and nausea. Reduction in serum calcium, magnesium, and potassium occur in ~15% of patients and may be associated with tetany, cardiac rhythm disturbances, or seizures.

Cidofovir is a nucleotide analogue that is effective in treating CMV retinitis and equivalent or better than ganciclovir in some experimental models of murine CMV encephalitis, although data concerning its efficacy in human CMV CNS disease are limited. The usual dose is 5 mg/kg intravenously once weekly for 2 weeks, then biweekly for 2 or more additional doses, depending on clinical response. Patients must be prehydrated with normal saline (e.g., 1 L over 1 to 2 h) prior to each dose and treated with probenecid (e.g., 1 g 3 h before cidofovir and 1 g 2 and 8 h after cidofovir). Nephrotoxicity is common; the dose should be reduced if renal function deteriorates.

Intravenous ribavirin (15 to 25 mg/kg per day in divided doses given every 8 h) has been reported to be of benefit in isolated cases of severe encephalitis due to California encephalitis (LaCrosse) virus. Ribavirin might be of benefit for the rare patients, typically infants or young children, with severe adenovirus or rotavirus encephalitis and in patients with encephalitis due to LCMV or other arenaviruses. However, clinical trials are lacking. Hemolysis, with resulting anemia, has been the major side effect limiting therapy.

No specific antiviral therapy of proven efficacy is currently available for treatment of WNV encephalitis. Small groups of patients have been treated with interferon α, ribavirin, and IVIg preparations of non-U.S. origin containing high-titer anti-WNV antibody. Evidence is insufficient to establish efficacy of any of these therapies.

SEQUELAE

There is considerable variation in the incidence and severity of sequelae in patients surviving viral encephalitis. In the case of Eastern equine encephalitis virus infection, nearly 80% of survivors have severe neurologic sequelae. At the other extreme are infections due to EBV, California encephalitis virus, and Venezuelan equine encephalitis virus, where severe sequelae are unusual. For example, ~5 to 15% of children infected with LaCrosse virus have a residual seizure disorder, and 1% have persistent hemiparesis. Detailed information about sequelae in patients with HSV encephalitis treated with acyclovir are available from the NIAID-CASG trials. Of 32 acyclovir-treated patients, 26 survived (81%). Of the 26 survivors, 12 (46%) had no or only minor sequelae, 3 (12%) were moderately impaired (gainfully employed but not functioning at their previous level), and 11 (42%) were severely impaired (requiring continuous supportive care). The incidence and severity of sequelae were directly related to the age of the patient and the level of consciousness at the time of initiation of therapy. Patients with severe neurologic impairment (Glasgow coma score 6) at initiation of therapy either died or survived with severe sequelae. Young patients (<30 years) with good neurologic function at initiation of therapy did substantially better (100% survival, 62% with no or mild sequelae) compared with their older counterparts (>30 years); (64% survival, 57% no or mild sequelae). Some recent studies using quantitative CSF PCR tests for HSV indicate that clinical outcome following treatment also correlates with the amount of HSV DNA present in CSF at the time of presentation. Many patients with WNV infection have acute sequelae including cognitive impairment; weakness; and hyper- or hypo-kinetic movement disorders including tremor, myoclonus, and parkinsonism. Improvement in these symptoms may occur over the subsequent 6 to 12 months, although detailed clinical studies of the duration and severity of WNV sequelae are still lacking.

SUBACUTE MENINGITIS

CLINICAL MANIFESTATIONS

Patients with subacute meningitis typically have an unrelenting headache, stiff neck, low-grade fever, and lethargy for days to several weeks before they present for evaluation. Cranial nerve abnormalities and night sweats may be present. This syndrome overlaps that of chronic meningitis discussed in detail in Chap. 30.

ETIOLOGY

Common causative organisms include *M. tuberculosis, C. neoformans, H. capsulatum, C. immitis,* and *T. pallidum.* Initial infection with *M. tuberculosis* is acquired by inhalation of aerosolized droplet nuclei. Tuberculous meningitis in adults does not develop acutely from hematogenous spread of tubercle bacilli to the meninges. Rather, millet seed–size (miliary) tubercles form in the parenchyma of the brain during hematogenous dissemination of tubercle bacilli in the course of primary infection. These tubercles enlarge and are usually caseating. The propensity for a caseous lesion to produce meningitis is determined by its proximity to the SAS and the rate at which fibrous encapsulation develops. Subependymal caseous foci cause meningitis via discharge of bacilli and tuberculous antigens into the SAS. Mycobacterial antigens produce an intense inflammatory reaction that leads to the production of a thick exudate that fills the basilar cisterns and surrounds the cranial nerves and major blood vessels at the base of the brain.

Fungal infections are typically acquired by the inhalation of airborne fungal spores. The initial pulmonary infection may be asymptomatic or present with fever, cough, sputum production, and chest pain. The pulmonary infection is often self-limited. A localized pulmonary fungal infection can then remain dormant in the lungs until there is an abnormality in cell-mediated immunity that allows the fungus to reactivate and disseminate to the CNS. The most common pathogen causing fungal meningitis is *C. neoformans.* This fungus is found worldwide in soil and bird excreta. *H. capsulatum* is endemic to the Ohio and Mississippi River valleys of the central United States and to parts of Central and South America. *C. immitis* is endemic to the desert areas of the southwest United States, northern Mexico, and Argentina.

Syphilis is a sexually transmitted disease that is manifest by the appearance of a painless chancre at the site of inoculation. *T. pallidum* invades the CNS early in the course of syphilis. Cranial nerves VII and VIII are most frequently involved.

LABORATORY DIAGNOSIS

The classic CSF abnormalities in tuberculous meningitis are as follows: (1) elevated opening pressure, (2) lymphocytic pleocytosis (10 to 500 cells/μL), (3) elevated protein concentration in the range of 1 to 5 g/L (10 to 500 mg/dL), and (4) decreased glucose concentration in the range of 1.1 to 2.2 mmol/L (20 to 40 mg/dL). *The combination of unrelenting headache, stiff neck, fatigue, night sweats, and fever with a CSF lymphocytic pleocytosis and a mildly decreased glucose concentration is highly suspicious for tuberculous meningitis.* The last tube of fluid collected at LP is the best tube to send for a smear for acid-fast bacilli (AFB). If there is a pellicle in the CSF or a cobweb-like clot on the surface of the fluid, AFB can best be demonstrated in a smear of the clot or pellicle. Positive smears are typically reported in only 10 to 40% of cases of tuberculous meningitis in adults. Cultures of CSF take 4 to 8 weeks to identify the organism and are positive in ~50% of adults. Culture remains the "gold standard" to make the diagnosis of tuberculous meningitis. PCR for the detection of *M. tuberculosis* DNA has a sensitivity of 70 to 80% but at the present time is limited by a high rate of false-positive results.

The characteristic CSF abnormalities in fungal meningitis are a mononuclear or lymphocytic pleocytosis, an increased protein concentration, and a decreased glucose concentration. There may be eosinophils in the CSF in *C. immitis* meningitis. Large volumes of CSF are often required to demonstrate the organism on India ink smear or grow the organism in culture. If spinal fluid obtained by LP on two separate occasions fails to yield an organism, CSF should be obtained by high-cervical or cisternal puncture.

The cryptococcal polysaccharide antigen test is a highly sensitive and specific test for cryptococcal meningitis. A reactive CSF cryptococcal antigen test establishes the diagnosis. The detection of the *histoplasma* polysaccharide antigen in CSF establishes the diagnosis of a fungal meningitis but is not specific for meningitis due to *H. capsulatum*. It may be falsely positive in coccidioidal meningitis. The CSF complement fixation antibody test is reported to have a specificity of 100% and a sensitivity of 75% for coccidioidal meningitis.

The diagnosis of syphilitic meningitis is made when a reactive serum treponemal test [fluorescent treponemal antibody, absorbed (FTA-ABS) or microhemagglutination–*T. pallidum* (MHA-TP)] is associated with a CSF lymphocytic or mononuclear pleocytosis and an elevated protein concentration, or when the CSF VDRL is positive. A reactive CSF-FTA-ABS is not definitive evidence of neurosyphilis. The CSF-FTA-ABS can be falsely positive from blood contamination. A negative CSF VDRL does not rule out neurosyphilis. A negative CSF FTA-ABS or MHA-TP rules out neurosyphilis.

TREATMENT FOR SUBACUTE MENINGITIS

Empirical therapy of tuberculous meningitis is often initiated on the basis of a high index of suspicion without adequate laboratory support. Initial therapy is a combination of isoniazid (300 mg/d), rifampin (10 mg/kg per day), pyrazinamide (30 mg/kg per day in divided doses), ethambutol (15 to 25 mg/kg per day in divided doses), and pyridoxine (50 mg/d). If the clinical response is good, pyrazinamide and ethambutol can be discontinued after 8 weeks and isoniazid and rifampin continued alone for the next 6 to 12 months. A 6-month course of therapy is acceptable, but therapy should be prolonged for 9 to 12 months in patients who have an inadequate resolution of symptoms of meningitis or who have positive mycobacterial cultures of CSF during the course of therapy. In addition to its use in hydrocephalus, adjunctive dexamethasone therapy was recently demonstrated to reduce risk of death in a cohort of patients with tuberculous meningitis in Vietnam.

Meningitis due to *C. neoformans* is treated with amphotericin B (0.7 mg/kg per day) and flucytosine (100 mg/kg per day in four divided doses) for 2 weeks, followed by an 8- to 10-week course of fluconazole (400 to 800 mg/d). If the CSF culture is sterile after 10 weeks of acute therapy, the dose of fluconazole is decreased to 200 mg/d for 6 months to a year. Patients with HIV infection may require indefinite maintenance therapy. Meningitis due to *H. capsulatum* is treated with amphotericin B (0.7 to 1.0 mg/kg per day) for 4 to 12 weeks followed by itraconazole (400 mg/d). Therapy with amphotericin B is not discontinued until fungal cultures are sterile. After completing a course of amphotericin B, maintenance therapy with itraconazole is initiated and continued for at least 6 months to a year. *C. immitis* meningitis is treated with intravenous amphotericin B (0.5 to 0.7 mg/kg per day) for ≥4 weeks until CSF fungal cultures are negative. Intrathecal amphotericin B may be required to eradicate the infection. Lifelong therapy with fluconazole is recommended to prevent relapse. Ambisome (4 mg/kg per day) or amphotericin B lipid complex (5 mg/kg per day) can be substituted for amphotericin B in patients who have or who develop significant renal dysfunction. The most common complication of fungal meningitis is hydrocephalus. Patients who develop hydrocephalus should receive a CSF diversion device. A ventriculostomy can be used until CSF fungal cultures are sterile, at which time the ventriculostomy is replaced by a ventriculoperitoneal shunt.

Syphilitic meningitis is treated with aqueous penicillin G in a dose of 3 to 4 million units intravenously every 4 h for 10 to 14 days. An alternative regimen is 2.4 million units of procaine penicillin G intramuscularly daily with 500 mg of oral probenecid four times daily for 10 to 14 days. Either regimen is followed with 2.4 million units of benzathine penicillin G intramuscularly once a week for 3 weeks. The standard criterion for treatment success is reexamination of the CSF. The CSF should be reexamined at 6-month intervals for 2 years. The cell count is expected to normalize within 12 months, and the VDRL titer to decrease by two dilutions or revert to nonreactive within 2 years of completion of therapy. Failure of the CSF pleocytosis to resolve or an increase in the CSF VDRL titer by two or more dilutions requires re-treatment.

CHRONIC ENCEPHALITIS

PROGRESSIVE MULTIFOCAL LEUKOENCEPHALOPATHY

Clinical Features and Pathology

Progressive multifocal leukoencephalopathy (PML) is a progressive disorder characterized pathologically by multifocal areas of demyelination of varying size distributed throughout the CNS. In addition to demyelination, there are characteristic cytologic alterations in both astrocytes and oligodendrocytes. Astrocytes are tremendously enlarged and contain hyperchromatic, deformed, and bizarre nuclei and frequent mitotic figures. Oligodendrocytes have enlarged, densely staining nuclei that contain viral inclusions formed by crystalline arrays of JC virus particles. Patients often present with visual deficits (45%), typically a homonymous hemianopia, and mental impairment (38%) (dementia, confusion, personality change). Motor weakness may not be present early but eventually occurs in 75% of cases.

Almost all patients have an underlying immunosuppressive disorder. Prior to the HIV epidemic, common associated diseases included lymphoproliferative disorders, immune deficiency states, myeloproliferative disease, and chronic infectious or granulomatous diseases. More than 60% of currently diagnosed PML cases occur in patients with AIDS. Conversely, it has been estimated that nearly 1% of AIDS patients will develop PML. The basic features of AIDS-associated and non-AIDS-associated PML are identical.

Diagnostic Studies

MRI reveals multifocal asymmetric, coalescing white matter lesions located periventricularly, in the centrum semiovale, in the parietal-occipital region, and in the cerebellum. These lesions have increased T2 and decreased T1 signal, are generally nonenhancing or show only minimal peripheral enhancement, and are not associated with edema or mass effect. CT scans, which are less sensitive than MRI for the diagnosis of PML, often show hypodense nonenhancing white matter lesions.

The CSF is typically normal, although mild elevation in protein and/or IgG may be found. Pleocytosis occurs in <25% of cases, is predominantly mononuclear, and rarely exceeds 25 cells/μL. PCR amplification of JC virus DNA from CSF has become an important diagnostic tool. CSF PCR for JC virus DNA has high specificity, but sensitivity has varied among studies. Rare cases of positive CSF PCR for JC virus DNA in the absence of clinical or radiographic evidence of PML have been described in HIV-infected patients. It remains to be established whether these results are false positives or indicate preclinical PML.

A positive CSF PCR for JC virus DNA in association with typical MRI lesions in the appropriate clinical setting is diagnostic of PML. Patients with negative CSF PCR studies may require brain biopsy for definitive diagnosis; JC virus antigen and nucleic acid can be detected by immunocytochemistry, in situ hybridization, or PCR amplification. Detection of JC virus antigen or genomic material should be considered diagnostic of PML only if accompanied by characteristic pathologic changes, since both antigen and genomic material have been found in the brains of normal patients.

TREATMENT FOR PML

No effective therapy is available. Recent trials in HIV-associated PML failed to show benefit from either cytarabine or cidofovir. Some patients with HIV-associated PML have shown dramatic clinical improvement associated with improvement in their immune status following institution of highly active antiretroviral therapy.

SUBACUTE SCLEROSING PANENCEPHALITIS

SSPE is a rare progressive demyelinating disease of the CNS associated with a chronic infection of brain tissue with measles virus. Most patients give a history of primary measles infection at an early age (2 years), which is followed after a latent interval of 6 to 8 years by the development of insidious intellectual decline and mood and personality changes. Typical signs of a CNS viral infection, including fever and headache, do not occur. Focal and/or generalized seizures, myoclonus, ataxia, and visual disturbances occur as the disease progresses. The EEG shows a characteristic periodic pattern with bursts every 3 to 8 s of high-voltage, sharp slow waves, followed by periods of attenuated ("flat") background. The CSF is acellular with a normal or mildly elevated protein level and a markedly elevated γ-globulin level (>20% of total CSF protein). CSF antimeasles antibody levels are invariably elevated, and oligoclonal antimeasles antibodies are often present. CT and MRI show evidence of multifocal white matter lesions and generalized atrophy. Measles virus can be cultured from brain tissue, and viral genome can be detected by in situ hybridization or PCR amplification. Treatment with isoprinosine (Inosiplex) (100 mg/kg per day), alone or in combination with intrathecal or intraventricular interferon, has been reported to prolong survival and produce clinical improvement in some patients but has never been subjected to a controlled clinical trial.

PROGRESSIVE RUBELLA PANENCEPHALITIS

This is an extremely rare disorder that primarily affects males with congenital rubella syndrome, although isolated cases have been reported following childhood rubella. After a latent period of 8 to 19 years, patients develop progressive neurologic deterioration. The manifestations are similar to those seen in SSPE. CSF shows a mild lymphocytic pleocytosis, slightly elevated protein level, markedly increased γ-globulin, and rubella virus–specific oligoclonal bands. No therapy is available.

BRAIN ABSCESS

DEFINITION

A brain abscess is a focal, suppurative infection within the brain parenchyma, typically surrounded by a vascularized capsule. The term *cerebritis* is often employed to describe a nonencapsulated brain abscess.

EPIDEMIOLOGY

A bacterial brain abscess is a relatively uncommon intracranial infection, with an incidence of ~1 in 100,000 persons per year. Predisposing conditions include otitis media and mastoiditis, paranasal sinusitis, pyogenic infections in the chest or other body sites, penetrating head trauma or neurosurgical procedures, and dental infections. In most modern series, an increasing proportion of brain abscesses are not caused by classic pyogenic bacteria, but rather by fungi and parasites including *Toxoplasma gondii, Aspergillus* spp., *Nocardia* spp., *Mycobacteria* spp., and *C. neoformans.* These organisms are almost exclusively restricted to immunocompromised hosts with underlying HIV infection, organ transplantation, cancer, or immunosuppressive therapy. In Latin America and in immigrants from Latin America, the most common cause of brain abscess is *Taenia solium* (neurocysticercosis). In India and the Far East, mycobacterial infection (tuberculoma) remains a major cause of focal CNS mass lesions.

ETIOLOGY

A brain abscess may develop (1) by direct spread from a contiguous cranial site of infection, such as paranasal sinusitis, otitis media, mastoiditis, or dental infection; (2) following head trauma or a neurosurgical procedure; or (3) as a result of hematogenous spread from a remote site of infection. In up to 25% of cases no obvious primary source of infection is apparent (cryptogenic brain abscess).

Up to one-third of brain abscesses are associated with otitis media and mastoiditis, often with an associated cholesteatoma. Otogenic abscesses occur predominantly in the temporal lobe (55 to 75%) and cerebellum (20 to 30%). In some series up to 90% of cerebellar abscesses are otogenic. Common organisms include streptococci, *Bacteroides* spp., *P. aeruginosa,* and Enterobacteriaceae. Abscesses that develop as a result of direct spread of infection from the frontal, ethmoidal, or sphenoidal sinuses and those that occur due to dental infections are usually located in the frontal lobes. Approximately 10% of brain abscesses are associated with paranasal sinusitis, and this association is particularly strong in young males in their second and third decades of life. The most common pathogens in brain abscesses associated with paranasal sinusitis are streptococci (especially *S. milleri*), *Haemophilus* spp., *Bacteroides* spp., *Pseudomonas* spp., and *S. aureus.* Dental infections are associated with ~2% of brain abscesses, although it is often suggested that many "cryptogenic" abscesses are in fact due to dental infections. The most common pathogens in this setting are streptococci, staphylococci, and *Bacteroides* and *Fusobacterium* spp.

Hematogenous abscesses account for ~25% of brain abscesses. These abscesses show a predilection for the territory of the middle cerebral artery (i.e., posterior frontal or parietal lobes). Hematogenous abscesses are often located at the junction of the gray and white matter and are often poorly encapsulated. Not surprisingly, hematogenous abscesses are often multiple, and multiple abscesses often have a hematogenous origin. The microbiology of these hematogenous abscesses is dependent on the primary source of infection. For example, brain abscesses that develop as a complication of infective endocarditis are often due to viridans streptococci or *S. aureus.* Abscesses associated with pyogenic lung infections such as lung abscess or bronchiectasis are often due to Streptococci, staphylococci, or *Bacteroides* or *Fusobacterium* spp. Enterobacteriaceae and *P. aeruginosa* are important causes of abscesses associated with urinary sepsis. Abscesses that follow penetrating head trauma or neurosurgical procedures are frequently due to staphylococci, Enterobacteriaceae, and *Pseudomonas* species. Congenital cardiac malformations that produce a right-to-left shunt (congenital cyanotic heart disease), such as tetralogy of Fallot, patent ductus arteriosus, and atrial and ventricular septal defects, allow bloodborne bacteria to bypass the pulmonary capillary bed and reach the brain. Similar phenomena can occur with pulmonary arteriovenous malformations. The decreased arterial oxygenation and saturation from the right-to-left shunt and polycythemia may cause focal areas of cerebral ischemia, thus providing a nidus for microorganisms that bypassed the pulmonary circulation to multiply and form an abscess. Streptococci are the most common pathogens in this setting.

PATHOGENESIS AND HISTOPATHOLOGY

The intact brain parenchyma is relatively resistant to infection; preexisting brain ischemia, necrosis, or hypoxia appears to be a prerequisite for effective bacterial invasion. Once infection is established, brain abscess frequently evolves through a series of stages, influenced by the nature of the infecting organism and by the immunocompetence of the host. The early cerebritis stage (days 1 to 3) is characterized by a perivascular infiltration of inflammatory cells, which surround a central core of coagulative necrosis. Marked edema surrounds the lesion at this stage. In the late cerebritis stage (days 4 to 9), pus formation leads to enlargement of the necrotic center, which is surrounded at its border by an inflammatory infiltrate of macrophages and fibroblasts. A thin capsule of fibroblasts and reticular fibers gradually develops, and the surrounding area of cerebral edema becomes more distinct than in the previous stage. The third stage, early capsule formation (days 10 to 13), is characterized by the formation of a capsule that is better developed on the cortical than on the ventricular side of the lesion. This stage correlates with the appearance of a ring-enhancing capsule on neuroimaging studies. The final stage, late capsule formation (day 14 and beyond), is defined by a well-formed necrotic center surrounded by a dense collagenous capsule. The surrounding area of cerebral edema has regressed, but marked gliosis with large numbers of reactive astrocytes has developed outside the capsule. This gliotic process may contribute to the development of seizures as a sequelae of brain abscess.

CLINICAL PRESENTATION

A brain abscess typically presents as an expanding intracranial mass lesion, rather than as an infectious process. Although the evolution of signs and symptoms is extremely variable, ranging from hours to weeks or even months, most patients present to the hospital 11 to 12 days following onset of symptoms. The classic clinical triad of headache, fever, and a focal neurologic deficit is present in <50% of cases. The most common symptom in patients with a brain abscess is headache, occurring in >75% of patients. The headache is often characterized as a constant, dull, aching sensation, either hemicranial or generalized, and it becomes progressively more severe and refractory to therapy. Fever is present in only 50% of patients at the time of diagnosis, and its absence should not exclude the diagnosis. The new onset of focal or generalized seizure activity is a presenting sign in 15 to 35% of patients. Focal neurologic deficits including hemiparesis, aphasia, or visual field defects are part of the initial presentation in >60% of patients.

The clinical presentation of a brain abscess depends on its location, the nature of the primary infection if present, and on the level of the ICP. Hemiparesis is the most common localizing sign of a frontal lobe abscess. A temporal lobe abscess may present with a disturbance of language (dysphasia) or an upper homonymous quadrantanopia. Nystagmus and ataxia are signs of a cerebellar abscess. Signs of raised ICP—papilledema, nausea and vomiting, and drowsiness or confusion—can be the dominant presentation of some abscesses, particularly those in the cerebellum. Meningismus is not present unless the abscess has ruptured into the ventricle or the infection has spread to the subarachnoid space.

DIAGNOSIS

Diagnosis is made by neuroimaging studies. MRI (**Fig. 29–3**) is better than CT for demonstrating abscesses in the early (cerebritis) stages and is superior to CT for identifying abscesses in the posterior fossa. A mature brain abscess appears on CT as a focal area of hypodensity

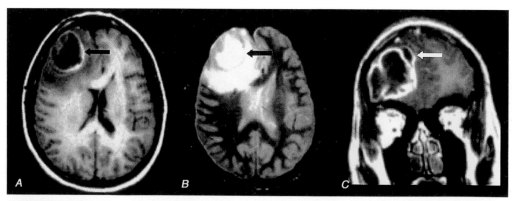

FIGURE 29-3
Pneumococcal brain abscess. Note that the abscess wall has hyperintense signal on the axial T1-weighted image (*A*, black arrow), hypointense signal on the axial proton density images (*B*, black arrow), and enhances prominently after gadolinium administration on the coronal T1-weighted image (*C*). The abscess is surrounded by a large amount of vasogenic edema and has a small "daughter" abscess (*C*, white arrow). (*Courtesy of Joseph Lurito, MD.*)

surrounded by ring enhancement. The CT and MRI appearance, particularly of the capsule, may be altered by treatment with glucocorticoids. The distinction between a brain abscess and other focal lesions such as tumors may be facilitated with diffusion-weighted imaging (DWI) sequences in which brain abscesses typically show increased signal and low apparent diffusion coefficient.

Microbiologic diagnosis of the etiologic agent is most accurately determined by Gram's stain and culture of abscess material obtained by stereotactic needle aspiration. Up to 10% of patients will also have positive blood cultures. LP should not be performed in patients with known or suspected focal intracranial infections such as abscess or empyema; CSF analysis contributes nothing to diagnosis or therapy, and LP increases the risk of herniation.

Additional laboratory studies may provide clues to the diagnosis of brain abscess in patients with a CNS mass lesion. About 50% of patients have a peripheral leukocytosis, 60% an elevated ESR, and 80% an elevated C-reactive protein.

DIFFERENTIAL DIAGNOSIS

Conditions that can cause headache, fever, focal neurologic signs, and seizure activity include brain abscess, subdural empyema, bacterial meningitis, viral meningoencephalitis, superior sagittal sinus thrombosis, and acute disseminated encephalomyelitis. When fever is absent, primary and metastatic brain tumors become the major differential diagnosis. Less commonly, cerebral infarction or hematoma can have an MRI or CT appearance resembling brain abscess.

TREATMENT FOR BRAIN ABSCESS

Optimal therapy of brain abscess involves a combination of high-dose parenteral antibiotics and neurosurgical drainage. Empirical therapy of community-acquired brain abscess in an immunocompetent patient typically includes a third-generation cephalosporin (e.g., cefotaxime or ceftriaxone) and metronidazole (see Table 29-2 for antibiotic dosages). In patients with penetrating head trauma or recent neurosurgical procedures, treatment should include ceftazidime as the third-generation cephalosporin to enhance coverage of *Pseudomonas* spp. and vancomycin for coverage of staphylococci. Meropenem plus vancomycin also provides good coverage in this setting.

Aspiration and drainage of the abscess under stereotaxic guidance are beneficial for both diagnosis

and therapy. Empirical antibiotic coverage should be modified based on the results of Gram's stain and culture of the abscess contents. Complete excision of a bacterial abscess via craniotomy or craniectomy is generally reserved for multiloculated abscesses or those in which stereotactic aspiration is unsuccessful.

Medical therapy alone is not optimal for treatment of brain abscess and should be reserved for patients whose abscesses are neurosurgically inaccessible, for patients with small nonencapsulated abscesses (cerebritis), and patients whose condition is too tenuous to allow performance of a neurosurgical procedure. All patients should receive a minimum of 6 to 8 weeks of parenteral antibiotic therapy. The role, if any, of supplemental oral antibiotic therapy following completion of a standard course of parenteral therapy has never been adequately studied.

Patients should also receive prophylactic anticonvulsant therapy because of the high risk of seizures. Anticonvulsant therapy is continued for at least 3 months after resolution of the abscess, and decisions regarding withdrawal are then based on the EEG. If the EEG is abnormal, anticonvulsant therapy should be continued. If the EEG is normal, anticonvulsant therapy can be slowly withdrawn, with close follow-up and repeat EEG after the medication has been discontinued.

Glucocorticoids should not be given routinely to patients with brain abscesses. Intravenous dexamethasone therapy (10 mg every 6 h) is usually reserved for patients with substantial periabscess edema and associated mass effect and increased ICP. Dexamethasone should be tapered as rapidly as possible to avoid delaying the natural process of encapsulation of the abscess.

Serial MRI or CT scans should be obtained on a monthly or twice-monthly basis to document resolution of the abscess. More frequent studies (e.g., weekly) are probably warranted in the subset of patients who are receiving antibiotic therapy alone. A small amount of enhancement may remain for months after the abscess has been successfully treated.

PROGNOSIS

The mortality of brain abscess has declined in parallel with the development of enhanced neuroimaging techniques, improved neurosurgical procedures for stereotactic aspiration, and improved antibiotics. In modern series the mortality is typically <15%. Significant sequelae including seizures, persisting weakness, aphasia, or mental impairment occur in ≥20% of survivors.

NONBACTERIAL CAUSES OF INFECTIOUS FOCAL CNS LESIONS

ETIOLOGY

Neurocysticercosis is the most common parasitic disease of the CNS worldwide. Humans acquire cysticercosis by the ingestion of food contaminated with the eggs of the parasite *T. solium*. Eggs are contained in undercooked pork or in drinking water or other foods contaminated with human feces. *T. gondii* is a parasite that is acquired from the ingestion of undercooked meat and from handling cat feces.

CLINICAL PRESENTATION

The most common manifestation of neurocysticercosis is new-onset partial seizures with or without secondary generalization. Cysticerci may develop in the brain parenchyma and cause seizures or focal neurologic deficits. When present in the subarachnoid or ventricular spaces, cysticerci can produce increased ICP by interference with CSF flow. Spinal cysticerci can mimic the presentation of intraspinal tumors. When the cysticerci first lodge in the brain, they frequently cause little in the way of an inflammatory response. As the cysticercal cyst degenerates, it elicits an inflammatory response that may present clinically as a seizure. Eventually the cyst dies, a process that may take several years, and is typically associated with resolution of the inflammatory response and often abatement of seizures.

Primary *Toxoplasma* infection is often asymptomatic. However, during this phase parasites may spread to the CNS, where they become latent. Reactivation of CNS infection is almost exclusively associated with immunocompromised hosts, particularly those with HIV infection. During this phase patients present with headache, fever, seizures, and focal neurologic deficits.

DIAGNOSIS

The lesions of neurocysticercosis are readily visualized by MRI or CT scans. Parenchymal brain calcifications are the most common finding. The scolex can often be visualized on MRI. A very early sign of cyst death is hypointensity of the vesicular fluid on T2-weighted images when compared with CSF. MRI findings consist of multiple lesions in the deep white matter, the thalamus, and basal ganglia and at the gray-white junction in the cerebral

hemispheres. With contrast administration, the majority of the lesions enhance in a ringed, nodular, or homogeneous pattern and are surrounded by edema. In the presence of the characteristic neuroimaging abnormalities of this parasitic infection, serum anti–*T. gondii* antibodies should be obtained; if positive, the patient should be treated.

TREATMENT FOR NEUROCYSTICERCOSIS AND CNS TOXOPLASMOSIS

Anticonvulsant therapy is initiated when the patient with neurocysticercosis presents with a seizure. There is controversy about whether or not antihelminthic therapy should be given to all patients. Such therapy does not necessarily reduce the risk of seizure recurrence, but the control of seizures is easier after treatment with cysticidal drugs than when the disease is untreated. Albendazole and praziquantel are used in the treatment of neurocysticercosis. Approximately 85% of parenchymal cysts are destroyed by a single course of albendazole and ~75% are destroyed by a single course of praziquantel. The dose of albendazole is 15 mg/kg per day in two doses for 8 days. The dose of praziquantel is 50 mg/kg per day for 15 days, although a number of other dosage regimens are also frequently cited. Antiepileptic therapy can be stopped once the follow-up CT scan shows resolution of the lesion. Long-term antiepileptic therapy is recommended when seizures occur after resolution of edema and resorption or calcification of the degenerating cyst.

CNS toxoplasmosis is treated with a combination of sulfadiazine, 1.5 to 2.0 g orally qid, plus pyrimethamine, 100 mg orally to load then 75 to 100 mg orally qd, plus folinic acid, 10 to 15 mg orally qd. Folinic acid is added to the regimen to prevent megaloblastic anemia. Therapy is continued until there is no evidence of active disease on neuroimaging studies, which typically takes at least 6 weeks, and then the dose of sulfadiazine is reduced to 2 to 4 g/d and pyrimethamine to 50 mg/d. Clindamycin plus pyrimethamine is an alternative therapy for patients who cannot tolerate sulfadiazine, but the combination of pyrimethamine and sulfadiazine is more effective.

SUBDURAL EMPYEMA

A subdural empyema (SDE) is a collection of pus between the dura and arachnoid membranes (**Fig. 29-4**).

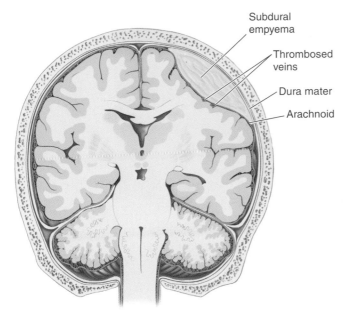

Subdural empyema

Thrombosed veins

Dura mater

Arachnoid

FIGURE 29-4

Subdural empyema is a collection of pus between the dura and arachnoid membranes

EPIDEMIOLOGY

SDE is a rare disorder that accounts for 15 to 25% of focal suppurative CNS infections. Sinusitis is the most common predisposing condition and typically involves the frontal sinuses, either alone or in combination with the ethmoid and maxillary sinuses. Sinusitis-associated empyema has a striking predilection for young males, possibly reflecting sex-related differences in sinus anatomy and development. It has been suggested that SDE may complicate 1 to 2% of cases of frontal sinusitis severe enough to require hospitalization. As a consequence of this epidemiology, SDE shows an ~3:1 male:female predominance, with 70% of cases occurring in the second and third decades of life. SDE may also develop as a complication of head trauma or neurosurgery. Secondary infection of a subdural effusion may also result in empyema, although secondary infection of hematomas, in the absence of a prior neurosurgical procedure, is rare.

ETIOLOGY

Aerobic and anaerobic streptococci, staphylococci, Enterobacteriaceae, and anaerobic bacteria are the most common causative organisms of sinusitis-associated SDE. Staphylococci and gram-negative bacilli are often the etiologic organisms when SDE follows neurosurgical procedures or head trauma. Up to one-third of cases are culture-negative, possibly reflecting difficulty in obtaining adequate anaerobic cultures.

PATHOPHYSIOLOGY

Sinusitis-associated SDE develops as a result of either retrograde spread of infection from septic thrombophlebitis of the mucosal veins draining the sinuses or contiguous spread of infection to the brain from osteomyelitis in the posterior wall of the frontal or other sinuses. SDE may also develop from direct introduction of bacteria into the subdural space as a complication of a neurosurgical procedure. The evolution of SDE can be extremely rapid because the subdural space is a large compartment that offers few mechanical barriers to the spread of infection. In patients with sinusitis-associated SDE, suppuration typically begins in the upper and anterior portions of one cerebral hemisphere and then extends posteriorly. SDE is often associated with other intracranial infections including epidural empyema (40%), cortical thrombophlebitis (35%), and intracranial abscess or cerebritis (>25%). Cortical venous infarction produces necrosis of underlying cerebral cortex and subcortical white matter, with focal neurologic deficits and seizures (see below).

CLINICAL PRESENTATION

A patient with SDE typically presents with fever and a progressively worsening headache. The diagnosis of SDE should always be suspected in a patient with known sinusitis who presents with new CNS signs or symptoms. Patients with underlying sinusitis frequently have symptoms related to this infection. As the infection progresses, focal neurologic deficits, seizures, nuchal rigidity, and signs of increased ICP commonly occur. Headache is the most common complaint at the time of presentation; initially it is localized to the side of the subdural infection but then becomes more severe and generalized. Contralateral hemiparesis or hemiplegia is the most common focal neurologic deficit and can occur from the direct effects of the SDE on the cortex or as a consequence of venous infarction. Seizures begin as partial motor seizures that then become secondarily generalized. Seizures may be due to the direct irritative effect of the SDE on the underlying cortex or result from cortical venous infarction (see above). In untreated SDE, the increasing mass effect and increase in ICP cause progressive deterioration in consciousness, leading ultimately to coma.

DIAGNOSIS

MRI (**Fig. 29-5**) is superior to CT in identifying SDE and any associated intracranial infections. The administration of

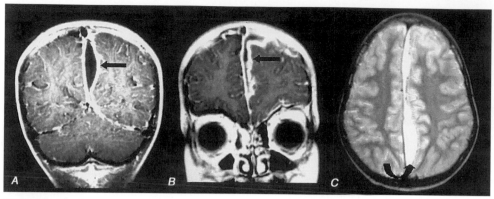

FIGURE 29-5

Subdural empyema. There is marked enhancement of the dura and leptomeninges (*A*, *B*, straight arrows) along the left medial hemisphere. The pus is hypointense on T1-weighted images (*A*, *B*), but markedly hyperintense on the proton density–weighted (*C*, curved arrow) image. (*Courtesy of Joseph Lurito, MD.*)

gadolinium greatly improves diagnosis by enhancing the rim of the empyema and allowing the empyema to be clearly delineated from the underlying brain parenchyma. Cranial MRI is also extremely valuable in identifying sinusitis, other focal CNS infections, cortical venous infarction, cerebral edema, and cerebritis. CT may show a crescent-shaped hypodense lesion over one or both hemispheres or in the interhemispheric fissure. Frequently the degree of mass effect, exemplified by midline shift, ventricular compression, and sulcal effacement, is far out of proportion to the mass of the SDE.

CSF examination should be avoided in patients with known or suspected SDE as it adds no useful information and is associated with the risk of cerebral herniation.

DIFFERENTIAL DIAGNOSIS

The differential diagnosis of the combination of headache, fever, focal neurologic signs, and seizure activity that progresses rapidly to an altered level of consciousness includes subdural hematoma, bacterial meningitis, viral encephalitis, brain abscess, superior sagittal sinus thrombosis, and acute disseminated encephalomyelitis. The presence of nuchal rigidity is unusual with brain abscess or epidural empyema and should suggest the possibility of SDE when associated with significant focal neurologic signs and fever. Patients with bacterial meningitis also have nuchal rigidity but do not typically have focal deficits of the severity seen with SDE.

TREATMENT FOR SDE

SDE is a medical emergency. Emergent neurosurgical evacuation of the empyema, either through burr-hole drainage or craniotomy, is the definitive step in the management of this infection. Empirical antimicrobial therapy should include a combination of a third-generation cephalosporin (e.g., cefotaxime or ceftriaxone), vancomycin, and metronidazole (see Table 29-2 for dosages). Parenteral antibiotic therapy should be continued for a minimum of 4 weeks. Specific diagnosis of the etiologic organisms is made based on Gram's stain and culture of fluid obtained via either burr holes or craniotomy; the initial empirical antibiotic coverage can be modified accordingly.

PROGNOSIS

Prognosis is influenced by the level of consciousness of the patient at the time of hospital presentation, the size of the empyema, and the speed with which therapy is instituted. Long-term neurologic sequelae, which include seizures and hemiparesis, occur in up to 50% of cases.

EPIDURAL ABSCESS

Cranial epidural abscess is a suppurative infection occurring in the potential space between the inner skull table and dura (**Fig. 29-6**).

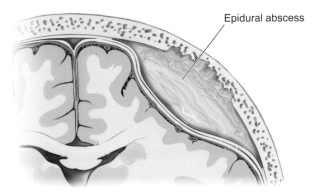

Epidural abscess

FIGURE 29-6
Cranial epidural abscess is a collection of pus between the dura and the inner table of the skull.

ETIOLOGY AND PATHOPHYSIOLOGY

Cranial epidural abscess is less common than either brain abscess or SDE and accounts for <2% of focal suppurative CNS infections. A cranial epidural abscess develops as a complication of a craniotomy or compound skull fracture or as a result of spread of infection from the frontal sinuses, middle ear, mastoid, or orbit. An epidural abscess may develop contiguous to an area of osteomyelitis, when craniotomy is complicated by infection of the wound or bone flap, or as a result of direct infection of the epidural space. Infection in the frontal sinus, middle ear, mastoid, or orbit can reach the epidural space through retrograde spread of infection from septic thrombophlebitis in the emissary veins that drain these areas or by way of direct spread of infection through areas of osteomyelitis. Unlike the subdural space, the epidural space is really a potential rather than an actual compartment. The dura is normally tightly adherent to the inner skull table, and infection must dissect the dura away from the skull table as it spreads. As a result, epidural abscesses are often smaller than SDEs. Cranial epidural abscesses, unlike brain abscesses, only rarely result from hematogenous spread of infection from extracranial primary sites. The bacteriology of a cranial epidural abscess is similar to that of SDE (see above). The etiologic organisms of an epidural abscess that arises from frontal sinusitis, middle ear infections, or mastoiditis are usually streptococci or anaerobic organisms. Staphylococci or gram-negative organisms are the usual cause of an epidural abscess that develops as a complication of craniotomy or compound skull fracture.

CLINICAL PRESENTATION

Patients present with fever (60%), headache (40%), nuchal rigidity (35%), seizures (10%), and focal deficits (5%). Periorbital edema and Potts puffy tumor, reflecting underlying associated frontal bone osteomyelitis, are present in ~40%. In patients with a recent neurosurgical procedure, wound infection is invariably present, but other symptoms may be subtle and can include altered mental status (45%), fever (35%), and headache (20%). The diagnosis should also be considered when fever and headache follow recent head trauma or occur in the setting of frontal sinusitis, mastoiditis, or otitis media.

DIAGNOSIS

Cranial MRI is the procedure of choice to demonstrate a cranial epidural abscess. The sensitivity of CT is limited by the presence of signal artifacts arising from the bone of the inner skull table. The CT appearance of an epidural empyema is that of a lens or crescent-shaped hypodense extraaxial lesion. On MRI, an epidural empyema appears as a lentiform or crescent-shaped fluid collection that is hyperintense compared to CSF on T2-weighted images. On T1-weighted images, the fluid collection has a signal intensity that is intermediate between that of brain tissue and CSF. Following the administration of gadolinium, a significant enhancement of the dura is seen on T1-weighted images. In distinction to subdural empyema, signs of mass effect or other parenchymal abnormalities are uncommon.

TREATMENT FOR EPIDURAL ABSCESS

Immediate neurosurgical drainage is indicated. Empirical antimicrobial therapy, pending the results of Gram's stain and culture of the purulent material obtained at surgery, should include a combination of a third-generation cephalosporin, nafcillin or vancomycin, and metronidazole (Table 29-2). Ceftazidime should be substituted for ceftriaxone or cefotaxime in neurosurgical patients. Meropenem and vancomycin also provide effective empirical therapy in postneurosurgical cases. When the organism has been identified, antimicrobial therapy can be modified accordingly. Antibiotics should be continued for at least 3 weeks after surgical drainage.

PROGNOSIS

Mortality is <5% in modern series, and full recovery is the rule in most survivors.

SUPPURATIVE THROMBOPHLEBITIS

DEFINITION

Suppurative intracranial thrombophlebitis is septic venous thrombosis of cortical veins and sinuses. This may occur as a complication of bacterial meningitis; SDE; epidural abscess; or infection in the skin of the face, paranasal sinuses, middle ear, or mastoid.

ANATOMY AND PATHOPHYSIOLOGY

The cerebral veins and venous sinuses have no valves; therefore, blood within them can flow in either direction. The superior sagittal sinus is the largest of the venous sinuses (**Fig. 29-7**). It receives blood from the frontal, parietal, and occipital superior cerebral veins and the diploic veins, which communicate with the meningeal veins. Bacterial meningitis is a common predisposing condition for septic thrombosis of the superior sagittal sinus. The diploic veins, which drain into the superior sagittal sinus, provide a route for the spread of infection from the meninges, especially in cases where there is purulent exudate near areas of the superior sagittal sinus. Infection can also spread to the superior sagittal sinus from nearby SDE or epidural abscess. Dehydration from vomiting, hypercoagulable states, and immunologic abnormalities, including the presence of circulating antiphospholipid antibodies, also contribute to cerebral venous sinus thrombosis. Thrombosis may extend from one sinus to another, and often at autopsy thrombi of different histologic ages can be detected in several sinuses. Thrombosis of the superior sagittal sinus is often associated with thrombosis of superior cortical veins and small parenchymal hemorrhages.

The superior sagittal sinus drains into the transverse sinuses (Fig. 29-7). The transverse sinuses also receive venous drainage from small veins from both the middle ear and mastoid cells. The transverse sinus becomes the sigmoid sinus before draining into the internal jugular vein. Septic transverse/sigmoid sinus thrombosis can be a complication of acute and chronic otitis media or mastoiditis. Infection spreads from the mastoid air cells to the transverse sinus via the emissary veins or by direct invasion. The cavernous sinuses are inferior to the superior sagittal sinus at the base of the skull. The cavernous sinuses receive blood from the facial veins via the superior and inferior ophthalmic veins. Bacteria in the facial veins enter the cavernous sinus via these veins. Bacteria in the sphenoid and ethmoid sinuses can spread to the cavernous sinuses via the small emissary veins. The sphenoid and ethmoid sinuses are the most common sites of primary infection resulting in septic cavernous sinus thrombosis.

CLINICAL MANIFESTATIONS

Septic thrombosis of the superior sagittal sinus presents with headache, fever, nausea and vomiting, confusion, and focal or generalized seizures. There may be a rapid development of stupor and coma. Weakness of the lower extremities with bilateral Babinski signs or hemiparesis is often present. When superior sagittal sinus thrombosis occurs as a complication of bacterial meningitis, nuchal rigidity and Kernig's and Brudzinski's signs may be present.

The oculomotor nerve, the trochlear nerve, the abducens nerve, the ophthalmic and maxillary branches of the trigeminal nerve, and the internal carotid artery all pass through the cavernous sinus. The symptoms of *septic cavernous sinus thrombosis* are fever, headache, frontal and retroorbital pain, and diplopia. The classic signs are ptosis, proptosis, chemosis, and extraocular dysmotility due to deficits of cranial nerves III, IV, and VI; hyperesthesia of the ophthalmic and maxillary divisions of the fifth cranial nerve and a decreased corneal reflex may be detected. There may be evidence of dilated, tortuous retinal veins and papilledema.

Headache and earache are the most frequent symptoms of *transverse sinus thrombosis.* A transverse sinus thrombosis may also present with otitis media, sixth nerve palsy, and retroorbital or facial pain (*Gradinego's syndrome*). Sigmoid sinus and internal jugular vein thrombosis may present with neck pain.

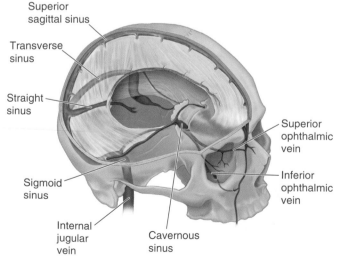

Superior
sagittal sinus

Transverse
sinus

Straight
sinus

Sigmoid
sinus

Internal
jugular
vein

Cavernous
sinus

Superior
ophthalmic
vein

Inferior
ophthalmic
vein

FIGURE 29-7
Anatomy of the cerebral venous sinuses.

DIAGNOSIS

The diagnosis of septic venous sinus thrombosis is suggested by an absent flow void within the affected venous sinus on MRI and confirmed by magnetic resonance venography or the venous phase of cerebral angiography. The diagnosis of thrombophlebitis of intracerebral and meningeal veins is suggested by the presence of intracerebral hemorrhage but requires cerebral angiography for definitive diagnosis.

TREATMENT FOR SUPPURATIVE THROMBOPHLEBITIS

Septic venous sinus thrombosis is usually treated with antibiotics and hydration. The choice of antimicrobial therapy is based on the bacteria responsible for the predisposing or associated condition. Optimal duration of therapy is unknown, but antibiotics are usually continued for 6 weeks or until there is radiographic evidence of resolution of thrombosis. Anticoagulation with dose-adjusted heparin has been reported to be beneficial in patients with aseptic venous sinus thrombosis; it is also used in the treatment of septic venous sinus thrombosis complicating bacterial meningitis in patients who are worsening despite antimicrobial therapy and intravenous fluids. The presence of a small intracerebral hemorrhage from septic thrombophlebitis is not an absolute contraindication to heparin therapy. Successful management of aseptic venous sinus thrombosis has been reported with urokinase therapy and with a combination of intrathrombus recombinant tissue plasminogen activator (rtPA) and intravenous heparin, but the efficacy of these therapies in septic venous sinus thrombosis is unknown.

FURTHER READINGS

☑ DEAN JL, PALERMO BJ: West Nile virus encephalitis. Curr Infect Dis Rep 7:292, 2005

   A review of neurologic complications of West Nile virus infection.

☑ DE GANS J, VAN DE BEEK D: Dexamethasone in adults with bacterial meningitis. N Engl J Med 347:1549, 2002

   Study establishing the role of corticosteroids in acute bacterial meningitis.

DWORKIN MS: A review of progressive multifocal leukoencephalopathy in persons with and without AIDS. Curr Clin Top Infect Dis 22:181, 2002

LU CH et al: Bacterial brain abscess: Microbiological features, epidemiological trends and therapeutic outcomes. QJM ed 95:501, 2002

ROOS KL: Acute bacterial meningitis. Semin Neurol 20:293, 2000

ROSENSTEIN NE et al: Meningococcal disease. N Engl J Med 344:1378, 2001

SOLOMON T et al: West Nile encephalitis, BMJ 326:865, 2003

THWAITES G et al: Dexamethasone for the treatment of tuberculous meningitis in adolescents and adults. New Engl J Med 351:1741, 2004

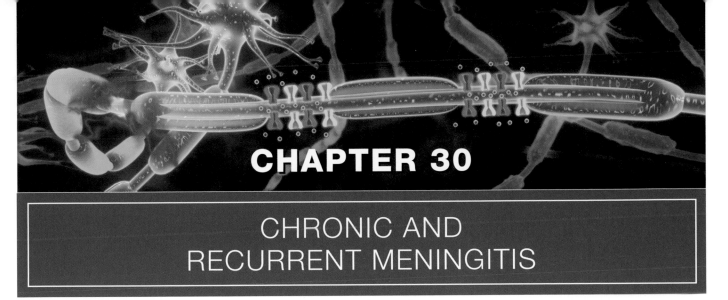

CHAPTER 30

CHRONIC AND RECURRENT MENINGITIS

Walter J. Koroshetz
Morton N. Swartz

Chronic inflammation of the meninges (pia, arachnoid, and dura) can produce profound neurologic disability and may be fatal if not successfully treated. The condition is most commonly diagnosed when a characteristic neurologic syndrome exists for >4 weeks and is associated with a persistent inflammatory response in the cerebrospinal fluid (CSF) (white blood cell count >5/μL). The causes are varied, and appropriate treatment depends on identification of the etiology. Five cat-

egories of disease account for most cases of chronic meningitis: (1) meningeal infections, (2) malignancy, (3) noninfectious inflammatory disorders, (4) chemical meningitis, and (5) parameningeal infections.

CLINICAL PATHOPHYSIOLOGY

Neurologic manifestations of chronic meningitis (**Table 30-1**) are determined by the anatomical location of the inflammation and its consequences. Persistent headache with or without stiff neck, and hydrocephalus, cranial neuropathies, radiculopathies, and cognitive or personality changes are the cardinal features. These can occur alone or in combination. When they appear in combination, widespread dissemination of the inflammatory process along CSF pathways has occurred. In some cases, the presence of

TABLE 30-1

SYMPTOMS AND SIGNS OF CHRONIC MENINGITIS	
SYMPTOM	**SIGN**
Chronic headache	+/− Papilledema
Neck or back pain	Brudzinski's or Kernig's sign of meningeal irritation
Change in personality	Altered mental status — drowsiness, inattention, disorientation, memory loss, frontal release signs (grasp, suck, snout), perseveration
Facial weakness	Peripheral seventh CN palsy
Double vision	Palsy of CNs III, IV, VI
Visual loss	Papilledema, optic atrophy
Hearing loss	Eighth CN palsy
Arm or leg weakness	Myelopathy or radiculopathy
Numbness in arms or legs	Myelopathy or radiculopathy
Sphincter dysfunction	Myelopathy or radiculopathy
	Frontal lobe dysfunction
Clumsiness	Ataxia

Note: CN, cranial nerve.

an underlying systemic illness points to a specific agent or class of agents as the probable cause. The diagnosis of chronic meningitis is usually made when the clinical presentation prompts the astute physician to examine the CSF for signs of inflammation. CSF is produced by the choroid plexus of the cerebral ventricles, exits through narrow foramina into the subarachnoid space surrounding the brain and spinal cord, circulates around the base of the brain and over the cerebral hemispheres, and is resorbed by arachnoid villi projecting into the superior sagittal sinus. CSF flow provides a pathway for rapid spread of infectious and malignant processes over the brain, spinal cord, and cranial and spinal nerve roots. Spread from the subarachnoid space into brain parenchyma may occur via the arachnoid cuffs that surround blood vessels that penetrate brain tissue (Virchow-Robin spaces).

INTRACRANIAL MENINGITIS

Nociceptive fibers of the meninges are stimulated by the inflammatory process, resulting in headache or neck or back pain. Obstruction of CSF pathways at foramina or arachnoid villi may produce *hydrocephalus* and symptoms of raised intracranial pressure (ICP), including headache, vomiting, apathy or drowsiness, gait instability, papilledema, visual loss, impaired upgaze, or palsy of the sixth cranial nerve (CN). Cognitive and behavioral changes during the course of chronic meningitis may also result from vascular damage, which may similarly produce seizures, stroke, or myelopathy. Inflammatory deposits seeded via the CSF circulation are often prominent around the brainstem and cranial nerves and along the undersurface of the frontal and temporal lobes. Such cases, termed *basal meningitis,* often present as multiple cranial neuropathies, with visual loss (CN II), facial weakness (CN VII), hearing loss (CN VIII), diplopia (CNs III, IV, and VI), sensory or motor abnormalities of the oropharynx (CNs IX, X, and XII), decreased olfaction (CN I), or facial sensory loss and masseter weakness (CN V).

SPINAL MENINGITIS

Injury may occur to motor and sensory roots as they traverse the subarachnoid space and penetrate the meninges. These cases present as multiple radiculopathies with combinations of radicular pain, sensory loss, motor weakness, and sphincter dysfunction. Meningeal inflammation can encircle the cord, resulting in myelopathy. Patients with slowly progressive involvement of multiple cranial nerves and/or spinal nerve roots are likely to have chronic meningitis. Electrophysiologic testing (electromyography, nerve conduction studies, and evoked response testing) may be helpful in determining whether there is involvement of cranial and spinal nerve roots.

SYSTEMIC MANIFESTATIONS

In some patients, evidence of systemic disease provides clues to the underlying cause of chronic meningitis. A careful history and physical examination are essential before embarking on a diagnostic workup, which may be costly, prolonged, and associated with risk from invasive procedures. A complete history of travel, sexual practice, and exposure to infectious agents should be sought. Infectious causes are often associated with fever, malaise, anorexia, and signs of localized or disseminated infection outside the nervous system. Infectious causes are of major concern in the immunosuppressed patient, especially in patients with AIDS, in whom chronic meningitis may present without headache or fever. Noninfectious inflammatory disorders often produce systemic manifestations, but meningitis may be the initial manifestation. Carcinomatous meningitis may or may not be accompanied by clinical evidence of the primary neoplasm.

APPROACH TO THE PATIENT WITH MENINGITIS

The occurrence of chronic headache, hydrocephalus, cranial neuropathy, radiculopathy, and/or cognitive decline in a patient should prompt consideration of a lumbar puncture for evidence of meningeal inflammation. On occasion the diagnosis is made when an imaging study [computed tomography (CT) or magnetic resonance imaging (MRI)] shows contrast enhancement of the meninges, always abnormal with the exception of dural enhancement after lumbar puncture, neurosurgical procedures, or spontaneous CSF leakage. Once chronic meningitis is confirmed by CSF examination, effort is focused on identifying the cause (**Tables 30-2** and **30-3**) by (1) further analysis of the CSF, (2) diagnosis of an underlying systemic infection or noninfectious inflammatory condition, or (3) pathologic examination of meningeal biopsy specimens.

Two clinical forms of chronic meningitis exist. In the first, the symptoms are chronic and persistent, whereas in the second there are recurrent, discrete episodes of illness. In the latter group, all symptoms, signs, and CSF parameters of meningeal inflammation resolve completely between episodes without specific therapy. In such patients, the likely etiologies include infection with herpes simplex virus (HSV) type 2; chemical meningitis due to leakage into CSF of contents from an epidermoid tumor, craniopharyngioma, or cholesteatoma; primary inflammatory conditions, including Vogt-

TABLE 30-2

INFECTIOUS CAUSES OF CHRONIC MENINGITIS

CAUSATIVE AGENT	CSF FORMULA	HELPFUL DIAGNOSTIC TESTS	RISK FACTORS AND SYSTEMIC MANIFESTATIONS
COMMON BACTERIAL CAUSES			
Partially treated suppurative meningitis	Mononuclear or mixed mononuclear-polymorphonuclear cells	CSF culture and Gram stain	History consistent with acute bacterial meningitis and incomplete treatment
Parameningeal infection	Mononuclear or mixed polymorphonuclear-mononuclear cells	Contrast-enhanced CT or MRI to detect parenchymal, subdural, epidural, or sinus infection	Otitis media, pleuropulmonary infection, right-to-left cardiopulmonary shunt for brain abscess; focal neurologic signs; neck, back, ear, or sinus tenderness
Mycobacterium tuberculosis	Mononuclear cells except polymorphonuclear cells in early infection (commonly <500 WBC/μL); low CSF glucose, high protein	Tuberculin skin test may be negative; AFB culture of CSF (sputum, urine, gastric contents if indicated); tuberculostearic acid detection in CSF; identify tubercle bacillus on acid-fast stain of CSF or protein pellicle; PCR	Exposure history; previous tuberculous illness; immunosuppressed or AIDS; young children; fever, meningismus, night sweats, miliary TB on x-ray or liver biopsy; stroke due to arteritis
Lyme disease (Bannwarth's syndrome) *Borrelia burgdorferi*	Mononuclear cells; elevated protein	Serum Lyme antibody titer; western blot confirmation; (patients with syphilis may have false-positive Lyme titer)	History of tick bite or appropriate exposure history; erythema chronicum migrans skin rash; arthritis, radiculopathy, Bell's palsy, meningoencephalitis–multiple sclerosis-like syndrome
Syphilis (secondary, tertiary) *Treponema pallidum*	Mononuclear cells; elevated protein	CSF VDRL; serum VDRL (or RPR); fluorescent treponemal antibody-absorbed (FTA) or MHA-TP; serum VDRL may be negative in tertiary syphilis	Appropriate exposure history; HIV seropositive individuals at increased risk of aggressive infection; "dementia"; cerebral infarction due to endarteritis
UNCOMMON BACTERIAL CAUSES			
Actinomyces	Polymorphonuclear cells	Anaerobic culture	Parameningeal abscess or sinus tract (oral or dental focus); pneumonitis
Nocardia	Polymorphonuclear; occasionally mononuclear cells; often low glucose	Isolation may require weeks; weakly acid fast	Associated brain abscess may be present
Brucella	Mononuclear cells (rarely polymorphonuclear); elevated protein; often low glucose	CSF antibody detection; serum antibody detection	Intake of unpasteurized dairy products; exposure to goats, sheep, cows; fever, arthralgia, myalgia, vertebral osteomyelitis
Whipple's disease *Tropheryma whipplei*	Mononuclear cells	Biopsy of small bowel or lymph node; CSF PCR for *T. whipplei;* brain and meningeal biopsy (with PAS stain and EM examination)	Diarrhea, weight loss, arthralgias, fever; dementia, ataxia, paresis, ophthalmoplegia, oculomasticatory myoclonus

(continued)

TABLE 30-2   *(Continued)*

INFECTIOUS CAUSES OF CHRONIC MENINGITIS

CAUSATIVE AGENT	CSF FORMULA	HELPFUL DIAGNOSTIC TESTS	RISK FACTORS AND SYSTEMIC MANIFESTATIONS
RARE BACTERIAL CAUSES			
Leptospirosis (occasionally if left untreated may last 3–4 weeks)			
FUNGAL CAUSES			
Cryptococcus neoformans	Mononuclear cells; count not elevated in some patients with AIDS	India ink or fungal wet mount of CSF (budding yeast); blood and urine cultures; antigen detection in CSF	AIDS and immune suppression; pigeon exposure; skin and other organ involvement due to disseminated infection
Coccidioides immitis	Mononuclear cells (sometimes 10–20% eosinophils); often low glucose	Antibody detection in CSF and serum	Exposure history — southwestern U.S.; increased virulence in dark-skinned races
Candida sp.	Polymorphonuclear or mononuclear	Fungal stain and culture of CSF	IV drug abuse; post surgery; prolonged intravenous therapy; disseminated candidiasis
Histoplasma capsulatum	Mononuclear cells; low glucose	Fungal stain and culture of large volumes of CSF; antigen detection in CSF, serum, and urine; antibody detection in serum, CSF	Exposure history — Ohio and central Mississippi River Valley; AIDS; mucosal lesions Midwestern and Southeastern USA; usually systemic infection; abscesses, draining sinus, ulcers
Blastomyces dermatitidis	Mononuclear cells	Fungal stain and culture of CSF; biopsy and culture of skin, lung lesions; antibody detection in serum	
Aspergillus sp.	Mononuclear or polymorphonuclear	CSF culture	Sinusitis; granulocytopenia or immunosuppression
Sporothrix schenckii	Mononuclear cells	Antibody detection in CSF and serum; CSF culture	Traumatic inoculation; IV drug use; ulcerated skin lesion
RARE FUNGAL CAUSES			
Xylohypha (formerly *Cladosporium*) *trichoides* and other dark-walled (demateaceous) fungi such as *Curvularia,*		*Drechslera; Mucor, Pseudallescheria boydii*	
PROTOZOAL CAUSES			
Toxoplasma gondii	Mononuclear cells	Biopsy or response to empirical therapy in clinically appropriate context (including presence of antibody in serum)	Usually with intracerebral abscesses common in HIV seropositive patients
Trypanosomiasis *Trypanosoma gambiense, T. rhodesiense*	Mononuclear cells, elevated protein	Elevated CSF IgM; identification of trypanosomes in CSF and blood smear	Endemic in Africa; chancre, lymphadenopathy; prominent sleep disorder
RARE PROTOZOAL CAUSES			
Acanthamoeba sp. causing granulomatous amebic encephalitis and meningoencephalitis in immunocompromised		and debilitated individuals	
HELMINTHIC CAUSES			
Cysticercosis (infection with cysts of *Taenia solium*)	Mononuclear cells; may have eosinophils; glucose level may be low	Indirect hemagglutination assay in CSF; ELISA immunoblotting in serum	Usually with multiple cysts in basal meninges and hydrocephalus; cerebral cysts, muscle calcification

(continued)

TABLE 30-2 *(Continued)*

INFECTIOUS CAUSES OF CHRONIC MENINGITIS

CAUSATIVE AGENT	CSF FORMULA	HELPFUL DIAGNOSTIC TESTS	RISK FACTORS AND SYSTEMIC MANIFESTATIONS
Gnathostoma spinigerum	Eosinophils, mononuclear cells	Peripheral eosinophilia	History of eating raw fish; common in Thailand and Japan; subarachnoid hemorrhage; painful radiculopathy
Angiostrongylus cantonensis	Eosinophils, mononuclear cells	Recovery of worms from CSF	History of eating raw shellfish; common in tropical Pacific regions; often benign
Baylisascaris procyonis (raccoon ascarid)	Eosinophils, mononuclear cells		Infection follows accidental ingestion of *B. procyonis* eggs from raccoon feces; fatal meningoencephalitis

RARE HELMINTHIC CAUSES

Trichinella spiralis (trichinosis); *Echinococcus* cysts; *Schistosoma* sp. The former may produce a lymphocytic pleocytosis whereas the latter two may produce an eosinophilic response in CSF associated with cerebral cysts (*Echinococcus*) or granulomatous lesions of brain or spinal cord

VIRAL CAUSES

Mumps	Mononuclear cells	Antibody in serum	No prior mumps or immunization; may produce meningoencephalitis; may persist for 3–4 weeks
Lymphocytic choriomeningitis	Mononuclear cells	Antibody in serum	Contact with rodents or their excreta; may persist for 3–4 weeks
Echovirus	Mononuclear cells; may have low glucose	Virus isolation from CSF	Congenital hypogammaglobulinemia; history of recurrent meningitis
HIV (acute retroviral syndrome)	Mononuclear cells	p24 antigen in serum and CSF; high level of HIV viremia	HIV risk factors; rash, fever, lymphadenopathy; lymphopenia in peripheral blood; syndrome may persist long enough to be considered "chronic meningitis"; or chronic meningitis may develop in later stages (AIDS) due to HIV
Herpes simplex (HSV)	Mononuclear cells	PCR for HSV DNA; CSF antibody	Recurrent meningitis due to HSV-2 (rarely HSV-1) often associated with genital recurrences

Abbreviations: AFB, acid-fast bacillus; CSF, cerebrospinal fluid; CT, computed tomography; ELISA, enzyme-linked immunosorbent assay; EM, electron microscopy; FTA, fluorescent treponemal antibody absorption test; MHA-TP, microhemagglutination *assay-T. pallidum*; MRI, magnetic resonance imaging; PAS, periodic acid–Schiff; PCR, polymerase chain reaction; RPR, rapid plasma reagin test; TB, tuberculosis; VDRL, Venereal Disease Research Laboratories test.

TABLE 30-3

NONINFECTIOUS CAUSES OF CHRONIC MENINGITIS

CAUSATIVE AGENTS	CSF FORMULA	HELPFUL DIAGNOSTIC TESTS	RISK FACTORS AND SYSTEMIC MANIFESTATIONS
Malignancy	Mononuclear cells elevated protein, low glucose	Repeated cytologic examination of large volumes of CSF; CSF exam by polarizing microscopy; clonal lymphocyte markers; deposits on nerve roots or meninges seen on myelogram or contrast-enhanced MRI; meningeal biopsy	Metastatic cancer of, breast, lung, stomach, or pancreas; melanoma, lymphoma, leukemia; meningeal gliomatosis; meningeal sarcoma; cerebral dysgerminoma; meningeal melanoma or B cell lymphoma
Chemical compounds (may cause recurrent meningitis)	Mononuclear or PMNs, low glucose, elevated protein; xanthochromia from subarachnoid hemorrhage in week prior to presentation with "meningitis"	Contrast-enhanced CT scan or MRI Cerebral angiogram to detect aneurysm	History of recent injection into the subarachnoid space; history of sudden onset of headache; recent resection of acoustic neuroma or craniopharyngioma; epidermoid tumor of brain or spine, sometimes with dermoid sinus tract; pituitary apoplexy
Primary inflammation			
CNS sarcoidosis	Mononuclear cells; elevated protein; often low glucose	Serum and CSF angiotensin-converting enzyme levels; biopsy of extraneural affected tissues or brain lesion/meningeal biopsy	CN palsy, especially of CN VII; hypothalamic dysfunction, especially diabetes insipidus; abnormal chest radiograph; peripheral neuropathy or myopathy
Vogt-Koyanagi-Harada syndrome (recurrent meningitis)	Mononuclear cells		Recurrent meningoencephalitis with uveitis, retinal detachment, alopecia, lightening of eyebrows and lashes, dysacousia, cataracts, glaucoma
Isolated granulomatous angiitis of the nervous system	Mononuclear cells, elevated protein	Angiography or meningeal biopsy	Subacute dementia; multiple cerebral infarctions; recent zoster ophthalmicus
Systemic lupus erythematosus	Mononuclear or PMNs	Anti-DNA antibody, antinuclear antibodies	Encephalopathy; seizures; stroke; transverse myelopathy; rash; arthritis
Behçet's syndrome (recurrent meningitis)	Mononuclear or PMNs, elevated protein		Oral and genital aphthous ulcers; iridocyclitis; retinal hemorrhages; pathergic lesions at site of skin puncture
Chronic benign lymphocytic meningitis	Mononuclear cells		Recovery in 2–6 months, diagnosis by exclusion
Mollaret's meningitis (recurrent meningitis)	Large endothelial cells and PMNs in first hours, followed by mononuclear cells	PCR for herpes; MRI/CT to rule out epidermoid tumor or dural cyst	Recurrent meningitis; exclude HSV-2; rare cases due to HSV-1; occasional case associated with dural cyst

(continued)

TABLE 30-3 *(Continued)*

NONINFECTIOUS CAUSES OF CHRONIC MENINGITIS

CAUSATIVE AGENTS	CSF FORMULA	HELPFUL DIAGNOSTIC TESTS	RISK FACTORS AND SYSTEMIC MANIFESTATIONS
Drug hypersensitivity	PMNs; occasionally mononuclear cells or eosinophils		Exposure to ibuprofen, sulfonamides, isoniazid, tolmetin, ciprofloxacin, phenazopyridine; improvement after discontinuation of drug; recurrent episodes with recurrent exposure
Wegener's granulomatosis	Mononuclear cells	Chest and sinus radiographs; urinalysis; ANCA antibodies in serum	Associated sinus, pulmonary, or renal lesions; CN palsies; skin lesions; peripheral neuropathy
Other: multiple sclerosis, Sjögren's syndrome, neonatal-onset multisystemic inflammatory disease (NOMID), and rarer forms of vasculitis (e.g., Cogan's syndrome)			

Abbreviations: ANCA, anti-neutrophil cytoplasmic antibodies; CN, cranial nerve; CSF, cerebrospinal fluid; CT, computed tomography; HSV, herpes simplex virus; MRI, magnetic resonance imaging; PCR, polymerase chain reaction; PMNs, polymorphonuclear cells.

Koyanagi-Harada syndrome, Behçet's syndrome, Mollaret's meningitis, and systemic lupus erythematosus; and drug hypersensitivity with repeated administration of the offending agent.

The epidemiologic history is of considerable importance and may provide direction for selection of laboratory studies. Pertinent features include a history of tuberculosis or exposure to a likely case; past travel to areas endemic for fungal infections (the San Joaquin Valley in California and southwestern states for coccidioidomycosis, midwestern states for histoplasmosis, southeastern states for blastomycosis); travel to the Mediterranean region or ingestion of imported unpasteurized dairy products (*Brucella*); time spent in areas endemic for Lyme disease (e.g., Connecticut, New York, Massachusetts); exposure to sexually transmitted disease (syphilis); exposure of an immunocompromised host to pigeons and their droppings (*Cryptococcus*); gardening (*Sporothrix schenckii*); ingestion of poorly cooked meat or contact with a household cat (*Toxoplasma gondii*); residence in Thailand or Japan (*Gnathostoma spinigerum*) or the South Pacific (*Angiostrongylus cantonensis*); rural residence and raccoon exposure (*Baylisascaris procyonis*); and residence in Latin America, the Philippines, or Southeast Asia when eosinophilic meningitis is present (*Taenia solium*).

The presence of focal cerebral signs in a patient with chronic meningitis suggests the possibility of a brain abscess or other parameningeal infection; identification of a potential source of infection (chronic draining ear, sinusitis, right-to-left cardiac or pulmonary shunt, chronic pleuropulmonary infection) supports this diagnosis. In some cases, diagnosis may be established by recognition and biopsy of unusual skin lesions (Behçet's syndrome, cryptococcosis, blastomycosis, SLE, Lyme disease, intravenous drug use, sporotrichosis, trypanosomiasis) or enlarged lymph nodes (lymphoma, tuberculosis, sarcoid, infection with HIV, secondary syphilis, or Whipple's disease). A careful ophthalmologic examination may reveal uveitis [Vogt-Koyanagi-Harada syndrome, sarcoid, or central nervous system (CNS) lymphoma], keratoconjunctivitis sicca (Sjögren's syndrome), or iridocyclitis (Behçet's syndrome) and is essential to assess visual loss from hydrocephalus. Aphthous oral lesions, genital ulcers, and hypopyon suggest Behçet's syndrome. Hepatosplenomegaly suggests lymphoma, sarcoid, tuberculosis, or brucellosis. Herpetic lesions in the genital area or on the thighs suggest HSV-2 infection. A breast nodule, a suspicious pigmented skin lesion, focal bone pain, or an abdominal mass directs attention to possible carcinomatous meningitis.

IMAGING

Once the clinical syndrome is recognized as a potential manifestation of chronic meningitis, proper analysis of the CSF is essential. However, if the possibility of raised ICP exists, a brain imaging study should be performed before lumbar puncture. If ICP is elevated because of a mass lesion, brain swelling, or a block in ventricular CSF outflow (obstructive hydrocephalus), then lumbar puncture carries the potential risk of brain herniation. Obstructive hydrocephalus usually requires direct ventricular drainage of CSF. In patients with open CSF flow pathways, elevated ICP can occur due to impaired resorption of CSF by arachnoid villi. In such patients, lumbar puncture is usually safe, but repetitive or continuous lumbar drainage may be necessary to prevent relatively sudden death from raised ICP. In some patients, especially with cryptococcal meningitis, life-threatening levels of ICP can occur without visible hydrocephalus on brain imaging.

Contrast-enhanced MRI or CT studies of the brain and spinal cord can identify meningeal enhancement, parameningeal infections (including brain abscess), encasement of the spinal cord (malignancy or inflammation and infection), or nodular deposits on the meninges or nerve roots (malignancy or sarcoidosis) (**Fig. 30-1**). Imaging studies are also useful to localize areas of meningeal disease prior to meningeal biopsy.

Cerebral angiography may be indicated in patients with chronic meningitis and stroke to identify cerebral arteritis (granulomatous angiitis, other inflammatory or infectious causes).

CEREBROSPINAL FLUID ANALYSIS

The CSF pressure should be measured and samples sent for bacterial culture, cell count and differential, Gram's stain, and measurement of glucose and protein. In cases without a known cause, CSF should be sent for the Venereal Disease Research Laboratories (VDRL) test, acid-fast bacillus (AFB) stain and culture, wet mount for fungus and parasites, India ink preparation and culture, culture for fastidious bacteria and fungi, assays for cryptococcal antigen and oligoclonal immunoglobulin bands, and cytology. Other specific CSF or blood tests and cultures (Tables 30-2 and 30-3) should be ordered as indicated on the basis of the history, physical examination, or preliminary CSF results (i.e., eosinophilic, mononuclear, or polymorphonuclear meningitis). Rapid diagnosis may be facilitated by serologic tests and polymerase chain reaction (PCR) testing to identify DNA sequences in the CSF that are specific for the suspected pathogen.

In most categories of chronic (not recurrent) meningitis, mononuclear cells predominate in the CSF. When neutrophils predominate after 3 weeks of illness, the principal considerations are *Nocardia asteroides, Actinomyces israelii, Brucella, Mycobacterium*

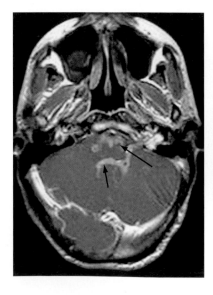
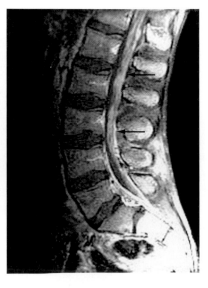

FIGURE 30-1

Primary central nervous system lymphoma. A 24-year-old man, immunosuppressed due to intestinal lymphangiectasia, developed multiple cranial neuropathies. CSF findings consisted of 100 lymphocytes/μL and a protein of 250 mg/dL; cytology and cultures were negative. Gadolinium-enhanced T1 MRI revealed diffuse, multifocal meningeal enhancement surrounding the brainstem (*left*) and spinal cord and cauda equina (*right*).

tuberculosis (5 to 10% of early cases only), various fungi (*Blastomyces dermatitidis, Candida albicans, Histoplasma capsulatum, Aspergillus* species, *Pseudallescheria boydii, Cladophialophora bantiana*), and noninfectious causes (SLE, exogenous chemical meningitis). When eosinophils predominate or are present in limited numbers in a primarily mononuclear cell response in the CSF, the differential diagnosis includes parasitic diseases (*A. cantonensis, G. spinigerum, B. procyonis,* or *Toxocara canis* infection, cysticercosis, schistosomiasis, echinococcal disease, *T. gondii* infection), fungal infections (6 to 20% eosinophils along with a predominantly lymphocyte pleocytosis, particularly with coccidioidal meningitis), neoplastic disease (lymphoma, leukemia, metastatic carcinoma), or other inflammatory processes (sarcoidosis, hypereosinophilic syndrome).

It is often necessary to broaden the number of diagnostic tests if the initial workup does not reveal the cause. In addition, repeated samples of large volumes of CSF may be required to diagnose certain infectious and malignant causes of chronic meningitis. For instance, lymphomatous or carcinomatous meningitis may be diagnosed by examination of sections cut from a cell block formed by spinning down the sediment from a large volume of CSF. The diagnosis of fungal meningitis may require large volumes of CSF for culture of sediment. If standard lumbar puncture is unrewarding, a cervical cisternal tap to sample CSF near to the basal meninges may be fruitful.

LABORATORY INVESTIGATION

In addition to the CSF examination, an attempt should be made to uncover pertinent underlying illnesses. Tuberculin skin test, chest radiograph, urine analysis and culture, blood count and differential, renal and liver function tests, alkaline phosphatase, sedimentation rate, antinuclear antibody, anti-Ro and anti-La antibody, and serum angiotensin-converting enzyme level are often indicated. Liver or bone marrow biopsy may be diagnostic in some cases of miliary tuberculosis, disseminated fungal infection, sarcoidosis, or metastatic malignancy. Abnormalities discovered on chest radiograph or chest CT can be pursued by bronchoscopy or transthoracic needle biopsy.

MENINGEAL BIOPSY

A diagnostic meningeal biopsy should be strongly considered in patients who are severely disabled,

who need chronic ventricular decompression, or whose illness is progressing rapidly. The activities of the surgeon, pathologist, microbiologist, and cytologist should be coordinated so that a large enough sample is obtained and the appropriate cultures and histologic and molecular studies, including electron microscopic and PCR studies, are performed. The diagnostic yield of meningeal biopsy can be increased by targeting regions that enhance with contrast on MRI or CT. With current microsurgical techniques, most areas of the basal meninges can be accessed for biopsy via a limited craniotomy. In a series from the Mayo Clinic reported by Cheng and colleagues, MRI demonstrated meningeal enhancement in 47% of patients undergoing meningeal biopsy. Biopsy of an enhancing region was diagnostic in 80% of cases; biopsy of nonenhancing regions was diagnostic in only 9%; sarcoid (31%) and metastatic adenocarcinoma (25%) were the most common conditions identified.

APPROACH TO THE ENIGMATIC CASE

In approximately one-third of cases, the diagnosis is not known despite careful evaluation of CSF and potential extraneural sites of disease. A number of the organisms that cause chronic meningitis may take weeks to be identified by cultures. In enigmatic cases several options are available, determined by the extent of the clinical deficits and rate of progression. It is prudent to wait until cultures are finalized if the patient is asymptomatic or symptoms are mild and not progressive. Unfortunately, in many cases progressive neurologic deterioration occurs, and rapid treatment is required. Ventricular-peritoneal shunts may be placed to relieve hydrocephalus, but the risk of disseminating the undiagnosed inflammatory process into the abdomen must be considered.

EMPIRICAL TREATMENT

Diagnosis of the causative agent is essential because effective therapies exist for many etiologies of chronic meningitis; if the condition is left untreated, however, progressive damage to the CNS and cranial nerves and roots is likely to occur. Occasionally, empirical therapy must be initiated when all attempts at diagnosis fail. In general, empirical therapy in the United States consists of antimycobacterial agents, amphotericin for fungal infection, or glucocorticoids for noninfectious inflammatory causes. It is important to direct empirical therapy of lymphocytic meningitis at tuberculosis, particularly if the condition is associated with hypoglycorrhachia and sixth and other CN palsies, since untreated disease is fatal in 4 to 8 weeks. In a series from the Mayo Clinic, the most useful empirical therapy was administration of glucocorticoids rather than antituberculous therapy. Carcinomatous or lymphomatous meningitis may be difficult to diagnose initially, but the diagnosis becomes evident with time.

THE IMMUNOSUPPRESSED PATIENT
(See Also Chap. 31)

Chronic meningitis is not uncommon in the course of HIV infection. Pleocytosis and mild meningeal signs often occur at the onset of HIV infection, and occasionally low-grade meningitis persists. Toxoplasmosis commonly presents as intracranial abscesses and may also be associated with meningitis. Other important causes of chronic meningitis in AIDS include infection with *Cryptococcus, Nocardia, Candida,* or other fungi; syphilis; and lymphoma (Fig. 30-1). Toxoplasmosis, cryptococcosis, nocardiosis, and other fungal infections are important etiologic considerations in individuals with immunodeficiency states other than AIDS, including those due to

immunosuppressive medications. Because of the increased risk of chronic meningitis and the attenuation of clinical signs of meningeal irritation in immunosuppressed individuals, CSF examination should be performed for any persistent headache or unexplained change in mental state.

FURTHER READINGS

Ginsberg L: Difficult and recurrent meningitis. J Neurol Neurosurg Psychiatry 75:i16, 2004

A review of recent studies guiding the treatment of tuberculous meningitis.

Lan SH et al: Cerebral infarction in chronic meningitis: A comparison of tuberculous meningitis and cryptococcal meningitis. Q J Med. 94:247, 2001

Liliang PC et al: Use of ventriculoperitoneal shunts to treat uncontrollable intracranial hypertension in patients who have cryptococcal meningitis without hydrocephalus. Clin Infect Dis. 34:E64, 2002

Thwaits G, Tran TH: Tuberculous meningitis: Many questions, too few answers. Lancet Neurol 4:160, 2005

Further information regarding the evaluation of the patient with unidentified chronic meningitis.

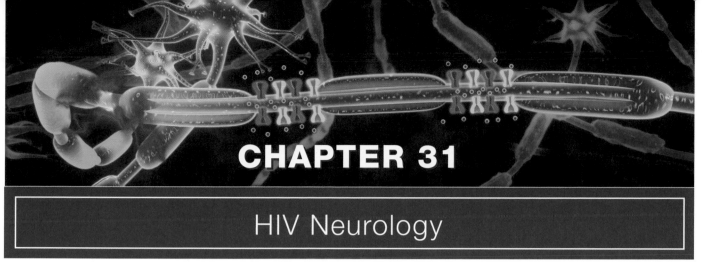

CHAPTER 31

HIV Neurology

Anthony S. Fauci
H. Clifford Lane

Clinical disease of the nervous system accounts for a significant degree of morbidity in a high percentage of patients with HIV infection. Neurologic problems occur throughout the course of disease and may be inflammatory, infectious, demyelinating, or degenerative in nature. These problems fall into four basic categories: neurologic disease caused by HIV itself, HIV-related neoplasms, opportunistic infections of the nervous system, and adverse effects of medical therapy (**Table 31–1**).

AIDS CLASSIFICATION

With the identification of HIV in 1983 and its proof as the etiologic agent of AIDS in 1984, and with the availability of sensitive and specific diagnostic tests for HIV infection, the case definition of AIDS has undergone several revisions over the years. The current U.S. Centers for Disease Control and Prevention (CDC) classification system for HIV-infected adolescents and adults categorizes persons on the basis of clinical conditions associated with HIV infection and CD4+ T lymphocyte counts. The system is based on three

ranges of CD4+ T lymphocyte counts and three clinical categories and is represented by a matrix of nine

TABLE 31-1

NEUROLOGIC DISEASES IN PATIENTS WITH HIV INFECTION
HIV infection
Aseptic meningitis
HIV-associated dementia (HIV encephalopathy, AIDS dementia complex)
Myelopathy
Vacuolar myelopathy
Pure sensory ataxia
Paresthesia/dysesthesia
Peripheral neuropathy
Distal symmetric polyneuropathy
Acute inflammatory demyelinating polyneuropathy (Guillain-Barré syndrome)
Chronic inflammatory demyelinating polyneuropathy (CIDP)
Mononeuritis multiplex
Myopathy
HIV-related neoplasms
Primary CNS lymphoma
Kaposi's sarcoma
Opportunistic infections
Cryptococcosis
Toxoplasmosis
Progressive multifocal leukoencephalopathy
Cytomegalovirus
Reactivation Chagas' disease
Syphilis
Mycobacterium tuberculosis
HTLV-I infection
Complications of HIV-related Medications
Zidovudine myopathy
NRTI-related polyneuropathy

Note: HTLV, human T lymphotropic virus; NRTI, nucleoside-analogue reverse transcriptase inhibitor.

mutually exclusive categories (**Tables 31-2** and **31-3**). Using this system, any HIV-infected individual with a CD4+ T cell count of <200/μL has AIDS by definition, regardless of the presence of symptoms or opportunistic diseases (Table 31-2). Once individuals have had a clinical condition in category B, their disease cannot again be classified as category A, even if the condition resolves; the same holds true for category C in relation to category B.

The definition of AIDS is indeed complex and comprehensive; however, the clinician should not focus on whether AIDS is present but should view HIV disease as a spectrum ranging from primary infection, with or without the acute syndrome, to the asymptomatic stage, to advanced disease (see below). The definition of AIDS was established not for the practical care of patients but for surveillance purposes.

ETIOLOGIC AGENT

The etiologic agent of AIDS is HIV, which belongs to the family of human retroviruses (Retroviridae) and the subfamily of lentiviruses. The four recognized human retroviruses belong to two distinct groups: the human T lymphotropic viruses (HTLV) I and HTLV-II, which are transforming retroviruses; and the human immunodeficiency viruses, HIV-1 and HIV-2, which are cytopathic viruses. The most common cause of HIV disease throughout the world, and certainly in the United States, is HIV-1, which comprises several subtypes with different geographic distributions. HIV-2 was first identified in 1986 in West African patients and was originally confined to West Africa. However, a number of cases that can be traced to West Africa or to sexual contacts with West Africans have been identified throughout the world. HIV-2 is more closely related phylogenetically to the simian immunodeficiency virus (SIV) found in sooty

mangabeys than it is to HIV-1. HIV-1 likely originated from the *Pan troglodytes troglodytes* species of chimpanzees in whom the virus had co-evolved over centuries.

MORPHOLOGY OF HIV

Electron microscopy shows that the HIV virion is an icosahedral structure (**Fig. 31-1***A*) containing numerous external spikes formed by the two major envelope proteins, the external gp120 and the transmembrane gp41. The virion buds from the surface of the infected cell and incorporates a variety of host proteins, including major histocompatibility complex (MHC) class I and II antigens, into its lipid bilayer. The structure of HIV-1 is schematically diagrammed in Fig. 31-1*B*.

REPLICATION CYCLE OF HIV

HIV is an RNA virus whose hallmark is the reverse transcription of its genomic RNA to DNA by the enzyme *reverse transcriptase*. The replication cycle of HIV begins with the high-affinity binding of the gp120 protein to its receptor on the host cell surface, the CD4 molecule (**Fig. 31-2**). The CD4 molecule is found predominantly on a subset of T lymphocytes that are responsible for helper or inducer function in the immune system. It is also expressed on the surface of monocytes/macrophages and dendritic/Langerhans cells. Once gp120 binds to CD4, the gp120 undergoes a conformational change that facilitates binding to one of a group of co-receptors. The two major co-receptors for HIV-1 are the chemokine receptors CCR5 and CXCR4. Following binding of the envelope protein to the CD4 molecule, the conformation of the viral envelope changes dramatically, and fusion with the host cell membrane occurs via the newly exposed gp41 molecule. Following fusion, the HIV genomic RNA is uncoated and internalized into the tar-

TABLE 31-2

1993 REVISED CLASSIFICATION SYSTEM FOR HIV INFECTION AND EXPANDED AIDS SURVEILLANCE CASE DEFINITION FOR ADOLESCENTS AND ADULTS			
	CLINICAL CATEGORIES		
CD4+ T CELL CATEGORIES	A: ASYMPTOMATIC, ACUTE (PRIMARY) HIV OR PGL[a]	B: SYMPTOMATIC, NOT A OR C CONDITIONS	C: AIDS-INDICATOR CONDITIONS
>500/μL	A1	B1	C1
200–499/μL	A2	B2	C2
<200/μL	A3	B3	C3

[a]PGL, progressive generalized lymphadenopathy.
Source: MMWR 42(No. RR-17), December 18, 1992.

TABLE 31-3

CLINICAL CATEGORIES OF HIV INFECTION

Category A: Consists of one or more of the conditions listed below in an adolescent or adult (>13 years) with documented HIV infection. Conditions listed in categories B and C must not have occurred.
Asymptomatic HIV infection
Persistent generalized lymphadenopathy
Acute (primary) HIV infection with accompanying illness or history of acute HIV infection

Category B: Consists of symptomatic conditions in an HIV-infected adolescent or adult that are not included among conditions listed in clinical category C and that meet at least one of the following criteria: (1) The conditions are attributed to HIV infection or are indicative of a defect in cell-mediated immunity; or (2) the conditions are considered by physicians to have a clinical course or to require management that is complicated by HIV infection. Examples include, but are not limited to, the following:
Bacillary angiomatosis
Candidiasis, oropharyngeal (thrush)
Candidiasis, vulvovaginal; persistent, frequent, or poorly responsive to therapy
Cervical dysplasia (moderate or severe)/cervical carcinoma in situ
Constitutional symptoms, such as fever (38.5°C) or diarrhea lasting >1 month
Hairy leukoplakia, oral
Herpes zoster (shingles), involving at least two distinct episodes or more than one dermatome
Idiopathic thrombocytopenic purpura
Listeriosis
Pelvic inflammatory disease, particularly if complicated by tuboovarian abscess
Peripheral neuropathy

Category C: Conditions listed in the AIDS surveillance case definition.
Candidiasis of bronchi, trachea, or lungs
Candidiasis, esophageal
Cervical cancer, invasive[a]
Coccidioidomycosis, disseminated or extrapulmonary
Cryptococcosis, extrapulmonary
Cryptosporidiosis, chronic intestinal (>1 month's duration)
Cytomegalovirus disease (other than liver, spleen, or nodes)
Cytomegalovirus retinitis (with loss of vision)
Encephalopathy, HIV-related
Herpes simplex: chronic ulcer(s) (>1 month's duration); or bronchitis, pneumonia, or esophagitis
Histoplasmosis, disseminated or extrapulmonary
Isosporiasis, chronic intestinal (>1 month's duration)
Kaposi's sarcoma
Lymphoma, Burkitt's (or equivalent term)
Lymphoma, primary, of brain
Mycobacterium avium complex or *M. kansasii,* disseminated or extrapulmonary
Mycobacterium tuberculosis, any site (pulmonary[a] or extrapulmonary)
Mycobacterium, other species or unidentified species, disseminated or extrapulmonary
Pneumocystis carinii pneumonia
Pneumonia, recurrent[a]
Progressive multifocal leukoencephalopathy
Salmonella septicemia, recurrent
Toxoplasmosis of brain
Wasting syndrome due to HIV

[a]Added in the 1993 expansion of the AIDS surveillance case definition.
Source: MMWR 42(No. RR-17), December 18, 1992.

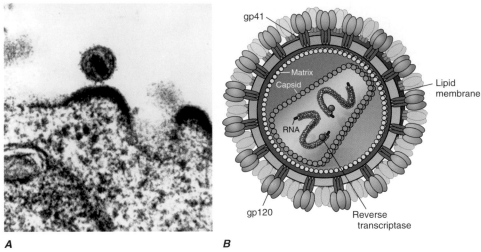

FIGURE 31-1

A. Electron micrograph of HIV. Figure illustrates a typical virion following budding from the surface of a CD4+ T lymphocyte, together with two additional incomplete virions in the process of budding from the cell membrane. **B**. Structure of HIV-1, including the gp120 outer membrane, gp41 transmembrane components of the envelope, genomic RNA, enzyme reverse transcriptase, p18(17) inner membrane (matrix), and p24 core protein (capsid) (copyright by George V. Kelvin). (*Adapted from RC Gallo: Sci Am 256:46, 1987.*)

get cell (Fig. 31-2). The reverse transcriptase enzyme, which is contained in the infecting virion, then catalyzes the reverse transcription of the genomic RNA into double-strand DNA. The DNA translocates to the nucleus, where it is integrated in a somewhat, but not completely, random fashion into the host cell chromosomes through the action of another virally encoded enzyme, *integrase*.

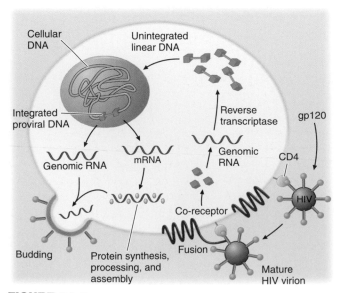

FIGURE 31-2

The replication cycle of HIV. See text for description. (*Adapted from AS Fauci: Nature 384:529, 1996.*)

Sites of HIV integration into the nuclear DNA are preferential for active genes and regional hotspots. This provirus may remain transcriptionally inactive (latent) or it may manifest varying levels of gene expression, up to active production of virus.

Cellular activation plays an important role in the life cycle of HIV and is critical to the pathogenesis of HIV disease. Following initial binding and internalization of virions into the target cell, incompletely reverse-transcribed DNA intermediates are labile in quiescent cells and will not integrate efficiently into the host cell genome unless cellular activation occurs shortly after infection. Furthermore, some degree of activation of the host cell is required for the initiation of transcription of the integrated proviral DNA into either genomic RNA or mRNA. This latter process may not necessarily be associated with the obvious expression of the classic cell surface markers of activation. In this regard, activation of HIV expression from the latent state depends on the interaction of a number of cellular and viral factors. Following transcription, HIV mRNA is translated into proteins that undergo modification through glycosylation, myristylation, phosphorylation, and cleavage. The viral particle is formed by the assembly of HIV proteins, enzymes, and genomic RNA at the plasma membrane of the cells. Budding of the progeny virion occurs through specialized regions in the lipid bilayer of the host cell membrane known as *lipid rafts,* where the core acquires its external envelope. The virally encoded protease then catalyzes the cleavage of the gag-pol precursor protein to yield the mature virion.

Progression through the virus replication cycle is profoundly influenced by a variety of viral regulatory gene products. Likewise, each point in the replication cycle of HIV is a real or potential target for therapeutic intervention. Thus far, the reverse transcriptase and protease enzymes have proven clinically to be susceptible to pharmacologic disruption. Recently, inhibitors of virus–target cell fusion have shown therapeutic promise, and inhibitors of the viral enzyme integrase are in clinical trials.

PATHOPHYSIOLOGY AND PATHOGENESIS

The hallmark of HIV disease is a profound immunodeficiency resulting primarily from a progressive quantitative and qualitative deficiency of the subset of T lymphocytes referred to as *helper T cells,* or *inducer T cells.* When the number of CD4+ T cells declines below a certain level, the patient is at high risk of developing a variety of opportunistic diseases, particularly the infections and neoplasms that are AIDS-defining illnesses. Some features of AIDS, such as Karposi sarcoma and neurologic abnormalities, cannot be explained completely by the immunosuppressive effects of HIV, since these complications may occur prior to the development of severe immunologic impairment.

NEUROPATHOGENESIS

Virtually all patients with HIV infection, including those without neuropsychiatric abnormalities, have some degree of nervous system involvement with the virus. This is evidenced by the fact that cerebrospinal fluid (CSF) findings are abnormal in ~90% of patients, even during the asymptomatic phase of HIV infection. CSF abnormalities include pleocytosis (50 to 65% of patients), detection of viral RNA (~75%), elevated CSF protein (35%), and evidence of intrathecal synthesis of anti-HIV antibodies (90%).

The main cell types that are infected in the brain in vivo are the perivascular macrophages and the microglial cells; monocytes that have already been infected in the blood can migrate into the brain, where they then reside as macrophages, or macrophages can be directly infected within the brain. The precise mechanisms whereby HIV enters the brain are unclear; however, they are felt to relate, at least in part, to the ability of virus-infected and immune-activated macrophages to induce adhesion molecules such as E-selectin and vascular cell adhesion molecule-1 (VCAM-1) on brain endothelium. Other studies have demonstrated that HIV gp120 enhances the expression of intercellular adhesion molecule-1 (ICAM-1) in glial cells; this effect may facilitate entry of HIV-infected cells into the central nervous system (CNS) and

may promote syncytia formation. Although there have been reports of infrequent HIV infection of neuronal cells and astrocytes, there is no convincing evidence that brain cells other than those of monocyte/macrophage lineage can be productively infected in vivo.

HIV-infected individuals may manifest white matter lesions as well as neuronal loss. Given the relative absence of evidence of HIV infection of neurons either in vivo or in vitro, it is unlikely that direct infection of these cells accounts for their loss. Rather, the HIV-mediated effects on neurons and oligodendrocytes are felt to involve indirect pathways whereby viral proteins, particularly gp120 and Tat, trigger the release of endogenous neurotoxins from macrophages and to a lesser extent from astrocytes. In addition, it has been demonstrated that certain HIV-1 proteins (Nef and Tat) can induce chemotaxis of leukocytes, including monocytes, into the CNS. Neurotoxins can be released from monocytes as a consequence of infection and/or immune activation. Astrocytes may play diverse roles in HIV neuropathogenesis. Reactive gliosis or astrocytosis has been demonstrated in the brains of HIV-infected individuals, and tumor necrosis factor (TNF) α and interleukin (IL) 6 have been shown to induce astrocyte proliferation.

CLINICAL MANIFESTATIONS

The overall systemic clinical consequences of HIV infection encompass a spectrum ranging from an acute syndrome associated with primary infection to a prolonged asymptomatic state to advanced disease. As noted above, the neurologic complications that occur in HIV-infected individuals may be either primary to the pathogenic processes of HIV infection itself or secondary to HIV-related neoplasms, opportunistic infections, or adverse effects of HIV medical therapies.

NEUROLOGIC DISEASE CAUSED BY HIV

Aseptic Meningitis and Encephalitis

Aseptic meningitis may be seen in any but the very late stages of HIV infection. In the setting of acute primary infection patients may experience a syndrome of headache, photophobia, and meningismus (**Table 31-4**). An acute encephalopathy due to encephalitis may occur. Rarely, acute infection can cause a myelopathy suggestive of transverse myelitis or neuropathy similar to the Guillain-Barré syndrome. Cranial nerve involvement may be seen, predominantly cranial nerve VII (mimicking Bell's palsy) but occasionally V and/or VIII. CSF findings include a lymphocytic pleocytosis, elevated protein level, and normal glucose level. This syndrome, which cannot be clinically differentiated from other

TABLE 31-4

CLINICAL FINDINGS IN THE ACUTE HIV SYNDROME

General
Fever
Pharyngitis
Lymphadenopathy
Headache/retroorbital pain
Arthralgias/myalgias
Lethargy/malaise
Anorexia/weight loss
Nausea/vomiting/diarrhea

Neurologic

Meningitis	Encephalitis
Peripheral neuropathy	Myelopathy

Dermatologic

Erythematous maculopapular rash	Mucocutaneous ulceration

Source: From B Tindall, DA Cooper: AIDS 5:1, 1991.

viral meningitides, usually resolves spontaneously within 2 to 4 weeks; however, in some patients, signs and symptoms may become chronic. Aseptic meningitis is rare following the development of AIDS, suggesting that clinical aseptic meningitis in the context of HIV infection is an immune-mediated disease.

HIV-Associated Dementia

HIV-associated dementia (HAD), also called HIV encephalopathy or AIDS dementia complex, affected up to 25% of AIDS patients prior to the availability of highly active antiretroviral therapy (HAART). Its incidence with HAART has been reduced greatly, but with prolonged overall survival the prevalence is now increasing. HAD is generally a late complication of HIV infection that progresses slowly over months, though it can be seen in patients with CD4 counts >350 cells/μL. It is the initial AIDS-defining illness in only ~3% of patients with HIV infection and thus only rarely precedes clinical evidence of immunodeficiency.

A cardinal feature of HAD is progressive cognitive slowing. This may present subtly at first, with mildly impaired ability to concentrate, increased forgetfulness, difficulty reading, or increased difficulty performing complex tasks. Initially these symptoms may be indistinguishable from findings of situational depression or fatigue. Behavioral problems include apathy and lack of initiative, with progression to a vegetative state in some instances. In contrast to "cortical" dementias (such as Alzheimer's disease), higher cortical dysfunction such as aphasia, apraxia, and agnosia are uncommon, leading some investigators to classify HAD as a "subcortical dementia."

In addition to cognitive decline, patients with HAD may also experience motor symptoms including unsteady gait, poor balance, tremor, and difficulty with rapid alternating movements. Increased tone and exaggerated deep tendon reflexes may be found in patients with spinal cord involvement. Late stages may be complicated by bowel and/or bladder incontinence.

Several classification schemes have been developed for grading HIV-associated dementia. A commonly used clinical staging system is outlined in **Table 31-5.**

There are no specific criteria for a diagnosis of HAD, and this syndrome must be differentiated from a number of other diseases that affect the CNS of HIV-infected patients (see below and also Table 31-1). Longitudinal screening for cognitive decline can be done objectively with the use of a Mini-Mental Status Examination (MMSE) (Table18-4). For this reason, it is advisable for all patients with a diagnosis of HIV infection to have a baseline MMSE. However, changes in MMSE scores may be absent in patients with early mild HAD.

Imaging studies of the CNS, by either magnetic resonance imaging (MRI) or computed tomography (CT), often demonstrate cerebral atrophy (**Fig. 31-3**). MRI may also reveal scattered punctate areas of abnormal signal in the subcortical white matter on T2-weighted images. Lumbar puncture is generally most helpful in ruling out or making a diagnosis of opportunistic infections. In HAD, patients may have the nonspecific findings of an increase in CSF cells and protein level. While HIV RNA can often be detected in the spinal fluid and HIV can be cultured from the CSF, there appears to be no correlation between the presence of HIV in the CSF and the presence of HAD.

The precise cause of HAD remains unclear, although the condition is thought to be a result of direct effects of HIV on the CNS. Multinucleated giant cells, macrophages, and microglial cells appear to be the main cell types harboring virus in the CNS. Histologically, the major changes are seen in the subcortical areas of the brain and include gliosis and multinucleated giant cell encephalitis. Less commonly, diffuse or focal spongiform changes occur in the white matter.

Multiple factors of both HIV and the patient influence the risk of developing HAD. Clinical risk factors include older age, high plasma viral load, and low CD4 count. HIV-infected individuals who are heterozygous for the chemokine receptor *CCR5-δ32* deletion appear to be relatively protected against the development of HAD, while those individuals with the E4 allele of apolipoprotein E appear to be at increased risk. Viral factors are also important, and distinct HIV envelope sequences are associated with the clinical expression of the AIDS dementia complex.

Combination antiretroviral therapy benefits many patients with HAD. Improvement in neuropsychiatric test scores has been noted for both adult and pediatric

TABLE 31-5

CLINICAL STAGING OF HIV-ASSOCIATED DEMENTIA (AIDS DEMENTIA COMPLEX)

STAGE	DEFINITION
Stage 0 (normal)	Normal mental and motor function
Stage 0.5 (equivocal/subclinical)	Absent, minimal, or equivocal symptoms without impairment of work or capacity to perform activities of daily living. Mild signs (snout response, slowed ocular or extremity movements) may be present. Gait and strength are normal.
Stage 1 (mild)	Able to perform all but the more demanding aspects of work or activities of daily living but with unequivocal evidence (signs or symptoms that may include performance on neuropsychological testing) of functional, intellectual, or motor impairment. Can walk without assistance.
Stage 2 (moderate)	Able to perform basic activities of self-care but cannot work or maintain the more demanding aspects of daily life. Ambulatory, but may require a single prop.
Stage 3 (severe)	Major intellectual incapacity (cannot follow news or personal events, cannot sustain complex conversation, considerable slowing of all output) or motor disability (cannot walk unassisted, usually with slowing and clumsiness of arms as well).
Stage 4 (end-stage)	Nearly vegetative. Intellectual and social comprehension and output are at a rudimentary level. Nearly or absolutely mute. Paraparetic or paraplegic with urinary and fecal incontinence.

Source: Adapted from JJ Sidtis, RW Price: Neurology 40:323, 1990

patients treated with antiretrovirals. The rapid improvement in cognitive function following the initiation of antiretroviral therapy supports the hypothesis that HIV or its products are involved in neuropathogenesis of HAD. There has been a remarkable decrease in the incidence of HIV encephalopathy in the era of successful combination antiretroviral therapy.

Finally, patients with HAD often have an increased sensitivity to the side effects of neuroleptic drugs. The use of these drugs for symptomatic treatment is associated with an increased risk of extrapyramidal side effects; therefore, patients with HAD who receive these agents must be monitored carefully.

HIV Myelopathy

Spinal cord disease, or myelopathy, is present in ~20% of patients with AIDS, often as part of HAD. In fact, 90% of patients with HIV-associated myelopathy have some evidence of dementia, suggesting that similar pathologic processes may be responsible for both conditions.

Three main types of spinal cord disease are seen in patients with AIDS. The first of these is a vacuolar myelopathy. This condition is pathologically similar to subacute combined degeneration of the cord such as occurs with pernicious anemia. Although vitamin B_{12} deficiency can be seen in patients with AIDS, it does not appear to be responsible for the myelopathy seen in the majority of patients. Vacuolar myelopathy is characterized by a subacute onset and often presents with gait disturbances, predominantly ataxia and spasticity; it may progress to include bladder and bowel dysfunction. Physical findings include evidence of increased deep tendon reflexes and extensor plantar responses. The second form of spinal cord disease involves the dorsal columns and presents as a pure sensory ataxia. The third form is also sensory in nature and presents

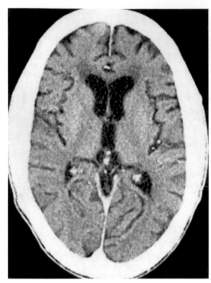

FIGURE 31-3

HIV-associated dementia. Postcontrast CT scan through the lateral ventricles of a 47-year-old man with AIDS, altered mental status, and dementia. The lateral and third ventricles and the cerebral sulci are abnormally prominent. Mild white matter hypodensity is also seen adjacent to the frontal horns of the lateral ventricles.

with paresthesias and dysesthesias of the lower extremities. In contrast to the cognitive problems seen in patients with HIV-associated dementia, these spinal cord syndromes do not respond well to antiretroviral drugs, and therapy is mainly supportive.

HIV Neuropathy

Two-thirds of patients with AIDS may be shown by electrophysiologic studies to have some evidence of peripheral nerve disease. This occurs at all stages of illness and may take a variety of forms.

Most common is a *distal sensory polyneuropathy* that may be a direct consequence of HIV infection. Presenting symptoms are usually the subacute onset of painful burning sensations in the feet and lower extremities. Findings on examination include a stocking-type sensory loss to pinprick, temperature, and touch sensation and a loss of ankle reflexes. Hyperpathia is common. Motor changes are mild and are usually limited to weakness of the intrinsic foot muscles. Nerve conduction studies may be normal or show only mild axonal changes.

In addition to primary HIV infection, other entities to consider in the differential diagnosis include diabetes mellitus, vitamin B_{12} deficiency, and side effects from dideoxynucleoside inhibitors, metronidazole or dapsone (see below). Response of this condition to antiretrovirals has been variable. For distal symmetric polyneuropathy

that fails to resolve following the discontinuation of dideoxynucleosides, therapy is symptomatic; gabapentin, carbamazepine, tricyclics, or analgesics may be effective for dysesthesias. Treatment-naive patients may respond to combination antiretroviral therapy, and preliminary data suggest that nerve growth factor may benefit some cases.

Early in the course of HIV infection, an acute inflammatory demyelinating polyneuropathy resembling the Guillain-Barré syndrome may occur (Chap. 35). In other patients, a progressive or relapsing-remitting inflammatory neuropathy resembling chronic inflammatory demyelinating polyneuropathy (CIDP) has been noted. Patients commonly present with progressive weakness, areflexia, and minimal sensory changes. CSF examination often reveals a mononuclear pleocytosis, and peripheral nerve biopsy demonstrates a perivascular infiltrate suggesting an autoimmune etiology. Plasma exchange or intravenous immunoglobulin has been tried with variable success. Because of the immunosuppressive effects of glucocorticoids, they should be reserved for severe cases of CIDP refractory to other measures.

HIV Myopathy

The clinical and histopathologic features of HIV-associated myopathy are indistinguishable from those of idiopathic polymyositis, and the condition is often referred to as *HIV polymyositis*. It may occur at any stage of HIV infection, but is rarely the first clinical presentation of HIV. HIV polymyositis may range in severity from an asymptomatic elevation in creatine kinase levels to a subacute syndrome characterized by proximal muscle weakness and myalgias. Quite pronounced elevations in creatine kinase may occur in asymptomatic patients, particularly after exercise; the clinical significance of this isolated laboratory finding is unclear.

Electromyography reveals abnormal spontaneous activity and short-duration polyphasic motor unit potentials. Muscle biopsy provides the best evidence for inflammatory muscle disease. A variety of both inflammatory and noninflammatory pathologic processes have been noted in patients with more severe myopathy, including myofiber necrosis with inflammatory cells, nemaline rod bodies, cytoplasmic bodies, and mitochondrial abnormalities.

The treatment of HIV polymyositis is similar to that of idiopathic polymyositis and includes glucocorticoids, azathioprine, cyclophosphamide, and intravenous immunoglobulin (IVIg). Immunosuppressants must be used cautiously in HIV patients. Prolonged administration of oral glucocorticoids has been associated with an increased risk of opportunistic infections, and pulse intravenous glucocorticoids may be a more attractive alternative.

HIV-RELATED NEOPLASMS

Systemic Lymphoma

Lymphomas occur with an increased frequency in patients with congenital or acquired T cell immunodeficiencies. AIDS is no exception; at least 6% of all patients with AIDS develop lymphoma at some time during the course of their illness. This is a 120-fold increase in incidence compared to the general population. In contrast to the situation with Kaposi's sarcoma (KS), primary CNS lymphoma, and most opportunistic infections, the incidence of AIDS-associated systemic lymphomas has not experienced as dramatic a decrease as a consequence of the widespread use of effective antiretroviral therapy. Lymphoma occurs in all risk groups, with the highest incidence in patients with hemophilia and the lowest incidence in patients from the Caribbean or Africa with heterosexually acquired infection. Lymphoma is a late manifestation of HIV infection, generally occurring in patients with CD4+ T cell counts <200/μL. As HIV disease progresses, the risk of lymphoma increases. In contrast to KS, which occurs at a relatively constant rate throughout the course of HIV disease, the attack rate for lymphoma increases exponentially with increasing duration of HIV infection and decreasing level of immunologic function. At 3 years following a diagnosis of HIV infection, the risk of lymphoma is 0.8% per year; by 8 years after infection, it is 2.6% per year. As persons with HIV infection live longer as a consequence of improved antiretroviral therapy and better treatment and prophylaxis of opportunistic infections, it is anticipated that the incidence of lymphomas may increase.

The clinical presentation of lymphoma in patients with HIV infection is quite varied, ranging from focal seizures to rapidly growing mass lesions in the oral mucosa to persistent unexplained fever. At least 80% of patients present with extranodal disease, and a similar percentage have B-type symptoms of fever, night sweats, or weight loss. Virtually any site in the body may be involved. The most common extranodal site is the CNS, which is involved in approximately one-third of all patients with lymphoma. Approximately 60% of these cases are primary CNS lymphoma.

CNS Lymphoma

Primary CNS lymphoma generally presents with focal neurologic deficits, including cranial nerve findings, headaches, and/or focal seizures. MRI or CT generally reveals a limited number (one to three) of 3- to 5-cm lesions (**Fig. 31-4**). CNS lymphoma lesions are classically seen in the deep white matter, often adjacent to the ventricular surface. They often show ring enhancement on contrast administration, but enhancement is usually less

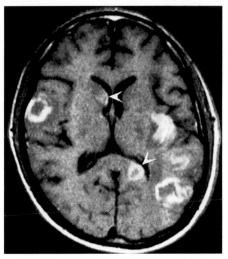

FIGURE 31-4

Central nervous system lymphoma. Postcontrast T1-weighted MR scan in a patient with AIDS, an altered mental status, and hemiparesis. Multiple enhancing lesions, some ring-enhancing, are present. The left Sylvian lesion shows gyral and subcortical enhancement, and the lesions in the caudate and splenium (*arrowheads*) show enhancement of adjacent ependymal surfaces.

pronounced than that seen with toxoplasmosis. The main diseases in the differential diagnosis are cerebral toxoplasmosis and cerebral Chagas' disease (see below).

In contrast to HIV-associated Burkitt's lymphoma, primary CNS lymphomas are usually positive for Epstein-Barr virus (EBV). In one study, the incidence of EBV positivity was 100%. This malignancy does not have a predilection for any particular age group. The median CD4+ T cell count at the time of diagnosis is ~50/μL. Thus, CNS lymphoma generally presents at a later stage of HIV infection than systemic lymphoma. This fact may at least in part explain the poorer prognosis for this subset of patients.

In addition to the 20% of lymphomas in HIV-infected individuals that are primary CNS lymphomas, CNS disease is also seen in HIV-infected patients with systemic lymphoma. Approximately 20% of patients with systemic lymphoma have CNS disease in the form of leptomeningeal involvement. This fact underscores the importance of lumbar puncture in the staging evaluation of patients with systemic lymphoma.

Both conventional and unconventional approaches have been employed in an attempt to treat HIV-related lymphomas. Treatment of primary CNS lymphoma remains a significant challenge. Treatment is complicated by the fact that this illness usually occurs in patients with advanced HIV disease. Palliative measures such as radiation therapy provide some relief. The prognosis remains poor in this group, with median survival <1 year.

HIV-RELATED OPPORTUNISTIC INFECTIONS

A broad spectrum of opportunistic infections secondary to bacterial, viral, fungal, mycobacterial, and parasitic microbes has been described in AIDS patients. The risk of many such infections correlates well with the CD4+ T cell count (**Fig. 31-5**). A selected group of common and important opportunistic infections of the nervous system in patients with HIV is discussed below.

Cryptococcosis

Cryptococcus neoformans is the leading infectious cause of meningitis in patients with AIDS. It is the initial AIDS-defining illness in ~2% of patients and generally occurs in patients with CD4+ T cell counts <100/μL. Cryptococcal meningitis is particularly common in patients with AIDS in Africa, occurring in ~20% of patients. Despite advances in the treatment of HIV, mortality from cryptococcal meningitis remains between 10 and 30%.

C. neoformans is an encapsulated yeastlike fungus found worldwide in soil contaminated by pigeon excreta. Infection is thought to be acquired by inhalation of the fungus into the lungs, although rare cases of cutaneous cryptococcosis appear to arise by minor trauma. Pulmonary infection has a tendency toward spontaneous resolution and is frequently asymptomatic, though severe pneumonia can develop. Silent hematogenous spread to the meninges and brain leads to clusters of cryptococci in the perivascular areas of cortical gray matter, in the basal ganglia, and, to a lesser extent, in other areas of the CNS. The inflammatory response around these foci is usually scant. In the more chronic cases, a dense basilar meningitis is typical.

Cryptococcal meningitis in AIDS patients is notable for the relative paucity of clinical symptoms and signs, even in severe disease. Headache is present in ~90% of cases and fever in ~75%. Meningeal signs are often mild or lacking. Other early manifestations include cognitive decline, irritability, nausea, and gait abnormalities. Blurred vision, cranial nerve palsies, lethargy, and confusion signal advanced infection. Papilledema is evident in one-third of cases at the time of diagnosis. Rapid and permanent loss of vision may occur, leaving a central scotoma or optic atrophy. Cranial nerve palsies, typically asymmetric, occur in about one-fourth of cases; sixth nerve palsies are common due to the association with elevated intracranial pressure (ICP). Other lateralized signs are rare. With progression of the infection, deepening coma and signs of brainstem compression appear.

Neuroimaging is most often normal. Focal lesions called *cryptococcomas* are more common in previously normal patients than in immunosuppressed patients. These

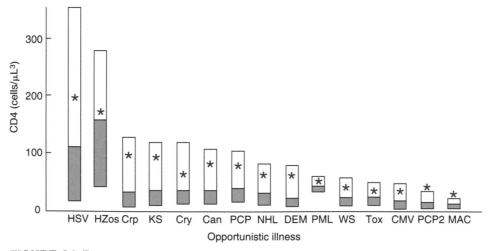

FIGURE 31-5

Relationship between CD4+ T cell counts and the development of opportunistic diseases. Boxplot of the median (line inside the box), first quartile (bottom of the box), third quartile (top of the box), and mean (asterisk) CD4+ lymphocyte count at the time of the development of opportunistic disease. Can, candidal esophagitis; CMV, cytomegalovirus infection; Crp, cryptosporidiosis; Cry, cryptococcal meningitis; DEM, HIV-associated dementia; HSV, herpes simplex virus infection; HZos, herpes zoster; KS, Kaposi's sarcoma; MAC, *Mycobacterium avium* complex bacteremia; NHL, non-Hodgkin's lymphoma; PCP, primary *Pneumocystis carinii* pneumonia; PCP2, secondary *P. carinii* pneumonia; PML, progressive multifocal leukoencephalopathy; Tox, *Toxoplasma gondii* encephalitis; WS, wasting syndrome. (*From RD Moore, RE Chaisson: Ann Intern Med 124:633, 1996.*)

lesions are commonly located in the basal ganglia, especially the head of the caudate nucleus. Cryptococcomas are best seen on MRI with T2 or FLAIR (fluid-attenuated inversion recovery) sequences and gadolinium enhancement. Edema around the mass disappears with successful therapy, but the cryptococcoma can persist for years. Autopsy often reveals cerebral edema in more acute cases and hydrocephalus in more chronic cases.

CSF abnormalities are modest, but an elevated opening pressure is characteristic. A CSF leukocyte count of $<10/\mu L$ and an opening pressure of >250 mmH_2O are poor prognostic signs. The specific diagnosis of cryptococcal meningitis depends upon the identification of organisms in spinal fluid with India ink examination, CSF fungal culture, or the detection of cryptococcal antigen in either serum or CSF. India ink examination is positive in 70 to 90% of AIDS patients with cryptococcal meningitis; ~90% of all patients have capsular antigen detectable in CSF or serum by latex agglutination. A biopsy may be needed to make a diagnosis of CNS cryptococcoma. The differential diagnosis of cryptococcal meningitis includes common bacterial and viral causes of meningitis, neurosyphilis, mycobacterial infections such as *Mycobacterium tuberculosis,* other fungi such as *Coccidioides immitis* and *Histoplasma capsulatum,* as well as HIV itself.

Most HIV patients have cryptococcal meningoencephalitis at the time of diagnosis. This form of cryptococcosis is invariably fatal without appropriate therapy; death occurs anytime from 2 weeks to several years after the onset of symptoms. Treatment is with intravenous amphotericin B, at a dose of 0.7 mg/kg daily, with flucytosine, 25 mg/kg qid for 2 weeks, followed by fluconazole, 400 mg/d orally for 10 weeks, and then fluconazole, 200 mg/d until the CD4+ T cell count has increased to >200 cells/μL for 6 months in response to HAART. Management of elevated ICP with serial lumbar punctures and removal of CSF to target a closing pressure of <200 mmH_2O is advocated by some, though few controlled studies are available to precisely guide this therapy.

Toxoplasmosis

Toxoplasmosis has been one of the most common causes of secondary CNS infections in patients with AIDS, but its incidence is decreasing in the era of HAART. It is most common in patients from the Caribbean and from France. Toxoplasmosis is generally a late complication of HIV infection and usually occurs in patients with CD4+ T cell counts $<200/\mu L$.

Cerebral toxoplasmosis, caused by the obligate intracellular parasite *Toxoplasma gondii,* is thought to represent a reactivation syndrome. It is 10 times more common in patients with antibodies to the organism than in patients who are seronegative. Patients diagnosed with HIV infection should be screened for IgG antibodies to *T. gondii* during the time of their initial workup. Those who are seronegative should be counseled about ways to minimize the risk of primary infection, including avoiding the consumption of undercooked meat and careful hand washing after contact with soil or changing the cat litter box.

The most common clinical presentation of cerebral toxoplasmosis in patients with HIV infection is fever, headache, and focal neurologic deficits. Patients may present with seizure, hemiparesis, or aphasia as a manifestation of these focal deficits or with a picture more influenced by the accompanying cerebral edema and characterized by confusion, dementia, and lethargy, which can progress to coma.

The diagnosis is usually suspected on the basis of MRI findings of lesions in multiple locations, although in some cases only a single lesion is seen. Pathologically, these lesions generally exhibit inflammation and central necrosis and, as a result, demonstrate ring enhancement on contrast MRI (**Fig. 31-6**) or, if MRI is unavailable or contraindicated, on double-dose contrast CT. There is usually evidence of surrounding edema.

In addition to toxoplasmosis, the differential diagnosis of single or multiple enhancing mass lesions in the HIV-infected patient includes primary CNS lymphoma (see above) and, less commonly, mycobacterial, fungal, or bacterial abscesses. The definitive diagnostic procedure is brain biopsy. However, given the morbidity that can accompany this procedure, it is usually reserved for the

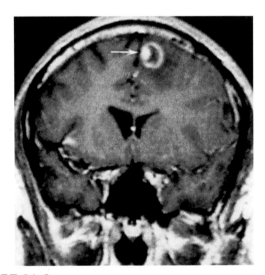

FIGURE 31-6

Central nervous system toxoplasmosis. A coronal postcontrast T1-weighted MR scan demonstrates a peripheral enhancing lesion in the left frontal lobe, associated with an eccentric nodular area of enhancement (*arrow*); this so-called "eccentric target sign" is typical of toxoplasmosis.

patient who has failed 2 to 4 weeks of empirical therapy. If the patient is seronegative for *T. gondii,* the likelihood that a mass lesion is due to toxoplasmosis is <10%. In that setting, one may choose to be more aggressive and perform a brain biopsy sooner. Standard treatment is sulfadiazine and pyrimethamine with leucovorin as needed for a minimum of 4 to 6 weeks. Alternative therapeutic regimens include clindamycin in combination with pyrimethamine; atovaquone plus pyrimethamine; and azithromycin plus pyrimethamine plus rifabutin. Relapses are common, and it is recommended that patients with a history of prior toxoplasmic encephalitis receive maintenance therapy with sulfadiazine, pyrimethamine, and leucovorin.

Patients with CD4+ T cell counts <100/μL and IgG antibody to *Toxoplasma* should receive primary prophylaxis for toxoplasmosis. Fortunately, the same daily regimen of a single double-strength tablet of trimethoprim/sulfamethoxazole (TMP/SMX) used for *Pneumocystis carinii* prophylaxis provides adequate primary protection against toxoplasmosis. Secondary prophylaxis for toxoplasmosis may be discontinued in the setting of effective antiretroviral therapy and increases in CD4+ T cell counts to >200/μL for 6 months.

Progessive Multifocal Leukoencephalopathy

JC virus, a human polyomavirus that is the etiologic agent of *progressive multifocal leukoencephalopathy* (PML), is an important opportunistic pathogen in patients with AIDS. While ~70% of the general adult population have antibodies to JC virus, indicative of prior infection, <10% of healthy adults show any evidence of ongoing viral replication. PML is the only known clinical manifestation of JC virus infection. It is a late manifestation of AIDS and is seen in ~4% of patients with AIDS.

The lesions of PML begin as small foci of demyelination in subcortical white matter that eventually coalesce. The cerebral hemispheres, cerebellum, and brainstem may all be involved. Patients typically have a protracted course with multifocal neurologic deficits, with or without changes in mental status. Ataxia, hemiparesis, visual field defects, aphasia, and sensory defects may occur.

MRI typically reveals multiple, nonenhancing white matter lesions that may coalesce and have a predeliction for the occipital and parietal lobes. The lesions show signal hyperintensity on T2-weighted images and hypointensity on T1-weighted images. Prior to the availability of potent antiretroviral combination therapy, the majority of patients with PML died within 3 to 6 months of the onset of symptoms. Paradoxical worsening of PML has been seen with initiation of HAART as an immune reactivation syndrome.

There is no specific treatment for PML; however, regressions of >2.5 years in duration have been reported in patients with PML treated with HAART for their HIV disease. Studies with antiviral agents such as cidofovir have failed to show clear benefit. Factors influencing a favorable prognosis for PML in the setting of HIV infection include a CD4+ T cell count >100/μL at baseline and the ability to maintain an HIV viral load of <500 copies per milliliter. Baseline viral load does not have independent predictive value of survival. PML is one of the few opportunistic infections that continues to occur with some frequency despite the widespread use of HAART.

Cytomegalovirus

In AIDS patients, infection with cytomegalovirus (CMV) can produce retinitis, encephalitis, myelitis, or polyradiculitis. Myelitis and polyradiculopathy secondary to CMV are typically seen late in the course of HIV infection (often with CD4 counts <50/μL) and is fulminant in onset, with lower extremity and sacral paresthesias, difficulty in walking, areflexia, ascending sensory loss, and urinary retention. The clinical course is rapidly progressive over a period of weeks. CSF examination reveals a predominantly neutrophilic pleocytosis, and CMV DNA can be detected by CSF polymerase chain reaction (PCR). Therapy with ganciclovir or foscarnet can lead to rapid improvement, and prompt initiation of foscarnet or ganciclovir therapy is important in minimizing the degree of permanent neurologic damage. Combination therapy with both drugs should be considered in patients who have been previously treated for CMV disease. Other diseases involving the spinal cord in patients with HIV infection include HTLV-I-associated myelopathy, neurosyphilis, herpes simplex or varicellazoster viruses, tuberculosis, and lymphoma.

Chagas' Disease

Reactivation American trypanosomiasis may present as acute meningoencephalitis with focal neurologic signs, fever, headache, vomiting, and seizures. In South America, reactivation of *Chagas' disease* is considered to be an AIDS-defining condition and may be the initial AIDS-defining condition. CNS lesions appear radiographically as single or multiple hypodense areas, typically with ring enhancement and edema. They are found predominantly in the subcortical areas, a feature that helps to differentiate them from the deeper lesions of toxoplasmosis and CNS lymphoma. *Trypanosoma cruzi* amastigotes, or trypanosomes, can be identified from biopsy specimens or CSF. Other CSF findings include elevated protein and a mild (<100 cells/μL) lymphocytic pleocytosis. Organisms can also be identified by direct examination of the blood. Treatment consists of benzimidazole (2.5 mg/kg bid) or nifurtimox (2 mg/kg qid) for at least 60 days, followed by maintenance therapy for life with either drug at a dose of 5 mg/kg three times a week. As is the case with cerebral toxoplasmosis, successful therapy with antiretrovirals may allow discontinuation of therapy for Chagas' disease.

COMPLICATIONS OF THERAPY

The most common neurologic complications of HIV-related medical therapy are polyneuropathy and myopathy.

Neuropathy

The successful evolution of HAART for HIV infection has greatly decreased many of the neurologic complications of the disease. With improved survival and the chronic use of neurotoxic medications, however, the incidence and prevalence of peripheral neuropathies in HIV-infected patients are increasing.

The nucleoside-analogue reverse transcriptase inhibitors [NRTIs, including didanosine (ddI), zalcitabine (ddC) and stavudine (d4T)] are all associated with a dose-dependent polyneuropathy. Clinically, symptoms are similar to those of HIV-associated polyneuropathy (see above). Painful burning parasthesias and hyperpathia typically begin in the feet and progress in a stocking and glove pattern. Examination reveals loss to pinprick, temperature, and touch sensation and a loss of ankle reflexes. As compared to HIV-associated neuropathy, NRTI-related neuropathy often follows a more fulminant course, with more abrupt onset and rapid progression, as well as increased severity of pain.

Patients with the clinical history suggestive of neuropathy due to either HIV or an NRTI should discontinue the potentially offending medication if at all possible. Symptomatic treatment for this small-fiber neuropathic pain often begins with gabapentin, as it is effective in diabetic neuropathic pain and does not interact with the metabolism of other medications. Amitryptyline and lamotrigine are also used for pain relief, though data supporting their efficacy are lacking.

Finally, a variety of other medications often used in HIV-infected patients are associated with neuropathy. These include isoniazid, metronidazole, and dapsone. Isoniazid (INH) neuropathy is a distal sensory polyneuropathy related to pyridoxine (vitamin B_6) depletion, and thus all patients taking INH should receive supplemental oral pyridoxine. Metronidazole is also associated with a distal symmetric sensory polyneuropathy. Dapsone-related neuropathy is a distal axonal neuropathy that selectively affects motor fibers. Treatment begins with removal of the offending drug if possible, and pain symptoms are approached as described above.

Myopathy

A myopathy similar to HIV polymyositis can be seen in patients following prolonged treatment with the NRTI zidovudine (AZT). (It is unclear if other NRTIs are also associated with myopathy.) This toxic side effect of the drug is dose-dependent and is related to its ability to interfere with the function of mitochondrial polymerases. It is usually reversible following discontinuation of the drug.

Patients present with progressive proximal weakness and profound muscle wasting, often with muscle pain. Serum levels of creatine kinase are usually elevated, and electromyography shows nonspecific myopathic changes. Muscle biopsy is most useful for distinguishing zidovudine myopathy from HIV polymyositis; whereas HIV polymyositis typically is associated with inflammatory changes, zidovudine myopathy has the histologic hallmark of red ragged fibers.

SPECIFIC NEUROLOGIC PRESENTATIONS
Focal Neurologic Deficits.

Patients with HIV infection may present with focal neurologic deficits from a variety of causes. The most common causes are toxoplasmosis, PML, and CNS lymphoma. Other causes include cryptococcal infections, reactivation Chagas' disease, transient postictal paralysis following a focal seizure, and stroke.

The onset of a stroke is usually sudden, in contrast to most other causes of focal neurologic deficits in patients with HIV infection. Among the secondary infectious diseases that may be associated with stroke in this setting, considerations include vasculitis due to cerebral varicella zoster or neurosyphilis and septic embolism in association with fungal infection. Other elements of the differential diagnosis of stroke in the patient with HIV infection include atherosclerotic cerebral vascular disease (especially with chronic lipid abnormalities seen with HAART), thrombotic thrombocytopenic purpura, and cocaine or amphetamine use.

Seizures

Seizures may be a consequence of opportunistic infections, neoplasms, or HIV-associated dementia (**Table 31-6**). The seizure threshold is often lower than

TABLE 31-6

CAUSES OF SEIZURES IN PATIENTS WITH HIV INFECTION

DISEASE	OVERALL CONTRIBUTION TO FIRST SEIZURE, %	PERCENT OF PATIENTS WHO HAVE SEIZURES, %
HIV-associated dementia	24–47	7–50
Cerebral toxoplasmosis	28	15–40
Cryptococcal meningitis	13	8
Primary CNS lymphoma	4	15–30
Progressive multifocal leukoencephalopathy	1	

Source: From DM Holtzman et al: Am J Med 87:173, 1989.

normal in these patients owing to the frequent presence of electrolyte abnormalities. Seizures are seen in 15 to 40% of patients with cerebral toxoplasmosis, 15 to 35% of patients with primary CNS lymphoma, 8% of patients with cryptococcal meningitis, and 7 to 50% of patients with HIV-associated dementia. Seizures may also be seen in patients with CNS tuberculosis, aseptic meningitis, and progressive multifocal leukoencephalopathy.

Seizures may also be the presenting clinical symptom of HIV disease. In one study of 100 patients with HIV infection presenting with a first seizure, cerebral mass lesions were the most common cause, responsible for 32 of the 100 new-onset seizures. Of these 32 cases, 28 were due to toxoplasmosis and 4 to lymphoma. HIV–related dementia accounted for an additional 24 new-onset seizures. Cryptococcal meningitis was the third most common diagnosis, responsible for 13 of the 100 seizures. In 23 cases, no cause could be found, and it is possible that these cases represent a subcategory of HIV-associated dementia. Of these 23 cases, 16 (70%) had two or more seizures, suggesting that anticonvulsant therapy is indicated in all patients with HIV infection and seizures unless a rapidly correctable cause is found. While phenytoin remains the initial treatment of choice, hypersensitivity reactions to this drug have been reported in >10% of patients with AIDS, and therefore the use of phenobarbital or valproic acid must be considered as alternatives. More recently, levetiracetam has been utilized, as it is cleared by the kidneys and has little interaction with HAART medications, although formal studies of its use in this setting are lacking.

FURTHER READINGS

Authier FJ et al: Skeletal muscle involvement in human immunodeficiency virus (HIV)-infected patients in the era of highly active antiretroviral therapy (HAART). Muscle Nerve 32:247, 2005

☑ Benson CA et al: Treating opportunistic infections among HIV-infected adults and adolescents. Recommendations from CDC, the National Institutes of Health, and the HIV Medicine Association/Infectious Diseases Society of America. MMWR Recomm Rep 53(RR-15):1, 2004. Updates available at *http://www.aidsinfo.nih.gov*

This website provides continuously updated guidelines for the treatment of AIDS-related opportunistic infections of the nervous system.

Bicanic T, Harrison TS: Cryptococcal meningitis. Br Med Bull 72:99, 2005

Dube B et al: Neuropsychiatric manifestations of HIV infection and AIDS. J Psychiatry Neurosci 30:237, 2005

Gonzalez-Scarano F, Martin-Garcia J: The neuropathogenesis of AIDS. Nat Rev Immunol 5:69, 2005

Kasamon YL, Ambinder RF: AIDS-related primary central nervous system lymphoma. Hematol Oncol Clin North Am 19:665, 2005

Keswani SC et al: HIV-associated sensory neuropathies. AIDS 16:2105, 2002

Koralnik IJ: New insights into progressive multifocal leukoencephalopathy. Curr Opin Neurol 17:365, 2004

Manji H, Miller R: The neurology of HIV infection. J Neurol Neurosurg Psychiatry 75(Suppl 1):i29, 2004

McArthur JC et al: Human immunodeficiency virus–associated dementia: An evolving disease. J Neurovirol 9:205, 2003

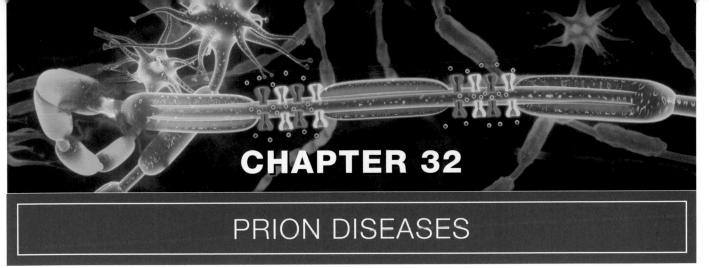

CHAPTER 32

PRION DISEASES

Stanley B. Prusiner
Bruce Miller

Prions are infectious proteins that cause degeneration of the central nervous system (CNS). Prion diseases are disorders of protein conformation, the most common of which in humans is called Creutzfeldt-Jakob disease (CJD). CJD typically presents with dementia and myoclonus, is relentlessly progressive, and generally causes death within a year of onset. Most CJD patients are between 50 and 75 years of age; however, patients as young as 17 years and as old as 83 years have been recorded.

In mammals, prions reproduce by binding to the normal, cellular isoform of the prion protein (PrP^C) and stimulating conversion of PrP^C into the disease-causing isoform (PrP^{Sc}). PrP^C is rich in α-helix and has little β-structure, while PrP^{Sc} has less α-helix and a high amount of β-structure (**Fig. 32–1**). This α-to-β structural transition in the prion protein (PrP) is the fundamental event underlying prion diseases (**Table 32–1**).

Four new concepts have emerged from studies of prions: (1) Prions are the only known infectious pathogens that are devoid of nucleic acid; all other infectious agents possess genomes composed of either RNA or DNA that direct the synthesis of their progeny. (2) Prion diseases may be manifest as infectious, genetic, and sporadic disorders; no other group of illnesses with a single etiology presents with such a wide spectrum of clinical manifestations. (3) Prion diseases result from the accumulation of PrP^{Sc}, the conformation of which differs substantially from that of its precursor PrP^C. (4) PrP^{Sc} can exist in a variety of different conformations, each of which seems to specify a particular disease phenotype. How a specific conformation of a PrP^{Sc} molecule is imparted to PrP^C during prion replication to produce nascent PrP^{Sc} with the same conformation is unknown. Additionally, it is unclear what factors determine where in the CNS a particular PrP^{Sc} molecule will be deposited.

SPECTRUM OF PRION DISEASES

The sporadic form of CJD is the most common prion disorder in humans. Sporadic CJD (sCJD) accounts for ~85% of all cases of human prion disease, while inherited prion diseases account for 10 to 15% of all cases (**Table 32–2**). Familial CJD (fCJD), Gerstmann-Sträussler-Scheinker (GSS) disease, and fatal familial insomnia (FFI) are all dominantly inherited prion diseases that are caused by mutations in the *PrP* gene.

Although infectious prion diseases account for <1% of all cases and infection does not seem to play an important role in the natural history of these illnesses, the transmissibility of prions is an important biologic feature. *Kuru* of the Fore people of New Guinea is thought to have resulted from the consumption of brains from dead relatives during ritualistic cannibalism. With the cessation of ritualistic cannibalism in the late 1950s, kuru has nearly disappeared with the exception of a few recent patients exhibiting incubation periods of >40 years. Iatrogenic CJD (iCJD) seems to be the result of the accidental inoculation of patients with prions. Variant CJD (vCJD) in teenagers and young adults in Europe is the

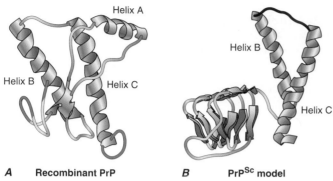

FIGURE 32-1

Structures of prion proteins. **A.** NMR structure of Syrian hamster recombinant (rec) PrP(90–231). Presumably, the structure of the α-helical form of recPrP(90–231) resembles that of PrP^C. recPrP(90–231) is viewed from the interface where PrP^{Sc} is thought to bind to PrP^C. The following are shown: α-helices A (residues 144–157), B (172–193), and C (200–227). Flat ribbons depict β-strands S1 (129–131) and S2 (161–163). (*Reprinted with permission from H Lui et al: Biochemistry 38:5362, 1999. Copyright American Chemical Society.*) **B.** Theoretical structural model of PrP^{Sc}. The 90–160 region has been modeled onto a β-helical architecture while the COOH terminal helices B and C are preserved as in PrP^C. (*Image prepared by C. Govaerts.*)

TABLE 32-1

GLOSSARY OF PRION TERMINOLOGY

Prion	*Proteinaceous infectious* particle that lacks nucleic acid. Prions are composed largely, if not entirely, of PrP^{Sc} molecules. They can cause scrapie in animals and related neurodegenerative diseases of humans such as Creutzfeldt-Jakob disease (CJD).
PrP^{Sc}	Disease-causing isoform of the prion protein. This protein is the only identifiable macromolecule in purified preparations of scrapie prions.
PrP^C	Cellular isoform of the prion protein. PrP^C is the precursor of PrP^{Sc}.
PrP 27-30	A fragment of PrP^{Sc}, generated by truncation of the NH$_2$-terminus by limited digestion with proteinase K. PrP 27-30 retains prion infectivity and polymerizes into amyloid.
PRNP	PrP gene located on human chromosome 20.
Prion rod	An aggregate of prions composed largely of PrP 27-30 molecules. Created by detergent extraction and limited proteolysis of PrP^{Sc}. Morphologically and histochemically indistinguishable from many amyloids.
PrP amyloid	Amyloid containing PrP in the brains of animals or humans with prion disease; often accumulates as plaques.

result of exposure to tainted beef from cattle with bovine spongiform encephalopathy (BSE).

Six diseases of animals are caused by prions (Table 32-2). Scrapie of sheep and goats is the prototypic prion disease. Mink encephalopathy, BSE, feline spongiform encephalopathy, and exotic ungulate encephalopathy are all thought to occur after the consumption of prion-infected foodstuffs. The BSE epidemic emerged in Britain in the late 1980s and was shown to be due to industrial cannibalism. Whether BSE began as a sporadic case of BSE in a cow or started with scrapie in sheep is unknown. The origin of chronic wasting disease (CWD), a prion disease endemic in deer and elk in regions of North America, is uncertain.

EPIDEMIOLOGY

CJD is found throughout the world. The incidence of sCJD is approximately one case per million population. Although many geographic clusters of CJD have been reported, each has been shown to segregate with a PrP gene mutation. Attempts to identify common exposure to some etiologic agent have been unsuccessful for both the sporadic and familial cases. Ingestion of scrapie-infected sheep or goat meat as a cause of CJD in humans has not been demonstrated by epidemiologic studies, although speculation about this potential route of inoculation continues. Of particular interest are deer hunters who develop CJD, because up to 90% of culled deer in some game herds have been shown to harbor CWD prions. Studies with Syrian hamsters demonstrate that oral infection with prions can occur, but the process is inefficient compared with intracerebral inoculation.

PATHOGENESIS

The human prion diseases were initially classified as neurodegenerative disorders of unknown etiology on the basis of pathologic changes being confined to the CNS. With the transmission of kuru and CJD to apes, investigators began to view these diseases as infectious CNS illnesses caused by slow viruses. Even though the familial nature of a subset of CJD cases was well described, the significance of this observation became more obscure with the transmission of CJD to animals. Eventually, the meaning of heritable CJD became clear with the discovery of mutations in the *PrP* gene of these patients. The prion concept explains how a disease can manifest as a heritable as well as an infectious illness. Moreover, the hallmark of all prion diseases, whether sporadic, dominantly inherited, or acquired by infection, is that they involve the aberrant metabolism of PrP.

TABLE 32-2

THE PRION DISEASES

DISEASE	HOST	MECHANISM OF PATHOGENESIS
Human		
Kuru	Fore people	Infection through ritualistic cannibalism
iCJD	Humans	Infection from prion-contaminated hGH, dura mater grafts, etc.
vCJD	Humans	Infection from bovine prions
fCJD	Humans	Germ-line mutations in *PRNP*
GSS	Humans	Germ-line mutations in *PRNP*
FFI	Humans	Germ-line mutation in *PRNP* (D178N, M129)
sCJD	Humans	Somatic mutation or spontaneous conversion of PrP^C into PrP^{Sc}?
sFI	Humans	Somatic mutation or spontaneous conversion of PrP^C into PrP^{Sc}?
Animal		
Scrapie	Sheep	Infection in genetically susceptible sheep
BSE	Cattle	Infection with prion-contaminated MBM
TME	Mink	Infection with prions from sheep or cattle
CWD	Mule deer, elk	Unknown
FSE	Cats	Infection with prion-contaminated beef
Exotic ungulate encephalopathy	Greater kudu, nyala, or oryx	Infection with prion-contaminated MBM

Abbreviations: BSE, bovine spongiform encephalopathy; CJD, Creutzfeldt-Jakob disease; fCJD, familial Creutzfeldt-Jakob disease; iCJD, iatrogenic Creutzfeldt-Jakob disease; sCJD, sporadic Creutzfeldt-Jakob disease; vCJD, variant Creutzfeldt-Jakob disease; CWD, chronic wasting disease; FFI, fatal familial insomnia; sFI, sporadic fatal insomnia; FSE, feline spongiform encephalopathy; GSS, Gerstmann-Sträussler-Scheinker disease; hGH, human growth hormone; MBM, meat and bone meal; TME, transmissible mink encephalopathy.

A major feature that distinguishes prions from viruses is the finding that both PrP isoforms are encoded by a chromosomal gene. In humans, the *PrP* gene is designated *PRNP* and is located on the short arm of chromosome 20. Limited proteolysis of PrP^{Sc} produces a smaller, protease-resistant molecule of ~142 amino acids designated PrP 27-30; PrP^C is completely hydrolyzed under the same conditions (**Fig. 32-2**). In the presence of detergent, PrP 27-30 polymerizes into amyloid. Prion rods formed by limited proteolysis and detergent extraction are indistinguishable from the filaments that aggregate to form PrP amyloid plaques in the CNS. Both the rods and the PrP amyloid filaments found in brain tissue exhibit similar ultrastructural morphology and green-gold birefringence after staining with Congo red dye.

SPECIES BARRIER

Studies on the role of the primary and tertiary structures of PrP in the transmission of prion disease have given new insights into the pathogenesis of these maladies. The amino acid sequence of PrP encodes the species of the prion, and the prion derives its PrP^{Sc} sequence from the last mammal in which it was passaged. While the primary structure of PrP is likely to be the most important or even sole determinant of the tertiary structure of PrP^C, PrP^{Sc} seems to function as a template in determining the tertiary structure of nascent PrP^{Sc} molecules as

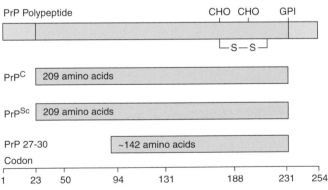

FIGURE 32-2

Prion protein isoforms. Bar diagram of Syrian hamster PrP, which consists of 254 amino acids. After processing of the NH$_2$ and COOH termini, both PrP^C and PrP^{Sc} consist of 209 residues. After limited proteolysis, the NH$_2$ terminus of PrP^{Sc} is truncated to form PrP 27–30 composed of ~142 amino acids. [*Reprinted from Les Prix Nobel T. Frängsmyr (ed), Stockholm, Norstedts Tryckeri, 1998, pp 268–323, with permission; © Nobel Foundation.*]

they are formed from PrP^C. In turn, prion diversity appears to be enciphered in the conformation of PrP^{Sc} and thus, prion strains seem to represent different conformers of PrP^{Sc}.

In general, transmission of prion disease from one species to another is inefficient, in that not all intracerebrally inoculated animals develop disease, and those that fall ill do so only after long incubation times that can approach the natural life span of the animal. This "species barrier" to transmission is correlated with the degree of similarity between the amino acid sequence of PrP^C in the inoculated host and of PrP^{Sc} in the prion inoculum. The importance of sequence similarity between the host and donor PrP argues that PrP^C directly interacts with PrP^{Sc} in the prion conversion process.

SPORADIC AND INHERITED PRION DISEASES

Several different scenarios might explain the initiation of sporadic prion disease: (1) A somatic mutation may be the cause and thus follow a path similar to that for germ-line mutations in inherited disease. In this situation, the mutant PrP^{Sc} must be capable of targeting wild-type PrP^C, a process known to be possible for some mutations but less likely for others. (2) The activation barrier separating wild-type PrP^C from PrP^{Sc} could be crossed on rare occasions when viewed in the context of a population. Most individuals would be spared, while presentations in the elderly with an incidence of ~1 per million would be seen. (3) PrP^{Sc} may be present at very low levels in some normal cells, where it performs some important, as yet unknown, function. The level of PrP^{Sc} in such cells is hypothesized to be sufficiently low as to be undetected by bioassay. In some altered metabolic states, the cellular mechanisms for clearing PrP^{Sc} might become compromised and the rate of PrP^{Sc} formation would then begin to exceed the capacity of the cell to clear it. The third possible mechanism is attractive since it suggests that PrP^{Sc} is not simply a misfolded protein, as proposed for the first and second mechanisms, but rather an alternatively folded molecule with a function. Studies in mice with the PrP^C gene knocked out do not, however, show an obvious phenotype, questioning why this protein has been so highly conserved across species.

More than 30 different mutations resulting in nonconservative substitutions in the human *PRNP* gene have been found to segregate with inherited human prion diseases. Missense mutations and expansions in the octapeptide repeat region of the gene are responsible for familial forms of prion disease. Five different mutations of the *PRNP* gene have been linked genetically to heritable prion disease.

Although phenotypes may vary dramatically within families, specific phenotypes tend to be observed with certain mutations. A clinical phenotype indistinguishable from typical sCJD is usually seen with substitutions at codons 180, 183, 200, 208, 210, and 232. Substitutions at codons 102, 105, 117, 198, and 217 are associated with the GSS variant of prion disease. The normal human PrP sequence contains five repeats of an eight-amino-acid sequence. Insertions from two to nine extra octarepeats frequently cause variable phenotypes ranging from a condition indistinguishable from sCJD to a slowly progressive dementing illness of many years' duration. A mutation at codon 178 resulting in substitution of asparagine for aspartic acid produces FFI if a methionine is encoded at the polymorphic 129 residue on the same allele. Typical CJD is seen if a valine is encoded at position 129 of the same allele.

HUMAN *PRNP* GENE POLYMORPHISMS

Polymorphisms influence the susceptibility to sporadic, inherited, and infectious forms of prion disease. The methionine/valine polymorphism at position 129 not only modulates the age of onset of some inherited prion diseases but can also determine the clinical phenotype. The finding that homozygosity at codon 129 predisposes to sCJD supports a model of prion production that favors PrP interactions between homologous proteins.

Substitution of the basic residue lysine at position 218 in mouse PrP produced dominant-negative inhibition of prion replication in transgenic mice. This same lysine at position 219 in human PrP has been found in 12% of the Japanese population, and this group appears to be resistant to prion disease. Dominant-negative inhibition of prion replication was also found with substitution of the basic residue arginine at position 171; sheep with arginine are resistant to scrapie prions but are susceptible to BSE prions that were inoculated intracerebrally.

INFECTIOUS PRION DISEASES

IATROGENIC CJD

Accidental transmission of CJD to humans appears to have occurred with corneal transplantation, contaminated electroencephalogram (EEG) electrode implantation, and surgical procedures. Corneas from donors with inapparent CJD have been transplanted to apparently healthy recipients who developed CJD after prolonged incubation periods. The same improperly decontaminated EEG electrodes that caused CJD in two young patients with intractable epilepsy caused CJD in a chimpanzee 18 months after their experimental implantation.

Surgical procedures may have resulted in accidental inoculation of patients with prions during their operations, presumably because some instrument or apparatus in the operating theater became contaminated when a CJD patient underwent surgery. Although the epidemiology of these studies is highly suggestive, no proof for such episodes exists.

Dura Mater Grafts

More than 120 cases of CJD after implantation of dura mater grafts have been recorded. All of the grafts were thought to have been acquired from a single manufacturer whose preparative procedures were inadequate to inactivate human prions. One case of CJD occurred after repair of an eardrum perforation with a pericardium graft.

Human Growth Hormone and Pituitary Gonadotropin Therapy

The possibility of transmission of CJD from contaminated human growth hormone (hGH) preparations derived from human pituitaries has been raised by the occurrence of fatal cerebellar disorders with dementia in >120 patients ranging in age from 10 to 41 years. These patients received injections of hGH every 2 to 4 days for 4 to 12 years. If it is assumed that these patients developed CJD from injections of prion-contaminated hGH preparations, the possible incubation periods range from 4 to 30 years. Even though several investigations argue for the efficacy of inactivating prions in hGH fractions prepared from human pituitaries with 6 M urea, it seems doubtful that such protocols will be used for purifying hGH because recombinant hGH is available. Four cases of CJD have occurred in women receiving human pituitary gonadotropin.

VARIANT CJD

The restricted geographic occurrence and chronology of vCJD raised the possibility that BSE prions have been transmitted to humans through the consumption of tainted beef. More than 140 cases of vCJD have occurred, with >90% of these in Britain. Since 2001 the incidence of vCJD has been declining. Although the eventual extent of this illness is still epidemiologically unclear, what is certain is that prion-tainted meat should be prevented from entering the human food supply.

The most compelling evidence that vCJD is caused by BSE prions was obtained from experiments in mice expressing the bovine PrP transgene. Both BSE and vCJD prions were efficiently transmitted to these transgenic mice and with similar incubation periods. In contrast to sCJD prions, vCJD prions did not transmit disease efficiently to mice expressing a chimeric human-mouse PrP

transgene. Earlier studies with nontransgenic mice suggested that vCJD and BSE might be derived from the same source because both inocula transmitted disease with similar but very long incubation periods.

NEUROPATHOLOGY

Frequently, the brains of patients with CJD have no recognizable abnormalities on gross examination. Patients who survive for several years have variable degrees of cerebral atrophy.

On light microscopy, the pathologic hallmarks of CJD are spongiform degeneration and astrocytic gliosis. The lack of an inflammatory response in CJD and other prion diseases is an important pathologic feature of these degenerative disorders. Spongiform degeneration is characterized by many 1- to 5-μm vacuoles in the neuropil between nerve cell bodies. Generally, the spongiform changes occur in the cerebral cortex, putamen, caudate nucleus, thalamus, and molecular layer of the cerebellum. Astrocytic gliosis is a constant but nonspecific feature of prion diseases. Widespread proliferation of fibrous astrocytes is found throughout the gray matter of brains infected with CJD prions. Astrocytic processes filled with glial filaments form extensive networks.

Amyloid plaques have been found in ~10% of CJD cases. Purified CJD prions from humans and animals exhibit the ultrastructural and histochemical characteristics of amyloid when treated with detergents during limited proteolysis. In first passage from some human Japanese CJD cases, amyloid plaques have been found in mouse brains. These plaques stain with antisera raised against PrP.

The amyloid plaques of GSS disease are morphologically distinct from those seen in kuru or scrapie. GSS plaques consist of a central dense core of amyloid surrounded by smaller globules of amyloid. Ultrastructurally, they consist of a radiating fibrillar network of amyloid fibrils, with scant or no neuritic degeneration. The plaques can be distributed throughout the brain but are most frequently found in the cerebellum. They are often located adjacent to blood vessels. Congophilic angiopathy has been noted in some cases of GSS disease.

In vCJD, a characteristic feature is the presence of "florid plaques." These are composed of a central core of PrP amyloid, surrounded by vacuoles in a pattern suggesting petals on a flower.

CLINICAL FEATURES OF CJD

Nonspecific prodromal symptoms occur in about a third of patients with CJD and may include fatigue, sleep disturbance, weight loss, headache, malaise, and ill-defined pain. Most patients with CJD present with deficits in higher cortical function. These deficits almost always progress over weeks or months to a state of profound dementia characterized by memory loss, impaired judgment, and a decline in virtually all aspects of intellectual function. A few patients present with either visual impairment or cerebellar gait and coordination deficits. Frequently, the cerebellar deficits are rapidly followed by progressive dementia. Visual problems often begin with blurred vision and diminished acuity, rapidly followed by dementia.

Other symptoms and signs include extrapyramidal dysfunction manifested as rigidity, masklike facies, or choreoathetoid movements; pyramidal signs (usually mild); seizures (usually major motor) and, less commonly, hypesthesia; supranuclear gaze palsy; optic atrophy; and vegetative signs such as changes in weight, temperature, sweating, or menstruation.

Myoclonus

Most patients (~90%) with CJD exhibit myoclonus that appears at various times throughout the illness. Unlike other involuntary movements, myoclonus persists during sleep. Startle myoclonus elicited by loud sounds or bright lights is frequent. It is important to stress that myoclonus is neither specific nor confined to CJD. Dementia with myoclonus can also be due to Alzheimer's disease (AD) (Chap. 18), to cryptococcal encephalitis, or to the myoclonic epilepsy disorder Unverricht-Lundborg disease (Chap. 14).

Clinical Course

In documented cases of accidental transmission of CJD to humans, an incubation period of 1.5 to 2.0 years preceded the development of clinical disease. In other cases, incubation periods of up to 30 years have been suggested. Most patients with CJD live 6 to 12 months after the onset of clinical signs and symptoms, whereas some live for up to 5 years.

DIAGNOSIS

The constellation of dementia, myoclonus, and periodic electrical bursts in an afebrile 60-year-old patient generally indicates CJD. Clinical abnormalities in CJD are confined to the CNS. Fever, elevated sedimentation rate, leukocytosis in blood, or a pleocytosis in cerebrospinal fluid (CSF) should alert the physician to another etiology to explain the patient's CNS dysfunction.

Variations in the typical course appear in inherited and transmitted forms of the disease. fCJD has an earlier mean age of onset than sCJD. In GSS disease, ataxia is usually a prominent and presenting feature, with dementia occurring late in the disease course. GSS disease typically presents earlier than CJD (mean age, 43 years) and is typically more slowly progressive than CJD; death usually occurs within 5 years of onset. FFI is characterized by insomnia and dysautonomia; dementia occurs only in the terminal phase of the illness. Rare sporadic cases have been identified. vCJD has an unusual clinical course, with a prominent psychiatric prodrome that may include visual hallucinations and early ataxia, while frank dementia is usually a late sign of vCJD.

DIFFERENTIAL DIAGNOSIS

Many conditions may mimic CJD superficially. AD is occasionally accompanied by myoclonus but is usually distinguished by its protracted course and lack of motor and visual dysfunction.

Intracranial vasculitides (Chap. 29) may produce nearly all of the symptoms and signs associated with CJD, sometimes without systemic abnormalities. Myoclonus is exceptional with cerebral vasculitis, but focal seizures may confuse the picture; furthermore, myoclonus is often absent in the early stages of CJD. Stepwise change in deficits, prominent headache, abnormal CSF, and focal magnetic resonance imaging (MRI) or angiographic abnormalities all favor vasculitis.

CNS lymphoma or less commonly a diffuse intracranial tumor (gliomatosis cerebri; Chap. 25) may be confused with CJD. Neurosyphilis may present with dementia and myoclonus that progresses in a relatively rapid fashion but is easily distinguished from CJD by CSF findings, as is cryptococcal meningoencephalitis. Adult-onset leukodystrophies (ceroid lipofuscinosis; Chap. 18) and myoclonic epilepsy with Lafora bodies (Chap. 14) may be responsible for dementia, myoclonus, and ataxia, but the less acute courses and prominent seizures distinguish them from CJD. A number of diseases that may simulate CJD are easily distinguished by the clinical setting in which they occur. These diseases include anoxic encephalopathy, subacute sclerosing panencephalitis, progressive rubella panencephalitis, herpes simplex encephalitis (in immunoincompetent hosts), dialysis dementia, uremia, and hepatic encephalopathy. When CJD begins atypically, it may for a short time resemble other disorders such as Parkinson's disease, progressive supranuclear palsy (Chap. 19), or progressive multifocal leukoencephalopathy (Chap. 29).

Certain drug intoxications, particularly lithium and bismuth, may produce encephalopathy and myoclonus. The rare condition known as Hashimoto's encephalopathy, which presents with a subacute progressive encephalopathy and myoclonus with periodic triphasic complexes on the EEG, should be excluded in cases of suspected CJD. It is diagnosed by the finding of high titers of antithyroglobulin or antithyroid peroxidase (antimicrosomal) antibodies in the blood, and improves with glucocorticoid therapy. Unlike CJD, fluctuations in severity typically occur in Hashimoto's encephalopathy.

The AIDS dementia complex (Chap. 31) may occasionally imitate CJD in onset, early course, physical signs, computed tomography (CT) findings, and lack of abnormalities on routine CSF studies. The few such patients without manifestations of systemic immunodeficiency (<10%) should be questioned about risk factors and should have serum antibodies to HIV determined.

LABORATORY TESTS

The only specific diagnostic tests for CJD and other human prion diseases measure PrP^{Sc}. The most widely used method involves limited proteolysis that generates PrP 27–30, which is detected by immunoassay after denaturation. The conformation-dependent immunoassay (CDI) is based on immunoreactive epitopes that are exposed in PrP^{C} but buried in PrP^{Sc}. The CDI is extremely sensitive and quantitative and is likely to find wide application in both the post- and antemortem detection of prions. In humans, the diagnosis of CJD can be established by brain biopsy if PrP^{Sc} is detected. If no attempt is made to measure PrP^{Sc}, but the constellation of pathologic changes frequently found in CJD is seen in a brain biopsy, then the diagnosis is reasonably secure (see "Neuropathology," above). Because PrP^{Sc} is not uniformly distributed throughout the CNS, the apparent absence of PrP^{Sc} in a limited sample such as a biopsy does not rule out prion disease. At autopsy, sufficient brain samples should be taken for both PrP^{Sc} immunoassay, preferably by the CDI, and immunohistochemistry of tissue sections.

Whether an antemortem test can be developed using the CDI to detect protease-sensitive forms of PrP^{Sc} in blood is uncertain. Another possibility is such a test based on PrP^{Sc} formation in muscle, lymphoid tissue, or olfactory mucosa.

To establish the diagnosis of either sCJD or familial prion disease, sequencing the *PRNP* gene must be performed. Finding the wild-type *PRNP* gene sequence permits the diagnosis of sCJD if there is no history to suggest exposure to an exogenous source of prions. The identification of a mutation in the *PRNP* gene sequence that encodes a nonconservative amino acid substitution argues for familial prion disease.

CT may be normal or show cortical atrophy. The MRI scan may show a subtle increased intensity in the basal ganglia with T2- or diffusion-weighted imaging, and this finding when present aids in diagnosis of sCJD (**Fig. 32-3**).

CSF is nearly always normal but may show minimal protein elevation. Although the stress protein 14-3-3 is elevated in the CSF of some patients with CJD, similar ele-

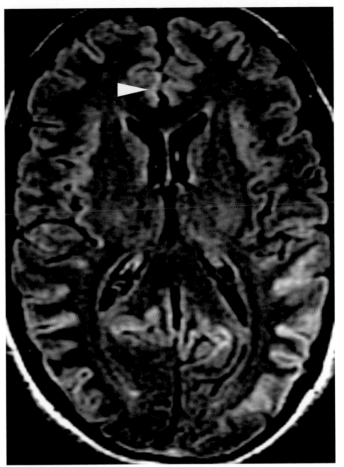

FIGURE 32-3

T2-weighted (FLAIR) MRI showing hyperintensity in the cortex in a patient with sporadic CJD. This so-called "cortical ribboning" along with increased intensity in the basal ganglia on T2 or diffusion-weighted imaging can aid in the diagnosis of CJD.

vations of 14-3-3 are found in patients with herpes simplex virus encephalitis, multi-infarct dementia, and stroke, and recent work questions the sensitivity of this test in CJD. In AD, 14-3-3 is generally not elevated. In the serum of some patients with CJD, the S-100 protein is elevated, but as with 14-3-3, this elevation is not specific.

The EEG is often useful in the diagnosis of CJD. During the early phase of CJD, the EEG is usually normal or shows only scattered theta activity. In most advanced cases, repetitive, high-voltage, triphasic, and polyphasic sharp discharges are seen, but in many cases their presence is transient. The presence of these stereotyped periodic bursts of <200 ms duration, occurring every 1 to 2 s, makes the diagnosis of CJD very likely. These discharges are frequently but not always symmetric; there may be a one-sided predominance in amplitude. As CJD progresses, normal background rhythms become fragmentary and slower.

CARE OF CJD PATIENTS

Although CJD should not be considered either a contagious or communicable disease, it is transmissible. The risk of accidental inoculation by aerosols is very small; nonetheless, procedures producing aerosols should be performed in certified biosafety cabinets. Biosafety level 2 practices, containment equipment, and facilities are recommended by the Centers for Disease Control and Prevention and the National Institutes of Health. The primary problem in caring for patients with CJD is the inadvertent infection of health care workers by needle and stab wounds. The transmission of prions through the air has never been documented. Electroencephalographic and electromyographic needles should not be reused after studies on patients with CJD have been performed.

There is no reason for pathologists or morgue dieners to resist performing autopsies on patients whose clinical diagnosis was CJD. Standard microbiologic practices outlined here, along with specific recommendations for decontamination, seem to be adequate precautions for the care of patients with CJD and the handling of infected specimens.

DECONTAMINATION OF CJD PRIONS

Prions are extremely resistant to common inactivation procedures, and there is some disagreement about the optimal conditions for sterilization. Some investigators recommend treating CJD-contaminated materials once with 1 N NaOH at room temperature, but we believe this procedure may be inadequate for sterilization. Autoclaving at 132°C for 5 h or treatment with 2 N NaOH for several hours is recommended for sterilization of prions. The term "sterilization" implies complete destruction of prions; any residual infectivity can be hazardous.

PREVENTION AND THERAPEUTICS

There is no known effective therapy for preventing or treating CJD. The finding that phenothiazines and acridines inhibit PrP^{Sc} formation in cultured cells led to clinical studies of quinacrine in CJD patients. Although quinacrine seems to slow the rate of decline in some CJD patients, no cure of the disease has been observed. In mice, the results of quinacrine treatment are mixed: some investigators report that treatment is ineffective, while others find that quinacrine prolongs the lives of prion-infected mice compared with untreated animals. Human studies on this compound are underway.

Like the acridines, anti-PrP antibodies have been shown to eliminate PrP^{Sc} from cultured cells. Additionally, such antibodies in mice either administered by injection or produced from a transgene have been shown to prevent prion disease when prions are introduced by a peripheral route, such as intraperitoneal inoculation. Unfortunately, the antibodies were ineffective in mice inoculated intracerebrally with prions. Several drugs delay the onset of disease in animals inoculated intracerebrally with prions if the drugs are given around the time of the inoculation.

Structure-based drug design predicated on dominant-negative inhibition of prion formation has produced several promising compounds. Modified quinacrine compounds that are more potent than the parent drug have been found. Whether improving the efficacy of such small molecules will provide general methods for developing novel therapeutics for other neurodegenerative disorders, including AD and Parkinson's disease, as well as amyotrophic lateral sclerosis (ALS), remains to be established. *Financial Disclosure: SBP has a financial interest in InPro Biotechnology, Inc.*

FURTHER READINGS

Bosque PJ et al: Prions in skeletal muscle. Proc Natl Acad Sci USA 99:3812, 2002

Geschwind MD et al: Challenging the clinical utility of the 14-3-3 protein for the diagnosis of sporadic Creutzfeldt-Jakob disease. Arch Neurol 60:813, 2003

May BCH et al: Potent inhibition of scrapie prion replication in cultured cells by bis-acridines. Proc Natl Acad Sci USA 100:3416, 2003

☑ Prusiner SB (ed): *Prion Biology and Diseases,* 2nd ed. Cold Spring Harbor, New York, Cold Spring Harbor Laboratory Press, 2004.

A comprehensive review of various prion disorders.

Shiga Y et al: Diffusion-weighted MRI abnormalities as an early diagnostic marker for Creutzfeldt-Jakob disease. N Engl J Med 348:711, 2003

Will RG et al: Diagnosis of new variant Creutzfeldt-Jakob disease. Ann Neurol 47:575, 2000

☑ Young GS et al: Diffusion-weighted and fluid-attenuated recovery imaging in Creutzfeldt-Jakob disease: High sensitivity and specificity for diagnosis. Am J Neuroradiol 26:1551, 2005

Review of MRI changes in sCJD and the accuracy of these findings.

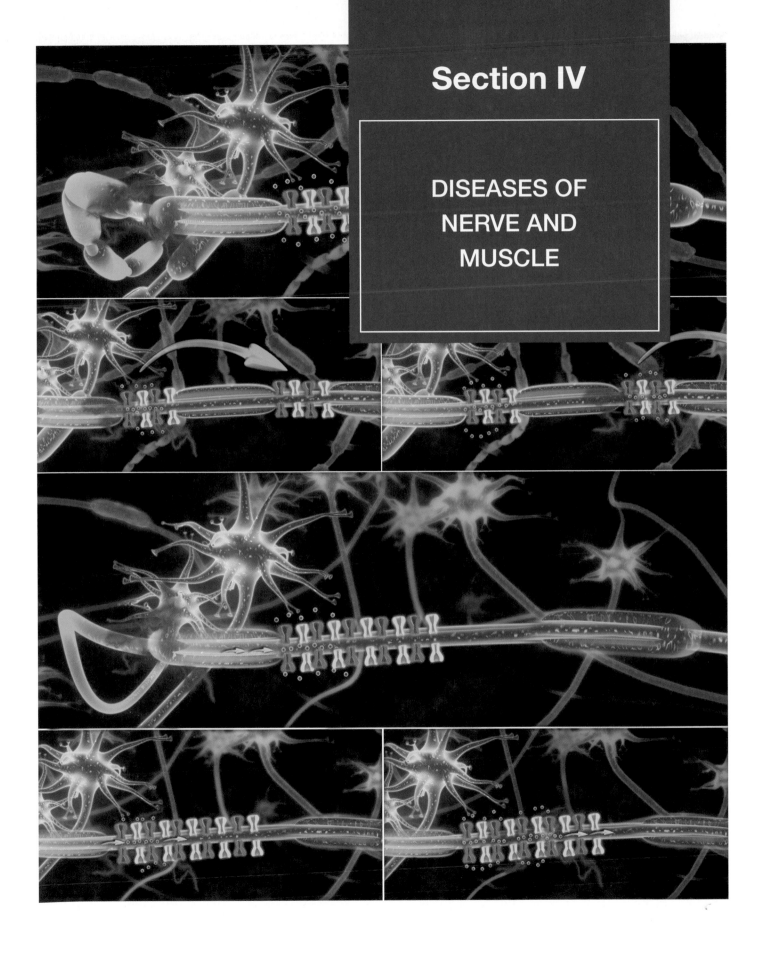

Section IV

DISEASES OF NERVE AND MUSCLE

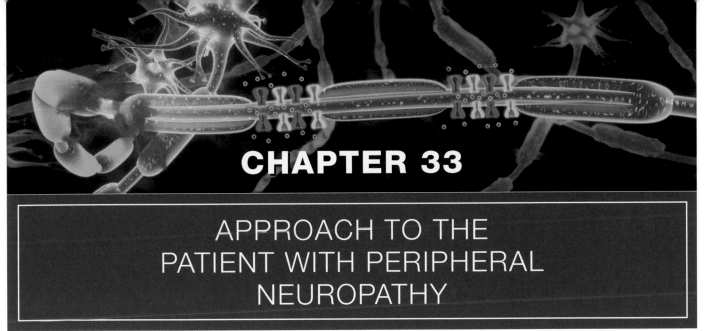

CHAPTER 33

APPROACH TO THE PATIENT WITH PERIPHERAL NEUROPATHY

Arthur K. Asbury

Peripheral neuropathy is a generic term for peripheral nerve disorders of any cause. Mononeuropathy refers to involvement of a single nerve, whereas polyneuropathy refers to involvement of multiple nerves (**Fig. 33–1**).

Focal weakness or sensory loss that follows the distribution of a single nerve characterizes a mononeuropathy. A typical distal, symmetric polyneuropathy is characterized by sensory loss and/or weakness that begins in the feet. The neuropathy is "length-dependent" because the longest axons are the most vulnerable; the deficits spread circumferentially up both legs to the knees from the feet, then simultaneously into the thighs and hands. The latter pattern is also termed a *stocking-glove* distribution. Deviations from this pattern of sensory deficit suggest other etiologies. For example, spread of a sensory deficit up the legs to the waist, without coincident involvement of the hands, likely reflects a spinal cord disorder (Chap. 24).

Electromyography (EMG) is an electrophysiologic method used to measure nerve and muscle function (see "Electrodiagnosis," below). In the nerve conduction study (NCS) portion of EMG, nerves are stimulated cutaneously with electric current and the induced electrical potentials are recorded over a distal or proximal segment of the same nerve, or over a muscle supplied by the nerve. The amplitude of the recorded signals correlates with axonal function, while the conduction velocity of the signal correlates with the function of peripheral nerve myelin. The potentials recorded can be sensory (sensory nerve action potentials, or SNAPs) or motor (compound motor action potentials, or CMAPs). Needle EMG allows for the assessment of function of a single motor nerve cell and the muscle cells it supplies (e.g., the motor unit). NCS and needle EMG together can be used to (1) determine if a nerve injury is present, (2) localize the site of injury along the course of the motor unit (e.g., anterior horn cell, nerve root, plexus, nerve, neuromuscular junction, or muscle), (3) suggest nerve pathology (axonal or demyelinating), or (4) provide information regarding prognosis. EMG is most helpful when used as an extension of the neurologic examination to resolve diagnostic and management questions that cannot be answered by the neurologic history and examination alone.

The clinical and electrodiagnostic (EDX) approach to evaluation and management of a neuropathic disorder is

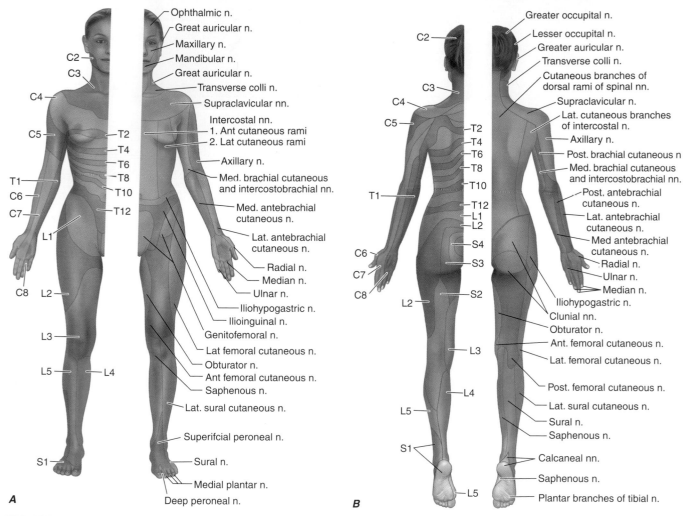

FIGURE 33-1

A. Anterior view of dermatomes (*left*) and cutaneous areas (*right*); *B.* posterior view of dermatomes (left) and cutaneous areas (right) supplied by individual peripheral nerves.

(Modified from MB Carpenter and J Sutin, in *Human Neuroanatomy*, 8th ed, Baltimore, Williams & Wilkins, 1983.)

summarized in **Fig. 33-2**. The examiner determines for each patient the tempo, distribution, and severity of the neuropathy and makes a judgment as to whether the problem represents a mononeuropathy, a mononeuropathy multiplex, or a polyneuropathy. Often this distinction is obvious. With the sum of clinical and EDX information in hand, the differential diagnostic possibilities and treatment options are usually narrowed to a manageable number.

MONONEUROPATHY

Mononeuropathy refers to focal involvement of a single nerve trunk and therefore implies a local cause. Direct trauma, compression, and entrapment are the usual causes. Ulnar neuropathies, due to lesions either at the ulnar groove or in the cubital tunnel, and median neuropathy due to compression in the carpal tunnel

constitute the great majority of mononeuropathies encountered in clinical practice. Common mononeuropathies are listed in **Table 33-1**. EDX examination is part of the evaluation of mononeuropathies, mainly to judge the nature of the focal lesion (demyelinating or axonal degeneration) and, in severe mononeuropathies, to determine whether any functioning nerve fibers remain.

In the absence of a history of trauma to the nerve trunk, factors favoring conservative management of a mononeuropathy include sudden onset, no motor deficit, few or no sensory findings (even though pain and sensory symptoms may be present), and no evidence of axonal degeneration by EDX criteria. Factors favoring active measures including surgical intervention are chronicity and worsening neurologic deficit on examination, particularly if motor and EDX evidence suggests that the lesion has resulted in axonal injury.

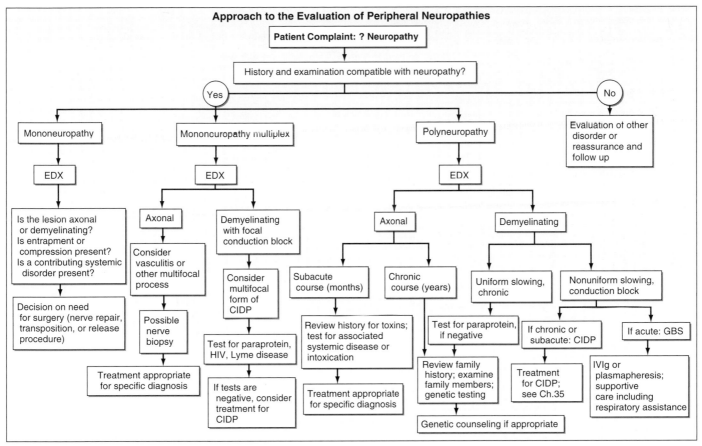

FIGURE 33-2

Approach to the evaluation of peripheral neuropathies. CIDP, chronic inflammatory demyelinating polyradiculoneuropathy; EDX, electrodiagnostic studies; GBS, Guillain-Barré syndrome; IVIg, intravenous immunoglobulin. For management and treatment considerations, see relevant sections of this chapter or of the two succeeding chapters on immune-mediated and on genetically determined neuropathies.

ULNAR NEUROPATHY

The most common site for ulnar nerve injury is at the elbow, either in the condylar groove proximally or the cubital tunnel distally. Severe, chronic ulnar paralysis results in a characteristic claw-hand deformity owing to wasting and weakness of the interossei and abductor digiti minimi muscles. The web space between the thumb and index finger is concave in appearance, highlighting the associated muscle wasting. Sensory loss occurs over the palmar aspect of the fifth finger and along the ulnar border of the palm. The superficial location of the nerve at the medial aspect of the elbow makes it vulnerable to trauma or compression. The ulnar nerve may also become entrapped just distal to the elbow in the cubital tunnel (cubital tunnel syndrome) formed by the aponeurotic arch linking the two heads of the flexor carpi ulnaris muscles. The differential diagnosis of ulnar neuropathy at the elbow includes a C8 radiculopathy or a brachial plexus lesion (lower trunk or medial cord).

The sensory loss associated with ulnar neuropathy at the elbow does not extend proximal to the wrist, but the sensory loss associated with brachial plexopathy or C8 radiculopathy frequently extends to the medial aspect of the foream. C8 radiculopathy is usually associated with neck pain that radiates into the arm. Neuroimaging of the cervical spine and EMG studies are helpful when the history and examination alone do not clearly distinguish between these common possibilities.

There are many causes of ulnar neuropathy at the elbow. Medical causes include diabetes mellitus, Paget's disease, rheumatoid arthritis, osteoarthritis, and leprosy. Recurrent pressure on the nerve (as in resting the elbow on a table, repetitive wrist flexion with compression of the ulnar nerve by the heads of the flexor carpi ulnaris muscle at the cubital tunnel) or a single episode (such as coma with compression of the nerve by a motionless arm) may cause ulnar neuropathy at the elbow. Trauma from fracture, dislocation, or recurrent prolapse of the ulnar nerve are other potential causes. Despite all at-

TABLE 33-1

COMMON MONONEUROPATHIES

NERVE	ORIGIN[a]	MUSCLES INNERVATED	USUAL SITE OF LESION	CLINICAL FEATURES	COMMENTS
UPPER EXTREMITY					
Suprascapular	C5, C6	Supraspinatus Infraspinatus	Suprascapular notch of scapula	Weakness of lateral rotation of the humerus	No sensory deficit
Long thoracic	C5–C7	Serratus anterior	Variable	Winging of scapula	No sensory deficit
Axillary	C5, C6	Deltoid, teres minor	Near shoulder joint	Weakness of shoulder abduction; atrophy of shoulder	Sensory deficit similar to C5 dorsal root lesion (see Fig. 33-1)
Radial	C5–T1	Triceps, brachioradialis, wrist, finger, and thumb extensors	Spiral groove of humerus	Wrist drop most obvious, also finger and thumb extensors paralyzed	Saturday night palsy (acute compression) is frequent cause
Posterior interosseous branch	C7, C8	Finger and thumb extensors	Edge of supinator muscle below elbow	Finger drop; wrist relatively spared	No sensory deficit
Ulnar	C8, T1	Ulnar flexor of the wrist, long flexors of 4th and 5th digits, and most intrinsic hand muscles	Ulnar groove at the elbow	Weakness of finger adduction and abduction and thumb adduction (see text); interosseous atrophy, claw-hand	May be acute or insidious; sensory symptoms/signs are distinctive (Fig. 33-1)
			Cubital tunnel	Same as above	Often pain over medial proximal forearm (cubital tunnel)
			Medial base of palm	Intrinsic hand muscles only, interosseous atrophy	No sensory deficit
Median	C6–T1	Abductor pollicis brevis, more proximal muscles include forearm pronator, long finger and thumb flexors	Carpal tunnel	Characteristic sensory symptoms and deficit and inability to make a circle with thumb and index finger	Sensory deficit as per (Fig. 33-1); known as carpal tunnel syndrome
Anterior interosseous branch	C7–T1	Long flexors of thumb and index and middle fingers	Anterior interosseus branch below the elbow	Weakness of pinch; pain in volar forearm	No sensory deficit
LOWER EXTREMITY					
Femoral	L2–L4	Iliopsoas (hip flexor) and quadriceps femoris (knee extensor)	Proximal to inguinal ligament	Knee buckling; absent knee jerk; weak anterior thigh muscles with atrophy	Association with diabetes mellitus; sensory disturbance as per Fig. 33-1
Lateral femoral cutaneous branch	L2, L3	None	Inguinal ligament	Dysesthetic hyperpathia of lateral thigh	Known as meralgia paresthetica
Obturator	L3, L4	Thigh adductors	Intrapelvic or at pubis	Weakness of hip adduction	Sensory deficit on medial thigh
Sciatic	L4–S3	Hamstring muscles, hip abductor, and all muscles below the knee	Near sciatic notch	Severe lower leg and hamstring weakness; flail foot; severe disability	Uncommon except from war wounds; sometimes after a misdirected injection
Posterior tibial	L5–S2	Calf muscles (proximally), toe flexors, and other intrinsic foot muscles	Tarsal tunnel, near medial malleolus	Pain and numbness of sole, weak toe flexors	Known as tarsal tunnel syndrome (see text)
Peroneal	L4–S1	Dorsiflexors of toes and foot, evertors of foot	At neck of fibula	Foot drop and weakness of foot eversion	Sensory deficit is similar in distribution to L5, S1 sensory roots

[a]Spinal segments.

tempts to identify a cause, some ulnar neuropathies remain idiopathic.

The wrist is a less common site of ulnar nerve injury. Traumatic injury at the wrist is usually due to prolonged pressure at the base of the palm, as occurs with repetitive use of hand tools or riding a bicycle. When the deep palmar branch of the ulnar nerve is affected, there is only weakness of ulnar-innervated muscles and no sensory loss. The lack of sensory loss in an apparent ulnar neuropathy should raise the possibility that the site of nerve injury is at the wrist. EMG can help localize the site of injury in unclear cases.

Management of ulnar neuropathy depends on the timing, site, and severity of the responsible focal lesion. In mild cases (e.g., a mild sensory deficit with minimal or no motor involvement), use of an elbow pad and avoidance of positions likely to traumatize the nerve may be sufficient. Follow-up assessment every 3 to 6 months for a year to assess recovery and make sure that the neuropathy has not worsened is advisable. When motor deficits are obvious, entrapment of the ulnar nerve within the cubital tunnel may be treated surgically by incising the aponeurosis of the flexor carpi ulnaris muscle (cubital tunnel release). Entrapment at the condylar groove may be treated surgically by an ulnar nerve transposition to move the nerve away from the site of recurrent trauma.

CARPAL TUNNEL SYNDROME

Entrapment of the median nerve at the wrist results in carpal tunnel syndrome (CTS). The most common symptoms of CTS are intermittent nocturnal paresthesias of the thumb, index, and middle fingers that awaken the patient from sleep and are relieved by shaking the hands. Pain is rarely, if ever, the predominant symptom. CTS can occur over a wide range of ages, but is most common in middle-aged women. The dominant hand is typically affected first, but the condition is bilateral to some degree in at least 50% of patients at the time of initial clinical evaluation. With worsening, symptoms extend into the day and eventually become constant. The examination reveals a decrease in pin or light touch sensation in the palmar aspect of the thumb, index, and third finger. Eventually, weakness and atrophy of the abductor pollicis brevis (thenar eminence) become evident. EMG is extremely helpful to localize early symptoms to the carpal tunnel, C6 nerve root, brachial plexus, or proximal median nerve.

There are many causes of CTS. Medical conditions that predispose to CTS include thyroid disease, diabetes mellitus, rheumatoid arthritis, chronic renal failure, amyloidosis, acromegaly, pregnancy, and myeloma, as well as mucopolysaccharidoses and mucolipidoses. Any patho-

logic process that occupies and limits space in the carpal tunnel (osteophytes, congenitally small canal, tophi due to gout, lipomas, ganglia) predisposes to CTS. Although CTS is often associated with repetitive use of the hands, it is also frequently idiopathic. Definitive confirmation of CTS can almost always be made with EMG studies.

The management of CTS includes the exclusion of secondary causes described above and selection of treatment appropriate for the severity of the median nerve involvement. Mild cases without sensory or motor weakness can occasionally be managed by the use of nocturnal wrist splints and the avoidance of activities or hand postures that trigger symptoms. A brief course of oral glucocorticoids or a glucocorticoid injection into the carpal tunnel may provide temporary symptomatic relief, but is rarely long-lasting. CTS associated with pregnancy often resolves following delivery. Surgical treatment (open carpal tunnel release) is performed under local anesthesia and is effective in relieving symptoms in 90 to 95% of patients with EMG-confirmed CTS. Patients with symptoms of >3 years' duration are less likely to respond. Endoscopic carpal tunnel release is an option for patients who need to return to work quickly or desire a smaller scar.

PERONEAL NEUROPATHY

Peroneal neuropathy is the most common mononeuropathy in the lower limbs. The nerve is typically injured at the neck of the fibula, usually from compression, traction, or trauma. The most notable deficit is weakness of foot dorsiflexion (foot drop); weakness of foot eversion is often present also. Sensory loss is found over the dorsum of the foot and the lateral calf. Peroneal neuropathy needs to be distinguished from sciatic neuropathy and L5 radiculopathy. Sciatic neuropathy produces weakness of the flexors of the toes and sensory loss over the sole of the foot. L5 radiculopathy is usually accompanied by back pain as well as radiating pain down the posterior or lateral aspect of the affected leg; weakness of L5-innervated proximal leg muscles such as hip abductors may also be present. EMG and neuroimaging of the spine are usually helpful in distinguishing among these possibilities. Common peroneal neuropathy may follow prolonged immobility (e.g., with coma or following general anesthesia), direct trauma (a bullet wound, fracture, laceration), or external pressure (from leg crossing, squatting, or a leg cast). Less common causes include focal masses (tumor, Baker's cyst, ganglia), diabetes mellitus, vasculitis, and leprosy. Many cases are idiopathic. Management usually consists of an ankle-foot orthosis (AFO) to prevent the patient from tripping due to the foot drop, and avoidance of situations or postures that predispose to additional trauma, pressure, or traction on the nerve at the fibular head.

TARSAL TUNNEL SYNDROME

The distal tibial nerve, along with several tendons and the posterior tibial artery, lies in the tarsal tunnel just posterior to the medial malleolus. Because of its superficial site, the distal tibial nerve is subject to compression or to direct trauma. Causes include sprain or fracture of the ankle, ill-fitting footwear, posttraumatic fibrosis, cysts or ganglia adjacent to the nerve, arthritis, and tenosynovitis. Characteristic symptoms are pain in the ankle and the sole of the foot with paresthesias, particularly while walking. On examination, the tibial nerve trunk in the tarsal tunnel is usually tender to palpation, sensory deficit should be demonstrable on the sole of the foot, and weakness of the toe plantar flexor muscles may be noted. EDX examination and also nerve block using local anesthetic are useful in establishing the diagnosis. Definitive treatment is extensive surgical decompression of the tibial nerve in the tarsal tunnel. Tarsal tunnel syndrome, in terms of its pathophysiology and management, is similar to carpal tunnel syndrome but is much less common (Table 33-1).

CRANIAL MONONEUROPATHY

Mononeuropathy affecting individual cranial nerves is discussed in Chap. 23.

POLYNEUROPATHY

The prototypical picture of polyneuropathy occurs with acquired toxic or metabolic states. The first symptoms tend to be sensory and consist of tingling, prickling, burning, or bandlike dysesthesias in the balls of the feet or tips of the toes, or in a general distribution over the soles. Symptoms and findings are usually symmetric and graded distally and often precede objective motor or sensory signs.

With progression, dysesthesias spread up the lower legs. Pansensory loss is usually found over both feet, ankle reflexes are lost, and weakness of dorsiflexion of the toes, best demonstrated in the great toe, is present. In some instances, the process begins with weakness in the feet, without preceding sensory symptoms. As worsening occurs, sensory loss moves centripetally in a graded "stocking" fashion, and the patient may complain that the feet have a numb or "wooden" feeling or may say "I feel as though I'm walking on stumps." Patients have difficulty walking on their heels during examination, and their feet may slap while walking. Later, the knee jerk reflex disappears and foot drop becomes more apparent. By the time sensory disturbance has reached the upper shin, dysesthesias are usually noticed in the tips of the fingers. The degree of spontaneous pain varies but is often considerable.

Light stimuli to hypesthetic areas, once perceived, may be experienced as extremely uncomfortable (*allodynia*). Unsteadiness of gait may be out of proportion to muscle weakness because of proprioceptive loss; in such cases, the imbalance may worsen in the dark and improve when the patient looks at the position of the feet.

Worsening is more severe in the legs than in the arms and proceeds in a centripetal, symmetrically graded manner with pansensory loss, areflexia, and muscle atrophy; motor weakness is usually greater in the extensor muscles than in corresponding flexor groups. When the sensory disturbance reaches the elbows and mid-thighs, a tent-shaped area of hypesthesia may often be demonstrated on the lower abdomen. This area will grow broader, and its apex will extend rostrally toward the sternum as the neuropathy worsens. By this time, patients generally cannot stand or walk or hold objects in their hands.

Overall, nerve fibers are affected according to axon length, without regard to root or nerve trunk distribution—hence the aptness of the term *stocking-glove* to describe the pattern of sensory deficit. In general, the motor deficit is also graded, distal, and symmetric.

Although *polyneuropathy* connotes a widespread symmetric process, usually distal and graded, polyneuropathies are quite diverse because of the variability of tempo, severity, mix of sensory and motor features, and presence or absence of positive symptoms (**Table 33-2**). For instance, a patient with a subacute, severely dysesthetic sensory polyneuropathy and alopecia who is in the early phases of thallium intoxication bears little similarity to the patient with a 40-year history of insidiously progressive clumsiness of gait whose findings are foot drop, lower leg atrophy, pes cavus, and minimal asymptomatic distal sensory deficit, all due to a hereditary polyneuropathy (Chap. 34). These two patients fall at opposite ends of the spectrum of polyneuropathy.

The classification of peripheral neuropathies has become increasingly complex as the capacity to discriminate new subgroups and identify new associations with toxins and systemic disorders improves. The important features of each major grouping of polyneuropathies are summarized in Table 33-2, and key aspects of specific polyneuropathies are given in **Tables 33-3** to Table **33-6**.

MONONEUROPATHY MULTIPLEX (MULTIFOCAL NEUROPATHY)

Mononeuropathy multiplex refers to simultaneous or sequential involvement of individual noncontiguous nerve trunks, either partially or completely, evolving over days to years. Since the disease process underlying mononeuropathy multiplex affects peripheral nerves in a multifocal and random fashion, progression of the disease favors

TABLE 33-2

MAJOR TYPES OF POLYNEUROPATHY

TYPE OF POLYNEUROPATHY	EVOLUTION	CAUSES	COMMENTS
Axonal			
Acute	Days to weeks	Porphyria	See Table 33-3
		Massive intoxications (arsenic; inhalants)	See Table 33-4
		Guillain-Barré syndrome—axonal form	See Chap. 35.
Subacute	Weeks to months	Mostly toxic or metabolic polyneuropathies; see Tables 33-3 and 33-4	Treatment involves eliminating the toxins or treating the associated systemic disorder
Chronic	Months to years	<5 years, consider toxic/metabolic causes; >5 years, consider hereditary basis, also diabetic and dysproteinemic causes	See Tables 33-3 and 33-4; also Chap. 34 on hereditary neuropathy
Demyelinating			
Acute	Days to weeks	Almost all are the common form of Guillain-Barré syndrome; see Chap. 35	Rare possibilities include diphtheritic polyneuritis or buckthorn berry intoxication
Subacute	Weeks to months	Mostly relapsing form of CIDP; see Chap. 35	Rarely, toxins mentioned above plus aurothioglucose and taxol (see Table 33-3)
Chronic	Months to years	Many possibilities including hereditary; inflammatory-autoimmune; dysproteinemias; other metabolic and toxic neuropathies	See Chaps. 34 and 35; also Tables 33-3 and 33-4

Note: CIDP, chronic inflammatory demyelinating polyneuropathy.

the neurologic deficit becoming less patchy and multifocal and more confluent and symmetric. As a result, some patients present with what appears to be a distal symmetric polyneuropathy. Attention to the pattern of early symptoms is therefore important in making the judgment that a particular neuropathy is indeed a mononeuropathy multiplex and not a polyneuropathy.

ASSESSMENT AND DIAGNOSIS OF POLYNEUROPATHY AND MONONEUROPATHY MULTIPLEX

Clues to the diagnosis of these neuropathies often lie in unnoticed or forgotten events occurring weeks or months prior to the onset of symptoms. Inquiry should be made about recent viral illnesses; other systemic symptoms; institution of new medications; exposures to solvents, pesticides, or heavy metals; the occurrence of similar symptoms in family members or co-workers; habits concerning alcohol; and the presence of preexisting medical disorders. Patients should be asked if they would feel well if free of their neuropathic symptoms; answers will suggest the presence or absence of an underlying systemic illness.

How did symptoms first appear? Even with distal polyneuropathies, symptoms may appear in the sole of one foot a few days or a week before the other, but usually the patient will describe a distal graded disturbance that moves evenly and symmetrically in centripetal fashion. Symptoms that first appear in the distribution of individual digital nerves, involving only half of a digit at a time, and then gradually spread and coalesce suggest a multifocal process (mononeuropathy multiplex), as might occur with a systemic vasculitis or cryoglobulinemia.

The evolution of neuropathy ranges from rapid worsening over a few days to an indolent process lasting decades. Polyneuropathies that progress slowly, over >5 years, are most likely to be genetically determined, particularly if the major manifestations are distal atrophy and weakness with few or no positive sensory symptoms. Diabetic polyneuropathy and paraproteinemic neuropathies also progress insidiously over 5 to 10 years. Axonal degenerations of toxic or metabolic origin tend to evolve over several weeks to a year or more, and the rate of progression of demyelinating neuropathies is highly variable, ranging from a few days in Guillain-Barré syndrome (GBS; Chap. 35) to many years in others.

TABLE 33-3

POLYNEUROPATHY ASSOCIATED WITH SYSTEMIC DISEASES

SYSTEMIC DISEASE (OCCURRENCE)	AXONAL[a]			DEMYELINATING[a]			SENSORY VS. MOTOR[b]	AUTONOMIC[a]	COMMENT
	ACUTE	SUBACUTE	CHRONIC	ACUTE	SUBACUTE	CHRONIC			
Diabetes mellitus (common)	−	±	+	−	±	+	S, SM, rarely M	± to +	See Table 33-5
Uremia (sometimes)	±	+	+	−	−	−	SM	±	Controllable with proper dialysis: curable with successful renal transplant
Porphyria (3 types) (rare)	+	±	−	−	−	−	M or SM	± to +	May be proximal > distal and may have atypical proximal sensory deficits
Hypoglycemia (rare)	±	+	±	−	−	−	M	−	Usually with insulinoma; arms often > legs
Vitamin deficiency, excluding B$_{12}$ (sometimes)	−	+	+	−	−	−	SM	±	Involves thiamine, pyridoxine, folate, pantothenic acid, and probably others
Vitamin B$_{12}$ deficiency (sometimes)	−	±	+	−	−	−	S	−	Neuropathy overshadowed by myelopathy
Critical illness (sepsis) (common)	−	+	±	−	−	−	M > S	−	Sepsis patients severely ill
Chronic liver disease (sometimes)	−	−	−	−	−	+	S or SM	−	Usually mild or subclinical
Primary biliary cirrhosis (rare)	−	±	+	−	−	−	S	−	Intraneural xanthomas; dysesthesias
Primary systemic amyloidosis (rare)	−	±	+	−	−	−	SM	+	Also in amyloidosis with myeloma or macroglobulinemia
Hypothyroidism (rare)	−	−	−	−	±	+	S	−	May respond to thyroid replacement
Chronic obstructive lung disease (rare)	−	±	+	−	−	−	S or SM	−	Severe pulmonary insufficiency
Acromegaly (rare)	−	−	+	−	−	−	S	−	Carpal tunnel syndrome also frequent
Malabsorption (sprue, celiac disease) (sometimes)	−	±	+	−	−	−	S or SM	±	Basis for neuropathy unclear; deficiency?
Carcinoma (sensory) (rare)	−	+	+	−	−	−	Pure S	−	Due to ganglionitis, mostly small cell lung or breast carcinoma; paraneoplastic
Carcinoma (sensorimotor) (sometimes)	−	+	+	−	−	−	SM	±	Sensorimotor axonal neuropathy; mostly with lung cancer
Carcinoma (late) (common)	−	+	+	−	−	−	S > M	±	Mild, probably related to weight loss and wasting
Carcinoma (demyelinating) (sometimes)	−	−	−	+	+	±	SM	−	Acute or relapsing demyelinating neuropathy
HIV infection (sometimes)	−	±	+	−	−	−	S ≫ M	−	Late stages of AIDS; other neuropathies occur; see text
Lyme disease (sometimes)	−	±	+	−	−	−	S > M	−	Variable picture: see text

(Continued)

TABLE 33-3   *(Continued)*

POLYNEUROPATHY ASSOCIATED WITH SYSTEMIC DISEASES

SYSTEMIC DISEASE (OCCURRENCE)	AXONAL[a]			DEMYELINATING[a]			SENSORY VS. MOTOR[b]	AUTONOMIC[a]	COMMENT
	ACUTE	SUBACUTE	CHRONIC	ACUTE	SUBACUTE	CHRONIC			
Lymphoma, including Hodgkin's (sometimes)	−	+	+	+	+	±	See above	±	Same as with carcinomatous types
Polycythemia vera (rare)	−	±	+	−	−	−	S	−	Also CNS manifestations; often shooting pains in limbs
Multiple myeloma, lytic type (sometimes)	−	±	+	−	−	−	S, M, or SM	±	Symptomatic neuropathy uncommon; subclinical neuropathy frequent
Multiple myeloma, osteosclerotic[c] (sometimes)	−	−	±	−	±	+	SM	−	May show severe slowing of nerve conduction velocity
MGUS[d] (sometimes):									
IgA	−	±	+	−	−		SM	−	IgM$_k$ mainly; may bind
IgG	−	±	+	−	−	−	SM	−	to myelin-associated
IgM	−	−	−	−	±	+	SM or S	−	glycoprotein (MAG) or other glycoconjugates
Cryoglobulinemia (rare)	−	±	+	−	−	−	SM	−	May be mononeuropathy multiplex in presentation

[a]+, Usually; ±, sometimes; −, rare, if ever.

[b]S, sensory; M, motor; SM, sensorimotor.

[c]Some cases associated with POEMS syndrome (*p*olyneuropathy, *o*rganomegaly, *e*ndo-crinopathy, *M* proteins, and *s*kin change.

[d]Monoclonal gammopathy of undetermined significance.

Major fluctuations in the course of neuropathy raise two possibilities: (1) relapsing forms of neuropathy and (2) repeated toxic exposures. Slow fluctuation in symptoms taking place over weeks or months (reflecting changes in the activity of neuropathy) should not be confused with day-to-day variation or diurnal undulation of symptoms. The latter are common to all neuropathic disorders. An example is carpal tunnel syndrome, in which dysesthesias may be prominent at night but absent during the day.

Palpation of the nerve trunk to detect enlargement is a frequently forgotten part of the neurologic examination. In mononeuropathy or mononeuropathy multiplex, the entire course of the nerve trunk in question should be explored manually for focal thickening, for the presence of neurofibroma, point tenderness, or Tinel's phenomenon (generation of a tingling sensation in the sensory territory of the nerve by tapping along the course of the nerve trunk); and for pain elicited by stretching of the nerve trunk. In leprous neuritis, fusiform thickening of nerve trunks is frequent; beading of nerve trunks may be encountered in amyloid polyneuropathy. In genetically determined hypertrophic neuropathies, uniform thickening of all nerve trunks may occur, often to the diameter of one's little finger.

Most neuropathies involve nerve fibers of all sizes, but damage is sometimes restricted either to large or to small fibers. In a polyneuropathy affecting mainly small fibers, diminished pinprick and temperature sensation, often with painful, burning dysesthesias, will predominate, along with autonomic dysfunction, but with relative sparing of motor power, balance, and tendon jerks. Some cases of amyloid and distal diabetic polyneuropathies fall into this category. In contrast, large-fiber polyneuropathy is characterized by areflexia, sensory ataxia, relatively minor cutaneous sensory deficit (even though distal dysesthesias are common), and variable degrees of motor dysfunction, sometimes severe.

For patients with distal polyneuropathy, standard tests for potentially treatable causes should include measurement of the erythrocyte sedimentation rate, thyroid-stimulating hormone (TSH), and vitamin B$_{12}$; serum protein electrophoresis; immunofixation electrophoresis; and measurement of blood urea nitrogen (BUN), creatinine, and fasting blood glucose or a postprandial glucose

TABLE 33-4

POLYNEUROPATHY ASSOCIATED WITH DRUGS AND ENVIRONMENTAL TOXINS

	AXONAL[a]			DEMYELINATING[a]			SENSORY VS. MOTOR[b]	AUTONOMIC[a]	CNS[a]	COMMENT
	ACUTE	SUBACUTE	CHRONIC	ACUTE	SUBACUTE	CHRONIC				
DRUGS[c]										
Amiodarone (antiarrhythmic)	−	−	+	−	−	+	SM	−	−	Dose-dependent neuropathy, reversible by decreasing dose
Aurothioglucose (antirheumatic)	±	±	−	+	+	−	SM	−	−	Idiosyncratic reaction; ? immune-mediated
Cisplatin (antineoplastic)	−	+	+	−	−	−	S	−	−	Severe sensory neuropathy, also ototoxicity; dose-related
Dapsone (dermatologic agent, e.g., for leprosy)	−	±	+	−	−	−	M	−	−	Dose-related pure motor neuropathy
Disulfiram (anti-alcoholism agent)	±	+	+	−	−	−	SM	−	±	Usually occurs after months of treatment
Hydralazine (antihypertensive)	−	±	+	−	−	−	S > M	−	−	A pyridoxine antagonist
Isoniazid	−	±	+	−	−	−	SM	±	−	A pyridoxine antagonist; neurotoxic in slow acetylators
Metronidazole (antiprotozoal)	−	−	±	−	−	−	S or SM	−	+	Dose-related central-peripheral distal axonopathy
Misonidazole (radiosensitizer)	−	±	+	−	−	−	S or SM	−	+	Neurotoxicity is the limiting factor
Nitrofurantoin (urinary antiseptic)	−	±	+	−	−	−	SM	−	−	Generally total dose-related; renal failure enhances toxicity
Nucleoside analogues (ddC, ddI, d4T) (antiretroviral agents)	±	+	+	−	−	−	S ≫ M	−	?	Dose-related; painful
Phenytoin (anticonvulsant)	−	−	+	−	−	−	S > M	−	−	After 20–30 years of phenytoin use
Pyridoxine (vitamin)	−	±	+	−	−	−	S	−	−	Occurs with large intake (>300 mg/d)
Statins (HMG CoA reductase inhibitors)	−	±	+	−	−	−	S > M	−	−	Cases reported for most statins
Suramin (antineoplastic)	+	+	−	+	+	−	M > S	−	−	Related to serum levels 350 μg/mL or above
Taxol (antineoplastic)	±	+	±	±	+	±	S > M	−	−	Dose-related
Vincristine (antineoplastic)	−	+	+	−	−	−	S > M	−	−	Sensory symptoms common, hands > feet; motor signs ominous; should stop treatment

(Continued)

TABLE 33-4 *(Continued)*

POLYNEUROPATHY ASSOCIATED WITH DRUGS AND ENVIRONMENTAL TOXINS

	AXONAL[a]			DEMYELINATING[a]			SENSORY VS. MOTOR[b]	AUTONOMIC[a]	CNS[a]	COMMENT
	ACUTE	SUBACUTE	CHRONIC	ACUTE	SUBACUTE	CHRONIC				
TOXINS[c]										
Acrylamide (flocculant; grouting agent)	−	±	+	−	−	−	S > M	±	+	Large-fiber neuropathy; sensory ataxia
Arsenic (herbicide; insecticide)	±	+	+	−	−	−	SM	±	±	Skin changes, Mees, lines in nails; painful; systemic effects
Diphtheria toxin	−	−	−	+	+	−	SM	−	−	Clinically very rare; can be confused with GBS
γ-Diketone hexacarbons (solvents)	−	±	+	−	−	+	SM	±	+	Neurofilamentous swelling of axons: these solvents now in restricted use
Inorganic lead	−	−	+	−	−	−	M > S or M	−	±	Selective motor neuropathy with prominent wrist drop
Organophosphates	−	±	+	−	−	−	SM	−	+	Brain and spinal cord also affected, the latter irreversibly
Thallium (rat poison)	−	+	+	−	−	−	SM	−	+	Also alopecia, Mees' lines in nails; painful

[a] +, Usually; ±, sometimes; −, rare, if ever.

[b] S, sensory; M, motor; SM, sensorimotor.

[c] The following drugs and environmental toxins are also neurotoxic, mainly to the peripheral nervous system:

Drugs: Allopurinol, amitriptyline, chloramphenicol, colchicines, ethambutol, flecainide, indomethacin, lithium, nitrous oxide, perhexiline maleate, podophyllin, sodium cyanate, thalidomide, L-tryptophan.

Environmental toxins: Allyl chloride, buckthorn berry, carbon disulfide, diglycols (either ethylene or propylene), dimethylaminoproprionitrile (DMAPN), ethylene oxide, metallic mercury, methyl bromide, polychlorinated biphenyls, styrene, trichlorethylene, vacor.

Note: CNS, central nervous system; GBS, Guillain-Barré syndrome.

tolerance test. For patients with mononeuropathy multiplex, tests for potentially treatable causes should include complete blood count with differential, urinalysis, chest x-ray or chest computed tomography (CT) scan, postprandial blood glucose, HIV antibody, and serum protein electrophoresis. Further tests are dictated by the combined results of the history and the physical and EDX examination (Fig. 33–2).

ELECTRODIAGNOSIS

EDX studies are an essential part of the evaluation of neuropathies, myopathies, and neuromuscular junction disorders, and can help to distinguish between these three categories of disease. As described above, the EDX

TABLE 33-5

CLASSIFICATION OF DIABETIC NEUROPATHIES

Symmetric
1. Distal, primarily sensory polyneuropathy
   a. Mainly large fibers affected
   b. Mixed[a]
   c. Mainly small fibers affected[a]
2. Autonomic neuropathy
3. Chronically evolving proximal motor neuropathy[a,b]

Asymmetric
1. Acute or subacute proximal motor neuropathy[a,b]
2. Cranial mononeuropathy[b]
3. Truncal neuropathy[a,b]
4. Entrapment neuropathy in the limbs

[a] Often painful.

[b] Recovery, partial or complete, is likely.

TABLE 33-6

SENSORY NEUROPATHIES

CAUSE OR ASSOCIATION	COURSE	NERVE FIBER SIZE AFFECTED		NEURONOPATHY	COMMENT
		SMALL	LARGE		
TOXINS/DRUGS					
Cisplatin (antineoplastic)	Sub/Chr	+	++	+	Dose-related
Pyridoxine (vitamin, in megadose amounts)	Sub/Chr	+	++	+/−	Dose-related
Taxol (antineoplastic)	Acu/Sub	++	+	−	NGF may be protective
SYSTEMIC DISEASES					
Paraneoplastic	Sub	+	++	++	Most SCLC and breast
Sjögren's syndrome	Sub/Chr	+/−	+	++	Variable presentation
Dysproteinemia (mainly IgM$_\kappa$)	Chr	+	++	−	Demyelinating; may bind to MAG and other myelin glycoproteins
IDIOPATHIC					
Acute sensory neuronopathy	Acu	+/−	++	++	Poor recovery; persistent deficit
Chronic ataxic neuropathy	Chr	+/−	++	Prob.	Gradual progression
HEREDITARY					
Many varieties (see Chap. 34)	Chr	Variable		Some	Progressive

Abbreviations: ++, most; +, some; ±, occasionally; Prob, probable; Acu, acute; Sub, subacute; Chr, chronic; NGF, nerve growth factor; MAG, myelin-associated glycoprotein; SCLC, small-cell lung carcinoma.

examination ordinarily comprises EMG and NCSs. EMG involves recording electrical potentials from a needle electrode in muscle both at rest and during voluntary contraction of the muscle. Resulting electromyographic patterns are displayed on a screen for analysis. EMG is generally most useful for distinguishing between and among myopathic and neuropathic disorders. Myopathic disorders are marked by small, short-duration, polyphasic motor unit action potentials recruited in excessive numbers for a given degree of voluntary muscle contraction. Other patterns characteristic of specific muscle abnormalities can also be observed, such as myotonia (high-frequency discharges that wax or wane).

By contrast, EMG findings in neuropathic disorders demonstrate a decrease in the number of motor units (denervation). A motor unit is, by definition, an anterior horn cell, its axon, and the motor end plates and muscle fibers it innervates. The number of muscle fibers in a normal motor unit varies widely, from as few as 20 in an extraocular muscle to over 1500 in a large leg muscle. In long-standing muscle denervation (months or years), motor unit potentials become large and polyphasic. This occurs as a result of collateral reinnervation of nearby denervated muscle fibers by axonal sprouts from surviving motor axons. In brief, when motor axons die

back, their muscle fiber domains are taken over by intact neighboring axons. Other EMG features that favor denervation include fibrillations (random, unregulated firing of individual denervated muscle fibers), fasciculations (random, spontaneous firing of motor units, which in chronic states can be markedly enlarged and polyphasic), positive sharp waves, and complex repetitive discharges.

NCSs are carried out by stimulating motor or sensory nerves electrically at two or more sites and recording from either the muscle innervated, for motor nerves, or from yet another site on the stimulated nerve trunk, for sensory nerves. From the data recorded, the velocity of conduction and other informative characteristics of the recorded waveforms can be determined. When a disorder of the neuromuscular junction is suspected, other more specialized techniques are used, including muscle response to repetitive stimulation of nerve and single-fiber EMG. Detailed discussion of the full range of EDX techniques and their application, use, and interpretation may be found in several recent monographs listed in the references.

It is generally not possible to distinguish between axonal and demyelinating disorders by clinical examination alone; here EDX analysis is particularly useful. EDX features of demyelination are slowing of nerve conduction velocity (NCV), dispersion of evoked compound action potentials, conduction block (major decrease in amplitude of muscle compound action potentials on proximal stimulation of the nerve, as compared to distal stimulation), and marked prolongation of distal latencies. In contrast, axonal neuropathies are characterized by a reduction in amplitude of evoked compound action potentials with relative preservation of NCV. The distinction between a primarily demyelinating neuropathy and an axonal neuropathy is crucial because of the differing approaches to diagnosis and management.

EDX studies also help to determine the presence or absence of a sensory involvement when that is not clear by clinical examination alone. It provides information about the distribution of subclinical findings, thus sharpening the diagnostic focus. Other issues that may be clarified by the electrodiagnostician include:

1. The distinction between disorders primary to nerve or to muscle (neuropathy versus myopathy)
2. The distinction between root or plexus involvement and more distal nerve trunk involvement
3. The distinction between generalized polyneuropathic processes and widespread multifocal nerve trunk involvement
4. The distinction between upper and lower motor neuron weakness
5. The distinction, in a given generalized polyneuropathic process, between primary demyelinating neuropathy and primary axonal degeneration
6. The assessment, in both primary axonal and demyelinating neuropathies, of features bearing on the nature, activity, and likely prognosis of the neuropathy, particularly the extent of primary or secondary axonal degeneration
7. The assessment, in mononeuropathies, of the site of the lesion and its major effect on nerve fibers, especially the distinction between demyelination vs. axonal loss
8. The characterization of disorders of the neuromuscular junction
9. The identification, often in muscle of normal bulk and strength, of important features such as chronic partial denervation, fasciculations, and myotonia
10. The analysis of cramp, and its distinction from physiologic contracture

If in a particular instance of progressive polyneuropathy of subacute or chronic evolution the EDX findings are those of an axonopathy, a long list of metabolic states and exogenous toxins comes under consideration (Tables 33-3 and 33-4). If the course is protracted over several years, it raises the likelihood of a hereditary neuropathy (Chap. 34); family members must be examined

and additional attention given to the family history. If the EDX findings indicate primary demyelination of nerve, the approach is entirely different. The possibilities then include acquired demyelinating neuropathy, thought to be immunologically mediated (Chap. 35), and genetically determined demyelinating neuropathies, many of which are marked by uniform and drastic slowing of nerve conduction velocities (Chap. 34).

If the clinical features indicate mononeuropathy multiplex, the EDX question is whether the process is primarily axonal or demyelinating. Almost one-third of all adults with the clinical syndrome of mononeuropathy multiplex have a clear-cut picture of a demyelinating disorder, often with foci of persistent conduction block on EDX examination. Multifocal demyelinating neuropathy may represent part of the spectrum of chronic inflammatory demyelinating polyneuropathy (CIDP) or, if multifocal and only motor, would fit into the related category of multifocal motor neuropathy. For further discussion of the management of multifocal motor neuropathy, see Chap. 35.

The remaining two-thirds of patients with mononeuropathy multiplex have a picture of patchy axonal involvement by EDX examination. Although ischemia should be suspected as the basis of neuropathy in these patients, only about one-half can be shown to have disease of the vasa nervorum, usually vasculitis. Management of those with proven vasculitis of vasa nervorum is often the same as treatment for systemic vasculitis (Chap. 35). If the cause of mononeuropathy multiplex remains undiagnosed even on follow-up, management should be conservative. In many patients the disease will stabilize or reverse, at least partially.

Mononeuropathy multiplex syndrome may also be seen as a manifestation of leprosy, sarcoidosis, certain types of amyloidosis, hypereosinophilia syndrome, cryoglobulinemia, neuroAIDS, and multifocal types of diabetic neuropathy.

NERVE BIOPSY

The sural nerve at the ankle is the preferred site for cutaneous nerve biopsy. There are few indications to employ this invasive technique. The main one is in asymmetric and multifocal neuropathic disorders producing a clinical picture of mononeuropathy multiplex, the basis of which is still unclear after other laboratory investigations are complete. Diagnostic considerations include vasculitis, multifocal demyelinating neuropathies, amyloidosis, leprosy, and occasionally sarcoidosis. Nerve biopsy is also helpful when one or more cutaneous nerves are palpably enlarged. Another clinical application is in establishing the diagnosis in some genetically determined childhood disorders such as metachromatic leukodystrophy, Krabbe's disease, giant axonal neuropa-

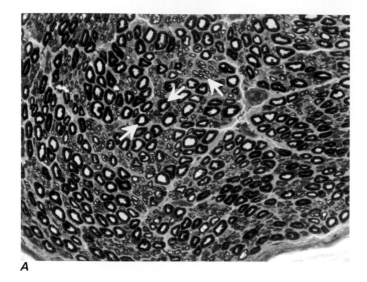

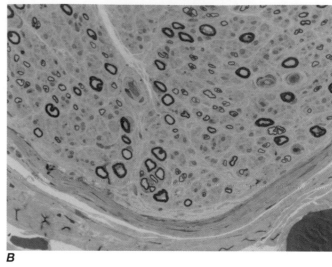

FIGURE 33-3

A. Normal sural nerve. This transverse section consists of multiple nerve fascicles invested by dense, collagenous perineurium. The nerve fascicle contains abundant myelinated axons of different calibers (*arrows*) (Toluidine blue, 400x; Courtesy of Dr. Joanna Phillips, Department of Pathology, University of California, San Francisco). *B.* Axonal polyneuropathy. This transverse section demonstrates significant loss of large and small diameter axons. The remaining axons have relatively uniform myelin coats (Toluidine blue, 400x); Courtesy of Dr. Andrew Bollen, Department of Pathology, University of California, San Francisco). *C.* The sural nerve biopsy demonstrates a necrotizing vasculitis with fibrinoid necrosis of the wall of a medium-sized blood vessel (*arrowheads*) and an associated lymphoplasmacytic inflammatory cell infiltrate (*arrows*) (hematoxylin and eosin, 200x; Courtesy of Dr. Andrew Bollen, Department of Pathology, University of California, San Francisco).

thy, and infantile neuroaxonal dystrophy. In all of these recessively inherited diseases, both the central nervous system and the peripheral nervous system are affected **(Fig. 33–3)**.

There is a tendency to carry out sural nerve biopsy in distal symmetric polyneuropathies of subacute or chronic evolution. This practice is discouraged because its yield is low and not worth the risk of wound infection, poor healing, or persistent pain. Nerve biopsy in this situation may be useful as part of an approved research protocol when the biopsy will provide crucial information not otherwise obtainable.

SPECIAL CATEGORIES OF NEUROPATHY

Some neuropathies require individual description because of their importance or distinctiveness.

DIABETIC NEUROPATHIES

The neuropathies of diabetes mellitus are classified in Table 33-5. A limitation of this classification is that most patients do not fit neatly into any single category but instead have overlapping clinical features of several. For instance, many diabetic patients with distal, primarily sensory polyneuropathy can also be shown to have autonomic dysfunction, usually in the form of vasomotor disturbance in the limbs and abnormalities of sweating. Similarly, patients who develop a proximal motor syndrome often have dysautonomic features (including sexual impotence in males) and some degree of distal sensory polyneuropathy. To compound matters, such patients appear at risk of developing a cranial mononeuropathy. Pain is a frequent feature of diabetic neuropathies (Table 33-5) but is variable in incidence and degree.

Neuropathies occur in the setting of long-standing hyperglycemia, the principal manifestation of the group of metabolic disorders comprising diabetes mellitus. By far the most common neuropathies related to diabetes mellitus are the diffuse sensory and autonomic types (categories 1 and 2 under "Symmetric" in Table 33-5). Sensory and autonomic polyneuropathy, chronic and indolent in evolution, may first be noticed in the third to fifth decades in patients with juvenile-onset diabetes (type 1) but tend to occur after age 50 in patients with adult-onset diabetes (type 2). Focal and multifocal types of neuropathy are less common but quite dramatic (categories 1, 2, and 3 under "Asymmetric" in Table 33-5). They rarely occur before the age of 45 and are usually subacute or acute in onset. Cranial mononeuropathies are mainly isolated sixth or third nerve palsies. The latter spares the pupil in three-fourths of cases, and some local pain or headache occurs in one-half. Truncal (thoracoabdominal) neuropathy is painful, involves one or more intercostal or lumbar nerves unilaterally, and frequently coexists with asymmetric proximal motor neuropathy in the legs. In asymmetric proximal motor neuropathy (diabetic amyotrophy), the most evident features are weakened muscles innervated by the femoral and obturator nerves (quadriceps femoris, iliopsoas, adductor magnus) and ipsilateral loss of the knee jerk reflex. Sensory deficit is minor, but pain in the hip and anterior thigh may be prominent. In all these multifocal and focal neuropathies, the pain usually subsides within weeks to a year, and function is usually partly or completely recovered. The same is true for symmetric proximal motor neuropathy (category 3 under "Symmetric" in Table 33-5).

Focal and multifocal diabetic neuropathies are considered to be ischemic in origin; ischemia may also underlie symmetric polyneuropathies, which are also thought to involve an abnormality of nerve metabolism.

Management of diabetic neuropathies is directed toward optimal glycemic control and symptomatic pain suppression. In the long-term Diabetes Control and Complications Trial, patients who controlled their diabetes meticulously showed significantly less neuropathy. Entrapment neuropathies are frequently amenable to surgical decompression. Medications helpful for the pain associated with diabetic polyneuropathy include tricyclic antidepressants (nortriptyline, amitriptyline), gabapentin, tramadol, and duloxetine.

NEUROPATHIES WITH HIV INFECTION
(See Chap. 31)

Neuropathies are common in infection with HIV; different types of neuropathy are seen according to the stage of the disease. GBS or CIDP (Chap. 35) are the neuropathies likely to occur following conversion to seropositivity and during the asymptomatic phase of HIV infection. Treatment is the same as for HIV-negative patients. In later, symptomatic stages, mononeuritis multiplex, axonal in nature, can occur; the course is typically subacute or chronic. In some cases, vasculitis of the vasa nervorum has been demonstrated.

A common neuropathy is a distal, symmetric, mainly sensory polyneuropathy, which evolves slowly in the late symptomatic stages of HIV infection and frequently coexists with symptomatic encephalopathy and myelopathy (Table 33-3; Chap. 31). The incidence of late-stage neurologic disorders, including sensory polyneuropathy, appears to be diminishing for HIV-positive individuals on effective highly active antiretroviral therapy (HAART) programs. Sensory polyneuropathy of late-stage HIV infection must be distinguished from toxic polyneuropathy that may result from the use of nucleoside analogue treatment (Table 33-4). At times, nucleoside analogues may precipitate a rapidly evolving, severe polyneuropathy with concurrent lactic acidemia. Clinically the neuropathy can be mistaken for GBS. Also in the late stages, a severe, destructive, subacute, asymmetric polyradiculopathy involving the cauda equina may be seen; it is caused by infection of the nerve roots with cytomegalovirus. Ganciclovir, started early, can arrest the disorder.

NEUROPATHIES WITH LYME DISEASE

A focal or multifocal radiculoneuropathy may occur weeks, months, or even years after primary infection by the tick-borne spirochete *Borrelia burgdorferi*. Although usually sensory and either dysesthetic or painful, the neuropathy is variable in distribution, affecting cranial nerves and spinal roots or nerves in a patchy, asymmetric fashion. Neuropathy is often chronic and persistent; cerebrospinal fluid pleocytosis is the rule. In many, improvement occurs spontaneously, but the course is shortened by treatment with antibiotics, usually intravenous ceftriaxone.

HERPES ZOSTER

This is a sensory neuritis due to infection with varicella-zoster virus (VZV) and is characterized by acute inflammation of one or more dorsal root ganglia. Lancinating pain and hyperalgesia over the skin surface supplied by the affected roots occur for 3 to 4 days, followed by the appearance in the same segment of a herpetic eruption characterized by painful raised vesicles on an erythematous base. Pain usually subsides in a few weeks. If the inflammatory process spreads to involve related motor roots, segmental motor weakness and wasting appear. Paralysis of the oculomotor nerves may occur in conjunction with involvement of the ophthalmic division of the trigeminal ganglion (ophthalmoplegic zoster). Facial paralysis may occur with involvement of the geniculate ganglion and herpetic eruption on the ipsilateral tympanic membrane or external ear canal (Ramsay Hunt syndrome).

In a small proportion of patients, neuropathic pain persists in the dermatomal distribution of the affected ganglia. This pain, known as *postherpetic neuralgia*, is intense, burning, hyperpathic and unrelenting; it often dominates the lives of those affected. Advancing age is a risk factor for this outcome. In some patients, blunting of the pain to tolerable levels is achieved by use of anticonvulsants such as carbamazepine or gabapentin or a tricyclic antidepressant such as nortriptyline. Postherpetic neuralgia may reflect active persistent VZV infection of the ganglion and may respond to intravenous antiviral therapy. A recent study found that administration of a live, attenuated virus vaccine to adults >60 years old reduced the incidence of postherpetic neuralgia by 66%, and the incidence of herpes zoster by half.

LEPROUS NEURITIS

This is a major worldwide cause of neuropathy. *Mycobacterium leprae* organisms readily invade Schwann cells in cutaneous nerve twigs, particularly those associated with unmyelinated nerve fibers. *M. leprae* thrives best in the coolest tissues in the body. Two major forms of leprous neuritis are recognized, tuberculoid and lepromatous, which actually represent the ends of a spectrum of disease, the middle of which is called borderline (dimorphous) leprosy (patchy and multifocal involvement of skin and nerve). The treatment of a given case depends on where it falls in this spectrum. Tuberculoid (high-resistance) leprosy consists of a single patch of hypesthetic or anesthetic skin in any location. The skin patch is frequently thickened, reddened, or hypopigmented. Few or no *M. leprae* bacilli may be demonstrated. If a superficially placed nerve trunk, typically a cutaneous nerve, courses just beneath the area of affected skin, it may be engulfed in the inflammatory reaction, resulting in an associated mononeuropathy. Such a nerve may be palpably enlarged and beaded. Lepromatous (low-resistance) leprosy is marked by immunologic tolerance; numerous bacilli; and widespread skin thickening, cutaneous anesthesia, and anhidrosis, which spare only the warmest parts of the body, notably the axilla, the groin, and beneath the scalp hair. Motor signs (focal weakness and atrophy) result from damage to mixed nerves lying close to the skin, particularly the median, ulnar, peroneal, and facial nerves.

SPECIAL NEUROPATHIC PRESENTATIONS

Some disorders selectively affect the peripheral nervous system, limiting dysfunction to specific systems or sites, such as motor nerves, brachial plexus, or the autonomic nervous system.

AUTONOMIC NEUROPATHY

The autonomic nervous system regulates the visceral organs and vegetative functions (Chap. 22). Many pharmacologic agents modify specific autonomic functions, but autonomic neuropathy (dysautonomia) with structural changes in pre- and postganglionic neurons can also occur. Usually autonomic neuropathy is a manifestation of a more generalized polyneuropathy, as in diabetic neuropathy, GBS, and alcoholic polyneuropathy, but occasionally syndromes of pure pandysautonomia are encountered. Symptoms of dysautonomia are mainly negative (i.e., loss of function) and include postural hypotension with faintness or syncope, anhidrosis, hypothermia, bladder atony, obstipation, dry mouth and dry eyes from failure of salivary and lacrimal glands to secrete, blurring of vision from lack of pupillary and ciliary regulation, and sexual impotence in males. Positive phenomena (hyperfunction) may also occur and include episodic hypertension, diarrhea, hyperhidrosis, and either tachycardia or bradycardia. Management is symptomatic and also directed at the underlying cause, if it can be identified.

PURE MOTOR NEUROPATHY

Disorders affecting any level of the motor unit—anterior horn cell, motor axon, or neuromuscular junction—can result in a purely lower motor syndrome without sensory disturbance. Distinguishing anterior horn cell disorders (motor neuronopathies) from motor axonopathies may be difficult clinically because they share manifestations (weakness, muscle denervation atrophy, hypo- or areflexia, fasciculations). EDX examination may also fail to localize the primary site of the lesion (neuropathic versus neuronopathic) unless the lesion is demyelinating in nature, in which case it is by definition neuropathic.

Examples of motor neuronopathies include the lower-motor form of amyotrophic lateral sclerosis (Chap. 21), poliomyelitis, hereditary spinal muscular atrophies, and adult variant of hexosaminidase A deficiency. Motor neuropathies may be seen with lead, dapsone, or suramin intoxication, occasionally with porphyria, and also with multifocal motor neuropathy. The latter is a chronic asymmetric disorder of mid-life associated with persistent conduction block on EDX examination, and often high titers of antiganglioside antibodies (particularly anti-GM$_1$) (Chap. 35). Neuromuscular junction disorders (e.g., Lambert-Eaton myasthenic syndrome, tick bite paralysis, other types of toxic neuromuscular blockade) are purely motor and can be recognized and localized electrodiagnostically. Some motor-sensory polyneuropathies have predominant motor symptoms and signs, such as hereditary motor-sensory neuropathies, GBS, and CIDP, but the subclinical sensory component is readily demonstrated electrodiagnostically or by quantitative sensory testing.

PURE SENSORY NEUROPATHY

Clinical presentations involving primary sensation only (Table 33-6) are common. Manifestations may (1) reflect mainly large afferent fiber involvement with deficits of vibratory and proprioceptive sense, areflexia, and sensory ataxia with or without tingling dysesthesias; (2) reflect mainly small afferent fiber involvement with numbness and cutaneous hypesthesia to pin-prick and temperature stimuli, often with painful, burning dysesthesias; or (3) be pansensory, with both large- and small-fiber manifestations. The pattern of distribution, although variable, is often distal and symmetric, particularly for large-fiber neuropathies.

The most severe and widespread of these pure sensory syndromes exhibits poor or no recovery, suggesting irreversible lesions of nerve cell bodies in dorsal root and trigeminal ganglia. These are referred to as *sensory neuronopathies*. Sensory deficits can be distal, but can also be patchy or multifocal depending on which dorsal root ganglia are affected. The differential diagnosis of sensory neuronopathy includes pyridoxine (vitamin B6) toxicity, connective tissue disease, and paraneoplastic etiologies (particulary in association with small cell carcinoma of the lung). With sensory neurotoxins, moderate doses lead to potentially reversible neuropathy, but high doses appear to cause irreversible neuronopathy.

PLEXOPATHY

This term refers to disorders of either the brachial or the lumbosacral plexus. Lesions of the brachial plexus are characterized by motor and sensory signs different from those expected in either mononeuropathies of the upper limb or polyneuropathies. The usual causes are direct trauma to the plexus, idiopathic brachial neuritis (also called *neuralgic amyotrophy*; Chap. 6), cervical rib or band, infiltration by malignant tumor, or prior radiation therapy. When the upper parts of the brachial plexus, arising from cervical roots 5 through 7, are affected, weakness and atrophy of shoulder girdle and upper arm muscles occur. Injuries to the lower brachial plexus, arising from the eighth cervical and first thoracic roots, produce distal arm weakness, atrophy, and focal sensory deficit in the forearm and hand. In general, idiopathic brachial

neuritis, irradiation with >60 Gy (6000 rad), and particular types of trauma (arm jerked downward) result in damage to the upper portions of the brachial plexus. In contrast, infiltration by malignant tumor, cervical rib or band, and certain other types of trauma (arm jerked upward) cause damage to the lower brachial plexus. Lumbosacral plexopathies are less common; they may be due to trauma, including intraoperative damage, retroperitoneal hemorrhage, idiopathic plexitis, or malignant tumor infiltration or may occur in association with long-standing diabetes mellitus.

COLD EFFECTS

Cold exerts direct deleterious effects on peripheral nerve, independent of ischemia. Cold injury to nerve occurs after prolonged exposure, usually of a limb, to moderately low temperatures, as with immersion of the feet in seawater; actual freezing of tissue is not required. Axonal degeneration of myelinated fibers is the pathologic expression of cold injury. Frequently, limbs affected by cold injury to nerve show sensory deficit and dysesthesias, cutaneous vasomotor instability, pain, and marked sensitivity to minimal cold exposure, which may persist for years. The pathophysiology of these phenomena is uncertain.

TROPHIC CHANGES

The array of observable changes in completely denervated muscle, bone, and skin, including hair and nails, is well known, if incompletely understood. It is unclear what portion of the changes is due purely to denervation versus what is due to disuse, immobility, lack of weight bearing, and particularly recurrent, unnoticed, painless trauma. Considerable evidence favors the view that ulceration of skin, poor healing, tissue resorption, neurogenic arthropathy, and mutilation are the result of repeated unheeded injury to insensitive parts. This sequence of events is avoidable with proper attention to and care of the insensitive parts by both patient and physician.

RECOVERY FROM NEUROPATHY

In contrast to axons in the central nervous system, peripheral nerve fibers have an excellent ability to regenerate under proper circumstances. The process of regeneration following axonal degeneration may take from 2 months to more than a year, depending on the severity of the neuropathy and the length of regeneration required. Regeneration can take place when the cause of the neuropathy has been eliminated, such as removal from contact with a neurotoxic substance or correction of an abnormal metabolic state. A deficit secondary to demyelination may recover rapidly, since intact axons may remyelinate in just a few weeks. For example, a patient with GBS, in whom demyelination but no secondary axonal degeneration has occurred, may recover to normal strength from bedfastness and paralysis of arms and legs in as little as 3 to 4 weeks.

PERIPHERAL NERVE TUMORS

These tumors are mostly benign and can arise on any nerve trunk or twig. Although peripheral nerve tumors can occur anywhere in the body, including the spinal roots and cauda equina, many are subcutaneous in location and present as a soft swelling, sometimes with a purplish discoloration of the skin. Two major categories of peripheral nerve tumors are recognized: neurilemmoma (schwannoma) and neurofibroma. Neurilemmomas are usually solitary and grow in the nerve sheath, rendering the tumor relatively easy to dissect free. In contrast, neurofibromas tend to be multiple, grow in the endoneurial substance, which renders them difficult to dissect, may undergo malignant changes, and are the hallmark of von Recklinghausen's neurofibromatosis (NF1).

FURTHER READINGS

Brown WF et al (eds): *Neuromuscular Function and Disease: Basic, Clinical and Electrodiagnostic Aspects*. Philadelphia, Saunders, 2002

☑ Dyck PJ, Thomas PK (eds): *Peripheral Neuropathy*, 4th ed. Philadelphia, Saunders, 2004

Comprehensive text covering clinical features, pathology, pathophysiology.

Goldstein DJ et al: Duloxetine versus placebo in patients with painful diabetic neuropathy. Pain 116(1–2):109, 2005

Katirji B et al (eds): *Neuromuscular Disorders in Clinical Practice*. Boston, Butterworth-Heinemann, 2002

Kuntzer T et al: Clinical features and pathophysiological basis of sensory neuronopathies (ganglionopathies). Muscle Nerve 30:255, 2004

Llewelyn JG: The diabetic neuropathies: Types, diagnosis and management. J Neurol Neurosurg Psychiatry 74(Suppl 2):15, 2003

Mendell JR, Sahenk Z: Painful sensory neuropathy. N Engl J Med 348:1243, 2003

☑ Oxman MN et al: A vaccine to prevent herpes zoster and postherpetic neuralgia in older adults. N Engl J Med 352:2271, 2005

Clinical trial showing effectiveness of a new vaccine.

Shapiro BE, Preston DC: Entrapment and compressive neuropathies. Med Clin North Am 87:663, 2003

☑ Stewart JD: *Focal Peripheral Neuropathies*, 3d ed. Philadelphia, Lippincott Williams & Wilkins, 1999

Comprehensive text with excellent tables for differential diagnosis.

Willison HJ, Winer JB: Clinical evaluation and investigation of neuropathy. J Neurol Neurosurg Psychiatry 74(Suppl 2):3, 8, 2003

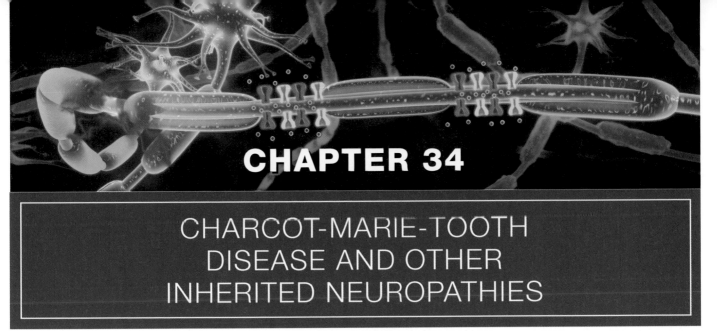

CHAPTER 34

CHARCOT-MARIE-TOOTH DISEASE AND OTHER INHERITED NEUROPATHIES

Phillip F. Chance
Thomas D. Bird

CHARCOT-MARIE-TOOTH DISEASE

GENERAL CLINICAL FEATURES

Charcot-Marie-Tooth (CMT) neuropathy comprises a heterogeneous group of inherited peripheral nerve diseases (**Table 34–1**). Transmission is most frequently autosomal dominant but may also be autosomal recessive or X-linked. An estimated 1 in 2500 persons has a form of CMT, making it one of the most frequently encountered inherited neurologic syndromes.

The neuropathy of CMT affects both motor and sensory nerves. Typical features consist of distal muscle weakness and atrophy, impaired sensation, and absent or hypoactive deep tendon reflexes. Common signs and symptoms are related to muscle weakness initially involving the feet and legs, and later progressing to the hands and forearms. A history of an abnormal high-stepped (steppage) gait with frequent tripping and falling is frequently elicited. Complaints related to foot deformity (pes cavus or high-arched feet) result from atrophy of intrinsic muscles of the feet. Despite the involvement of sensory nerves in CMT, complaints of limb pain or sensory disturbances are unusual.

Onset is most often during the first or second decade of life, although presentation in mid–adult life is not unusual. The variation in clinical presentation is exceptionally wide, ranging from individuals whose only clinical finding is pes cavus and minimal or no distal muscle weakness to those with severe distal atrophy and marked hand and foot deformity.

TREATMENT FOR CMT

It is unusual for patients with CMT to lose ambulation. There are no therapies that can prevent the onset or delay progression of disability associated with CMT. Patients frequently benefit from physical therapy, use of ankle-foot orthoses (AFOs) to alleviate foot drop, and occasionally surgical procedures to the foot. Surgery should be undertaken only when pain or difficulty walking due to severe foot deformity cannot be managed by more conservative means.

CLASSIFICATION BY PHENOTYPE

A widely accepted classification system distinguishes demyelinating forms of CMT (also designated as CMT type 1, or CMT1) from those due to axonal degeneration (CMT type 2, or CMT2). Individuals with CMT1 have electrophysiologic findings of reduced motor and sensory nerve conduction velocities (NCVs; typically <38 to 40 m/s). The pathologic findings on nerve biopsy are those of hypertrophic demyelinating neuropathy; "onion bulbs" are common (**Fig. 34-1**). By

TABLE 34-1

FORMS OF CHARCOT-MARIE-TOOTH DISEASE (HEREDITARY MOTOR AND SENSORY NEUROPATHY) AND RELATED DISORDERS

	LOCUS	GENE	MECHANISM
CHARCOT-MARIE-TOOTH TYPE 1			
(HMSNI)			
CMT1A	17p11.2-p12	*PMP22*	AD
CMT1B	1q22-q23	*P$_0$*	AD
CMT1C	16p12-p13	*SIMPLE*	AD
CMT1D	10q21-q22	*EGR2*	AD/AR
CMTX	Xq13.1	*CX32*	X-linked
CMT4A	8q13-q21	*GDAP1*	AR
CMT4B1	11q22	*MTMR2*	AR
CMT4B2	11p15	*SBF2*	AR
CMT4D (HMSN-Lom)	8q24	*NDRG1*	AR
CMT4F	19q13	*PRX*	AR
CHARCOT-MARIE-TOOTH TYPE 2			
(HMSNII)			
CMT2A	1p35-p36	*KIF1B*	AD
CMT2B	3q13-q22	*RAB7*	AD
CMT2C	12q23-q24	*Unknown*	AD
CMT2D	7p14	*GARS*	AD
CMT2E	8p21	*NEF-L*	AD
CMT2B1	11q21	*LMNA*	AR
DÉJERINE-SOTTAS			
(HMSNIII)			
DSS	17p11.2-p12	*PMP22*	AD
	1q22-p23	*P$_0$*	AD
	10q21-q22	*EGR2*	AD/AR
	19q13	*PRX*	AD
CONGENITAL HYPOMYELINATION			
CHN	1q22-23	*P$_0$*	AD
	10q21-q22	*EGR2*	AR/AD
HEREDITARY NEUROPATHY WITH PRESSURE PALSIES			
HNPP	17p11.2-p12	*PMP22*	AD

Abbreviations: *PMP22*, peripheral myelin protein 22; *P$_0$*, myelin protein zero; *SIMPLE*, small integral membrane protein of late endosome; *Cx32*, connexin32; *EGR2* (Krox-20), early growth response 2 gene; *GDAP1*, ganglioside-induced differentiation-associated protein-1; *MTMR2*, myotubularin-related protein-2; *SBF2*, SET binding factor 2; *NDRG1*, N-myc downstream regulated gene1; *PRX*, periaxin; *KIF1B*, kinesin family member 1B; *RAB7*, Ras-associated protein 7; *GARS*, Glycyl-tRNA synthetase; *NEFL*, neurofilament, light polypeptide; *LMNA*, lamin A.

contrast, in CMT2 there is relative preservation of the myelin sheath and these individuals have normal or near-normal NCVs. CMT3 refers to Déjerine–Sottas disease (DSD; see below), CMT4 to autosomal recessive forms of CMT, and CMTX to X-linked varieties.

An alternative classification system designates these disorders as hereditary motor and sensory neuropathies (HMSN); HMSNI refers to CMT1, HMSNII to CMT2, HMSNIII to DSD, and HMSNIV to Refsum disease (see below).

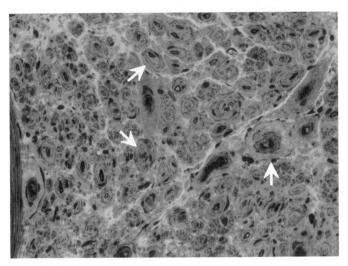

FIGURE 34-1

Transverse section of sural nerve showing numerous large onion bulbs consisting of concentric layers of basal lamina, connective tissue, and Schwann cells. There is also loss of large myelinated axons, endoneurial fibrosis, and perineurial fibrosis. (Toluidine blue, 400x; Courtesy of Dr. Joanna Phillips, Department of Pathology, University of California, San Francisco.)

APPROACH TO THE PATIENT WITH CMT

A clinical diagnosis of an inherited peripheral neuropathy consistent with a form of CMT (CMT1 or CMT2) should be established prior to undertaking specific genetic tests. Other causes of peripheral neuropathy (e.g., diabetes mellitus, alcoholism, heavy metal poisoning, immune neuropathies) should be considered and excluded. An environmental exposure may affect multiple family members, thereby potentially mimicking a hereditary illness. CMT is usually a chronic, slowly progressive condition. One should be suspicious of cases that seem to have a rapid course of deterioration. The neurologic findings show great variability in patients with CMT; mild pes cavus and depressed deep tendon reflexes may be the only signs of disease.

Although symptoms related to sensory disturbances are uncommon in CMT, a careful sensory examination is nonetheless essential. In patients who have no objective signs of sensory impairment and no evidence of sensory nerve dysfunction on electrophysiologic studies, alternative diagnoses including primary motor system disorders (e.g., distal spinal muscle atrophy, juvenile amyotrophic lateral sclerosis) should be considered.

The pedigree is of paramount importance in the diagnosis of CMT. Examination of multiple family members, particularly parents, for subtle signs of neuropathy may help to establish a diagnosis. If possible, it is also important to obtain NCVs and needle electromyography from all at-risk family members.

 GENETIC CONSIDERATIONS

CMT Neuropathy Type 1A (CMT1A)

Approximately three-quarters of pedigrees with autosomal dominant CMT1 demonstrate linkage to chromosome 17p11.2-12 (CMT1A) and are associated with a tandem 1.5-megabase (Mb) DNA duplication. The duplication is usually inherited as a stable Mendelian trait; however, it may also arise as a de novo event. The de novo duplication is responsible for many sporadic cases of CMT1 and may also account for some cases previously thought to be autosomal recessive. When present as a de novo event, the duplication results more commonly from an error in spermatogenesis; however, ~10% of de novo cases have been found to result from an error in oogenesis.

The critical gene for CMT1A is the peripheral myelin protein-22 (*PMP22*), which is expressed in Schwann cells. The level of expression of *PMP22* is crucial for proper myelination of peripheral nerves. The neuropathy in patients with the duplication results from the presence of three copies of *PMP22* leading to increased expression at this locus. In rare cases, patients homozygous for the CMT1A duplication have been identified, and in some cases these individuals exhibit a more severe phenotype than their heterozygous siblings or parents. As discussed below, monosomic underexpression of *PMP22* results in hereditary neuropathy with liability to pressure palsies (HNPP).

Rare CMT1 pedigrees that are linked to chromosome 17p11.2-p12, yet lack the duplication, may harbor missense mutations within the *PMP22* gene.

DNA testing for CMT1A (including the duplication and sequencing to detect point mutations in *PMP22*) is available and now an accepted part of the evaluation of patients with suspected hereditary neuropathies (see below).

CMT Neuropathy Type 1B (CMT1B)

CMT1B is less common than CMT1A; it results from mutations in the human myelin protein zero gene (*MPZ* or P_0). P_0 is the major structural protein component of peripheral nervous system myelin (quantitatively 50% by weight). P_0 is a member of the immunoglobulin gene superfamily of cell adhesive molecules and localizes to the compact portion of peripheral nerve myelin. Many different point mutations in the P_0 gene have been found in patients with CMT1B, and these mutations predominantly map to the extracellular domain of its gene product.

At the clinical level it is not possible to differentiate patients with CMT1A from those with CMT1B. Molecular genetic testing is available.

Déjerine-Sottas Disease (CMT3)

Patients who never ambulate (or lose the ability to ambulate in infancy or childhood) are sometimes diagnosed with DSD (also called HMSNIII) or congenital hypomyelinating neuropathy (CHN). These disorders are severe, infantile- or childhood-onset, hypertrophic demyelinating polyneuropathies. NCVs are substantially slowed (typically 10 m/s), and elevations in the cerebrospinal fluid (CSF) protein level are typically present. The clinical features of DSD and CHN overlap those of severe CMT1, and for this reason the continued clinical separation of CMT1 and DSD/CHN is perhaps unwarranted. Many cases of DSD or CHN appear to be sporadic.

Molecular genetic studies indicate that DSD and CHN may be associated with point mutations in the P_0 or the *PMP22* genes, although pedigrees have been described that lack mutations in the P_0, *PMP22*, or *Cx32* gene (see below). Most DSD mutations identified to date are dominant genetic traits.

Hereditary Neuropathy with Liability to Pressure Palsies

HNPP (also called *tomaculous neuropathy*) is an autosomal dominant disorder that produces an episodic, recurrent demyelinating neuropathy. HNPP typically develops during adolescence and may cause attacks of numbness, muscular weakness, and atrophy. Peroneal palsies, carpal tunnel syndrome, and other entrapment neuropathies are manifestations of HNPP. Motor and sensory NCVs are mildly reduced in affected patients as well as in asymptomatic gene carriers. Pathologic changes observed in HNPP include segmental demyelination and tomaculous, or sausage-like, formations in peripheral nerves. Due to overlap of clinical features between HNPP and CMT1, some HNPP patients may be misdiagnosed as having CMT1. Approximately 10% of patients with HNPP present with a brachial plexopathy that is typically painless. Rare patients with HNPP have been found by magnetic resonance imaging (MRI) to have central nervous system (CNS) demyelination.

The HNPP locus maps to chromosome 17p11.2-p12 and is associated with a 1.5-Mb deletion. The duplicated CMT1A chromosome (described earlier) and the deleted HNPP chromosome are the reciprocal products of unequal crossing-over during meiosis. In the case of HNPP, loss of a copy of the *PMP22* gene and underexpression of this critical myelin gene lead to demyelination. Most HNPP patients have the associated chromosome 17 deletion; however, rare patients with HNPP have been found to have point mutations in the *PMP22* gene. Molecular genetic testing is clinically available.

Treatment for HNPP is largely supportive. Surgical decompression of nerves has been proposed but is controversial. There is some evidence that surgical repair of carpal tunnel syndrome in HNPP is of little benefit and that transposition of the ulnar nerve at the elbow may produce poor results because the nerves are especially sensitive to manipulation and minor trauma.

CMT Neuropathy Type 2

CMT2 is less common than CMT1 and, in general, has a later age of onset, produces less involvement of the intrinsic muscles of the hands, and lacks palpably enlarged nerves. Extensive demyelination with "onion bulb" formation is not present in CMT2. Motor NCVs are normal or only slightly reduced in affected persons. The CMT2A locus maps to chromosome 1p35-p36, and in one pedigree a mutation in KIF1B, an axonal motor protein, was found. Limb ulceration is a notable feature of CMT2B. CMT2B maps to chromosome 3q13-q22 and results from mutations in the *RAB7* gene, a member of the Rab family of ras-related GTPases that function in intracellular membrane trafficking. Further genetic heterogeneity within CMT2 is evidenced by the identification of kindreds with the features of axonal neuropathy, weakness of the diaphragm, and vocal cord paralysis. Such pedigrees carry the designation of CMT2C, which has been mapped to chromosome 12q23-q24. Yet another form of CMT2, designated CMT2D, maps to chromosome 7p14 and results from mutations in the glycyl tRNA synthetase gene (*GARS*). In a large Russian pedigree having an autosomal dominant axonopathy, a CMT2 gene was mapped to chromosome 8p21 (and designated CMT2E), and a mutation was found in the neurofilament-light (*NEFL*) gene.

Additionally, certain P_0 or connexin32 (*Cx32*, see below) mutations have been found to be the underlying genetic defect in a subset of patients with CMT1 or CMTX who were initially thought to have CMT2 because of only mild slowing of NCVs. With these exceptions, DNA testing is not widely available for any form of apparent CMT2.

X-Linked CMT Neuropathy

The clinical features of X-linked CMT disease (CMTX) include demyelinating neuropathy, absence of male-to-male transmission, and an earlier age of onset and faster rate of progression in males. NCVs vary widely in CMTX from nearly normal to moderately slowed. CMTX accounts for ~10% of all patients thought to have a form of demyelinating CMT (i.e., CMT1). CMTX should be suspected when the commonly associated chromosome 17 duplication is not present and there is no history of father-to-son transmission of the neuropathy.

Typical CMTX results from point mutations in the *Cx32* gene. *Cx32* encodes a major component of gap junctions and is structurally similar to PMP22, as both of these proteins contain four putative transmembrane domains in similar orientation. Unlike PMP22 and P_0, which are present in compact myelin, Cx32 is located at uncompacted folds of Schwann cell cytoplasm around the nodes of Ranvier and at Schmidt-Lanterman incisures. This localization suggests a role for gap junctions composed of Cx32 in providing a pathway for the transfer of ions and nutrients around and across the myelin sheath of peripheral nerves. Mutations in the Cx32 protein have been suggested to alter its cellular localization and its trafficking and interfere with cell-to-cell communication. Over 200 different mutations in the *Cx32* gene have been described in patients with CMTX, and the distribution pattern of these mutations suggests that all parts of the Cx32 protein are functionally important. DNA testing is available.

Other X-linked genes can result in CMT; a fifth gene has recently been mapped and proposed as CMTX5.

Rare Forms of CMT

Mutations in the putative zinc finger domain of the early growth response 2 gene (*EGR2*, or *Krox-20*) or in the small integral membrane protein of the lysosome/late endosome (*SIMPLE*) gene have been found in CMT1 families that were found to be negative for the CMT1A duplication, as well as for mutations in *PMP22*, P_0, or *Cx32*. *EGR2* mutations have also been reported in CHN. EGR2 acts as a direct transactivator of myelination genes in differentiating Schwann cells. SIMPLE has been proposed to play a role in myelin protein degradation and turnover. Mutations have also been found in periaxin (PRX), an important structural myelin protein, in demyelinating forms of neuropathy clinically diagnosed as CMT1 or DSD. DNA testing is available for EGR2 and PRX.

Rare families with autosomal recessive motor and sensory neuropathy have been reported, particularly Tunisian families with parental consanguinity. Both demyelinating and axonal types of neuropathy have been described and given the designation CMT4. One form of autosomal recessive demyelinating neuropathy, CMT4A, has been mapped to chromosome 8q13-q21 and is associated with mutations in the ganglioside-induced differentiation-associated protein (GDAP1). CMT4B is characterized by focally folded myelin sheaths and maps to chromosome 11q23. CMT4B is caused by mutations in the myotubularin-related protein-2 (*MTMR2*), which is thought to be a transcriptional regulator. Additional loci for other rare forms of CMT4 have been found, and in some cases causal genes are known (Table 34-1).

Genetic Evaluation of CMT and HNPP

An approach for evaluating a patient suspected of having an inherited peripheral neuropathy is presented in **Fig. 34-2**. If the proband has evidence for CMT1, NCVs are a useful screening tool for parents and other at-risk family members. The *CMT1* gene is penetrant in early life, and correct disease status can probably be determined by age 5 by screening with NCVs. However, if a proband's nerve conduction is normal or only mildly slowed, the diagnosis may be CMT2. In this case the screening examination will need to focus on determination of motor unit amplitudes and other electrical signs of denervation and reinnervation. Rare patients have been found to have point mutations in either P_0 or *Cx32*, resulting in very mild demyelination and misclassification as CMT2.

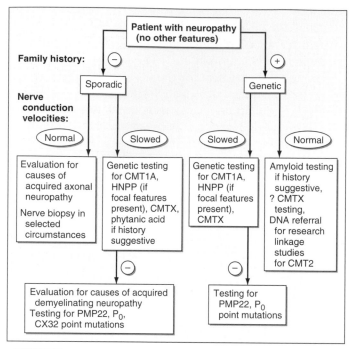

FIGURE 34-2

Evaluation of patients suspected of having an inherited peripheral neuropathy. CMT, Charcot-Marie-Tooth; HNPP, hereditary neuropathy with liability to pressure palsies. (*Modified from Lynch and Chance.*)

Most CMT1 and CMT2 pedigrees have autosomal dominant inheritance. CMTX should be suspected in pedigrees lacking male-to-male transmission, when males are more severely affected than females and have an earlier onset. Determination of autosomal dominant versus X-linked CMT is important as the genetic counseling for these two modes of inheritance is different. For any form of autosomal dominant CMT, the likelihood of an affected parent (of either sex) having an affected child is 50% for each pregnancy, regardless of the sex of the child. For CMTX, all daughters of an affected father will inherit the gene, and none of the sons will be affected. For a woman with CMTX, there is a 50% likelihood that her children will be affected regardless of their sex.

Sporadic cases in males can be especially difficult to evaluate, as the neuropathy could be nongenetic or the pattern of inheritance could be autosomal dominant, X-linked, or even autosomal recessive. Sporadic cases may also represent de novo duplications (CMT1A) or de novo deletions (HNPP). False paternity is another explanation for apparent sporadic CMT or HNPP.

Molecular genetic testing is currently available for the DNA duplication (or deletion) associated with CMT1A or HNPP and for point mutations in the *PMP22*, P_0, *EGR2*, *PRX*, and *Cx32* genes associated with other forms of CMT1 and CMTX.

CHEMOTHERAPY IN PATIENTS WITH CMT

Chemotherapeutic agents known to affect peripheral nerves should be used with great caution in patients with inherited neuropathies. In the case of vincristine, total avoidance is strongly advised. A number of reports have documented the serious consequences of vincristine treatment administered in standard oncologic dosages in patients with CMT, including CMT1A and CMT2. The complications included the precipitation of severe neuropathies in clinically asymptomatic at-risk individuals, induction of marked worsening in symptomatic patients, and even death due to respiratory collapse. The extent to which these concerns extend to other neurotoxic chemotherapeutic agents is unclear, but severe toxicity has been reported with the use of paclitaxel for ovarian cancer.

OTHER INHERITED NEUROPATHIES

HEREDITARY SENSORY NEUROPATHIES

Hereditary sensory neuropathies (HSNs) are a heterogeneous group of disorders affecting sensory neurons. The most common form of HSN, HSN type I, is an autosomal degenerative disorder of sensory and motor neurons. Distal sensory loss, distal muscle wasting and weakness, and variable neural deafness are observed. The disease involves progressive loss of dorsal root ganglion cells and axons in peripheral nerves. Age of onset is the second decade of life or later. The HSN-I locus maps to chromosome 9q22.1-q22.3 and results from mutations in the serine palmityl transferase (*SPTLC1*) gene. Because of the presence of muscular weakness in some patients with HSN, this disorder may be clinically confused with CMT.

FAMILIAL AMYLOID NEUROPATHY

Familial amyloid polyneuropathy (FAP) is an autosomal dominant disorder that classically presents as progressive sensory peripheral neuropathy, with early involvement of the autonomic nervous system and an associated cardiomyopathy. When the family history is positive, vitreous opacities and renal or gastrointestinal disease may be present also. Postmortem studies have shown extensive amyloid deposition in multiple organs throughout the body. Transthyretin (TTR) is the most common constituent amyloid fibril protein deposited in FAP. Several different point mutations in the *TTR* gene have been described in TTR–related FAP, and DNA testing for these mutations is clinically available. Cardiac transplantation in selected cases has been successful.

REFSUM DISEASE

This autosomal recessive disorder is characterized by a progressive sensorimotor demyelinating polyneuropathy associated with cerebellar ataxia and retinitis pigmentosa. Neural deafness, cardiomyopathy, cataracts, and ichthyosis are additional features. Onset is in late childhood or early adulthood. Patients often complain of night blindness as the earliest symptom. The CSF protein is typically elevated. Diagnosis is made by demonstration of elevated levels of phytanic acid (a 20-carbon branched-chain fatty acid) in the serum and urine. The disorder appears to be due to a deficiency of a peroxisomal enzyme, phytanic acid oxidase, responsible for alpha oxidation of phytanic acid. Therapy, consisting of avoidance of dietary sources of phytanic acid and plasmapheresis in some cases, is partially effective.

FURTHER READINGS

Bennett CL, Chance PF: Molecular pathogenesis of hereditary motor, sensory and autonomic neuropathies. Curr Opin Neuro 14:621, 2001

Chance PF, Shapiro BE: Charcot-Marie-Tooth disease and related disorders, in *Neuromuscular Disorders in Clinical Practice,* B Katirji et al (eds). Philadelphia, Butterworth-Heinemann, pp 513–525, 2002

Ellegala DB et al: Characterization of genetically defined types of Charcot-Marie-Tooth neuropathies by using magnetic resonance neurography. J Neurosurg 102:242, 2005

Kamholz J et al: Charcot-Marie-Tooth disease type 1: Molecular pathogenesis to gene therapy. Brain 123:222, 2000

Kim HJ et al: A novel locus for X-linked recessive CMT with deafness and optic neuropathy maps to Xq21.32–q24. Neurology 64:1964, 2005

Lynch D, Chance PF: Inherited peripheral neuropathies. Neurologist 3:277, 1997

☑ Martino MA et al: The administration of chemotherapy in a patient with Charcot-Marie-Tooth and ovarian cancer. Gynecol Oncol 97:710, 2005

Predisposition of patients with CMT to severe chemotherapy-related polyneuropathy.

Meuleman JR, Chance PF: Hereditary pressure palsy, in *Neurological Therapeutics: Principles and Practice,* J Noseworthy (ed). London, Martin Dunitz, 2003

☑ Scherer SS et al: Peripheral neuropathies, in *The Molecular and Genetic Basis of Neurological Disease,* RN Rosenberg et al (eds). Oxford, Butterworth-Heinemann, pp 435–453, 2003

Comprehensive review of genetics, pathology, phenotype of inherited neuropathies.

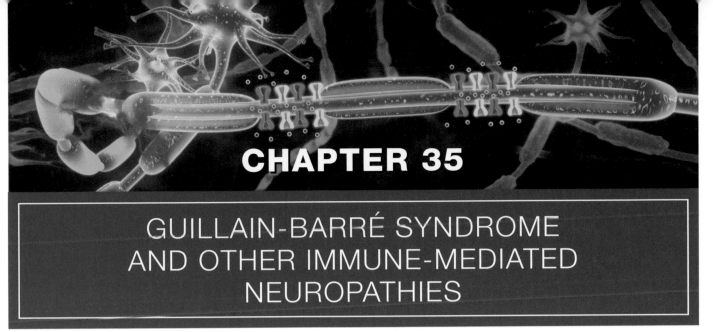

CHAPTER 35

GUILLAIN-BARRÉ SYNDROME AND OTHER IMMUNE-MEDIATED NEUROPATHIES

Stephen L. Hauser
Arthur K. Asbury

GUILLAIN-BARRÉ SYNDROME

Guillain-Barré syndrome (GBS) is an acute, frequently severe, and fulminant polyradiculoneuropathy that is autoimmune in nature. It occurs year-round at a rate of about one case per million per month, or ~3500 cases per year in the United States and Canada. Males and females are equally at risk, and in western countries adults are more frequently affected than children.

CLINICAL MANIFESTATIONS

GBS manifests as rapidly evolving areflexic motor paralysis with or without sensory disturbance. The usual pattern is an ascending paralysis that may be first noticed as rubbery legs. Weakness typically evolves over hours to a few days and is frequently accompanied by tingling dysesthesias in the extremities. The legs are usually more affected than the arms, and facial diparesis is present in 50% of affected individuals. The lower cranial nerves also are frequently involved, causing bulbar weakness and difficulty with handling secretions and maintaining an airway; the diagnosis in these patients may initially be mistaken for brainstem ischemia. Most patients require hospitalization, and almost 30% require ventilatory assistance at some time during the illness. Fever and constitutional symptoms are absent at the onset and, if present, cast doubt on the diagnosis. Deep tendon reflexes usually disappear within the first few days of onset. Cutaneous sensory deficits (e.g., loss of pain and temperature sensation) are usually relatively mild, but functions subserved by large sensory fibers, such as deep tendon reflexes and proprioception, are more severely affected. Bladder dysfunction may occur in severe cases but is usually transient. If bladder dysfunction is a prominent feature and comes early in the course, diagnostic possibilities other than GBS should be considered, particularly spinal cord disease. Once clinical worsening stops and the patient reaches a plateau (almost always over 4 weeks), further progression is unlikely.

In severe cases of GBS requiring critical care management, autonomic involvement is common. Usual features are loss of vasomotor control with wide fluctuation in blood pressure, postural hypotension, and cardiac dysrhythmias. These features require close monitoring and management and can be fatal. Pain is another common feature of GBS; several types are encountered. Most common is deep aching pain in weakened muscles that patients liken to having overexercised the previous

TABLE 35-1

SUBTYPES OF GUILLAIN-BARRÉ SYNDROME (GBS)

SUBTYPE	FEATURES	ELECTRODIAGNOSIS	PATHOLOGY
Acute inflammatory demyelinating polyneuropathy (AIDP)	Adults affected more than children; 90% of cases in western world; recovery rapid; anti-GM1 antibodies (<50%)	Demyelinating	First attack on Schwann cell surface; widespread myelin damage, macrophage activation, and lymphocytic infiltration; variable secondary axonal damage
Acute motor axonal neuropathy (AMAN)	Children and young adults; prevalent in China and Mexico; may be seasonal; recovery rapid; anti-GD1a antibodies	Axonal	First attack at motor nodes of Ranvier; macrophage activation, few lymphocytes, frequent periaxonal macrophages; extent of axonal damage highly variable
Acute motor sensory axonal neuropathy (AMSAN)	Mostly adults; uncommon; recovery slow, often incomplete; closely related to AMAN	Axonal	Same as AMAN, but also affects sensory nerves and roots; axonal damage usually severe
M. Fisher syndrome (MFS)	Adults and children; uncommon; ophthalmoplegia, ataxia, and areflexia; anti-GQ1b antibodies (90%)	Demyelinating	Few cases examined; resembles AIDP

day. Other pains in GBS include back pain involving the entire spine and sometimes dysesthetic pain in the extremities as a manifestation of sensory nerve fiber involvement. These pains are self-limited and should be treated with standard analgesics.

Several subtypes of GBS are now recognized, as determined primarily by electrodiagnostic and pathologic distinctions (**Table 35-1**). A range of limited or regional GBS syndromes may be encountered, although uncommonly. These include (1) the Miller Fisher syndrome (Table 35-1 and see "Immunopathogenesis," below); (2) pure sensory forms; (3) ophthalmoplegia with anti-GQ1b antibodies (see "Immunopathogenesis," below) as part of severe motor-sensory GBS; (4) GBS with severe bulbar and facial paralysis, sometimes associated with antecedent cytomegalovirus (CMV) infection and anti-GM2 antibodies; and (5) acute pandysautonomia.

ANTECEDENT EVENTS

Some 75% of cases of GBS are preceded 1 to 3 weeks by an acute infectious process, usually respiratory or gastrointestinal. Culture and seroepidemiologic techniques show that 20 to 30% of all cases occurring in North America, Europe, and Australia are preceded by infection or reinfection with *Campylobacter jejuni*. A similar proportion is preceded by a human herpes virus infection, often CMV or Epstein-Barr virus. Other viruses and also *Mycoplasma*

pneumoniae have been identified as agents involved in antecedent infections, as have recent immunizations. The swine influenza vaccine, administered widely in the United States in 1976, is the most notable example; influenza vaccines in use from 1992 to 1994, however, resulted in only one additional case of GBS per million persons vaccinated. Older type rabies vaccine, prepared in nervous system tissue, is implicated as a trigger of GBS in developing countries where it is still used; the mechanism is presumably immunization against neural antigens. GBS also occurs more frequently than can be attributed to chance alone in patients with lymphoma, including Hodgkin's disease, in HIV-seropositive individuals, and in patients with systemic lupus erythematosus.

IMMUNOPATHOGENESIS

Several lines of evidence support an autoimmune basis for acute inflammatory demyelinating polyneuropathy (AIDP), the most common and best studied type of GBS; the concept extends to all of the subtypes of GBS (Table 35-1).

It is likely that both cellular and humoral immune mechanisms contribute to tissue damage in AIDP. T cell activation is suggested by the finding that elevated levels of cytokines and cytokine receptors are present in serum [interleukin (IL) 2, soluble IL-2 receptor] and in cerebrospinal fluid (CSF) (IL-6, tumor necrosis factor α, interferon γ). AIDP is also closely analogous to an experimental T cell–mediated immunopathy designated *experimental allergic neuritis* (EAN); EAN is induced in laboratory animals by immune sensitization against protein fragments derived from peripheral nerve proteins, and in particular against the P2 protein. Based on analogy to EAN, it was initially thought that AIDP was likely to be primarily a T cell–mediated disorder; however, abundant data now suggest that autoantibodies directed against nonprotein determinants may be central to many cases.

Circumstantial evidence suggests that all GBS results from immune responses to nonself antigens (infectious agents, vaccines) that misdirect to host nerve tissue through a resemblance-of-epitope (molecular mimicry) mechanism (**Fig. 35-1**). The neural targets are likely to be glycoconjugates, specifically gangliosides (**Table 35-2**; **Fig. 35-2**). Gangliosides are complex glycosphingolipids that contain one or more sialic acid residues; various gangliosides participate in cell-cell interactions (including those between axons and glia), modulation of receptors,

and regulation of growth. They are typically exposed on the plasma membrane of cells, rendering them susceptible to an antibody-mediated attack. Gangliosides and other glycoconjugates are present in large quantity in human nervous tissues and in key sites, such as nodes of Ranvier. Antiganglioside antibodies, most frequently to GM1, are common in GBS (20 to 50% of cases), particularly in those cases preceded by *C. jejuni* infection. Furthermore, isolates of *C. jejuni* from stool cultures of patients with GBS have surface glycolipid structures that antigenically cross-react with gangliosides, including GM1, concentrated in human nerves. Another line of evidence is derived from experience in Europe with parenteral use of purified bovine brain gangliosides for treatment of various neuropathic disorders. Between 5 and 15 days after injection some recipients developed acute motor axonal GBS with high titers of anti-GM1 antibodies that recognized epitopes at nodes of Ranvier and motor endplates.

Particularly noteworthy is the Miller Fisher syndrome (MFS), which presents as rapidly evolving ataxia and

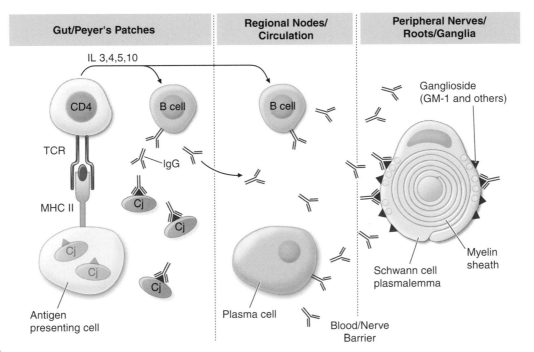

FIGURE 35-1

Postulated immunopathogenesis of GBS associated with *C. jejuni* infection. B cells recognize glycoconjugates on *C. jejuni* (Cj) (triangles) that cross-react with ganglioside present on Schwann cell surface and subjacent peripheral nerve myelin. Some B cells, activated via a T cell–independent mechanism, secrete primarily IgM (not shown). Other B cells (upper left side) are activated via a partially T cell–dependent route and secrete primarily IgG; T cell help is provided by CD4 cells activated locally by fragments of Cj proteins that are presented on the surface of antigen-presenting cells (APC). A critical event in the development of GBS is the escape of activated B cells from Peyers patches into regional

lymph nodes. Activated T cells probably also function to assist in opening of the blood-nerve barrier, facilitating penetration of pathogenic autoantibodies. The earliest changes in myelin (right) consist of edema between myelin lamellae and vesicular disruption (shown as circular blebs) of the outermost myelin layers. These effects are associated with activation of the C5b-C9 membrane attack complex and probably mediated by calcium entry; it is possible that the macrophage cytokine tumor necrosis factor (TNF) also participates in myelin damage. B, B cell; MHC II, class II major histocompatibility complex molecule; TCR, T cell receptor; A, axon.

TABLE 35-2

PRINCIPAL ANTI-GLYCOLIPID ANTIBODIES IMPLICATED IN IMMUNE NEUROPATHIES

CLINICAL PRESENTATION	ANTIBODY TARGET	USUAL ISOTYPE
Acute Immune Neuropathies (Guillain Barré Syndromes)		
Acute inflammatory demyelinating polyneuropathy (AIDP)	No clear patterns GM1 most common	IgG (polyclonal)
Acute motor axonal neuropathy (AMAN)	GD1a, GM1, GM1b, Ga1NAc–GD1a (<50% for any)	IgG (polyclonal)
Miller Fisher Syndrome (MFS)	GQ1b (>90%)	IgG (polyclonal)
Acute pharyngeal cervicobrachial neuropathy (APCBN)	GT1a (? Most)	IgG (polyclonal)
Chronic Immune Neuropathies		
Chronic inflammatory demyelinating polyneuropathy (CIDP); 75% of cases	Po in some	No clear pattern
CIDPa (MGUS associated); 25% of cases	Neural binding sites	IgG, IgA (monoclonal)
Chronic sensory > motor neuropathy	SPGP, SGLPG (on MAG) (50%)	IgM (monoclonal)
	Uncertain (50%)	IgM (monoclonal)
Multifocal motor neuropathy (MMN)	GM1, Ga1NAc–GD1a, others (25–50%)	IgM (polyclonal, monoclonal)
Chronic sensory atoxic neuropathy	GD1b, GQ1b and other b-series gangliosides	IgM (monoclonal)

Note: MGUS, monoclonal gammopathy of undetermined significance; MAG, myelin-associated glycoprotein. Modified from HJ Willison, N Yuki: Brain 125:2591, 2002.

areflexia of limbs without weakness, and ophthalmoplegia often with pupillary paralysis. The MFS variant accounts for ~5% of all GBS cases. Anti-GQ1b IgG antibodies are found in >90% of patients with MFS (Tables 35-1 and 35-2; Fig. 35-2), and titers of IgG are highest early in the course. Anti-GQ1b antibodies are not found in other forms of GBS unless there is extraocular motor nerve involvement. Extraocular motor nerves are enriched in GQ1b gangliosides in comparison to limb nerves. Furthermore, a monoclonal anti-GQ1b antibody raised against *C. jejuni* isolated from a patient with MFS blocked neuromuscular transmission experimentally.

Taken together, these observations provide strong but still inconclusive evidence that autoantibodies play an important pathogenic role in GBS. Although antiganglioside antibodies have been studied most intensively, other antigenic targets also may be important. One recent report identified IgG antibodies against Schwann cells and neurons (nerve growth cone region) in some GBS cases. Proof that these antibodies are pathogenic requires that they be capable of mediating disease following direct passive transfer to naive hosts; this has not yet been demonstrated, although a case of apparent maternal-fetal transplacental transfer of GBS has been described.

PATHOPHYSIOLOGY

In the demyelinating forms of GBS, the basis for flaccid paralysis and sensory disturbance is conduction block. This finding, demonstrable electrophysiologically, implies that the axonal connections remain intact. Hence, recovery can take place rapidly as remyelination occurs. In severe cases of demyelinating GBS, secondary axonal degeneration usually occurs; its extent can be estimated electrophysiologically. More secondary axonal degeneration correlates with a slower rate of recovery and a greater degree of residual disability. When a severe primary axonal pattern is encountered electrophysiologically, the implication is that axons have degenerated and become disconnected from their targets, specifically the

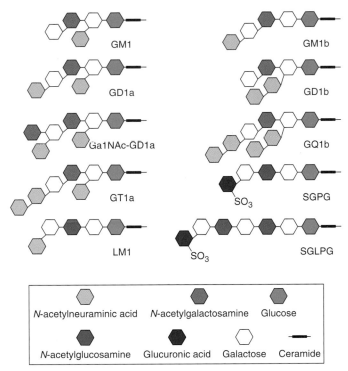

FIGURE 35-2

Glycolipids implicated as antigens in immune-mediated neuropathies. (*Modified from HJ Willison, N Yuki: Brain 125:2591, 2002. By permission of Oxford University Press.*)

neuromuscular junctions, and must therefore regenerate for recovery to take place. In motor axonal cases in which recovery is rapid, the lesion is thought to be localized to preterminal motor branches, allowing regeneration and reinnervation to take place quickly. Alternatively, in mild cases, collateral sprouting and reinnervation from

surviving motor axons near the neuromuscular junction may begin to reestablish physiologic continuity with muscles cells over a period of several months.

LABORATORY FEATURES

CSF findings are distinctive, consisting of an elevated CSF protein level [1 to 10 g/L (100 to 1000 mg/dL)] without accompanying pleocytosis. The CSF is often normal when symptoms have been present for ≤48 h; by the end of the first week the level of protein is usually elevated. A transient increase in the CSF white cell count (10 to 100/μL) occurs on occasion in otherwise typical GBS; however, a sustained CSF pleocytosis suggests an alternative diagnosis (viral myelitis) or a concurrent diagnosis such as unrecognized HIV infection. Electrodiagnostic features are mild or absent in the early stages of GBS and lag behind the clinical evolution. In cases with demyelination (Table 35-1), prolonged distal latencies, conduction velocity slowing, evidence of conduction block, and temporal dispersion of compound action potential are the usual features. In cases with primary axonal pathology, the principal electrodiagnostic finding is reduced amplitude of compound action potentials without conduction slowing or prolongation of distal latencies.

DIAGNOSIS

GBS is a descriptive entity. The diagnosis is made by recognizing the pattern of rapidly evolving paralysis with areflexia, absence of fever or other systemic symptoms, and characteristic antecedent events (**Table 35-3**).

TABLE 35-3

DIAGNOSTIC CRITERIA FOR GUILLAIN-BARRÉ SYNDROME

REQUIRED

1. Progressive weakness of 2 or more limbs due to neuropathy[a]
2. Areflexia
3. Disease course <4 weeks
4. Exclusion of other causes [e.g., vasculitis (polyarteritis nodosa, systemic lupus erythematosus, Churg-Strauss syndrome), toxins (organophosphates, lead), botulism, diphtheria, porphyria, localized spinal cord or cauda equina syndrome]

SUPPORTIVE

1. Relatively symmetric weakness
2. Mild sensory involvement
3. Facial nerve or other cranial nerve involvement
4. Absence of fever
5. Typical CSF profile (acellular, increase in protein level)
6. Electrophysiologic evidence of demyelination

[a]Excluding M. Fisher and other variant syndromes.
Note: CSF, cerebrospinal fluid.
Modified from AK Asbury, DR Cornblath: Ann Neurol 27:S21, 1990.

TABLE 35-4

MAJOR CLINICAL TRIALS OF TREATMENT FOR GUILLAIN-BARRÉ SYNDROME (GBS)

TRIAL/SITE	REFERENCE	NO. PATIENTS (N)/FOLLOW-UP (FU)/TRIAL ARMS	ENDPOINTS	RESULTS/P VALUE	COMMENT
GBS Study Group; USA/Canada (18 centers)	Neurology 35:1096, 1985	N = 245 FU = 6 months PE vs. none	1. % improved 1 grade at 4 weeks	1. 59% (PE) vs. 39% (none) p<.001	First major trial showing efficacy — prior smaller trials showed conflicting results
			2. Days to improve 1 grade	2. 19 days (PE) vs. 40 days (none) p<.001	
			3. Days to reach grade 2	3. 53 days (PE) vs. 85 days (none) p<.001	
French Coop. Group on PE in GBS; France/Switzerland (28 centers)	Ann Neurol 22:753, 1987; Ann Neurol 32:94, 1992	N = 220 FU = 1 year PE vs. none;	1. Days to walk with assistance	1. 30 days (PE) vs. 44 days (none) p<.01	At 1 year, full strength recovery in 71% (PE) vs. 52% (none); p = .007
			2. Days to positive Δ score	2. 4 days (PE) vs. 12 days (none) p<.001	
		Albumin vs. FFP in PE arm	3. Albumin vs. FFP	3. No significant difference	
Dutch GB Study Group; The Netherlands (15 centers)	N Engl J Med 326:1123, 1992	N = 150 FU = 6 months IVIg vs. PE	1. % improved 1 grade at 4 weeks	1. 53% (IVIg) vs. 34% (PE) p = .024	Patient assignment inadvertently favored IVIg group
			2. Days to reach grade 2	2. 55 days (IVIg) vs. 70 days (PE) p>= .07	
Plasma Exchange/Sando-globulin GBS Trial (38 centers in 11 countries)	Lancet 349:225, 1997	N = 329 FU = 48 weeks	1. % improved 1 grade at 4 weeks	No significant difference between the 3 groups for any endpoints	Nonsignificant trends favoring combined therapy
		IVIg vs. PE vs. both (3 arms)	2. Secondary endpoints: days to reach grade 2; days to off-respirator; disability at 48 weeks		

Abbreviations: PE, plasma exchange; IVIg, intravenous immunoglobulin; FFP, fresh-frozen plasma

Note: All studies except the French Coop. Group used the London grade scale: 0, healthy; 1, minor symptoms/signs; 2, walk 5 m unassisted; 3, walk 5 m with assistance; 4, bed/chairbound; 5, requiring assisted respiration; 6, dead.

Other disorders that may enter into the differential diagnosis include acute myelopathies (especially with prolonged back pain and sphincter disturbances); botulism (pupillary reactivity lost early); diphtheria (early oropharyngeal disturbances); Lyme polyradiculitis and other tick-borne paralyses; porphyria (abdominal pain, seizures, psychosis); vasculitic neuropathy (check erythrocyte sedimentation rate, described below); poliomyelitis (fever and meningismus common); CMV polyradiculitis (in immunocompromised patients); critical illness neuropathy; neuromuscular disorders such as myasthenia gravis; poisonings with organophosphates, thallium, or arsenic; tick paralysis; paralytic shellfish poisoning; or severe hypophosphatemia (rare). Laboratory tests are helpful primarily to exclude mimics of GBS. Electrodiagnostic features may be minimal, and the CSF protein level may not rise until the end of the first week. If the diagnosis is strongly suspected, treatment should be initiated without waiting for evolution of the characteristic electrodiagnostic and CSF findings to occur. GBS patients with risk factors for HIV or with CSF pleocytosis should have a serologic test for HIV.

TREATMENT FOR GBS

In the vast majority of patients with GBS, treatment should be initiated as soon after diagnosis as possible. Each day counts; ~2 weeks after the first motor symptoms, immunotherapy is no longer effective. Either high-dose intravenous immune globulin (IVIg) or plasmapheresis can be initiated, as they are equally effective (**Table 35-4**). A combination of the two therapies is not significantly better than either alone. IVIg is often the initial therapy chosen because of its ease of administration and good safety record. IVIg is administered as five daily infusions for a total dose of 2 g/kg body weight. There is some evidence that GBS autoantibodies are neutralized by anti-idiotypic antibodies present in IVIg preparations, perhaps accounting for the therapeutic effect. A course of plasmapheresis, consisting of ~40 to 50 mL/kg plasma exchange (PE) four times over a week, is usually employed. In patients who are treated early in the course of GBS and improve, relapse may occur in the second or third week. Brief re-treatment with the original therapy is usually effective. Glucocorticoids have not been found to be effective in GBS. Occasional patients with very mild forms of GBS, especially those who appear to have already reached a plateau when initially seen, may

be managed conservatively without IVIg or plasma exchange.

In the worsening phase of GBS, most patients require monitoring in a critical care setting, with particular attention to vital capacity, heart rhythm, blood pressure, nutrition, deep-vein thrombosis prophylaxis, cardiovascular status, early consideration (after 2 weeks of intubation) of tracheotomy, and chest physiotherapy. As noted, ~30% of patients with GBS require ventilatory assistance, sometimes for prolonged periods of time (several weeks or longer). Frequent turning and assiduous skin care are important, as are daily range-of-motion exercises to avoid joint contractures, and daily reassurance as to the generally good outlook for recovery.

PROGNOSIS AND RECOVERY

Approximately 85% of patients with GBS achieve a full functional recovery within several months to a year, although minor findings on examination (such as areflexia) may persist. The mortality rate is <5% in optimal settings; death usually results from secondary pulmonary complications. The outlook is worst in patients with severe proximal motor and sensory axonal damage. Such axonal damage may be either primary or secondary in nature (see "Pathophysiology," above), but in either case successful regeneration cannot occur. Other factors that worsen the outlook for recovery are advanced age, a fulminant or severe attack, and a delay in the onset of treatment. Some 5 to 10% of patients with typical GBS have one or more late relapses; such cases are then classified as chronic inflammatory demyelinating polyneuropathy (CIDP).

CHRONIC INFLAMMATORY DEMYELINATING POLYNEUROPATHY

CIDP is distinguished from GBS by its chronic course. In other respects, this neuropathy shares many features with GBS, including elevated CSF protein levels and the electrodiagnostic findings of acquired demyelination. Most cases occur in adults, and males are affected slightly more often than females. The incidence of CIDP is lower than that of GBS, but due to the protracted course the prevalence is greater.

CLINICAL MANIFESTATIONS

Onset is usually gradual, sometimes subacute; in a few, the initial attack is indistinguishable from that of GBS. It has recently been suggested that an acute-onset form of CIDP be considered when GBS deteriorates more than 9 weeks after onset or relapses at least three times. Symptoms are both motor and sensory in most cases. Weakness of the limbs is usually symmetric but can be strikingly asymmetric. There is considerable variability from case to case. Some patients experience a chronic progressive course, whereas others, usually younger patients, have a relapsing and remitting course. Some have only motor findings, and a small proportion present with a relatively pure syndrome of sensory ataxia. Tremor occurs in ~10% and may become more prominent during periods of subacute worsening or improvement. A small proportion have cranial nerve findings, including external ophthalmoplegia. CIDP tends to ameliorate over time with treatment; the result is that many years after onset nearly 75% of patients have reasonable functional status. Death from CIDP is uncommon.

DIAGNOSIS

The diagnosis rests on characteristic clinical, CSF, and electrophysiologic findings. The CSF is usually acellular with an elevated protein level, sometimes several times normal. Electrodiagnostically, variable degrees of conduction slowing, prolonged distal latencies, temporal dispersion of compound action potentials, and conduction block are the principal features. In particular, the presence of conduction block is a certain sign of an acquired demyelinating process. Evidence of axonal loss, presumably secondary to demyelination, is present in >50% of patients. Serum protein electrophoresis with immunofixation is indicated to search for monoclonal gammopathy and associated conditions (see "Monoclonal Gammopathy of Undetermined Significance," below). In all patients with presumptive CIDP, it is also reasonable to exclude collagen vascular disease (especially systemic lupus erythematosus), chronic hepatitis, HIV infection, and diabetes mellitus. Other associated conditions include inflammatory bowel disease and Hodgkin's lymphoma.

PATHOGENESIS

Although there is evidence of immune activation in CIDP, the precise mechanisms of pathogenesis are unknown. Biopsy typically reveals little inflammation and onion-bulb changes (imbricated layers of attenuated Schwann cell processes surrounding an axon) that result from recurrent demyelination and remyelination (Fig. 35-1). The response to therapy suggests that CIDP is immune-mediated; interestingly, CIDP responds to glucocorticoids whereas GBS does not. Passive transfer of demyelination into experimental animals was recently accomplished using IgG

purified from the serum of some patients with CIDP, lending support for a humoral autoimmune pathogenesis. Although the target antigen or antigens in CIDP have not yet been identified, one recent study implicated the myelin protein Po as a potential autoantigen in some patients. Approximately 25% of patients with clinical features of CIDP also have a monoclonal gammopathy of undetermined significance (MGUS). Cases associated with monoclonal IgA or IgG usually respond to treatment as favorably as cases without a monoclonal gammopathy. Patients with IgM monoclonal gammopathy tend to have more sensory findings and a more protracted course, and may have a less satisfactory response to treatment, although this is an area of controversy.

TREATMENT FOR CIDP

Most authorities initiate treatment for CIDP when progression is rapid or walking is compromised. If the disorder is mild, management can be expectant, awaiting spontaneous remission. Controlled studies have shown that high-dose IVIg, PE, and glucocorticoids are all more effective than placebo. Initial therapy is usually either IVIg or PE, which appear to be equally effective. IVIg is administered as 0.4 g/kg body weight daily for 5 days; most patients require periodic re-treatment at ~6-week intervals. PE is initiated at two to three treatments per week for 6 weeks; periodic re-treatment also may be required. Treatment with oral glucocorticoids is another option (60 to 80 mg prednisone daily for 1 to 2 months, followed by a gradual dose reduction of 10 mg per month as tolerated), but long-term adverse effects including bone demineralization, gastrointestinal bleeding, and cushingoid changes are problematic. Approximately one-half of patients with CIDP fail to respond adequately to the initial therapy chosen; a different treatment should then be tried. Patients who fail therapy with IVIg, PE, and glucocorticoids may benefit from treatment with immunosuppressive agents such as azathioprine, methotrexate, cyclosporine, and cyclophosphamide, either alone or as adjunctive therapy. Use of these therapies requires periodic reassessment of their risks and benefits.

MULTIFOCAL MOTOR NEUROPATHY

Multifocal motor neuropathy (MMN) is a distinctive but uncommon neuropathy that presents as slowly progressive motor weakness and atrophy evolving over years in the distribution of selected nerve trunks, associated with sites of persistent focal motor conduction block in the same nerve trunks. Sensory fibers are relatively spared. The arms are affected more frequently than the legs, and >75% of all patients are male. Some cases have been confused with lower motor neuron forms of amyotrophic lateral sclerosis (Chap. 21). Approximately 50% of patients present with high titers of polyclonal IgM antibody to the ganglioside GM1. It is uncertain how this finding relates to the discrete foci of persistent motor conduction block, but high concentrations of GM1 gangliosides are normal constituents of nodes of Ranvier in peripheral nerve fibers. Pathology reveals demyelination and mild inflammatory changes at the sites of conduction block.

Most patients with MMN respond to high-dose IVIg (dosages as for CIDP, above), and some refractory patients have responded to cyclophosphamide. Glucocorticoids and PE are not effective.

NEUROPATHIES WITH MONOCLONAL GAMMOPATHY

MULTIPLE MYELOMA

Clinically overt polyneuropathy occurs in ~5% of patients with the commonly encountered type of multiple myeloma, which exhibits either lytic or diffuse osteoporotic bone lesions. These neuropathies are sensorimotor, are usually mild but may be severe, and generally do not reverse with successful suppression of the myeloma. In most cases, electrodiagnostic and pathologic features are consistent with a process of axonal degeneration.

In contrast, myeloma with osteosclerotic features, although representing only 3% of all myelomas, is associated with polyneuropathy in one-half of cases. These neuropathies, which may also occur with solitary plasmacytoma, are distinct because they (1) are usually demyelinating in nature; (2) often respond to radiation therapy or removal of the primary lesion; (3) are associated with different monoclonal proteins and light chains (almost always lambda as opposed to primarily kappa in the lytic type of multiple myeloma); and (4) may occur in association with other systemic findings including thickening of the skin, hyperpigmentation, hypertrichosis, organomegaly, endocrinopathy, anasarca, and clubbing of fingers. These are features of the POEMS syndrome (*p*olyneuropathy, *o*rganomegaly, *e*ndocrinopathy, *M* protein, and *s*kin changes). The pathogenesis of this uncommon syndrome and the explanation for its association with lambda light chains are unknown. Treatment of the neuropathy is best directed at the osteosclerotic myeloma using surgery, radiotherapy, or chemotherapy, as indicated.

Neuropathies are also encountered in other systemic conditions with gammopathy including Waldenström's macroglobulinemia, primary systemic amyloidosis, and cryoglobulinemic states (mixed essential cryoglobulinemia, some cases of hepatitis C).

MONOCLONAL GAMMOPATHY OF UNDETERMINED SIGNIFICANCE

Chronic polyneuropathies occurring in association with MGUS are usually associated with the immunoglobulin isotypes IgG, IgA, and IgM. From a clinical standpoint, many of these patients are indistinguishable from patients with CIDP without monoclonal gammopathy (see "Chronic Inflammatory Demyelinating Polyneuropathy," above), and their response to immunosuppressive agents also is similar. An exception is the syndrome of IgM kappa monoclonal gammopathy associated with an indolent, longstanding, sometimes static sensory neuropathy, frequently with tremor and sensory ataxia. Most patients are male and over age 50. In the majority, the monoclonal IgM immunoglobulin binds to a normal peripheral nerve constituent, myelin-associated glycoprotein (MAG), found in the paranodal regions of Schwann cells. Binding appears to be specific for a polysaccharide epitope that is also found in other normal peripheral nerve myelin glycoproteins, P_0 and PMP22, and also in other normal nerve-related glycosphingolipids (Fig. 35-1). In the MAG-positive cases, IgM paraprotein is incorporated into the myelin sheaths of affected patients and widens the spacing of the myelin lamellae, thus producing a distinctive ultrastructural pattern. Demyelination and remyelination are the hallmarks of the lesions. The chronic demyelinating neuropathy appears to result from a destabilization of myelin metabolism rather than activation of an immune response. Therapy with chlorambucil or cyclophosphamide often results in improvement of the neuropathy associated with a prolonged reduction in the levels in the circulating paraprotein; chronic use of these alkylating agents is associated with significant risks. In a small proportion of patients (30% at 10 years), MGUS will in time evolve into frankly malignant conditions such as multiple myeloma or lymphoma.

VASCULITIC NEUROPATHY

Peripheral nerve involvement is common in polyarteritis nodosa (PAN), appearing in half of all cases clinically and in 100% of cases at postmortem studies. The most common pattern is multifocal (asymmetric) motor-sensory neuropathy (mononeuropathy multiplex) due to ischemic lesions of nerve trunks and roots; however, some cases of vasculitic neuropathy present as a distal, symmetric sensorimotor polyneuropathy. Symptoms of neuropathy are a common presenting complaint in patients with PAN. The electrodiagnostic findings are those of an axonal process. Small- to medium-sized arteries of the vasa nervorum, particularly the epineural vessels, are affected in PAN, resulting in a widespread ischemic neuropathy. A high frequency of neuropathy is also present in allergic angiitis and granulomatosis (Churg-Strauss syndrome).

Systemic vasculitis should always be considered when a subacute or chronically evolving mononeuropathy multiplex occurs in conjunction with constitutional symptoms (fever, anorexia, weight loss, loss of energy, malaise, and nonspecific pains). Diagnosis of suspected vasculitic neuropathy is made by a combined nerve and muscle biopsy, with serial section or skip-serial techniques (Chap. 33).

Approximately one-third of biopsy-proven cases of vasculitic neuropathy are "nonsystemic" in that the vasculitis appears to affect only peripheral nerve. Constitutional symptoms are absent, and the course is more indolent than that of PAN. The erythrocyte sedimentation rate may be elevated, but other tests for systemic disease are negative. Nevertheless, clinically silent involvement of other organs is likely, and vasculitis is frequently found in muscle biopsied at the same time as nerve.

Vasculitic neuropathy may also be seen as part of the vasculitis syndrome occurring in the course of other connective tissue disorders. The most frequent is rheumatoid arthritis, but ischemic neuropathy due to involvement of vasa nervorum may also occur in mixed cryoglobulinemia, Sjögren's syndrome, Wegener's granulomatosis, hypersensitivity angiitis, and progressive systemic sclerosis. Management of these neuropathies, including the "nonsystemic" vasculitic neuropathy, consists of treatment of the underlying condition as well as the aggressive use of glucocorticoids and other immunosuppressant drugs, usually cyclophosphamide.

ANTI-HU PARANEOPLASTIC NEUROPATHY

This uncommon immune-mediated disorder manifests as a sensory neuronopathy (i.e., selective damage to sensory nerve bodies in dorsal root ganglia). The onset is often asymmetric with dysesthesias and sensory loss in the limbs that soon progress to affect all limbs, the torso, and face. Marked sensory ataxia, pseudoathetosis, and in-

ability to walk, stand, or even sit unsupported are frequent features and are secondary to the extensive deafferentation. Subacute sensory neuronopathy is often idiopathic; ~25% of cases are paraneoplastic, primarily related to lung cancer, and most of those are small-cell lung cancer (SCLC). The target antigens are a family of RNA binding proteins (HuD, HuC, and Hel-N1) that in normal tissues are expressed only by neurons. The same proteins are usually expressed by SCLC, triggering in some patients an immune response characterized by antibodies and cytotoxic T cells that cross-react with the Hu proteins of the dorsal root ganglion neurons, resulting in immune-mediated neuronal destruction. An encephalomyelitis may accompany the sensory neuronopathy and presumably has the same pathogenesis. Neurologic symptoms usually precede, by 1 year on average, the identification of SCLC. The sensory neuronopathy runs its course in a few weeks or months and stabilizes, leaving the patient disabled. Most cases are unresponsive to treatment with glucocorticoids, IVIg, PE, or immunosuppressant drugs.

FURTHER READINGS

Gong Y et al: Localization of major gangliosides in the PNS: Implications for immune neuropathies. Brain 125:2491, 2002

☑ Hughes RAC et al: Practice parameter: Immunotherapy for Guillain-Barré syndrome. Report of the Quality Standards Subcommittee of the American Academy of Neurology. Neurology 61:736, 2003

Role of IVIg or plasma exchange in the treatment of GBS in adults or children.

Olney RK et al: Consensus criteria for the diagnosis of multifocal motor neuropathy. Muscle Nerve 27:117, 2003

☑ Ruts L et al: Distinguishing acute-onset CIDP from Guillain-Barre syndrome with treatment related fluctuations. Neurology 65:138, 2005

Clinical features separating CIDP from relapsing GBS.

Willison HJ, Yuki N: Peripheral neuropathies and anti-glycolipid antibodies. Brain 125:2591, 2002

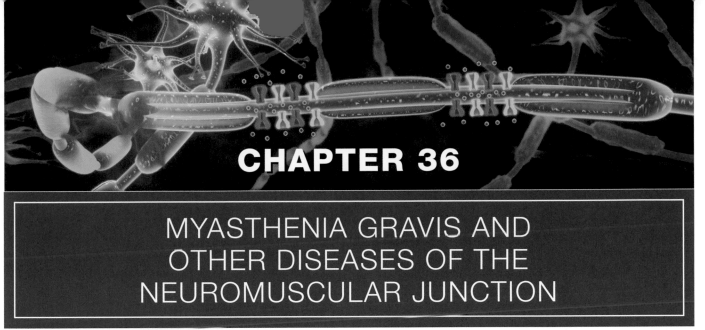

CHAPTER 36

MYASTHENIA GRAVIS AND OTHER DISEASES OF THE NEUROMUSCULAR JUNCTION

Daniel B. Drachman

Myasthenia gravis (MG) is a neuromuscular disorder characterized by weakness and fatigability of skeletal muscles. The underlying defect is a decrease in the number of available acetylcholine receptors (AChRs) at neuromuscular junctions due to an antibody-mediated autoimmune attack. Treatment now available for MG is highly effective, although a specific cure has remained elusive.

PATHOPHYSIOLOGY

In the neuromuscular junction (**Fig. 36-1**), acetylcholine (ACh) is synthesized in the motor nerve terminal and stored in vesicles (quanta). When an action potential travels down a motor nerve and reaches the nerve terminal, ACh from 150 to 200 vesicles is released and combines with AChRs that are densely packed at the peaks of postsynaptic folds. The structure of the AChR has been fully elucidated; it consists of 5 subunits (2 α, 1 β, 1 δ, and 1 γ or ε) arranged around a central pore. When ACh combines with the binding sites on the AChR, the channel in the AChR opens, permitting the rapid entry of cations, chiefly sodium, which produces depolarization at the end-plate region of the muscle fiber. If the depolarization is sufficiently large, it initiates an action potential that is propagated along the muscle fiber, triggering muscle contraction. This process is rapidly terminated by hydrolysis of ACh by acetylcholinesterase (AChE), which is present within the synaptic folds, and by diffusion of ACh away from the receptor.

In MG, the fundamental defect is a decrease in the number of available AChRs at the postsynaptic muscle membrane. In addition, the postsynaptic folds are flattened, or "simplified." These changes result in decreased efficiency of neuromuscular transmission. Therefore, although ACh is released normally, it produces small end-plate potentials that may fail to trigger muscle action potentials. Failure of transmission at many neuromuscular junctions results in weakness of muscle contraction.

The amount of ACh released per impulse normally declines on repeated activity (termed *presynaptic rundown*). In the myasthenic patient, the decreased efficiency of neuromuscular transmission combined with the normal rundown results in the activation of fewer and fewer muscle fibers by successive nerve impulses and hence increasing weakness, or *myasthenic fatigue*. This mechanism also accounts for the decremental response to repetitive nerve stimulation seen on electrodiagnostic testing.

The neuromuscular abnormalities in MG are brought about by an autoimmune response mediated by specific anti-AChR antibodies. The anti-AChR antibodies reduce the number of available AChRs at neuromuscular junctions by three distinct mechanisms: (1) accelerated turnover of AChRs, by a mechanism involving cross-linking and rapid endocytosis of the receptors; (2) blockade of the active site of the AChR, i.e., the site that normally binds ACh; and (3) damage to the postsynaptic muscle membrane by the antibody in collaboration with complement. The pathogenic antibodies are IgG and T cell dependent.

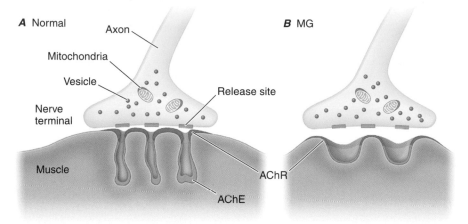

FIGURE 36-1

Diagrams of (**A**) normal and (**B**) myasthenic neuromuscular junctions. V, vesicles; M, mitochondria; AChE, acetylcholinesterase. See text for description of normal neuromuscular transmission. The MG junction shows a normal nerve terminal; a reduced number of AChRs (stippling); flattened, simplified postsynaptic folds; and a widened synaptic space.

Thus, immunotherapeutic strategies directed against T cells are effective in this antibody-mediated disease.

How the autoimmune response is initiated and maintained in MG is not completely understood. However, the thymus appears to play a role in this process. The thymus is abnormal in ~75% of patients with MG; in about 65% there is thymic hyperplasia and in another 10% there are thymic tumors (thymomas). Muscle-like cells within the thymus (myoid cells), which bear AChRs on their surface, may serve as a source of autoantigen and trigger the autoimmune reaction within the thymus gland.

CLINICAL FEATURES

MG is not rare, having a prevalence of at least 1 in 7500. It affects individuals in all age groups, but peaks of incidence occur in women in their twenties and thirties and in men in their fifties and sixties. Overall, women are affected more frequently than men, in a ratio of ~3:2. The cardinal features are *weakness* and *fatigability* of muscles. The weakness increases during repeated use (fatigue) and may improve following rest or sleep. The course of MG is often variable. Exacerbations and remissions may occur, particularly during the first few years after the onset of the disease. Remissions are rarely complete or permanent. Unrelated infections or systemic disorders often lead to increased myasthenic weakness and may precipitate "crisis" (see below).

The distribution of muscle weakness often has a characteristic pattern. The cranial muscles, particularly the eyelids and extraocular muscles, are often involved early in the course of MG, and diplopia and ptosis are common initial complaints. Facial weakness produces a "snarling" expression when the patient attempts to smile. Weakness in chewing is most noticeable after prolonged effort, as in chewing meat. Speech may have a nasal quality caused by weakness of the palate or a dysarthric "mushy" quality due to tongue weakness. Difficulty in swallowing may occur as a result of weakness of the palate, tongue, or pharynx, giving rise to nasal regurgitation or aspiration of liquids or food. In ~85% of patients, the weakness becomes generalized and affects the limb muscles as well. Limb weakness in MG is often proximal and may be asymmetric. Despite the muscle weakness, deep tendon reflexes are preserved. If weakness of respiration becomes so severe as to require respiratory assistance, the patient is said to be in *crisis*.

DIAGNOSIS AND EVALUATION
(Table 36-1)

The diagnosis is suspected on the basis of weakness and fatigability in the typical distribution described above, without loss of reflexes or impairment of sensation or other neurologic function. The suspected diagnosis should always be confirmed definitively before treatment is undertaken; this is essential because (1) other treatable conditions may closely resemble MG, and (2) the treatment of MG may involve surgery and the prolonged use of drugs with adverse side effects.

ANTICHOLINESTERASE TEST

Drugs that inhibit the enzyme AChE allow ACh to interact repeatedly with the limited number of AChRs, producing improvement in the strength of myasthenic

TABLE 36-1

DIAGNOSIS OF MYASTHENIA GRAVIS (MG)

History
  Diplopia, ptosis, weakness
  Weakness in characteristic distribution
  Fluctuation and fatigue: worse with repeated activity,
    improved by rest
  Effects of previous treatments
Physical examination
  Ptosis, diplopia
  Motor power survey: quantitative testing of muscle
    strength
  Forward arm abduction time (5 min)
  Vital capacity
  Absence of other neurologic signs
Laboratory testing
  Anti-AChR radioimmunoassay: ~85% positive in
    generalized MG; 50% in ocular MG; definite diagnosis
    if positive; negative result does not exclude MG.
    ~40% of AChR antibody-negative patients with gener-
    alized MG have anti-MuSK antibodies.
  Edrophonium chloride (Tensilon) 2 mg + 8 mg IV; highly
    probable diagnosis if unequivocally positive
  Repetitive nerve stimulation; decrement of >15% at
    3 Hz: highly probable
  Single-fiber electromyography: blocking and jitter, with
    normal fiber density; confirmatory, but not specific
  For ocular or cranial MG: exclude intracranial lesions by
    CT or MRI

Note: AChR, acetylcholine receptor; CT, computed tomography; MRI, magnetic resonance imaging; MuSK, muscle specific tyrosine kinase.
Source: From DB Drachman: N Engl J Med 330:1797, 1994.

muscles. Edrophonium is used most commonly for diagnostic testing because of the rapid onset (30 s) and short duration (about 5 min) of its effect. An objective endpoint must be selected to evaluate the effect of edrophonium. The examiner should focus on one or more unequivocally weak muscle groups and evaluate their strength objectively. For example, weakness of extraocular muscles, impairment of speech, or the length of time that the patient can maintain the arms in forward abduction may be useful measures. An initial dose of 2 mg of edrophonium is given intravenously. If definite improvement occurs, the test is considered positive and is terminated. If there is no change, the patient is given an additional 8 mg intravenously. The dose is administered in two parts because some patients react to edrophonium with unpleasant side effects such as nausea, diarrhea, urge to defecate, salivation, fasciculations, and rarely with severe symptoms of syncope or bradycardia. Atropine (0.6 mg) should be drawn up in a syringe, ready for intravenous administration if these symptoms become troublesome.

False-positive tests occur occasionally in patients with other neurologic disorders, such as amyotrophic lateral sclerosis (ALS) or mitochondrial myopathy. False-negative or equivocal tests also may occur. In virtually all instances, it is desirable to carry out further testing to establish the diagnosis of MG definitively.

ELECTRODIAGNOSTIC TESTING

Repetitive nerve stimulation often provides helpful diagnostic evidence of MG. Anti-AChE medication is stopped 6 to 24 h before testing. It is best to test weak muscles or proximal muscle groups. Electric shocks are delivered at a rate of two or three per second (low-frequency repetitive stimulation) to the appropriate nerves, and action potentials are recorded from the muscles. In normal individuals, the amplitude of the evoked muscle action potentials does not change at these rates of stimulation. However, in myasthenic patients there is a rapid reduction in the amplitude of the evoked responses of >10 to 15%.

ANTIACETYLCHOLINE RECEPTOR ANTIBODY

As noted above, anti-AChR antibodies are detectable in the serum of ~85% of all myasthenic patients but in only ~50% of patients with weakness confined to the ocular muscles. The presence of anti-AChR antibodies is virtually diagnostic of MG, but a negative test does not exclude the disease. The measured level of anti-AChR antibody does not correspond well with the severity of MG in different patients. However, in an individual patient, a treatment-induced fall in the antibody level often correlates with clinical improvement. Recently, antibodies to muscle-specific kinase (MuSK) have been found to be present in ~40% of AChR antibody–negative patients with generalized MG, and their presence is a useful diagnostic test in these patients. MuSK antibodies are not present in AChR antibody–positive patients or in patients with MG limited to ocular muscles. The role of these antibodies in the pathogenesis of MG is as yet uncertain. MuSK is known to participate in clustering of AChRs at neuromuscular junctions during development.

INHERITED MYASTHENIC SYNDROMES

The congenital myasthenic syndromes (CMS) are a heterogeneous group of disorders of the neuromuscular junction that are not autoimmune but rather are due to genetic mutations in which virtually any component of the neuromuscular junction may be affected. Alterations in function of the presynaptic nerve terminal or in the various subunits of the AChR or AChE have been identified in the various forms of CMS. These disorders share many of the clinical features of autoimmune MG, including weakness and fatigability of skeletal muscles, in some cases involving extraocular muscles (EOMs), lids, and proximal muscles, similar to the distribution in autoimmune MG. CMS should be suspected when symptoms of myasthenia have begun in infancy or childhood and AChR antibody tests are consistently negative. Features of four of the most common forms of CMS are summarized in **Table 36–2**. Although clinical features and electrodiagnostic and pharmacologic tests may suggest the correct diagnosis, sophisticated electrophysiologic and molecular analyses are required for precise elucidation of the defect; this may lead to helpful treatment as well as genetic counseling. In the forms that involve the AChR, a wide variety of mutations have been identified in each of the subunits, but the α subunit is affected in ~75% of these cases. In most of the recessively inherited forms of CMS, the mutations are heteroallelic—that is, different mutations affecting each of the two alleles are present.

DIFFERENTIAL DIAGNOSIS

Many other conditions can cause weakness of the cranial and/or somatic musculature, superficially resembling

MG. These include myopathies (especially mitochondrial and some dystrophies), diabetes mellitus, basilar meningitis, Guillain-Barré syndrome, vasculitis, ALS, drug-induced myasthenia, Lambert-Eaton myasthenic syndrome (LEMS), neurasthenia, hyperthyroidism, and botulism. Skull base tumors and lesions of the superior orbital fissure, cavernous sinus, or brainstem are additional causes. Drug treatment with penicillamine (used for scleroderma or rheumatoid arthritis) may result in true MG, but the weakness is usually mild, and recovery occurs within weeks or months after discontinuing its use. Aminoglycoside antibiotics or procainamide can cause exacerbation of weakness in myasthenic patients.

LEMS is a presynaptic disorder of the neuromuscular junction that can cause weakness similar to that of MG. The proximal muscles of the lower limbs are most commonly affected, but other muscles may be involved as well. Cranial nerve findings, including ptosis of the eyelids and diplopia, occur in up to 70% of patients and resemble features of MG. However, the two conditions are readily distinguished, since patients with LEMS have depressed or absent reflexes, show autonomic symptoms such as dry mouth and impotence, and show incremental

TABLE 36–2

THE CONGENITAL MYASTHENIC SYNDROMES

TYPE	CLINICAL FEATURES	ELECTRO-PHYSIOLOGY	GENETICS	END-PLATE EFFECTS	TREATMENT
Slow channel	Most common; weak forearm extensors; onset 2d to 3d decade; variable severity	Repetitive muscle response on nerve stimulation; prolonged channel opening and MEPP duration	Antosomal dominant; α, β, ε AChR mutations	Excitotoxic end-plate myopathy; decreased AChRs; postsynaptic damage	Quinidine: decreases end-plate damage; made worse by anti-AChE
Low-affinity fast channel	Onset early: moderately severe; ptosis, EOM involvement; weakness and fatigue	Brief and infrequent channel openings; opposite of slow channel syndrome	Autosomal recessive; may be heteroallelic	Normal end-plate structure	3, 4-DAP; anti-AChE
Severe AChR deficiencies	Early onset, variable severity; fatigue; typical MG features	Decremental response to repetitive nerve stimulation; decreased MEPP amplitudes	Autosomal recessive ε; mutations most common; many different mutations	Increased length of end plates; variable synaptic folds	Anti-AchE; ?3, 4-DAP
AChE deficiency	Early onset; variable severity; scoliosis; may have normal EOMs, absent pupillary responses	Decremental response to repetitive nerve stimulation	Mutant gene for AChE's collagen anchor	Small nerve terminals; degenerated junctional folds	Worse with anti-AChE drugs

Abbreviations: AChR, acetylcholine receptor; AChE, acetylcholinesterase; EOMs, extraocular muscles; MEPP, miniature end-plate potentials; 3, 4-DAP, 3-4-Diaminopyridine.

rather than decremental responses on high-frequency (e.g., 50-Hz) repetitive nerve stimulation. LEMS is caused by autoantibodies directed against P/Q-type calcium channels at the motor nerve terminals, which can be detected in ~85% of LEMS patients by radioimmunoassay. These autoantibodies result in impaired release of ACh from nerve terminals. A majority of patients with this syndrome have an associated malignancy, most commonly small-cell carcinoma of the lung, which is thought to trigger the autoimmune response. The diagnosis of LEMS may signal the presence of the tumor long before it would otherwise be detected, permitting early removal. Treatment of the neuromuscular disorder involves plasmapheresis and immunosuppression, as for MG. 3,4 Diaminopyridine (3,4-DAP) and pyridostigmine may be symptomatically helpful in LEMS. 3,4-DAP acts by blocking potassium channels; this results in prolonged depolarization of the motor nerve terminals and thereby enhances ACh release. Pyridostigmine prolongs the action of ACh, allowing repeated interactions with AChRs.

Botulism is due to a potent bacterial toxin produced by Clostridium botulinum. The toxin interferes with the release of acetylcholine from the presynaptic neuromuscular junction thereby interfering with neuromuscular transmission. The most common form is food-borne botulism from ingestion of food containing toxin; in wound and intestinal botulism, spores germinate and give rise to organisms that produce toxin. Patients present with bulbar weakness (e.g., diplopia, dysarthria, dysphagia) but lack sensory symptoms and signs; deep tendon reflexes are preserved early in the disease course. Weakness generalizes to the limbs and may result in respiratory failure; reflexes may be diminished as the disease progresses. Mentation is normal. Autonomic findings include paralytic ileus, constipation, urinary retention, dilated or poorly reactive pupils, and dry mouth. The differential diagnosis includes brainstem stroke, myasthenia gravis, toxin ingestion (e.g., organophosphates), Lambert-Eaton syndrome, tick paralysis, and Guillain-Barré syndrome. The demonstration of toxin in serum by bioassay is definitive but may be negative. Nerve conduction studies reveal findings of presynaptic neuromuscular blockade with reduced compound muscle action potentials (CMAPs) that increase in amplitude following high frequency repetitive stimulation. Treatment may include intubation for airway protection, ventilatory support, or aggressive inpatient supportive care (e.g., nutrition, DVT prophylaxis). Equine antitoxin is given rapidly before the results of laboratory studies are available. The prognosis is better among patients with type B infection who are <60 years old. A vaccine is available for highly exposed individuals.

Neurasthenia is the historic term for a myasthenia-like fatigue syndrome without an organic basis. These patients may present with subjective symptoms of weakness and fatigue, but muscle testing usually reveals the "give-away weakness" characteristic of nonorganic disorders; the complaint of fatigue in these patients means tiredness or apathy rather than decreasing muscle power on repeated effort. Hyperthyroidism is readily diagnosed or excluded by tests of thyroid function. Abnormalities of thyroid function (hyper- or hypothyroidism) may increase myasthenic weakness. Botulism can cause myasthenic-like weakness, but the pupils are often dilated, and repetitive nerve stimulation gives an incremental response. Diplopia that mimics the symptoms of MG may occasionally be due to an intracranial mass lesion that compresses nerves to the EOMs (e.g., sphenoid ridge meningioma), but magnetic resonance imaging (MRI) of the head and orbits usually reveals the lesion.

Progressive external ophthalmoplegia is a rare condition resulting in weakness of the EOMs, which may be accompanied by weakness of the proximal muscles of the limbs and other systemic features. Most patients with this condition have mitochondrial disorders that can be detected on muscle biopsy (Chap. 38).

SEARCH FOR ASSOCIATED CONDITIONS (Table 36-3)

Myasthenic patients have an increased incidence of several associated disorders. Thymic abnormalities occur in ~75% of patients, as noted above. Neoplastic change (thymoma) may produce enlargement of the thymus, which is detected by computed tomography (CT) or MRI scanning of the anterior mediastinum. A thymic shadow on CT scan may normally be present through young adulthood, but enlargement of the thymus in a patient >40 years old is highly suspicious of thymoma. Hyperthyroidism occurs in 3 to 8% of patients and may aggravate the myasthenic weakness. Tests of thyroid function should be obtained. Because of the association of MG with other autoimmune disorders, blood tests for rheumatoid factor and antinuclear antibodies should be carried out in all patients. Chronic infection of any kind can exacerbate MG and should be sought carefully. Measurements of ventilatory function are valuable because of the frequency and seriousness of respiratory impairment in myasthenic patients.

Because of the side effects of glucocorticoids and other immunosuppressive agents used in the treatment of MG, a thorough medical investigation should be undertaken, searching specifically for evidence of chronic or latent infection (such as tuberculosis or hepatitis), hypertension, diabetes, renal impairment, and glaucoma.

TABLE 36-3

DISORDERS ASSOCIATED WITH MYASTHENIA GRAVIS AND RECOMMENDED LABORATORY TESTS

Associated disorders

Disorders of the thymus: thymoma, hyperplasia
Other autoimmune disorders: Hashimoto's thyroiditis, Graves' disease, rheumatoid arthritis, lupus erythematosus, skin disorders, family history of autoimmune disorder
Disorders or circumstances that may exacerbate myasthenia gravis: hyperthyroidism or hypothyroidism, occult infection, medical treatment for other conditions (aminoglycoside antibiotics, quinine, antiarrhythmic agents)
Disorders that may interfere with therapy: tuberculosis, diabetes, peptic ulcer, gastrointestinal bleeding, renal disease, hypertension, asthma, osteoporosis, obesity

Recommended laboratory tests or procedures

CT or MRI of mediastinum
Test for lupus erythematosus, antinuclear antibody, rheumatoid factor, antithyroid antibodies
Thyroid-function tests
PPD skin test
Chest radiography
Fasting blood glucose measurement
Pulmonary-function tests
Bone densitometry in older patients

Note: CT, computed tomography; MRI, magnetic resonance imaging; PPD, purified protein derivative.
Source: From RT Johnson, JW Griffin (eds): *Current Therapy in Neurologic Disease*, 4th ed. St. Louis, Mosby Year Book, 1993, p 379.

TREATMENT FOR MG

The prognosis has improved strikingly as a result of advances in treatment; virtually all myasthenic patients can be returned to full productive lives with proper therapy. The most useful treatments for MG include anticholinesterase medications, immunosuppressive agents, thymectomy, and plasmapheresis or intravenous immunoglobulin (IVIg). See **Fig. 36-2**.

Anticholinesterase Medications

Anticholinesterase medication produces at least partial symptomatic improvement in most myasthenic patients, although improvement is rarely complete. Oral pyridostigmine is the most widely used anticholinesterase medication in the United States. As a rule, the beneficial action of oral pyridostigmine begins within 15 to 30 min and lasts for 3 to 4 h, but individual responses vary. Treatment is begun with a moderate dose, e.g., 60 mg three to five times daily. The frequency and

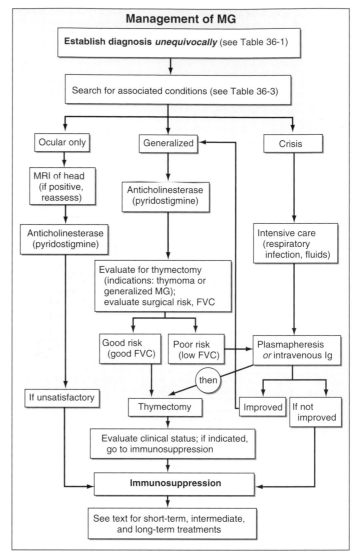

FIGURE 36-2
Algorithm for the management of myasthenia gravis. MRI, magnetic resonance imaging; FVC, forced vital capacity.

amount of the dose should be tailored to the patient's individual requirements throughout the day. For example, patients with weakness in chewing and swallowing may benefit by taking the medication before meals so that peak strength coincides with mealtime. Long-acting pyridostigmine may occasionally be useful to get the patient through the night but should never be used for daytime medication because of variable absorption. The maximum useful dose of pyridostigmine rarely exceeds 120 mg every 3 to 6 h during daytime. Overdosage with anticholinesterase medication may cause increased weakness and other side effects. In some patients, muscarinic side effects of the anticholinesterase medication (diarrhea, abdominal cramps, salivation, nausea) may limit the dose tolerated. Atropine/diphenoxylate or loperamide is useful for the treatment of GI symptoms.

Thymectomy

Two separate issues should be distinguished: (1) surgical removal of thymoma, and (2) thymectomy as a treatment for MG. Surgical removal of a thymoma is necessary because of the possibility of local tumor spread, although most thymomas are benign. In the absence of a tumor, the available evidence suggests that up to 85% of patients experience improvement after thymectomy; of these, ~35% achieve drug-free remission. However, the improvement is typically delayed for months to years. The advantage of thymectomy is that it offers the possibility of long-term benefit, in some cases diminishing or eliminating the need for continuing medical treatment. In view of these potential benefits and of the negligible risk in skilled hands, thymectomy has gained widespread acceptance in the treatment of MG. It is the consensus that thymectomy should be carried out in all patients with generalized MG who are between the ages of puberty and at least 55 years. Whether thymectomy should be recommended in children, in adults >55 years of age, and in patients with weakness limited to the ocular muscles is still a matter of debate. Thymectomy must be carried out in a hospital where it is performed regularly and where the staff is experienced in the pre- and postoperative management, anesthesia, and surgical techniques of total thymectomy.

Immunosuppression

Immunosuppression using glucocorticoids, azathioprine, and other drugs is effective in nearly all patients with MG. The choice of drugs or other immunomodulatory treatments should be guided by the relative benefits and risks for the individual patient and the urgency of treatment. It is helpful to develop a treatment plan based on short-term, intermediate-term, and long-term objectives. For example, if immediate improvement is essential either because of the severity of weakness or because of the patient's need to return to activity as soon as possible, IVIg or plasmapheresis are reasonable choices. For the intermediate term, glucocorticoids and cyclosporine generally produce clinical improvement within a period of 1 to 3

months. The beneficial effects of azathioprine and mycophenolate mofetil usually begin after many months (up to a year), but these drugs have advantages for the long-term treatment of patients with MG. For the occasional patient with MG that is genuinely refractory to optimal treatment with conventional immunosuppressive agents, a course of high-dose cyclophosphamide may induce long-lasting (possibly permanent) benefit by "rebooting" the immune system. At high doses, cyclophosphamide eliminates mature lymphocytes, but hematopoietic precursors (stem cells) are spared because they express the enzyme aldehyde dehydrogenase, which hydrolyzes cyclophosphamide. This procedure should be reserved for truly refractory patients and administered only in a facility fully familiar with this approach.

GLUCOCORTICOID THERAPY

Glucocorticoids, when used properly, produce improvement in myasthenic weakness in the great majority of patients. To minimize adverse side effects, prednisone should be given in a single dose rather than in divided doses throughout the day. The initial dose should be relatively low (15 to 25 mg/d) to avoid the early weakening that occurs in about one-third of patients treated initially with a high-dose regimen. The dose is increased stepwise, as tolerated by the patient (usually by 5 mg/d at 2- to 3-day intervals), until there is marked clinical improvement or a dose of 50 to 60 mg/d is reached. This dose is maintained for 1 to 3 months and then is gradually modified to an alternate-day regimen over the course of an additional 1 to 3 months; the goal is to reduce the dose on the "off day" to zero or to a minimal level. Generally, patients begin to improve within a few weeks after reaching the maximum dose, and improvement continues to progress for months or years. The prednisone dosage may gradually be reduced, but usually months or years may be needed to determine the minimum effective dose, and close monitoring is required. Few patients are able to do without immunosuppressive agents entirely. Patients on long-term glucocorticoid therapy must be followed carefully to prevent or treat adverse side effects. The most common errors in glucocorticoid treatment of myasthenic patients include (1) insufficient persistence—improvement may be delayed and gradual; (2) too early, too rapid, or excessive tapering of dosage; and (3) lack of attention to prevention and treatment of side effects.

OTHER IMMUNOSUPPRESSIVE DRUGS

Azathioprine, cyclosporine, mycophenolate mofetil, or occasionally cyclophosphamide are effective in many patients, either alone or in combination with glucocorticoid therapy. Azathioprine has been the most widely used of these drugs because of its relative safety in most patients and long track record. Its therapeutic effect may add to that of glucocorticoids and/or allow the glucocorticoid dose to be reduced. However, up to 10% of patients are unable to tolerate azathioprine because of idiosyncratic reactions consisting of flulike symptoms of fever and malaise, bone marrow depression, or abnormalities of liver function. An initial dose of 50 mg/d should be used to test for adverse side effects. If this dose is tolerated, it is increased gradually until the white blood count falls to ~3000 to 4000/μL. In patients who are receiving glucocorticoids concurrently, leukocytosis precludes the use of this measure. A reduction of the lymphocyte count to <1000/μL and/or an increase of the mean corpuscular volume of red blood cells may be used as indications of adequacy of azathioprine dosage. The typical dosage range is 2 to 3 mg/kg total body weight. The beneficial effect of azathioprine takes at least 3 to 6 months to begin and even longer to peak. In patients taking azathioprine, allopurinol should never be used to treat hyperuricemia, because the two drugs share a common degradation pathway; the result may be severe bone marrow depression due to increased effects of the azathioprine.

Cyclosporine is approximately as effective as azathioprine and is being used increasingly in the management of MG. Its beneficial effect appears more rapidly than that of azathioprine. It may be used alone but is usually used as an adjunct to glucocorticoids to permit reduction of the glucocorticoid dose. The usual dose of cyclosporine is 4 to 5 mg/kg per day, given in two equally divided doses (to minimize side effects). Side effects of cyclosporine include hypertension and nephrotoxicity, which must be closely monitored. "Trough" blood levels of cyclosporine are measured 12 h after the evening dose. The therapeutic range, as measured by radioimmunoassay, is 150 to 200 ng/L.

Mycophenolate mofetil also is useful in the treatment of MG. A dose of 1 g to 1.5 g bid is recommended. Its mechanism of action involves inhibition of purine synthesis by the de novo pathway. Since lymphocytes lack the alternative salvage pathway that is present in all other cells, mycophenolate inhibits proliferation of lymphocytes but not proliferation of other cells. It does not kill or eliminate preexisting autoreactive lymphocytes, and therefore clinical improvement may be delayed for many months to a year, until the preexisting autoreactive lymphocytes die spontaneously. The advantage of mycophenolate lies in its relative lack of adverse side effects, with only occasional production of diarrhea and rare development of leukopenia. This drug may become the choice for long-term treatment of myasthenic patients, but the present cost of mycophenolate is prohibitively high.

Cyclophosphamide is reserved for occasional patients refractory to the other drugs (see above for discussion of high-dose cyclophosphamide treatment).

Plasmapheresis and Intravenous Immunoglobulin

Plasmapheresis has been used therapeutically in MG. Plasma, which contains the pathogenic antibodies, is mechanically separated from the blood cells, which are returned to the patient. A course of five exchanges (3 to 4 L per exchange) is generally administered over a 2-week period. Plasmapheresis produces a short-term reduction in anti-AChR antibodies, with clinical improvement in many patients. It is useful as a temporary expedient in seriously affected patients or to improve the patient's condition prior to surgery (e.g., thymectomy).

The indications for the use of IVIg are the same as those for plasma exchange: to produce rapid improvement to help the patient through a difficult period of myasthenic weakness or prior to surgery. This treatment has the advantage of not requiring special equipment or large-bore venous access. The usual dose is 2 g/kg, which is typically administered over 5 days (400 mg/kg per day). If tolerated, the course of IVIg can be shortened to administer the entire dose over a 3-day period. Improvement occurs in about 70% of patients, beginning during treatment, or within 4 to 5 days thereafter, and continuing for weeks to months. The mechanism of action of IVIg is not known; the treatment has no consistent effect on the measurable amount of circulating AChR antibody. Adverse reactions are generally not serious but include headache, fluid overload, and rarely aseptic meningitis or renal shutdown. IVIg should rarely be used as a long-term treatment in place of rationally managed immunosuppressive therapy. The intermediate and long-term treatment of myasthenic patients requires other methods of therapy outlined earlier in this chapter.

Management of Myasthenic Crisis

Myasthenic crisis is defined as an exacerbation of weakness sufficient to endanger life; it usually consists of respiratory failure caused by diaphragmatic and intercostal muscle weakness. Crisis rarely occurs in properly managed patients. Treatment should be carried out in an intensive care unit staffed with physicians experienced in the management of MG, respiratory insufficiency, infectious disease, and fluid and electrolyte therapy. The possibility that the deterioration could be due to excessive anticholinesterase medication ("cholinergic crisis") is best excluded by temporarily stopping anticholinesterase drugs. The most common cause of crisis is intercurrent infection. This should be treated immediately, because the mechanical and immunologic defenses of the patient can be assumed to be compromised. Early and effective antibiotic therapy, respiratory assistance, and pulmonary physiotherapy are essential. Plasmapheresis or IVIg is frequently helpful in hastening recovery.

Myasthenia Gravis Worksheet

History				
General	Normal	Good	Fair	Poor
Diplopia	None	Rare	Occasional	Constant
Ptosis	None	Rare	Occasional	Constant
Arms	Normal	Slightly limited	Some ADL impairment	Definitely limited
Legs	Normal	Walks/runs fatigues	Can walk limited distances	Minimal walking
Speech	Normal	Dysarthric	Severely dysarthric	Unintelligible
Voice	Normal	Fades	Impaired	Severely impaired
Chew	Normal	Fatigue on normal foods	Fatigue on soft foods	Feeding tube
Swallow	Normal	Normal foods	Soft foods only	Feeding tube
Respiration	Normal	Dyspnea on unusual effort	Dyspnea on any effort	Dyspnea at rest

Examination

BP _____ Pulse _____ Wt _____
Edema _____
Vital capacity _____
Cataracts? R _____ L _____
EOMS _____
Ptosis time _____
Face _____

Arm abduction time R_____ L_____
Deltoids   R_____ L_____
Biceps   R_____ L_____
Triceps   R_____ L_____
Grip   R_____ L_____
Iliopsoas   R_____ L_____
Quadriceps   R_____ L_____
Hamstrings   R_____ L_____
Other   R_____ L_____

FIGURE 36-3

Abbreviated interval assessment form for use in evaluating treatment for myasthenia gravis.

PATIENT ASSESSMENT

In order to evaluate the effectiveness of treatment as well as drug-induced side effects, it is important to assess the patient's clinical status at baseline and on repeated interval examinations in a systematic manner. The most useful clinical tests include forward arm abduction time (up to a full 5 min), forced vital capacity, range of eye movements, and time to development of ptosis on upward gaze. Manual muscle testing or, preferably, quantitative dynamometry of limb muscles, especially proximal muscles, also is important. An interval form can provide a succinct summary of the patient's status and a guide to treatment results; an abbreviated form is shown in **Fig. 36-3.** A progressive reduction in the patient's AChR antibody level also provides clinically valuable confirmation of the effectiveness of treatment; conversely, a rise in AChR antibody levels during tapering of immunosuppressive medication may predict clinical exacerbation. For reliable quantitative measurement of AChR antibody levels, it is best to compare antibody levels from prior frozen serum aliquots with current serum samples in simultaneously run assays.

FURTHER READINGS

☑ CARESS JB et al: Anti-MuSK myasthenia gravis presenting with purely ocular findings. Arch Neurol 62:1002, 2005

First report of MuSK antibodies in ocular MG.

☑ DRACHMAN DB et al: Treatment of refractory myasthenia gravis: "Rebooting" with high dose cyclophosphamide. Ann Neurol 53:29, 2003

Aggressive treatment for patients who do not respond to conventional agents.

☑ KAMINSKI HJ: *Myasthenia Gravis and Related Disorders.* Totowa, NJ, Humana Press, 2003

Recent comprehensive review text covering clinical and scientific aspects.

KUPERSMITH MJ et al: Development of generalized disease at 2 years in patients with ocular myasthenia gravis. Arch Neurol 60:243, 2003

Lindstrom JM: Acetylcholine receptors and myasthenia. Muscle Nerve 23:453, 2000

▨ Maddison P, Newsom-Davis J: Treatment for Lambert-Eaton myasthenic syndrome. Cochrane Database Syst Rev (2):CD003279, 2005

Evidence-based review of treatment options for Lambert-Eaton syndrome.

▨ Shiraishi H et al: Acetylcholine receptor loss and postsynaptic damage in MuSK antibody-positive myasthenia gravis. Ann Neurol 57:289, 2005

Highlights microscopic pathology differences in MuSK-mediated MG versus classic MG.

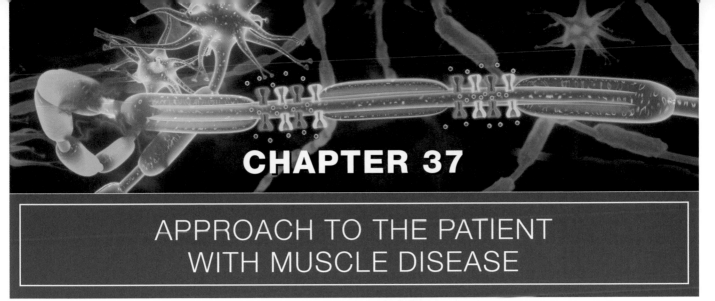

CHAPTER 37

APPROACH TO THE PATIENT WITH MUSCLE DISEASE

Jerry R. Mendell

Skeletal muscle diseases, or myopathies, are disorders with structural changes or functional impairment of muscle. These conditions can be differentiated from other diseases of the motor unit (e.g., lower motor neuron or neuromuscular junction pathologies) by characteristic clinical and laboratory findings. Myasthenia gravis and related disorders are discussed in Chap. 36; muscular dystrophies and inherited, metabolic, and toxic myopathies in Chap. 38; inflammatory muscle diseases and inclusion body myositis in Chap. 39.

CLINICAL FEATURES

The most common clinical findings of a myopathy are proximal, symmetric limb weakness (arms or legs) with preserved reflexes and sensation. An associated sensory loss suggests injury to peripheral nerve or the central nervous system rather than myopathy. On occasion, disorders affecting the motor nerve cell bodies in the spinal cord (anterior horn cell disease), the neuromuscular junction, or peripheral nerves can mimic findings of myopathy.

MUSCLE WEAKNESS

Symptoms of muscle weakness can be either intermittent or persistent. Disorders causing *intermittent weakness*

(**Fig. 37-1**) include myasthenia gravis, periodic paralyses (hypokalemic, hyperkalemic, and paramyotonia congenita), defects of glycolysis (especially myophosphorylase deficiency), and fatty acid utilization (carnitine palmitoyltransferase deficiency). Defects in glycolysis cause activity-related muscle breakdown accompanied by myoglobinuria, appearing as light or dark brown urine.

Most muscle disorders cause *persistent weakness* (**Fig. 37-2**). In the majority, the proximal muscles are weaker than the distal muscles, and the facial muscles are spared; the latter pattern is referred to as *limb-girdle*.

There are some characteristic patterns of weakness. Facial weakness (difficulty with eye closure and impaired smile) and scapular winging (**Fig. 37-3**) are characteristic of *facioscapulohumeral dystrophy (FSH)*. Facial and distal limb weakness associated with hand grip myotonia is virtually diagnostic of *myotonic dystrophy*. Ptosis and extraocular muscle weakness without diplopia suggests *oculopharyngeal muscular dystrophy, mitochondrial myopathies, or myotubular myopathy*. Loss of strength in both proximal and distal muscles, hand grip weakness, and wasting of quadriceps muscles is pathognomonic for *inclusion body myositis*. Dropped head syndrome indicates selective neck extensor muscle weakness. The most common neuromuscular diseases causing this pattern of weakness include *myasthenia gravis, polymyositis, or amyotrophic lateral sclerosis (ALS)*. Preferential distal extremity weakness is typical of the *distal myopathies* (Chap. 38).

It is important to examine functional capabilities to help disclose certain patterns of weakness (**Table 37-1**). The Gowers' sign (**Fig. 37-4**) is particularly useful. Observing the gait of an individual may disclose a lordotic posture caused by combined trunk and hip weakness, frequently exaggerated by toe walking (**Fig. 37-5**). A waddling gait is caused by the inability of weak hip muscles to prevent hip drop or hip dip. Hyperextension of the knee (genu recurvatum) is characteristic of quadriceps muscle

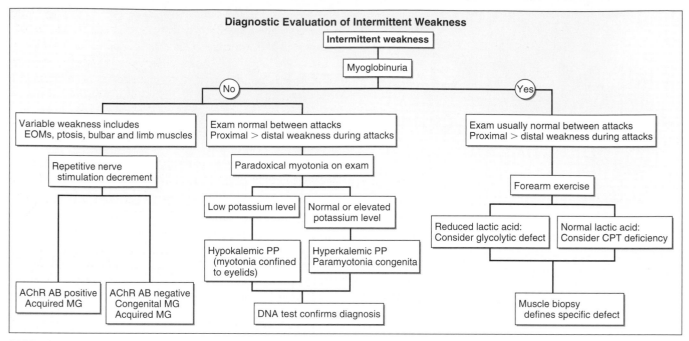

FIGURE 37-1

Diagnostic evaluation of intermittent weakness. EOMs, extraocular muscles; AChR AB, acetylcholine receptor antibody; PP, periodic paralysis; CPT, carnitine palmitoyltransferase; MG, myasthenia gravis.

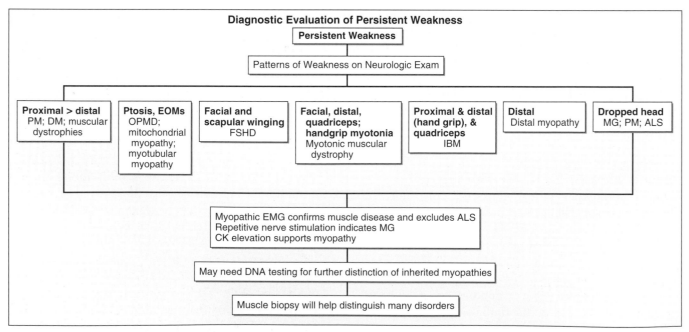

FIGURE 37-2

Diagnostic evaluation of persistent weakness. Examination reveals one of seven patterns of weakness. The pattern of weakness in combination with the laboratory evaluation leads to a diagnosis. EOMs, extraocular muscles; OPMD, oculopharyngeal muscular dystrophy; FSHD, facioscapulohumeral muscular dystrophy; IBM, inclusion body myositis; DM, dermatomyositis; PM, polymyositis; MG, myasthenia gravis, ALS, amyotrophic lateral sclerosis; CK, creatine kinase.

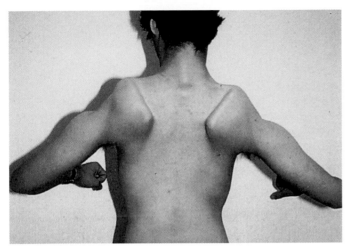

FIGURE 37-3
Facioscapulohumeral dystrophy with prominent scapular winging.

weakness. A steppage gait, due to footdrop, accompanies distal weakness.

Any disorder causing muscle weakness may be accompanied by *fatigue,* referring to an inability to maintain or sustain a force (pathologic fatigability). Pathologic fatigability must be differentiated from asthenia, a type of fatigue caused by excess tiredness or lack of energy. When excessive mental effort is associated with initiation of a motor task, the term *neurasthenia* is used. Associated symptoms may help differentiate asthenia and pathologic fatigability. Asthenia is often accompanied by a tendency to avoid physical activities, complaints of daytime sleepiness, necessity for frequent naps, and difficulty concentrating on activities such as reading. There may be feelings of overwhelming stress or depression. In short, asthenia is not a myopathy. In contrast, pathologic fatigability occurs in disorders of neuromuscular transmission and in disorders altering energy production, including defects in glycolysis, lipid metabolism, or mitochondrial energy production.

TABLE 37-1

OBSERVATIONS ON EXAMINATION THAT DISCLOSE MUSCLE WEAKNESS	
FUNCTIONAL IMPAIRMENT	**MUSCLE WEAKNESS**
Inability to forcibly close eyes	Upper facial muscles
Impaired pucker	Lower facial muscles
Inability to raise head from prone position	Neck extensor muscles
Inability to raise head from supine position	Neck flexor muscles
Inability to raise arms above head	Proximal arm muscles (may be only scapular stabilizing muscles)
Inability to walk without hyperextending knee (backkneeing or genu recurvatum)	Knee extensor muscles
Inability to walk with heels touching the floor (toe walking)	Shortening of the Achilles tendon
Inability to lift foot while walking (steppage gait or footdrop)	Anterior compartment of leg
Inability to walk without a waddling gait	Hip muscles
Inability to get up from the floor without climbing up the extremities (Gowers' sign)	Hip muscles
Inability to get up from a chair without using arms	Hip muscles

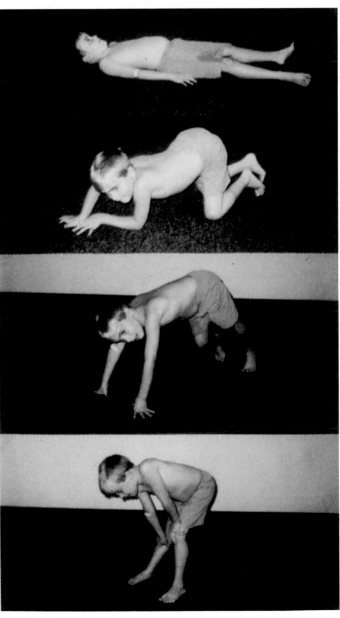

FIGURE 37-4
Gowers' sign showing a patient using arms to climb up the legs in attempting to get up from the floor.

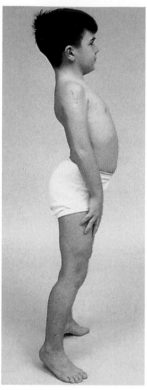

FIGURE 37-5
Lordotic posture, exaggerated by standing on toes, associated with trunk and hip weakness.

TABLE 37-2

DRUGS THAT CAUSE TRUE MYALGIA	
Statins[a]	Emetine
Gemfibrozil	Labetalol
Vincristine	Nifedipine
Zidovudine	D-Penicillamine
Cyclosporine	L-Tryptophan
Gold	Epsilon aminocaproic acid
Danazol	Heroin
Cimetidine	Cocaine
	Methadone

[a]3-Hydroxy-3-methylglutaryl coenzyme A reductase inhibitors.

Pathologic fatigability also occurs in chronic myopathies because of difficulty accomplishing a task with less muscle. Pathologic fatigability is accompanied by abnormal clinical or laboratory findings. Fatigue without those supportive features almost never indicates a primary muscle disease.

MUSCLE PAIN (MYALGIAS), CRAMPS, AND STIFFNESS

Muscle pain can be associated with cramps, spasms, contractures, and stiff or rigid muscles. In distinction, true myalgia (muscle aching) may be accompanied by weakness, tenderness to palpation, or swelling. Certain drugs cause true myalgia (**Table 37-2**).

There are two painful muscle conditions of particular importance, neither of which is associated with muscle weakness. *Fibromyalgia* is a common, yet poorly understood type of myofascial pain syndrome. Patients complain of severe muscle pain and tenderness and have specific painful trigger points, sleep disturbances, and easy fatigability. Serum creatine kinase (CK) and erythrocyte sedimentation rate (ESR) are normal. *Polymyalgia rheumatica (PMR)* occurs mainly in patients >50 years and is characterized by stiffness and pain in the shoulders, lower back, hips, and thighs. The ESR is elevated, but serum CK, electromyography (EMG), and muscle biopsy are normal. Temporal arteritis, an inflammatory disorder of medium- and large-sized arteries, often involves one or more branches of the carotid artery and may accompany PMR. Vision is threatened due to ischemic optic neuritis. Glucocorticoids can relieve the myalgias and protect against visual loss.

Localized muscle pain is most often traumatic. A common cause of sudden abrupt-onset pain is a ruptured tendon, which leaves the muscle belly appearing rounded and shorter in appearance compared to the normal side. The biceps brachii and Achilles tendons are particularly vulnerable to rupture. Infection or neoplastic infiltration of the muscle is a rare cause of localized muscle pain.

A *muscle cramp* or *spasm* is a painful, involuntary, localized muscle contraction with a visible or palpable hardening of the muscle. Cramps are abrupt in onset and short in duration; they may cause abnormal posturing of the joint. The EMG shows firing of motor units, reflecting an origin from spontaneous neural discharge. Muscle cramps often occur in neurogenic disorders, especially motor neuron disease (Chap. 21), radiculopathies, and polyneuropathies (Chap. 33), but are not a feature of most primary muscle diseases. Duchenne muscular dystrophy (Chap. 38) is an exception since calf muscle complaints are common. Muscle cramps are also common during pregnancy.

A *muscle contracture* is different from a muscle cramp. In both conditions, the muscle becomes hard, but a contracture is associated with energy failure in glycolytic disorders. The muscle is unable to relax after an active muscle contraction. The EMG shows electrical silence. Confusion is created because contracture also refers to a muscle that cannot be passively stretched to its proper length (fixed contracture) because of fibrosis. In some muscle disorders, especially Emery-Dreifuss muscular dystrophy (Chap. 38), fixed contractures occur early and represent distinctive features of the disease.

Muscle stiffness refers to various phenomena. Some patients with inflammation of joints and periarticular surfaces feel stiff. Disorders of hyperexcitable motor nerves cause stiff or rigid muscles. In *stiff-person syndrome* spontaneous discharges of the motor neurons of the spinal cord cause involuntary muscle contractions mainly involving the axial (trunk) and proximal lower extremity muscles. The gait becomes stiff and labored, with hyperlordosis of the lumbar spine. Superimposed episodic muscle spasms are precipitated by sudden movements, unexpected noises, and emotional upset. The muscles relax during sleep. Serum antiglutamic acid decarboxylase antibodies are present in approximately two-thirds of cases. In *neuromyotonia (Isaac's syndrome)* there is hyperexcitability of the peripheral nerves manifesting as continuous muscle fiber activity. *Myokymia* (continuous undulations of muscle) and impaired muscle relaxation are the result. Muscles of the leg are stiff, and the constant muscle contractions cause increased sweating of the extremities. This peripheral nerve hyperexcitability is antibody-mediated, targeted against voltage-gated potassium channels. The site of origin of the spontaneous nerve discharges is principally in the distal portion of the motor nerves.

Myotonia is a condition of prolonged muscle contraction followed by slow muscle relaxation that always follows muscle activation, usually voluntary, but may be elicited by mechanical stimulation (percussion myotonia) of the muscle. Myotonia results in difficulty releasing objects after a firm grasp. In myotonic muscular dystrophy, weakness accompanies myotonia. Myotonia also occurs with *myotonia congenita* (a chloride channel disorder), but in this condition muscle weakness is not prominent. *Paramyotonia congenita* (a sodium channel disorder more closely aligned with hyperkalemic periodic paralysis) is named for a paradoxical phenomenon whereby the prolonged muscle contraction is exacerbated by repeated muscle contractions (Chap. 38). In hypokalemic periodic paralysis, myotonia of the eyelids may be present but limb muscles are usually spared.

MUSCLE ENLARGEMENT AND ATROPHY

In most myopathies muscle tissue is replaced by fat and connective tissue, but muscle size is usually not affected. However, enlarged calf muscles are typical of Duchenne and Becker muscular dystrophies. In these patients, the muscle enlargement represents true muscle hypertrophy; hence the term "pseudohypertrophy" should be avoided. The calf muscles remain very strong even late in the course of these disorders. Muscle enlargement can also result from infiltration by sarcoid granulomas, amyloid deposits, bacterial and parasitic infections, and focal myositis.

LABORATORY EVALUATION

A limited battery of tests can be used to evaluate a suspected myopathy. Nearly all patients require serum enzyme level measurements and electrodiagnostic studies as screening tools to differentiate muscle disorders from other motor unit diseases. The other tests described—DNA studies, the forearm exercise test, and muscle biopsy—are used to diagnose specific types of myopathies.

SERUM ENZYMES

CK is the preferred muscle enzyme to measure in the evaluation of myopathies. Damage to muscle causes the CK to leak from the muscle fiber to the serum. The MM isoenzyme predominates in skeletal muscle, while CK-MB is the marker for cardiac muscle. Serum CK can be elevated in normal individuals without provocation, presumably on a genetic basis or after strenuous activity, minor trauma (including the EMG needle), a prolonged muscle cramp, or a generalized seizure. Aspartate aminotransferase (AST), alanine aminotransferase (ALT), and lactate dehydrogenase (LDH) are enzymes sharing an origin in both muscle and liver. Problems arise when the levels of these enzymes are found to be elevated in a routine screening battery, leading to the erroneous assumption that liver disease is present when in fact muscle could be the cause. An elevated gamma-glutamyl transferase (GGT) helps to establish a liver origin since this enzyme is not found in muscle. Aldolase is often thought to be a muscle-specific enzyme but is also present in liver.

ELECTRODIAGNOSTIC STUDIES

EMG, repetitive nerve stimulation, and nerve conduction studies (Chap. 33) provide information necessary to differentiate myopathies from neuropathies and neuromuscular junction diseases. Certain features of the EMG (e.g., fibrillation potentials) will point to muscle membrane instability that occurs in a more limited range of myopathies (inflammatory myopathy, dystrophy). A myopathic EMG is characterized on needle electromyography by early or rapid recruitment of low-amplitude and short-duration motor unit action potentials. The rapid recruitment is necessary to compensate for loss of muscle fibers related to the underlying myopathic process. The EMG can also help in choosing an appropriately affected muscle to sample for biopsy. The EMG can be used to fully characterize suspected involuntary activity seen during the examination, such as myokymia and myotonia.

DNA ANALYSIS

Advances in molecular diagnosis over the past decade have given rise to new important tools for diagnosis. Certain muscle disorders can be definitively diagnosed by DNA analysis; these are fully discussed in Chap. 38. Nevertheless, important limitations need to be mentioned in seeking a molecular diagnosis. For example, in Duchenne and Becker dystrophies, two-thirds of patients have deletion or duplication mutations that are easy to detect, while the remainder have point mutations that are much more difficult to find. For patients without identifiable gene defects, the muscle biopsy remains the main diagnostic tool.

FOREARM EXERCISE TEST

In myopathies with intermittent symptoms, and especially those associated with myoglobinuria, there may be a defect in glycolysis. Many variations of the forearm exercise test exist. For safety, the test should not be performed under ischemic conditions to avoid an unnecessary insult to the muscle, causing rhabdomyolysis. The test is performed by placing a small indwelling catheter into an antecubital vein. A baseline blood sample is obtained for lactic acid and ammonia. The forearm muscles are exercised by asking the patient to vigorously squeeze a sphygmomanometer bulb for 1 min. Blood is then obtained at intervals of 1, 2, 4, 6, and 10 min for comparison with the baseline sample. Normal controls must be established for each laboratory. A three- to fourfold rise of lactic acid is typical. The simultaneous measurement of ammonia serves as a control, since it should also rise with exercise. In patients with myophosphorylase deficiency or other glycolytic defects (Chap. 38), the lactic acid rise will be absent or below normal, while the rise in ammonia will reach control values. If there is lack of effort, neither lactic acid nor ammonia will rise. Patients with selective failure to increase ammonia may have myoadenylate deaminase deficiency. This condition has been reported to be a cause of myoglobinuria, but deficiency of this enzyme in asymptomatic individuals makes interpretation controversial.

MUSCLE BIOPSY

Muscle biopsy analysis is an important step in establishing the diagnosis of a myopathy. The biopsy is usually obtained from a quadriceps or biceps brachii muscle, less commonly from a deltoid muscle (**Figs. 37–6**, 38-1, and 39-3). The microscopic evaluation uses a combination of techniques—classic histochemistry, immunocytochemistry with a battery of antibodies, and electron microscopy. Not all techniques need to be used on every case. A specific diagnosis can be established for many

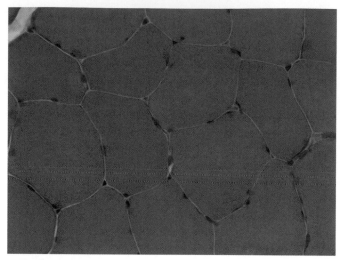

FIGURE 37-6

Normal quadriceps muscle. The muscle fibers are of relatively uniform size with multiple small peripherally located nuclei, minimal endomysial connective tissue, and a thin perimysium composed of loose collagenous tissue. Contrast this appearance with Figs. 38-1 and 39-3. (Hematoxylin and eosin, 400x; Courtesy of Dr. Joanna Phillips, Department of Pathology, University of California, San Francisco.)

disorders. A combination of stains to identify mononuclear cells (polymyositis), complement (dermatomyositis), and amyloid (inclusion body myositis) helps to distinguish the inflammatory myopathies. Mitochondrial and metabolic (e.g., myophosphorylase and acid maltase deficiencies) myopathies demonstrate distinctive histochemical and electron-microscopic profiles. A battery of antibodies is available for the identification of missing components of the dystrophin-glycoprotein complex and related proteins to help diagnose specific types of muscular dystrophies. In addition, the congenital myopathies have distinctive histologic features essential for diagnosis.

TREATMENT FOR MYOPATHY

Treatable causes of acquired myopathy include hypokalemia, hyperthyroidism, vitamin D deficiency, alcoholic myopathy, Cushing's disease, polymyositis, and dermatomyositis. The most common medication-induced myopathies are due to chronic steroid or statin use. Discontinuation of exposure to an offending drug or toxin (e.g., alcohol) will limit further muscle injury and provide an opportunity for recovery. Selective use of adaptive strategies (e.g., braces, steering column controls for driving), physical therapy, or occupational therapy can help patients adapt to their physical limitations and maximize daily function. Genetic counseling can be helpful for family planning or discussion of prognosis in circumstances where definitive DNA diagnosis is possible.

FURTHER READINGS

COLDING-JORGENSEN E: Phenotypic variability in myotonia congenita. Muscle Nerve 32:19, 2005.

Current review of the influence of genetic variants on disease expression.

DAUBE JR: Myokymia and neuromyotonia. Muscle Nerve 24:1711, 2001

MEINCK HM, THOMPSON PD: Stiff man syndrome and related conditions. Mov Disord 17:853, 2002

Review of clinical features and possible pathophysiology.

THOMPSON PD ET AL: Statin-associated myopathy. JAMA 289:1681, 2003

Review of statin-associated myopathy and skeletal muscle symptoms.

VERNINO S, LENNON VA: Ion channel and striational antibodies define a continuum of autoimmune neuromuscular hyperexcitability. Muscle Nerve 26:70, 2002

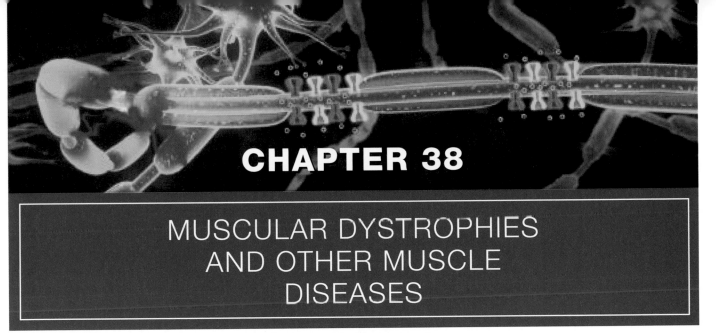

CHAPTER 38

MUSCULAR DYSTROPHIES AND OTHER MUSCLE DISEASES

Robert H. Brown, Jr.
Jerry R. Mendell

The muscle disorders discussed in this chapter include diseases that cause acute, subacute, and chronic muscle weakness. Some cause pain in addition to or instead of weakness. Dermatomyositis and polymyositis are discussed in Chap. 39.

HEREDITARY MYOPATHIES

Muscular dystrophy refers to a group of hereditary progressive diseases each with unique phenotypic and genetic features (**Table 38–1**).

DUCHENNE MUSCULAR DYSTROPHY

This X-linked recessive disorder, sometimes also called *pseudohypertrophic muscular dystrophy,* has an incidence of ~30 per 100,000 live-born males.

TABLE 38-1

PROGRESSIVE MUSCULAR DYSTROPHIES

TYPE	INHERITANCE	DEFECTIVE GENE/PROTEIN	ONSET AGE	CLINICAL FEATURES	OTHER ORGAN SYSTEMS INVOLVED
Duchenne	XR	Dystrophin	Before 5 years	Progressive weakness of girdle muscles Unable to walk after age 12 Progressive kyphoscoliosis Respiratory failure in 2d or 3d decade	Cardiomyopathy Mental impairment
Becker	XR	Dystrophin	Early childhood to adult	Progressive weakness of girdle muscles Able to walk after age 15 Respiratory failure may develop by 4th decade	Cardiomyopathy
Limb-girdle	AD/AR	Several (Tables 38–2, 38–3)	Early childhood to early adult	Slow progressive weakness of shoulder and hip girdle muscles	±Cardiomyopathy
Emery-Dreifuss	XR/AD	Emerin/Lamins A/C	Childhood to adult	Elbow contractures, humeral and peroneal weakness	Cardiomyopathy
Congenital	AR	Several	At birth or within first few months	Hypotonia, contractures, delayed milestones Progression to respiratory failure in some; static course in others	CNS abnormalities (hypomyelination, malformation) Eye abnormalities
Myotonic[a] (DM1, DM2)	AD	DM1: Expansion CTG repeat DM2: Expansion CCTG repeat	Usually 2d decade May be infancy if mother affected (DM1 only)	Slowly progressive weakness of face, shoulder girdle, and foot dorsiflexion Preferential proximal weakness in DM2	Cardiac conduction defects Mental impairment Cataracts Frontal baldness Gonadal atrophy
Facioscapulo-humeral	AD	Deletion, distal 4q	Before age 20	Slowly progressive weakness of face, shoulder girdle, and foot dorsiflexion	Deafness Coats' (eye) disease
Oculopharyn-geal	AD	Expansion, poly-A RNA binding protein	5th to 6th decade	Slowly progressive weakness of pharyngeal, and limb muscles	—

[a]Two forms of myotonic dystrophy, DM1 and DM2, have been identified. Many features overlap (see text).

Abbreviations: XR, X-linked recessive; AD, autosomal dominant; AR, autosomal recessive; CNS, central nervous system.

Clinical Features

Duchenne dystrophy is present at birth, but the disorder usually becomes apparent between ages 3 and 5. The boys fall frequently and have difficulty keeping up with friends when playing. Running, jumping, and hopping are invariably abnormal. By age 5, muscle weakness is obvious by muscle testing. On getting up from the floor, the patient uses his hands to climb up himself [Gowers' maneuver (Fig. 37-4)]. Contractures of the heel cords and iliotibial bands become apparent by age 6, when toe walking is associated with a lordotic posture. Loss of muscle strength is

progressive, with predilection for proximal limb muscles and the neck flexors; leg involvement is more severe than arm involvement. Between ages 8 and 10 walking may require the use of braces; joint contractures and limitations of hip flexion, knee, elbow, and wrist extension are made worse by prolonged sitting. By age 12, most patients are wheelchair dependent. Contractures become fixed, and a progressive scoliosis often develops that may be associated with pain. The chest deformity with scoliosis impairs pulmonary function, which is already diminished by muscle weakness. By age 16 to 18, patients are predisposed to serious, sometimes fatal pulmonary infections. Other causes of death include aspiration of food and acute gastric dilation.

A cardiac cause of death is uncommon despite the presence of a cardiomyopathy in almost all patients. Congestive heart failure seldom occurs except with severe stress such as pneumonia. Cardiac arrhythmias are rare. The typical electrocardiogram (ECG) shows an increase net RS in lead V_1; deep, narrow Q waves in the precordial leads; and tall right precordial R waves in V_1. Intellectual impairment in Duchenne dystrophy is common; the average intelligence quotient (IQ) is approximately one standard deviation below the mean. Impairment of intellectual function appears to be nonprogressive and affects verbal ability more than performance.

Laboratory Features

Serum creatine kinase (CK) levels are invariably elevated to between 20 and 100 times normal. The levels are abnormal at birth but decline late in the disease because of inactivity and loss of muscle mass. Electromyography (EMG) demonstrates features typical of myopathy. Muscle biopsy features are demonstrated in **Fig. 38-1**A, B, C. A definitive diagnosis of Duchenne dystrophy can be established on the basis of dystrophin deficiency in a biopsy of muscle tissue (Fig. 38-1B and 1C) or mutation analysis on peripheral blood leukocytes, as discussed below.

Duchenne dystrophy is caused by a mutation of the gene that encodes dystrophin, a 427-kDa protein localized to the inner surface of the sarcolemma of the muscle fiber. The dystrophin gene is >2000 kb in size and thus is one of the largest identified human genes. It is localized to the short arm of the X chromosome at Xp21. The most common gene mutation is a deletion. Less often, Duchenne dystrophy is caused by a gene duplication or point mutation. Identification of a specific mutation allows for an unequivocal diagnosis, makes possible accurate testing of potential carriers, and is useful for prenatal diagnosis.

A diagnosis of Duchenne dystrophy can also be made by Western blot analysis of muscle biopsy specimens, revealing abnormalities on the quantity and molecular

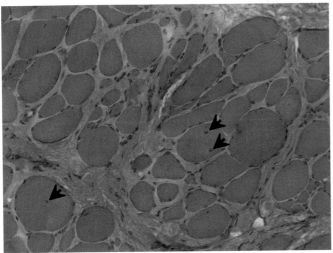

A.

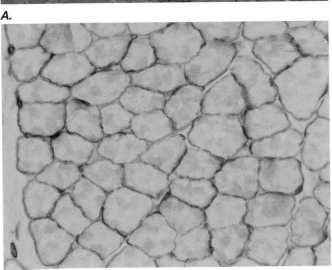

C.

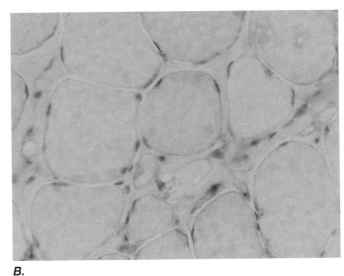

B.

FIGURE 38-1

A.This vastus lateralis biopsy shows severe dystrophic features including dramatic variation in muscle fiber diameter, numerous large-diameter fibers, marked expansion and fibrosis of the endomysium, and increased numbers of central nuclei (hematoxylin and eosin 200×). **B** and **C**. The immunohistochemical stain for dystrophin shows complete absence of dystrophin staining of the sarcolemma and scattered fibers with partial or complete membrane positivity. The normal control muscle shows strong sarcolemmal staining for dystrophin (dystrophin and control dystrophin 400×). (Courtesy of Dr. Joanna Phillips, Department of Pathology, University of California, San Francisco.)

weight of dystrophin protein. In addition, immunocyto-chemical staining of muscle with dystrophin antibodies can be used to demonstrate absence or deficiency of dystrophin localizing to the sarcolemmal membrane. Carriers of the disease may demonstrate a mosaic pattern, but dystrophin analysis of muscle biopsy specimens for carrier detection is not reliable.

Pathogenesis

Dystrophin is part of a large complex of sarcolemmal proteins and glycoproteins (**Fig. 38-2**). The dystrophin-glycoprotein complex appears to confer stability to the sarcolemma, although the function of each individual component of the complex is incompletely understood. Deficiency of one member of the complex may cause abnormalities in other components. For example, a primary deficiency of dystrophin (Duchenne dystrophy)

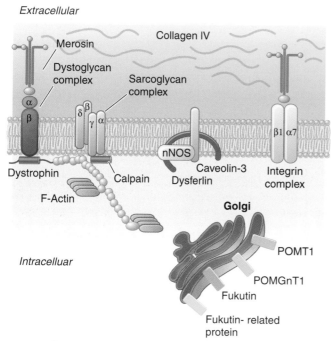

FIGURE 38-2
Selected muscular dystrophy–associated proteins in the cell membrane and Golgi complex. Dystrophin localizes to the cytoplasmic face of the muscle cell membrane. It complexes with two transmembrane protein complexes, the dystroglycans and the sarcoglycans. The dystroglycans bind to the extracellular matrix protein merosin, which is also complexed with α1 and α7 integrins (Tables 38-1, 38-2, 38-3). Dysferlin complexes with caveolin-3 (which binds to neuronal nitric oxide synthase, or nNOS) but not with the dystrophin-associated proteins or the integrins. In each of four congenital dystrophies, there is loss of function of different Golgi-associated proteins: POMT1, POMGnT1, Fukutin, and Fukutin-related protein.

may lead to secondary loss of the sarcoglycans and dystroglycan. The primary loss of a single sarcoglycan (see "Limb-Girdle Muscular Dystrophy," below) results in a secondary loss of other sarcoglycans in the membrane without uniformly affecting dystrophin. In either instance, disruption of the dystrophin-glycoprotein complexes weakens the sarcolemma, causing membrane tears and a cascade of events leading to muscle fiber necrosis. This sequence of events occurs repeatedly during the life of a patient with muscular dystrophy.

TREATMENT FOR DUCHENNE MUSCULAR DYSTROPHY

Glucocorticoids, administered as prednisone in a dose of 0.75 mg/kg per day, significantly slow progression of Duchenne dystrophy for up to 3 years. Some patients cannot tolerate glucocorticoid therapy; weight gain in particular represents a significant deterrent for some boys.

BECKER MUSCULAR DYSTROPHY

This less severe form of X-linked recessive muscular dystrophy results from allelic defects of the same gene responsible for Duchenne dystrophy. Becker muscular dystrophy is approximately 10 times less frequent than Duchenne, with an incidence of about 3 per 100,000 live-born males.

Clinical Features

The pattern of muscle wasting in Becker muscular dystrophy closely resembles that seen in Duchenne. Proximal muscles, especially of the lower extremities, are prominently involved. As the disease progresses, weakness becomes more generalized. Significant facial muscle weakness is not a feature. Hypertrophy of muscles, particularly in the calves, is an early and prominent finding.

Most patients with Becker dystrophy first experience difficulties between ages 5 and 15 years, although onset in the third or fourth decade or even later can occur. By definition, patients with Becker dystrophy walk beyond age 15, while patients with Duchenne dystrophy are typically in a wheelchair by the age of 12. Patients with Becker dystrophy have a reduced life expectancy, but most survive into the fourth or fifth decade.

Mental retardation may occur in Becker dystrophy, but it is not as common as in Duchenne. Cardiac involvement occurs in Becker dystrophy and may result in heart failure.

Laboratory Features

Serum CK levels, results of EMG, and muscle biopsy findings closely resemble those in Duchenne dystrophy. The diagnosis of Becker muscular dystrophy requires Western blot analysis of muscle biopsy samples demonstrating a reduced amount or abnormal size of dystrophin. Mutation analysis of DNA from peripheral blood leukocytes reveals deletions or duplications of the dystrophin gene in 65% of patients with Becker dystrophy, approximately the same percentage as in Duchenne dystrophy. In both Becker and Duchenne dystrophies, the size of the DNA deletion does not predict clinical severity; however, in ~95% of patients with Becker dystrophy, the DNA deletion does not alter the translational reading frame of messenger RNA. These "in-frame" mutations allow for production of some dystrophin, which accounts for the presence of altered rather than absent dystrophin on Western blot analysis.

TREATMENT FOR BECKER DYSTROPHY

The use of glucocorticoids has not been adequately studied in Becker dystrophy.

LIMB-GIRDLE MUSCULAR DYSTROPHY

The syndrome of limb-girdle muscular dystrophy (LGMD) represents more than one disorder. Both males and females are affected, with onset ranging from late in the first decade to the fourth decade. The LGMDs typically manifest with progressive weakness of pelvic and shoulder girdle musculature. Respiratory insufficiency from weakness of the diaphragm may occur, as may cardiomyopathy. Unlike Duchenne dystrophy, intellectual function is unaffected.

A systematic classification of LGMD is based on autosomal dominant (LGMD1) and autosomal recessive (LGMD2) inheritance. Superimposed on the backbone of LGMD1 and LGMD2, the classification employs a sequential alphabetical lettering system (LGMD1A, LGMD2A, etc.). Disorders receive letters in the order in which they are found to have chromosomal linkage. This results in an ever-expanding list of conditions. Presently there are 5 autosomal dominant and 10 autosomal recessive disorders, summarized in **Tables 38–2** and **38–3**. None of the conditions is as common as the dystrophinopathies; however, prevalence data for the LGMDs have not been systematically gathered for any large heterogeneous population. In referral-based clinical populations, the sarcoglycan deficiencies (LGMD2C, 2D, 2E, 2F) and dysferlinopathies (LGMD2B) have

TABLE 38-2

AUTOSOMAL DOMINANT LIMB-GIRDLE MUSCULAR DYSTROPHIES (LGMDs)			
DISEASE	**CLINICAL FEATURES**	**LABORATORY FEATURES**	**LOCUS OR GENE**
LGMD1A	Onset 3d to 4th decade Muscle weakness affects distal limb muscles, vocal cords, and pharyngeal muscles	Serum CK 2 × normal EMG mixed myopathy/neuropathy NCS normal	Myotilin
LGMD1B	Onset 1st or 2d decade Proximal lower limb weakness and cardiomyopathy with conduction defects Some cases indistinguishable from Emery-Dreifuss muscular dystrophy with joint contractures	Serum CK 3–5 × normal NCS normal EMG myopathic	Lamin A/C
LGMD1C	Onset in early childhood Proximal weakness Gowers' sign, calf hypertrophy Exercise-related muscle cramps	Serum CK 4–25 × normal NCS normal EMG myopathic	Caveolin-3
LGMD1D	Onset 3d to 5th decade Proximal muscle weakness Cardiomyopathy and arrhythmias	Serum CK 2–4 × normal NCS normal EMG myopathic	Linked to chromosome 7q Gene unidentified
LGMD1E	Childhood onset Proximal muscle weakness	Serum CK usually normal NCS normal EMG myopathic	Linked to chromosome 6q23 Gene unidentified

Abbreviations: CK, creatine kinase; NCS, nerve conduction studies; EMG, electromyography.

TABLE 38-3

AUTOSOMAL RECESSIVE LIMB-GIRDLE MUSCULAR DYSTROPHIES (LGMDs)

DISEASE	CLINICAL FEATURES	LABORATORY FEATURES	LOCUS OR GENE
LGMD2A	Onset 1st or 2d decade Tight heel cords Contractures at elbows, wrists, and fingers; rigid spine in some Proximal and distal weakness	Serum CK 3–15 × normal NCS normal EMG myopathic	Calpain-3
LGMD2B	Onset 2d or 3d decade Proximal muscle weakness at onset, later distal (calf) muscles affected Miyoshi myopathy is variant of LGMD2B with calf muscles affected at onset	Serum CK 3–100 × normal NCS normal EMG myopathic Inflammation on muscle biopsy may simulate polymyositis	Dysferlin
LGMD2C–F	Onset in childhood to teenage yrs Clinical condition similar to Duchenne and Becker muscular dystrophies Cardiomyopathy uncommon Cognitive function normal	Serum CK 5–100 × normal NCS normal EMG myopathic	$\gamma, \alpha, \beta, \delta$ sarcoglycans
LGMD2G	Onset age 10 to 15 Proximal and distal muscle weakness	Serum CK 3–17 × normal NCS normal EMG myopathic	Telethonin
LGMD2H	Onset 1st to 3d decade Proximal muscle weakness	Serum CK 2–25 × normal NCS normal EMG myopathic	TRIM32 gene
LGMD2I	Onset 1st to 3d decade Clinical condition similar to Duchenne or Becker dystrophies Cardiomyopathy (some not all) Cognitive function normal	Serum CK 10–30 × normal NCS normal EMG myopathic	Fukutin-related protein
LGMD2J[a]	Onset 1st to 3d decade Proximal lower limb weakness Mild distal weakness Progressive weakness causes loss of ambulation	Serum CK 1.5–2 × normal NCS normal EMG myopathic	Titin

[a]Tibial muscular dystrophy is a form of titin deficiency with only distal muscle weakness (see Table 38–4).

Abbreviations: CK, creatine kinase; NCS, nerve conduction studies; EMG, electromyography.

emerged as the most common disorders. Some small group analyses predict that calpain-3 deficiency (LGMD2A) and Fukutin-related protein (FKRP) deficiency (LGMD2I) may rival others for prevalence.

EMERY-DREIFUSS MUSCULAR DYSTROPHY

There are two genetically distinct forms of Emery-Dreifuss muscular dystrophy (EDMD). One is inherited as an X-linked disorder, while the other is autosomal dominant. The latter is classified under the rubric of LGMD1B, but clinically the conditions are closely related.

Clinical Features

Prominent contractures can be recognized in early childhood and teenage years, often preceding muscle weakness. The contractures persist throughout the course of the disease and are present at the elbows and neck. Muscle weakness affects humeral and peroneal muscles at first and later spreads to a limb-girdle distribution. The cardiomyopathy is potentially life threatening and may result in sudden death. A spectrum of atrial rhythm and conduction defects includes atrial fibrillation and paralysis and atrioventricular heart block. Some patients have a dilated cardiomyopathy. Female carriers of the X-linked variant may have cardiac manifestations that become clinically significant.

Laboratory Features

Serum CK may be elevated two- to tenfold. EMG is myopathic. Muscle biopsy shows nonspecific dystrophic features. ECGs demonstrate atrial and atrioventricular rhythm disturbances.

X-linked EDMD arises from defects in the emerin gene encoding a nuclear envelope protein. The autosomal dominant disease is caused by mutations of the *LMNA* gene on chromosome 1q21.2 encoding the lamin proteins A and C. Loss of structural integrity of the nuclear envelope from defects in emerin or lamin A/C accounts for overlapping phenotypes.

TREATMENT FOR EDMD

Supportive care should be offered for neuromuscular disability, including ambulatory aids, if necessary. Stretching of contractures is difficult. Management of cardiomyopathy and arrhythmias can save lives.

MYOTONIC DYSTROPHY

Myotonic dystrophy is also known as *dystrophia myotonica* (DM). The condition is composed of at least two clinical disorders with overlapping phenotypes and distinct molecular genetic defects: myotonic dystrophy type 1 (DM1), the classic disease originally described by Steinert, and myotonic dystrophy type 2 (DM2), also called *proximal myotonic myopathy* (PROMM).

Clinical Features

The clinical expression of myotonic dystrophy varies widely and involves many systems other than muscle. Affected patients have a typical "hatchet-faced" appearance due to temporalis, masseter, and facial muscle atrophy and weakness. Frontal baldness is characteristic of men with the disease. Neck muscles, including flexors and sternocleidomastoids, and distal limb muscles are involved early. Weakness of wrist extensors, finger extensors, and intrinsic hand muscles impairs function. Ankle dorsiflexor weakness may cause footdrop. Proximal muscles remain stronger throughout the course, although preferential atrophy and weakness of quadriceps muscles occur in many patients. Palatal, pharyngeal, and tongue involvement produce a dysarthric speech, nasal voice, and swallowing problems. Some patients have diaphragm

and intercostal muscle weakness, resulting in respiratory insufficiency.

Myotonia, when present, appears by age 5 and is demonstrable by percussion of the thenar eminence, the tongue, and wrist extensor muscles. Myotonia causes a slow relaxation of hand grip after a forced voluntary closure. Advanced muscle wasting makes myotonia more difficult to detect.

Cardiac disturbances occur commonly in patients with DM1. ECG abnormalities include first-degree heart block and more extensive conduction system involvement. Complete heart block and sudden death can occur. Congestive heart failure occurs infrequently but may result from cor pulmonale secondary to respiratory failure. Mitral valve prolapse also occurs commonly. Other associated features include intellectual impairment, hypersomnia, posterior subcapsular cataracts, gonadal atrophy, insulin resistance, and decreased esophageal and colonic motility.

Congenital myotonic dystrophy is a more severe form of DM1 and occurs in ~25% of infants of affected mothers. It is characterized by severe facial and bulbar weakness, transient neonatal respiratory insufficiency, and mental retardation.

DM2, or PROMM, has a distinct pattern of muscle weakness affecting mainly proximal muscles. Other features of the disease overlap with DM1, including cataracts, testicular atrophy, insulin resistance, constipation, hypersomnia, and cognitive defects. Cardiac conduction defects occur but are less common, and the hatchet face and frontal baldness are less consistent features. A very striking difference is the failure to clearly identify a congenital form of DM2.

Laboratory Features

The diagnosis of myotonic dystrophy can usually be made on the basis of clinical findings. Serum CK levels may be normal or mildly elevated. EMG evidence of myotonia is present in most cases. Muscle biopsy shows muscle atrophy, which selectively involves type 1 fibers in 50% of cases. Typically, increased numbers of central nuclei can be seen. Necrosis of muscle fibers and increased connective tissue, common in other muscular dystrophies, do not usually occur in myotonic dystrophy (Fig. 38-1).

DM1 and DM2 are both autosomal dominant disorders. New mutations do not appear to contribute to the pool of affected individuals. DM1 is transmitted by an intronic mutation consisting of an unstable expansion of a CTG trinucleotide repeat in a serine-threonine protein kinase gene (named *DMPK*) on chromosome 19q13.3. An increase in the severity of the disease phenotype in successive generations (genetic anticipation) is accompanied by an increase in the number of trinucleotide repeats. A similar type of mutation has been identified in fragile X syndrome. The unstable triplet repeat in myotonic dystrophy can be used for prenatal diagnosis. Congenital disease occurs almost exclusively in infants born to affected mothers; it is possible that sperm with greatly expanded triplet repeats do not function well.

DM2 has been linked to chromosome 3q13.3-q24. At this locus, a DNA expansion mutation consists of a CCTG repeat in intron 1 of the *ZNF9* gene. The gene is believed to encode an RNA binding protein expressed in many different tissues, including skeletal and cardiac muscle.

How the DNA expansions in DM1 and DM2 impair function of muscle and other cells is not well understood. They may alter expression of an adjacent protein kinase gene (DM1), inactivate an important RNA binding protein (DM2), or influence other neighboring genes. In both DM1 and DM2, the mutant RNA appears to form intranuclear inclusions composed of aberrant RNA.

TREATMENT FOR MYOTONIC DYSTROPHY

The myotonia in myotonic dystrophy occasionally warrants treatment. Phenytoin is the preferred agent for the occasional patient who requires an antimyotonia drug; other agents, particularly quinine and procainamide, may worsen cardiac conduction. Cardiac pacemaker insertion should be considered for patients with unexplained syncope or advanced conduction system abnormalities with evidence of second-degree heart block, or trifascicular conduction disturbances with marked prolongation of the PR interval. Molded ankle-foot orthoses help prevent footdrop in patients with distal lower extremity weakness.

FACIOSCAPULOHUMERAL (FSH) MUSCULAR DYSTROPHY

This form of muscular dystrophy has a prevalence of ~1 in 20,000. It is distinct from a similar disorder known as scapuloperoneal dystrophy.

Clinical Features

The condition typically has an onset in childhood or young adulthood. In most cases, facial weakness is the initial manifestation, appearing as an inability to smile, whis-

tle, or fully close the eyes. Weakness of the shoulder girdles, rather than the facial muscles, usually brings the patient to medical attention. Loss of scapular stabilizer muscles makes arm elevation difficult. Scapular winging (Fig. 37-3) becomes apparent with attempts at abduction and forward movement of the arms. Biceps and triceps muscles may be severely affected, with relative sparing of the deltoid muscles. Weakness is invariably worse for wrist extension than for wrist flexion, and weakness of the anterior compartment muscles of the legs may lead to footdrop.

In most patients, the weakness remains restricted to facial, upper extremity, and distal lower extremity muscles. In 20% of patients, weakness progresses to involve the pelvic girdle muscles, and severe functional impairment and possible wheelchair dependency result.

Characteristically, patients with FSH dystrophy do not have involvement of other organ systems, although labile hypertension is common, and there is an increased incidence of nerve deafness. *Coats' disease,* a disorder consisting of telangiectasia, exudation, and retinal detachment, also occurs.

Laboratory Features

The serum CK level may be normal or mildly elevated. EMG usually indicates a myopathic pattern. The muscle biopsy shows nonspecific features of a myopathy. A prominent inflammatory infiltrate, which is often multifocal in distribution, is present in some biopsy samples. The cause or significance of this finding is unknown.

An autosomal dominant inheritance pattern with almost complete penetrance has been established, but each family member should be examined for the presence of the disease, since ~30% of those affected are unaware of involvement. FSH dystrophy is caused by deletions of tandem 3.3-kb repeats at 4q35. The deletion reduces the number of repeats to a fragment of <35 kb in most patients. This mutation results in an overexpression of upstream genes and a loss of DNA binding of a multiprotein complex mediating transcriptional repression of 4q35 genes. The mutation permits carrier detection and prenatal diagnosis. Most sporadic cases represent new mutations.

TREATMENT FOR FSH MUSCULAR DYSTROPHY

No specific treatment is available; ankle-foot orthoses are helpful for footdrop. Scapular stabilization procedures improve scapular winging but may not improve function.

OCULOPHARYNGEAL DYSTROPHY

This form of muscular dystrophy represents one of several disorders characterized by progressive external ophthalmoplegia, which consists of slowly progressive ptosis and limitation of eye movements with sparing of pupillary reactions for light and accommodation. Patients usually do not complain of diplopia, in contrast to patients having conditions with a more acute onset of ocular muscle weakness (e.g., myasthenia gravis).

Clinical Features

Oculopharyngeal muscular dystrophy has a late onset; it usually presents with ptosis and/or dysphagia in the fourth to sixth decade. The extraocular muscle impairment is less prominent in the early phase but may be severe later. Swallowing difficulties may become debilitating and result in pooling of secretions and repeated episodes of aspiration. Mild weakness of the neck and extremities also occurs.

Laboratory Features

The serum CK level may be two to three times normal. Myopathic EMG findings are typical. On biopsy, muscle fibers are found to contain vacuoles, which by electron microscopy are shown to contain membranous whorls, accumulation of glycogen, and other nonspecific debris related to lysosomes. A distinct feature of oculopharyngeal dystrophy is the presence of tubular filaments, 8.5 nm in diameter, in muscle cell nuclei.

Oculopharyngeal dystrophy has an autosomal dominant inheritance pattern with complete penetrance. The incidence is high in French-Canadians and in Spanish-American families of the southwestern United States. Large kindreds of Italian and of eastern European Jewish descent have been reported. The molecular defect in oculopharyngeal muscular dystrophy is a subtle expansion of a modest polyanine repeat tract in a poly-RNA binding protein (PABP2) in muscle.

℞
TREATMENT FOR OCULOPHARYNGEAL DYSTROPHY

Dysphagia can cause inanition, making oculopharyngeal muscular dystrophy a potentially life-threatening disease. Cricopharyngeal myotomy may improve swallowing, although it does not prevent aspiration. Eyelid crutches can improve vision in patients in whom ptosis obstructs vision; candidates for ptosis surgery must be carefully selected—those with severe facial weakness are not suitable.

DISTAL MYOPATHIES

A group of muscle diseases, the distal myopathies, are notable for their preferential distal distribution of muscle weakness in contrast to most muscle conditions associated with proximal weakness. The major distal myopathies are summarized in **Table 38-4**.

Clinical Features

Two of the conditions, *Welander distal myopathy* and *tibial muscular dystrophy,* are late-onset disorders, usually manifesting after age 40. *Nonanka distal myopathy* and *Miyoshi myopathy* are distinguished by their early onset in the late teens or twenties. Only Welander disease begins in the hands; all others start in the lower limbs. Miyoshi myopathy is unique in that gastrocnemius muscles are preferentially affected at onset. A clinical feature that makes all of these disorders confusing is that proximal muscles can be affected as the disorders progress (less so for Welander disease than others), perhaps diminishing the entire concept of the distal myopathy. In contrast to many genetic muscle diseases, the distal myopathies are for the most part limited to skeletal muscle.

Laboratory Features

Serum CK is particularly helpful in diagnosing Miyoshi myopathy since it is very elevated. In the other conditions serum CK is only slightly increased. EMGs are myopathic. Muscle biopsy shows nonspecific dystrophic features. In Nonanka distal myopathy rimmed vacuoles, which contain 15- to 19-nm filaments, are common findings. Immune staining for gene product can be helpful in demonstrating titin abnormalities in tibial muscular dystrophy and reduced dysferlin in Miyoshi myopathy.

Welander and tibial muscular dystrophy are inherited as autosomal dominant disorders, while Nonanka and Miyoshi myopathies are autosomal recessive conditions. The affected genes and their gene products are listed in Table 38-4. The gene for Welander disease has been mapped to chromosome 2.

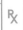
TREATMENT FOR DISTAL MYOPATHIES

Occupational therapy can help patients adapt to loss of hand function; ankle-foot orthoses can support distal leg muscles.

TABLE 38-4

DISTAL MYOPATHIES

DISEASE	CLINICAL FEATURES	LABORATORY FEATURES	LOCUS/GENE
Welander distal myopathy	Onset in fifth decade Weakness begins in hands Slow progression with spread to distal lower extremities Lifespan normal	Serum CK 2–3 × normal EMG myopathic NCS normal Muscle biopsy shows dystrophic features	AD inheritance Linked to chromosome 2p13
Tibial muscular dystrophy (Markesbery/ Griggs/Udd)	Onset 4th to 8th decade Distal lower extremity weakness (tibial distribution) Upper extremities usually normal Lifespan normal	Serum CK 2–4 × normal EMG myopathic NCS normal Muscle biopsy shows dystrophic features Titin absent in M-line of muscle	AD inheritance Titin
Nonanka distal myopathy (distal myopathy with rimmed vacuoles)	Onset 2d to 3d decade Lower extremity distal weakness Mild distal upper limb weakness may be present early Progression to other muscles sparing quadriceps Ambulation may be lost in 10–15 years	Serum CK 3–10 × normal EMG myopathic NCS normal Dystrophic features on muscle biopsy plus rimmed vacuoles 15–19-nm filaments within vacuoles	AR Allelic to hereditary inclusion body myopathy GNE gene: UDP-*N*-acetylglucosamine 2-epimerase/*N*-acetylmannosamine kinase
Miyoshi myopathy	Onset 2d to 3d decade Lower extremity weakness in posterior compartment muscles Progression leads to weakness in other muscle groups Ambulation lost after 10–15 years in about one-third of cases	Serum CK 20–100 × normal EMG myopathic NCS normal Muscle biopsy shows nonspecific dystrophic features	AR Allelic to LGMD2B (see Table 38–3). Dysferlin

Abbreviations:: CK, creatine kinase; AD, autosomal dominant; AR, autosomal recessive; EMG, electromyography; NCS, nerve conduction studies.

CONGENITAL MYOPATHIES

These rare disorders are distinguished from muscular dystrophies by the presence of specific histochemical and structural abnormalities in muscle. Although primarily disorders of infancy or childhood, three forms that may present in adulthood are described here: central core disease, nemaline (rod) myopathy, and centronuclear (myotubular) myopathy. Other types, such as minicore myopathy (multi-minicore disease), fingerprint body myopathy, and sarcotubular myopathy, are not discussed.

CENTRAL CORE DISEASE

Patients with central core disease may have decreased fetal movements. Hypotonia and delay in motor milestones, particularly in walking, are common. Later in childhood, patients develop problems with stair climbing, running, and getting up from the floor. On examination, there is mild facial, neck-flexor, and proximal-extremity muscle weakness. Legs are more affected than arms. Skeletal abnormalities include congenital hip dislocation, scoliosis, and pes cavus; clubbed feet also occur. Most cases are nonprogressive, but exceptions are well documented. Susceptibility to malignant hyperthermia must be considered as a potential risk for patients with central core disease.

The serum CK level is usually normal. Needle EMG demonstrates a myopathic pattern. Muscle biopsy shows fibers with single or multiple central or eccentric discrete zones (*cores*) devoid of oxidative enzymes. Cores occur preferentially in type 1 fibers and represent poorly aligned sarcomeres associated with Z disk streaming.

Autosomal dominant inheritance is characteristic; sporadic cases also occur. The disease is caused by point mutations of the ryanodine receptor gene on chromosome 19q, encoding the calcium-release channel of the sarcoplasmic reticulum of skeletal muscle. Mutations of this gene also account for some cases of inherited malignant hyperthermia. Malignant hyperthermia is an allelic condition; C-terminal mutations of the *RYR1* gene predispose to this complication.

Specific treatment is not required, but establishing a diagnosis of central core disease is extremely important because these patients have a known predisposition to malignant hyperthermia during anesthesia.

NEMALINE MYOPATHY

The term *nemaline* refers to the distinctive presence in muscle fibers of rods or threadlike structures (Greek *nema,* "thread"). Nemaline myopathy is clinically heterogeneous. A severe neonatal form presents with hypotonia and feeding and respiratory difficulties, leading to early death. Nemaline myopathy usually presents in infancy or childhood with delayed motor milestones. The course is nonprogressive or slowly progressive. The physical appearance is striking because of the long, narrow facies, high-arched palate, and open-mouthed appearance due to a prognathous jaw. Other skeletal abnormalities include pectus excavatum, kyphoscoliosis, pes cavus, and clubfoot deformities. Facial and generalized muscle weakness, including respiratory muscle weakness, is common. An adult-onset disorder with progressive proximal weakness may be seen. Myocardial involvement is occasionally present in both the childhood and adult-onset forms. The serum CK level is usually normal or slightly elevated. The EMG demonstrates a myopathic pattern. Muscle biopsy shows clusters of small rods (nemaline bodies), which occur preferentially, but not exclusively, in type 1 muscle fibers. The muscle often shows type 1 muscle fiber predominance. Rods originate from the Z disk material of the muscle fiber.

Five genes have been associated with nemaline myopathy. All code for thin filament–associated proteins, suggesting disturbed assembly or interplay of these structures as a pivotal mechanism. Mutations of the nebulin (*NEB*) gene account for most cases, including both severe neonatal and early childhood forms, inherited as autosomal recessive disorders. Neonatal and childhood cases, inherited as predominantly autosomal dominant disorders, are caused by mutations of the skeletal muscle α-actinin (*ACTA1*) gene. In milder forms of the disease with autosomal dominant inheritance, mutations have been identified in both the slow α-tropomyosin (*TPM3*) and β-tropomyosin (*TPM2*) genes accounting for <3% of cases. No specific treatment is available.

MYOTUBULAR (CENTRONUCLEAR) MYOPATHY

Three distinct variants of centronuclear myopathy occur. A neonatal form, also known as *myotubular myopathy,* presents with severe hypotonia and weakness at birth. The late infancy–early childhood form presents with delayed motor milestones. Later, difficulty with running and stair climbing becomes apparent. A marfanoid, slender body habitus, long narrow face, and high-arched palate are typical. Scoliosis and clubbed feet may be present. Most patients exhibit progressive weakness, some requiring wheelchairs. Progressive external ophthalmoplegia with ptosis and varying degrees of extraocular muscle impairment are characteristic of both the neonatal and the late-infantile forms. A third variant, the late childhood–adult form, has an onset in the second or third decade. Patients have full extraocular muscle movements and rarely exhibit ptosis. There is mild, nonprogressive limb weakness and no associated skeletal abnormalities.

Normal or slightly elevated CK levels occur in each of the forms. EMG studies often give distinctive results, showing positive sharp waves and fibrillation potentials, complex and repetitive discharges, and rarely myotonic discharges. Muscle biopsy specimens in longitudinal section demonstrate rows of central nuclei, often surrounded by a halo. In transverse sections, central nuclei are found in 25 to 80% of muscle fibers.

A gene for the neonatal form of centronuclear myopathy has been localized to Xq28; this gene encodes myotubularin, a protein tyrosine phosphatase. Missense, frameshift, and splice-site mutations predict loss of myotubularin function in affected individuals. Carrier identification and prenatal diagnosis are possible. The inheritance pattern for the late infancy–early childhood disorder is probably autosomal recessive, and for the late childhood–adult form is probably autosomal dominant. No specific treatment is available.

DISORDERS OF MUSCLE ENERGY METABOLISM

There are two principal sources of energy for skeletal muscle—fatty acids and glucose. Abnormalities in either glucose or lipid utilization can be associated with distinct clinical presentations that can range from an acute, painful syndrome with rhabdomyolysis and myoglobinuria to a chronic, progressive muscle weakness simulating muscular dystrophy.

GLYCOGEN STORAGE AND GLYCOLYTIC DEFECTS

Disorders of Glycogen Storage Causing Progressive Weakness

Acid Maltase Deficiency Three clinical forms of acid maltase deficiency (*type II glycogenosis*) can be distinguished. The infantile form is the most common, with onset of symptoms in the first 3 months of life.

Infants develop severe muscle weakness, cardiomegaly, hepatomegaly, and respiratory insufficiency. Glycogen accumulation in motor neurons of the spinal cord and brainstem contributes to muscle weakness. Death usually occurs by 1 year of age. In the childhood form, the picture resembles muscular dystrophy. Delayed motor milestones result from proximal limb muscle weakness and involvement of respiratory muscles. The heart may be involved, but the liver and brain are unaffected. The adult form begins in the third or fourth decade. Respiratory failure and diaphragmatic weakness are often initial manifestations, heralding progressive proximal muscle weakness. The heart and liver are not involved.

In all forms of acid maltase deficiency, the serum CK level is 2 to 10 times normal. EMG examination demonstrates a myopathic pattern, but other distinctive features include myotonic discharges, trains of fibrillation and positive waves, and complex repetitive discharges. EMG discharges are very prominent in the lumbosacral paraspinal muscles. The muscle biopsy shows vacuoles containing glycogen and the lysosomal enzyme acid phosphatase. Electron microscopy reveals membrane-bound and free tissue glycogen. Definitive diagnosis is established by enzyme determination in muscle.

Acid maltase deficiency is inherited as an autosomal recessive disorder caused by mutations of the acid maltase gene. Recombinant human α-glucosidase infused intravenously is well tolerated. Clinical benefits in the infantile disease include reduced heart size, improved muscle tone, and longer life.

Other Glycogen Storage Diseases With Progressive Weakness In *debranching enzyme deficiency (type III glycogenosis)*, a slowly progressive form of muscle weakness can develop after puberty. Rarely, myoglobinuria may be seen. Patients are usually diagnosed in infancy with hypotonia and delayed motor milestones, hepatomegaly, growth retardation, and hypoglycemia. *Branching enzyme deficiency (type IV glycogenosis)* is a rare and fatal glycogen storage disease characterized by failure to thrive and hepatomegaly. Hypotonia and muscle wasting may be present, but the skeletal muscle manifestations are minor compared to liver failure.

Disorders of Glycolysis Causing Exercise Intolerance

Five glycolytic defects are associated with recurrent myoglobinuria: *myophosphorylase deficiency (type V glycogenosis), phosphofructokinase deficiency (type VII glycogenosis), phosphoglycerate kinase deficiency (type IX glycogenosis), phosphoglycerate mutase deficiency (type X glycogenosis)*, and *lactate dehydrogenase deficiency (glycogenosis type XI)*. Myophosphorylase deficiency, also known as *McArdle's disease*, is by far the most common of the glycolytic defects associated with exercise intolerance. These five glycolytic defects result in a common failure to support energy production at the initiation of exercise, although the exact site of energy failure remains controversial.

Clinical muscle manifestations in these five conditions usually begin in adolescence. Symptoms are precipitated by brief bursts of high-intensity exercise, such as running or lifting heavy objects. A history of myalgia and muscle stiffness usually precedes the intensely painful muscle contractures, which may be followed by myoglobinuria. Acute renal failure accompanies significant pigmenturia. Exercise tolerance can be enhanced by a slow induction phase (warm-up) or brief periods of rest, allowing for the start of the "second-wind" phenomenon (switching to utilization of fatty acids).

Certain features help distinguish some enzyme defects. Varying degrees of hemolytic anemia accompany deficiencies of both phosphofructokinase (mild) and phosphoglycerate kinase (severe). In phosphoglycerate kinase deficiency, the usual clinical presentation is a seizure disorder associated with mental retardation; exercise intolerance is an infrequent manifestation.

In all of these conditions, the serum CK levels fluctuate widely and may be elevated even during symptom-free periods. CK levels >100 times normal are expected, accompanying myoglobinuria. All patients with suspected glycolytic defects leading to exercise intolerance should undergo a forearm exercise test (Chap. 37). An impaired rise in venous lactate is highly indicative of a glycolytic defect. In lactate dehydrogenase deficiency, venous levels of lactate do not increase, but pyruvate rises to normal. A definitive diagnosis of glycolytic disease is made by muscle biopsy.

Myophosphorylase deficiency, phosphofructokinase deficiency, and phosphoglycerate mutase deficiency are inherited as autosomal recessive disorders. Phosphoglycerate kinase deficiency is X-linked recessive. Mutations can be found in the respective genes encoding the abnormal proteins in each of these disorders.

Training may enhance the second-wind phenomenon, but attempts to raise blood glucose or to modify these disorders through diet have not proved beneficial.

LIPID AS AN ENERGY SOURCE AND ASSOCIATED DEFECTS

Lipid is an important muscle energy source during rest and during prolonged, submaximal exercise. Fatty acids are derived from circulating very low density lipoprotein (VLDL) in the blood or from triglycerides stored in muscle fibers. Oxidation of fatty acids occurs in the mitochondria. To enter the mitochondria, a fatty acid must first be converted to an "activated fatty acid," acyl-CoA.

The acyl-CoA must be linked with carnitine by the enzyme carnitine palmitoyltransferase (CPT) I for transport into the mitochondria. CPT I is present on the inner side of the outer mitochondrial membrane. Carnitine is removed by CPT II, an enzyme attached to the inside of the inner mitochondrial membrane, allowing transport of acyl-CoA into the mitochondrial matrix for β-oxidation.

Carnitine Palmitoyltransferase Deficiency

CPT II deficiency is the most common recognizable cause of recurrent myoglobinuria, more common than the glycolytic defects. Onset is usually in the teenage years or early twenties. Muscle pain and myoglobinuria typically occur after prolonged exercise, but a recent study found that up to 20% of patients do not exhibit myoglobinuria. Strength is normal between attacks. Fasting predisposes to the development of symptoms. In contrast to disorders caused by defects in glycolysis, in which muscle cramps follow short, intense bursts of exercise, the muscle pain in CPT II deficiency does not occur until the limits of utilization have been exceeded and muscle breakdown has already begun. Episodes of rhabdomyolysis may produce severe weakness. In young children and newborns, CPT II deficiency can present with a very severe clinical picture including hypoketotic hypoglycemia, cardiomyopathy, liver failure, and sudden death.

Serum CK levels and EMG findings are both usually normal between episodes. A normal rise of venous lactate during forearm exercise distinguishes this condition from glycolytic defects, especially myophosphorylase deficiency. Muscle biopsy does not show lipid accumulation and is usually normal between attacks. The diagnosis requires direct measurement of muscle CPT.

CPT II deficiency is much more common in men than women (5:1); nevertheless, all evidence indicates autosomal recessive inheritance. A mutation in the gene for CPT II (chromosome 1p36) causes the disease in some individuals. It has been suggested that frequent meals and a low-fat, high-carbohydrate diet can prolong exercise tolerance. Others suggest substituting medium-chain triglycerides in the diet. Neither approach has proved beneficial.

Myoadenylate Deaminase Deficiency

The muscle enzyme myoadenylate deaminase converts adenosine 5'-monophosphate (5'-AMP) to inosine monophosphate (IMP) with liberation of ammonia. Myoadenylate deaminase may play a role in regulating adenosine triphosphate (ATP) levels in muscles. Most individuals with myoadenylate deaminase deficiency have no symptoms. There have been a few reports of patients with this disorder who have exercise-exacerbated myalgia and myoglobinuria. Many questions have been raised about the clinical effects of myoadenylate deaminase deficiency, and, specifically, its relationship to exertional myalgia and fatigability, but there is no consensus.

MITOCHONDRIAL MYOPATHIES

In 1972, Olson and colleagues recognized that muscle fibers with significant numbers of abnormal mitochondria could be highlighted with the modified trichrome stain; the term *ragged red fibers* was coined. By electron microscopy, the mitochondria in ragged red fibers are enlarged and often bizarrely shaped and have crystalline inclusions. Since that seminal observation, the understanding of these disorders of muscle and other tissues has expanded.

Mitochondria play a key role in energy production. Oxidation of the major nutrients derived from carbohydrate, fat, and protein leads to the generation of reducing equivalents. The latter are transported through the respiratory chain via *oxidative phosphorylation*. The energy generated by the oxidation-reduction reactions of the respiratory chain is stored in an electrochemical gradient coupled to ATP synthesis.

A novel feature of mitochondria is their genetic composition. Each mitochondrion possesses a DNA genome that is distinct from that of the nuclear DNA. Human mitochondrial DNA (mtDNA) consists of a double-stranded, circular molecule comprising 16,569 base pairs. It codes for 22 transfer RNAs, 2 ribosomal RNAs, and 13 polypeptides of the respiratory chain enzymes. The genetics of mitochondrial diseases differ from the genetics of chromosomal disorders. The DNA of mitochondria is directly inherited from the cytoplasm of the gametes, mainly from the oocyte. The sperm contributes very little of its mitochondria to the offspring at the time of fertilization. Thus, mitochondrial genes are derived almost exclusively from the mother, accounting for maternal inheritance of some mitochondrial disorders.

Patients with mitochondrial disorders have clinical manifestations that fall into three groups: chronic progressive external ophthalmoplegia (CPEO), skeletal muscle–central nervous system syndromes, and pure myopathy simulating muscular dystrophy.

PROGRESSIVE EXTERNAL OPHTHALMOPLEGIA SYNDROMES WITH RAGGED RED FIBERS

The single most common sign of a mitochondrial myopathy is CPEO, occurring in >50% of all mitochondrial myopathies. Varying degrees of ptosis and weakness of extraocular muscles are seen, usually in the absence of diplopia, a point of distinction from disorders with fluctuating eye weakness (e.g., myasthenia gravis).

KEARNS-SAYRE SYNDROME (KSS)

KSS is a widespread multiorgan system disorder with a defined triad of clinical findings—onset before age 20, CPEO, pigmentary retinopathy—and one or more of the following features: complete heart block, cerebrospinal fluid protein >1.0 g/L (100 mg/dL), or cerebellar ataxia. Some patients with CPEO and ragged red fibers may not fulfill all of the criteria for KSS. The cardiac disease includes syncopal attacks and cardiac arrest related to the abnormalities in the cardiac conduction system: prolonged intraventricular conduction time, bundle branch block, and complete atrioventricular block. Death attributed to heart block occurs in about 20% of patients. Varying degrees of progressive limb muscle weakness and easy fatigability affect activities of daily living. Endocrine abnormalities are common including gonadal dysfunction in both sexes with delayed puberty, short stature, and infertility. Diabetes mellitus is a cardinal sign of mitochondrial disorders and is estimated to occur in 13% of KSS patients. Other less common endocrine disorders include thyroid disease, hyperaldosteronism, Addison's disease, and hypoparathyroidism. Both mental retardation and dementia are common accompaniments to this disorder. Serum CK levels are normal or slightly elevated. Serum lactate and pyruvate levels may be elevated. EMG is myopathic. Nerve conduction studies may be abnormal related to an associated neuropathy. Muscle biopsies reveal ragged red fibers, highlighted in oxidative enzyme stains, many showing defects in cytochrome oxidase. On electron microscopy, there are increased numbers of mitochondria that appear enlarged and contain paracrystalline inclusions.

KSS is a sporadic disorder. The disease is caused by single mtDNA deletions presumed to arise spontaneously in the ovum or zygote. The most common deletion, occurring in about one-third of patients, removes 4977 bp of contiguous mtDNA. Monitoring for cardiac conduction defects is critical. Prophylactic pacemaker implantation is indicated when electrocardiograms demonstrate a bifascicular block. In KSS no benefit has been shown for supplementary therapies, including multivitamins or coenzyme Q10. Of all the proposed options, exercise might be the most applicable but must be approached cautiously because of defects in the cardiac conduction system.

AUTOSOMAL DOMINANT PROGRESSIVE EXTERNAL OPHTHALMOPLEGIA

This condition is caused by nuclear DNA mutations affecting mtDNA copy number and integrity, and is inherited in a Mendelian fashion. Onset is usually after puberty. Fatigue, exercise intolerance, and complaints of muscle weakness are typical. Some patients notice swallowing problems. The neurologic examination confirms the ptosis and ophthalmoplegia, usually asymmetric in distribution. A sensorineural hearing loss may be encountered. Mild facial, neck flexor, and proximal weakness are typical. Rarely, respiratory muscles may be progressively affected and may be the direct cause of death. Serum CK is normal or mildly elevated. The resting lactates are normal or slightly elevated but may rise excessively after exercise. Spinal fluid protein is normal. The EMG is myopathic, and nerve conduction studies are usually normal. Ragged red fibers are prominently displayed in the muscle biopsy.

This autosomal dominant form of CPEO has been linked to loci on three chromosomes: 4q35, 10q24, and 15q22-26. In the chromosome 4q–related form of disease, mutations of the gene encoding the heart and skeletal muscle–specific isoform of the adenine nucleotide translocator 1 (*ANT1*) gene are found. This highly abundant mitochondrial protein forms a homodimeric inner mitochondrial channel through which ADP enters and ATP leaves the mitochondrial matrix. In the chromosome 10q–related disorder, mutations of the gene *C10orf2* are found. Its gene product, *twinkle,* co-localizes with the mtDNA and is named for its punctate, starlike staining properties. The function of twinkle is presumed to be critical for lifetime maintenance of mitochondrial integrity. In the cases mapped to chromosome 15q, a mutation affects the gene encoding mtDNA polymerase (*POLG*), an enzyme important in mtDNA replication.

Exercise may improve function but will depend on the patients' ability to participate.

AUTOSOMAL RECESSIVE CARDIOMYOPATHY AND OPHTHALMOPLEGIA (ARCO)

ARCO is a rare mitochondrial disorder clinically important because of an associated life-threatening cardiomyopathy. CPEO is the initial manifestation, occurring between ages 8 and 10. Exercise intolerance and fatigue follow the early symptoms, accompanied by palpitations and chest pain. Examination reveals extraocular muscle weakness, ptosis, facial weakness, reduced muscle bulk, and limb weakness, which is greater in proximal muscles. A dilated cardiomyopathy is typical, and some patients have conduction system involvement. Death from congestive heart failure occurs as early as age 13. Serum lactate is normal at rest but increases with mild exercise. Serum CK is increased by two- to fourfold. EMG is normal or myopathic. Muscle biopsy demonstrates typical ragged red fibers. Multiple mtDNA deletions are seen. Echocardiograms show reduced ejection fraction. Conduction block is seen on electrocardiograms. The disease is inherited as an autosomal recessive disorder. The gene has not been identified. Heart failure may require orthotopic cardiac transplantation. Cardiac pacemakers are appropriate for patients with heart block.

MTDNA SKELETAL MUSCLE–CENTRAL NERVOUS SYSTEM SYNDROMES

Myoclonic Epilepsy with Ragged Red Fibers (MERRF)

The onset of MERRF is variable, ranging from late childhood to middle adult life. Characteristic features include myoclonic epilepsy, cerebellar ataxia, and progressive muscle weakness. The seizure disorder is an integral part of the disease and may be the initial symptom. Cerebellar ataxia precedes or accompanies epilepsy. It is slowly progressive, affects both trunk and limbs, and impairs gait and extremity functions. The third major feature of the disease is muscle weakness in a limb-girdle distribution. Other more variable features include dementia, peripheral neuropathy, optic atrophy, hearing loss, and diabetes mellitus.

Serum CK levels are normal or slightly increased. The serum lactate may be elevated. EMG is myopathic, and in some patients nerve conduction studies show a neuropathy. The electroencephalogram is abnormal, corroborating clinical findings of epilepsy. Typical ragged red fibers are seen on muscle biopsy. MERRF is caused by maternally inherited point mutations of mitochondrial transfer RNA (tRNA) genes. The most common mutation found in 80% of MERRF patients is an A to G substitution at nucleotide 8344 of tRNA lysine (A8344G tRNA^{lys}). Only supportive treatment is possible, with special attention to epilepsy.

MITOCHONDRIAL MYOPATHY, ENCEPHALOPATHY, LACTIC ACIDOSIS, AND STROKE-LIKE EPISODES (MELAS)

MELAS is the most common mitochondrial encephalomyopathy. The term *stroke-like* is appropriate because the cerebral lesions do not conform to a strictly vascular distribution. The onset in the majority of patients is before age 20. Seizures, usually partial motor or generalized, are common and may represent the first clearly recognizable sign of disease. The cerebral insults that resemble strokes cause hemiparesis, hemianopia, and cortical blindness. A presumptive stroke occurring before age 40 should place this mitochondrial encephalomyopathy high in the differential diagnosis. Associated conditions include hearing loss, diabetes mellitus, hypothalamic pituitary dysfunction causing growth hormone deficiency, hypothyroidism, and absence of secondary sexual characteristics. In its full expression MELAS leads to dementia, a bedridden state, and a fatal outcome. Serum lactic acid is typically elevated. The spinal fluid protein is also increased but is usually ≤1.0 g/L (100 mg/dL). Muscle biopsies show ragged red fibers. Neuroimaging demonstrates basal ganglia calcification in a high percentage of cases. Focal lesions that mimic infarction are present predominantly in the occipital and parietal lobes. Strict vascular territories are not respected, and cerebral angiography fails to demonstrate lesions of the major cerebral blood vessels.

MELAS is caused by maternally inherited point mutations of mitochondrial tRNA genes. Most of the tRNA mutations are lethal, accounting for the paucity of multigeneration families with this syndrome. The A3243G point mutation in tRNA$^{Leu(UUR)}$ is the most common, occurring in ~80% of MELAS cases. About 10% of MELAS patients have other mutations of the tRNA$^{Leu(UUR)}$ gene including 3252G, 3256T, 3271C, and 3291C. Other tRNA gene mutations have also been reported in MELAS including G583A tRNA^{Phe}, G1642A tRNA^{Val}, G4332A tRNA^{Glu}, and T8316C tRNA^{Lys}. Mutations have also been reported in mtDNA polypeptide-coding genes. Two mutations were found in the ND5 subunit of complex I of the respiratory chain. A missense mutation has been reported at mtDNA position 9957 in the gene for subunit III of cytochrome C oxidase. No specific treatment is available. Supportive treatment is essential for the stroke-like episodes, seizures, and endocrinopathies.

PURE MYOPATHY SYNDROMES

Muscle weakness and fatigue can be the predominant manifestations of mtDNA mutations. When the condition affects exclusively muscle (pure myopathy), the disorder becomes difficult to recognize.

Mitochondrial DNA Depletion Myopathy

This disorder, clinically indistinguishable from muscular dystrophy, usually presents in the neonatal period with weakness, hypotonia, and delayed motor milestones. Some cases are rapidly fatal, with death before age 2. A milder form affects patients at a slightly later age. These patients have slowly evolving proximal muscle weakness simulating Duchenne muscular dystrophy. In some, seizures and cardiomyopathy may be present. Serum CK can reach levels of 20 to 30 times normal. Resting lactates vary from normal to mildly elevated. The EMG is myopathic, and ragged red fibers are seen on muscle biopsy. The mtDNA depletion syndrome is inherited as an autosomal recessive condition. Mutations have been identified in the *TK2* gene on chromosome 16q22 encoding thymidine kinase-2. The affected gene controls the supply of deoxyribonucleotides used for the synthesis of mtDNA. No specific treatment is available. Supportive care follows the approaches outlined for muscular dystrophy.

DISORDERS OF MUSCLE MEMBRANE EXCITABILITY

Muscle membrane excitability is affected in a group of disorders referred to as *channelopathies*. The heart may also be involved, resulting in life-threatening complications (**Table 38–5**).

CALCIUM CHANNEL DISORDERS OF MUSCLE

Hypokalemic Periodic Paralysis (HypoKPP)

Onset occurs at adolescence. Men are more often affected because of decreased penetrance in women. Episodic weakness with onset after age 25 is almost never due to periodic paralyses with the exception of thyrotoxic periodic paralysis (see below). Attacks are often provoked by meals high in carbohydrates or sodium and may accompany rest following prolonged exercise. Weakness usually affects proximal limb muscles more than distal. Ocular and bulbar muscles are less likely to be affected. Respiratory muscles are usually spared, but when they are involved the condition may prove fatal. Weakness may take as long as 24 h to resolve. Life-threatening cardiac arrhythmias related to hypokalemia may occur during attacks. Myotonia, if present, is confined to the eyelids. As a late complication, patients commonly develop severe, disabling proximal lower extremity weakness.

Attacks of thyrotoxic periodic paralysis resemble those of primary hypoKPP. Despite a higher incidence of thyrotoxicosis in women, men, particularly those of Asian descent, are more likely to manifest this complication. Attacks abate with treatment of the underlying thyroid condition.

A low serum potassium level during an attack, excluding secondary causes, establishes the diagnosis. Interattack muscle biopsies show the presence of single or multiple centrally placed vacuoles. Provocative tests with glucose and insulin to establish a diagnosis are usually not necessary and are potentially hazardous. HypoKPP is inherited as an autosomal dominant disorder with incomplete penetrance. Mutations in the voltage-sensitive, skeletal muscle calcium channel (**Fig. 38–3**) cause the disease.

TABLE 38-5

CLINICAL FEATURES OF PERIODIC PARALYSIS AND NONDYSTROPHIC MYOTONIAS

	CALCIUM CHANNEL	SODIUM CHANNEL		POTASSIUM CHANNEL
FEATURE	HYPOKALEMIC PP	HYPERKALEMIC PP	PARAMYOTONIA CONGENITA	ANDERSON'S SYNDROME[b]
Mode of inheritance	AD	AD	AD	AD
Age of onset	Adolescence	Early childhood	Early childhood	Early childhood
Myotonia[a]	No	Yes	Yes	No
Episodic weakness	Yes	Yes	Yes	Yes
Frequency of attacks of weakness	Daily to yearly	May be 2–3/d	With cold, usually rare	Daily to yearly
Duration of attacks of weakness	2–12 h	From 1–2 h to >1 day	2–24 h	2–24 h
Serum K+ level during attacks of weakness	Decreased	Increased or normal	Usually normal	Variable
Effect of K+ loading	No change	Increased myotonia, then weakness	Increased myotonia	No change
Effect of muscle cooling	No change	Increased myotonia	Increased myotonia, then weakness	No change
Fixed weakness	Yes	Yes	Yes	Yes

[a]May be paradoxical in paramyotonia congenita.
[b]Dysmorphic features and cardiac arrhythmias are distinguishing features (see text).
Abbreviations: AD, autosomal dominant; AR, autosomal recessive; PP, periodic paralysis.

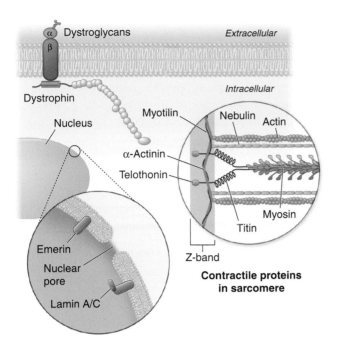

FIGURE 38-3

Selected muscular dystrophy–associated proteins in the nuclear membrane and sarcomere. As shown in the exploded view, emerin and laminin A/C are constitutents of the inner nuclear membrane. Several dystrophy-associated proteins are represented in the sarcomere including titin, nebulin, calpain, telethonin, actinin, and myotilin. The position of the dystrophin-dystroglycan complex is also illustrated.

The acute paralysis improves after the administration of potassium. Muscle strength and electrocardiogram should be monitored. Oral KCl (0.2 to 0.4 mmol/kg) should be given every 30 min. Only rarely is intravenous therapy necessary (e.g., swallowing problems or vomiting present). Administration of potassium in glucose or saline, which may further lower potassium, should be avoided. Mannitol is the preferred vehicle for administration of intravenous potassium. The long-term goal of therapy is to avoid attacks. This may reduce late-onset, fixed weakness. Patients should be made aware of the importance of a low-carbohydrate, low-sodium diet and consequences of intense exercise. Prophylactic administration of acetazolamide (125 to 1000 mg/d in divided doses) reduces or may abolish attacks. Paradoxically the potassium is lowered, but this is offset by the beneficial effect of metabolic acidosis. If attacks persist on acetazolamide, oral KCl should be added. Some patients require treatment with triamterine (25 to 100 mg/d) or spironolactone (25 to 100 mg/d).

SODIUM CHANNEL DISORDERS OF MUSCLE

Hyperkalemic Periodic Paralysis (HyperKPP)

The term *hyperkalemic* is misleading since patients are often normokalemic during attacks. The fact that attacks are precipitated by potassium administration best defines the disease. The onset is in the first decade. Attacks are brief and mild, usually lasting 30 min to 4 h. Weakness affects proximal muscles, sparing bulbar muscles. Attacks are precipitated by rest following exercise and fasting. In a variant of this disorder, the predominant symptom is myotonia without weakness (*potassium-aggravated myotonia*). The symptoms are aggravated by cold, and myotonia makes the muscles stiff and painful. This disorder can be confused with paramyotonia and myotonia congenita (described below).

Potassium may be slightly elevated but may also be normal during an attack. The EMG will often demonstrate myotonia during and between attacks. The muscle biopsy shows vacuoles that are smaller, less numerous, and more peripheral compared to the hypokalemic form. Provocative tests by administration of potassium can induce weakness but are usually not necessary to establish the diagnosis. HyperKPP and potassium-aggravated myotonia are inherited as autosomal dominant disorders. Mutations of the voltage-gated sodium channel SCN4A (**Fig. 38-4**) cause these conditions. For patients with frequent attacks acetazolamide (125 to 100 mg/d) is helpful.

Paramyotonia Congenita

In paramyotonia congenita (PC) the attacks of weakness are cold-induced or occur spontaneously and are mild. Myotonia is a prominent feature but worsens with muscle activity (paradoxical myotonia). This is in contrast to classic myotonia in which exercise alleviates the condition. Attacks of weakness are seldom severe enough to require emergency room treatment. Over time patients develop interattack weakness as they do in other forms of periodic paralysis. PC is usually associated with normokalemia or hyperkalemia. Other features are similar to those of hyperKPP. PC is inherited as an autosomal dominant condition; voltage-gated sodium channel mutations (Fig. 38-4) are responsible. Patients with PC seldom seek treatment during attacks. Oral administration of glucose or other carbohydrates hastens recovery. Since interattack weakness may develop after repeated episodes, prophylactic treatment is usually indicated. Thiazide diuretics (e.g., chlorothiazide 250 to 1000 mg/d) and mexiletine (slowly increase dose from 450 mg/d) are reported to be helpful. Patients should be advised to increase carbohydrates in their diet.

POTASSIUM CHANNEL DISORDERS

Andersen's Syndrome

This rare disease is characterized by episodic weakness, cardiac arrhythmias, and dysmorphic features (short stature, scoliosis, clinodactyly, hypertelorism, small or

Sodium channel α subunit

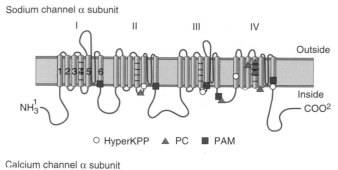

○ HyperKPP   ▲ PC   ■ PAM

Calcium channel α subunit

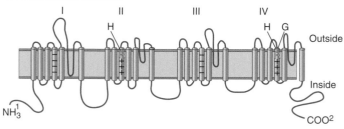

Chloride channel

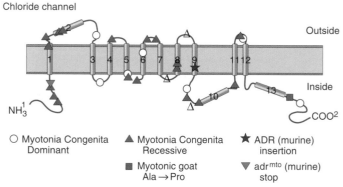

○ Myotonia Congenita   ▲ Myotonia Congenita   ★ ADR (murine)
  Dominant   Recessive   insertion

■ Myotonic goat   ▼ adr^mto (murine)
  Ala → Pro   stop

FIGURE 38-4

The sodium and calcium channels are depicted here as containing four homologous domains, each with six membrane-spanning segments. The fourth segment of each domain bears positive charges and acts as the "voltage sensor" for the channel. The association of the four domains is thought to form a pore through which ions pass. Sodium channel mutations are shown along with the phenotype that they confer. HyperKPP, hyperkalemic periodic paralysis; PC, paramyotonia congenita; PAM, potassium-aggravated myotonia. See text for details. The chloride channel is envisioned to have ten membrane-spanning domains. The positions of mutations causing dominantly and recessively inherited myotonia congenita are indicated, along with mutations that cause this disease in mice and goats.

prominent low set ears, micrognathia, and broad forehead). The cardiac arrhythmias are potentially serious and life threatening. They include long QT, ventricular ectopy, bidirectional ventricular arrhythmias, and tachycardia. For many years the classification of this disorder was uncertain because episodes of weakness are associated with elevated, normal, or reduced levels of potassium during an attack. In addition, the potas-

sium levels differ among kindreds but are consistent within a family. Inheritance is autosomal dominant with incomplete penetrance and variable expressivity. The disease is caused by mutations of the inwardly rectifying potassium channel (*kir*) gene. The treatment is similar to that for other forms of periodic paralysis and must include cardiac monitoring. The episodes of weakness may differ between patients because of potassium variability. Acetazolamide will decrease the attack frequency and severity.

CHLORIDE CHANNEL DISORDERS

Two forms of this disorder, autosomal dominant (*Thomsen's disease*) and autosomal recessive (*Becker's disease*) are related to the same gene abnormality. Symptoms are noted in infancy and early childhood. The severity lessens in the third to fourth decade. Myotonia is worsened by cold and improved by activity. The gait may appear slow and labored at first but improves with walking. In Thomsen's disease muscle strength is normal, but in Becker's, which is usually more severe, there may be muscle weakness. Muscle hypertrophy is usually present. Myotonia is prominently displayed by EMG recordings. Serum CK is normal or mildly elevated. The muscle biopsy shows hypertrophied fibers. The disease is inherited as dominant or recessive and is caused by mutations of the chloride channel gene (Fig. 38-4). Many patients will not require treatment and learn that the symptoms improve with activity. Medications that can be used to decrease myotonia include quinine, phenytoin, and mexilitene.

ENDOCRINE AND METABOLIC MYOPATHIES

Many endocrine disorders cause weakness. Muscle fatigue is more common than true weakness. The cause of weakness in these disorders is not well defined. It is not even clear that weakness results from disease of muscle as opposed to another part of the motor unit, since the serum CK level is often normal (except in hypothyroidism) and the muscle histology is characterized by atrophy rather than destruction of muscle fibers. Nearly all endocrine myopathies respond to treatment.

THYROID DISORDERS

Abnormalities of thyroid function can cause a wide array of muscle disorders. These conditions relate to the important role of thyroid hormones in regulating the metabolism of carbohydrates and lipids as well as the rate of protein synthesis and enzyme production. Thyroid hormones also stimulate calorigenesis in muscle, increase muscle demand for vitamins, and enhance muscle sensitivity to circulating catecholamines.

Hypothyroidism

Patients with hypothyroidism have frequent muscle complaints, and proximal muscle weakness occurs in about one-third of them. Muscle cramps, pain, and stiffness are common. Features of slow muscle contraction and relaxation occur in 25% of patients; the relaxation phase of muscle stretch reflexes is characteristically prolonged and best observed at the ankle or biceps brachii reflexes. The serum CK level is often elevated (up to 10 times normal), even when there is minimal clinical evidence of muscle disease. *Hoffman's syndrome* results in prominent muscle enlargement and weakness with muscle stiffness. The cause of muscle enlargement has not been determined, and muscle biopsy shows no distinctive morphologic abnormalities.

Hyperthyroidism

Patients who are thyrotoxic commonly have proximal muscle weakness and atrophy on examination, but they rarely complain of the deficit. Muscle stretch reflexes are preserved and often brisk. Bulbar, respiratory, and even esophageal muscles may occasionally be affected, causing dysphagia, dysphonia, and aspiration. When bulbar involvement occurs, it is usually accompanied by chronic proximal limb weakness, but occasionally it presents in the absence of generalized thyrotoxic myopathy. Other neuromuscular disorders occur in association with hyperthyroidism, including hypokalemic periodic paralysis, myasthenia gravis, and a progressive ocular myopathy associated with proptosis (*Graves' ophthalmopathy*). Serum CK levels are not elevated in thyrotoxic myopathy. The muscle histology usually shows only atrophy of muscle fibers.

PARATHYROID DISORDERS

Hyperparathyroidism

Muscle weakness is an integral part of primary and secondary hyperparathyroidism. Proximal muscle weakness, muscle wasting, and brisk muscle stretch reflexes are the main features of this endocrinopathy. Serum CK levels are usually normal or slightly elevated. Serum calcium and phosphorus levels show no correlation with the clinical neuromuscular manifestations. Muscle biopsies show only varying degrees of atrophy without muscle fiber degeneration.

Hypoparathyroidism

An overt myopathy due to hypocalcemia rarely occurs. Neuromuscular symptoms are usually related to local-ized or generalized tetany. Serum CK levels may be increased secondary to muscle damage from sustained tetany. Hyporeflexia or areflexia is usually present and contrasts with the hyperreflexia in hyperparathyroidism.

ADRENAL DISORDERS

Conditions associated with glucocorticoid excess cause a myopathy; in fact, steroid myopathy is the most commonly diagnosed endocrine muscle disease. Glucocorticoid excess, either endogenous or exogenous, produces various degrees of proximal limb weakness. Muscle wasting may be striking. A cushingoid appearance usually accompanies clinical signs of myopathy. Histologic sections demonstrate muscle fiber atrophy rather than degeneration or necrosis of muscle fibers. Adrenal insufficiency commonly causes muscle fatigue. The degree of weakness may be difficult to assess but is typically mild. In primary hyperaldosteronism (*Conn's syndrome*), neuromuscular complications are due to potassium depletion. The clinical picture is one of persistent muscle weakness. Long-standing hyperaldosteronism may lead to proximal limb weakness and wasting. Serum CK levels may be elevated, and a muscle biopsy may demonstrate degenerating fibers, some with vacuoles. These changes relate to hypokalemia and are not a direct effect of aldosterone on skeletal muscle.

PITUITARY DISORDERS

Patients with acromegaly usually have mild proximal weakness without muscle atrophy. Muscles often appear enlarged but exhibit decreased force generation. The duration of acromegaly, rather than the serum growth hormone levels, correlates with the degree of myopathy.

DIABETES MELLITUS

Neuromuscular complications of diabetes mellitus are most often related to neuropathy, with cranial and peripheral nerve palsies or distal sensorimotor polyneuropathy. *Diabetic amyotrophy* is a clumsy term since the condition represents a neuropathy affecting the proximal major nerve trunks and lumbosacral plexus. More appropriate terms for this disorder include *diabetic proximal neuropathy* and *lumbosacral radiculoplexus neuropathy*.

The only notable myopathy of diabetes mellitus is ischemic infarction of thigh muscles. This condition occurs in patients with poorly controlled diabetes and presents with abrupt onset of pain, tenderness, and edema of one thigh. The area of muscle infarction is hard and indurated. The muscles most often affected include the vastus lateralis, thigh adductors, and biceps femoris. Computed tomography or magnetic resonance imaging can demonstrate focal abnormalities in the affected muscle. Diagnosis by imaging is preferable to muscle biopsy, if possible.

VITAMIN DEFICIENCY

Vitamin D deficiency due to either decreased intake, decreased absorption, or impaired vitamin D metabolism (as occurs in renal disease) may lead to chronic muscle weakness. Pain reflects the underlying bone disease (*osteomalacia*). Vitamin E deficiency may result from malabsorption. Clinical manifestations include ataxic neuropathy due to loss of proprioception and myopathy with proximal weakness. Progressive external ophthalmoplegia is a distinctive finding. It has not been established that deficiency of other vitamins causes a myopathy.

MYOPATHIES OF SYSTEMIC ILLNESS

Systemic illnesses such as chronic respiratory, cardiac, or hepatic failure are frequently associated with severe muscle wasting and complaints of weakness. Fatigue is usually a more significant problem than weakness, which is typically mild.

Myopathy may be a manifestation of chronic renal failure, independent of the better known uremic polyneuropathy. Abnormalities of calcium and phosphorus homeostasis and bone metabolism in chronic renal failure result from a reduction in 1,25-dihydroxyvitamin D, leading to decreased intestinal absorption of calcium. Hypocalcemia, further accentuated by hyperphosphatemia due to decreased renal phosphate clearance, leads to secondary hyperparathyroidism. Renal osteodystrophy results from the compensatory hyperparathyroidism, which leads to osteomalacia from reduced calcium availability and to osteitis fibrosa from the parathyroid hormone excess. The clinical picture of the myopathy of chronic renal failure is identical to that of primary hyperparathyroidism and osteomalacia. There is proximal limb weakness with bone pain.

Gangrenous calcification represents a separate, rare, and sometimes fatal complication of chronic renal failure. In this condition, widespread arterial calcification occurs and results in ischemia. Extensive skin necrosis may occur, along with painful myopathy and even myoglobinuria.

DRUG-INDUCED MYOPATHIES

Drug-induced myopathies are relatively uncommon in clinical practice with the exception of those caused by the cholesterol-lowering agents and glucocorticoids. Others impact practice to a lesser degree but are important to consider in specific situations. **Table 38–6** provides a comprehensive list of drugs that induce toxic myopathies with their distinguishing features.

MYOPATHY FROM LIPID-LOWERING AGENTS

All classes of lipid-lowering agents have been implicated in muscle toxicity including fibrates (clofibrate, gemfibrozil), HMG-COA reductase inhibitors (referred to as *statins*), and niacin (nicotinic acid). Myalgia, malaise, and muscle tenderness are the most common manifestations. Muscle pain may be related to exercise. Patients may exhibit proximal weakness. Varying degrees of muscle necrosis are seen, and in severe reactions there are rhabdomyolysis and myoglobinuria. Patients improve with drug cessation. Concomitant use of statins with fibrates and cyclosporine is more likely to cause adverse reactions than use of one agent alone. Elevated serum CK is an important indication of toxicity. Muscle weakness is accompanied by a myopathic EMG, and muscle necrosis is observed by muscle biopsy. Myopathic reactions are indications for stopping the drug.

GLUCOCORTICOID-RELATED MYOPATHIES

Glucocorticoid myopathy occurs with chronic treatment or as "acute quadriplegic" myopathy secondary to high-dose, intravenous glucocorticoids. Chronic administration produces proximal weakness accompanied by cushingoid manifestations, which can be quite debilitating; the chronic use of prednisone at a daily dose of ≥30 mg/d is most often associated with toxicity. Patients taking fluorinated glucocorticoids (triamcinolone, betamethasone, dexamethasone) appear to be at especially high risk for myopathy. Patients receiving high-dose, intravenous glucocorticoids for status asthmaticus, chronic obstructive pulmonary disease, or other indications may develop severe generalized weakness. Involvement of the diaphragm and intercostal muscles causes respiratory failure and requires ventilatory support. In this setting, the use of glucocorticoids in combination with nondepolarizing neuromuscular blocking agents to further decrease airway resistance is particularly likely to lead to this complication. In chronic steroid myopathy the serum CK is usually normal. Serum potassium may be low. The muscle biopsy in chronic cases shows preferential type 2 muscle fiber atrophy; the EMG is usually normal as it measures type I fiber function only. In acute cases with quadraplegic myopathy, the muscle biopsy is abnormal and shows a distinctive loss of thick filaments by electron microscopy. By light microscopy there is focal loss of ATPase staining in central or paracentral areas of the muscle fiber. Calpain stains show diffusely reactive atrophic fibers. Withdrawal of glucocorticoids will improve the chronic myopathy. In acute quadriplegic myopathy, recovery is slow. Patients require supportive care and rehabilitation.

TABLE 38-6

DRUG-INDUCED MYOPATHIES

DRUGS	MAJOR TOXIC REACTION
Lipid-lowering agents Fibric acid derivatives HMG-CoA reductase inhibitors Niacin (nicotinic acid)	Drugs belonging to all three of the major classes of lipid-lowering agents can produce a spectrum of toxicity: asymptomatic serum creatine kinase elevation, myalgias, exercised-induced pain, rhabdomyolysis, and myoglobinuria.
Glucocorticoids	Acute, high-dose glucocorticoid treatment can cause acute quadriplegic myopathy. These high doses of steroids are often combined with nondepolarizing neuromuscular blocking agents but the weakness can occur without their use. Chronic steroid administration produces predominantly proximal weakness.
Nondepolarizing neuromuscular blocking agents	Acute quadriplegic myopathy can occur with or without concomitant glucocorticoids.
Zidovudine	Mitochondrial myopathy with ragged red fibers.
Drugs of abuse Alcohol Amphetamines Cocaine Heroin Phencyclidine Meperidine	All drugs in this group can lead to widespread muscle breakdown, rhabdomyolysis, and myoglobinuria. Local injections cause muscle necrosis, skin induration, and limb contractures.
D-Penicillamine	Autoimmune toxic myopathy; use of this drug may cause polymyositis and myasthenia gravis.
Amphophilic cationic drugs Amiodarone Chloroquine Hydroxychloroquine	All amphophilic drugs have the potential to produce painless, proximal weakness associated with autophagic vacuoles in the muscle biopsy.
Antimicrotubular drugs Colchicine	This drug produces painless, proximal weakness especially in the setting of renal failure. Muscle biopsy shows autophagic vacuoles.

MYOPATHY OF NONDEPOLARIZING NEUROMUSCULAR BLOCKING AGENTS

Patients may receive nondepolarizing neuromuscular blocking agents because of life-threatening airway resistance. Acute quadriplegic myopathy may result, with or without glucocorticoid use. The clinical features are identical to acute quadriplegic myopathy secondary to glucocorticoids.

DRUG-INDUCED MITOCHONDRIAL MYOPATHY

Zidovudine, used in the treatment of HIV infection, is a thymidine analogue that inhibits viral replication by interrupting reverse transcriptase. Myopathy is a well-established complication of this agent. Patients present with myalgias, muscle weakness, and atrophy affecting the thigh and calf muscles. The complication occurs in about 17% of patients treated with doses of 1200 mg/d for 6 months. The introduction of protease inhibitors for treatment of HIV infection has led to lower doses of zidovudine therapy and a decreased incidence of myopathy. Serum CK is elevated and EMG is myopathic. Muscle biopsy shows ragged red fibers with minimal inflammation; the lack of inflammation serves to distinguish zidovudine toxicity from HIV-related myopathy. If the myopathy is thought to be drug related, then the medication should be stopped or the dosage reduced.

DRUGS OF ABUSE AND RELATED MYOPATHIES

Myotoxicity is a potential consequence of addiction to alcohol and illicit drugs. Ethanol is one of the most commonly abused substances with potential to damage muscle. Other potential toxins include cocaine, heroin, and amphetamines. The most deleterious reactions occur from overdosing leading to coma and seizures, causing rhabdomyolysis, myoglobinuria, and renal failure. Direct toxicity can occur from cocaine, heroin, and amphetamines causing muscle breakdown and varying degrees of weakness. The effects of alcohol are more controversial. Direct muscle damage is less certain, since toxicity usually occurs in the setting of poor nutrition and possible contributing factors such as hypokalemia and hypophosphatemia. Alcoholics are also prone to neuropathy and a variety of central nervous system disorders (Chap. 42).

Focal myopathies from self-administration of meperidine, heroin, and pentazocine can cause pain, swelling, muscle necrosis, and hemorrhage. The cause is multifactorial: needle trauma, direct toxicity of the drug or vehicle, and infection. When severe, there may be overlying skin induration and contractures with replacement of muscle by connective tissue. Elevated serum CK and myopathic EMG are characteristic of these reactions. The muscle biopsy shows widespread or focal areas of necrosis. In conditions leading to rhabdomyolysis, patients need adequate hydration to reduce serum myoglobin and protect renal function. In all of these conditions, counseling is essential to limit drug abuse.

DRUG-INDUCED AUTO IMMUNE MYOPATHIES

The most consistent drug-related inflammatory or antibody-mediated myopathy is caused by D-penicillamine. This drug chelates copper and is used in the treatment of Wilson's disease. It is also used to treat other disorders including scleroderma, rheumatoid arthritis, and primary biliary cirrhosis. Adverse events include drug-induced polymyositis indistinguishable from the spontaneous disease. The incidence of this inflammatory muscle disease is about 1%. Myasthenia gravis is also induced by D-penicillamine, with a higher incidence estimated at 7%. These disorders resolve with drug withdrawal, although immunosuppressive therapy may be warranted in severe cases.

Scattered reports of other drugs causing an inflammatory myopathy are rare and include a heterogeneous group of agents: cimetidine, phenytoin, procainamide, and propylthiouracil. In most cases, a cause-and-effect relationship is uncertain. A complication of interest was related to L-tryptophan. In 1989 an epidemic of eosinophilia-myalgia syndrome (EMS) in the United States was caused by a contaminant in the product from one manufacturer. The product was withdrawn, and incidence of EMS diminished abruptly following this action.

OTHER DRUG-INDUCED MYOPATHIES

Certain drugs produce painless, largely proximal, muscle weakness. These drugs include the amphophilic cationic drugs (amiodarone, chloroquine, hydroxychloroquine) and antimicrotubular drugs (colchicine). Muscle biopsy can be useful in the identification of toxicity since autophagic vacuoles are prominent pathologic features of these toxins.

FURTHER READINGS

☑ BANSAL D et al: Defective membrane repair in dysferlin-deficient muscular dystrophy. Nature 423:168, 2003

   Normal dysferlin plays an essential role in muscle-membrane repair.

CHINNERY PF et al: Risk of developing a mitochondrial DNA deletion disorder. Lancet 364:592, 2004

☑ DESCHAUER, M et al: Muscle carnitine palmitoyltransferase II deficiency. Arch Neurol 62:37, 2005

   Discusses clinical features, molecular genetics, and diagnostic approach.

FAN X, ROULEAU GA: Progress in understanding the pathogenesis of oculopharyngeal muscular dystrophy. Can J Neurol Sci 30:8, 2003

☑ FINSTERER J, STOLLBERGER C: The heart in human dystrophinopathies. Cardiology 99:1, 2003

   Reviews the anatomic, electrocardiographic, and pathologic changes in the heart in dystrophinopathies.

Jurkat-Rott K et al: Skeletal muscle channelopathies. J Neurol 249:1493, 2002

KULLMANN DM, HANNA MG: Neurological disorders caused by inherited ion-channel mutations. Lancet Neurol 1:157, 2002

LENNON N et al: Dysferlin interacts with Annexins A1 and A2 and mediates sarcolemmal wound-healing. J Biol Chem 278(50):50466, 2003

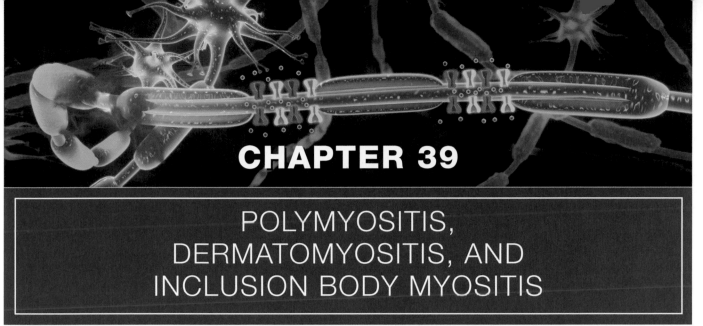

CHAPTER 39

POLYMYOSITIS, DERMATOMYOSITIS, AND INCLUSION BODY MYOSITIS

Marinos C. Dalakas

The inflammatory myopathies represent the largest group of acquired and potentially treatable causes of skeletal muscle weakness. They are classified into three major groups: polymyositis (PM), dermatomyositis (DM), and inclusion body myositis (IBM).

CLINICAL FEATURES

The prevalence of the inflammatory myopathies is estimated at 1 in 100,000. PM as a stand-alone entity is a rare disease affecting adults. DM affects both children and adults, and women more often than men. IBM is three times more frequent in men than in women, more common in Caucasians than blacks, and most likely to affect persons >50 years of age.

These disorders present as progressive and often symmetric muscle weakness. Patients usually report increasing difficulty with everyday tasks requiring the use of proximal muscles, such as getting up from a chair, climbing steps, stepping onto a curb, lifting objects, or combing hair. Fine-motor movements that depend on the strength of distal muscles, such as buttoning a shirt, sewing, knitting, or writing, are affected only late in the course of PM and DM, but fairly early in IBM. Falling is common in IBM because of early involvement of the quadriceps muscle with buckling of the knees. Ocular muscles are spared, even in advanced, untreated cases; if these muscles are affected, the diagnosis of inflammatory myopathy should be questioned. Facial muscles are unaffected in PM and DM, but mild facial muscle weakness is common in patients with IBM. In all forms of inflammatory myopathy, pharyngeal and neck-flexor muscles are often involved, causing dysphagia or difficulty in holding up the head (*head drop*). In advanced and rarely in acute cases, respiratory muscles also may be affected. Severe weakness, if untreated, is almost always associated with muscle wasting. Sensation remains normal. The tendon reflexes are preserved but may be absent in severely weakened or atrophied muscles, especially in IBM where atrophy of the quadriceps and the distal muscles is common and severe. Myalgia and muscle tenderness may occur in a small number of patients, usually early in the disease, and particularly in DM associated with connective tissue disorders. Weakness in PM and DM progresses subacutely over a period of weeks or months and rarely acutely; by contrast, IBM progresses very slowly, over years, simulating a late-life muscular dystrophy

(Chap. 38) or slowly progressive motor neuron disorder (Chap. 21).

SPECIFIC FEATURES (Table 39-1)

POLYMYOSITIS

The onset of PM is often insidious, and patients typically delay seeking medical advice for several months. The rash facilitates early recognition of DM (see below). PM mimics many other myopathies and is a diagnosis of exclusion. It is a subacute inflammatory myopathy affecting adults, and rarely children, who *do not have* any of the following: rash, involvement of the extraocular and facial muscles, family history of a neuromuscular disease, history of exposure to myotoxic drugs or toxins, endocrinopathy, neurogenic disease, muscular dystrophy, biochemical muscle disorder (deficiency of a muscle enzyme), or IBM (excluded by muscle biopsy). As an isolated entity, PM is rare and overdiagnosed; more commonly, PM occurs in association with a systemic autoimmune or connective tissue disease, or a known viral or bacterial infection. Drugs, especially D-penicillamine or zidovudine (AZT), also may produce an inflammatory myopathy similar to PM.

DERMATOMYOSITIS

DM is a distinctive entity identified by a characteristic rash accompanying, or more often preceding, muscle weakness. The rash may consist of a blue–purple discoloration on the upper eyelids with edema (heliotrope rash), a flat red rash on the face and upper trunk, and erythema of the knuckles with a raised violaceous scaly eruption (*Gottron rash*). The erythematous rash can also occur on other body surfaces, including the knees, elbows, malleoli, neck and anterior chest (often in a *V sign*), or back and shoulders (*shawl sign*), and may worsen after sun exposure. In some patients the rash is pruritic, especially on the scalp, chest, and back. Dilated capillary loops at the base of the fingernails also are characteristic. The cuticles may be irregular, thickened, and distorted. The lateral and palmar areas of the fingers may become rough and cracked, with irregular, "dirty" horizontal lines, resembling *mechanic's hands*. The weakness can be mild, moderate, or severe enough to lead to quadriparesis. At times, muscle strength appears normal, hence the term *dermatomyositis sine myositis*. When muscle biopsy is performed in such cases, significant perivascular and perimysial inflammation is seen.

DM usually occurs alone but may overlap with scleroderma and mixed connective tissue disease. Fasciitis and thickening of the skin, similar to that seen in

TABLE 39-1

FEATURES ASSOCIATED WITH INFLAMMATORY MYOPATHIES

CHARACTERISTIC	POLYMYOSITIS	DERMATOMYOSITIS	INCLUSION BODY MYOSITIS
Age at onset	>18 years	Adulthood and childhood	>50 years
Familial association	No	No	Yes, in some cases
Extramuscular manifestations	Yes	Yes	Yes
Associated conditions			
Connective tissue diseases	Yes[a]	Scleroderma and mixed connective tissue disease (overlap syndromes)	Yes, in up to 20% of cases[a]
Systemic autoimmune diseases[b]	Frequent	Infrequent	Infrequent
Malignancy	No	Yes, in up to 15% of cases	No
Viruses	Yes[c]	Unproven	Yes[c]
Drugs[d]	Yes	Yes, rarely	No
Parasites and bacteria[e]	Yes	No	No

[a]Systemic lupus erythematosus, rheumatoid arthritis, Sjögren's syndrome, systemic sclerosis, mixed connective tissue disease.
[b]Crohn's disease, vasculitis, sarcoidosis, primary biliary cirrhosis, adult celiac disease, chronic graft-versus-host disease, discoid lupus, ankylosing spondylitis, Behçet's syndrome, myasthenia gravis, acne fulminans, dermatitis herpetiformis, psoriasis, Hashimoto's disease, granulomatous diseases, agammaglobulinemia, monoclonal gammopathy, hypereosinophilic syndrome, Lyme disease, Kawasaki disease, autoimmune thrombocytopenia, hypergammaglobulinemic purpura, hereditary complement deficiency, IgA deficiency.
[c]HIV (human immunodeficiency virus) and HTLV-I (human T cell lymphotropic virus type I).
[d]Drugs include penicillamine (dermatomyositis and polymyositis), zidovudine (polymyositis), and contaminated tryptophan (dermatomyositis-like illness). Other myotoxic drugs may cause myopathy but not an inflammatory myopathy (see text for details).
[e]Parasites (protozoa, cestodes, nematodes), tropical and bacterial myositis (pyomyositis).

chronic cases of DM, have occurred in patients with the *eosinophilia-myalgia syndrome* associated with the ingestion of contaminated L-tryptophan.

INCLUSION BODY MYOSITIS

In patients ≥50 years of age, IBM is the most common of the inflammatory myopathies. It is often misdiagnosed as PM and suspected only later when a patient with presumed PM does not respond to therapy. Weakness and atrophy of the distal muscles, especially foot extensors and deep finger flexors, occur in almost all cases of IBM and may be a clue to early diagnosis. Some patients present with falls because their knees collapse due to early quadriceps weakness. Others present with weakness in the small muscles of the hands, especially finger flexors, and complain of inability to hold objects such as golf clubs or perform tasks such as turning keys or tying knots. On occasion, the weakness and accompanying atrophy can be asymmetric and selectively involve the quadriceps, iliopsoas, triceps, biceps, and finger flexors, resembling a lower motor neuron disease. Dysphagia is common, occurring in up to 60% of IBM patients, and may lead to episodes of choking. Sensory examination is generally normal, but some patients have mildly diminished vibratory sensation at the ankles that may be age-related. The pattern of distal weakness, which superficially resembles motor neuron or peripheral nerve disease, results from the myopathic process affecting distal muscles selectively. Disease progression is slow but steady, and most patients require an assistive device such as a cane, walker, or wheelchair within several years of onset.

In at least 20% of cases, IBM is associated with systemic autoimmune or connective tissue diseases. Familial aggregation of typical IBM may occur; such cases have been designated as *familial inflammatory IBM*. Clinical features, other than family history, cannot be used to distinguish familial from sporadic cases. This disorder is distinct from *hereditary inclusion body myopathy* (h-IBM), which describes a heterogeneous group of recessive, and less frequently dominant, inherited syndromes; the h-IBMs are noninflammatory myopathies. A subset of h-IBM that spares the quadriceps muscles has emerged as a distinct entity. This disorder, originally described in Iranian Jews and now seen in many ethnic groups, is linked to chromosome 9p1 and results from mutations in the UDP-*N*-acetylglucosamine 2-epimerase/*N*-acetylmannosamine kinase (*GNE*) gene.

ASSOCIATED CLINICAL FINDINGS

EXTRAMUSCULAR MANIFESTATIONS

These may be present to a varying degree in patients with PM or DM including the following:

1. *Systemic symptoms* such as fever, malaise, weight loss, arthralgia, and Raynaud's phenomenon, especially when inflammatory myopathy is associated with a connective tissue disorder.
2. *Joint contractures,* mostly in DM and especially in children.
3. *Dysphagia and gastrointestinal symptoms,* due to involvement of oropharyngeal and upper esophagus striated muscles, especially in DM and IBM.
4. *Cardiac disturbances,* including atrioventricular conduction defects, tachyarrhythmias, dilated cardiomyopathy, and a low ejection fraction. Congestive heart failure and myocarditis also may occur from the disease itself or from hypertension associated with long-term use of glucocorticoids.
5. *Pulmonary dysfunction* due to weakness of the thoracic muscles, interstitial lung disease, or drug-induced pneumonitis (e.g., from methotrexate) that may cause dyspnea, nonproductive cough, and aspiration pneumonia. Interstitial lung disease may precede myopathy or occur early in the disease, and develops in up to 10% of patients with PM or DM; most have antibodies to t-RNA synthetases, as described below.
6. *Subcutaneous calcifications* in DM sometimes extruding on the skin and causing ulcerations and infections.

ASSOCIATION WITH MALIGNANCIES

Although all the inflammatory myopathies can have a chance association with malignant lesions, especially in older age groups, the incidence of malignant conditions appears to be specifically increased only in patients with DM and not in PM or IBM. The most common tumors associated with DM are ovarian cancer, breast cancer, melanoma, colon cancer, and non-Hodgkin's lymphoma. The extent of the search that should be conducted for an occult neoplasm in adults with DM depends on the clinical circumstances. Tumors in these patients are usually uncovered by abnormal findings in the medical history and physical examination, and not through an extensive blind search. The weight of evidence argues against performing expensive, invasive, and nondirected tumor searches. A complete annual physical examination with pelvic, breast (mammogram, if indicated), and rectal examinations (with colonoscopy according to age and family history); urinalysis; complete blood count; blood chemistry tests; and a chest film should suffice in most cases. In Asians, nasopharyngeal cancer is common, and a careful examination of ears, nose, and throat is indicated.

OVERLAP SYNDROMES

The association of inflammatory myopathies with connective tissue diseases defines the overlap syndromes. A well-characterized overlap syndrome occurs in patients with DM who also have manifestations of systemic sclerosis or mixed connective tissue disease including sclerotic thickening of the dermis, contractures, esophageal hypomotility, microangiopathy, and calcium deposits (Table 39-1). By contrast, signs of rheumatoid arthritis, systemic lupus erythematosus, or Sjögren's syndrome are very rare in patients with DM. Patients with the overlap syndrome of DM and systemic sclerosis may have a specific antinuclear antibody, the anti-PM/Scl, directed against a nucleolar-protein complex.

PATHOGENESIS

An autoimmune etiology of the inflammatory myopathies is indirectly supported by an association with other autoimmune or connective tissue diseases, the presence of various autoantibodies, an association with specific major histocompatibility complex (MHC) genes, demonstration of T cell–mediated myocytotoxicity or complement-mediated microangiopathy, and a response to immunotherapy.

AUTOANTIBODIES AND IMMUNOGENETICS

Various autoantibodies against nuclear antigens (antinuclear antibodies) and cytoplasmic antigens are found in up to 20% of patients with inflammatory myopathies. The antibodies to cytoplasmic antigens are directed against ribonucleoproteins involved in protein synthesis (anti-synthetases) or translational transport (anti-signal-recognition particles). The antibody directed against the histidyl-transfer RNA synthetase, called *anti-Jo-1*, accounts for 75% of all the anti-synthetases and is clinically useful because up to 80% of patients with anti-Jo-1 antibodies have interstitial lung disease. Some patients with the anti-Jo-1 antibody also have Raynaud's phenomenon or non-erosive arthritis.

IMMUNOPATHOLOGIC MECHANISMS

In DM, humoral immune mechanisms result in a microangiopathy and muscle ischemia (**Fig. 39-1**). Endomysial inflammatory infiltrates are composed of B cells located in proximity to CD4 T cells and macrophages; there is a relative absence of lymphocytic invasion of nonnecrotic muscle fibers. Activation of the complement C5b-9 membranolytic attack complex is thought to be a critical early event. Necrosis of the endothelial cells, reduced numbers of endomysial capillaries, ischemia, and muscle-fiber destruction resembling microinfarcts occur. The remaining capillaries often have dilated lumens in response to the ischemic process. Larger intramuscular blood vessels also may be affected

in the same pattern. Residual perifascicular atrophy reflects the endofascicular hypoperfusion that is prominent in the periphery of the muscle fascicles.

By contrast, in PM and IBM a mechanism of T cell–mediated cytotoxicity is likely. CD8 T cells, along with macrophages, initially surround and eventually invade and destroy healthy, nonnecrotic muscle fibers that aberrantly express class I MHC molecules. MHC-I expression, absent from the sarcolemma of normal muscle fibers, is probably induced by cytokines secreted by activated T cells and macrophages. The CD8/MHC-I complex is characteristic of PM and IBM; its detection has now become necessary to confirm the histologic diagnosis of PM. Key molecules involved in T cell–mediated cytotoxicity are depicted in **Fig. 39-2**.

THE ROLE OF NONIMMUNE FACTORS IN IBM

In IBM, the presence of rimmed vacuoles (almost always in fibers not invaded by T cells) together with β-amyloid deposits within the vacuolated muscle fibers and abnormal mitochondria with cytochrome oxidase–negative fibers suggest that, in addition to the autoimmune component, there is also a degenerative process. Similar to Alzheimer's disease, the amyloid deposits in IBM are immunoreactive against amyloid precursor protein (APP), chymotrypsin, apolipoprotein E, and phosphorylated tau, but it is unclear whether these deposits are directly pathogenic or represent secondary phenomena.

ASSOCIATION WITH VIRAL INFECTIONS AND THE ROLE OF RETROVIRUSES

Several viruses, including coxsackieviruses, influenza, paramyxoviruses, mumps, cytomegalovirus, and Epstein-Barr virus, have been indirectly associated with myositis. For the coxsackieviruses, an autoimmune myositis triggered by molecular mimicry has been proposed because of structural homology between histidyl-transfer RNA synthetase that is the target of the Jo-1 antibody (see above) and genomic RNA of an animal picornavirus, the encephalomyocarditis virus. Sensitive polymerase chain reaction (PCR) studies, however, have repeatedly failed to confirm the presence of such viruses in muscle biopsies.

The best evidence of a viral connection in PM and IBM is with the retroviruses. Some individuals infected with HIV or with human T cell lymphotropic virus I (HTLV-1) develop PM or IBM; a similar disorder has been described in nonhuman primates infected with the simian immunodeficiency virus. The inflammatory myopathy may occur as the initial manifestation of a retroviral infection, or myositis may develop later in the disease course. Retroviral antigens have been detected

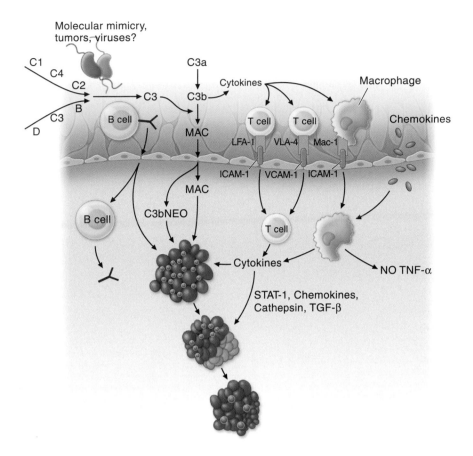

FIGURE 39-1

Immunopathogenesis of dermatomyositis. Autoantibodies (Y), possibly against endothelial cells, induce activation of complement and formation of C3 via the classic or alternative pathway. Activated C3 leads to formation of C3b, C3bNEO, and membrane attack complexes (MAC), which are deposited in and around the endothelial cell wall of the endomysial capillaries. Deposition of MAC leads to destruction of capillaries, ischemia, or microinfarcts most prominent in the periphery of the fascicles, and perifascicular atrophy. B cells, CD4 T cells, and macrophages (Mφ) traffic from the circulation to the muscle.

only in occasional endomysial macrophages and not within the muscle fibers themselves, suggesting that persistent infection and viral replication within the muscle do not occur. Histologic findings are identical to retroviral-negative PM or IBM. This disorder should be distinguished from a toxic myopathy related to long-term therapy with AZT, characterized by fatigue, myalgia, mild muscle weakness, and mild elevation of creatine kinase (CK). AZT-induced myopathy, which generally improves when the drug is discontinued, is a mitochondrial disorder characterized histologically by "ragged-red" fibers.

DIFFERENTIAL DIAGNOSIS

The clinical picture of the typical skin rash and proximal or diffuse muscle weakness has few causes other than DM. However, proximal muscle weakness without skin involvement can be due to many conditions other than PM or IBM.

SUBACUTE OR CHRONIC PROGRESSIVE MUSCLE WEAKNESS

This may be due to denervating conditions such as the spinal muscular atrophies or amyotrophic lateral sclerosis (Chap. 21). In addition to the muscle weakness, upper motor neuron signs in the latter and signs of denervation by electromyography (EMG) aid in the diagnosis. The muscular dystrophies (Chap. 38) are possible considerations, but these disorders usually develop over years rather than weeks or months and rarely present after the age of 30. It may be difficult, even with a muscle biopsy, to distinguish chronic PM from a rapidly advancing muscular dystrophy. This is particularly true of facioscapulohumeral muscular dystrophy, dysferlin myopathy, and the dystrophinopathies where inflammatory cell infiltration is often found early in the disease. Such doubtful cases should always be given an adequate trial of glucocorticoid therapy and be screened for the respective genetic defect. Search for the MHC/CD8 lesion by immunocytochemistry is helpful to identify

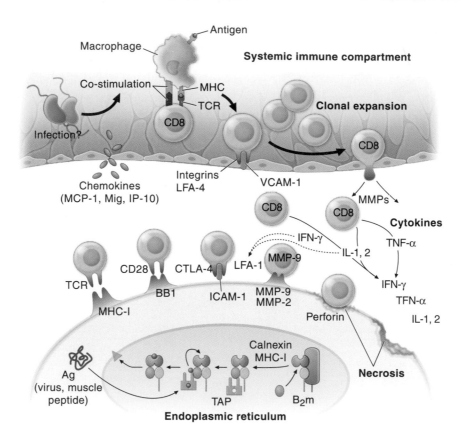

FIGURE 39-2

Cell-mediated mechanisms of muscle damage in polymyositis (PM) and inclusion body myositis (IBM). Antigen-specific CD8 cells are expanded in the periphery, cross the endothelial barrier, and bind directly to muscle fibers via T cell receptor (TCR) molecules that recognize aberrantly expressed MHC-I. Engagement of co-stimulatory molecules (BB1 and ICOSL) with their ligands (CD28, CTLA-4, and ICOS), along with ICAM-1/LFA-1, stabilize the CD8–muscle fiber interaction. Metalloproteinases (MMP) facilitate the migration of T cells and their attachment to the muscle surface. Muscle fiber necrosis occurs via perforin granules released by the autoaggressive T cells. A direct myocytotoxic effect exerted by the cytokines interferon (IFN) γ, interleukin (IL) 1, or tumor necrosis factor (TNF) α also may play a role. Death of the muscle fiber is mediated by necrosis.

cases of PM as mentioned above. Some metabolic myopathies, including glycogen storage disease due to myophosphorylase or acid maltase deficiency, lipid storage myopathies due to carnitine deficiency, and mitochondrial diseases, produce weakness that is often associated with other characteristic clinical signs; diagnosis rests upon histochemical and biochemical studies of the muscle biopsy. The endocrine myopathies such as those due to hypercorticosteroidism, hyper- and hypothyroidism, and hyper- and hypoparathyroidism require the appropriate laboratory investigations for diagnosis. Muscle wasting in patients with an underlying neoplasm may be due to disuse, cachexia, or rarely to a paraneoplastic neuromyopathy.

Diseases of the neuromuscular junction, including myasthenia gravis or Lambert-Eaton myasthenic syndrome, cause fatiguing weakness that also affects the eye and cranial muscles (Chap. 37). Repetitive nerve stimulation and single-fiber EMG studies aid in diagnosis.

ACUTE MUSCLE WEAKNESS

This may be caused by an acute neuropathy such as Guillain-Barré syndrome (Chap. 35), transverse myelitis (Chap. 24), a neurotoxin (Chap. 38), or a viral infection such as poliomyelitis or West Nile virus (Chap. 29). When acute weakness is associated with painful muscle cramps, rhabdomyolysis, and myoglobinuria, it may be due to metabolic disorders including a glycogen storage disease such as myophosphorylase deficiency or carnitine palmityltransferase deficiency (Chap. 38). Acute viral infections may cause a similar syndrome. Several animal parasites, such as protozoa (*toxoplasma, trypanosoma*), cestodes (cysticerci), and nematodes (trichinae), may produce a focal or diffuse inflammatory myopathy known as *parasitic polymyositis*. *Staphylococcus aureus, Yersinia, Streptococcus,* or other anaerobic bacteria may produce a suppurative myositis, known as *tropical polymyositis,* or *pyomyositis.* Pyomyositis, previously rare in the west, is now occasionally seen in AIDS patients. Other bacteria, such as *Borrelia burgdorferi* (Lyme disease) and *Legionella pneumophila* (Legionnaire's disease) may infrequently cause myositis.

Patients with periodic paralysis develop acute episodes of recurrent, painless muscle weakness, always beginning in childhood. Chronic alcoholics may develop painful myopathy with myoglobinuria after a bout of heavy drinking or present with a painless, acute hypokalemic myopathy that is completely reversible with replacement therapy; other times they show an asymptomatic elevation of serum CK and myoglobin. Acute muscle weakness with myoglobinuria may occur with prolonged severe hypokalemia, hypophosphatemia, or hypomagnesemia that is seen in chronic alcoholics and patients on nasogastric suction receiving parenteral hyperalimentation.

MACROPHAGIC MYOFASCIITIS

This distinctive inflammatory muscle disorder presents as diffuse myalgias, fatigue, and mild muscle weakness. Muscle biopsy reveals pronounced infiltration of the connective tissue around the muscle by sheets of periodic acid–Schiff-positive macrophages and occasional CD8 T cells. The CK or erythrocyte sedimentation rate is variably elevated. Most patients respond to glucocorticoid therapy, and the overall prognosis seems favorable. Histologic involvement is focal and limited to sites of vaccinations that may have been administered months or years earlier. This disorder, which to date has not been observed outside of France, has been linked to an aluminum-containing substrate used in vaccine preparation.

DRUG-INDUCED MYOPATHIES

D-Penicillamine and procainamide may produce a true myositis resembling PM, and a DM-like illness has been associated with the contaminated preparations of L-tryptophan. As noted above, AZT causes a mitochondrial myopathy. Other drugs may elicit a toxic noninflammatory myopathy that is histologically different from DM, PM, or IBM. These include the cholesterol-lowering agents such as clofibrate, lovastatin, simvastatin, or pravastatin, especially when combined with cyclosporine or gemfibrozil. Acute alcohol intoxication superimposed on chronic use, or chronic administration of corticosteroids also may result in a myopathy. Rhabdomyolysis and myoglobinuria have been rarely associated with amphotericin B, α-aminocaproic acid, fenfluramine, heroin, and phencyclidine. The use of amiodarone, chloroquine, colchicine, carbimazole, emetine, etretinate, ipecac syrup, chronic laxative or licorice use resulting in hypokalemia, and glucocorticoids or

growth hormone administration also have been associated with myopathic muscle weakness. Some neuromuscular blocking agents such as pancuronium, in combination with glucocorticoids, may cause the acute critical illness myopathy. A careful drug history is essential for diagnosis of these drug-induced myopathies, which do not require immunosuppressive therapy.

PAIN ON MOVEMENT AND MUSCLE TENDERNESS

A number of conditions including *polymyalgia rheumatica* and arthritic disorders of adjacent joints may enter into the differential diagnosis of inflammatory myopathy, even though they do not cause myositis. The muscle biopsy either is normal or discloses type II muscle fiber atrophy. Patients with *fibrositis* and *fibromyalgia* complain of focal or diffuse muscle tenderness, fatigue, and aching that is sometimes poorly differentiated from joint pain. In other patients there may be suggestive signs of a collagen vascular disorder, such as an increased erythrocyte sedimentation rate, antinuclear antibody, or rheumatoid factor. Occasionally, there is slight but transient elevation of the serum CK. The muscle biopsy is usually normal and the prognosis favorable. Many such patients show some response to nonsteroidal anti–inflammatory agents, though most continue to have indolent complaints. *Chronic fatigue syndrome,* which may follow a viral infection, can present with debilitating fatigue, fever, sore throat, painful lymphadenopathy, myalgia, arthralgia, sleep disorder, and headache. These patients do not have muscle weakness, and the muscle biopsy is normal.

DIAGNOSIS

The clinically suspected diagnosis of PM, DM, or IBM is confirmed by examining the serum muscle enzymes, EMG findings, and muscle biopsy (**Table 39–2**).

The most sensitive enzyme is CK, which in active disease can be elevated as much as 50-fold. Although the CK level usually parallels disease activity, it can be normal in some patients with active IBM or DM, especially when associated with a connective tissue disease. The CK is always elevated in patients with active PM. Along with the CK, the serum glutamic–oxaloacetic and glutamate pyruvate transaminases, lactate dehydrogenase, and aldolase may be elevated.

Needle EMG shows myopathic potentials characterized by short-duration, low-amplitude polyphasic units on voluntary activation and increased spontaneous activity with fibrillations, complex repetitive discharges, and positive sharp waves. Mixed potentials (polyphasic units of short and long duration) indicating a chronic process and muscle fiber regeneration are often present in IBM.

TABLE 39-2

CRITERIA FOR DIAGNOSIS OF INFLAMMATORY MYOPATHIES

CRITERION	POLYMYOSITIS		DERMATOMYOSITIS	INCLUSION BODY MYOSITIS
	DEFINITE	PROBABLE		
Myopathic muscle weakness[a]	Yes	Yes	Yes[b]	Yes; slow onset, early involvement of distal muscles, frequent falls
Electromyographic findings	Myopathic	Myopathic	Myopathic	Myopathic with mixed potentials
Muscle enzymes	Elevated (up to 50-fold)	Elevated (up to 50-fold)	Elevated (up to 50-fold) or normal	Elevated (up to 10-fold) or normal
Muscle biopsy findings[c]	Primary inflammation with the CD8/MHC-I complex and no vacuoles	Ubiquitous MHC-I expression but minimal inflammation and no vacuoles[d]	Perifascicular, perimysial, or perivascular infiltrates, perifascicular atrophy	Primary inflammation with CD8/MHC-I complex; vacuolated fibers with β-amyloid deposits; cytochrome oxygenase–negative fibers; signs of chronic myopathy[e]
Rash or calcinosis	Absent	Absent	Present[f]	Absent

[a]Myopathic muscle weakness, affecting proximal muscles more than distal ones and sparing eye and facial muscles, is characterized by a subacute onset (weeks to months) and rapid progression in patients who have no family history of neuromuscular disease, no endocrinopathy, no exposure to myotoxic drugs or toxins, and no biochemical muscle disease (excluded on the basis of muscle-biopsy findings).

[b]In some cases with the typical rash, the muscle strength is seemingly normal (dermatomyositis sine myositis); these patients often have new onset of easy fatigue and reduced endurance. Careful muscle testing may reveal mild muscle weakness.

[c]See text for details.

[d]An adequate trial of prednisone or other immunosuppressive drugs is warranted in probable cases. If, in retrospect, the disease is unresponsive to therapy, another muscle biopsy should be considered to exclude other diseases or possible evolution in inclusion body myositis.

[e]If the muscle biopsy does not contain vacuolated fibers but shows chronic myopathy with hypertrophic fibers, primary inflammation with the CD8/MHC-I complex and cytochrome oxygenase–negative fibers, then the diagnosis is probable inclusion body myositis.

[f]If rash is absent but muscle biopsy findings are characteristic of dermatomyositis, the diagnosis is probable DM.

Note: MHC, major histocompatibility complex.

These EMG findings are not diagnostic of an inflammatory myopathy but are useful to identify the presence of active or chronic myopathy and to exclude neurogenic disorders.

Magnetic resonance imaging is not routinely used for the diagnosis of PM, DM, or IBM, but it may guide the location of the muscle biopsy in certain clinical settings.

Muscle biopsy is the definitive test for establishing the diagnosis of inflammatory myopathy and for excluding other neuromuscular diseases (**Fig. 39-3**). Inflammation is the histologic hallmark for these diseases, but additional features are characteristic of each subtype.

In PM the inflammation is *primary*, a term used to indicate that T cell infiltrates, located primarily within the muscle fascicles (endomysially), surround individual healthy muscle fibers and result in phagocytosis and necrosis. The MHC-I molecule is ubiquitously expressed on the sarcolemma, even in fibers not invaded by CD8+ cells. The CD8/MHC-I lesion is now fundamental for confirming or establishing the diagnosis and to exclude disorders with secondary, nonspecific inflammation.

In DM the endomysial inflammation is predominantly perivascular or in the interfascicular septae and around, rather than within, the muscle fascicles. The intramuscular blood vessels show endothelial hyperplasia with tubuloreticular profiles, fibrin thrombi, and obliteration of capillaries. The muscle fibers undergo necrosis, degeneration, and phagocytosis, often in groups involving a portion of a muscle fascicle in a wedgelike shape or at the periphery of the fascicle, due to microinfarcts within the muscle. This results in perifascicular atrophy, characterized by 2 to 10 layers of atrophic fibers at the periphery of the fascicles. The presence of perifascicular atrophy is diagnostic of DM, *even in the absence of inflammation.*

The histologic features of IBM include endomysial inflammation with T cells invading MHC-I-expressing nonvacuolated muscle fibers; basophilic granular deposits distributed around the edge of slitlike vacuoles (rimmed vacuoles); loss of muscle fibers that are replaced by fat and connective tissue, hypertrophic fibers, and angulated or round fibers; eosinophilic cytoplasmic inclusions; abnormal mitochondria characterized by the

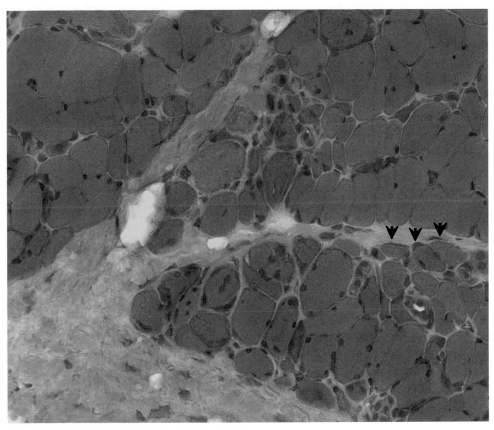

A

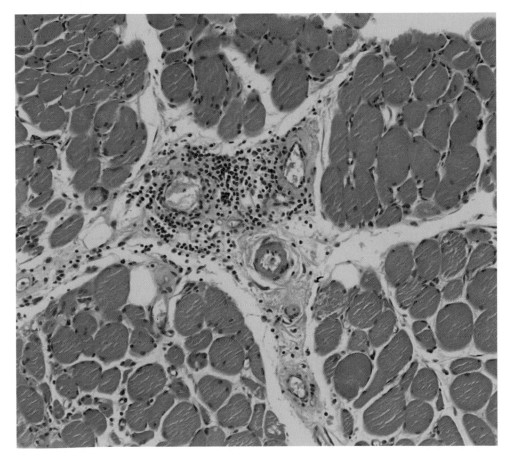

B

FIGURE 39-3

Dermatomyositis. **A**. Quadriceps muscle biopsy revealing myopathic features: (1) internal nuclei, (2) variation in muscle fiber size; *arrowheads* highlight small fibers, and (3) increased connective tissue between myocytes and in the perimysium. There is a predominant perifascicular pattern of muscle fiber atrophy and injury. **B**. Mononuclear inflammatory cell infiltrate within the perimysium with no involvement of the endomysium. (Hematoxylin and eosin, 200X; Courtesy of Dr. Andrew Bollen, Department of Pathology, University of California, San Francisco.)

presence of ragged-red fibers or cytochrome oxidase–negative fibers; amyloid deposits within or next to the vacuoles; and filamentous inclusions seen by electron microscopy in the vicinity of the rimmed vacuoles.

TREATMENT OF PM, DM, AND IBM

The goal of therapy is to improve muscle strength, increase function in activities of daily living, and ameliorate the extramuscular manifestations (rash, dysphagia, dyspnea, fever). When strength improves, the serum CK falls concurrently; however, the reverse is not always true. The common tendency to "chase" or treat the CK level instead of the muscle weakness has led to prolonged and unnecessary use of immunosuppressive drugs and erroneous assessment of their efficacy. It is prudent to discontinue these drugs if, after an adequate trial, there is no objective improvement in muscle strength whether or not CK levels are reduced. A recent Cochrane database review concluded that there is a "lack of high quality randomised controlled trials that assess the efficacy and toxicity of immunosuppressants in inflammatory myositis." Agents used in the treatment of PM and DM include the following:

1. **Glucocorticoids.** Oral prednisone is the initial treatment of choice; the effectiveness and side effects of this therapy determine the future need for stronger immunosuppressive drugs. High-dose prednisone, at least 1 mg/kg per day, is initiated as early in the disease as possible. After 3 to 4 weeks, prednisone is tapered slowly over a period of 10 weeks to 1 mg/kg every other day. If there is evidence of efficacy and no serious side effects, the dosage is then further reduced by 5 or 10 mg every 3 to 4 weeks until the lowest possible dose that controls the disease is reached. The efficacy of prednisone is determined by an objective increase in muscle strength and activities of daily living, which almost always occur by the third month of therapy. A feeling of increased energy or a reduction of the CK level without a concomitant increase in muscle strength is not a reliable sign of improvement. If prednisone provides no objective benefit after ~3 months of high-dose therapy, the disease is probably unresponsive to the drug and tapering should be accelerated while the next-in-line immunosuppressive drug is started. Although controlled

trials have not been performed, almost all patients with true PM or DM respond to glucocorticoids to *some degree and for some period of time*; in general, DM responds better than PM.

The long-term use of prednisone may cause increased weakness associated with a normal or unchanged CK level; this effect is referred to as *steroid myopathy*. In a patient who previously responded to high doses of prednisone, the development of new weakness may be related to steroid myopathy or to disease activity that either will respond to a higher dose of glucocorticoids or has become glucocorticoid-resistant. In uncertain cases, the prednisone dosage can be adjusted arbitrarily: the cause of the weakness is usually evident in 2 to 8 weeks.

2. **Other immunosuppressive drugs.** Approximately 75% of patients ultimately require additional treatment. This occurs when a patient fails to respond adequately to glucocorticoids after a 3-month trial, the patient becomes glucocorticoid-resistant, glucocorticoid-related side effects appear, attempts to lower the prednisone dose repeatedly result in a new relapse, or rapidly progressive disease with evolving severe weakness and respiratory failure develops.

The following drugs are commonly used: (1) *Azathioprine* is well tolerated, has few side effects, and appears to be as effective for long-term therapy as other drugs. The dose is up to 3 mg/kg daily. (2) *Methotrexate* has a faster onset of action than azathioprine. It is given orally starting at 7.5 mg weekly for the first 3 weeks (2.5 mg every 12 h for 3 doses), with gradual dose escalation by 2.5 mg per week to a total of 25 mg weekly. A rare side effect is methotrexate pneumonitis, which can be difficult to distinguish from the interstitial lung disease of the primary myopathy associated with Jo-1 antibodies (described above). (3) *Cyclophosphamide* (0.5 to 1 g IV monthly for 6 months) has limited success and significant toxicity. (4) *Chlorambucil* has variable results. (5) *Cyclosporine* has inconsistent and mild benefit. (6) *Mycophenolate mofetil* has recently shown some effectiveness.

3. **Immunomodulation.** In a controlled trial of patients with refractory DM, intravenous immunoglobulin (IVIg) improved not only strength and rash but also the underlying immunopathology. The benefit is often short-lived (≤8 weeks); repeated infusions every 6 to 8 weeks are generally required to maintain im-

provement. A dose of 2 g/kg divided over 2 to 5 days per course is recommended. Uncontrolled observations suggest that IVIg may also be beneficial for patients with PM. Neither plasmapheresis nor leukapheresis appears to be effective in PM and DM.

The following sequential empirical approach to the treatment of PM and DM is suggested: *step 1*: high-dose prednisone; *step 2*: azathioprine or methotrexate; *step 3*: IVIg; *step 4*: a trial, with guarded optimism, of one of the following agents, chosen according to the patient's age, degree of disability, tolerance, experience with the drug, and general health: cyclosporine, chlorambucil, cyclophosphamide, mycophenolate. Patients with interstitial lung disease may benefit from aggressive treatment with cyclophosphamide.

A patient with presumed PM who has not responded to any form of immunotherapy most likely has IBM or another disease, usually a metabolic myopathy, a muscular dystrophy, a drug-induced myopathy, or an endocrinopathy. In these cases, a repeat muscle biopsy and a renewed search for another cause of the myopathy are indicated.

Calcinosis, a manifestation of DM, is difficult to treat. New calcium deposits may be prevented if the primary disease responds to the available therapies. Diphosphonates, aluminum hydroxide, probenecid, colchicine, low doses of warfarin, calcium blockers, and surgical excision have all been tried without success.

IBM is generally resistant to immunosuppressive therapies. Prednisone together with azathioprine or methotrexate is often tried for a few months in newly diagnosed patients, although results are generally disappointing. Because occasional patients may feel subjectively weaker after these drugs are discontinued, some clinicians prefer to maintain some patients on low-dose, every-other-day prednisone or weekly methotrexate in an effort to halt disease progression, even though there is no objective evidence or controlled study to support this practice. In two controlled studies of IVIg in IBM, minimal benefit in up to 30% of patients was found; the strength gains were not of sufficient magnitude to justify its routine use. Another trial of IVIg combined with prednisone was ineffective. Nonetheless, many experts believe that a 2- to 3-month trial with IVIg may be reasonable for selected patients with IBM who experience rapid progression of muscle weakness or choking episodes due to worsening dysphagia.

PROGNOSIS

The 5-year survival rate for treated patients with PM and DM is ~95% and the 10-year survival 84%; death is usually due to pulmonary, cardiac, or other systemic complications. Patients severely affected at presentation or treated after long delays, those with severe dysphagia or respiratory difficulties, older patients, and those with associated cancer have a worse prognosis. DM responds more favorably to therapy than PM and thus has a better prognosis. Most patients improve with therapy, and many make a full functional recovery that is often sustained with maintenance therapy. Up to 30% may be left with some residual muscle weakness. Relapses may occur at any time.

IBM has the least favorable prognosis of the inflammatory myopathies. Most patients will require the use of an assistive device such as a cane, walker, or wheelchair within 5 to 10 years of onset. In general, the older the age of onset in IBM, the more rapidly progressive the course.

FURTHER READINGS

ASKANAS V, ENGEL WK: Inclusion body myopathies: Different etiologies, possibly similar pathogenic mechanisms. Curr Opin Neurol 15:525, 2002

CHOY E et al: Immunosuppressant and immunomodulatory treatment for dermatomyositis and polymyositis. Cochrane Database Syst Rev (3):CD003643, 2005.

Evidence-based review of current treatments for polymyositis and dermatomyositis.

DALAKAS MC: The molecular and cellular pathology of inflammatory muscle diseases. Curr Opin Pharmacol 1:300, 2001
————: Understanding the immunopathogenesis of inclusion body myositis: Present and future prospects. Rev Neurol 158:948, 2002

————, HOHLFELD R: Polymyositis and dermatomyositis. Lancet. 362:971, 2003

Comprehensive review of clinical features, pathology, and pathogenesis.

HILTON-JONES D: Inflammatory myopathies. Curr Opin Neurol 14:591, 2001
MARIE I et al: Polymyositis and dermatomyositis: Short term and long term outcome and predictive factors of prognosis. J Rheumatol 28:2230, 2001

◪ Mastaglia FL et al: Inflammatory myopathies: Clinical, diagnostic and therapeutic aspects. Muscle Nerve 27:407, 2003

Review of clinical aspects, including genetics, associated conditions, diagnostic assessment.

Ranque-Francois B et al: Familial inflammatory inclusion body myositis. Ann Rheum Dis 64:634, 2005

Sontheimer RD: Dermatomyositis: An overview of recent progress with emphasis on dermatologic aspects. Dermatol Clin 20:387, 2002

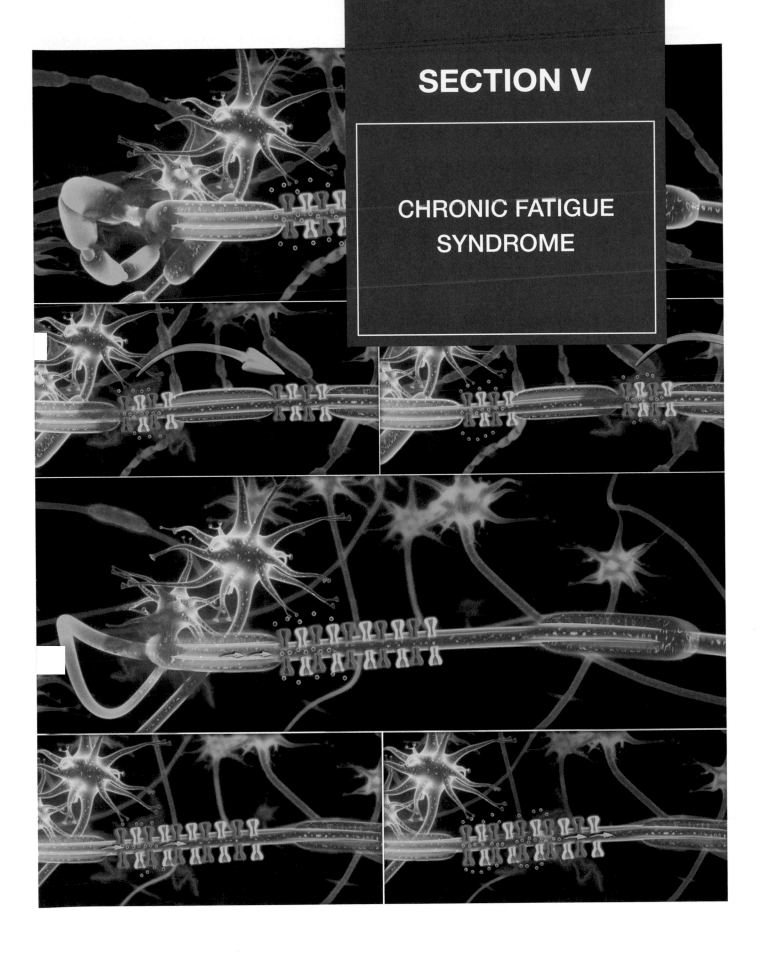

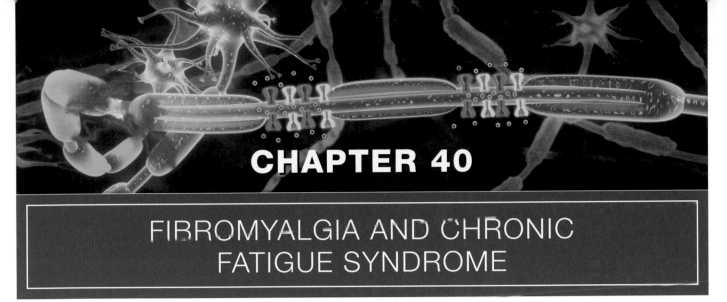

CHAPTER 40

FIBROMYALGIA AND CHRONIC FATIGUE SYNDROME

Bruce C. Gilliland
Stephen E. Straus

FIBROMYALGIA

Fibromyalgia is a commonly encountered disorder characterized by chronic widespread musculoskeletal pain, stiffness, paresthesias, disturbed sleep, and easy fatigability along with multiple painful tender points that are widely and symmetrically distributed. Fibromyalgia affects predominantly women in a ratio of 9 to 1 compared with men. This disorder is found in most countries, in most ethnic groups, and in all types of climates. The prevalence of fibromyalgia in the general population of a community in the United States using the 1990 American College of Rheumatology (ACR) classification criteria (see below) was reported to be 3.4% in women and 0.5% in men. Contrary to some previous reports, fibromyalgia was not found to be present mainly in young women but, rather, to be most prevalent in women ≥ 50 years. The prevalence increased with age, being 7.4% in women between the ages of 70 and 79. Fibromyalgia also occurs in children, although not commonly. The reported prevalence of fibromyalgia in some rheumatology clinics has been as high as 20%. Most patients present with fibromyalgia between the ages of 30 and 50 years.

CLINICAL MANIFESTATIONS

Symptoms are generalized musculoskeletal aching and stiffness and fatigue. Patients may complain of low back pain, which may radiate into the buttocks and legs. Others complain of pain and tightness in the neck and across the upper posterior shoulders. Patients complain of muscle pain after even mild exertion, and some degree of pain is always present. The pain has been described as a burning or gnawing pain or as soreness, stiffness, or aching. Pain may begin in one region, such as the shoulders, neck, or lower back, before it eventually becomes widespread. Patients may complain of joint pain and perceive that their joints are swollen; however, joint examination yields normal findings. Stiffness is usually present on arising in the morning; usually it improves during the day, but in some patients it lasts all day. Patients may complain of numbness of their hands and feet. They may also feel colder overall than others in the home, and some may experience Raynaud's-like phenomena or actual Raynaud's phenomenon. Patients complain of feeling fatigued and exhausted and wake up tired. They also awaken frequently at night and have trouble falling back to sleep. Patients may experience cognitive impairment with difficulty thinking and loss of short-term memory. Headaches, including migraine type, also are common symptoms. Others experience episodes of light-headedness, dizziness, anxiety, or depression. Symptoms are made worse by stress or anxiety, cold, damp weather, and overexertion. Patients often feel better during warmer weather and vacations.

The characteristic feature on physical examination is the demonstration of specific sites or points that are more tender or painful than the same sites in normal individuals. The ACR Criteria for Fibromyalgia define 18 tender points. These points of tenderness are remarkably constant in location. A moderate and consistent degree of pressure should be used in digital palpation of these tender points. As a guideline to reduce variability in the interpretation of point tenderness, the amount of force applied should be 4 kg (~9 lb), which is the degree of force required to just blanch the examiner's thumbnail. This amount of pressure does not produce significant tenderness or pain in normal subjects. Some workers recommend that the tender site be palpated using a rolling motion, which may be more effective in eliciting the tenderness. The tender sites can also be examined using a dolorimeter, which is a spring-loaded pressure gauge; however, digital palpation appears to be as effective and accurate. Some investigators have quantitated the degree of tenderness or pain, but the number of tender point sites is more diagnostic. Some patients are tender all over although still more tender or painful at the specific tender point sites.

Skinfold tenderness may be present, particularly over the upper scapular region. Subcutaneous nodules may be felt at sites of tenderness. Nodules in similar locations are present in normal persons but are not tender.

Fibromyalgia may be triggered by emotional stress, infections and other medical illness, surgery, hypothyroidism, and trauma. It has appeared in some patients with hepatitis C infection, HIV infection, parvovirus B19 infection, or Lyme disease. In the latter situation, fibromyalgia may persist despite adequate antibiotic treatment for Lyme disease, and especially anxious patients may believe that they still have Lyme disease. Disorders commonly associated with fibromyalgia include irritable bowel syndrome, irritable bladder, headaches (including migraine headaches), dysmenorrhea, premenstrual syndrome, restless leg syndrome, temporomandibular joint pain, noncardiac chest pain, Raynaud's phenomenon, and sicca syndrome.

The course of fibromyalgia is variable. Symptoms wax and wane in some patients, while in others pain and fatigue are persistent regardless of therapy. Studies from tertiary medical centers indicate a poor prognosis for most patients. The prognosis may be better in community-treated patients. In a community-based study reported after 2 years of treatment, 24% of patients were in remission, and 47% no longer fulfilled the ACR criteria for fibromyalgia.

DIAGNOSIS

Fibromyalgia is diagnosed by a history of widespread musculoskeletal pain present for at least 3 months and the demonstration of significant tenderness or pain in at least 11 of the 18 tender point sites on digital palpation. The ACR criteria are useful for standardizing the diagnosis; however, not all patients with fibromyalgia meet these criteria (**Table 40-1**). Some patients have fewer tender sites and more regional pain and may be considered to have fibromyalgia.

The musculoskeletal and neurologic examinations are normal in fibromyalgia patients, and there are no laboratory abnormalities. Fibromyalgia may occur in patients with rheumatoid arthritis, systemic lupus erythematosus (SLE), other connective tissue diseases,

TABLE 40-1

THE AMERICAN COLLEGE OF RHEUMATOLOGY 1990 CRITERIA FOR THE CLASSIFICATION OF FIBROMYALGIA[a]

1. History of widespread pain. Pain is considered widespread when all of the following are present:
   a. Pain in the left side of the body
   b. Pain in the right side of the body
   c. Pain above the waist
   d. Pain below the waist
   e. Axial skeletal pain (cervical spine or anterior chest or thoracic spine or low back)
2. Pain on digital palpation in at least 11 of the following 18 tender point sites:
   a. Occiput: bilateral, at the suboccipital muscle insertion
   b. Low cervical: bilateral, at the anterior aspect of the intertransverse spaces at C5–7
   c. Trapezius: bilateral, at the midpoint of the upper border
   d. Supraspinatus: bilateral, at the origin, above the scapular spine near the medial border
   e. Second rib: bilateral, at the second costochondral junction, just lateral to the junction on the upper surface
   f. Lateral epicondyle: bilateral, 2 cm distal to the epicondyle
   g. Gluteal: bilateral, in the upper outer quadrant of the buttock
   h. Greater trochanter: bilateral, posterior to the trochanteric prominence
   i. Knee: bilateral, at the medial fat pad proximal to the joint line

Digital palpation should be performed with a moderate degree of pressure. For a tender point to be considered positive, the subject must state that the palpation was painful. "Tender" is not to be considered painful.

[a]For purposes of classification, patients will be said to have fibromyalgia if both criteria are satisfied. Widespread pain must have been present for at least 3 months. The presence of a second clinical disorder does not exclude the diagnosis of fibromyalgia.
Source: Modified from F Wolfe et al: Arthritis Rheum 33:171, 1990.

or other medical illness. A distinction is no longer made between primary and secondary fibromyalgia (concomitant with other disease), as the signs and symptoms are similar. Patients with fibromyalgia may be misdiagnosed with SLE or Sjögren's syndrome as these disorders have in common symptoms of musculoskeletal pain, dry eyes, cold hands, and fatigue. The antinuclear antibody (ANA) test may be positive. The frequency of a positive ANA test in fibromyalgia patients, however, is the same as sex- and age-matched normal controls. The predictive value of a positive ANA test in patients without characteristic symptoms and objective features of a connective tissue disease is quite low. Discretion is advised before ordering an ANA test. Patients with fibromyalgia may complain of muscle weakness, but on muscle strength testing, they have "giveaway" weakness secondary to pain. Proximal muscle weakness and elevated muscle enzymes distinguish patients with polymyositis. Polymyalgia rheumatica is distinguished from fibromyalgia in an elderly patient by the presence of more proximal muscle stiffness and pain and an elevated erythrocyte sedimentation rate. Patients should be evaluated for hypothyroidism, which may have symptoms similar to fibromyalgia or may accompany fibromyalgia. Disturbed sleep, musculoskeletal pain, and fatigue occur in patients with sleep apnea and restless leg syndrome. A distinguishing feature of sleep apnea is the presence of significant daytime somnolence. These patients should be referred to a sleep laboratory for evaluation and treatment. Myofascial pain syndrome, which involves an area such as the shoulder or neck, may represent a localized form of fibromyalgia. Some patients with this syndrome progress to fibromyalgia.

The diagnosis of fibromyalgia has taken on a more complex significance in regard to labor and industry issues. This has become a significant issue since it has been reported that 10 to 25% of patients are not able to work in any capacity, while others require modification of their work. Disability evaluation in fibromyalgia is controversial. The diagnosis of fibromyalgia is not accepted by all. It is hard to evaluate patients' perceptions of their inability to function. The determination of tender points can be subjective, on the part of both the physician and the patient, particularly when issues of compensation are pending. Patients also encounter difficulty in having their illness recognized as a disability. Physicians have been placed in the inappropriate role of assessing the patient's disability. Physicians are not in a position to quantitate disability at the workplace; that is better done by a work evaluation specialist. Better instruments are clearly needed for measuring disability, particularly in patients with fibromyalgia.

TREATMENT FOR FIBROMYALGIA

Patients should be informed that they have a condition that is not crippling, deforming, or degenerative, and that treatment is available. The initial step in treatment is to improve the quality of sleep. The use of tricyclics such as amitriptyline (10 to 50 mg), nortriptyline (10 to 75 mg), and doxepin (10 to 25 mg) or a pharmacologically similar drug, cyclobenzaprine (10 to 40 mg), 1 to 2 h before bedtime will give the patient restorative sleep (stage 4 sleep), resulting in clinical improvement. Patients should be started on a low dose, which is increased gradually as needed. Side effects of these tricyclics and cyclobenzaprine limit their use; these include constipation, dry mouth, weight gain, drowsiness, and difficulty thinking. Trazodone or zolpidem also improves sleep quality. In patients with restless leg syndrome, clonazepam may be effective. Depression and anxiety should next be treated with appropriate drugs and, when indicated, with psychiatric counseling. Fluoxetine, sertraline, paroxetine, citalopram, or other newer selective serotonin reuptake inhibitors can be used as antidepressants. Other useful antidepressants are trazodone and venlafaxine. Alprazolam and lorazepam are effective for anxiety. Patients may also benefit by regular aerobic exercises, which are started after patients begin to have improved sleep and less pain and fatigue. Exercise should be of a low-impact type and begun at a low level. Eventually, the patient should be exercising 20 to 30 min 3 to 4 days a week. Regular stretching exercises also are very important. Salicylates or other nonsteroidal anti-inflammatory drugs (NSAIDs) only partially improve symptoms. Glucocorticoids have been of little benefit and should not be used in these patients. Opiate analgesics should be avoided. For pain, acetaminophen or tramadol may be useful. Gabapentin (300 to 1200 mg/d in divided doses) also may reduce pain. Local measures such as heat, massage, injection of tender sites with steroids or lidocaine, and acupuncture provide only temporary relief of symptoms. Other therapies that may help to varying degrees include biofeedback, behavioral modification, hypnotherapy, and stress management and relaxation response training. Life stresses should be identified and discussed with the patient, and the patient should be provided with help on how to cope with these stresses. Patients may benefit from a multidisciplinary team approach involving a mental health professional, a physical therapist, and a physical medicine and rehabilitation specialist. Group therapy may be beneficial. Patients should be well educated about their disorder and taught the importance of self-help. There are patient support groups in many communities. While treatment of fibromyalgia is effective in some patients, others continue to have chronic disease that is relieved only partially if at all.

CHRONIC FATIGUE SYNDROME

DEFINITION

Chronic fatigue syndrome (CFS) is the current name for a disorder characterized by debilitating fatigue and several associated physical, constitutional, and neuropsychological complaints. This syndrome is not new; in the past, patients diagnosed with conditions such as the vapors, neurasthenia, effort syndrome, chronic brucellosis, epidemic neuromyasthenia, myalgic encephalomyelitis, hypoglycemia, multiple chemical sensitivity syndrome, chronic candidiasis, chronic mononucleosis, chronic Epstein-Barr virus infection, and postviral fatigue syndrome may have had what is now called CFS. A subset of ill veterans of military campaigns suffer from CFS. The U.S. Centers for Disease Control and Prevention (CDC) has developed diagnostic criteria for CFS based on symptoms and the exclusion of other illnesses (**Table 40–2**).

EPIDEMIOLOGY

Patients with CFS are twice as likely to be women as men and are generally 25 to 45 years old, although cases in childhood and in later life have been described.

Estimates of the prevalence of CFS have depended on the case definition used and the method of study. Chronic fatigue itself is a common symptom, occurring in as many as 20% of patients attending general medical clinics; CFS is far less common. Community-based studies find that 100 to 300 individuals per 100,000 population in the United States meet the current CDC case definition.

PATHOGENESIS

The diverse names for the syndrome reflect the many and controversial hypotheses about its etiology. Several common themes underlie attempts to understand the disorder: it is often postinfectious, it is associated with

TABLE 40-2

CDC CRITERIA FOR DIAGNOSIS OF CHRONIC FATIGUE SYNDROME

A case of chronic fatigue syndrome is defined by the presence of

1. Clinically evaluated, unexplained, persistent or relapsing fatigue that is of new or definite onset; is not the result of ongoing exertion; is not alleviated by rest; and results in substantial reduction of previous levels of occupational, educational, social, or personal activities; and
2. Four or more of the following symptoms that persist or recur during 6 or more consecutive months of illness and that do not predate the fatigue:
   - Self-reported impairment in short-term memory or concentration
   - Sore throat
   - Tender cervical or axillary nodes
   - Muscle pain
   - Multijoint pain without redness or swelling
   - Headaches of a new pattern or severity
   - Unrefreshing sleep
   - Postexertional malaise lasting ≥ 24 h

Note: CDC, U.S. Centers for Disease Control and Prevention.
Source: Adapted from K Fukuda et al: Ann Intern Med 121:953, 1994; with permission.

immunologic disturbances, and it is commonly accompanied or even preceded by neuropsychological complaints, somatic preoccupation, and/or depression.

Many studies in the 1980s and 1990s attempted to link CFS to infection with Epstein-Barr virus, a retrovirus, or an enterovirus. In many patients with chronic fatigue, titers of antibodies to several viruses are elevated. Reports that viral antigens and nucleic acids could be specifically identified in patients with CFS have not been confirmed.

Mild to moderate depression is present in half to two-thirds of patients. Much of this depression may be reactive, but its prevalence exceeds that seen in other chronic medical illnesses. Some propose that CFS is fundamentally a psychiatric disorder and that the various neuroendocrine and immune disturbances arise secondarily.

MANIFESTATIONS

Typically, CFS arises suddenly in a previously active individual. An otherwise unremarkable flulike illness or some other acute stress leaves unbearable exhaustion in its wake. Other symptoms, such as headache, sore throat, tender lymph nodes, muscle and joint aches, and frequent feverishness, lead to the belief that an infection persists, and medical attention is sought. Over several weeks, despite reassurances that nothing serious is wrong, the symptoms persist and other features of the syndrome become evident—disturbed sleep, difficulty in concentration, and depression.

DIAGNOSIS

A thorough history, physical examination, and judicious use of laboratory tests are required to exclude other causes of the patient's symptoms. Prominent abnormalities argue strongly in favor of alternative diagnoses. No laboratory test, however, can diagnose this condition or measure its severity. In most cases, elaborate, expensive workups are not helpful. The dilemma for patient and clinician alike is that CFS has no pathognomonic features and remains a constellation of symptoms and a diagnosis of exclusion. Often the patient presents with features that also meet criteria for other subjective disorders such as fibromyalgia and irritable bowel syndrome.

TREATMENT FOR CFS

After other illnesses have been excluded, there are several points to address in the long-term care of a patient with chronic fatigue.

The patient should be informed about the illness and what is known of its pathogenesis; its potential impact on the physical, psychological, and social dimensions of life; and its prognosis. Patients are relieved when their complaints are taken seriously. Periodic reassessment is appropriate to identify a possible underlying process that is late in declaring itself and to address intercurrent symptoms that should not be simply dismissed as yet another subjective complaint.

Many symptoms of CFS respond to treatment. NSAIDs alleviate headache, diffuse pain, and feverishness. Allergic rhinitis and sinusitis are common; antihistamines or decongestants may be helpful. Although the patient may be averse to psychiatric diagnoses, depression and anxiety are often prominent and should be treated. Expert psychiatric assessment is sometimes advisable. Nonsedating antidepressants improve mood and disordered sleep and may attenuate the fatigue. Even modest improvements in symptoms can make an important difference in the patient's degree of self-sufficiency and ability to appreciate life's pleasures.

Practical advice should be given regarding lifestyle. Sleep disturbances are common; con-

sumption of heavy meals with alcohol and caffeine at night can make sleep even more elusive, compounding fatigue. Total rest leads to further deconditioning and the self-image of being an invalid, whereas overexertion may worsen exhaustion and lead to total avoidance of exercise. A moderate, carefully graded regimen should be encouraged and has been proven to relieve symptoms and enhance exercise tolerance.

Controlled therapeutic trials have established that acyclovir, fludrocortisone, and intravenous immunoglobulin, among others, are of little or no value in CFS. Low doses of hydrocortisone provide modest benefit, but they may lead to adrenal suppression. Countless anecdotes circulate regarding other traditional and nontraditional therapies. It is important to guide patients away from those therapeutic modalities that are toxic, expensive, or unreasonable.

The physician should promote the patient's efforts to recover. Controlled trials in the United Kingdom, in Australia, and in the Netherlands showed cognitive-behavioral therapy to be helpful. This approach aims to dispel misguided beliefs and fears about CFS that can contribute to inactivity and despair. For CFS, as for many other conditions, a comprehensive approach to physical, psychological, and social aspects of well-being is in order.

FURTHER READINGS

Alfari N, Buchwald D: Chronic fatigue syndrome: A review. Am J Psychiatry 160:221, 2003

☑ Goldenberg DL et al: Management of fibromyalgia syndrome. JAMA 19:2388, 2004

A good comprehensive review detailing the evidence for pharmacologic and nonpharmacologic treatment of fibromyalgia.

Mannerkorpi K: Exercise in fibromyalgia. Curr Opin Rheumatol 17:190, 2005

Reid S et al: Chronic fatigue syndrome. Clin Evid 12:1578, 2004

☑ Whiting P et al: Interventions for the treatment and management of chronic fatigue syndrome: A systematic review. JAMA 286:1360, 2001

Nicely summarizes the evidence for various proposed treatments of CFS.

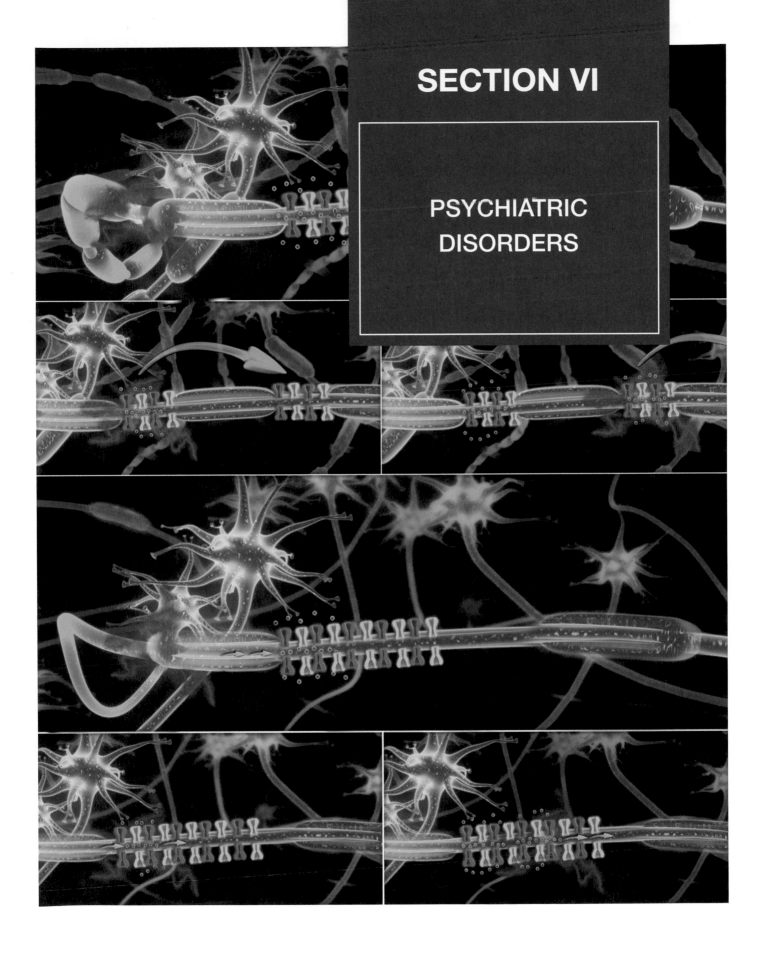

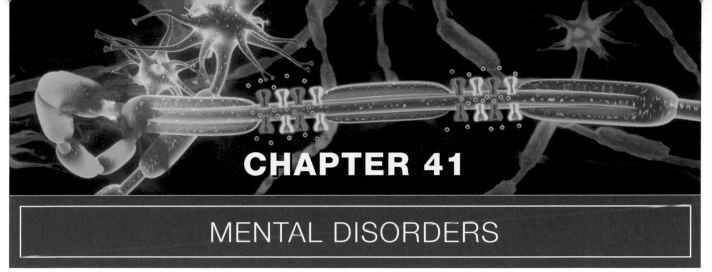

CHAPTER 41

MENTAL DISORDERS

Victor I. Reus

Mental disorders are common in medical practice and may present either as a primary disorder or as a comorbid condition. The prevalence of mental or substance use disorders in the United States is 18.5%, resulting in an annual cost of $148 billion, only slightly less than the costs of cardiovascular diseases. Only 15% of these individuals are currently receiving treatment.

The revised 4th edition for use by primary care physicians of the *Diagnostic and Statistical Manual* (DSM-IV-PC) provides a useful synopsis of mental disorders most likely to be seen in primary care practice. The current system of classification is multiaxial and includes the presence or absence of a major mental disorder (axis I), any underlying personality disorder (axis II), general medical condition (axis III), psychosocial and environmental problems (axis IV), and overall rating of general psychosocial functioning (axis V).

ANXIETY DISORDERS

Anxiety disorders, the most prevalent psychiatric illnesses in the general community, are present in 15 to 20% of medical clinic patients. Anxiety, defined as a subjective sense of unease, dread, or foreboding, can indicate a primary psychiatric condition or can be a component of, or reaction to, a primary medical disease. The primary anxiety disorders are classified according to their duration and course and the existence and nature of precipitants.

When evaluating the anxious patient, the clinician must first determine whether the anxiety antedates or postdates a medical illness or is due to a medication side effect. Approximately one-third of patients presenting with anxiety have a medical etiology for their psychiatric symptoms, but an anxiety disorder can also present with somatic symptoms in the absence of a diagnosable medical condition.

PANIC DISORDER

Clinical Manifestations

Panic disorder is defined by the presence of recurrent and unpredictable panic attacks, which are distinct episodes of intense fear and discomfort associated with a variety of physical symptoms, including palpitations, sweating, trembling, shortness of breath, chest pain, dizziness, and a fear of impending doom or death (**Table 41-1**). Paresthesias, gastrointestinal distress, and feelings of unreality also are common. Diagnostic criteria also require at least 1 month of concern or worry about the attacks or a change in behavior related to them. The lifetime prevalence of panic disorder is 1 to 3%. Panic attacks have a sudden onset, developing within 10 min and usually resolving over the course of an hour, and they occur in an unexpected fashion. The frequency and severity of panic attacks vary, ranging from once a week to clusters of attacks separated by months of well-being. The first attack is usually outside the home, and onset is typically in late adolescence to early adulthood. In some individuals, anticipatory anxiety develops over time and results in a generalized fear and a progressive avoidance of places or situations in which a panic attack might recur. *Agoraphobia,* which occurs commonly in patients

TABLE 41-1

DIAGNOSTIC CRITERIA FOR PANIC ATTACK

A discrete period of intense fear or discomfort, in which four or more of the following symptoms developed abruptly and reached a peak within 10 min:

1. Palpitations, pounding heart, or accelerated heart rate
2. Sweating
3. Trembling or shaking
4. Sensations of shortness of breath or smothering
5. Feeling of choking
6. Chest pain or discomfort
7. Nausea or abdominal distress
8. Feeling dizzy, unsteady, lightheaded, or faint
9. Derealization (feelings of unreality) or depersonalization (being detached from oneself)
10. Fear of losing control or going crazy
11. Fear of dying
12. Paresthesias (numbness or tingling sensations)
13. Chills or hot flushes

Source: Reprinted with permission from the Diagnostic and Statistical Manual of Mental Disorders, Fourth Edition, Text Revision (Copyright 2000). American Psychiatric Association.

with panic disorder, is an acquired irrational fear of being in places where one might feel trapped or unable to escape (**Table 41–2**). Typically, it leads the patient into a progressive restriction in lifestyle and, in a literal sense, in geography. Frequently, patients are embarrassed that they

TABLE 41-2

DIAGNOSTIC CRITERIA FOR AGORAPHOBIA

1. Anxiety about being in places or situations from which escape might be difficult (or embarrassing) or in which help may not be available in the event of having an unexpected or situationally predisposed panic attack or panic-like symptoms. Agoraphobic fears typically involve characteristic clusters of situations that include being outside the home alone; being in a crowd or standing in a line; being on a bridge; and traveling in a bus, train, or automobile.
2. The situations are avoided (e.g., travel is restricted) or else are endured with marked distress or with anxiety about having a panic attack or panic-like symptoms, or require the presence of a companion.
3. The anxiety or phobic avoidance is not better accounted for by another mental disorder, such as social phobia (e.g., avoidance limited to social situations because of fear of embarrassment), specific phobia (e.g., avoidance limited to a single situation like elevators), obsessive-compulsive disorder (e.g., avoidance of dirt in someone with an obsession about contamination), posttraumatic stress disorder (e.g., avoidance of stimuli associated with a severe stressor), or separation anxiety disorder (e.g., avoidance of leaving home or relatives).

Source: Reprinted with permission from the Diagnostic and Statistical Manual of Mental Disorders, Fourth Edition, Text Revision (Copyright 2000). American Psychiatric Association.

are housebound and dependent on the company of others to go out into the world and do not volunteer this information; thus physicians will fail to recognize the syndrome if direct questioning is not pursued.

Differential Diagnosis

A diagnosis of panic disorder is made after a medical etiology for the panic attacks has been ruled out. A variety of cardiovascular, respiratory, endocrine, and neurologic conditions can present with anxiety as the chief complaint. Patients with true panic disorder will often focus on one specific feature to the exclusion of others. For example, 20% of patients who present with syncope as a primary medical complaint have a primary diagnosis of a mood, anxiety, or substance-abuse disorder, the most common being panic disorder. The differential diagnosis of panic disorder is complicated by a high rate of comorbidity with other psychiatric conditions, especially alcohol and benzodiazepine abuse, which patients initially use in an attempt at self-medication. Some 75% of panic disorder patients will also satisfy criteria for major depression at some point in their illness.

When the history is nonspecific, physical examination and focused laboratory testing must be used to rule out anxiety states resulting from medical disorders such as pheochromocytoma, thyrotoxicosis, or hypoglycemia. Electrocardiogram (ECG) and echocardiogram may detect some cardiovascular conditions associated with panic, such as paroxysmal atrial tachycardia and mitral valve prolapse. In two studies, panic disorder was the primary diagnosis in 43% of patients with chest pain who had normal coronary angiograms and was present in 9% of all outpatients referred for cardiac evaluation. Panic disorder has also been diagnosed in many patients referred for pulmonary function testing or with symptoms of irritable bowel syndrome.

TREATMENT FOR PANIC DISORDER

Achievable goals of treatment are to decrease the frequency of panic attacks and to reduce their intensity. The cornerstone of drug therapy is antidepressant medication (**Tables 41-3, 41-4,** and **41-5**). The tricyclic antidepressants (TCAs) imipramine and clomipramine benefit 75 to 90% of panic disorder patients. Low doses (e.g., 10 to 25 mg/d) are given initially to avoid transient increased anxiety associated with heightened monoamine levels. Selective serotonin reuptake inhibitors (SSRIs) are equally effective and do not have the adverse effects of TCAs. SSRIs should be started at one-third to

TABLE 41-3

ANTIDEPRESSANTS

NAME	USUAL DAILY DOSE, MG	SIDE EFFECTS	COMMENTS
SSRIs			
Fluoxetine (Prozac)	10–80	Headache; nausea and other GI effects; jitteriness; insomnia; sexual dysfunction; can affect plasma levels of other meds (except sertraline); akathisia rare; caution in children and adolescents given possible increased risk of suicidal ideation after therapy initiation	Once daily dosing, usually In A.M.; fluoxetine has very long half-life; must not be combined with MAOIs
Sertraline (Zoloft)	50–200		
Paroxetine (Paxil)	20–60		
Fluvoxamine (Luvox)	100–300		
Citalopram (Celexa)	20–60		
Escitalopram (Lexapro)	10–30		
Duloxetine (Cymbalta)	40-60		
TCAs			
Amitriptyline (Elavil)	150–300	Anticholinergic (dry mouth, tachycardia, constipation, urinary retention, blurred vision); sweating; tremor; postural hypotension; cardiac conduction delay; sedation; weight gain	Once daily dosing, usually qhs; blood levels of most TCAs available; can be lethal in O.D (lethal dose = 2 g); nortriptyline best tolerated, especially by elderly
Nortriptyline (Pamelor)	50–200		
Imipramine (Tofranil)	150–300		
Desipramine (Norpramin)	150–300		
Doxepin (Sinequan)	150–300		
Clomipramine (Anafranil)	150–300		
MIXED NOREPINEPHRINE/ SEROTONIN REUPTAKE INHIBITORS			
Venlafaxine (Effexor)	75–375	Nausea; dizziness; dry mouth; headaches; increased blood pressure; anxiety and insomnia	Bid-tid dosing (extended release available); lower potential for drug interactions than SSRIs; contraindicated with MAOIs
Mirtazapine (Remeron)	15–45	Somnolence; weight gain; neutropenia rare	Once daily dosing
MIXED-ACTION DRUGS			
Bupropion (Wellbutrin)	250–450	Jitteriness; flushing; seizures in at-risk patients; anorexia; tachycardia; psychosis	Tid dosing, but sustained release also available; fewer sexual side effects than SSRIs or TCAs; may be useful for adult ADD
Trazodone (Desyrel)	200–600	Sedation; dry mouth; ventricular irritability; postural hypotension; priapism rare	Useful in low doses for sleep because of sedating effects with no anticholinergic side effects
Nefazodone (Serzone)	300–600	Sedation; headache; dry mouth; nausea; constipation	Once daily dosing; no effect on REM sleep unlike other antidepressants
Amoxapine (Asendin)	200–600	Sexual dysfunction	Lethality in overdose; EPS possible
MAOIs			
Phenelzine (Nardil)	45–90	Insomnia; hypotension; anorgasmia; weight gain; hypertensive crisis; tyramine cheese reaction; lethal reactions with SSRIs; serious reactions with narcotics	May be more effective in patients with atypical features or treatment-refractory depression
Tranylcypromine (Parnate)	20–50		
Isocarboxazid (Marplan)	20–60		

Note: ADD, attention deficit disorder; EPS, extrapyramidal symptoms; MAOI, monoamine oxidase inhibitor; REM, rapid eye movement; SSRI, selective serotonin reuptake inhibitor; TCA, tricyclic antidepressant.

TABLE 41-4

MANAGEMENT OF ANTIDEPRESSANT SIDE EFFECTS

SYMPTOMS	COMMENTS AND MANAGEMENT STRATEGIES
Gastrointestinal	
Nausea, loss of appetite	Usually short-lived and dose-related; consider temporary dose reduction or administration with food and antacids
Diarrhea	Famotidine, 20–40 mg/d
Constipation	Wait for tolerance; try diet change, stool softener, exercise; avoid laxatives
Sexual dysfunction	Consider dose reduction; drug holiday
Anorgasmia/impotence; impaired ejaculation	Bethanechol, 10–20 mg, 2 h before activity, or cyproheptadine, 4–8 mg 2 h before activity, or bupropion, 100 mg bid or amantadine, 100 mg bid/tid
Orthostasis	Tolerance unlikely; increase fluid intake, use calf exercises/support hose; fludrocortisone, 0.025 mg/d
Anticholinergic	Wait for tolerance
Dry mouth, eyes	Maintain good oral hygiene; use artificial tears, sugar-free gum
Tremor/jitteriness	Antiparkinsonian drugs not effective; use dose reduction/slow increase; lorazepam, 0.5 mg bid, or propranolol, 10–20 mg bid
Insomnia	Schedule all doses for the morning; trazodone, 50–100 mg qhs
Sedation	Caffeine; schedule all dosing for bedtime; bupropion, 75–100 mg in afternoon
Headache	Evaluate diet, stress, other drugs; try dose reduction; amitriptyline, 50 mg/d
Weight gain	Decrease carbohydrates; exercise; consider fluoxetine
Loss of therapeutic benefit over time	Related to tolerance? Increase dose or drug holiday; add amantadine, 100 mg bid, buspirone, 10 mg tid, or pindolol, 2.5 mg bid

TABLE 41-5

POSSIBLE DRUG INTERACTIONS WITH SELECTIVE SEROTONIN REUPTAKE INHIBITORS

AGENT	EFFECT
Monoamine oxidase inhibitors	Serotonin syndrome—absolute contraindication
Serotonergic agonists, e.g., tryptophan, fenfluramine	Potential serotonin syndrome
Drugs that are metabolized by P450 isoenzymes: tricyclics, other SSRIs, antipsychotics, beta blockers, codeine, terfenadine, astemizole, triazolobenzodiazepines, calcium channel blockers	Delayed metabolism resulting in increased blood levels and potential toxicity—possible fatality secondary to QT prolongation with terfenadine or astemizole
Drugs that are bound tightly to plasma proteins, e.g., warfarin	Increased bleeding secondary to displacement
Drugs that inhibit the metabolism of SSRIs by P450 isoenzymes, e.g., quinidine	Increased SSRI side effects

Note: SSRI, selective serotonin reuptake inhibitor.

one-half of their usual antidepressant dose (e.g., 5 to 10 mg fluoxetine, 25 to 50 mg sertraline, 10 mg paroxetine). Monoamine oxidase inhibitors (MAOIs) also are effective and may specifically benefit patients who have comorbid features of atypical depression (i.e., hypersomnia and weight gain). Insomnia, orthostatic hypotension, and the need to maintain a low-tyramine diet (avoidance of cheese and wine) have limited their use, however. Antidepressants typically take 2 to 6 weeks to become effective, and doses may need to be adjusted based on the clinical response.

Because of anticipatory anxiety and the need for immediate relief of panic symptoms, benzodiazepines are useful early in the course of treatment and sporadically thereafter (**Table 41-6**). For example, alprazolam, starting at 0.5 mg qid and increasing to 4 mg/d in divided doses, is effective, but patients must be monitored closely, as some develop dependence and begin to escalate the dose of this medication. Clonazepam, at a final maintenance dose of 2 to 4 mg/d, also is helpful; its longer half-life permits twice-daily dosing, and patients appear less likely to develop dependence on this agent.

Early psychotherapeutic intervention and education aimed at symptom control enhances the effectiveness of drug treatment. Patients can be taught breathing techniques, can be educated about physiologic changes that occur with panic, and can learn to expose themselves voluntarily to precipitating events in a treatment program spanning 12 to 15 sessions. Homework assignments and monitored compliance are important components of successful treatment. Once patients have achieved a satisfactory response, drug treatment should be maintained for 1 to 2 years to prevent relapse. Controlled trials indicate a success rate of 75 to 85%, although the likelihood of complete remission is somewhat lower.

GENERALIZED ANXIETY DISORDER

Clinical Manifestations

Patients with generalized anxiety disorder (GAD) have persistent, excessive, and/or unrealistic worry associated with muscle tension, impaired concentration, autonomic arousal, feeling "on edge" or restless, and insomnia (**Table 41-7**). Onset is usually before age 20, and a history of childhood fears and social inhibition may be present. The lifetime prevalence of GAD is 5 to 6%; the risk is higher in first-degree relatives of patients with the

diagnosis. Interestingly, family studies indicate that GAD and panic disorder segregate independently. More than 80% of patients with GAD also suffer from major depression, dysthymia, or social phobia. Comorbid substance abuse is common in these patients, particularly alcohol and/or sedative/hypnotic abuse. Patients with GAD worry excessively over minor matters, with life-disrupting effects; unlike in panic disorder, complaints of shortness of breath, palpitations, and tachycardia are relatively rare.

TREATMENT FOR GAD

A combination of pharmacologic and psychotherapeutic interventions is most effective in GAD, but complete symptomatic relief is rare. A short course of a benzodiazepine is usually indicated, preferably lorazepam, oxazepam, or temazepam. (The first two of these agents are metabolized via conjugation rather than oxidation and thus do not accumulate if hepatic function is altered.) Administration should be initiated at the lowest dose possible and prescribed on an as-needed basis as symptoms warrant. Benzodiazepines differ in their milligram per kilogram potency, half-life, lipid solubility, metabolic pathways, and presence of active metabolites. Agents that are absorbed rapidly and are lipid soluble, such as diazepam, have a rapid onset of action and a higher abuse potential. Benzodiazepines should generally not be prescribed for >4 to 6 weeks because of the development of tolerance and the risk of abuse and dependence. It is important to warn patients that concomitant use of alcohol or other sedating drugs may be neurotoxic and impair their ability to function. An optimistic approach that encourages the patient to clarify environmental precipitants, anticipate his or her reactions, and plan effective response strategies is an essential element of therapy.

Adverse effects of benzodiazepines generally parallel their relative half-lives. Longer-acting agents, such as diazepam, chlordiazepoxide, flurazepam, and clonazepam, tend to accumulate active metabolites, with resultant sedation, impairment of cognition, and poor psychomotor performance. Shorter-acting compounds, such as alprazolam and oxazepam, can produce daytime anxiety, early morning insomnia, and, with discontinuation, rebound anxiety and insomnia. Although patients develop tolerance to the sedative effects of benzodiazepines, they are less

TABLE 41-6

ANXIOLYTICS

NAME	EQUIVALENT PO DOSE, MG	ONSET OF ACTION	HALF-LIFE, H	COMMENTS
BENZODIAZEPINES				
Diazepam (Valium)	5	Fast	20–70	Active metabolites; quite sedating
Flurazepam (Dalmane)	15	Fast	30–100	Flurazepam is a prodrug; metabolites are active; quite sedating
Triazolam (Halcion)	0.25	Intermediate	1.5–5	No active metabolites; can induce confusion and delirium, especially in elderly
Lorazepam (Ativan)	1	Intermediate	10–20	No active metabolites; direct hepatic glucuronide conjugation; quite sedating
Alprazolam (Xanax)	0.5	Intermediate	12–15	Active metabolites; not too sedating; may have specific antidepressant and antipanic activity; tolerance and dependence develop easily
Chlordiazepoxide (Librium)	10	Intermediate	5–30	Active metabolites; moderately sedating
Oxazepam (Serax)	15	Slow	5–15	No active metabolites; direct glucuronide conjugation; not too sedating
Temazepam (Restoril)	15	Slow	9–12	No active metabolites; moderately sedating
Clonazepam (Klonopin)	0.5	Slow	18–50	No active metabolites; moderately sedating
NON-BENZODIAZEPINES				
Buspirone (BuSpar)	7.5	2 weeks	2–3	Active metabolites; tid dosing—usual daily dose 10–20 mg tid; nonsedating; no additive effects with alcohol; useful for agitation in demented or brain-injured patients

likely to habituate to the adverse psychomotor effects. Withdrawal from the longer-half-life benzodiazepines can be accomplished through gradual, stepwise dose reduction (by 10% every 1 to 2 weeks) over 6 to 12 weeks. It is usually more difficult to taper patients off shorter-acting benzodiazepines. Physicians may need to switch the patient to a benzodiazepine with a longer half-life or use an adjunctive medication, such as a beta blocker or carbamazepine, before attempting to discontinue the benzodiazepine. Withdrawal reactions vary in severity and duration; they can include depression, anxiety, delirium, lethargy, diaphoresis, tinnitus, autonomic arousal, adventitious movements, and, rarely, seizures.

Buspirone is a nonbenzodiazepine anxiolytic agent. It is nonsedating, does not produce tolerance or dependence, does not interact with benzodiazepine receptors or alcohol, and has no abuse or disinhibition potential. However, it requires several weeks to take effect and requires thrice-daily dosing. Patients who were previously responsive to

TABLE 41-7

DIAGNOSTIC CRITERIA FOR GENERALIZED ANXIETY DISORDER

A. There is excessive anxiety and worry (apprehensive expectation), occurring more days than not for at least 6 months, about a number of events or activities (such as work or school performance).

B. The person finds it difficult to control the worry.

C. The anxiety and worry are associated with three (or more) of the following six symptoms (with at least some symptoms present for more days than not for the past 6 months): (1) restlessness or feeling keyed up or on edge; (2) being easily fatigued; (3) difficulty concentrating or mind going blank; (4) irritability; (5) muscle tension; (6) sleep disturbance (difficulty falling or staying asleep, or restless unsatisfying sleep).

D. The focus of the anxiety and worry is not confined to features of an Axis I disorder, e.g., the anxiety or worry is not about having a panic attack (as in panic disorder), being embarrassed in public (as in social phobia), being contaminated (as in obsessive-compulsive disorder), being away from home or close relatives (as in separation anxiety disorder), gaining weight (as in anorexia nervosa), having multiple physical complaints (as in somatization disorder), or having a serious illness (as in hypochondriasis), and the anxiety and worry do not occur exclusively during posttraumatic stress disorder.

E. The anxiety, worry, or physical symptoms cause clinically significant distress or impairment in social, occupational, or other important areas of functioning.

F. The disturbance is not due to the direct physiologic effects of a substance (e.g., a drug of abuse, a medication) or a general medical condition (e.g., hyperthyroidism) and does not occur exclusively during a mood disorder, a psychotic disorder, or a pervasive developmental disorder.

Source: Reprinted with permission from the Diagnostic and Statistical Manual of Mental Disorders, Fourth Edition, Text Revision (Copyright 2000). American Psychiatric Association.

a benzodiazepine are unlikely to rate buspirone as equally effective, but patients with head injury or dementia who have symptoms of anxiety and/or agitation may do well with this agent.

Administration of benzodiazepines to geriatric patients requires special care. Such patients have increased drug absorption; decreased hepatic metabolism, protein binding, and renal excretion; and an increased volume of distribution. These factors, together with the likely presence of comorbid medical illnesses and medication, dramatically increase the likelihood of toxicity. Iatrogenic psychomotor impairment can result in falls and fractures, confusional states, or motor vehicle acci-

dents. If used, agents in this class should be started at the lowest possible dose, and effects should be monitored closely. Benzodiazepines are contraindicated during pregnancy and breast-feeding.

Anticonvulsants with GABAergic properties also may be effective against anxiety. Gabapentin, oxcarbazepine, tiagabine, pregabalin, and divalproex have all shown some degree of benefit in a variety of anxiety-related syndromes. Agents that selectively target $GABA_A$ receptor subtypes are currently under development; it is hoped that these will lack the sedating, memory-impairing, and addicting properties of benzodiazepines.

PHOBIC DISORDERS

Clinical Manifestations

The cardinal feature of phobic disorders is a marked and persistent fear of objects or situations, exposure to which results in an immediate anxiety reaction. The patient avoids the phobic stimulus, and this avoidance usually impairs occupational or social functioning. Panic attacks may be triggered by the phobic stimulus or may occur spontaneously. Unlike patients with other anxiety disorders, individuals with phobias usually experience anxiety only in specific situations. Common phobias include fear of closed spaces (claustrophobia), fear of blood, and fear of flying. Social phobia is distinguished by a specific fear of social or performance situations in which the individual is exposed to unfamiliar individuals or to possible examination and evaluation by others. Examples include having to converse at a party, use public restrooms, and meet strangers. In each case, the affected individual is aware that the experienced fear is excessive and unreasonable given the circumstance. The specific content of a phobia may vary across gender, ethnic, and cultural boundaries.

Phobic disorders are common, affecting ~10% of the population. Full criteria for diagnosis are usually satisfied first in early adulthood, but behavioral avoidance of unfamiliar people, situations, or objects dating from early childhood is common.

In one study of female twins, concordance rates for agoraphobia, social phobia, and animal phobia were found to be 23% for monozygotic twins and 15% for dizygotic twins. A twin study of fear conditioning, a model for the acquisition of phobias, demonstrated a heritability of 35 to 45%, and a genome-wide linkage scan has identified a risk locus on chromosome 14 in a region previously implicated in a mouse model of fear. Animal studies of fear conditioning have indicated that processing of the fear stimulus occurs through the lateral nucleus of the amygdala, extending through the central nucleus and projecting to the periaqueductal gray region, lateral hypothalamus, and paraventricular hypothalamus.

TREATMENT FOR PHOBIC DISORDERS

Beta blockers (e.g., propranolol, 20 to 40 mg orally 2 h before the event) are particularly effective in the treatment of "performance anxiety" (but not general social phobia) and appear to work by blocking the peripheral manifestations of anxiety, such as perspiration, tachycardia, palpitations, and tremor. MAOIs alleviate social phobia independently of their antidepressant activity, and SSRIs appear to be effective also. Benzodiazepines can be helpful in reducing fearful avoidance, but the chronic nature of phobic disorders limits their usefulness.

Behaviorally focused psychotherapy is an important component of treatment, as relapse rates are high when medication is used as the sole treatment. Cognitive-behavioral strategies are based on the finding that distorted perceptions and interpretations of fear-producing stimuli play a major role in perpetuation of phobias. Individual and group therapy sessions teach the patient to identify specific negative thoughts associated with the anxiety-producing situation and help to reduce the patient's fear of loss of control. In desensitization therapy, hierarchies of feared situations are constructed and the patient is encouraged to pursue and master gradual exposure to the anxiety-producing stimuli.

Patients with social phobia, in particular, have a high rate of comorbid alcohol abuse, as well as of other psychiatric conditions (e.g., eating disorders), necessitating the need for parallel management of each disorder if anxiety reduction is to be achieved.

STRESS DISORDERS

Clinical Manifestations

Patients may develop anxiety after exposure to extreme traumatic events such as the threat of personal death or injury or the death of a loved one. The reaction may occur shortly after the trauma (*acute stress disorder*) or be delayed and subject to recurrence [posttraumatic stress disorder (PTSD)] (**Table 41-8**). In both syndromes,

individuals experience associated symptoms of detachment and loss of emotional responsivity. The patient may feel depersonalized and unable to recall specific aspects of the trauma, though typically it is reexperienced through intrusions in thought, dreams, or flashbacks, particularly when cues of the original event are present. Patients often actively avoid stimuli that precipitate recollections of the trauma and demonstrate a resulting increase in vigilance, arousal, and startle response. Patients with stress disorders are at risk for the development of other disorders related to anxiety, mood, and substance abuse (especially alcohol). Between 5 and 10% of Americans will at some time in their life satisfy criteria for PTSD, with women more likely to be affected than men.

Risk factors for the development of PTSD include a past psychiatric history and personality characteristics of high neuroticism and extroversion. Twin studies show a substantial influence of genetics on all symptoms associated with PTSD, with less evidence for environment effect.

TREATMENT FOR STRESS DISORDERS

Acute stress reactions are usually self-limited, and treatment typically involves the short-term use of benzodiazepines and supportive/expressive psychotherapy. The chronic and recurrent nature of PTSD, however, requires a more complex approach employing drug and behavioral treatments. PTSD is highly correlated with peritraumatic dissociative symptoms and the development of an acute stress disorder at the time of the trauma. TCAs such as imipramine and amitriptyline, the MAOI phenelzine, and the SSRIs (fluoxetine, sertraline, citalopram, paroxetine) can all reduce anxiety, symptoms of intrusion, and avoidance behaviors, as can prazosin, an α_1 antagonist. Trazodone, a sedating antidepressant, is frequently used at night to help with insomnia (50 to 150 mg qhs). Carbamazepine, valproic acid, or alprazolam have also independently produced improvement in uncontrolled trials. Psychotherapeutic strategies for PTSD help the patient overcome avoidance behaviors and demoralization and master fear of recurrence of the trauma; therapies that encourage the patient to dismantle avoidance behaviors through stepwise focusing on the experience of the traumatic event are the most effective.

TABLE 41-8

DIAGNOSTIC CRITERIA FOR POSTTRAUMATIC STRESS DISORDER

A. The person has been exposed to a traumatic event in which both of the following were present:
1. The person experienced, witnessed, or was confronted with an event or events that involved actual or threatened death or serious injury, or a threat to the physical integrity of self or others.
2. The person's response involved intense fear, helplessness, or horror.

B. The traumatic event is persistently reexperienced in one (or more) of the following ways:
1. Recurrent and intrusive distressing recollections of the event, including images, thoughts, or perceptions.
2. Recurrent distressing dreams of the event.
3. Acting or feeling as if the traumatic event were recurring (includes a sense of reliving the experience, illusions, hallucinations, and dissociative flashback episodes, including those that occur on awakening or when intoxicated).
4. Intense psychological distress at exposure to internal or external cues that symbolize or resemble an aspect of the traumatic event.
5. Physiologic reactivity on exposure to internal or external cues that symbolize or resemble an aspect of the traumatic event.

C. Persistent avoidance of stimuli associated with the trauma and numbing of general responsiveness (not present before the trauma), as indicated by three or more of the following:
1. Efforts to avoid thoughts, feelings, or conversations associated with the trauma
2. Efforts to avoid activities, places, or people that arouse recollections of the trauma
3. Inability to recall an important aspect of the trauma
4. Markedly diminished interest or participation in significant activities
5. Feeling of detachment or estrangement from others
6. Restricted range of affect (e.g., unable to have loving feelings)
7. Sense of a foreshortened future (e.g., does not expect to have a career, marriage, children, or a normal life span)

D. Persistent symptoms of increased arousal (not present before the trauma), as indicated by two (or more) of the following:
1. Difficulty falling or staying asleep
2. Irritability or outbursts of anger
3. Difficulty concentrating
4. Hypervigilance
5. Exaggerated startle response

E. Duration of the disturbance (symptoms in criteria B, C, and D) is more than 1 month.

F. The disturbance causes clinically significant distress or impairment in social, occupational, or other important areas of functioning.

Source: Reprinted with permission from the Diagnostic and Statistical Manual of Mental Disorders, Fourth Edition, Text Revision (Copyright 2000). American Psychiatric Association.

OBSESSIVE-COMPULSIVE DISORDER

Clinical Manifestations

Obsessive-compulsive disorder (OCD) is characterized by obsessive thoughts and compulsive behaviors that impair everyday functioning. Fears of contamination and germs are common, as are handwashing, counting behaviors, and having to check and recheck such actions as whether a door is locked. The degree to which the disorder is disruptive for the individual varies, but in all cases obsessive-compulsive activities take up >1 h/d and are undertaken to relieve the anxiety triggered by the core fear. Patients often conceal their symptoms, usually because they are embarrassed by the content of their thoughts or the nature of their actions. Physicians must ask specific questions regarding recurrent thoughts and behaviors, particularly if physical clues such as chafed and reddened hands or patchy hair loss (from repetitive hair pulling, or trichotillomania) are present. Comorbid conditions are common, the most frequent being depression, other anxiety disorders, eating disorders, and tics. OCD has a lifetime prevalence of 2 to 3% worldwide. Onset is usually gradual, beginning in early adulthood, but childhood onset is not rare. The disorder usually has a waxing and waning course, but some cases may show a steady deterioration in psychosocial functioning.

TREATMENT FOR OCD

Clomipramine, fluoxetine, and fluvoxamine are approved for the treatment of OCD. Clomipramine is a TCA that is often tolerated poorly owing to anticholinergic and sedative side effects at the doses required to treat the illness (150 to 250 mg/d). Its efficacy in OCD is unrelated to its antidepressant activity. Fluoxetine (40 to 60 mg/d) and fluvoxamine (100 to 300 mg/d) are as effective as clomipramine and have a more benign side-effect profile. Only 50 to 60% of patients with OCD show adequate improvement with pharmacotherapy alone. In treatment-resistant cases, augmentation with other serotonergic agents, such as buspirone, or with a neuroleptic or benzodiazepine may be beneficial. When a therapeutic response is achieved, long-duration maintenance therapy is usually indicated.

For many individuals, particularly those with time-consuming compulsions, behavior therapy will result in as much improvement as that afforded by medication. Effective techniques include the gradual increase in exposure to stressful situations, maintenance of a diary to clarify stressors, and homework assignments that substitute new activities for compulsive behaviors.

MOOD DISORDERS

Mood disorders are characterized by a disturbance in the regulation of mood, behavior, and affect. Mood disorders are subdivided into (1) depressive disorders, (2) bipolar disorders, and (3) depression in association with medical illness or alcohol and substance abuse (Chaps. 42 and 43). Depressive disorders are differentiated from bipolar disorders by the absence of a manic or hypomanic episode. The relationship between pure depressive syndromes and bipolar disorders is not well understood; depression is more frequent in families of bipolar individuals, but the reverse is not true. In the Global Burden of Disease Study conducted by the World Health Organization, unipolar major depression

ranked fourth among all diseases in terms of disability-adjusted life years and was projected to rank second by year 2020. In the United States, lost productivity directly related to depression has been estimated at $44 billion per year.

DEPRESSION IN ASSOCIATION WITH MEDICAL ILLNESS

Depression occurring in the context of medical illness is difficult to evaluate. Depressive symptomatology may reflect the psychological stress of coping with the disease, may be caused by the disease process itself or by the medications used to treat it, or may simply coexist in time with the medical diagnosis.

Virtually every class of *medication* includes some agent that can induce depression. Antihypertensive drugs, anticholesterolemic agents, and antiarrhythmic agents are common triggers of depressive symptoms. Among the antihypertensive agents, β-adrenergic blockers and, to a lesser extent, calcium channel blockers are the most likely to cause depressed mood. Iatrogenic depression should also be considered in patients receiving glucocorticoids, antimicrobials, systemic analgesics, antiparkinsonian medications, and anticonvulsants. To decide whether a causal relationship exists between pharmacologic therapy and a patient's change in mood, it may sometimes be necessary to undertake an empirical trial of an alternative medication.

Between 20 and 30% of cardiac patients manifest a depressive disorder; an even higher percentage experience depressive symptomatology when self-reporting scales are used. Depressive symptoms following unstable angina, myocardial infarction, or heart transplant impair rehabilitation and are associated with higher rates of mortality and medical morbidity. Depressed patients often show decreased variability in heart rate (an index of reduced parasympathetic nervous system activity), and this has been proposed as one mechanism by which depression may predispose individuals to ventricular arrhythmia and increased morbidity. Depression also appears to increase the risk of developing coronary heart disease; increased serotonin-induced platelet aggregation has been implicated as a possible cause. TCAs are contraindicated in patients with bundle branch block, and TCA-induced tachycardia is an additional concern in patients with congestive heart failure. SSRIs appear not to induce ECG changes or adverse cardiac events and thus are reasonable first-line drugs for patients at risk for TCA-related complications. SSRIs may interfere with hepatic metabolism of anticoagulants, however, causing increased anticoagulation.

In patients with cancer, the mean prevalence of depression is 25%, but depression occurs in 40 to 50% of patients with cancers of the pancreas or oropharynx. Extreme cachexia, common with some cancers, may be misinterpreted as part of the symptom complex of depression; the higher prevalence of depression in patients with pancreatic cancer nevertheless persists when compared to those with advanced gastric cancer. Initiation of antidepressant medication in cancer patients has been shown to improve quality of life as well as mood. Psychotherapeutic approaches, particularly group therapy, may have some effect on short-term depression, anxiety, and pain symptoms and, speculatively, on recurrence rates and long-term survival.

Depression occurs frequently in patients with *neurologic disorders,* particularly cerebrovascular disorders, Parkinson's disease, dementia, multiple sclerosis, and traumatic brain injury. One in five patients with left-hemisphere stroke involving the dorsal lateral frontal cortex experiences major depression. Late-onset depression in otherwise cognitively normal individuals increases the risk of a subsequent diagnosis of Alzheimer's disease. Both TCA and SSRI agents are effective against these depressions, as are stimulant compounds and, in some patients, MAOIs.

The reported prevalence of depression in patients with *diabetes mellitus* varies from 8 to 27%, with the severity of the mood state correlating with the level of hyperglycemia and the presence of diabetic complications. Treatment of depression may be complicated by effects of antidepressive agents on glycemic control. MAOIs can induce hypoglycemia and weight gain. TCAs can produce hyperglycemia and carbohydrate craving. SSRIs, like MAOIs, may reduce fasting plasma glucose, but they are easier to use and may also improve dietary and medication compliance.

Hypothyroidism is frequently associated with features of depression, most commonly depressed mood and memory impairment. Hyperthyroid states also may present in a similar fashion, usually in geriatric populations. Improvement in mood usually follows normalization of thyroid function, but adjunctive antidepressant medication is sometimes required. Patients with subclinical hypothyroidism can also experience symptoms of depression and cognitive difficulty that respond to thyroid replacement.

The lifetime prevalence of depression in HIV-positive individuals has been estimated at 22 to 45%. The relationship between depression and disease progression is multifactorial and likely to involve psychological and social factors, alterations in immune function, and central nervous system disease. Chronic hepatitis C infection also is associated with depression, which may worsen with interferon α treatment.

Some chronic disorders of uncertain etiology, such as chronic fatigue syndrome and fibromyalgia (Chap. 40), are strongly associated with depression and anxiety and may partially benefit from antidepressant treatment, usually at lower than normal dosing.

DEPRESSIVE DISORDERS

Clinical Manifestations

Major depression is defined as depressed mood on a daily basis for a minimum duration of 2 weeks (**Table 41-9**). An episode may be characterized by sadness, indifference, apathy, or irritability and is usually associated with the following: changes in sleep patterns, appetite, and weight; motor agitation or retardation; fatigue; impaired concentration and decision-making; feelings of shame or guilt; and thoughts of death or dying. Patients with depression have a profound loss of pleasure in all enjoyable activities, exhibit early morning awakening, feel that the dysphoric mood state is qualitatively different from sadness, and often notice a diurnal variation in mood (worse in morning hours).

Approximately 15% of the population experiences a major depressive episode at some point in life, and 6 to 8% of all outpatients in primary care settings satisfy diagnostic criteria for the disorder. Depression is often undiagnosed, and, even more frequently, it is treated inadequately. If a physician suspects the presence of a major depressive episode, the initial task is to determine whether it represents unipolar or bipolar depression or is one of the 10 to 15% of cases that are secondary to general medical illness or substance abuse. Physicians should also assess the risk of suicide by direct questioning, as patients are often reluctant to verbalize such thoughts without prompting. If specific plans are uncovered or if significant risk factors exist (e.g., a past history of suicide attempts, profound hopelessness, concurrent medical illness, substance abuse, or social isolation), the patient must be referred to a mental health specialist for immediate care. The physician should specifically probe each of these areas in an empathic and hopeful manner, being sensitive to denial and possible minimization of distress. The presence of anxiety, panic, or agitation significantly increases near-term suicidal risk. Approximately 4 to 5% of all depressed patients will commit suicide; most will have sought help from a physician within 1 month of their death.

In some depressed patients, the mood disorder does not appear to be episodic and is not clearly associated with either psychosocial dysfunction or change from the individual's usual experience in life. *Dysthymic disorder* consists of a pattern of chronic (at least 2 years), ongoing, mild depressive symptoms that are less severe and less disabling than those found in major depression; the two conditions are sometimes difficult to separate, however, and can occur together ("double depression"). Many patients who exhibit a profile of pessimism, disin-

TABLE 41-9

CRITERIA FOR MAJOR DEPRESSIVE EPISODE

A. Five (or more) of the following symptoms have been present during the same 2-week period and represent a change from previous functioning; at least one of the symptoms is either (1) depressed mood or (2) loss of interest or pleasure. **Note:** Do not include symptoms that are clearly due to a general medical condition, or mood-incongruent delusions or hallucinations.

1. Depressed mood most of the day, nearly every day, as indicated by either subjective report (e.g., feels sad or empty) or observation made by others (e.g., appears tearful)
2. Markedly diminished interest or pleasure in all, or almost all, activities most of the day, nearly every day (as indicated by either subjective account or observation made by others)
3. Significant weight loss when not dieting or weight gain (e.g., a change of >5% of body weight in a month), or decrease or increase in appetite nearly every day
4. Insomnia or hypersomnia nearly every day
5. Psychomotor agitation or retardation nearly every day (observable by others, not merely subjective feelings of restlessness or being slowed down)
6. Fatigue or loss of energy nearly every day
7. Feelings of worthlessness or excessive or inappropriate guilt (which may be delusional) nearly every day (not merely self-reproach or guilt about being sick)
8. Diminished ability to think or concentrate, or indecisiveness, nearly every day (either by subjective account or as observed by others)
9. Recurrent thoughts of death (not just fear of dying), recurrent suicidal ideation without a specific plan, or a suicide attempt or a specific plan for committing suicide

B. The symptoms do not meet criteria for a mixed episode

C. The symptoms cause clinically significant distress or impairment in social, occupational, or other important areas of functioning

D. The symptoms are not due to the direct physiologic effects of a substance (e.g., a drug of abuse, a medication) or a general medical condition (e.g., hypothyroidism)

E. The symptoms are not better accounted for by bereavement—i.e., after the loss of a loved one, the symptoms persist for >2 months or are characterized by marked functional impairment, morbid preoccupation with worthlessness, suicidal ideation, psychotic symptoms, or psychomotor retardation

Source: Reprinted with permission from the Diagnostic and Statistical Manual of Mental Disorders, Fourth Edition, Text Revision (Copyright 2000). American Psychiatric Association.

terest, and low self-esteem respond to antidepressant treatment. Dysthymic disorder exists in ~5% of primary care patients. The term *minor depression* is used for individuals who experience at least two depressive symptoms for 2 weeks, but who do not meet the full criteria for major depression. Despite its name, minor depression is associated with significant morbidity and disability and also responds to pharmacologic treatment.

Depression is approximately twice as common in women as in men, and the incidence increases with age in both sexes. Twin studies indicate that the liability to major depression in adult women is largely genetic in origin. Negative life events can precipitate and contribute to depression, but genetic factors influence the sensitivity of individuals to these stressful events. In most cases, both biologic and psychosocial factors are involved in the precipitation and unfolding of depressive episodes. The most potent stressors appear to involve death of a relative, assault, or severe marital or relationship problems.

Unipolar depressive disorders usually begin in early adulthood and recur episodically over the course of a lifetime. The best predictor of future risk is the number of past episodes; 50 to 60% of patients who have a first episode have at least one or two recurrences. Some patients experience multiple episodes that become more severe and frequent over time. The duration of an untreated episode varies greatly, ranging from a few months to ≥1 year. The pattern of recurrence and clinical progression in a developing episode also is variable. Within an individual, the nature of attacks (e.g., specific presenting symptoms, frequency and duration of episodes) may be similar over time. In a minority of patients, a severe depressive episode may progress to a psychotic state; in elderly patients, depressive symptoms may be associated with cognitive deficits mimicking dementia ("pseudodementia"). A seasonal pattern of depression, called *seasonal affective disorder,* may manifest with onset and remission of episodes at predictable times of the year. This disorder is more common in women, whose symptoms are anergy, fatigue, weight gain, hypersomnia, and episodic carbohydrate craving. The prevalence increases with distance from the equator, and improvement may occur by altering light exposure.

TREATMENT FOR DEPRESSIVE DISORDERS

Treatment planning requires coordination of short-term symptom remission with longer-term maintenance strategies designed to prevent recurrence. The most effective intervention for achieving remission and preventing relapse is medication, but combined treatment, incorporating psychotherapy to help the patient cope with decreased self-esteem and demoralization, improves outcome (**Fig. 41-1**). About 40% of primary care patients with depression drop out of treatment and discontinue medication if symptomatic improvement is not noted within a month, unless additional support is provided. Outcome improves with (1) increased intensity and frequency of visits during the first 4 to 6 weeks of treatment, (2) supplemental educational materials, and (3) psychiatric consultation as indicated. Despite the widespread use of SSRIs, there is no convincing evidence that this class of antidepressant is more efficacious than TCAs. Between 60 and 70% of all depressed patients respond to any drug chosen, if it is given in a sufficient dose for 6 to 8 weeks. There is no ideal antidepressant; no current compound combines rapid onset of action, moderate half-life, a meaningful relationship between dose and blood level, a low side-effect profile, minimal interaction with other drugs, and safety in overdose. A rational approach to selecting which antidepressant to use involves matching the patient's preference and medical history with the metabolic and side effect profile of the drug (Tables 41-4 and 41-5). A previous response, or a family history of a positive response, to a specific antidepressant would suggest that that drug be tried first. Before initiating antidepressant therapy, the physician should evaluate the possible contribution of comorbid illnesses and consider their

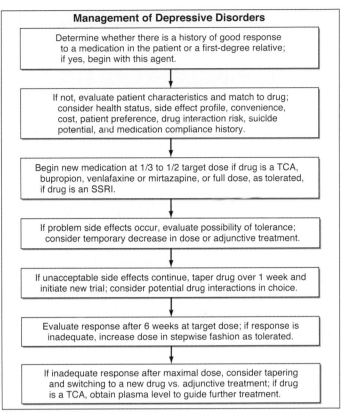

Management of Depressive Disorders

Determine whether there is a history of good response to a medication in the patient or a first-degree relative; if yes, begin with this agent.

If not, evaluate patient characteristics and match to drug; consider health status, side effect profile, convenience, cost, patient preference, drug interaction risk, suicide potential, and medication compliance history.

Begin new medication at 1/3 to 1/2 target dose if drug is a TCA, bupropion, venlafaxine or mirtazapine, or full dose, as tolerated, if drug is an SSRI.

If problem side effects occur, evaluate possibility of tolerance; consider temporary decrease in dose or adjunctive treatment.

If unacceptable side effects continue, taper drug over 1 week and initiate new trial; consider potential drug interactions in choice.

Evaluate response after 6 weeks at target dose; if response is inadequate, increase dose in stepwise fashion as tolerated.

If inadequate response after maximal dose, consider tapering and switching to a new drug vs. adjunctive treatment; if drug is a TCA, obtain plasma level to guide further treatment.

FIGURE 41-1

A guideline for the medical management of major depressive disorders. SSRI, selective serotonin reuptake inhibitor; TCA, tricyclic antidepressant.

specific treatment. In individuals with suicidal ideation, particular attention should be paid to choosing a drug with low toxicity if taken in overdose. The SSRIs and other newer antidepressant drugs are distinctly safer in this regard; nevertheless, the advantages of TCAs have not been completely superseded. The existence of generic equivalents makes TCAs relatively inexpensive, and for several tricyclics, particularly nortriptyline, imipramine, and desipramine, well-defined relationships among dose, plasma level, and therapeutic response exist. The steady-state plasma level achieved for a given drug dose can vary more than tenfold between individuals. Plasma levels may help in interpreting apparent resistance to treatment and/or unexpected drug toxicity. The principal side effects of TCAs are antihistamine (sedation) and anticholinergic (constipation, dry mouth, urinary hesitancy, blurred vision). Cardiac toxicity due to conduction block or arrhythmias also can occur but is uncommon at therapeutic levels. TCAs are probably contraindicated in patients with serious cardiovascular risk factors. Overdoses of tricyclic agents can be lethal, with desipramine carrying the greatest risk. It is judicious to prescribe only a 10-day supply when suicide is a risk. Most patients require a daily dose of 150 to 200 mg of imipramine or amitriptyline or its equivalent to achieve a therapeutic blood level of 150 to 300 ng/mL and a satisfactory remission; some patients show a partial effect at lower doses. Geriatric patients may require a low starting dose and slow escalation. Ethnic differences in drug metabolism are significant; Hispanic, Asian, and African-American patients generally require lower doses than Caucasians to achieve a comparable blood level.

Second-generation antidepressants include amoxapine, maprotiline, trazodone, and bupropion. Amoxapine is a dibenzoxazepine derivative that blocks norepinephrine and serotonin reuptake and has a metabolite that shows a degree of dopamine blockade. Long-term use of this drug carries a risk of tardive dyskinesia. Maprotiline is a potent noradrenergic reuptake blocker that has little anticholinergic effect but may produce seizures. Bupropion is a novel antidepressant whose mechanism of action is thought to involve enhancement of noradrenergic function. It has no anticholinergic, sedating, or orthostatic side effects and has a low incidence of sexual side effects. It may, however, be associated with stimulant-like side effects, may lower seizure threshold, and has an exceptionally short half-life, requiring frequent dosing. An extended-release preparation is available.

SSRIs such as fluoxetine, sertraline, paroxetine, citalopram, escitalopram, and duloxetine cause a lower frequency of anticholinergic, sedating, and cardiovascular side effects but a possibly greater incidence of gastrointestinal complaints, sleep impairment, and sexual dysfunction than do TCAs. Akathisia, involving an inner sense of restlessness and anxiety in addition to increased motor activity, also may be more common, particularly during the first week of treatment. A concern is the risk of "serotonin syndrome," thought to result from hyperstimulation of brainstem $5HT_{1A}$ receptors and characterized by myoclonus, agitation, abdominal cramping, hyperpyrexia, hypertension, and potentially death. Serotonergic agonists taken in combination should be monitored closely for this reason. Considerations such as half-life, compliance, toxicity, and drug-drug interactions may guide the choice of a particular SSRI. Fluoxetine and its principal active metabolite, norfluoxetine,

for example, have a combined half-life of almost 7 days, resulting in a delay of 5 weeks before steady-state levels are achieved and a similar delay for complete drug excretion once its use is discontinued. All the SSRIs may impair sexual function, resulting in diminished libido, impotence, or difficulty in achieving orgasm. Sexual dysfunction frequently results in noncompliance and should be asked about specifically. Sexual dysfunction can sometimes be ameliorated by lowering the dose, by instituting weekend drug holidays (two or three times a month), or by treatment with amantadine (100 mg tid), bethanechol (25 mg tid), buspirone (10 mg tid), or bupropion (100–150 mg/d). Paroxetine appears to be more anticholinergic than either fluoxetine or sertraline, and sertraline carries a lower risk of producing an adverse drug interaction than the other two. Rare side effects of SSRIs include angina due to vasospasm and prolongation of the prothrombin time. Escitalopram is the most specific of currently available SSRIs and appears to have no specific inhibitory effects on the P450 system.

Recently, case-control studies have shown an association between initiation of SSRI medications for depression and an increased risk of suicidal ideation. This risk has been demonstrated mainly in children and adolescents and is highest just after beginning therapy. Based on these data, the U.S. Food and Drug Administration (FDA) in 2004 issued a warning urging physicians to carefully monitor suicidal symptoms in their pediatric as well as adult patients after initiation of these medicines.

Venlafaxine, like imipramine, blocks the reuptake of both norepinephrine and serotonin, but it produces relatively little in the way of traditional tricyclic side effects. Unlike the SSRIs, it has a relatively linear dose-response curve. Patients should be monitored for a possible increase in diastolic blood pressure, and multiple daily dosing is required because of the drug's short half-life. An extended-release form is available and has a somewhat lower incidence of gastrointestinal side effects. Nefazadone is a selective $5HT_2$ receptor antagonist that also inhibits the presynaptic reuptake of serotonin and norepinephrine. Its side effects are similar to those of the SSRIs, and twice-daily dosing produces a steady state within 4 to 5 days. The drug is related structurally to trazodone, which is currently used more for its sedative than its antidepressant properties.

Nefazadone appears to produce a lower incidence of sexual side effects than do the SSRIs. Mirtazapine is a tetracyclic antidepressant that has a unique spectrum of activity. It increases noradrenergic and serotonergic neurotransmission through a blockade of central α_2-adrenergic receptors and postsynaptic $5HT_2$ and $5HT_3$ receptors. It is also strongly antihistaminic and, as such, may produce sedation.

With the exception of citalopram and escitalopram, each of the SSRIs, as well as nefazadone, may inhibit one or more cytochrome P450 enzymes. Depending on the specific isoenzyme involved, the metabolism of a number of concomitantly administered medications can be dramatically affected. Fluoxetine and paroxetine, for example, by inhibiting 2D6, can cause dramatic increases in the blood level of type 1C antiarrhythmics, while sertraline and nefazadone, by acting on 3A4, may alter blood levels of terfenadine, carbamazepine, and astemizole. Many of these compounds have a narrow therapeutic window and can cause iatrogenic ventricular arrhythmias at toxic levels; thus, the possibility of an adverse drug interaction should always be considered.

The MAOIs are highly effective, particularly in atypical depression, but the risk of hypertensive crisis following intake of tyramine-containing food or sympathomimetic drugs makes them inappropriate as first-line agents. Common side effects include orthostatic hypotension, weight gain, insomnia, and sexual dysfunction. MAOIs should not be used concomitantly with SSRIs, because of the risk of serotonin syndrome, or with TCAs, because of possible hyperadrenergic effects.

Electroconvulsive therapy is at least as effective as medication, but its use is reserved for treatment-resistant cases and delusional depressions. Transcranial magnetic stimulation (TMS) is an investigational treatment of depression that has been shown to have efficacy in several controlled trials; it is uncertain whether the observed benefits were clinically meaningful, however. Vagus nerve stimulation (VNS) appeared to be effective in treatment-resistant depression in an initial open study, only to fail in a controlled trial.

Regardless of the treatment undertaken, the response should be evaluated after $\sim$2 months. Three-quarters of patients show improvement by this time, but if remission is inadequate the patient should be questioned about compliance and an increase in medication dose should be considered if side effects are not troublesome. If this approach is unsuccessful, referral to a mental health specialist is advised. Strategies for treatment then include selection of an alternative drug, combinations of antidepressants, and/or adjunctive treatment with other classes of drugs, including lithium, thyroid hormone, and dopamine agonists. Patients whose response to an SSRI wanes over time may benefit from the addition of buspirone (10 mg tid) or pindolol (2.5 mg tid) or small amounts of a TCA such as desipramine (25 mg bid or tid). Once significant remission is achieved, drug treatment should be continued for at least 6 to 9 months to prevent relapse. In patients who have had two or more episodes of depression, indefinite maintenance treatment should be considered.

It is essential to educate patients about both depression and the benefits and side effects of medications they are receiving. Advice about stress reduction and cautions that alcohol may exacerbate depressive symptoms and impair drug response are helpful. Patients should be given time to describe their experience, their outlook, and the impact of the depression on them and their families. Occasional empathic silence may be as helpful for the treatment alliance as verbal reassurance. Controlled trials have shown that cognitive-behavioral and interpersonal therapies are effective in improving psychological and social adjustment and that a combined treatment approach is more successful than medication alone for many patients.

BIPOLAR DISORDER

Clinical Manifestations

Bipolar disorder is characterized by unpredictable swings in mood from mania (or hypomania) to depression. Some patients suffer only from recurrent attacks of *mania,* which in its pure form is associated with increased psychomotor activity; excessive social extroversion; decreased need for sleep; impulsivity and impairment in judgment; and expansive, grandiose, and sometimes irritable mood (**Table 41–10**). In severe mania, patients may experience delusions and paranoid thinking indistinguishable from schizophrenia. Half of patients with bipolar disorder present with a mixture of psychomotor agitation and activation with dysphoria, anxiety, and irritability. It may be difficult to distinguish *mixed mania* from *agitated depression.* In some bipolar patients (*bipolar II disorder*), the full criteria for mania are lacking, and the requisite recurrent depressions are separated by periods of mild activation and increased energy

TABLE 41-10

CRITERIA FOR A MANIC EPISODE

A. A distinct period of abnormally and persistently elevated, expansive, or irritable mood, lasting at least 1 week (or any duration if hospitalization is necessary)

B. During the period of mood disturbance, three (or more) of the following symptoms have persisted (four if the mood is only irritable) and have been present to a significant degree:
  1. Inflated self-esteem or grandiosity
  2. Decreased need for sleep (e.g., feels rested after only 3 hours of sleep)
  3. More talkative than usual or pressure to keep talking
  4. Flight of ideas or subjective experience that thoughts are racing
  5. Distractibility (i.e., attention too easily drawn to unimportant or irrelevant external stimuli)
  6. Increase in goal-directed activity (either socially, at work or school, or sexually) or psychomotor agitation
  7. Excessive involvement in pleasurable activities that have a high potential for painful consequences (e.g., engaging in unrestrained buying sprees, sexual indiscretions, or foolish business investments)

C. The symptoms do not meet criteria for a mixed episode.

D. The mood disturbance is sufficiently severe to cause marked impairment in occupational functioning or in usual social activities or relationships with others, or to necessitate hospitalization to prevent harm to self or others, or there are psychotic features.

E. The symptoms are not due to the direct physiologic effects of a substance (e.g., a drug of abuse, a medication, or other treatment) or a general medical condition (e.g., hyperthyroidism).

Note: Manic-like episodes that are clearly caused by somatic antidepressant treatment (e.g., medication, electroconvulsive therapy, light therapy) should not count toward a diagnosis of bipolar I disorder.

Source: Reprinted with permission from the Diagnostic and Statistical Manual of Mental Disorders, Fourth Edition, Text Revision (Copyright 2000). American Psychiatric Association.

(hypomania). In *cyclothymic disorder,* there are numerous hypomanic periods, usually of relatively short duration, alternating with clusters of depressive symptoms that fail, either in severity or duration, to meet the criteria of major depression. The mood fluctuations are chronic and should be present for at least 2 years before the diagnosis is made.

Manic episodes typically emerge over a period of days to weeks, but onset within hours is possible, usually in the early morning hours. An untreated episode of either depression or mania can be as short as several weeks or last as long as 8 to 12 months, and rare patients have an unremitting chronic course. The term *rapid cycling* is used for patients who have four or more episodes of either depression or mania in a given year. This pattern

occurs in 15% of all patients, almost all of whom are women. In some cases, rapid cycling is linked to an underlying thyroid dysfunction and, in others, it is iatrogenically triggered by prolonged antidepressant treatment. Approximately half of patients have sustained difficulties in work performance and psychosocial functioning.

Bipolar disorder is common, affecting ~1% of the population in the United States. Onset is typically between 20 and 30 years of age, but many individuals report premorbid symptoms in late childhood or early adolescence. The prevalence is similar for men and women; women are likely to have more depressive and men more manic episodes over a lifetime.

Differential Diagnosis

The differential diagnosis of mania includes toxic effects of stimulant or sympathomimetic drugs as well as secondary mania induced by hyperthyroidism, AIDS, or neurologic disorders, such as Huntington's or Wilson's disease, or cerebrovascular accidents. Comorbidity with alcohol and substance abuse is common, either because of poor judgment and increased impulsivity or because of an attempt to self-treat the underlying mood symptoms and sleep disturbances.

TREATMENT FOR BIPOLAR DISORDER

Lithium carbonate is the mainstay of treatment in bipolar disorder, although sodium valproate and olanzapine are equally effective in acute mania, as is lamotrigine in the depressed phase. The response rate to lithium carbonate is 70 to 80% in acute mania, with beneficial effects appearing in 1 to 2 weeks. Lithium also has a prophylactic effect in prevention of recurrent mania and, to a lesser extent, in the prevention of recurrent depression. A simple cation, lithium is rapidly absorbed from the gastrointestinal tract and remains unbound to plasma or tissue proteins. Some 95% of a given dose is excreted unchanged through the kidneys within 24 h. See **Table 41-11**.

Serious side effects from lithium administration are rare, but minor complaints such as gastrointestinal discomfort, nausea, diarrhea, polyuria, weight gain, skin eruptions, alopecia, and edema are common. Over time, urine-concentrating ability may be decreased, but significant nephrotoxicity does not usually occur. Lithium exerts an antithyroid effect by interfering with the synthesis and release of thyroid hormones. More serious

TABLE 41-11

CLINICAL PHARMACOLOGY OF MOOD STABILIZERS

AGENT AND DOSING	SIDE EFFECTS AND OTHER EFFECTS

Lithium
  Starting dose: 300 mg bid or tid
  Therapeutic blood level: 0.8–1.2 meq/L
	Common side effects:
	Nausea/anorexia/diarrhea, fine tremor, thirst, polyuria, fatigue, weight gain, acne, folliculitis, neutrophilia, hypothyroidism
	Blood level is increased by thiazides, tetracyclines, and NSAIDs
	Blood level is decreased by bronchodilators, verapamil, and carbonic anhydrase inhibitors
	Rare side effects: Neurotoxicity, renal toxicity, hypercalcemia, ECG changes

Valproic acid
  Starting dose: 250 mg tid
  Therapeutic blood level: 50–125 μg/mL
	Common side effects:
	Nausea/anorexia, weight gain, sedation, tremor, rash, alopecia
	Inhibits hepatic metabolism of other medications
	Rare side effects: Pancreatitis, hepatotoxicity, Stevens-Johnson syndrome

Carbamazepine/oxcarbazepine
  Starting dose: 200 mg bid for carbamazepine, 150 bid for oxcarbazepine
  Therapeutic blood level: 4–12 μg/mL for carbamazepine
	Common side effects: Nausea/anorexia, sedation, rash, dizziness/ataxia
	Carbamazepine, but not oxcarbazepine, induces hepatic metabolism of other medications
	Rare side effects: Hyponatremia, agranulocytosis, Stevens-Johnson syndrome

Lamotrigine Starting dose: 25 mg/d	*Common side effects:* Rash, dizziness, headache, tremor, sedation, nausea *Rare side effect:* Stevens-Johnson syndrome

Note: NSAID, nonsteroidal anti-inflammatory drug; ECG, electrocardiogram.

side effects include tremor, poor concentration and memory, ataxia, dysarthria, and incoordination. There is suggestive, but not conclusive, evidence that lithium is teratogenic, inducing cardiac malformations in the first trimester.

In the treatment of acute mania, lithium is initiated at 300 mg bid or tid, and the dose is then increased by 300 mg every 2 to 3 days to achieve blood levels of 0.8 to 1.2 meq/L. Because the therapeutic effect of lithium may not appear until after 7 to 10 days of treatment, adjunctive usage of lorazepam (1 to 2 mg every 4 h) or clonazepam (0.5 to 1 mg every 4 h) may be beneficial to control agitation. Antipsychotics are indicated in patients with severe agitation who respond only partially to benzodiazepines. Patients using lithium should be monitored closely, since the blood levels required to achieve a therapeutic benefit are close to those associated with toxicity.

Valproic acid is an alternative in patients who cannot tolerate lithium or respond poorly to it. Valproic acid may be better than lithium for patients who experience rapid cycling (i.e., more than four episodes a year) or who present with a mixed or dysphoric mania. Tremor and weight gain are the most common side effects; hepatotoxicity and pancreatitis are rare toxicities.

Carbamazepine and oxcarbazepine, although not formally approved by the FDA for bipolar disorder, have clinical efficacy in the treatment of acute mania. Preliminary evidence also suggests that other anticonvulsant agents such as levetirac-etam, zonisamide, and topiramate may possess some therapeutic benefit.

The recurrent nature of bipolar mood disorder necessitates maintenance treatment. A sustained blood lithium level of at least 0.8 meq/L is impor-tant for optimal prophylaxis and has been shown to reduce risk of suicide, a finding not yet apparent for other mood stabilizers. Compliance is fre-quently an issue and often requires enlistment and education of concerned family members. Efforts to identify and modify psychosocial factors that may trigger episodes are important, as is an emphasis on lifestyle regularity. Antidepressant medications are sometimes required for the treat-ment of severe breakthrough depressions, but their use should generally be avoided during mainte-nance treatment because of the risk of precipitat-ing mania or accelerating the cycle frequency. Loss of efficacy over time may be observed with any of the mood-stabilizing agents. In such situations, an alternative agent or combination therapy is usually helpful.

Consensus guidelines for the treatment of acute mania and bipolar depression are described in **Table 41–12.**

SOMATOFORM DISORDERS

Clinical Manifestations

Patients with multiple somatic complaints that cannot be explained by a known medical condition or by the effects of alcohol or of recreational or prescription drugs are commonly seen in primary care practice; one survey indicates a prevalence of such complaints of 5%. In *soma-tization disorder,* the patient presents with multiple physi-cal complaints referable to different organ systems (**Table 41–13**). Onset is usually before age 30, and the disorder is persistent. Formal diagnostic criteria require the recording of at least four pain, two gastrointestinal, one sexual, and one pseudoneurologic symptom. Pa-tients with somatization disorder often present with dra-matic complaints, but the complaints are inconsistent. Symptoms of comorbid anxiety and mood disorder are common and may be the result of drug interactions due to regimens initiated independently by different physi-cians. Patients with somatization disorder may be impul-sive and demanding and frequently qualify for a formal comorbid psychiatric diagnosis. In *conversion disorder,* the symptoms focus on deficits that involve motor or sen-sory function and on psychological factors that initiate or exacerbate the medical presentation. Like somatiza-tion disorder, the deficit is not intentionally produced or simulated, as is the case in factitious disorder (malingering). In *hypochondriasis,* the essential feature is a belief of seri-ous medical illness that persists despite reassurance and

TABLE 41-12

CONSENSUS GUIDELINES ON THE DRUG TREATMENT OF ACUTE MANIA AND BIPOLAR DEPRESSION	
CONDITION	**PREFERRED AGENTS**
Euphoric mania	Lithium
Mixed/dysphoric mania	Valproic acid
Mania with psychosis	Valproic acid with olanzapine, conventional antipsychotic, or risperidone
Hypomania	Lithium, lamotrigine, or valproic acid alone
Severe depression with psychosis	Venlafaxine, bupropion, or paroxetine *plus* lithium *plus* olanzapine, *or* risperidone; consider ECT
Severe depression without psychosis	Bupropion, paroxetine, sertraline, venlafaxine, *or* citalopram *plus* lithium
Mild to moderate depression	Lithium *or* lamotrigine alone; add bupropion if needed

Note: ECT, electroconvulsive therapy.
Source: *From GS Sachs et al: Postgrad Med April, 2000.*

TABLE 41-13

DIAGNOSTIC CRITERIA FOR SOMATIZATION DISORDER

A. A history of many physical complaints beginning before age 30 years that occur over a period of several years and result in treatment being sought or significant impairment in social, occupational, or other important areas of functioning.

B. Each of the following criteria must have been met, with individual symptoms occurring at any time during the course of the disturbance:

1. *Four pain symptoms:* a history of pain related to at least four different sites or functions (e.g., head, abdomen, back, joints, extremities, chest, rectum, during menstruation, during sexual intercourse, or during urination)

2. *Two gastrointestinal symptoms:* a history of at least two gastrointestinal symptoms other than pain (e.g., nausea, bloating, vomiting other than during pregnancy, diarrhea, or intolerance of several different foods)

3. *One sexual symptom:* a history of at least one sexual or reproductive symptom other than pain (e.g., sexual indifference, erectile or ejaculatory dysfunction, irregular menses, excessive menstrual bleeding, vomiting throughout pregnancy)

4. *One pseudoneurologic symptom:* a history of at least one symptom or deficit suggesting a neurologic condition not limited to pain (conversion symptoms such as impaired coordination or balance, paralysis or localized weakness, difficulty swallowing or lump in throat, aphonia, urinary retention, hallucinations, loss of touch or pain sensation, double vision, blindness, deafness, seizures; dissociative symptoms such as amnesia; or loss of consciousness other than fainting)

C. Either of the following:

1. After appropriate investigation, each of the symptoms in criterion B cannot be fully explained by a known general medical condition or the direct effects of a substance (e.g., a drug of abuse, a medication)

2. When there is a related general medical condition, the physical complaints or resulting social or occupational impairment are in excess of what would be expected from the history, physical examination, or laboratory findings

D. The symptoms are not intentionally produced or feigned (as in factitious disorder or malingering).

Source: Reprinted with permission from the *Diagnostic and Statistical Manual of Mental Disorders, Fourth Edition, Text Revision* (Copyright 2000). American Psychiatric Association.

appropriate medical evaluation. As with somatization disorder, patients with hypochondriasis have a history of poor relationships with physicians stemming from their sense that they have been evaluated and treated inappropriately or inadequately. Hypochondriasis can be disabling in intensity and is persistent, with waxing and waning symptomatology.

In *factitious illnesses,* the patient consciously and voluntarily produces physical symptoms of illness. The term *Munchausen's syndrome* is reserved for individuals with particularly dramatic, chronic, or severe factitious illness. In true factitious illness, the sick role itself is gratifying. A variety of signs, symptoms, and diseases have been either simulated or caused by factitious behavior, the most common including chronic diarrhea, fever of unknown origin, intestinal bleeding or hematuria, seizures, and hypoglycemia. Factitious disorder is usually not diagnosed until 5 to 10 years after its onset, and it can produce significant social and medical costs. In *malingering,* the fabrication derives from a desire for some external reward, such as a narcotic medication or disability reimbursement.

TREATMENT FOR SOMATOFORM DISORDERS

Patients with somatization disorders are frequently subjected to multiple diagnostic testing and exploratory surgeries in an attempt to find their "real" illness. Such an approach is doomed to failure and does not address the core issue. Successful treatment is best achieved through behavior modification, in which access to the physician is tightly regulated and adjusted to provide a sustained and predictable level of support that is less clearly contingent on the patient's level of presenting distress. Visits can be brief and should not be associated with a need for a diagnostic or treatment action. Although the literature is limited, some patients with somatization disorder may benefit from antidepressant treatment. Fluoxetine and MAOIs have both been found to be useful in reducing obsessive ruminations, dysphoria, and anxious preoccupation in patients with multiple somatic complaints.

The treatment of factitious disorder is complicated in that any attempt to confront the patient usually only creates a sense of humiliation and causes the patient to abandon treatment from that caregiver. A better strategy is to introduce psychological causation as one of a number of possible explanations and to include factitious illness as an option in the differential diagnoses that are discussed. Without directly linking psychotherapeutic intervention to the diagnosis, the patient can be offered a face-saving means by which the pathologic relationship with the health care system can be examined and alternative approaches to life stressors developed.

PERSONALITY DISORDERS

Clinical Manifestations

Personality disorders are characteristic patterns of thinking, feeling, and interpersonal behavior that are relatively inflexible and cause significant functional impairment or subjective distress for the individual. The observed behaviors are not secondary to another mental disorder, nor are they precipitated by substance abuse or a general medical condition. This distinction is often difficult to make in clinical practice, as personality change may be the first sign of serious neurologic, endocrine, or other medical illness. Patients with frontal lobe tumors, for example, can present with changes in motivation and personality while the results of the neurologic examination remain within normal limits. Individuals with personality disorders are often regarded as "difficult patients" in clinical medical practice because they are seen as excessively demanding and/or unwilling to follow recommended treatment plans. Although DSM-IV portrays personality disorders as qualitatively distinct categories, there is an alternative perspective that personality characteristics vary as a continuum between normal functioning and formal mental disorder.

Personality disorders have been grouped into three overlapping clusters. *Cluster A* includes paranoid, schizoid, and schizotypal personality disorders. It includes individuals who are odd and eccentric and who maintain an emotional distance from others. Individuals have a restricted emotional range and remain socially isolated. Patients with schizotypal personality disorder frequently have unusual perceptual experiences and express magical beliefs about the external world. The essential feature of paranoid personality disorder is a pervasive mistrust and suspiciousness of others to an extent that is unjustified by available evidence. *Cluster B* disorders include antisocial, borderline, histrionic, and narcissistic types and describe individuals whose behavior is impulsive, excessively emotional, and erratic. *Cluster C* incorporates avoidant, dependent, and obsessive-compulsive personality types; enduring traits are anxiety and fear. The boundaries between cluster types are to some extent artificial, and many patients who meet criteria for one personality disorder also meet criteria for aspects of another. The risk of a comorbid major mental disorder is increased in patients who qualify for a diagnosis of personality disorder.

TREATMENT FOR PERSONALITY DISORDERS

Dialectical behavior therapy (DBT) is a cognitive-behavioral approach that focuses on behavioral change while providing acceptance, compassion, and validation of the patient. Several randomized trials have demonstrated the efficacy of DBT in the treatment of personality disorders. Antidepressant medications and low-dose antipsychotic drugs have some efficacy in cluster A personality disorders, while anticonvulsant mood-stabilizing agents and MAOIs may be considered for patients with cluster B diagnoses who show marked mood reactivity, behavioral dyscontrol, and/or rejection hypersensitivity. Anxious or fearful cluster C patients often respond to medications used for axis I anxiety disorders (see above). It is important that the physician and the patient have reasonable expectations vis-á-vis the possible benefit of any medication used and its side effects. Improvement may be subtle and observable only over time.

SCHIZOPHRENIA

Clinical Manifestations

Schizophrenia is a heterogeneous syndrome characterized by perturbations of language, perception, thinking, social activity, affect, and volition. There are no pathognomonic features. The syndrome commonly begins in late adolescence, has an insidious (and less commonly acute) onset, and, classically, has a poor outcome, progressing from social withdrawal and perceptual distortions to a state of chronic delusions and hallucinations. Patients may present with positive symptoms (such as conceptual disorganization, delusions, or hallucinations) or negative symptoms (loss of function, anhedonia, decreased emotional expression, impaired concentration, and diminished social engagement) and must have at least two of these for a 1-month period and continuous signs for at least 6 months to meet formal diagnostic criteria. "Negative" symptoms predominate in one-third of the schizophrenic population and are associated with a poor long-term outcome and a poor response to drug treatment. However, marked variability in the course and individual character of symptoms is typical.

The four main subtypes of schizophrenia are catatonic, paranoid, disorganized, and residual. Many individuals have symptoms of more than one type. *Catatonic-type* describes patients whose clinical presentation is dominated by profound changes in motor activity, negativism, and echolalia or echopraxia. *Paranoid-type* describes patients who have a prominent preoccupation with a specific delusional system and who otherwise do not qualify as having *disorganized-type* disease, in which disorganized speech and behavior are accompanied by a superficial or silly affect. In *residual-type* disease, negative symptomatology exists in the absence of delusions, hallucinations, or motor disturbance. The term *schizophreniform disorder* describes patients who meet the symptom requirements but not the duration requirements for schizophrenia, and *schizoaffective disorder* is used for those who manifest symptoms of schizophrenia and independent periods of mood disturbance. Prognosis depends not on symptom severity but on the response to antipsychotic medication. A permanent remission without recurrence does occasionally occur. About 10% of schizophrenic patients commit suicide.

Schizophrenia is present in 0.85% of individuals worldwide, with a lifetime prevalence of ~1 to 1.5%. An estimated 300,000 episodes of acute schizophrenia occur annually in the United States, resulting in direct and indirect costs estimated at >$33 billion.

Differential Diagnosis

The diagnosis is principally one of exclusion, requiring the absence of significant associated mood symptoms, any relevant medical condition, and substance abuse. Drug reactions that cause hallucinations, paranoia, confusion, or bizarre behavior may be dose-related or idiosyncratic; β-adrenergic blockers, clonidine, cycloserine, quinacrine, and procaine derivatives are the most common prescription medications associated with these symptoms. Drug causes should be ruled out in any case

of newly emergent psychosis. The general neurologic examination in patients with schizophrenia is usually normal, but motor rigidity, tremor, and dyskinesias are noted in one-quarter of untreated patients.

Epidemiology

Epidemiologic surveys identify several risk factors for schizophrenia including genetic susceptibility, early developmental insults, winter birth, and increasing parental age. Genetic factors are involved in at least a subset of individuals who develop schizophrenia. Schizophrenia is observed in ~6.6% of all first-degree relatives of an affected proband. If both parents are affected, the risk for offspring is 40%. The concordance rate for monozygotic twins is 50%, compared to 10% for dizygotic twins. Schizophrenia-prone families are also at risk for other psychiatric disorders, including schizoaffective disorder and *schizotypal* and *schizoid personality disorders,* the latter terms designating individuals who show a lifetime pattern of social and interpersonal deficits characterized by an inability to form close interpersonal relationships, eccentric behavior, and mild perceptual distortions.

Despite evidence for a genetic causation, the results of molecular genetic linkage studies in schizophrenia are inconclusive. Major gene effects appear unlikely. Possible susceptibility genes include neuroregulin-1 at chromosome 8p21, dysbindin at 6p22.3, proline dehydrogenase at 22q11, and G72 at 13q34. Several of these may be involved in glutamatergic regulation, increasing interest in N-methyl-D-aspartate (NMDA)-mediated glutamate signaling as a possible therapeutic target for treatment. One group has reported risk variants in the $\alpha7$ nicotinic acetylcholine receptor subunit gene and linked it to a specific auditory processing deficit.

Schizophrenia is also associated with gestational and perinatal complications, including Rh factor incompatibility, fetal hypoxia, prenatal exposure to influenza during the second trimester, and prenatal nutritional deficiency. Studies of monozygotic twins discordant for schizophrenia have reported neuroanatomical differences between affected and unaffected siblings, supporting a "two-strike" etiology involving both genetic susceptibility and an environmental insult. The latter might involve localized hypoxia during critical stages of brain development.

The *dopamine hypothesis* of schizophrenia is based on the discovery that agents that diminish dopaminergic activity also reduce the acute symptoms and signs of psychosis, specifically agitation, anxiety, and hallucinations. Amelioration of delusions and social withdrawal is less dramatic. Thus far, however, evidence for increased dopaminergic activity in schizophrenia is indirect, although decreased D_2 receptor occupancy by dopamine has recently been shown in drug-naive patients. An increase in the activity of nigrostriatal and mesolimbic systems and a decrease in mesocortical tracts innervating the prefrontal cortex is hypothesized, although it is likely that other neurotransmitters, including serotonin, acetylcholine, glutamate, and GABA, also contribute to the pathophysiology of the illness. Possible involvement of excitatory amino acids is based on the genetic data cited above and the finding that NMDA receptor antagonists and channel blockers, such as phencyclidine (PCP) and ketamine, produce characteristic signs of schizophrenia in normal individuals; cycloserine, an NMDA receptor agonist, can decrease the negative symptoms of psychosis.

TREATMENT FOR SCHIZOPHRENIA

Antipsychotic agents (**Table 41-14**) are the cornerstone of acute and maintenance treatment of schizophrenia, and are effective in the treatment of hallucinations, delusions, and thought disorders, regardless of etiology. The mechanism of action involves, at least in part, blockade of dopamine receptors in the limbic system and basal ganglia; the clinical potencies of traditional antipsychotic drugs parallel their affinities for the D_2 receptor, and even the newer "atypical" agents exert some degree of D_2 receptor blockade. All neuroleptics induce expression of the immediate-early gene *c-fos* in the nucleus accumbens, a dopaminergic site connecting prefrontal and limbic cortices. The clinical efficacy of newer atypical neuroleptics, however, may involve D_1, D_3, and D_4 receptor blockade, α_1- and α_2-noradrenergic activity, and/or altering the relationship between $5HT_2$ and D_2 receptor activity, as well as faster dissociation of D_2 binding.

Conventional neuroleptics differ in their potency and side-effect profile. Older agents, such as chlorpromazine and thioridazine, are more sedating and anticholinergic and more likely to cause orthostatic hypotension, while higher-potency antipsychotics, such as haloperidol, perphenazine, and thiothixene, are more likely to induce extrapyramidal side effects. The model atypical antipsychotic agent is *clozapine,* a dibenzodiazepine that has a greater potency in blocking the $5HT_2$ than the D_2 receptor and a much higher affinity for the D_4 than the D_2 receptor. Its principal disadvantage is a risk of blood dyscrasias. Unlike

other antipsychotics, clozapine does not cause a rise in prolactin level. Approximately 30% of patients have a better response to these agents than to traditional neuroleptics, suggesting that they will increasingly displace the older-generation drugs. Clozapine appears to be the most effective member of this class and has demonstrated superiority to other atypical agents in preventing suicide; however, its side-effect profile makes it most appropriate for treatment-resistant cases. *Risperidone,* a benzisoxazole derivative, is more potent at $5HT_2$ than D_2 receptor sites, like clozapine, but it also exerts significant α_2 antagonism, a property that may contribute to its perceived ability to improve mood and increase motor activity. Risperidone is not as effective as clozapine in treatment-resistant cases but does not carry a risk of blood dyscrasias. *Olanzapine* is similar neurochemically to clozapine but has a significant risk of inducing weight gain. *Quetiapine* is distinct in having a weak D_2 effect but potent α_1 and histamine blockade. Ziprasidone causes minimal weight gain and is unlikely to increase prolactin, but may increase QT prolongation. Aripiprazole also has little risk of weight gain or prolactin increase but may increase anxiety, nausea, and insomnia as a result of its partial agonist properties.

Conventional antipsychotic agents are effective in 70% of patients presenting with a first episode. Improvement may be observed within hours or days, but full remission usually requires 6 to 8 weeks. The choice of agent depends principally on the side-effect profile and cost of treatment or on a past personal or family history of a favorable response to the drug in question. Atypical agents appear to be more effective in treating negative symptoms and improving cognitive function. An equivalent treatment response can usually be achieved with relatively low doses of any drug selected, e.g., 4 to 6 mg/d of haloperidol, 10 to 15 mg of olanzapine, or 4 to 6 mg/d of risperidone. Doses in this range result in >80% D_2 receptor blockade, and there is little evidence that higher doses increase either the rapidity or degree of response. Maintenance treatment requires careful attention to the possibility of relapse and monitoring for the development of a movement disorder. Intermittent drug treatment is less effective than regular dosing, but gradual dose reduction is likely to improve social functioning in many schizophrenic patients who have been maintained at high doses. If medications are completely

TABLE 41-14

ANTIPSYCHOTIC AGENTS

NAME	USUAL PO DAILY DOSE, MG	SIDE EFFECTS	SEDATION	COMMENTS
TYPICAL ANTIPSYCHOTICS				
Low-potency				
Chlorpromazine (Thorazine)	100–600	Anticholinergic effects;	+ + +	EPSEs usually not
Thioridazine (Mellaril)	100–600	orthostasis; photosensitivity;		prominent; can cause
		cholestasis; QT prolongation		anticholinergic delirium
				in elderly patients
Mid-potency				
Trifluoperazine (Stelazine)	2–15	Fewer anticholinergic side	+ +	Well tolerated by most
		effects; fewer EPSEs than		patients
		with higher-potency		
Perphenazine (Trilafon)	4–32	agents	+ +	
Loxapine (Loxitane)	20–250	Frequent EPSEs	+ +	
Molindone (Moban)	50–225	Frequent EPSEs	0	Little weight gain
High-potency		No anticholinergic side effects;		Often prescribed in
Haloperidol (Haldol)	0.5–10	EPSEs often prominent	0/+	doses that are too high;
Fluphenazine (Prolixin)	1–10	Frequent EPSEs	0/+	long-acting injectable
Thiothixene (Navane)	2–20	Frequent EPSEs	0/+	forms of haloperidol and
				fluphenazine available
NOVEL ANTIPSYCHOTICS				
Clozapine (Clozaril)	200–600	Agranulocytosis (1%); weight gain; seizures; drooling; hyperthermia	+ +	Requires weekly WBC
Risperidone (Risperdal)	2–6	Orthostasis	+	Requires slow titration; EPSEs observed with doses >6 mg qd
Olanzapine (Zyprexa)	10–20	Weight gain	+ +	Mild prolactin elevation
Quetiapine (Seroquel)	350–700	Sedation; weight gain; anxiety	+ + +	Bid dosing
Ziprasidone (Geodon)	40–60	Orthostatic hypotension	+/+ +	Minimal weight gain; increases QT interval
Aripiprazole (Abilify)	10–30	Nausea, anxiety, insomnia	0/+	Mixed agonist/antagonist

Note: EPSEs, extrapyramidal side effects; WBC, white blood count.

discontinued, however, the relapse rate is 60% within 6 months. Long-acting injectable preparations are considered when noncompliance with oral therapy leads to relapses. In treatment-resistant patients, a transition to clozapine usually results in rapid improvement, but a prolonged delay in response in some cases necessitates a 6- to 9-month trial for maximal benefit to occur.

Antipsychotic medications can cause a broad range of side effects, including lethargy, weight gain, postural hypotension, constipation, and dry mouth. Extrapyramidal symptoms such as dystonia, akathisia, and akinesia also are frequent with traditional agents and may contribute to poor compliance if not specifically addressed. Anticholinergic and parkinsonian symptoms respond well to trihexyphenidyl, 2 mg bid, or benztropine mesylate, 1 to 2 mg bid. Akathisia may respond to beta blockers. In rare cases, more serious and occasionally life-threatening side effects may emerge, including ventricular arrhythmias, gastrointestinal obstruction, retinal pigmentation, obstructive jaundice, and neuroleptic malignant syndrome (characterized by hyperthermia, autonomic dysfunction, muscular rigidity, and elevated creatine phosphokinase levels). The most serious adverse effects of clozapine are agranulocytosis, which has an incidence of 1%, and induction of seizures, which has an incidence of 10%. Weekly white blood cell counts are required, particularly during the first 3 months of treatment.

The risk of type 2 diabetes mellitus appears to be increased in schizophrenia, and atypical agents as a group produce greater adverse effects on glucose regulation, independent of effects on obesity, than traditional agents. Clozapine, olanzapine, and quetiapine seem more likely to cause hyperglycemia, weight gain, and hypertriglyceridemia than other atypical antipsychotic drugs. Close monitoring of plasma glucose and lipid levels are indicated with the use of these agents.

A serious side effect of long-term use of the classic antipsychotic agents is *tardive dyskinesia,* characterized by repetitive, involuntary, and potentially irreversible movements of the tongue and lips (bucco-linguo-masticatory triad), and, in approximately half of cases, choreoathetosis (Chap. 19). Tardive dyskinesia has an incidence of 2 to 4% per year of exposure, and a prevalence of 20% in chronically treated patients. The prevalence increases with age, total dose, and duration of drug administration. The risk associated with the newer atypical agents appears to be much lower. The cause may involve formation of free radicals and perhaps mitochondrial energy failure. Vitamin E may reduce abnormal involuntary movements if given early in the syndrome.

Drug treatment of schizophrenia is by itself insufficient. Educational efforts directed toward families and relevant community resources have proved to be necessary to maintain stability and optimize outcome. A treatment model involving a multidisciplinary case-management team that seeks out and closely follows the patient in the community has proved particularly effective.

ASSESSMENT AND EVALUATION OF VIOLENCE

Primary care physicians may encounter situations in which family, domestic, or societal violence is discovered or suspected. Such an awareness can carry legal and moral obligations; many state laws mandate reporting of child, spousal, and elder abuse. Physicians are frequently the first point of contact for both victim and abuser. Between 1 and 2 million older Americans and 1.5 million U.S. children are thought to experience some form of physical maltreatment each year. Spousal abuse is thought to be even more prevalent. One survey of internal medicine practices found that 5.5% of all female patients had experienced domestic violence in the previous year, and that these individuals were more likely to suffer from depression, anxiety, somatization disorder, and substance abuse and to have attempted suicide. When domestic violence is suspected, direct but nonjudgmental questioning should be pursued with each party separately—"Do you feel safe at home?" and "If there's a disagreement or a conflict between the two of you, how is it worked out?" Individuals who are abused may have signs of obvious or suspected physical injury; in addition, abused individuals frequently express low self-esteem, vague somatic symptomatology, social isolation, and a passive feeling of loss of control. Although it is essential to treat these elements in the victim, the first obligation is to ensure that the perpetrator has taken responsibility for preventing any further violence. Substance abuse and/or dependence and serious mental illness in the abuser may contribute to the risk of harm and require direct intervention. Depending on the situation, law enforcement agencies, community resources such as support groups and shelters, and individual and family counseling can be appropriate components of a treatment plan. A safety plan should be formulated with the victim, in addition to providing information about abuse, its likelihood of recurrence, and its tendency to increase in severity and frequency. Antianxiety and antidepressant medications may sometimes be useful in treating the acute symptoms, but only if independent evidence for an appropriate psychiatric diagnosis exists. Antidepressants are generally not indicated when the diagnosis is linked to the social situation, such as an adjustment disorder with depressed mood. The most important element in treatment is the development of a supportive doctor-patient relationship that avoids further blame of the victim. In certain circumstances, a significant potential for societal violence may be discovered. Sympathetic, but direct, questioning about potential violent impulses, access to weapons, recreational drug use, and specific homicidal ideation is necessary and is sometimes therapeutic in its own right. The existence and possible contribution of such medical conditions as delirium and/or intoxication should be evaluated. Available disposition options for potentially violent patients include police custody, psychiatric hospitalization, and referral to home care, with involvement of family, friends, and caregivers. In deciding which treatment option is most appropriate, clinicians should endeavor to establish an empathic interaction with the patient, while avoiding interventions or stimuli that might precipitate or increase the risk of violent behavior.

MENTAL HEALTH PROBLEMS IN THE HOMELESS

There is a high prevalence of mental disorders and substance abuse among homeless and impoverished people. The total number of homeless individuals in the United States is estimated at 2 to 3 million, one-third of whom qualify as having a serious mental disorder. Poor hygiene and nutrition, substance abuse, psychiatric illness, physical trauma, and exposure to the elements combine to make the provision of medical care challenging. Only a minority of these individuals receive formal mental health care; the main points of contact are outpatient medical clinics and emergency departments. Primary care settings represent a critical site in which housing needs, treatment of substance dependence, and evaluation and treatment of psychiatric illness can most efficiently take place. Successful intervention is dependent on breaking down traditional administrative barriers to health care and recognizing the physical constraints and emotional costs imposed by homelessness. Simplifying health care instructions and follow-up, allowing frequent visits, and dispensing medications in limited amounts that require ongoing contact are possible techniques for establishing a successful therapeutic relationship.

FURTHER READINGS

ABLON JS, JONES EEJ: Validity of controlled clinical trials of psychotherapy: Findings from the NIMH treatment of depression collaborative research program. Am J Psychiatry 159:775, 2002

COYLE JT, DUMAN RS: Finding the intracellular signaling pathways affected by mood disorder treatments. Neuron 38:157, 2003

FISCHHOFF B, WESSELY S: Managing patients with inexplicable health problems. BMJ 326:595, 2003

GOFF DC ET AL: Medical morbidity and mortality in schizophrenia: Guidelines for psychiatrists. J Clin Psychiatry 66:183, 2005

KESSLER RC ET AL: The epidemiology of major depressive disorder: Results from the National Comorbidity Survey Replication (NCSR). JAMA 289:3095, 2003

WATHEN CN, MACMILLAN HL: Interventions for violence against women: Scientific review. JAMA 289:589, 2003

◪ LIEBERMAN JA ET AL: Effectiveness of antipsychotic drugs in patients with chronic schzophrenia. N. Engl J Med. 353:1209,2005

A trial comparing typical versus atypical antipsychotic drugs for schizophrenic patients.

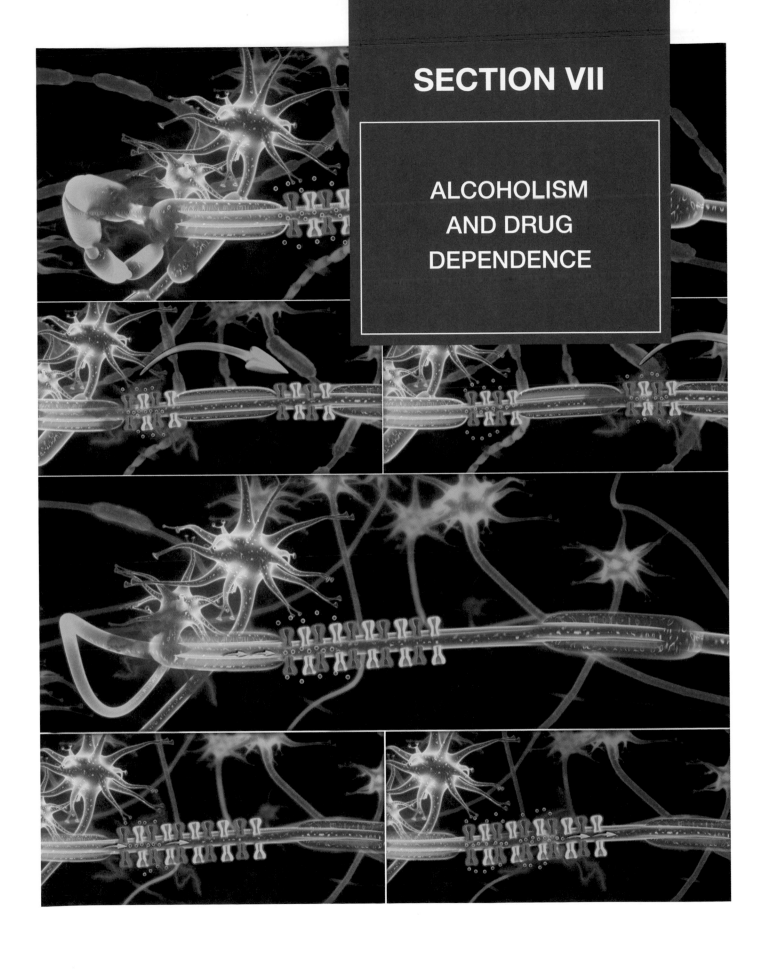

SECTION VII

ALCOHOLISM AND DRUG DEPENDENCE

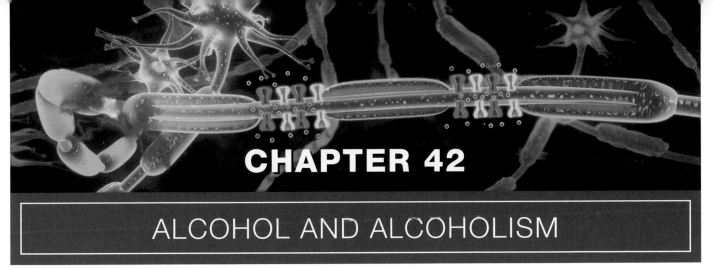

CHAPTER 42

ALCOHOL AND ALCOHOLISM

Marc A. Schuckit

Alcohol, a drug, is consumed at some time by up to 80% of the population. At low doses alcohol can have some beneficial effects such as decreased rates of myocardial infarction, stroke, gallstones, and possibly vascular or Alzheimer's dementias, but the consumption of more than two standard drinks per day increases the risk for health problems in many organ systems. Heavy repetitive drinking, as is seen in alcohol abuse and dependence, cuts short the life span by an estimated decade in both genders, all cultural groups, and all socioeconomic strata. Even low doses of alcohol have a significant effect on many organ systems, adversely affecting most preexisting disease states and altering the effectiveness or blood levels of most over-the-counter and prescribed medications.

PHARMACOLOGY AND NUTRITIONAL IMPACT OF ETHANOL

Ethanol is a weakly charged molecule that moves easily through cell membranes, rapidly equilibrating between blood and tissues. The level of alcohol in the blood is expressed as milligrams or grams of ethanol per deciliter (e.g., 100 mg/dL or 0.10 g/dL); a level of 0.02 to 0.03 results from the ingestion of one to two typical drinks. In round figures, 340 mL (12 oz) of beer, 115 mL (4 oz) of nonfortified wine, and 43 mL (1.5 oz) (a shot) of 80-proof beverage each contain ~10 to 15 g of ethanol; 0.5

L (~1 pint) of 86-proof beverage contains ~160 g (about 16 standard drinks), and 1 L of wine contains ~80 g of ethanol. Congeners found in alcoholic beverages, including low-molecular-weight alcohols (e.g., methanol and butanol), aldehydes, esters, histamine, phenols, tannins, iron, lead, and cobalt, may contribute to the adverse health consequences associated with heavy drinking.

Ethanol is a central nervous system (CNS) depressant that decreases neuronal activity, although some behavioral stimulation is observed at low blood levels. This drug has cross-tolerance with other depressants, including benzodiazepines and barbiturates, and all produce similar behavioral alterations. Alcohol is absorbed from mucous membranes of the mouth and esophagus (in small amounts), from the stomach and large bowel (in modest amounts), and from the proximal portion of the small intestine (the major site). The rate of absorption is increased by rapid gastric emptying; by the absence of proteins, fats, or carbohydrates (which interfere with absorption); by the absence of congeners; by dilution to a modest percentage of ethanol (maximum at about 20% by volume); and by carbonation (e.g., champagne).

Between 2% (at low blood alcohol concentrations) and 10% (at high blood alcohol concentrations) of ethanol is excreted directly through the lungs, urine, or sweat, but the greater part is metabolized to acetaldehyde, primarily in the liver. The most important pathway occurs in the cell cytosol where alcohol dehydrogenase (ADH) produces acetaldehyde, which is then rapidly destroyed by aldehyde dehydrogenase (ALDH) in the cytosol and mitochondria (**Fig. 42–1**). A second pathway in the microsomes of the smooth endoplasmic reticulum (the microsomal ethanol-oxidizing system, or MEOS), is responsible for ≥10% of ethanol oxidation at high blood alcohol concentrations.

While alcohol supplies calories (a drink contains ~300 kJ, or 70 to 100 kcal), these are devoid of nutrients such as minerals, proteins, and vitamins. Alcohol can also interfere with absorption of vitamins in the small

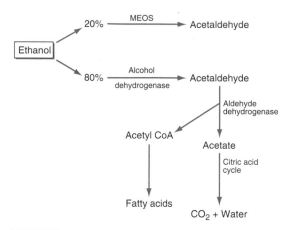

FIGURE 42-1

The metabolism of alcohol.

intestine and decreases their storage in the liver with effects on folate (folacin or folic acid), pyridoxine (B_6), thiamine (B_1), nicotinic acid (niacin, B_3), and vitamin A.

An ethanol load in a fasting, healthy individual is likely to produce transient hypoglycemia within 6 to 36 h, secondary to the acute actions of ethanol on gluconeogenesis. This can result in glucose intolerance until the alcoholic has abstained for 2 to 4 weeks. Alcohol ketoacidosis, probably reflecting a decrease in fatty acid oxidation coupled with poor diet or recurrent vomiting, should not be misdiagnosed as diabetic ketosis. With the former, patients show an increase in serum ketones along with a mild increase in glucose but a large anion gap, a mild to moderate increase in serum lactate, and a β-hydroxybutyrate/lactate ratio of between 2:1 and 9:1 (with normal being 1:1).

BEHAVIORAL EFFECTS, TOLERANCE, AND DEPENDENCE

The effects of any drug depend on the dose, the rate of increase in plasma, the concomitant presence of other drugs, and the past experience with the agent. With alcohol, an additional factor is whether blood alcohol levels are rising or falling; the effects are more intense during the former period.

Even though "legal intoxication" requires a blood alcohol concentration of at least 80 to 100 mg/dL, behavioral, psychomotor, and cognitive changes are seen at levels as low as 20 to 30 mg/dL (i.e., after one to two drinks) (**Table 42–1**). Deep but disturbed sleep can be seen at twice the legal intoxication level, and death can occur with levels between 300 and 400 mg/dL. Beverage alcohol is probably responsible for more overdose deaths than any other drug.

The intoxicating effects of alcohol appear to be due to actions at a number of neurotransmitter receptors and transporters. Alcohol enhances γ-aminobutyric acid A (GABA$_A$) receptors and inhibits N-methyl-D-aspartate

TABLE 42-1

EFFECTS OF BLOOD ALCOHOL LEVELS IN THE ABSENCE OF TOLERANCE

BLOOD LEVEL, MG/DL	USUAL EFFECT
20	Decreased inhibitions, a slight feeling of intoxication
80	Decrease in complex cognitive functions and motor performance
200	Obvious slurred speech, motor incoordination, irritability, and poor judgment
300	Light coma and depressed vital signs
400	Death

(NMDA) receptors. In vitro studies suggest that additional effects involve inhibition of adenosine uptake and a translocation of the cyclic AMP-dependent protein kinase catalytic subunit from the cytoplasm to the nucleus. Neurons adapt quickly to these actions, and thus different effects may be present during chronic administration and withdrawal.

At least three types of compensatory changes develop after repeated exposure to the drug, producing tolerance of higher ethanol levels. First, after 1 to 2 weeks of daily drinking, *metabolic or pharmacokinetic tolerance* can be seen, with a 30% increase in the rate of hepatic ethanol metabolism. This alteration disappears almost as rapidly as it develops. Second, *cellular or pharmacodynamic tolerance* develops through neurochemical changes that may also contribute to physical dependence. Third, individuals can learn to adapt their behavior so that they can function better than expected under drug influence (*behavioral tolerance*).

The cellular changes caused by chronic ethanol exposure may not resolve for several weeks or longer following cessation of drinking. In the interim, the neurons require ethanol to function optimally, and the individual can be said to be physically dependent. This is distinct from psychological dependence, a concept indicating that the person is psychologically uncomfortable without the drug.

THE EFFECTS OF ETHANOL ON ORGAN SYSTEMS

Although one to two drinks per day in an otherwise healthy and nonpregnant individual can have some beneficial cardiovascular effects, at higher doses alcohol is toxic to most organ systems. Knowledge about the deleterious effects of alcohol helps the physician to identify alcoholic patients and provides information that can be used to help motivate them to abstain. It is important to remember that the typical white- or blue-collar alcoholic functions at a fairly high level for years, and that not everyone develops each problem.

CENTRAL AND PERIPHERAL NERVOUS SYSTEM EFFECTS

Approximately 35% of drinkers may experience a *blackout,* an episode of temporary anterograde amnesia, in which the person forgets all or part of what occurred during a drinking evening. Another common problem, one seen after as few as several drinks, is that alcohol causes alterations between sleep stages and a deficiency in rapid eye movement and deep sleep with resulting prominent and sometimes disturbing dreams later in the night. Finally, alcohol relaxes muscles in the pharynx, which can cause snoring and exacerbate sleep apnea, with symptoms of the latter in 75% of alcoholic men over age 60. As a consequence of alcohol-related impairment in judgment and coordination, at least half of patients with physical trauma have evidence of substance-related impairment, a finding reflecting the fact that 40% of drinkers in the United States have at some time driven while intoxicated.

The effect of alcohol on the nervous system is even more pronounced among alcohol-dependent individuals. Chronic high doses cause *peripheral neuropathy* in 5 to 15% of alcoholics due to either alcohol itself or thiamine deficiency: patients experience bilateral limb numbness, tingling, and paresthesias, all of which are more pronounced distally. A proximal, symmetric alcoholic *myopathy* also may develop in some patients. *Wernicke's syndrome* (ophthalmoparesis, ataxia, and encephalopathy) and *Korsakoff's syndrome* are seen in <10% of alcoholics as the result of thiamine deficiency, especially in persons with transketolase deficiency (Chap. 15). Approximately 1% of alcoholics develop *cerebellar degeneration,* a syndrome of progressive unsteady stance and gait often accompanied by mild nystagmus; neuroimaging studies reveal atrophy of the cerebellar vermis.

Alcoholics can manifest severe *cognitive problems* including impairment in recent and remote memory for weeks to months after an alcoholic binge. Increased size of the brain ventricles and cerebral sulci are seen in ≥50% of chronic alcoholics, but these changes are often reversible, returning toward normal within a year or so of abstinence. There is no single alcoholic dementia syndrome; rather, this label is used to describe patients who have apparently irreversible cognitive changes (possibly from diverse causes) and chronic alcoholism.

Finally, almost every psychiatric syndrome can be seen temporarily during heavy drinking or subsequent withdrawal. These include intense *sadness* lasting for days to weeks in the midst of heavy drinking in 40% of alcoholics, which is classified as an alcohol-induced mood disorder; temporary severe *anxiety* in 10 to 30% of alcoholics, often beginning during alcohol withdrawal, which can persist for many months after cessation of drinking (alcohol-induced anxiety disorder); and auditory *hallucinations* and/or paranoid delusions in a clear sensorium (*alcohol-induced psychotic disorder*) seen temporarily in 1 to 10% of alcoholics. Treatment of all forms of alcohol-induced psychopathology includes abstinence and supportive care, with the likelihood of full recovery within several days to 4 weeks. A history of alcohol intake is an important consideration in any patient with one of these psychiatric symptoms.

NONNEUROLOGIC SYSTEMS

In the gastrointestinal system, acute alcohol intake can result in inflammation of the esophagus and stomach resulting in gastrointestinal bleeding and, in cases of heavy vomiting, Mallory-Weiss tears. Acute and chronic pancreatitis as well as fatty liver disease also can result from chronic alcoholism. In the cardiovascular system, chronic alcohol use can result in mild to moderate hypertension. Binge drinking can lead occasionally to atrial and ventricular arrhythmias termed "holiday heart." Hematopoietic effects include mild thrombocytopenia and a megaloblastic anemia in patients with folate deficiency. Heavy drinking during pregnancy results in the rapid placental transfer of both ethanol and acetaldehyde, which may have serious consequences for fetal development. The *fetal alcohol syndrome* can include any of the following: facial changes with epicanthal eye folds, poorly formed concha, and small teeth with faulty enamel; cardiac atrial or ventricular septal defects; an aberrant palmar crease and limitation in joint movement; and microcephaly with mental retardation. The amount of ethanol and/or time of vulnerability during pregnancy have not been defined, making it advisable for pregnant women to abstain completely.

ALCOHOLISM (ALCOHOL ABUSE OR DEPENDENCE)

Because many drinkers occasionally imbibe to excess, temporary alcohol-related pathology is common in nonalcoholics, especially those in the late teens to the late twenties. When repeated problems in multiple life areas develop, the person is likely to meet criteria for alcohol abuse or dependence.

DEFINITIONS AND EPIDEMIOLOGY

Alcohol dependence is defined in the Fourth Diagnostic and Statistical Manual (DSM-IV) of the American Psychiatric Association as repeated alcohol-related difficulties in at least three of seven areas of functioning that cluster together over any 12-month period. A special emphasis is placed on tolerance and/or withdrawal, a condition referred to as "dependence with a physiological component," which is associated with a more severe clinical course. Dependence occurs in both men and women and in individuals from all socioeconomic strata and of all racial backgrounds. The diagnosis predicts a course of recurrent problems with the use of alcohol and the consequent shortening of the life span by a decade or more. In the absence of alcohol dependence, an individual can be given a diagnosis of *alcohol abuse* if he or she demonstrates repetitive problems with alcohol in any one of four life areas that include social, interpersonal, legal, and occupational problems, or repeated use in hazardous situations such as driving.

The lifetime risk for alcohol dependence in most western countries is about 10 to 15% for men and 5 to 8% for women. When alcohol abuse also is considered, the rates are even higher. The typical alcoholic is a blue- or white-collar worker or homemaker and not the stereotypical homeless individual.

GENETICS OF ALCOHOLISM *Alcoholism* is a complex genetically influenced disorder; genes explain about 60% of the risk. The importance of genetic influences is supported by a higher risk in the identical versus fraternal twin of an alcoholic and a fourfold increased risk in children of alcoholics even if adopted at birth and raised without knowledge of their biologic parents.

A variety of independent genetically influenced characteristics likely combine to explain the contribution of hereditary factors. For alcoholism and other substance dependencies, some families appear to carry an enhanced risk through high levels of impulsivity, as can be seen in the antisocial personality disorder. In other families the risk is associated with vulnerability for several independent psychiatric disorders such as schizophrenia and manic-depressive disease. A diminished alcoholism risk is seen in approximately half of Asian men and women; this is due to an inactive form of the enzyme ALDH, which results in higher levels of acetaldehyde following alcohol ingestion. A significant proportion of the vulnerability for alcoholism appears to relate to genes that affect the intensity of the response to alcohol. Most studies have shown that 40% of some subgroups at high risk for future alcoholism (e.g., offspring of alcoholics) require higher blood alcohol concentrations to produce the effects seen at lower blood levels in most other people. This relatively low response to alcohol predicts the risk for alcohol-related problems over the next decade, including alcohol use disorders.

NATURAL HISTORY

For the "average" alcoholic, the age of first drink and first problems (e.g., an alcoholic blackout) are similar to those in the general population. However, by the early to mid-twenties, most men and women moderate their drinking (perhaps learning from minor problems), whereas difficulties for alcoholics are likely to escalate, with the first major life problem from alcohol appearing in the mid-twenties. Once established, the course of alcoholism is likely to be one of exacerbations and remissions. As a rule, there is little difficulty in stopping alcohol use when problems develop, and this step is often followed by days to months of carefully controlled drinking. Unless abstinence is maintained, these periods almost inevitably give way to escalations in alcohol intake and subsequent problems. The course is not hopeless, because between half and two-thirds of alcoholics maintain abstinence for years, and often permanently after treatment. Even without formal treatment or self-help groups there is at least a 20% chance of long-term abstinence. However, should the alcoholic continue to drink, the life span is shortened by an average of 10 years, with the leading causes of death, in decreasing order, the result of heart disease, cancer, accidents, and suicide.

IDENTIFICATION OF THE ALCOHOLIC AND INTERVENTION

Physicians even in affluent areas should recognize that ~20% of patients have alcoholism. Therefore, it is important to pay attention to the alcohol-related symptoms and signs as well as laboratory tests that are likely to be abnormal in the context of regular consumption of 6 to 8 or more drinks per day. The two blood tests with between 70% and 80% sensitivity and specificity are γ-glutamyl transferase (GGT) ($>$30 U) and carbohydrate-deficient transferrin (CDT) ($>$20 U/L); the combination of the two is likely to be more accurate than either alone. Physicians should consider these tests when screening patients for high levels of alcohol intake. These serologic markers of heavy drinking can also be useful in monitoring abstinence as they are likely to return toward normal within several weeks of the cessation of drinking; thus, increases in values of as little as 10% are likely to indicate a resumption of heavy alcohol intake. Other blood tests that can be useful in identifying individuals consuming six or more standard drinks per day include high normal mean corpuscular volumes (MCVs) ($>$91 μm^3) and serum uric acid ($>$416 mol/L, or 7 mg/dL). Physical signs and symptoms that can be useful in identifying alcoholism include mild and fluctuating hypertension (e.g., 140/95), repeated infections such as pneumonia, and otherwise unexplained cardiac arrhythmias. Other disorders suggestive of dependence include cancer of the head and neck, esophagus, or stomach as well as cirrhosis, unexplained hepatitis, pancreatitis, bilateral parotid gland swelling, and peripheral neuropathy.

The clinical diagnosis of alcohol abuse or dependence ultimately rests on the documentation of a pattern of difficulties associated with alcohol use; the definition is not based on the quantity and frequency of alcohol consumption. Thus, in screening it is important to probe for life problems and then attempt to tie in use of alcohol or another substance. Information regarding marital or job problems, legal difficulties, histories of accidents, medical problems, evidence of tolerance, etc., is important. While all physicians should be able to take the time needed to gather such information, some standardized questionnaires can be helpful, including the 10-item Alcohol Use Disorder Screening Test (AUDIT). However, these are only screening tools, and a careful face-to-face interview is still required for a meaningful diagnosis. Shorter questionnaires have limited usefulness.

After alcoholism is identified, the diagnosis must be shared with the patient as part of an intervention. The presenting complaint can be used as an entrée to the alcohol problem. For instance, the patient complaining of insomnia or hypertension could be told that these are clinically important symptoms and that physical findings and laboratory tests indicate that alcohol appears to have contributed to the complaints and is increasing the risk for further medical and psychological problems. The physician should share information about the course of alcoholism and explore possible avenues of addressing the problem. This process has been codified under the names of *brief interventions* and *motivational interviewing.* The former has been shown to be effective in decreasing alcohol use and problems when instituted as two 15-min sessions 1 month apart, along with a telephone follow-up reminder. Motivational interviewing uses the clinician's level of concern and understanding of the need for patients to progress through their own stages of enhanced understanding of their problems to optimize their ability to alter their drinking behaviors.

The process of intervention is rarely accomplished in one session. For the person who refuses to stop drinking at the first intervention, a logical step is to "keep the door open," establishing future meetings so that help is available as problems escalate. In the meantime the family may benefit from counseling or referral to self-help groups such as Al-Anon (the Alcoholics Anonymous group for family members) and Alateen (for teenage children of alcoholics).

THE ALCOHOL WITHDRAWAL SYNDROME

Once the brain has been repeatedly exposed to high doses of alcohol, any sudden decrease in intake can produce withdrawal symptoms, many of which are the opposite of those produced by intoxication. Features include tremor of the hands (shakes or jitters); agitation and anxiety; autonomic nervous system overactivity including an increase in pulse, respiratory rate, and body temperature; insomnia, possibly accompanied by bad dreams; and gastrointestinal upset. These withdrawal symptoms generally begin within 5 to 10 h of decreasing ethanol intake, peak in intensity on day 2 or 3, and improve by day 4 or 5. Anxiety, insomnia, and mild levels of autonomic dysfunction may persist to some degree for ≥ 6 months as a protracted abstinence syndrome, which may contribute to the tendency to return to drinking.

At some point in their lives, between 2 and 5% of alcoholics experience withdrawal seizures, often within 48 h of stopping drinking. These rare events usually involve a single generalized seizure, and electroencephalographic abnormalities generally return to normal within several days.

The term *delirium tremens* (DTs) refers to delirium (mental confusion, agitation, and fluctuating levels of consciousness) associated with a tremor and autonomic overactivity (e.g., marked increases in pulse, blood pressure, and respirations). Fortunately, this serious and potentially life-threatening complication of alcohol withdrawal is seen in <5% of alcohol-dependent individuals, with the result that the chance of DTs during any single withdrawal is <1%. DTs are most likely to develop in patients with concomitant severe medical disorders and can usually be avoided by identifying and treating medical conditions.

TREATMENT FOR ALCOHOLISM

Acute Intoxication

The first priority is to be certain that the vital signs are relatively stable without evidence of respiratory depression, cardiac arrhythmia, or potentially dangerous changes in blood pressure. The possibility of intoxication with other drugs should be considered, and a blood or urine sample is indicated to screen for opioids or other CNS depressants such as benzodiazepines or barbiturates. Other medical conditions that must be evaluated include hypoglycemia, hepatic failure, or diabetic ketoacidosis.

Patients who are medically stable should be placed in a quiet environment and asked to lie on their side if fatigued in order to minimize the risk of aspiration. When the behavior indicates an increased likelihood of violence, hospital procedures should be followed, including planning for the possibility of a show of force with an intervention team. In the context of aggressiveness, patients should be clearly reminded in a nonthreatening way that it is the goal of the staff to help them to feel better and to avoid problems. If the aggressive behavior continues, relatively low doses of a short-acting benzodiazepine such as lorazepam (e.g., 1 mg orally) may be used and can be repeated as needed, but care must be taken so that the addition of this second CNS depressant does not destabilize vital signs or worsen confusion. An alternative approach is to use an antipsychotic medication (e.g., 5 mg of haloperidol), but this has the potential danger of lowering the seizure threshold. If aggression escalates, the patient might require a short-term admission to a locked ward, where medications can be used more safely and vital signs more closely monitored.

Withdrawal

The first step is to perform a thorough physical examination in all alcoholics who are considering stopping drinking, including a search for evidence of liver failure, gastrointestinal bleeding, cardiac arrhythmia, and glucose or electrolyte imbalance.

The second step in treating withdrawal for even the typical well-nourished alcoholic is to offer adequate nutrition and rest. All patients should be given oral multiple B vitamins, including 50 to 100 mg of thiamine daily for a week or more. Most patients enter withdrawal with normal levels of body water or mild overhydration, and intravenous fluids should be avoided unless there is evidence of significant recent bleeding, vomiting, or diarrhea. Medications can usually be administered orally.

The third step in treatment is to recognize that most withdrawal symptoms are caused by the rapid removal of a CNS depressant. Patients can be weaned by administering any drug of this class and gradually decreasing the levels over 3 to 5 days. While many CNS depressants are effective, benzodiazepines have the highest margin of safety and lowest cost and are, therefore, the preferred class of drugs. Benzodiazepines with short half-lives (Chap. 41) are especially useful for patients with serious liver impairment or evidence of preexisting encephalopathy or brain damage, but they result in rapidly changing drug blood levels and must be given every 4 h to avoid abrupt fluctuations in blood levels that may increase the risk for seizures. Therefore, most clinicians use drugs with longer half-lives, such as diazepam or chlordiazepoxide,

administering enough drug on day 1 to alleviate most of the symptoms of withdrawal (e.g., the tremor and elevated pulse) and then decreasing the dose by 20% on successive days over a period of 3 to 5 days. The approach is flexible; the dose is increased if signs of withdrawal escalate, and the medication is withheld if the patient is sleeping or shows signs of increasing orthostatic hypotension. The average patient requires 25 to 50 mg of chlordiazepoxide or 10 mg of diazepam given orally every 4 to 6 h on the first day.

Treatment of the patient with DTs can be difficult, and the condition is likely to run a course of 3 to 5 days regardless of the therapy employed. The focus of care is to identify medical problems and correct them and to control behavior and prevent injuries. Many clinicians recommend the use of high doses of a benzodiazepine (as much as 800 mg/d of chlordiazepoxide have been reported), a treatment that will decrease the agitation and raise the seizure threshold but probably does little to improve the confusion. Other clinicians recommend the use of antipsychotic medications, such as haloperidol, 20 mg or more per day, an approach less likely to exacerbate confusion but which may increase the risk of seizures. Antipsychotic drugs have no place in the treatment of mild withdrawal symptoms.

Generalized withdrawal seizures rarely require aggressive pharmacologic intervention beyond that given to the usual patient undergoing withdrawal, i.e., adequate doses of benzodiazepines. There is little evidence that anticonvulsants such as phenytoin are effective in drug-withdrawal seizures, and the risk of seizures has usually passed by the time effective drug levels are reached. The rare patient with status epilepticus must be treated aggressively (Chap. 14).

While alcohol withdrawal is often treated in a hospital, efforts at reducing costs have resulted in the development of outpatient detoxification for relatively mild abstinence syndromes. This is appropriate for patients in good physical condition who demonstrate mild signs of withdrawal despite low blood alcohol concentrations and for those without prior history of DTs or withdrawal seizures. Such individuals still require a careful physical examination, evaluation of blood tests, and vitamin supplementation. Benzodiazepines can be given in a 1- to 2-day supply to be administered to the patient by a spouse or other family member four times a day. Patients are asked to return daily for evaluation of vital signs and to come to the emergency room if signs and symptoms of withdrawal escalate.

Rehabilitation of Alcoholics

After completing alcoholic rehabilitation, 60% or more of alcoholics maintain abstinence for at least a year, and many achieve lifetime abstinence. Considering the lack of evidence for the superiority of any specific treatment type, it is best to keep interventions simple.

Maneuvers in rehabilitation fall into several general categories, which are applied to all patients regardless of age or ethnic group. However, the manner in which the treatments are used should be sensitive to the practices and needs of specific populations. First are attempts to help the alcoholic achieve and maintain a high level of motivation toward abstinence. These include education about alcoholism and instructing family and/or friends to stop protecting the person from the problems caused by alcohol. The second step is to help the patient to readjust to life without alcohol and to reestablish a functional lifestyle through counseling, vocational rehabilitation, and self-help groups such as Alcoholics Anonymous (AA). The third component, called *relapse prevention,* helps the person to identify situations in which a return to drinking is likely, formulate ways of managing these risks, and develop coping strategies that increase the chances of a return to abstinence if a slip occurs.

There is no convincing evidence that inpatient rehabilitation is always more effective than outpatient care. However, more intense interventions work better than less intensive measures, and some alcoholics do not respond to outpatient approaches. The decision to hospitalize or place into residential care can be made if (1) the patient has medical problems that are difficult to treat outside a hospital; (2) depression, confusion, or psychosis interferes with outpatient care; (3) there is a severe life crisis that makes it difficult to work in an outpatient setting; (4) outpatient treatment has failed; or (5) the patient lives far from the treatment center. The best predictors of continued abstinence include evidence of higher levels of life stability (e.g., supportive family and friends) and higher levels of functioning (e.g., job skills, higher levels of education, and absence of crimes unrelated to alcohol).

Whether the treatment begins in an inpatient or an outpatient setting, subsequent outpatient contact should be maintained for a minimum of 6 months and preferably a full year after abstinence is achieved. Counseling with an individual physician or through groups focuses on day-to-day living—emphasizing areas of improved functioning in the absence of alcohol (i.e., why it is a good idea to continue to abstain) and helping the patient to manage free time without alcohol, develop a nondrinking peer group, and handle stresses on the job.

The physician serves an important role in identifying the alcoholic, treating associated medical or psychiatric syndromes, overseeing detoxification, referring the patient to rehabilitation programs, and providing counseling. The physician is also responsible for selecting which (if any) medication might be appropriate during alcoholism rehabilitation. Patients often complain of continuing sleep problems or anxiety when acute withdrawal treatment is over, problems that may be a component of protracted withdrawal. Unfortunately, there is no place for hypnotics or antianxiety drugs in the treatment of most alcoholics after acute withdrawal has been completed. Patients should be reassured that the trouble sleeping is normal after alcohol withdrawal and will improve over the subsequent weeks and months. Patients should follow a rigid bedtime and awakening schedule and avoid any naps or the use of caffeine in the evenings. The sleep pattern will improve rapidly. Anxiety can be addressed by helping the person to gain insight into the temporary nature of the symptoms and to develop strategies to achieve relaxation as well as by using forms of cognitive therapy.

While the mainstay of alcoholic rehabilitation involves counseling, education, and cognitive approaches, several medications might be useful. The first is the opioid-antagonist drug naltrexone, 50 to 150 mg/d, which has been reported in several small-scale, short-term studies to decrease the probability of a return to drinking and to shorten periods of relapse. A recent trial showed that a long-acting monthly injectable form of naltrexone was effective compared with placebo. A second medication, acamprosate (2 g/d), has been tested in >5000 patients in Europe, with results that appear similar to those reported for naltrexone. A third medication, topiramate, was shown to be superior to placebo in a randomized trial. A fourth medication, which has historically been used in the treatment of alcoholism, is the ALDH inhibitor disulfiram. In doses of 250 mg/d this drug produces an unpleasant (and potentially dangerous) reaction in the presence of alcohol, a phenomenon related to rapidly rising blood levels of the first metabolite of alcohol, acetaldehyde. However, few adequate controlled trials have demonstrated the superiority of disulfiram over placebo. Disulfiram has many side effects, and the reaction with alcohol can be dangerous, especially for patients with heart disease, stroke, diabetes mellitus, and hypertension. Thus, most clinicians reserve this medication for patients who have a clear history of longer-term abstinence associated with prior use of disulfiram and for those who might take the drug under the supervision of another individual (such as a spouse), especially during discrete periods that they have identified as representing high-risk drinking situations for them (such as the Christmas holiday).

Additional support for alcoholics and their relatives and friends is available through self-help groups such as AA. These groups, which typically consist of recovering alcoholics, offer an effective model of abstinence, provide a sober peer group, and make crisis intervention available when the urge to drink escalates. This can help patients optimize their chances for recovery, especially when incorporated into a more structured treatment milieu.

FURTHER READINGS

FLEMING MF ET AL: Brief physician advice for problem drinkers: Long-term efficacy and benefit-cost analysis. Alcohol Clin Exp Res 26:36, 2002

GARBUTT JC ET AL: Efficacy and tolerability of long-acting injectable naltrexone for alcohol dependence: A randomized controlled trial. JAMA 293:617, 2005

Recent trial demonstrating the efficacy of a long-acting alternative to traditional naltrexone administration for chronic alcoholism.

JOHNSON BA ET AL: Oral topiramate for treatment of alcohol dependence: A randomised controlled trial. Lancet 361:1677, 2003

Initial success treating alcoholism with a common oral antiepileptic drug.

KIEFER F ET AL: Comparing and combining naltrexone and acamprosate in relapse prevention of alcoholism. Arch Gen Psychiatry 60:92, 2003

SCHUCKIT MA ET AL: A 5-year prospective evaluation of DSM-IV alcohol dependence with and without a physiological component. Alcohol Clin Exp Res 27:818, 2003

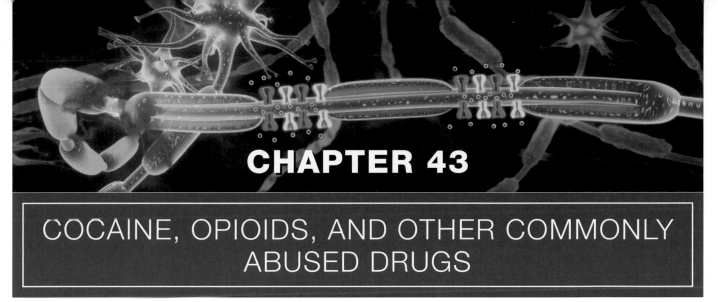

CHAPTER 43

COCAINE, OPIOIDS, AND OTHER COMMONLY ABUSED DRUGS

Jack H. Mendelson
Nancy K. Mello
Marc A. Schuckit
David S. Segal

Cocaine and other psychostimulant drug abuse remains a major public health problem in the United States and throughout the world; its prevalence appears to be increasing in some metropolitan areas for both college students and adults ages 19 to 40. Drug abuse by women continues to parallel abuse of cocaine and other psychostimulant drugs by men; psychostimulant abuse among youth in the United States is a special concern.

Chronic cocaine and psychostimulant abuse may cause a number of adverse health consequences, ranging from pulmonary disease to reproductive dysfunction. Preexisting disorders such as hypertension and cardiac disease may be exacerbated by drug abuse, and the combined use of two or more drugs may accentuate medical complications associated with abuse of one of them.

Drug abuse increases the risk of exposure to HIV. Cocaine and psychostimulant abuse contribute to the risk for HIV infection in part by suppression of immune function. In addition, concurrent use of cocaine and opiates (the "speedball") is frequently associated with needle-sharing by intravenous drug users. Intravenous drug abusers continue to represent the largest single group of persons with HIV infection in several major metropolitan areas in the United States as well as in urban areas in Scotland, Italy, Spain, Thailand, and China.

COCAINE

Cocaine is a stimulant and local anesthetic with potent vasoconstrictor properties. The leaves of the *coca* plant (*Erythroxylon coca*) contain ~0.5 to 1% cocaine. The drug produces physiologic and behavioral effects when administered orally, intranasally, intravenously, or via inhalation following pyrolysis (smoking). Cocaine increases synaptic concentrations of the monoamine neurotransmitters dopamine, norepinephrine, and serotonin by binding to transporter proteins in presynaptic neurons and blocking reuptake. The reinforcing effects of cocaine appear to be related to effects on dopaminergic neurons in the mesolimbic system.

PREVALENCE OF USE

Cocaine is widely available throughout the United States, and cocaine abuse occurs in virtually all social and economic strata of society. The prevalence of cocaine abuse in the general population has been accompanied by an increase in cocaine abuse by heroin-dependent persons, including those in methadone maintenance programs.

ACUTE AND CHRONIC INTOXICATION

There has been an increase in both intravenous administration and inhalation of pyrolyzed cocaine via smoking. Following intranasal administration, changes in mood and sensation are perceived within 3 to 5 min, and peak effects occur at 10 to 20 min. The effects rarely last more than 1 h. Inhalation of pyrolyzed materials includes inhaling crack/cocaine or smoking coca paste, a product made by extracting cocaine preparations with flammable solvents, and cocaine free-base smoking. Free-base cocaine, including the free base prepared with sodium bicarbonate (crack), has become increasingly popular because of the relative high potency of the compound and its rapid onset of action (8 to 10 s following smoking).

Cocaine produces a brief, dose-related stimulation and enhancement of mood and an increase in cardiac rate and blood pressure. Body temperature usually increases following cocaine administration, and high doses of cocaine may induce lethal pyrexia or hypertension. Because cocaine inhibits reuptake of catecholamines at adrenergic nerve endings, the drug potentiates sympathetic nervous system activity. Cocaine has a short plasma half-life of ~45 to 60 min. Cocaine is metabolized by plasma esterases, and cocaine metabolites are excreted in urine. The very short duration of the euphorigenic effects of cocaine observed in chronic abusers is probably due to both acute and chronic tolerance. Frequent self-administration of the drug (two to three times per hour) is often reported by chronic cocaine abusers.

The prevalent assumption that cocaine inhalation or intravenous administration is relatively safe is contradicted by reports of death from respiratory depression, cardiac arrhythmias, and convulsions associated with cocaine use. In addition to generalized seizures, neurologic complications may include headache, ischemic or hemorrhagic stroke, or subarachnoid hemorrhage. Disorders of cerebral blood flow and perfusion in cocaine-dependent persons have been detected with magnetic resonance spectroscopy (MRS) studies. Severe pulmonary disease may develop in individuals who inhale crack cocaine; this effect is attributed both to the direct effects of cocaine and to residual contaminants in the smoked material. Hepatic necrosis has been reported to occur following crack cocaine use.

Although men and women who abuse cocaine may report that the drug enhances libidinal drive, chronic cocaine use causes significant loss of libido and adversely affects reproductive function. Impotence and gynecomastia have been observed in male cocaine abusers, and these abnormalities often persist for long periods following cessation of drug use. Women who abuse cocaine have reported major derangements in menstrual cycle function including galactorrhea, amenorrhea, and infertility. Chronic cocaine abuse may cause persistent hyperpro-

lactinemia as a consequence of disordered dopaminergic inhibition of prolactin secretion by the anterior pituitary. Cocaine abuse by pregnant women, particularly the smoking of crack, has been associated with both an increased risk of congenital malformations in the fetus and perinatal cardiovascular and cerebrovascular disease in the mother. However, cocaine abuse per se is probably not the sole cause of these perinatal disorders, since many problems associated with maternal cocaine abuse, including poor nutrition and health care status as well as polydrug abuse, also contribute to risk for perinatal disease.

Protracted cocaine abuse may cause paranoid ideation and visual and auditory hallucinations, a state that resembles alcoholic hallucinosis. Psychological dependence on cocaine, indicated by inability to abstain from frequent compulsive use, also has been reported. Although the occurrence of withdrawal syndromes involving psychomotor agitation and autonomic hyperactivity remains controversial, severe depression ("crashing") following cocaine intoxication may accompany drug withdrawal.

TREATMENT FOR COCAINE OVERDOSE AND CHRONIC ABUSE

Treatment of cocaine overdose is a medical emergency that is usually best managed in an intensive care unit. Cocaine toxicity produces a hyperadrenergic state characterized by hypertension, tachycardia, tonic-clonic seizures, dyspnea, and ventricular arrhythmias. Intravenous diazepam in doses up to 0.5 mg/kg administered over an 8-h period has been shown to be effective for control of seizures. Ventricular arrhythmias have been managed successfully by administration of 0.5 to 1.0 mg of propranolol intravenously. Since many instances of cocaine-related mortality have been associated with concurrent use of other illicit drugs (particularly heroin), the physician must be prepared to institute effective emergency treatment for multiple drug toxicities.

Treatment of chronic cocaine abuse requires combined efforts of primary care physicians, psychiatrists, and psychosocial care providers. A number of medications and psychotherapeutic interventions used for the treatment of various medical and psychiatric disorders have been administered to reduce the duration and severity of cocaine abuse and dependence. However, no available medication or intervention is both safe and highly effective for either cocaine detoxification or maintenance of abstinence.

OPIOIDS AND RELATED COMPOUNDS

It is difficult to imagine modern medical practice without the use of opioid analgesics. These drugs have been part of health care since 300 B.C. Opium and codeine were isolated in the early nineteenth century, opioid-like substances produced by the body were recognized in the 1970s, and the first endogenous opioid was isolated in 1995. As important as these substances are to modern medicine, opioid drugs have many disadvantages, including overdosage and dependency; close to 1 million individuals in the United States are opioid-dependent. All opioid drugs are capable of producing a heroin-like intoxication, as well as tolerance and withdrawal.

PHARMACOLOGY

The prototypic opiates, morphine and codeine (3-methoxymorphine), are derived from the milky juice of the poppy *Papaver somniferum*. The semisynthetic drugs produced from the morphine or thebaine molecules include hydromorphone, diacetylmorphine (heroin), and oxycodone. The purely synthetic opioids and their cousins include meperidine, propoxyphene, diphenoxylate, fentanyl, buprenorphine, tramadol, methadone, and pentazocine.

Endogenous opioid peptides (i.e., enkephalins, endorphins, dynorphins, and others) have distinct distributions in the central nervous system (CNS) and appear to be natural ligands for opioid receptors. The receptors with which opioid peptides interact differentially produce analgesia, respiratory depression, constipation, euphoria, and other actions. Substances capable of antagonizing one or more of these actions include nalorphine, levallorphan, cyclazocine, butorphanol, buprenorphine, and pentazocine, each of which has mixed agonist and antagonist properties, as well as naloxone, nalmefene, and naltrexone, which are pure opiate antagonists.

The most rapid and pronounced effects of opioids occur following intravenous administration, with only slightly less efficient absorption after smoking or inhaling the vapor ("chasing the dragon"). The least intense effects occur after oral consumption. Most of the metabolism of opioids occurs in the liver, primarily through conjugation with glucuronic acid, and only small amounts are excreted directly in the urine or feces. The plasma half-lives of these drugs range from 2.5 to 3 h for morphine to more than 22 h for methadone and even longer for levomethadyl acetate (LAAM).

Street heroin is typically only 5 to 10% pure, mixed with sugars, quinine, powdered milk, phenacetin, caffeine, antipyrine, and strychnine. Unexpected increases in the purity of street drugs can cause unintentional lethal overdoses.

ACUTE AND CHRONIC EFFECTS OF OPIOIDS

With the exception of overdose and physical dependence, most opioid effects are rapidly reversible. A major danger, however, comes through the use of contaminated needles by intravenous users, which increases the risk of hepatitis B and C, bacterial endocarditis, and infection with HIV.

Opioid Toxicity and Overdosage

High doses of opioids can result in a potentially lethal overdose, which may occur in >60% of opioid-dependent persons, especially with the more potent drugs such as fentanyl (80 to 100 times more powerful than morphine). The typical syndrome, which occurs immediately with intravenous overdose, includes shallow and slow respirations, pupillary miosis (with mydriasis once brain anoxia develops), bradycardia, hypothermia, and stupor or coma. If not treated rapidly, respiratory depression, cardiorespiratory arrest, and death can ensue. Postmortem examination reveals few specific changes except for diffuse cerebral edema. An "allergic-like" reaction to intravenous heroin, perhaps in part related to adulterants, also can occur and is characterized by decreased alertness, frothy pulmonary edema, and an elevation in the blood eosinophil count.

The first step in managing overdose is to support vital signs, using intubation if needed. Definitive treatment is the administration of a narcotic antagonist such as 0.4 mg to 2 mg intravenous or intramuscular naloxone. A response should occur in 1 to 2 min; the dose should be repeated every 2 to 3 min up to 10 mg. Except with buprenorphene overdoses, no response after 10 mg makes an opioid toxic reaction unlikely. It is important to titrate the dose relative to the patient's symptoms to ameliorate the respiratory depression but not provoke a severe withdrawal state; the latter cannot be aggressively treated until overdose-related vital signs are relatively stable. Because the effects of naloxone diminish within 2 to 3 h, the individual must be monitored for at least 24 h after a heroin overdose and 72 h after an overdose of a longer-acting drug such as methadone. For methadone overdose, the substitution of the longer acting naltrexone should be considered. If there is little response to an opioid antagonist, the possibility of a concomitant overdose with a benzodiazepine should be considered and a challenge with intravenous flumazenil, 0.2 mg/min up to a maximum of 3 mg in an hour, might be used.

Treatment of either the typical or the "allergic" type of opioid toxic reaction often requires continued respiratory support (often with oxygen supplementation and positive-pressure breathing for the "allergic" type of overdose), intravenous fluids, pressor agents when needed to support blood pressure, and gastric lavage to remove any remaining drug. Intubation is often required to prevent aspiration in the stuporous or comatose patient. Cardiac arrhythmias and/or seizures also may be part of the opioid toxic reaction, especially with codeine, propoxyphene, or meperidine.

Symptoms of Withdrawal

Withdrawal symptoms, generally the opposite of the acute effects of the drug, include nausea and diarrhea, coughing, lacrimation, mydriasis, rhinorrhea, profuse sweating, twitching of muscles, and piloerection (or "goose bumps") as well as mild elevations in body temperature, respiratory rate, and blood pressure. In addition, diffuse body pain, insomnia, and yawning occur, along with intense drug craving. Drugs with shorter half-lives, such as morphine or heroin, usually cause symptoms within 8 to 16 h of the last dose; intensity peaks within 36 to 72 h after discontinuation of the drug; and the acute syndrome disappears within 5 to 8 days. A protracted abstinence phase of mild moodiness, autonomic dysfunction, and changes in pain threshold and sleep patterns may persist for ≥6 months and probably contributes to relapse.

TREATMENT FOR OPIOID WITHDRAWAL SYNDROME

A thorough physical examination, including an assessment of neurologic function and a search for focal and systemic infections, especially abscesses, is mandatory. Laboratory testing includes assessment of liver function and, in intravenous users, HIV and hepatitis B and C status. Proper nutrition and rest must be initiated as soon as possible.

One treatment of withdrawal requires administration of any opioid (e.g., 10 to 25 mg of methadone bid) on day 1 to decrease symptoms. After several days of a stabilized drug dose, the opioid is then decreased by 10 to 20% of the original day's dose each day. However, detoxification with opioids is proscribed or limited in most states. Thus, pharmacologic treatments often center on relief of symptoms of diarrhea with loperamide, of "sniffles" with decongestants, and pain with

nonopioid analgesics (e.g., ibuprofen). Comfort can be enhanced with administration of the α_2-adrenergic agonist clonidine in doses up to 0.3 mg given two to four times a day to decrease sympathetic nervous system overactivity. Blood pressure must be closely monitored. Some clinicians augment this regimen with low to moderate doses of benzodiazepines for 2 to 5 days to decrease agitation. An ultra-rapid detoxification procedure using deep sedation and withdrawal precipitated by naltrexone has been proposed, but it has many inherent dangers and little evidence of efficacy.

A special case of opioid withdrawal is seen in the newborn made passively dependent through the mother's drug abuse during pregnancy; withdrawal consists of irritability, crying, a tremor, increased reflexes, increased respiratory rate, diarrhea, vomiting, and sneezing/yawning/hiccupping. Treatment follows the same general steps used in the treatment of the physically dependent adult but using paregoric (0.2 mL orally every 3 to 4 h), methadone (0.1 to 0.5 mg/kg per day), phenobarbital (8 mg/kg per day), or diazepam (1 to 2 mg/kg every 8 h) in decreasing dosages for 10 to 20 days. Dependent infants of mothers on methadone maintenance also benefit by breast feeding while the mother continues to take methadone.

Opioid Maintenance

Maintenance programs with methadone and the longer-acting LAAM should be used only in combination with education and counseling. The goal is to provide a substitute drug that is legally accessible and safer, can be taken orally, and has a long half-life so that it can be taken once a day. This can help persons who have repeatedly failed in drug-free programs to improve functioning within the family and job, to decrease legal problems, and to improve health. Individuals who stay in methadone maintenance are likely to show improvement in antisocial behavior and employment status.

Methadone is a long-acting opioid optimally dosed at 80 to 120 mg/d (a goal met through slow, careful increases over time). This level is optimally effective in blocking heroin-induced euphoria, decreasing craving, and maintaining abstinence from illegal opioids. More than three-quarters of patients in well-supervised methadone clinics are likely to remain heroin-free for ≥6 months. Methadone is administered as an oral liquid given once a day at the program, with weekend doses taken at home. The longer-acting analogues, such as LAAM, can be given in doses up to 80 mg two or three times a week. After a period of maintenance (usually 6 months to ≥1 year), the clinician can work to slowly decrease the dose by about 5% per week.

An additional medication that has been used for maintenance treatment involves the μ opioid agonist and κ antagonist buprenorphine. Administered as either a sublingual liquid or a tablet, doses of 8 to 12 mg per day (up to 32 mg in some patients) are usually given between 3 and 7 days per week. This drug has several advantages including low overdose danger, easier detoxification than that seen with methadone, and a probable ceiling effect in which higher doses do not increase euphoria. While many studies report equal effectiveness of buprenorphine and methadone, others suggest higher dropout rates or concomitant drug use with buprenorphine. As with all opioids, there is still a danger of misuse.

Opioid Antagonists

The opiate antagonists (e.g., naltrexone) compete with heroin and other opioids at receptors, reducing the effects of the opioid agonists. Administered over long periods with the intention of blocking the opioid "high," these drugs can be useful as part of an overall treatment approach that includes counseling and support. Naltrexone doses of 50 mg/d antagonize 15 mg of heroin for 24 h, and the possibly more effective higher doses (125 to 150 mg) block the effects of 25 mg of intravenous heroin for up to 3 days. To avoid precipitating a withdrawal syndrome, patients must be free of opioids for a minimum of 5 days before beginning treatment with naltrexone and should first be challenged with 0.4 or 0.8 mg of the shorter-acting agent naloxone to be certain they can tolerate the long-acting antagonist. A test dose of 10 mg of naltrexone is then given, which can produce withdrawal symptoms in 0.5 to 2 h. If none appears, the patient can begin with the usual dose of 40 to 150 mg three times per week.

One randomized, controlled trial established the safety and efficacy of an office-based treatment of opiate addiction with a sublingual tablet administration of buprenorphine and naloxone. Further study is needed to definitively establish the role for this approach.

Drug-Free Programs

Most opioid-dependent individuals enter treatment programs based primarily on the cognitive behavioral approaches of enhancing commitment to abstinence, helping individuals to rebuild their lives without substances, and preventing relapse. Whether these programs are carried out in inpatient or outpatient settings, patients do not receive medications.

MARIJUANA AND CANNABIS COMPOUNDS

Cannabis sativa contains >400 compounds in addition to the psychoactive substance delta-9-tetrahydrocannabinol (THC). Marijuana cigarettes are prepared from the leaves and flowering tops of the plant, and a typical marijuana cigarette contains 0.5 to 1 g of plant material. Although the usual THC concentration varies between 10 and 40 mg, concentrations >100 mg per cigarette have been detected. Hashish is prepared from concentrated resin of *C. sativa* and contains a THC concentration of between 8 to 12% percent by weight. "Hash oil," a lipid-soluble plant extract, may contain a THC concentration of 25 to 60% percent and may be added to marijuana or hashish to enhance its THC concentration. Smoking is the most common mode of marijuana or hashish use. During pyrolysis, >150 compounds in addition to THC are released in the smoke. Although most of these compounds do not have psychoactive properties, they do have potential physiologic effects.

THC is quickly absorbed from the lungs into blood and is then rapidly sequestered in tissues. It is metabolized primarily in the liver, where it is converted to 11-hydroxy-THC, a psychoactive compound, and >20 other metabolites. Many THC metabolites are excreted through the feces at a rate of clearance that is relatively slow in comparison to that of most other psychoactive drugs.

Specific cannabinoid receptors (CB_1 and CB_2) have been identified in the central nervous system, including the spinal cord, and in the peripheral nervous system. High densities of these receptors have been found in the cerebral cortex, basal ganglia, and hippocampus. B lymphocytes also appear to have cannabinoid receptors. A naturally occurring THC-like ligand has been identified in the nervous system, where it is widely distributed.

PREVALENCE OF USE

Marijuana is the most commonly used illegal drug in the United States. Use is particularly prevalent among adolescents; studies suggest that ~37% of high school students in the United States have used marijuana. Marijuana is relatively inexpensive and is often considered to be less hazardous than other controlled drugs and substances. Very potent forms of marijuana (sinsemilla) are now available in many communities, and concurrent use of marijuana with crack/cocaine and phencyclidine is increasing. Marijuana abuse by individuals from all social strata has been increasing.

ACUTE AND CHRONIC INTOXICATION

Acute intoxication from marijuana and cannabis compounds is related to both the dose of THC and the route of administration. THC is absorbed more rapidly from marijuana smoking than from orally ingested cannabis compounds. Acute marijuana intoxication usually consists of a subjective perception of relaxation and mild euphoria resembling mild to moderate alcohol intoxication. This condition is usually accompanied by some impairment in thinking, concentration, and perceptual and psychomotor function. Higher doses of cannabis may produce behavioral effects analogous to severe alcohol intoxication. Although the effects of acute marijuana intoxication are relatively benign in normal users, the drug can precipitate severe emotional disorders in individuals who have antecedent psychotic or neurotic problems. As with other psychoactive compounds, both set (user's expectations) and setting (environmental context) are important determinants of the type and severity of behavioral intoxication.

As with abuse of cocaine, opioids, and alcohol, chronic marijuana abusers may lose interest in common socially desirable goals and steadily devote more time to drug acquisition and use. However, THC does not cause a specific and unique "amotivational syndrome." The range of symptoms sometimes attributed to marijuana use is difficult to distinguish from mild to moderate depression and the maturational dysfunctions often associated with protracted adolescence. Chronic marijuana use has also been reported to increase the risk of psychotic symptoms in individuals with a past history of schizophrenia. Persons who initiate marijuana smoking before the age of 17 may subsequently develop severe cognitive and neuropsychological disorders, and may be at higher risk for later polydrug and alcohol abuse problems.

PHYSICAL EFFECTS

Conjunctival injection and tachycardia are the most frequent immediate physical concomitants of smoking marijuana. Tolerance for marijuana-induced tachycardia develops rapidly among regular users. However, marijuana smoking may precipitate angina in persons with a history of coronary insufficiency. Exercise-induced angina may be increased after marijuana use to a greater extent than after tobacco cigarette smoking. Patients

with cardiac disease should be strongly advised not to smoke marijuana or use cannabis compounds.

Significant decrements in pulmonary vital capacity have been found in regular daily marijuana smokers. Because marijuana smoking typically involves deep inhalation and prolonged retention of marijuana smoke, marijuana smokers may develop chronic bronchial irritation. Impairment of single-breath carbon monoxide diffusion capacity (DL_{CO}) is greater in persons who smoke both marijuana and tobacco than in tobacco smokers.

TOLERANCE AND PHYSICAL DEPENDENCE

Habitual marijuana users rapidly develop tolerance to the psychoactive effects of marijuana and often smoke more frequently and try to secure more potent cannabis compounds. Tolerance for the physiologic effects of marijuana develops at different rates; e.g., tolerance develops rapidly for marijuana-induced tachycardia but more slowly for marijuana-induced conjunctival injection. Tolerance to both behavioral and physiologic effects of marijuana decreases rapidly upon cessation of marijuana use.

Withdrawal signs and symptoms have been reported in chronic cannabis users, with the severity of symptoms related to dosage and duration of use. These include tremor, nystagmus, sweating, nausea, vomiting, diarrhea, irritability, anorexia, and sleep disturbances. Withdrawal signs and symptoms observed in chronic marijuana users are usually relatively mild in comparison to those observed in heavy opiate or alcohol users and rarely require medical or pharmacologic intervention. More severe and protracted abstinence syndromes may occur after sustained use of high-potency cannabis compounds.

THERAPEUTIC USE

Marijuana, administered as cigarettes or as a synthetic oral cannabinoid (dronabinol), has been proposed to have a number of properties that may be clinically useful in some situations. These include antiemetic effects in chemotherapy recipients, appetite-promoting effects in AIDS, reduction of intraocular pressure in glaucoma, and reduction of spasticity in multiple sclerosis and other neurologic disorders. With the possible exception of AIDS-related cachexia, none of these attributes of marijuana compounds is clearly superior to other readily available therapies.

METHAMPHETAMINE

The abuse of methamphetamine, also referred to as "meth," "speed," "crank," "chalk," "ice," "glass," or "crystal," is prevalent in many metropolitan areas and communities throughout the United States.

Most persons who abuse methamphetamine self-administer the drug orally, although there have been reports of methamphetamine administration by inhalation and intravenous injection. Individuals who abuse or become dependent on methamphetamine state that use of this drug induces feelings of euphoria and decreases fatigue associated with difficult life situations. Adverse physiologic effects observed as a consequence of methamphetamine abuse include headache, difficulty concentrating, diminished appetite, abdominal pain, vomiting or diarrhea, disordered sleep, paranoid or aggressive behavior, and psychosis. Severe, life-threatening toxicity may present as hypertension, cardiac arrhythmia or failure, subarachnoid hemorrhage, ischemic stroke, intracerebral hemorrhage, convulsions, or coma. Methamphetamines increase the release of monoamine neurotransmitters (dopamine, norepinephrine, and serotonin) from presynaptic neurons.

Therapy of acute methamphetamine overdose is largely symptomatic. Ammonium chloride may be useful to acidify the urine and enhance clearance of the drug. Hypertension may respond to sodium nitroprusside or α-adrenergic antagonists. Sedatives may reduce agitation and other signs of central nervous system hyperactivity. Treatment of chronic methamphetamine dependence may be accomplished in either an inpatient or outpatient setting using strategies similar to those described above for cocaine abuse.

MDMA (3,4-methylenedioxymethamphetamine), or *Ecstasy*, is a derivative of methamphetamine. Ecstasy is usually taken orally but may be injected or inhaled. In addition to amphetamine-like effects, MDMA can induce hyperthermia and vivid hallucinations and other perceptual distortions. Hyponatremia with life-threatening cerebral edema is a rare but important life-threatening complication of use.

LYSERGIC ACID DIETHYLAMIDE (LSD)

The discovery of the psychedelic effects of LSD in 1947 led to an epidemic of LSD abuse during the 1960s. Imposition of stringent constraints on the manufacture and distribution of LSD (classified as a Schedule I substance by the U.S. Food and Drug Administration), as well as public recognition that psychedelic experiences induced by LSD were a health hazard, have resulted in a reduction in LSD abuse. The drug still retains some popularity among adolescents and young adults, however, and there are indications that LSD use among young persons has been increasing in some communities in the United States.

LSD is a very potent drug; oral doses as low as 20 μg may induce profound psychological and physiologic effects. Tachycardia, hypertension, pupillary dilation, tremor, and hyperpyrexia occur within minutes following oral administration of 0.5 to 2 $\mu g/kg$. A variety of bizarre and often conflicting perceptual and mood changes, including visual illusions, synesthesias, and extreme lability of mood, usually occur within 30 min after LSD intake. These effects of LSD may persist for 12 to 18 h, even though the half-life of the drug is only 3 h.

Tolerance develops rapidly for LSD-induced changes in psychological function when the drug is used one or more times per day for >4 days. Abrupt abstinence following continued use does not produce withdrawal signs or symptoms. There have been no clinical reports of death caused by the direct effects of LSD.

The most frequent acute medical emergency associated with LSD use is panic episode (the "bad trip"), which may persist up to 24 h. Management of this problem is best accomplished by supportive reassurance ("talking down") and, if necessary, administration of small doses of anxiolytic drugs. Adverse consequences of chronic LSD use include enhanced risk for schizophreniform psychosis and derangements in memory function, problem solving, and abstract thinking. Treatment of these disorders is best carried out in specialized psychiatric facilities.

PHENCYCLIDINE

Phencyclidine (PCP), a cyclohexylamine derivative, is widely used in veterinary medicine to briefly immobilize large animals and is sometimes described as a dissociative anesthetic. PCP binds to ionotropic *n*-methyl-*d*-aspartate (NMDA) receptors in the nervous system, blocking ion current through these channels. PCP is easily synthesized; its abusers are primarily young people and polydrug users. It is used orally, by smoking, or by intravenous injection. It is also used as an adulterant in THC, LSD, amphetamine, or cocaine. The most common street preparation, *angel dust*, is a white granular powder that contains 50 to 100% percent of the drug. Low doses (5 mg) produce agitation, excitement, impaired motor coordination, dysarthria, and analgesia. Users may have horizontal or vertical nystagmus, flushing, diaphoresis, and hyperacusis. Behavioral changes include distortions of body image, disorganization of thinking, and feelings of estrangement. Higher doses of PCP (5 to 10 mg) may produce profuse salivation, vomiting, myoclonus, fever, stupor, or coma. PCP doses of ≥ 10 mg cause convulsions, opisthotonos, and decerebrate posturing, which may be followed by prolonged coma.

The diagnosis of PCP overdose is difficult because the patient's initial symptoms may suggest an acute schizophrenic reaction. Confirmation of PCP use is possible by determination of PCP levels in serum or urine. PCP assays are available at most toxicologic centers. PCP remains in urine for 1 to 5 days following high-dose intake.

PCP overdose requires life-support measures, including treatment of coma, convulsions, and respiratory depression in an intensive care unit. There is no specific antidote or antagonist for PCP. PCP excretion from the body can be enhanced by gastric lavage and acidification of urine. Death from PCP overdose may occur as a consequence of some combination of pharyngeal hypersecretion, hyperthermia, respiratory depression, severe hypertension, seizures, hypertensive encephalopathy, and intracerebral hemorrhage.

Acute psychosis associated with PCP use should be considered a psychiatric emergency since patients may be at high risk for suicide or extreme violence toward others. Phenothiazines should not be used for treatment because these drugs potentiate PCP's anticholinergic effects. Haloperidol (5 mg intramuscularly) has been administered on an hourly basis to induce suppression of psychotic behavior. PCP, like LSD and mescaline, produces vasospasm of cerebral arteries at relatively low doses. Chronic PCP use has been shown to induce insomnia, anorexia, severe social and behavioral changes, and, in some cases, chronic schizophrenia.

POLYDRUG ABUSE

Although drug abusers often report a preference for a particular drug, such as alcohol or opiates, the concurrent use of other drugs is common. Multiple drug use often involves substances that may have different pharmacologic effects from the preferred drug. Concurrent use of such dissimilar compounds as stimulants and opiates or stimulants and alcohol is not unusual. There are many examples of situationally determined drug use patterns. For example, alcohol abuse, with its attendant medical complications, is one of the most serious problems encountered in former heroin addicts participating in methadone maintenance programs.

℞ TREATMENT OF POLYDRUG ABUSE

Adequate treatment of polydrug abuse, as well as other forms of drug abuse, requires innovative pro-

grams of intervention. The first step in successful treatment is detoxification, a process that may be difficult because of the abuse of several drugs with different pharmacologic actions (e.g., alcohol, opiates, and cocaine). Since patients may not recall or may deny simultaneous multiple drug use, diagnostic evaluation should always include urinalysis for qualitative detection of psychoactive substances and their metabolites. Treatment of polydrug abuse often requires hospitalization or inpatient residential care during detoxification and the initial phase of drug abstinence. When possible, specialized facilities for the care and treatment of chemically dependent persons should be used. Outpatient detoxification of polydrug abuse patients is likely to be ineffective and may be dangerous.

Polydrug abuse is a chronic disorder with an unpredictable pattern of remission and recrudescence. Definitive "cures" rarely occur. The physician should continue to assist polydrug abuse patients throughout the cyclic oscillations of this complex behavior disorder, recognizing that resumption of drug use is the rule rather than the exception.

FURTHER READINGS

CAMI J, FARRE M: Drug addiction. N Engl J Med 349:975, 2003

FUDALA PJ et al: Office-based treatment of opiate addiction with a sublingual-tablet formulation of buprenorphine and naloxone. New Engl J Med 349:949, 2003

LYNSKEY MT et al: Escalation of drug use in early-onset cannabis users vs co-twin controls. JAMA 289:427, 2003

MATTICK RP et al: Buprenorphine versus methadone maintenance therapy: A randomized double-blind trial with 405 opioid-dependent patients. Addiction 98:441, 2003

MAYET S et al: Psychosocial treatment for opiate abuse and dependence. Cochrane Database Syst Rev 25:CD004330, 2005

A systemic review of nonpharmacologic treatment of opiate dependence.

WEBER JE et al: Validation of a brief observation period for patients with cocaine-associated chest pain. N Engl J Med 348:510, 2003

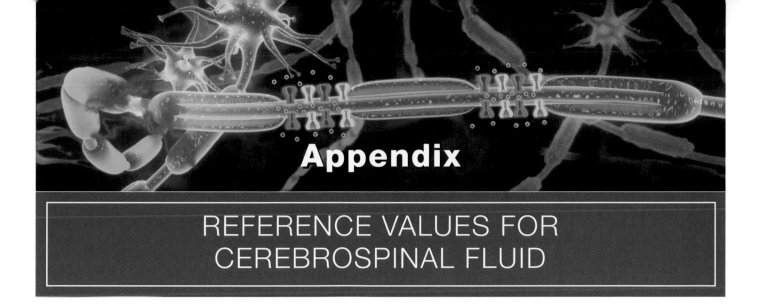

Appendix

REFERENCE VALUES FOR CEREBROSPINAL FLUID

TABLE A-1

CEREBROSPINAL FLUID[a]		
CONSTITUENT	**SI UNITS**	**CONVENTIONAL UNITS**
Glucose	2.22–3.89 mmol/L	40–70 mg/dL
Lactate	1–2 mmol/L	10–20 mg/dL
Total protein		
Lumbar	0.15–0.5 g/L	15–50 mg/dL
Cisternal	0.15–0.25 g/L	15–25 mg/dL
Ventricular	0.06–0.15 g/L	6–15 mg/dL
Albumin	0.066–0.442 g/L	6.6–44.2 mg/dL
IgG	0.009–0.057 g/L	0.9–5.7 mg/dL
IgG index[b]	0.29–0.59	
Oligoclonal bands (OGB)	<2 bands not present in matched serum sample	
Ammonia	15–47 μmol/L	25–80 μg/dL
CSF pressure		50–180 mmH$_2$O
CSF volume (adult)	~150 mL	
Red blood cells	0	0
Leukocytes		
Total	0–5 mononuclear cells per mm^3	
Differential		
Lymphocytes	60–70%	
Monocytes	30–50%	
Neutrophils	None	

[a]Since cerebrospinal fluid concentrations are equilibrium values, measurements of the same parameters in blood plasma obtained at the same time are recommended. However, there is a time lag in attainment of equilibrium, and cerebrospinal levels of plasma constituents that can fluctuate rapidly (such as plasma glucose) may not achieve stable values until after a significant lag phase.
[b]IgG index = CSF IgG(mg/dL) $\times$ serum albumin(g/dL)/Serum IgG(g/dL) $\times$ CSF albumin(mg/dL)

QUESTIONS

DIRECTIONS: Each question below contains five suggested responses. Choose the **one best** response to each question.

1. A 32-year-old male presents to the emergency department complaining of a painful red eye. The redness began abruptly with pain that the patient first noticed upon awakening from bed. He wears contact lenses and occasionally sleeps in them. He has not had any fevers, chills, viral symptoms, joint pain, rashes, or bowel symptoms. An ophthalmologic examination reveals the following as shown below. How should the patient be treated?

   A. Intraocular gentamicin
   B. Oral clindamycin
   C. Oral glucocorticoids
   D. Topical ciprofloxacin
   E. Topical clotrimazole

2. A 27-year-old female presents to the emergency department for evaluation of a painful red left eye. The redness began late in the afternoon. She notes pain when looking at bright lights. The patient has had no viral symptoms or fevers but recently has noticed dyspnea with exertion and a dry cough. She was treated for a single episode of acute cystitis 10 weeks ago. Slit-lamp examination of the eye shows inflammation in the aqueous humor and inflammatory deposits on the corneal epithelium. Head and neck examination shows lymphadenopathy. There are a few dry crackles at the bases. Occasional wheezes are heard. There is no joint inflammation. Pulmonary function tests show a combined obstructive and restrictive defect. What is the diagnosis of this patient's eye disease?

   A. Conjunctivitis
   B. Episcleritis
   C. Keratitis
   D. Keratoconjunctivitis sicca
   E. Uveitis

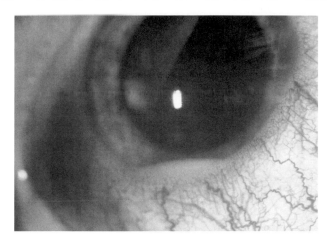

3. What is the most likely underlying disorder?

   A. Ankylosing spondylitis
   B. Inflammatory bowel disease
   C. Reiter's syndrome
   D. Sarcoidosis
   E. Sjögren's syndrome

4. A 62-year-old female presents to her primary care doctor complaining of gradual visual loss. She feels as if she has to turn her head slightly to one side to get a full field of view. There is a past history of diabetes mellitus. She currently takes insulin glargine 16 units at night, with an insulin aspartate sliding scale. The last hemoglobin A_{1C} was 7.4%. The most recent eye examination was 1 year ago. She wears bifocal lenses for presbyopia and myopia with astigmatism. Currently, intraocular pressure is 14 mmHg. The red reflex to light is normal. She has several discrete yellow lesions that are irregularly shaped. No vitreal hemorrhage or vascular proliferation is seen. There is a normal disc-to-cup ratio. What is the most likely diagnosis?

   A. Age-related macular degeneration
   B. Cataracts
   C. Diabetic retinopathy
   D. Glaucoma
   E. Orbital pseudotumor

5. All the following types of cancer commonly metastasize to the central nervous system (CNS) *except*

   A. ovarian
   B. breast
   C. hypernephroma
   D. melanoma
   E. acute lymphoblastic leukemia (ALL)

6. For the last 5 weeks a 35-year-old female has had episodes of intense vertigo that last several hours. Each episode is associated with tinnitus and a sense of fullness in the right ear; during the attacks she prefers to lie on the left side. Examination during an attack shows that she has fine rotary nystagmus that is maximal on gaze to the left. There are no ocular palsies, cranial nerve signs, or long-tract signs. An audiogram shows high-tone hearing loss in the right ear, with recruitment but no tone decay. The most likely diagnosis in this case is

   A. labyrinthitis
   B. Méniére's disease
   C. vertebral-basilar insufficiency
   D. acoustic neuroma
   E. multiple sclerosis

7. A 45-year-old male presents with a daily headache. He describes two attacks per day over the last 3 weeks. Each attack lasts about an hour and awakens the patient from sleep. The patient has noted associated tearing and reddening of the right eye as well as nasal stuffiness. The pain is deep, excruciating, and limited to the right side of the head. The neurologic examination is non-focal. The most likely diagnosis of this patient's headache is

   A. migraine heache
   B. cluster headache
   C. tension headache
   D. brain tumor
   E. giant cell arteritis

8. A 65-year-old male presents with severe right-sided eye and facial pain, nausea, vomiting, colored halos around lights, and loss of visual acuity. His right eye is quite red, and that pupil is dilated and fixed. Which of the following diagnostic tests would confirm the diagnosis?

   A. CT of the head
   B. MRI of the head
   C. Cerebral angiography
   D. Tonometry
   E. Slit-lamp examination

9. A 24-year-old college student is brought to the emergency department by friends from his dormitory for altered mental status. They state that he recently returned from a trip to South America and that many colleagues have upper respiratory tract infections. His physical examination is notable for confusion, fever, and a rigid neck. CSF examination reveals a white blood cell count of 1800 cells/μL with 98% neutrophils, glucose of 35 mg/dL, and protein of 100 mg/dL. He is placed on empirical treatment for meningitis. Which of the following statements about the CSF examination is true?

   A. A negative latex agglutination test for *Staphylococcus pneumoniae* rules out this organism as a cause of the meningitis.
   B. A negative latex agglutination test for *Neisseria meningitidis* rules out this organism as a cause of the meningitis.
   C. Meningeal enhancement on MRI is diagnostic of meningitis.
   D. A positive limulus amebocyte lysate assay is diagnostic of protozoal meningitis.
   E. A positive latex agglutination test for *S. pneumoniae* is diagnostic of *S. pneumoniae* meningitis.

10. A 19-year-old college student is brought to the emergency department by friends from his dormitory for confusion and altered mental status. They state that many colleagues have upper respiratory tract infections. He does not use alcohol or illicit drugs. His physical examination is notable for confusion, fever, and a rigid neck. CSF examination reveals a white blood cell count of 1800 cells/μL with 98% neutrophils, glucose of 35 mg/dL, and protein of 100 mg/dL. Which of the following antibiotic regimens is most appropriate as initial therapy?

    A. Ampicillin plus vancomycin
    B. Ampicillin plus gentamicin
    C. Cefazolin plus doxycycline
    D. Cefotaxime plus doxycycline
    E. Cefotaxime plus vancomycin

11. In addition to antibiotics, which of the following adjunctive therapies should be administered to improve the chance of a favorable neurologic outcome?

    A. Dexamethasone
    B. Dilantin
    C. Gabapentin
    D. L-Dopa
    E. Parenteral nutrition

12. A 24-year-old previously healthy office worker comes to the emergency department complaining of a severe bilateral headache, malaise, and photophobia for 1 day. Her physical examination is notable for a temperature of 38.8°C (101.8°F) and neck pain on extreme flexion. She is lethargic but fully oriented. CSF is clear with a white blood cell count of 50 cells/μL with 80% lymphocytes. CSF glucose is 80 mg/dL, and protein is 40 mg/dL. Which of the following tests is most likely to be diagnostic?

    A. Cerebral angiogram
    B. Cerebral MRI with gadolinium
    C. CSF acid-fast stain
    D. CSF india ink stain
    E. CSF PCR for enterovirus species.

13. A 64-year-old female is admitted to the hospital with altered mental status. She recently returned from a summer white-water rafting trip in Colorado. Her husband reports increasing confusion, alternating lethargy and agitation, and visual hallucinations over the last 3 days. There is no history of drug abuse or psychiatric illness. She takes no medications. Her physical examination is notable for a temperature of 39°C (102.2°F), myoclonic jerks, and hyperreflexia. She is delirious and oriented to person only when aroused. There is no nuchal rigidity. CSF examination reveals clear fluid with a white blood cell count of 15 cells/μL with 100% lymphocytes, protein of 100 mg/dL, and glucose of 80 mg/dL. Gram stain of the CSF shows no organisms. You suspect infection with West Nile virus. Which of the following studies will be most useful in making that diagnosis?

    A. CSF culture
    B. CSF IgM antibodies
    C. CSF PCR
    D. CNS MRI
    E. Stool culture

14. A 44-year-old male is undergoing evaluation for altered mental status. His wife reports increasing confusion, forgetfulness, and decreased vision over the last month. She also notes that his mood has become very labile with frequent outbursts of anger. He has a history of intravenous drug abuse but quit 4 years ago. He is on no medications. Physical examination is notable for a normal temperature and vital signs, cachexia, and a left homonymous hemianopia. He is oriented only to person, cannot follow complex commands, and has marked short-term memory loss. A brain MRI shows bilateral periven-

14. (Continued)
    tricular white matter lesions on T2 imaging. There are no masses, and the ventricles are of normal size. CSF testing is notable for the presence of JC viral DNA on PCR testing. Additional testing most likely will be positive for

    A. Anti-Hu antibody
    B. Antinuclear antibodies
    C. c-ANCA
    D. Hepatitis B antibody
    E. HIV antibody

15. A 40-year-old male presents with an insidious onset of fatigue, headaches, muscle weakness, and paresthesia. Physical examination reveals hypertension, an enlarged tongue, wide spacing of the teeth, and a doughy appearance to the skin. Which of the following laboratory results would be consistent with the expected diagnosis?

    A. Elevated serum thyroxine level
    B. Fasting serum glucose of 3.3 mmol/L (60 mg/dL)
    C. Elevated insulin-like growth factor 1 (IGF-1)
    D. Growth hormone concentration of 0.2 μg/L (0.2 ng/mL) 1 h after oral administration of 100 g glucose
    E. Decreased IGF binding protein 3

16. All the following are associated with a decreased sense of smell *except*

    A. head trauma
    B. HIV infection
    C. influenza B infection
    D. Kallmann syndrome
    E. parainfluenza virus type 3 infection

17. A 56-year-old male presents to your clinic complaining of hearing loss in the right ear. On exami-

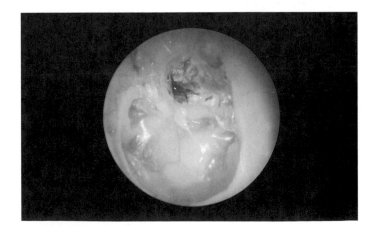

17. *(Continued)*

nation, the Rinne test at 256 Hz reveals louder conduction through placement on the mastoid process and the Weber test best localizes the sound to the right ear. The otologic examination is shown below. What is the diagnosis?

A. Otitis externa
B. Otosclerosis
C. Cholesteatoma
D. Acoustic neuroma
E. Presbycusis

18. A 34-year-old female complains of lower extremity weakness for the last 3 days. She has noted progressive weakness in the lower extremities with loss of sensation "below the belly button" and incontinence. She had had some low-grade fevers for the last week. She denies recent travel. Past medical history is unremarkable. Physical examination is notable for a sensory level at the level of the umbilicus. The lower extremities show +3/5 strength bilaterally proximally and distally. Reflexes, cerebellar examination, and mental status are normal. All the following are appropriate steps in evaluating this patient *except*

A. antinuclear antibodies
B. electromyography
C. lumbar puncture
D. MRI of the spine
E. viral serologies

19. Which of the following statements about syringomyelia is true?

A. More than half the cases are associated with Chiari malformations.
B. Symptoms typically begin in middle age.
C. Vibration and position sensation are usually diminished.
D. Syrinx cavities are always congenital.
E. Neurosurgical decompression is usually effective in relieving the symptoms.

20. A 50-year-old male complains of weakness and numbness in the hands for the last month. He describes paresthesias in the thumb and the index and middle fingers. The symptoms are worse at night. He also describes decreased grip strength bilaterally. He works as a mechanical engineer. The patient denies fevers, chills, or weight loss. The examination is notable for atrophy of the thenar eminences bilaterally and decreased sensation in a median nerve distribution. All the following are causes of carpal tunnel syndrome *except*

20. *(Continued)*

A. amyloidosis
B. chronic lymphocytic leukemia
C. diabetes mellitus
D. hypothyroidism
E. rheumatoid arthritis

21. A 62-year-old male with a history of hypertension and diabetes presents to the emergency department with a left facial droop and left-sided hemiparesis. He is not sure when the symptoms began. His wife noted that 4 h before he arrived at the hospital he was "normal" but did not see him again until 20 min before presentation. Past medical history is significant for reflux esophagitis seen on endoscopy 1 year ago. His medications include hydrochlorothiazide and omeprazole. Family history is noncontributory. Physical examination is notable for a blood pressure of 152/74 mmHg and an oxygen saturation of 98% on room air. He has an obvious left facial droop and has left-sided hemiparesis. Sensation is intact. The patient's stool is heme-negative. A complete blood count is normal, and coagulation studies are within normal limits. A computed tomography scan of the head shows a right middle cerebral artery territory infarct. There is no hemorrhage. What is the most appropriate next management step?

A. Aspirin
B. Clopidogrel
C. Intraarterial catheter-based thrombolytic therapy
D. Intravenous thrombolytic therapy
E. Intravenous heparin

22 The most common cause of a cerebral embolism is

A. cardiac prosthetic valves
B. rheumatic heart disease
C. dilated cardiomyopathy
D. endocarditis
E. atrial fibrillation

23. A 54-year-old male is referred to your clinic for evaluation of atrial fibrillation. He first noted the irregular heartbeat 2 weeks ago and presented to his primary care physician. He denies chest pain, shortness of breath, nausea, or gastrointestinal symptoms. Past medical history is unremarkable. There is no history of hypertension, diabetes, or tobacco use. His medications include metoprolol. The examination is notable for a blood pressure of 126/74 mmHg and a pulse of 64 beats/min. The jugular venous pressure is not elevated. His heart is irregularly

23. *(Continued)*

irregular, with normal S_1 and S_2. The lungs are clear, and there is no peripheral edema. An echocardiogram shows a left atrial size of 3.6 cm. Left ventricular ejection fraction is 60%. There are no valvular or structural abnormalities. Which of the following statements regarding his atrial fibrillation and stroke risk is true?

A. He requires no antiplatelet therapy or anticoagulation because the risk of embolism is low.

B. Lifetime warfarin therapy is indicated for atrial fibrillation in this situation to reduce the risk of stroke.

C. He should be admitted to the hospital for intravenous heparin and undergo electrical cardioversion; afterward there is no need for anticoagulation.

D. His risk of an embolic stroke is less than 1%, and he should take a daily aspirin.

E. He should be started on subcutaneous low-molecular-weight heparin and transitioned to warfarin.

24. All but which of the following statements regarding amyotrophic lateral sclerosis (ALS) are true?

A. Dementia occurs in the late stages of the disease.

B. The main cause of death is respiratory failure.

C. Familial ALS is inherited in an autosomal dominant fashion.

D. Glutamate plays a key role in the death of motor neurons in patients with ALS.

E. Riluzole improves survival in patients with ALS.

25. A 71-year-old male presents to your clinic to receive routine medical care. On examination you notice a left carotid bruit. You order a carotid ultrasound that shows a 60% stenosis of the left internal carotid artery. All but which of the following statements are true?

A. If this patient has symptoms of transient ischemic attacks (TIAs), he will receive a significant benefit from a carotid endarterectomy.

B. Without symptoms, his risk of stroke is approximately 2% a year.

C. Balloon angioplasty with stenting has been shown to be equivalent to carotid endarterectomy.

D. There is evidence that this patient will benefit from carotid endarterectomy (CEA) even in the absence of symptoms.

E. Surgery is recommended only in centers with perioperative complication rates under 6%.

26. All the following have been shown to reduce the risk of atherothrombotic stroke in primary or secondary prevention *except*

26. *(Continued)*

A. aspirin

B. blood pressure control

C. clopidogrel

D. statin therapy

E. warfarin

27. All the following cause primarily a sensory neuropathy *except*

A. acromegaly

B. critical illness

C. HIV infection

D. hypothyroidism

E. vitamin B_{12} deficiency

28. All but which of the following statements about Guillain-Barré syndrome are true?

A. Up to 30% of cases are associated with *Escherichia coli* infection.

B. Ascending areflexic motor paralysis is the typical clinical pattern.

C. Cerebrospinal fluid protein is often elevated.

D. The effectiveness of treatment diminishes if it is initiated more than 2 weeks after the onset of symptoms.

E. The main cause of mortality is pulmonary complications.

29. All but which of the following statements regarding neuropathy are true?

A. Neurologic symptoms often precede the diagnosis of small-cell lung cancer in patients with anti-Hu paraneoplastic neuropathy.

B. Twenty-five percent of patients with chronic inflammatory demyelinating polyradiculoneuropathy (CIDP) have a monoclonal gammopathy of undetermined significance (MGUS).

C. Polyneuropathy is associated with less than 5% of cases of myeloma with osteosclerotic features.

D. Multifocal motor neuropathy (MMN) is associated with polyclonal anti-GM1 antibodies in a majority of cases.

E. The most common pattern of neuropathy in patients with vasculitis is a mononeuritis multiplex.

30. All but which of the following statements regarding prion diseases are true?

A. Prions are the only known infectious agent that is devoid of DNA or RNA.

B. The majority of human cases are familial and have an autosomal dominant pattern.

C. Variant Creutzfeldt-Jakob (vCJD) disease has been associated with bovine spongiform encephalopathy (BSE) infection in cattle.

30. *(Continued)*
   D. The median age of presentation for sporadic CJD (sCJD) is 50 to 70 years of age.
   E. Histologically, the brain of a patient with CJD is characterized by spongiform degeneration and astrocytic gliosis with an absence of inflammation.

31. A 21-year-old man presents to your clinic complaining of progressive weakness in the feet for the last 2 years. He describes slowly progressive difficulty in lifting his feet off the ground when walking. The legs have "gotten smaller" in bulk. Past medical history is unremarkable. The family history is significant for his father, brother, and paternal grandmother all having similar "weaknesses." The examination is notable for distal atrophy below the mid-calves and for prominent high arches. There is obvious footdrop, and dorsiflexion of the foot is severely diminished bilaterally. You suspect a form of Charcot-Marie-Tooth disease and order nerve conduction studies. Which of the following statements about CMT disease is true?

   A. CMT disease is usually a motor neuropathy; sensory features are rare and should prompt an alternative diagnosis.
   B. Immunotherapy with intravenous immune globulin and/or plasmapheresis may slow the progression of CMT disease.
   C. CMT disease affects approximately 1 in 100,000 individuals.
   D. Transmission is most commonly autosomal dominant but may be autosomal recessive or X-linked.
   E. The age of this patient at presentation is atypical; patients usually present in the fourth and fifth decades of life.

32. An 18-year-old male is brought to your clinic by his mother for evaluation of his "strange behavior." Over the last week he has had four witnessed episodes of "staring spells," with each one preceded by the smell of lemons. A few seconds after the strange smell the patient is noted to appear dazed and unresponsive, but with his eyes open. These episodes typically last 20 to 30 s; afterward he is noted to make lip-smacking movements and remain confused. The confusion lasts up to an hour. The patient has no recollection of these events, and they are described in detail only by his mother. This presentation is consistent with which of the following diagnoses?

   A. Absence seizure
   B. Atonic seizure
   C. Complex partial seizure
   D. Grand mal seizure
   E. Simple partial seizure

33. All the following are common causes of seizures in adults older than 50 years of age *except*

   A. cerebrovascular disease
   B. central nervous system (CNS) neoplasia
   C. degenerative disease
   D. mesial temporal sclerosis
   E. subdural hematoma

34. All but which of the following statements regarding epilepsy are true?

   A. The incidence of suicide is higher in epileptic patients than it is in the general population.
   B. Mortality is no different in patients with epilepsy than it is in age-matched controls.
   C. A majority of patients with epilepsy that is completely controlled with medication eventually will be able to discontinue therapy and remain seizure-free.
   D. Surgery for mesial temporal lobe epilepsy (MTLE) decreases the number of seizures in over 70% of patients.
   E. Tricyclic antidepressants lower the seizure threshold and may precipitate seizures.

35. All the following are side effects of phenytoin *except*

   A. ataxia
   B. gum hyperplasia
   C. hirsutism
   D. leukopenia
   E. lymphadenopathy

36. A 34-year-old female complains of weakness and double vision for the last 3 weeks. She has also noted a change in her speech, and her friends tell her that she is "more nasal." She has noticed decreased exercise tolerance and difficulty lifting objects and getting out of a chair. The patient denies pain. The symptoms are worse at the end of the day and with repeated muscle use. You suspect myasthenia gravis. All the following are useful in the diagnosis of myasthenia gravis *except*

   A. acetylcholine receptor (AChR) antibodies
   B. edrophonium
   C. electrodiagnostic testing
   D. muscle-specific kinase (MuSK) antibodies
   E. voltage-gated calcium channel antibodies

37. In the patient described in Question 36 you confirm the diagnosis of myasthenia gravis. The patient's symptoms improve markedly after an initial dose of glucocorticoids and pyridostigmine. What is the best next treatment option for this patient?

37. *(Continued)*
    A. Surgical consultation
    B. Glucocorticoids
    C. Glucocorticoids and azathioprine
    D. Intravenous immunoglobulin
    E. Cyclosporine

38. A 29-year-old female who uses oral contraceptives comes to the emergency room because when she looked in the mirror this morning, her face was twisted. It felt numb and swollen. While eating breakfast, she found that the food tasted different and that she drooled out of the right side of her mouth when swallowing. Neurologic examination discloses only a dense right facial paresis equally involving the frontalis, orbicularis oculi, and orbicularis oris. Finger rubbing is appreciated as louder in the right ear than in the left. The physician should

    A. instruct the patient in using a patch over the right eye during sleep
    B. recommend that she discontinue oral contraceptives
    C. order brainstem auditory evoked potentials to assess the hearing asymmetry
    D. inform her that her chances of substantial improvement within several weeks are only about 40%
    E. order an echocardiogram to rule out mitral valve prolapse as a source of emboli

39. The most common presenting finding or symptom of multiple sclerosis is

    A. internuclear ophthalmoplegia
    B. transverse myelitis
    C. cerebellar ataxia
    D. optic neuritis
    E. urinary retention

40. A 68-year-old female presents with an 18-month history of progressive loss of recent memory and inattentiveness. At this time she is having difficulty speaking, her judgment appears to be impaired, and she occasionally evidences paranoid behavior. In addition to neurofibrillary tangles, the neuropathologic findings in this condition include plaques made of

    A. low-density lipoprotein
    B. unesterified cholesterol
    C. β-amyloid protein
    D. immunoglobulin proteins
    E. protease inhibitor

41. A 72-year-old female presents with brief, intermittent excruciating episodes of lancinating pain in the lips, gums, and cheek. These intense spasms of pain may be initiated by touching the lips or moving the

41. *(Continued)*
    tongue. The results of a physical examination are normal. MRI of the head is also normal. The most likely cause of this patient's pain is

    A. acoustic neuroma
    B. meningioma
    C. temporal lobe epilepsy
    D. trigeminal neuralgia
    E. facial nerve palsy

42. A 45-year-old male complains of severe right arm pain. He gives a history of having slipped on the ice and severely contusing his right shoulder approximately 1 month ago. At this time he has sharp knifelike pain in the right arm and forearm. Physical examination reveals a right arm that is more moist and hairy than the left arm. There is no specific weakness or sensory change. However, the right arm is clearly more edematous than the left, and the skin appears somewhat atrophic in the affected limb. The patient's pain most likely is due to

    A. subclavian vein thrombosis
    B. brachial plexus injury
    C. reflex sympathetic dystrophy
    D. acromioclavicular separation
    E. cervical radiculopathy

43. A 72-year-old right-handed male with a history of atrial fibrillation and chronic alcoholism is evaluated for dementia. His son gives a history of a stepwise decline in the patient's function over the last 5 years with the accumulation of mild focal neurologic deficits. On examination he is found to have a pseudobulbar affect, mildly increased muscle tone, and brisk deep tendon reflexes in the right upper extremity and an extensor plantar response on the left. The history and examination are most consistent with which of the following?

    A. Binswanger's disease
    B. Alzheimer's disease
    C. Creutzfeldt-Jakob disease
    D. Vitamin B_{12} deficiency
    E. Multi-infarct dementia

44. In addition to progressive memory loss, which of the following clinical findings is helpful in suggesting the diagnosis of Alzheimer's disease?

    A. Onset of symptoms before age 40
    B. Episodes of altered consciousness
    C. Neurofibrillary tangles
    D. Diminished independence in activities of daily living
    E. Absence of a family history of a similar disorder

ANSWERS

1. The answer is D.

Discussion: (*Chap. 11*) The photo shows a hypopyon, which is diagnostic of keratitis. A hypopyon is a collection of pus that is seen layering in the bottom portion of the anterior chamber of the eye. Keratitis can cause blindness if it is not treated properly and promptly. Worldwide, the most common causes of keratitis are vitamin A deficiency and trachoma, a chlamydial infection. In the United States, contact lens wear is associated with an increased risk of keratitis. A superficial infection is called keratoconjunctivitis and must be distinguished from keratitis, which is accompanied by greater visual loss, increased pain, photophobia, and discharge. Slit-lamp examination is helpful in the diagnosis, showing disruption of corneal epithelium, a cloudy infiltrate, and an inflammatory cellular reaction in the anterior chamber. At its most serious, hypopyon will appear. Empirical antibiotics should be started while one awaits the results of cultures from corneal scrapings. Fortified topical antibiotics are the treatment of choice. Fluoroquinolones have a broad spectrum of activity and are considered first-line therapy. They may be combined with aminoglycosides. Occasionally, they have to be supplemented with subconjunctival antibiotics. Fungal infection should be considered if there is failure to improve.

2. and 3. The answers are E and D.

Discussion: (*Chap. 11*) This patient has evidence of anterior uveitis that is associated with sarcoidosis. Anterior uveitis is usually marked by the abrupt onset of pain and photophobia. Specifically anterior uveitis causes iritis and iridocyclitis. Constriction of the pupil causes increased pain. Slit-lamp examination is diagnostic, showing inflammatory cells in the aqueous humor or deposited along the corneal endothelium. These deposits on the corneal endothelium are called keratic precipitates. Many diseases are associated with anterior uveitis, including sarcoidosis and the seronegative spondyloarthropathies, including ankylosing spondylitis, psoriasis, inflammatory bowel disease, and Behçet's disease. Infectious disease may also cause uveitis. Some of the associated infections include herpesviruses, tuberculosis, onchocerciasis, and leprosy. In the majority of cases, uveitis is idiopathic. Treatment should include topical glucocorticoids to decrease inflammation and mydriatics because dilation of the pupil decreases pain and the formation of synechiae.

4. The answer is A.

Discussion: (*Chap. 11*) Age-related macular degeneration is a common cause of blindness in older individuals. Visual loss is gradual and affects central vision. The most common form of macular degeneration is dry, or non-exudative. The hallmark of macular degeneration is the finding of drusen around the maculae. Drusen is the accumulation of pleomorphic extracellular deposits underneath the retinal pigment epithelium. These yellow deposits are initially small and are seen clustered around the maculae. Over time, they coalesce into large deposits. The retinal pigment epithelium becomes focally detached and atrophic, interfering with photoreceptor function. Treatment with multivitamin therapy may retard visual loss. In the exudative form of macular degeneration, neovascularization is prominent and starts at the choroid plexus. The neovascularization leaks into the potential space beneath the retinal pigment epithelium, causing blurring of vision.

5. The answer is A.

Discussion: (*Chap. 88, HPIM, 16e*) About 25% of patients with cancer die with intracranial metastases. Symptoms may relate to parenchymal or leptomeningeal involvement. The signs and symptoms of metastatic brain tumor are similar to those of other intracranial expanding lesions: headache, nausea, vomiting, behavioral changes, seizures, and focal neurologic deficits. Three percent to 8% of patients with cancer develop a tumor involving the leptomeninges. These patients typically present with multifocal neurologic signs and symptoms. Signs include cranial nerve palsies, extremity weakness, paresthesias, and loss of deep tendon reflexes. CT and MRI are useful in establishing the diagnosis of intraparenchymal lesions. The treatment of choice is radiotherapy. Solitary lesions in selected patients may be resected to achieve improved disease-free survival. The diagnosis of leptomeningeal disease is made by demonstrating tumor cells in the cerebrospinal fluid (CSF). Each attempt has limited sensitivity, and so patients with clinical features suggestive of leptomeningeal disease should undergo three serial CSF samplings. Neoplastic meningitis usually occurs in the setting of uncontrolled cancer outside the CNS. Therefore, the prognosis is typically dismal, with a median survival between 10 and 12 weeks.

6. The answer is B.

Discussion: (*Chap. 9*) The symptoms and signs described in this question are most consistent with Méniére's disease. In this disorder paroxysmal vertigo resulting from labyrinthine lesions associated with nausea, vomiting, rotary nystagmus, tinnitus, hightone hearing loss with recruitment, and, most characteristically, fullness in the ear. Labyrinthitis would be an unlikely diagnosis in this case because of the hearing loss and multiple episodes. Vertebral-basilar insufficiency and multiple sclerosis typically are associated with brainstem signs. Acoustic neuroma only rarely causes vertigo as the initial symptom, and the vertigo it does cause is mild and intermittent.

7. The answer is B.

Discussion: *(Chap. 5)* Cluster headaches, which can cause excruciating hemicranial pain, are notable for their occurrence during characteristic episodes. Usually attacks occur during a 4- to 8-week period in which the patient experiences one to three severe brief headaches daily. There may then be a prolonged pain-free interval before the next episode. Men between ages 20 and 50 are most commonly affected. The unilateral pain is usually associated with lacrimation, eye reddening, nasal stuffiness, ptosis, and nausea. During episodes alcohol may provoke the attacks. Even though the pain caused by brain tumors may awaken a patient from sleep, the typical history and normal neurologic examination do not mandate evaluation for a neoplasm of the central nervous system. Acute therapy for a cluster headache attack consists of oxygen inhalation, although intranasal lidocaine and subcutaneous sumatriptan may also be effective. Prophylactic therapy with prednisone, lithium, methysergide, ergotamine, or verapamil can be administered during an episode to prevent further cluster headache attacks.

8. The answer is D.

Discussion: *(Chap. 11)* This patient has acute angle-closure glaucoma resulting from obstruction of the outflow of aqueous humor at the iris. The buildup of intraocular pressure can be confirmed by measurement and requires urgent treatment with hyperosmotic agents. Permanent treatment requires laser or surgical iridotomy. Angle-closure glaucoma is less common than is primary open-angle glaucoma, which is asymptomatic and is usually detectable only through measurements of intraocular pressure at a routine eye examination.

9. The answer is E.

Discussion: *(Chap. 29)* The sensitivity of the latex agglutination (LA) test for *S. pneumoniae* is 70 to 100%. The LA test for *N. meningitides* is substantially lower at 33 to 70%. Thus, a negative test does not rule out disease. The specificity of these tests is 95 to 100%, and so a positive test is virtually diagnostic. MRI will be abnormal in most patients with bacterial meningitis, but the findings of cerebral edema, ischemia, and diffuse meningeal enhancement are not diagnostic. Meningeal enhancement occurs in any disease process that increases permeability of the blood-brain barrier. The limulus amebocyte lysate assay tests for endotoxin, and a positive test suggests gram-negative meningitis.

10. and 11. The answers are E and A.

Discussion: *(Chap. 29)* In a previously healthy student, particularly one living in a dormitory, *Staphylococcus pneumoniae* and *Neisseria meningitides* are the pathogens most likely to be causing community-acquired bacterial meningitis. As a result of the increasing prevalence of penicillin- and cephalosporin-resistant streptococci, initial empirical therapy should include a third- or fourth-generation cephalosporin plus vancomycin. Dexamethasone has been shown in children and adults to decrease meningeal inflammation and unfavorable outcomes in acute bacterial meningitis. In a recent study of adults the effect on outcome was most notable in patients with *S. pneumoniae* infection. The first dose (10 mg intravenous) should be administered 15 to 20 min before or with the first dose of antibiotics and is unlikely to be of benefit unless it is begun 6 h after the initiation of antibiotics. Dexamethasone may decrease the penetration of vancomycin into the CSF.

12. The answer is E.

Discussion: *(Chap. 29)* This patient has viral (aseptic) meningitis. The CSF showing mild pleocytosis with predominant lymphocytes and normal CSF glucose and protein is typical. Enteroviruses cause over 75% of cases of viral meningitis when a specific etiology is found. Enteroviral (coxsackievirus, echovirus, poliovirus, and human enterovirus 68-71) meningitis typically occurs in the summer and early fall but may occur year-round. PCR of CSF is useful for the identification of enteroviruses, herpes simplex virus (HSV), Epstein-Barr virus, varicella virus, and cytomegalovirus infection. MRI and cerebral angiography are useful for the diagnosis of subarachnoid hemorrhage; however, the CSF findings make this unlikely. The CSF findings in this case are less likely to be due to bacterial, fungal, or tuberculosis meningitis.

13. The answer is B.

Discussion: *(Chap. 29)* In 2002 West Nile virus (WNV) caused over 4000 cases of encephalitis with approximately 300 deaths. Cases typically occur in the summer, often in community outbreaks, associated with dead crows. WNV cannot be cultured, and there is not yet a PCR test. IgM antibodies normally do not cross the blood-brain barrier, and so their presence in the CSF is due to intrathecal production during acute infection with WNV. MRI is abnormal in only 30% of cases of WNV, significantly less often than is the case in HSV encephalitis. Stool culture may be useful in the diagnostic evaluation of enteroviral meningitis or encephalitis but not in cases of WNV.

14. The answer is D.

Discussion: *(Chap. 29)* This patient has progessive multifocal leukoencephalopathy (PML). The combination of MRI findings and the presence of JC virus in the CSF is diagnostic. The CSF may have a mild pleocytosis (25%) and a slightly elevated protein. PML almost always is seen in patients with advanced immunosuppression. Over 60% of cases are seen in patients with HIV, but PML can also be seen in patients with other conditions, such as lymphoproliferative and myeloproliferative disorders. There is no effective specific therapy. Patients with HIV may be treated with antiretroviral therapy to reduce the degree of immunosuppression.

15. The answer is C.

Discussion: *(Chap. 26)* Growth hormone excess in adults results in a clinical syndrome known as *acromegaly*, an insidious disease characterized by bony and soft tissue overgrowth, enlargement of the jaw and tongue, wide spacing of the teeth, and coarsened facial features. Hypertension may result from expansion of plasma volume and total body sodium. Laryngeal hypertrophy leads to a hollow-sounding voice. A moist, oily, doughy handshake is also characteristic. Because of the slow onset, relatives and friends who see the patient daily may not notice these changes. The diagnosis is more likely to be made by those who have not seen the patient before or for many years.

Laboratory abnormalities include abnormal glucose tolerance and mild hyperprolactinemia. The reason for growth hormone excess in virtually all patients with acromegaly is a pituitary adenoma. Useful screening tests for the diagnosis of acromegaly include measurements of glucose-suppressed growth hormone concentrations (60 min after the oral administration of 100 g glucose, growth hormone normally should be suppressed to a value <1 μg/L) and IGF binding protein 3. IGF-1 concentrations are elevated secondary to the high levels of growth hormone. Once a laboratory test has confirmed the clinical suspicion of acromegaly, magnetic resonance imaging (MRI) or CT should be done to define the presumptive pituitary adenoma. Thyroid function, gonadotropins, and sex steroids may be decreased because of tumor mass effect.

16. The answer is C.

Discussion: *(Chap. 12)* Head trauma is the most common etiology of a decreased sense of smell in young adults and children. In most cases this is permanent, with only 10% of these patients experiencing recovery. In older adults viral infections predominate. Parainfluenza virus type 3 is the most common associated virus. Patients with HIV also frequently have a distorted sense of smell, and this is associated with HIV wasting syndrome. Although rare, genetic defects such as Kallmann syndrome and albinism are also causes of anosmia. Influenza virus is not a cause of anosmia.

17. The answer is C.

Discussion: *(Chap. 12)* This patient exhibits conductive hearing loss as manifested by the Rinne and Weber tests. In the Rinne test, the vibrating tines of a 256- or 512-Hz tuning fork are placed near the opening of the external auditory canal, and then the stem is placed on either the

mastoid process or the teeth. If the sound is heard loudest when the fork is placed on bone, this is evidence of conductive hearing loss. The Weber test is performed by placing a vibrating tuning fork on the midline of the forehead. The sound is heard loudest in the affected ear if conductive hearing loss is present and in the unaffected ear if sensorineural hearing loss is present. This patient thus has evidence of conductive hearing loss. The picture reveals a rupture of the tympanic membrane filled with cheesy white squamous debris that is typical of cholesteatoma. The pathogenesis of this lesion is unclear but pathologically is defined by the presence of stratified squamous epithelium in the middle ear or mastoid. Surgery is required to prevent further hearing loss from erosion of the ossicles. Otosclerosis would have a normal appearance on examination. Otitis externa should not cause hearing loss and would be associated with pain on examination. Both presbycusis and acoustic neuroma cause sensorineural hearing loss.

18. The answer is B.

Discussion: *(Chap. 24)* This patient has a history and examination consistent with a myelopathy. The rapidity of onset and the lack of other antecedent symptoms (e.g., pain) make a noncompressive etiology most likely. An MRI is the initial test of choice and will easily identify a structural lesion such as a neoplasm or subluxation. Noncompressive myelopathies result from five basic causes: spinal cord infarction; systemic disorders such as vasculitis, systemic lupus erythematosus (SLE), and sarcoidosis; infections (particularly viral); demyelinating disease such as multiple sclerosis; and idiopathic. Therefore, serologies for antinuclear antibodies, viral serologies such as HIV and HTLV-I, and lumbar puncture are all indicated. Because the clinical scenario is consistent with a myelopathy, an electromyogram is not indicated.

19. The answer is A.

Discussion: *(Chap. 24)* Syringomyelia is a developmental, slowly enlarging cavitary expansion of the cervical cord that produces a progressive myelopathy. Symptoms typically begin in adolescence or early adulthood. They may undergo spontaneous arrest after several years. More than half are associated with Chiari malformations. Acquired cavitations of the spinal cord are referred to as syrinx cavities. They may result from trauma, myelitis, infection, or tumor. The classic presentation is that of a central cord syndrome with sensory loss of pain and temperature sensation and weakness of the upper extremities. Vibration and position sensation are typically preserved. Muscle wasting in the lower neck, shoulders, arms, and hands with asymmetric or absent reflexes reflects extension of the cavity to the anterior horns. With progression, spasticity and weakness of the lower extremities and bladder and bowel dysfunction may occur. MRI scans are the diagnostic modality of choice. Surgical therapy is generally unsatisfactory. Syringomyelia associated with Chiari malformations may require extensive decompressions of the posterior fossa. Direct decompression of the cavity is of debatable benefit. Syringomyelia secondary to trauma or infection is treated with decompression and a drainage procedure, with a shunt often inserted that drains into the subarachnoid space. Although relief may occur, recurrence is common.

20. The answer is B.

Discussion: *(Chap. 33)* Carpal tunnel syndrome is caused by entrapment of the median nerve at the wrist. Symptoms begin with paresthesias in the median nerve distribution. With worsening, atrophy and weakness may develop. This condition is most commonly caused by excessive use of the wrist. Rarely, systemic disease may result in carpal tunnel syndrome. This may be suspected when bilateral disease is apparent. Tenosynovitis with arthritis as in the case of rheumatoid arthritis and thickening of the connective tissue as in the case of amyloid or acromegaly are also causes. Other systemic diseases, such as hypothyroidism and diabetes mellitus, are also possible etiologies. Leukemia is not typically associated with carpal tunnel syndrome.

21. The answer is C.

Discussion: *(Chap. 17)* Cerebrovascular diseases account for up to 200,000 deaths a year in the United States and are a major cause of morbidity. Acute ischemic stroke results from an acute occlusion of an intracranial vessel from in situ thrombosis or an embolic source. The magnitude of the flow reduction is a function of the collateral blood flow, and this depends largely on the vascular anatomy of the individual patient. Brain tissue dies within minutes of a fall in cerebral blood flow. Therefore, reestablishment of flow and prevention of widening of the territory of infarction are two of the major goals of stroke therapy. A pivotal National Institute of Neurological Disorders and Stroke (NINDS) study showed that patients who received intravenous recombinant tissue plasminogen activator (rTPA) within 3 h of the onset of symptoms had a significant clinical benefit. This was the case despite a 6.4% risk of intracerebral hemorrhage. Other, more recent trials have looked at intraarterial delivery of rTPA by a catheter-based approach within a 6-h time frame for middle cerebral artery (MCA) territory infarctions, and there appears to be a significant benefit. Although this has not been approved by the U.S. Food and Drug Administration, based on early clinical trials, it is rapidly becoming the standard of care for patients with MCA strokes that fall out of the 3-h window for intravenous rTPA. Numerous studies have shown the benefit of aspirin administered within 48 h of stroke onset. Aspirin offers a modest benefit in regard to further stroke recurrence. Some literature supports a benefit of clopidogrel in ischemic stroke patients as a means of secondary prevention. Although frequently used, heparin remains unproven as a beneficial agent in the treatment of acute stroke. Because this patient

has no contraindication to thrombolytic therapy but falls outside the 3-h window for intravenous rTPA, catheter-delivered rTPA is the next best option if the support facilities exist and should be recommended for this patient.

22. The answer is E.

Discussion: *(Chap. 17)* Cardioembolism accounts for up to 20% of all ischemic strokes. Stroke caused by heart disease is due to thrombotic material forming on the atrial or ventricular wall or the left heart valves. If the thrombus lyses quickly, only a transient ischemic attack may develop. If the arterial occlusion lasts longer, brain tissue may die and a stroke will occur. Emboli from the heart most often lodge in the middle cerebral artery (MCA), the posterior cerebral artery (PCA), or one of their branches. Atrial fibrillation is the most common cause of cerebral embolism overall. Other significant causes of cardioembolic stroke include myocardial infarction, prosthetic valves, rheumatic heart disease, and dilated cardiomyopathy. Furthermore, paradoxical embolization may occur when an atrial septal defect or a patent foramen ovale exists. This may be detected by bubble-contrast echocardiography. Bacterial endocarditis may cause septic emboli if the vegetation is on the left side of the heart or if there is a paradoxical source.

23. The answer is D.

Discussion: *(Chap. 17)* Nonrheumatic atrial fibrillation is the most common cause of cerebral embolism overall. The presumed stroke mechanism is thrombus formation in the fibrillating atrium or atrial appendage. The average annual risk of stroke is around 5%. However, the risk varies with certain factors: age, hypertension, left ventricular function, prior embolism, diabetes, and thyroid function. Patients younger than 60 years of age without structural heart disease or without one of these risk factors have a very low annual risk of cardioembolism: less than 0.5%. Therefore, it is recommended that these patients only take aspirin daily for stroke prevention. Older patients with numerous risk factors may have annual stroke risks of 10 to 15% and must take warfarin indefinitely. Cardioversion is indicated for symptomatic patients who want an initial opportunity to remain in sinus rhythm. However, studies have shown that there is an increased stroke risk for weeks to months after a successful cardioversion, and these patients must remain on anticoagulation for a long period. Similarly, recent studies have shown that patients who do not respond to cardioversion and do not want catheter ablation have mortality and morbidity with rate control and anticoagulation similar to those of patients who opt for cardioversion. Low-molecular-weight heparin may be used as a bridge to warfarin therapy and may facilitate outpatient anticoagulation in selected patients.

24. The answer is A.

Discussion: *(Chap. 21)* ALS is the most common form of progressive motor neuron disease. It is characterized by degeneration of both upper and lower motor neurons. Destruction of peripheral motor neurons results in denervation and consequent atrophy of the corresponding muscle fibers. This results in the "amyotrophy" seen on muscle biopsy. The loss of cortical motor neurons results in thinning of the corticospinal tracts that travel via the internal capsule and brainstem to the lateral and anterior white matter columns of the spinal cord. The loss of fibers in these lateral columns results in the "lateral sclerosis." The etiology is thought to be related to the excitotoxicity of glutamate, which may accumulate as a result of certain transporter defects or as a result of defective superoxide dismutase. Most cases are sporadic, but a small percentage are familial and are inherited in an autosomal dominant fashion. Clinically, these patients may present with weakness in any muscle group. The initial phase is usually asymmetric and starts in the limbs. Denervation results in spontaneous twitching of motor units, or fasciculations. Involvement of the bulbar muscles results in difficulty swallowing. Eventually these patients develop respiratory failure. This is the eventual cause of death in ALS patients. One hallmark of sporadic disease is the preservation of cognitive function. There is no cure for this disease. Riluzole was recently approved for ALS secondary to evidence that it improves survival by an average of approximately 3 months. The mechanism is unclear and may be related to a reduction in excitotoxicity by diminishing glutamate release.

25. The answer is C.

Discussion: (Chap. 17) Carotid atherosclerosis frequently occurs in the common carotid bifurcation and the proximal internal carotid artery. Five percent of ischemic strokes result from carotid atherosclerosis. The decision to perform surgery in a patient with carotid disease depends on the presence of symptoms and the degree of stenosis. In symptomatic patients two large trials—the North American Symptomatic Carotid Endarterectomy Trial (NASCET) and the European Carotid Surgery Trial—showed a substantial benefit from surgery in patients with stenosis greater than 70%. There was a 17% absolute reduction in ipsilateral stroke in the NASCET trial. That trial also showed benefit in the group with 50 to 70% stenosis. Neither study showed a benefit for patients with symptomatic stenosis less than 50%. Another finding of the studies was that the outcome was heavily dependent on institutional experience with the procedure. Institutions with perioperative complication rates above or equal to 6% did not have the benefits of the CEA procedure. Therefore, the recommendation is that in symptomatic patients with carotid stenosis, CEA is the procedure of choice provided that it is done at an experienced center. In asymptomatic patients the situation is a bit more controversial. A recent study—the Asymptomatic Carotid Atherosclerosis Study (ACAS)—randomized asymptomatic patients with stenosis greater than 60% to surgery versus medical therapy. Although there was a relative risk

reduction of ipsilateral stroke of 53% over 5 years in the surgical group, the absolute risk reduction ended up being only 1.2% per year. It is unclear whether newer medical therapies with statins and antiplatelet agents will change this situation in favor of medical therapy. Asymptomatic patients have a stroke risk of about 2% per year, and aspirin and statin therapy are recommended for those patients. Interest in balloon angioplasty with stenting has increased. Although distal embolization has been a concern, newer devices designed to reduce this complication make this procedure an exciting potential alternative to surgery.

26. The answer is E.

Discussion: (Chap. 17) Numerous studies have identified key risk factors for ischemic stroke. Old age, family history, diabetes, hypertension, tobacco smoking, and cholesterol are all risk factors for atherosclerosis and therefore stroke. Hypertension is the most significant among these risk factors. All cases of hypertension must be controlled in the setting of stroke prevention. Antiplatelet therapy has been shown to reduce the risk of vascular atherothrombotic events. The overall relative risk reduction of nonfatal stroke is about 25 to 30% across most large clinical trials. The "true" absolute benefit is dependent on the individual patient's risk; therefore, patients with a low risk for stroke (e.g., younger, with minimal cardiovascular risk factors) may have a relative risk reduction with antiplatelet therapy but a meaningless "benefit." Numerous studies have shown the benefit of statin therapy in the reduction of stroke risk even in the absence of hypercholesterolemia. Although anticoagulation is the treatment of choice for atrial fibrillation and cardioembolic causes of stroke, there is no proven benefit in regard to the prevention of atherothrombotic stroke; therefore, warfarin cannot be recommended.

27. The answer is B.

Discussion: (Chap. 33) Peripheral neuropathy is a general term indicating peripheral nerve disorders of any cause. The causes are legion, but peripheral neuropathy can be classified by a number of means: axonal versus demyelinating, mononeuropathy versus polyneuropathy versus mononeuritis multiplex, sensory versus motor, and the tempo of the onset of symptoms. Mononeuropathy typically results from local compression, trauma, or entrapment of a nerve. Polyneuropathy often results from a more systemic process. The distinction between axonal and demyelinating can often be made only with nerve conduction studies. HIV infection causes a common, distal, symmetric, mainly sensory polyneuropathy. Vitamin B_{12} deficiency typically causes a sensory neuropathy that predominantly involves the dorsal columns. Hypothyroidism and acromegaly may both cause compression and swelling of nerve fibers, resulting first in sensory symptoms and later in disease with motor symptoms. Critical illness polyneuropathy is predominantly motor in presentation. These patients may recover over the course of weeks to months. The etiology is unknown, but an association may exist with neuromuscular blockade and glucocorticoids.

28. **The answer is A.**

Discussion: *(Chap. 35)* Guillain-Barré syndrome (GBS) is a rare acute fulminant polyradiculoneuropathy that is autoimmune in etiology. Approximately 3500 cases occur per year in the United States and Canada. The majority of cases are preceded by an acute infectious process, usually respiratory or gastrointestinal in origin. *Campylobacter jejuni* is associated with up to 30% of cases in North America, Europe, and Australia. Other etiologic agents include cytomegalovirus and Epstein-Barr virus, mycoplasma, and vaccination. GBS occurs more frequently in patients with lymphoma and HIV infection. Clinically, patients develop a rapidly evolving areflexic motor paralysis with or without sensory disturbance. It is classically ascending in nature. Patients may notice rubbery legs first. Symptoms may evolve over the course of hours to a few days. The legs are usually more involved than are the arms, and facial paresis is present in 50% of these patients. Involvement of lower cranial nerves may cause difficulty with handling secretions and maintaining an airway. Thirty percent of these patients require mechanical ventilation at some point during their illness. Autonomic involvement is common in severe cases. Pain is also a common feature of GBS, ranging from a deep aching pain in the muscles to a shocklike paresthesia. Subtypes of GBS include the Miller Fisher variant, pure sensory forms, ophthalmoplegia with anti-GQ1b antibodies, and bulbar and facial paralysis. CSF findings are distinctive, consisting of an elevated CSF protein level without pleocytosis. Electrodiagnostic features vary, depending on the stage of clinical symptoms. Treatment includes immunotherapy with intravenous immune globulin or plasmapheresis. Treatment must be initiated as soon as possible as the effectiveness diminishes the later it is after the onset of symptoms. Outcomes are good, with the majority of patients having a good recovery within a year. However, many will have persistent minor neurologic sequelae. The main cause of morbidity and mortality is infection, often from pulmonary complications that result from mechanical ventilation. Enteropathic strains of *E. coli* have been associated with hemolytic-uremic syndrome, not with GBS.

29. **The answer is C.**

Discussion: *(Chap. 35)* In addition to Guillain-Barré syndrome, there are many other immune-mediated neuropathies. CIDP is distinguished from GBS by its chronic course. Symptoms may be asymmetric and may show considerable variability from case to case. CSF protein may be elevated as it is in GBS. Electrodiagnostically, there are variable degrees of conduction slowing, prolonged distal latencies, and conduction block. This is consistent with a demyelinating process. The etiology is unknown, and collagen vascular disease, HIV infection, and other systemic diseases

must be ruled out. Approximately 25% of these patients have an MGUS present. MMN is an uncommon neuropathy that involves a slowly progressive motor weakness and atrophy in the distribution of selected nerve trunks. This occurs slowly over the course of years. Sensory fibers are relatively spared. Most of these patients are male, and the upper extremities are affected more than the lower extremities are. Fifty percent of these patients have a high titer of IgM antibodies to ganglioside GM1. Electrodiagnostic studies and pathology are consistent with an inflammatory demyelinating process. Polyneuropathy occurs in a minority of patients with multiple myeloma except in the rare case of those with osteosclerotic myeloma. This entity is associated with polyneuropathy in half the cases. In addition to polyneuropathy, other systemic findings may include thickening of the skin, hyperpigmentation, hypertrichosis, organomegaly, endocrinopathy, anasarca, and clubbing of the fingers. This constitutes the POEMS syndrome (polyneuropathy, organomegaly, endocrinopathy, M protein, and skin changes). Peripheral nerve involvement is common in some types of vasculitis, particularly polyarteritis nodosa. The most common pattern is mononeuritis multiplex caused by ischemic lesions of nerve trunks and roots. However, some types of vasculitic neuropathy present as a distal, symmetric motor-sensory neuropathy. Anti-Hu antibodies are associated with an autoimmune neuronopathy, resulting in an asymmetric sensory loss in the limbs, torso, and face. Marked sensory ataxia, pseudoathetosis, and inability to walk or stand are common features. Most cases are idiopathic, but in 25% of cases an underlying cancer, particularly small cell lung cancer, is detected. Interestingly, the neurologic symptoms often precede the diagnosis of cancer by approximately 1 year.

30. **The answer is B.**

Discussion: *(Chap. 32)* Prions are the only known infectious agent that is devoid of DNA or RNA. They are infectious proteins that cause degeneration of the central nervous system. Prions reproduce by binding to the normal cellular isotype of the prion protein and causing a conformational change to a pathogenic isoform of the prion protein. The mechanism is unknown. Patients may have sporadic disease or may have a familial form. Sporadic cases account for the vast majority, with sCJD accounting for 85% of human cases. The median age of presentation is the sixth decade. Variant CJD is associated with BSE infection epidemiologically and may present at any age. Histologically, these patients have spongiform degeneration without inflammation. Clinically, CJD patients may have nonspecific prodromal symptoms, including fatigue, sleep disturbance, weight loss, headache, malaise, and pain. Most of these patients develop higher cortical deficits. These deficits progress over the course of weeks to months to a state of profound dementia characterized by memory loss, impaired judgment, and a total decline in intellectual function. There is no known treatment.

31. The answer is D.

Discussion: *(Chap. 34)* CMT disease is a heterogeneous group of inherited peripheral neuropathies. Transmission is usually autosomal dominant but may be recessive or X-linked. Numerous genetic defects are associated with CMT disease. It is very common, affecting up to 1 in 2500 persons. Clinically, patients usually present in the first or second decade of life, but later presentations may occur. The neuropathy affects both motor and sensory nerves. Symptoms may vary, ranging from distal muscle weakness and severe atrophy and disability to only pes cavus and minimal weakness. Although sensory findings and involvement are common, these patients often do not have dominant sensory complaints. However, if patients have no evidence of sensory involvement on detailed neurologic examination or electrodiagnostic studies, an alternative diagnosis should be considered. There is no known effective therapy for CMT disease. Orthotics and physical therapy are mainstays for preserving function.

32. The answer is C.

Discussion: *(Chap. 14)* The classification of a seizure is important in determining the etiology and potential treatment options. The main characteristic that distinguishes the different categories of seizures is whether a seizure is partial or generalized. Partial seizures are seizures in which the activity is restricted to discrete regions of the brain. Generalized seizures involve diffuse regions of the brain simultaneously. Partial seizures are usually associated with structural abnormalities of the brain, whereas generalized seizures may result from cellular, biochemical, or structural abnormalities that have a more widespread distribution. With simple partial seizures, consciousness is maintained. With complex partial seizures, consciousness is impaired. Simple partial seizures may cause motor, sensory, autonomic, or psychic symptoms without an obvious impairment in consciousness. Motor seizures may include typical clonic activity that corresponds to a particular part of the brain on electroencephalography (EEG). Other forms may involve somatic sensation, equilibrium, and impairment in olfaction, hearing, or higher cortical functions (e.g., emotions). When these symptoms precede a complex partial or secondarily generalized seizure, these simple partial seizures are termed auras. Complex partial seizures are characterized by focal seizure activity accompanied by a transient impairment of the ability to maintain normal contact with the environment. The behavioral arrest is often accompanied by automatisms, which are involuntary automatic behaviors that may include chewing, lip smacking, swallowing, or more elaborate movements. Absence seizures often start in childhood. They are characterized by sudden brief lapses of consciousness without loss of postural control. There is no postictal confusion, and the episodes usually last only seconds. Generalized tonic-clonic, or grand mal, seizures involve generalized motor activity with loss of consciousness and a postictal

phase. Atonic seizures are characterized by a sudden loss of postural muscle tone that lasts 1 to 2 s. There is no postictal confusion, and the loss of consciousness is brief. Myoclonic seizures involve sudden and brief muscle contraction. They usually coexist with other forms of generalized seizure disorders but are the predominant feature in juvenile myoclonic epilepsy.

33. The answer is D.

Discussion: *(Chap. 14)* The causes of seizures vary with the age at presentation. In neonates, prepartum and peripartum factors predominate. Perinatal hypoxia or trauma, acute infection, maternal use of cocaine or opiates, and genetic disorders are the most common causes of seizure in that age group. In children older than 1 year through early adolescence (10 to 12 years of age), febrile seizures, genetic disorders, developmental disorders, trauma, and infection are common. In older patients (over 35 years of age), cerebrovascular disease, neoplasia, trauma (particularly subdural hematoma or intracranial hemorrhage), and degenerative diseases (e.g., Alzheimer's dementia) predominate. Mesial temporal lobe epilepsy (MTLE) is the syndrome most commonly associated with complex partial seizures. It is characterized by hippocampal sclerosis that is best seen on magnetic resonance imaging. Anticonvulsants are usually ineffective, but surgery may be curative. It usually presents in childhood or adolescence. It is uncommon for it to present in late adulthood.

34. The answer is B.

Discussion: *(Chap. 14)* Optimal medical therapy for epilepsy depends on the underlying cause, type of seizure, and patient factors. The goal is to prevent seizures and minimize the side effects of therapy. The minimal effective dose is determined by trial and error. In choosing medical therapies, drug interactions are a key consideration. Certain medications, such as tricyclic antidepressants, may lower the seizure threshold and should be avoided. Patients who respond well to medical therapy and have completely controlled seizures are good candidates for the discontinuation of therapy, with about 70% of children and 60% of adults being able to discontinue therapy eventually. Patient factors that aid in this include complete medical control of seizures for 1 to 5 years, a normal neurologic examination, a normal EEG, and single seizure type. On the other end of the spectrum, about 20% of these patients are completely refractory to medical therapy and should be considered for surgical therapy. In the best examples, such as mesial temporal sclerosis, resection of the temporal lobe may result in about 70% of these patients becoming seizure-free and an additional 15 to 25% having a significant reduction in the incidence of seizures. In patients with epilepsy other considerations are critical. Psychosocial sequelae such as depression, anxiety, and behavior problems may occur. Approximately 20% of epileptic patients have depression, with their suicide rate being higher than that of age-matched controls. There is an impact on the ability to drive, perform certain jobs, and function in social situations. Furthermore, there is a twofold to threefold increase in mortality for patients with epilepsy compared with age-matched controls. Although most of the increased mortality results from the underlying etiology of epilepsy, a significant number of these patients die from accidents, status epilepticus, and a syndrome known as sudden unexpected death in epileptic patients (SUDEP). The cause is unknown, but research has centered on brainstem-mediated effects of seizures on cardiopulmonary function.

35. The answer is D.

Discussion: (Chap. 14) Phenytoin is a commonly used anticonvulsant. Its principal use is in patients with tonic-clonic seizures. It may be given either orally or intravenously. Typical dosing is about 300 to 400 mg/d in adults. The therapeutic range is between 10 and 20 μg/mL. Neurologic side effects include dizziness, ataxia, diplopia, and confusion. Systemic side effects include gum hyperplasia, hirsutism, facial coarsening, and osteomalacia. These patients may develop lymphadenopathy and Stevens-Johnson syndrome. Toxicity may be enhanced by liver disease and competition with other medications. Phenytoin alters folate metabolism and is teratogenic. Leukopenia is not a typical side effect and is seen more often with carbamazepine.

36. The answer is E.

Discussion: (Chap. 36) Myasthenia gravis (MG) is a neuromuscular disorder characterized by weakness and fatigability of skeletal muscles. The primary defect is a decrease in the number of acetylcholine receptors at the neuromuscular junction secondary to autoimmune antibodies. MG is not rare, affecting at least 1 in 7500 individuals. Women are affected more frequently than are men. Women present typically in the second and third decades of life, and men present in the fifth and sixth decades. The key features of MG are weakness and fatigability. Clinical features include weakness of the cranial muscles, particularly the lids and extraocular muscles. Diplopia and ptosis are common initial complaints. Weakness in chewing is noticeable after prolonged effort. Speech may be affected secondary to weakness of the palate or tongue weakness. Swallowing may result from weakness of the palate, tongue, or pharynx. In the majority of patients the weakness becomes generalized. The diagnosis is suspected after the appearance of the characteristic symptoms and signs. Edrophonium is an acetylcholinesterase inhibitor that allows ACh to interact repeatedly with the limited number of AChRs, producing improvement in the strength of myasthenic muscles. False-positive tests may occur in patients with other neurologic diseases. Electrodiagnostic testing may show evidence of reduction in the amplitude of the evoked muscle action potentials with repeated stimulation. Testing for the specific antibodies to AChR

are diagnostic. In addition to anti-AChR antibodies, antibodies to MuSK have been found in some patients with clinical MG. Antibodies to voltage-gated calcium channels are found in patients with the Lambert-Eaton syndrome.

37. The answer is A.

Discussion: (Chap. 36) The pathophysiology of myasthenia gravis is thought to be autoimmune in nature, with the thymus playing a central role. Patients with MG often have an abnormal thymus. The incidence of thymoma is markedly increased in patients with MG. Although all the other treatment options are useful at varying points in the treatment of MG, clinical trials show that 85% of patients exhibit benefit from removal of the thymus as part of the treatment of myasthenia gravis. Up to 35% of these patients may attain long-term drug-free remission of disease. Therefore, all patients with MG between the ages of puberty and 55 years should undergo thymectomy as a possibly definitive treatment. There is concern that very young patients may experience long-term immunologic dysfunction as a result of early thymectomy. The benefit in older patients is less clear.

38. The answer is A.

Discussion: (Chap. 23) The abrupt appearance of an isolated peripheral facial palsy, which may include ipsilateral hyperacusis resulting from involvement of fibers to the stapedius and loss of taste on the anterior two-thirds of the tongue resulting from involvement of the fibers of the chorda tympani, is most often idiopathic, as in patients with Bell's palsy. If the patient is unable to close the eye, artificial tears may be helpful during the day to prevent drying, and the eye should be patched at night to prevent corneal abrasion. Excellent recovery occurs in 80% of these cases. Oral contraceptives and mitral valve prolapse are not associated with the causes of this clinical picture. Evoked potentials are not helpful diagnostically.

39. The answer is D.

Discussion: (Chap. 28) Optic neuritis is the initial symptom in approximately 40% of persons who are eventually diagnosed with multiple sclerosis. This rapidly developing ophthalmologic disorder is associated with partial or total loss of vision, pain on motion of the involved eye, scotoma affecting macular vision, and a variety of other visual field defects. Ophthalmoscopically visible optic papillitis occurs in about half these patients.

40. The answer is C.

Discussion: (Chap. 18; Yankner, N Engl J Med 325:1849–1857, 1991.) Alzheimer's disease is the most common cause of dementia in the elderly. It is highly prevalent, affecting up to 45% of those over age 85. In a relatively small percentage of cases the disease occurs in a familial pattern; this is thought to be due to autosomal dominant inheritance with linkage to chromosome 21 or

19. The clinical beginnings of the disease tend to be subtle. The initial symptoms are usually limited to loss of recent memory. Psychiatric symptoms may then supervene and can include depression, anxiety, delusions, and paranoid behavior. An extrapyramidal component exists so that patients walk in a shuffling manner with short steps. Radiographic evaluation usually reveals neuronal atrophy. Neuropathologically, the disease is characterized by neurofibrillary tangles, which may contain an abnormally phosphorylated form of a microtubular protein known as *tau* as well as spherical deposits known as *senile plaques*. A protein known as β-amyloid can be found in these plaques. Certain families with inherited Alzheimer's disease have been found to have a point mutation in the amyloid precursor protein. From a neurotransmitter standpoint, acetylcholine, a neurotransmitter that is important in memory formation, is synthesized at abnormally low levels. The current model for the pathogenesis of Alzheimer's disease is that altered cleavage of the amyloid precursor protein generates the so-called β-amyloid protein, which then binds to a protease inhibitor-enzyme complex, in turn preventing the normal inactivation of extracellular proteases. It is these abnormally activated extracellular proteases that may mediate the neuronal degeneration characteristic of Alzheimer's disease. Therapeutic strategies that could inhibit the generation of β-amyloid are of potential therapeutic interest.

41. **The answer is D.**
Discussion: *(Chap. 23)* Brief paroxysms of severe, sharp pains in the face without demonstrable lesions in the jaw, teeth, or sinuses are called tic douloureux, or trigeminal neuralgia. The pain may be brought on by stimuli applied to the face, lips, or tongue or by certain movements of those structures. Aneurysms, neurofibromas, and meningiomas impinging on the fifth cranial nerve at any point during its course typically present with trigeminal neuropathy, which will cause sensory loss on the face, weakness of the jaw muscles, or both; neither symptom is demonstrable in this patient. The treatment for this idiopathic condition is carbamazepine or phenytoin if carbamazepine is not tolerated. When drug treatment is not successful, surgical therapy, including the commonly applied percutaneous retrogasserian rhizotomy, may be effective. A possible complication of this procedure is partial facial numbness with a risk of corneal anesthesia, which increases the potential for ulceration.

42. **The answer is C.**
Discussion: *(Chap. 23)* Pain, loss of function (without clear-cut sensory or motor deficits), and a localized autonomic impairment are called reflex sympathetic dystrophy (also known as shoulder-hand syndrome or causalgia). Precipitating events in this unusual syndrome include myocardial infarction, shoulder trauma, and limb paralysis. In addition to the neuropathic-type pain, autonomic dysfunction,

possibly resulting from neuroadrenergic and cholinergic hypersensitivity, produces localized sweating, changes in blood flow, and abnormal hair and nail growth as well as edema or atrophy of the affected limb. Treatment is difficult; however, anticonvulsants such as phenytoin and carbamazepine may be effective, as they are in other conditions in which neuropathic pain is a major problem.

43. **The answer is E.**
Discussion: *(Chaps. 7 and 18)* All the choices given in the question are causes of or may be associated with dementia. Binswanger's disease, the cause of which is unknown, often occurs in patients with long-standing hypertension and/or atherosclerosis; it is associated with diffuse subcortical white matter damage and has a subacute insidious course. Alzheimer's disease, the most common cause of dementia, is also slowly progressive and can be confirmed at autopsy by the presence of amyloid plaques and neurofibrillary tangles. Creutzfeldt-Jakob disease, a prion disease, is associated with a rapidly progressive dementia, myoclonus, rigidity, a characteristic EEG pattern, and death within 1 to 2 years of onset. Vitamin B_{12} deficiency, which often is seen in the setting of chronic alcoholism, most commonly produces a myelopathy that results in loss of vibration and joint position sense and brisk deep tendon reflexes (dorsal column and lateral corticospinal tract dysfunction). This combination of pathologic abnormalities in the setting of vitamin B_{12} deficiency is also called subacute combined degeneration. Vitamin B_{12} deficiency may also lead to a subcortical type of dementia. Multi-infarct dementia, as in this case, presents with a history of sudden stepwise declines in function associated with the accumulation of bilateral focal neurologic deficits. Brain imaging demonstrates multiple areas of stroke.

44. **The answer is D.**
Discussion: *(Chap. 18; Mayeux, Sano, N Engl J Med 341:1670–1679, 1999.)* The definitive diagnosis of Alzheimer's disease remains elusive. Dementia is established by examination as well as by documentation of subjective testing. All patients with Alzheimer's disease have memory impairment and have at least one other cognitive function that is impaired, such as language or perception. These patients typically have worsening of their memory loss. Patients should not have an alteration of consciousness. The onset of Alzheimer's disease occurs between ages 40 and 90, and the absence of other brain disorders or systemic disease that may cause dementia should be established. In addition, the diagnosis of Alzheimer's disease is supported by the loss of motor skills, diminished independence and activities of daily living, altered patterns of behavior, a positive family history, and cerebral atrophy on CT. The presence of neurofibrillary tangles and senile plaques is made at postmortem examination; it confirms the diagnosis of clinical Alzheimer's disease but is not part of the clinical diagnostic criteria.

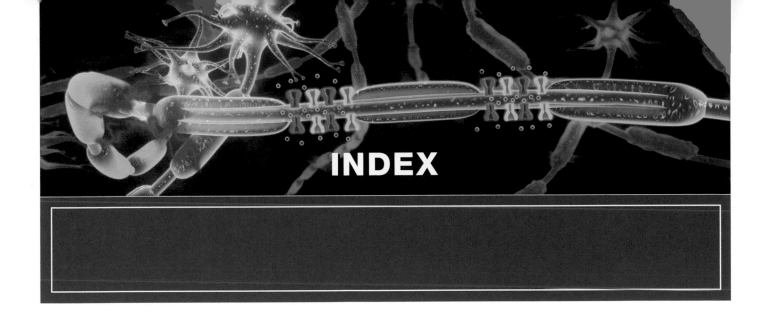

INDEX

Bold number indicates the start of the main discussion of the topic; numbers with "f" and "t" refer to figure and table pages.